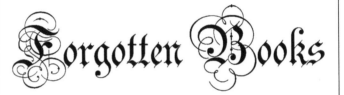

ISBN 978-1-5278-7887-7
PIBN 10899723

1 MONTH OF
FREE
READING

at

www.ForgottenBooks.com

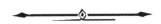

By purchasing this book you are eligible for one month membership to ForgottenBooks.com, giving you unlimited access to our entire collection of over 1,000,000 titles via our web site and mobile apps.

To claim your free month visit:
www.forgottenbooks.com/free899723

THE

PRINCIPLES OF PATHOLOGY

BY

J. GEORGE ADAMI, M.A., M.D., LL.D., F.R.S.

PROFESSOR OF PATHOLOGY IN MC GILL UNIVERSITY, AND PATHOLOGIST-IN-CHIEF TO THE ROYAL VICTORIA
HOSPITAL, MONTREAL; LATE FELLOW OF JESUS COLLEGE, CAMBRIDGE, ENGLAND

AND

ALBERT G. NICHOLLS, M.A., M.D., D.Sc., F.R.S. (Can.)

ASSISTANT PROFESSOR OF PATHOLOGY AND LECTURER IN MEDICINE IN MC GILL UNIVERSITY;
OUT-PATIENT PHYSICIAN TO THE MONTREAL GENERAL HOSPITAL; ASSISTANT
PHYSICIAN AND PATHOLOGIST TO THE WESTERN HOSPITAL.

———

VOLUME II
SYSTEMIC PATHOLOGY

———

SECOND EDITION, REVISED AND ENLARGED
WITH 301 ENGRAVINGS AND 15 PLATES

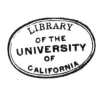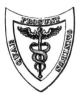

LEA & FEBIGER
PHILADELPHIA AND NEW YORK
1911

TO

WILLIAM H. WELCH

TO WHOM MEDICAL RESEARCH IN NORTH AMERICA OWES ITS DEEPEST DEBT

AND TO

THEIR PREDECESSOR

WILLIAM OSLER

WHO INITIATED THE TEACHING OF PATHOLOGY AT McGILL UNIVERSITY

THIS VOLUME

IS AFFECTIONATELY DEDICATED BY

ITS AUTHORS.

PREFACE.

LITTLE in the way of preface is here needed by those who have made themselves familiar with the first volume of this work. In that we dealt with the causes of disease and the morbid and reactive processes; now we pass forward to discuss the results of disease as it affects the different systems and, through them, the body as a whole.

We will not pretend that our first volume was other than bulky; to many readers it may have seemed that the treatment of the various sections was unnecessarily full. These same readers may be inclined to consider that, working upon the same scale, the subject matter of special pathology demands at least twice the space now afforded, or, put otherwise, that our treatment of systemic pathology is as condensed as that of general pathology was diffuse. A little consideration will, we trust, show that our method, if unusual, is, nevertheless, rational. Provided that the student has acquired a good grasp of the principles of general pathology, he has but to apply those principles in order to become possessed of a sound basis of special pathology. If, to cite examples, he be well acquainted with the modifications of the inflammatory process as it affects parenchymatous and connective tissues, epithelial and serous membranes, respectively; with the different forms of tumors originating from the different orders of cells; with the particular orders of degeneration likely to affect cells of one type or another; then his familiarity with the histology of the different organs gives him the key to special pathological histology. Taking this knowledge for granted, it becomes unnecessary to describe in detail the different conditions of inflammation, tumor growth, and degeneration that affect the different organs. Where these conditions are typical in their manifestations their existence alone need be cited. It is only when their manifestations present peculiarities that extended description is demanded; as also are the details of the gross morbid anatomy, or naked eye appearances, of the various organs under various conditions of disease.

We have proceeded, therefore, upon the assumption of a knowledge of the main data of general pathology as afforded in our first volume, and this second volume would have had relatively small dimensions had we not, in the first place, included the pathology of the blood and organs of circulation (usually and erroneously included under general pathology), and, in the second place, had we not endeavored to make our treatment more complete by dealing with the disturbances of function, as well as those of structure. We would reiterate that pathological anatomy (and histology) is but one division of our subject, and that from the pathologist of today there is equally demanded an acquaintance with the effects of disease upon the *function* of organs. Upon this we would lay particular stress, because it is this department or aspect of pathology which, for the clinician and practitioner, if not the more important, is assuredly that capable of the more immediate application. It is, indeed, interesting to note the extent to which, nowadays, the advanced teaching in medicine is based upon what we would term functional pathology, nay, has become teaching in this and little more; to observe, for example, the prominence given in the modern Systems of Medicine to the preliminary chapters upon the "physiological pathology" of the different organs. As a connecting link, therefore, between theory and practice this functional pathology is of prime importance. Realizing the attention that this branch of pathology receives from our colleagues, we have not attempted an exhaustive treatment; instead, remembering that the inclusion is more or less of a novelty, we have taken into consideration the functional pathology of the more important systems only.

In presenting this, the second edition of our volume on "Systemic Pathology," we would be ungracious were we not to acknowledge our high appreciation of the cordial manner in which our first effort was received. Cognizant as we are of its defects, it is perhaps but human that we have experienced relief in finding that those who have been good enough to study and criticise the work have convicted us of sins of omission rather than of commission. We know that it would be possible to produce a work which, in certain respects, would have been much more complete. We know that some such, dealing with special pathological anatomy, for example, are actually on the market. But with us the problem has been to impress upon the reader that systemic pathology is much more than special pathological anatomy, and so to indicate fairly this wider pathology as at the same time to afford a work within the covers of a single volume. And keeping in mind the main title of our work, our object has been, while affording what seemed to us an adequate substratum of necessary facts, to indicate the bearing of those facts and, generally, to link theory to its practical application. In short, to pro-

duce a work which, if not exhaustive, would yet be suggestive and help-
ful. In the second edition the general plan and scope of the work
have, therefore, been maintained. Nevertheless, we have strengthened
it in certain points where, in our judgment, it seemed lacking. Unnecessary repetition has been avoided. Where conflicting opinions had
inadvertently been expressed, these have been modified in harmony
with what we believe to be the trend of the latest investigation. Some
few subjects which were overlooked and omitted in the former edition
are dealt with now. Others, which possibly were handled with scant
courtesy, are discussed in more detail. Realizing that in a book which
does not attempt to be exhaustive its defects may to some extent be
compensated by the inclusion of a good bibliography, this phase of the
subject has received fuller recognition. To facilitate handy reference,
the index has been greatly amplified and the cross-references are much
more numerous. To save space, some few illustrations which were not
effective and some which were repeated have been omitted. What
to our minds were the characteristic features of the book, the introductions, in which we attempt to apply the facts of embryology, anatomy,
and physiology to the elucidation of disease processes, have been re-
arranged and have received much more adequate treatment. The
introductory chapters on the disorders of the Ductless Glands and
Nervous System have been rewritten, the latter, indeed, being almost
recreated. That on the Urinary System has been greatly amplified
by the addition of some chemistry, a discussion of the function of urination, and a consideration of the relationship of urinary disease to general
metabolic process and lesions elsewhere. The chapters preliminary to
the discussion of the Circulatory and Respiratory Systems are sub-
stantially unaltered, save for the addition of some points in embryology
and anatomy, which have been transferred from other parts of the
book. Thus, altogether, this portion of the subject has been rendered
more logical and coherent, and is much more adequate than before.
In view of these changes, we feel that the usefulness of the book has
been greatly enhanced. As it stands now, practically the whole of the
introductions to the Circulatory and Respiratory Systems and to the
Ductless Glands, and about half of that on Urinary Function are from
the pen of the senior author, together with sundry comments throughout
the text, while the junior author is responsible for the special descriptive
pathology, the preliminary chapters on the Digestive Functions, the
Nervous System, and the newly added portion on the Urinary Function.
Both have collaborated over the general arrangement of the subjects and

have criticised and emended harmoniously each other's work. way we have attempted to avoid "patchiness" and the other dual authorship.

In conclusion, we desire to thank our publishers for the coöperation in the production of this edition of our work.

J.
A.

Montreal, 1911.

CONTENTS.

SECTION II.

THE RESPIRATORY SYSTEM.

SECTION III.

THE ALIMENTARY SYSTEM.

————

SECTION IV.

THE NERVOUS SYSTEM.

————

SECTION V.

THE DUCTLESS GLANDS.

SECTION VI.

THE URINARY SYSTEM.

SECTION VII.

THE REPRODUCTIVE SYSTEM.

SECTION VIII.

THE TEGUMENTARY SYSTEM

SECTION IX.

THE MUSCULAR SYSTEM.

CHAPTER XLII

SECTION X.

THE OSSEOUS SYSTEM.

CHAPTER XLIII.

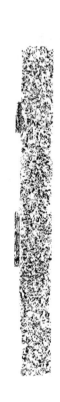

SYSTEMIC PATHOLOGY.

INTRODUCTORY.

In the first volume of this work, after having, if we may so express it, excavated with the endeavor to lay bare so far as possible the foundations of Cellular Pathology, we proceeded to discuss what is commonly known as General Pathology, inquiring first into the causes of disease and next into the general morbid and reactive processes. Doing this, we passed from a study of the cells to that of the tissues which they form, and ended by considering the progressive and regressive changes which may affect those tissues. Thence we pass naturally to a study of the yet larger aggregates, namely, of the organs and different systems of the body, and engage in the study of what we would term Systemic Pathology. Moreover, just as in the first volume we departed from custom and, instead of making our treatment mainly histological, based ourselves to a considerable extent upon the physiology, embryology, and chemistry of the cell and tissue, so here we have endeavored to present to the reader something more than the time-honored Special Pathology, by which has come to be understood the study of Morbid Anatomy and Histology, and of that alone.

We would once again emphasize that our subject has undergone material development, and that to-day something more than this is demanded. Inevitably, the study of Special Pathology forms the bulk of our work, but inevitably also the study of the anatomical changes occurring in the various organs leads to an inquiry into the significance of these changes and the influence they exert upon the function of those organs, and, what is more, upon the organism as a whole. Some knowledge of Functional Pathology, or, as some would express it, Physiological Pathology (although this designation involves a contradiction in terms), is now requisite, and, indeed, forms a most important link between the labors of the pathologist and the clinician. To indicate modern requirements we need but mention the popularity of Professor Krehl's well-known work, and the many editions it has undergone, despite the fact that its teaching covers no particular university course. We have thus thought it wise to preface our treatment of the individual systems with a consideration of the bearings of morbid changes in the component parts of that system upon function. The vast array of data that have accumulated in connection with the Morbid Anatomy and Histology of the different organs make any adequate modern text-book of Special Pathology necessarily a large volume. Hence, in adding these further chapters it has been indispensable to deal with these matters of Functional Pathology from a broad rather than a detailed standpoint. We can only hope that these additional chapters will render the work of additional service.

As regards the order of procedure there are two systems having ramifications which spread throughout the whole organism, namely, the vascular and the nervous; the others, if perhaps equally essential, are structurally more restricted and localized. Considering their intimate relationship with every region of the body, it would be appropriate to consider these two universal systems first. But here certain practical difficulties present themselves. For many reasons the nervous system should be given pride of place; its functions are so important, so sharply defined from those of all the other systems, that it might well be treated first and, as it were, dismissed before discussing the other systems which functionally appear to be more intimately connected. But this course is inadvisable, and that because the study of its pathology, if the most interesting, is also the most abstruse, and because that study is so specialized that it throws little light upon and does not naturally lead up to the other branches of systemic pathology. It is, therefore, most practical and most wise to study first the disturbances of the vascular system and their effect upon the body at large, the blood and lymph and the vessels which bear these; from this almost inevitably we pass on to consider the blood-forming organs. And this is additionally advisable when it is recalled that hitherto it has been customary to take up the more important disturbances affecting the distribution of the blood and its constituents (anemia, plethora, thrombosis, embolism, hemorrhage, œdema, etc.) as part of the course in General Pathology. By dealing with these matters first we make a compromise between that more usual and this, we believe, more logical method of procedure. To repeat, we see no reason, save prescription and convenience, why hemal and vascular disturbances—and not nervous and respiratory also —should be treated as portions of the course in General Pathology. Intimately associated with one of the main functions of the blood, the respiratory system next demands attention; and following this the digestive system, through which the blood is supplied with nutrient matter. Following this natural system, it becomes inevitable that, great as is its importance in the economy, the nervous system can only be discussed late in our course.

We begin then with a study of the pathology of the cardiovascular system, and first consider the pathology of the blood.

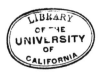

SECTION I.

THE CARDIOVASCULAR SYSTEM.

CHAPTER I.

THE BLOOD—QUANTITATIVE ALTERATIONS—ANEMIA—HYPEREMIA.

In discussing the circulation, we have to consider (1) the circulating medium, the blood, and with it the lymph, for this, as regards its fluid constituent at least, is drawn from the blood, and like that, circulates, even if slowly and imperfectly; and (2) the circulatory apparatus, the heart, bloodvessels, and lymphatic system. It is difficult often to separate these, disturbances in the distribution of the blood, for example, being now dependent upon primary disturbances in the bloodvessels, and now the reverse being the case. Remembering this, and being prepared to find that a certain amount of overlapping is inevitable, it is, on the whole, conducive to greater clearness if first the circulating medium be taken into consideration, and later the circulatory apparatus.

That the blood is the life is an old saying; that it ministers to the life of the constituent cells forming man's body, and is essential for the continuance of the same, more nearly states the facts of the case as we understand them at the present time. If this be so, if through diffusion, osmosis, and active or selective assimilation or excretion the cells gain their nourishment from it, and directly or indirectly discharge into it the products of their activity, then obviously the well-being of the organism as a whole, as of each constituent part, is liable to be affected by changes of two orders, namely, changes in quantity and changes in quality of the blood, either present in the body as a whole, or supplied to a particular region or organ. Whence it follows that we have to consider:

I. Quantitative alterations in:
    1. The amount of blood as a whole.
    2. The amount supplied to particular regions.
Closely allied to these, the further alterations in the amount and distribution of the blood caused by:
    3. Products of disorganization (thrombi and thrombosis).
    4. Presence of abnormal constituents and their effects (emboli and embolism).
    5. Escape of blood out of the vessels—hemorrhage.

II. Qualitative alterations in:
  1. The fluid menstruum of the blood.
  2. The corpuscular elements.

We have written above as though the blood came into immediate contact with the constituent cells of the body. Save in the case of the endothelial lining of the vessels, the cells of the splenic sinuses and those of the hemolymph glands, and certain cells of certain tissues, *e. g.*, the Kupfer cells of the liver parenchyma, this is not the case. It is not the blood as such that directly affords nourishment to the vast majority of the cells of the organism, nor do these cells, as a rule, discharge their products directly into the blood stream. It is the lymph derived from the blood that is the essential medium of interchange for most of the cells of the body. Hence, therefore, we have to consider also:

III. The lymph, both as regards quantitative and qualitative changes.

QUANTITATIVE ALTERATIONS.

1. **In the Total Quantity of Circulating Blood.**—We are apt to accept too freely that the total amount of blood in the body is about one-thirteenth of the body weight. This estimate we owe to Bischoff[1] more than a half century ago. His method consisted in taking two condemned criminals, weighing them before decapitation, collecting the blood, washing, so far as possible, all the remaining blood out of the vessels, washing their chopped-up organs, and finally deducting the weight of the washed residuum from the original weight. The method was, to say the least, somewhat crude and lacking in accuracy. As shown by Haldane and Lorrain Smith,[2] his results were excessive. They found that the amount varies between one-thirtieth and one-sixteenth of the body weight, the average given being roughly one-twentieth ($\frac{1}{20.5}$), or 4.78 grams per 100 grams of body weight. The method employed by those observers was ingenious, and based upon previous observations by Welcker and Grehant and Quinquaud.[3] The hemoglobin of the corpuscles takes up carbon monoxide (carbonic oxide) with very much greater avidity than it takes up oxygen (according to Nasmyth and Graham[4] the affinity is 140 times as great), and by colorimetric methods the proportion taken up by a given blood can be accurately determined. Thus, if, for example, an individual be made to inhale during a short period a *known amount* of the gas, well below the amount necessary to saturate the blood, and then a few drops of the blood be removed, and the percentage of CO present in this sample be determined, then it is a simple matter to determine how much has been absorbed per cubic centimeter and what ratio this bears to the total amount of

---

[1] Zeitschr. f. wiss. Zool., 7 : 1855 : 331, and 9 : 1857 : 65.
[2] Jour. of Physiol., 25: 1900: 331.
[3] Jour. de l'Anat. et de Physiol., 1882: 564
[4] Jour. of Physiol., 35: 1906: 32.

CO absorbed, and from this to estimate the amount of the total circulating blood. The figures gained by these two observers demonstrated that in fairly healthy individuals there may be close upon twice as much blood in one as in another. Making accurate observations upon series of members of different species of animals, Bollinger[1] arrived at similar conclusions. He, too, found marked variations in the amount of blood proportional to the body weight where there was no indication of disease. These observations are fully borne out by the current observations of any pathologist who performs a long series of autopsies. Often in elderly people, as again in those who had suffered from progressive wasting disease, the tissues and vessels are characteristically exsuccous (to employ old Sir Thomas Browne's expression); other corpses, on the contrary, ooze abundant blood at every cut; this last is particularly noticeable, it has seemed to us, in cases of obstructive heart disease.

Thus, it must be kept in mind that departures from the normal, not only in the specific gravity of a sample of blood taken from the finger or lobe of the ear, but also in the number of erythrocytes per c.mm., do not by any means necessarily mean only qualitative, but also may indicate quantitative changes. A heightened specific gravity, or an increase in the number of corpuscles, may mean a reduction in the fluid of the blood—a reduction in the amount circulating—and not an increased production of corpuscles; a lowered specific gravity, or decrease in the number of corpuscles, may indicate an actual or relative increase in the quantity of the blood plasma, and not an increased destruction of the erythrocytes. In short, the mere study of a blood film and enumeration of corpuscles is incapable of instructing us either as to variations in amount of the circulating blood, or (as is too often held) variations in the production or destruction of the erythrocytes. Hitherto, we have been reasoning on totally inadequate data. Thus, as Lorrain Smith has pointed out, not a few conditions which hitherto have been classed among the anemias or conditions of lack of blood are truly states of *hydremia,* of dilution and increase in actual amount of blood. We admit freely that the organism possesses, as shown by Sherrington, Lloyd Jones, and Cobbett, a singularly delicate mechanism to counteract any sudden change in the amount of circulating blood, and so to insure the due supply to all the tissues—a mechanism so delicate that within a very few minutes after a withdrawal of blood the specific gravity of that remaining within the vessels undergoes a decided fall, indicating a pouring of fluid.from the lymph spaces and tissue cells in order to restore the quantity of the circulating medium. But this admission does not oppose the fact that different individuals need very different amounts of blood. Your elderly maiden lady living sparely, and exercising her muscles with equal economy, has very different circulatory needs from those of the vigorous athlete in the prime of manhood, in whom the assimilative and disintegrative processes proceed apace. And if this be so in conditions of relative health, the variations in the quantity of blood in states

<hr />

[1] Münch. med. Woch., 1886 : Nos. 5 and 6.

of disease must be even more marked. We are bound, therefore, to recognize the existence of conditions of oligemia, or diminution in the amount of circulating blood, and of plethora, or increased amount.

Oligemia (Ischemia, Anemia).—Where, as may happen in secondary anemias and in pernicious anemia, during life the individual has been so bloodless that it has been difficult to secure a drop of blood from the finger, and where at autopsy the amount of blood in the heart and vessels is noticeably small in addition to being thin and of pale color, there can be no doubt that a condition of oligemia has been present.[1] Similar reduction in quantity may follow extreme or repeated hemorrhage, or great loss of the fluid part of the blood, as from cholera or pernicious vomiting. We are here speaking of quantitative changes, but it must be remembered that these conditions may produce profound qualitative changes also. Thus, within a very few minutes after a considerable hemorrhage there is a great drain of fluid from the tissues into the bloodvessels, whereby the quantity of blood is brought toward the normal. If the hemorrhage be repeated, the tissues may no longer be able to afford more fluid; what blood there is left in the vessels may be both thin and small in amount; the corpuscle count will be greatly lowered. In cholera, on the other hand, there is no loss of corpuscles; what blood there is left is thick and so concentrated as to be almost tarry.

Plethora.—For long years the teaching of Cohnheim[2] has influenced pathologists to disbelieve in the existence of plethora. Cohnheim showed that if saline solutions were injected into the vessels, they underwent a rapid excretion by the kidneys and removal from the blood into the lymph spaces of the body; the failure to produce plethora by this method led him to realize the remarkable regulative power of the vessels and tissues whereby the organism in health preserves a constant blood ratio. He neglected to take into account that, as with all other mechanisms of the organism, this also might be thrown out of order in disease. The observations of Lorrain Smith[3] by his carbon monoxide method have completely overthrown this older teaching. It would seem, as a general rule, that ample nutrition, coupled with active development of the muscular system, is associated with increase in the amount of blood above the normal. Take two individuals of the same age and height, the one a city clerk, the other a university athlete, and the large heart and full pulse of the latter can only mean a large amount of circulating blood. The rate of heart beat may not be faster in the muscular man, indeed it may be slower, but one has only to examine the heart of such a case to determine the large size of the cavities, which, with the

---

[1] The term anemia has unfortunately come to mean not what it should signify, "want of blood," but diminution in the hemoglobin content, or in the number of red corpuscles. It tends to greater precision to refer to this condition as oligemia, or small quantity of blood (ὀλίγος, few).

[2] Lectures on General Pathology, cap. 7.

[3] For an epitome of Lorrain Smith's work see his Appendix to Graham Steele's Diseases of the Heart, Manchester, University Press, 1906: 361

associated greater size of the aorta, can only indicate a larger volume of blood to be propelled. There is such a condition as simple plethora, *i. e.*, actual increase in the amount of normal blood.

But as with oligemia, so here: conditions of abnormal plethora are more recognizable, conditions in which there is increase in the fluid of the blood in excess of actual increase in the actual number of corpuscles. There can be no question regarding the existence of watery or hydremic plethora. Such occurs, as already noted, in many cases of obstructive heart and liver disease. There, from the increased venosity of the blood, it may be mistaken for true plethora, although study of the blood serum in these cases has, in general, shown that it is of lessened specific gravity, *i. e.*, that the serum is diluted, and, as Grawitz has pointed out, a coincident early sign of failure of compensation is reduction in the number of erythrocytes per c.mm. Lorrain Smith's observations[1] show that in these cases the volume of blood becomes increased two and three times above the normal; they show that at first, to antagonize its dilution and the slowing of the pulmonary circulation, the reduction in the number of red corpuscles is not proportional to the hydremia, and further, that the color index of the corpuscles is increased with indications of a compensatory hematopoiesis. Many more studies are needed before we are fully conversant with the changes in the blood accompanying heart disease.

What is the cause of this form of cardiac plethora it is difficult to say, whether it is due to the associated impaired circulation through the kidneys, and disturbance of their function, or to heightened venous and capillary pressure, dilatation and widening of the stream bed necessitating a larger amount of fluid in order to keep the blood in movement. A similar hydremic plethora has been noted in connection with obstructive lung disease. Closely allied is the plethora accompanying the Munich beer heart, ably studied by Bollinger. The hypertrophy and dilatation of the heart that follows the conscientious daily consumption of many liters of light beer would indicate that with absorption of this beer there is a daily considerable increase in the amount of the circulating blood.

Yet another form of hydremic plethora is associated with parenchymatous nephritis. It used to be thought that the accompanying albuminuria and drain of serum albumin from the blood was the cause of its more watery condition. That, however, would not account for the observed increase in amount in many of the cases, and for the absence of the plethora in other types of nephritis. Frènch observers have of late indicated a more probable cause, both of the hydremia and of the plethora. They have called attention to the deficient discharge of sodium chloride from the kidneys, and it is now gaining increasing acceptance that the accumulation of the chlorides in the blood and tissues attracts an increased amount of water leading to both hydremia and œdema. Re-

[1] Trans. Path. Soc. London, 53 : 1900: 136.

striction of chlorides has been found to be followed by material improvement.[1]

2. Local Alterations in the Quantity of Blood Supplied to a Part.—It is one of the commonplaces of physiological knowledge that the blood supply of a part varies according to circumstances; that increased activity of an organ is accompanied by increased passage of blood to the same; that such increase is largely controlled by the central nervous system through the vasodilator and vasoconstrictor nerves, although at the same time conditions within an organ, and again, the composition of the blood—the presence, for example, of acids or alkalies—directly affect the walls of the smaller arteries and capillaries, causing dilatation or contraction of the same, and, in consequence, variation in the blood supply to the organ.

Where there is excess of blood in a part we speak of (local) **hyperemia**, where deficiency, of (local) **anemia**.

In the above rapid statement we have by no means exhausted the list of conditions leading to a physiological alteration of the blood supply of a part. The tone, or state of partial contraction of the vessels, has to be kept in mind; the fact that the amount of blood is much below the capacity of the vessels that carry it; that hyperemia and dilatation of the vessels of one region demand a compensatory relative anemia of the rest of the body, or of some region of the same; that there is evidence of a special nervous control whereby, under normal conditions, the supply of blood to that region which in the erect position should be the first region to suffer from diversion of blood to other parts, namely, the cranium and brain, becomes the last to be seriously affected. A knowledge of the data upon which these conclusions are founded must be taken for granted.

Local Hyperemia.—Three conditions, it will be seen, determine the presence of an excessive amount of blood in an organ or part, namely: (1) the passage of an increased amount of blood into it, the outflow remaining the same; (2) diminished outflow, the inflow being unaltered; (3) no change in the caliber of the entering vessels or in the arterial blood pressure, and no resistance or obstruction to the outflow through the veins, but a widening of the capillary channels in the organ. The first of these we term *active* or arterial hyperemia, the second *passive* hyperemia or venous congestion; the existence of the third is largely neglected; we may refer to it as capillary hyperemia, and discuss it first.

Capillary Hyperemia.—The clearest physiological and, we are inclined to think, pathological examples of this condition are afforded by an organ which, it is true, does not so much possess capillaries as blood sinuses. As shown by Roy in his well-known oncometric observations upon this organ, the normal spleen exhibits a slow pulsation of its own, gradually expanding independently of any change in the general

---

[1] Vaguez et Digne, Études sur la Retention et l'Elimination des Chlorures, Paris, 1905; Ambard, Les Retentions Chlorures, Paris, 1905. This matter, however, must be regarded as still *sub judice*.

blood pressure, and then gradually contracting. This pulsation is attributed to the expansion and contraction of the plain muscle fibers contained in the capsule. With each act of contraction the capillaries and blood spaces of the organ are compressed and blood is driven out of them; with each expansion these become filled again. To some extent this must be true of all viscera possessing muscular walls; expansion of that muscle, or loss of tone of the same, must passively permit a hyperemia of the capillary areas within the muscle layer. It may well be that the enlarged hyperemic condition of the spleen in typhoid and other infections is not so much an example of arterial or active hyperemia as of the capillary hyperemia due to paresis and giving way of the muscular elements of the capsule, although with this another probable factor is the actual obstruction to onflow of the blood encountered in the sinuses themselves, through the arrest and accumulation there of the red corpuscles. But even in this latter case it will be seen that the hyperemia is of neither arterial nor venous origin. It will be recalled that a similar capillary obstruction has been noted, answerable for the obstruction to the passage forward of the blood and for the hyperemia seen in acute inflammation (vol. i, p. 423), which thus, save in its first stages, can scarce be regarded as truly of the active type. What may be regarded as almost physiological examples of this order are seen in the effects of cupping and hyperemia induced by suction.

Active Hyperemia.—This may be either *direct*, due to changes telling directly upon the arteries passing to a part, and leading to their dilatation, whereby a wider bed is afforded, and more blood enters the part; or *collateral*, due to contraction of other arteries, whereby, other things being equal, the blood pressure is raised and more blood is poured into the arteries under consideration, and so into the region supplied by them. Little need be said regarding the latter condition; we rarely encounter well-marked pathological examples save in the development of collateral circulation in a limb or other region. The direct form is relatively frequent, and may be due either to (1) stimulation of the vasodilators, (2) paralysis, or inhibition of the vasoconstrictors, or (3) direct local action of physical or chemical agents (warmth, temporary ligature, atropine, croton oil, etc.) upon the walls of the arterioles, leading to a giving way or expansion of the musculature. Diminution of external pressure acting upon an artery has a similar effect.[1]

The appearances of the affected part in true, active hyperemia are characteristic; it is enlarged and swollen, the color is a bright, arterial red; superficial parts, from the more abundant and freely circulating blood, are warmer than the surrounding regions, and in not a few cases it has been noted that the blood passing from the veins of the part is arterial in character. In extreme cases there may be a sensation of

[1] It may be urged that the example afforded by us to illustrate capillary hyperemia may be explained in this way, and that so this condition may be placed among the active hyperemias. There seems, however, to be a distinct difference between widening the capillary bed by reduction of pressure or active expansion of the organ itself, and removal of pressure from the afferent vessel.

throbbing in the affected part, together with visible pulsation of the smaller arteries or even of the capillaries, as, for example, at the base of the nail. The reddening may be distinguished from that due to hemorrhage by (in general) its brighter color, and more particularly by its temporary disappearance when pressure is applied.

Examples of these different forms of active hyperemia may here be rapidly passed in review.

Neuroparalytic hyperemia, due to removal of vasoconstrictor influences.—The type example of this form was afforded by Cl. Bernard in his well-known experiment of dividing the cervical sympathetic nerve in the rabbit. In man it has been noted that similar section of the cervical sympathetic, or destruction of the same by tumors, etc., leads to hyperemia of the side of the face, and dilatation of the retinal vessels, with heightened temperature. A like unilateral reddening, seen in some forms of migraine or hemicrania, has been attributed to inhibitory disturbance of the same nerve. It has, however, to be noted that not all the paralytic hyperemias observed in the lower animals as the result of nerve-section are to be encountered in man.

Neurotonic hyperemia, due to stimulation of the vasodilators.—The type example by which this is demonstrated is the intense hyperemia of the submaxillary gland which ensues upon stimulation of the chorda tympani, a hyperemia so intense that the blood in the emergent veins is of arterial character. To this order probably belong many of the fugitive erythemas of particular areas seen in neuralgic and hysterical conditions, as again in food and drug idiosyncrasies (vol. i, p. 410). Here also probably belongs that striking condition, **herpes zoster,** in which the cutaneous distribution of one or more nerves is sharply picked out to be the site of acute hyperemia followed by exudation and vesicle formation. We have already discussed the relationship of events of this kind to inflammation (vol. i, p. 449). Of the same order would seem to be **erythromelalgia,** a condition in which, suddenly, restricted areas, often symmetrically situated on the feet or hands, present a burning pain, with pronounced redness, heat, and pulsation. Closely allied are the *reflex hyperemias,* of which **blushing** affords the familiar example. Characteristic instances of this order are seen in certain cases of referred hyperemia or inflammation, *e. g.,* in the reddening and swelling of the side of the face which may accompany acute inflammation of a tooth. The rash upon the cheeks of infants when teething (**roseola infantilis**) is of the same order.

Myoparalytic hyperemia (Lubarsch), due to influences acting directly on the arterial wall.—Of influences which directly induce arterial expansion may be mentioned warmth, temporary ligature or compression (the active congestion which follows the use of Esmarch's bandage is a well-marked example), the presence of acids in the circulating blood, which, as Gaskell has shown, causes dilatation of the cerebral vessels (whereas alkalies bring about contraction), atropine, etc. In the experimental production of inflammation it has been demonstrated that croton oil applied to the rabbit's ear acts so slowly that the arterial dilatation can only be due to direct action and not reflex. In bacterial inflammation the toxins must act similarly.

Effects of Local Hyperemia.—Where this is fugitive no effects may be detected; where prolonged, the increased blood flow is inevitably accompanied by increased transudation from the distended capillaries, with, as a result, some swelling (œdema) of the part and increased flow of lymph from the same. Such increased flow signifies also increased nutrition. We have already discussed whether increased nutrition in itself leads to increased growth, concluding that, unless there be some coincident strain or demand for increased work, cells subjected to increased nourishment do not of necessity take on growth (vol. i, p. 597). We did not then take into account the undoubted influence of increased warmth in stimulating activities and growth. Such increased warmth is present in active hyperemia of a superficial area, and we would suggest that this may help to explain an apparent exception to the rule that has been noted, namely, that after section of the cervical sympathetic in the rabbit, the ear and the hair on the affected side grow more than do those on the sound side.

Extreme arterial hyperemia in an organ provided with a limiting capsule may, by compression of the specific cells, cause definite disturbance of function, as also in loosely constructed organs, by overfilling, it may lead to capillary hemorrhages.

Passive Congestion, or Venous Hyperemia.—As already laid down, passive congestion is brought about by obstruction or closure of a vein, so that the blood, propelled forward through the arteries, accumulates behind the point of arrest. There is this striking difference between active and passive hyperemia, that the former can only affect a relatively restricted area, the latter may be widespread. A little consideration shows why this is the case. Normally there is considerable tone or partial contraction of the arteries. Removal of this tone over a wide area renders the bed too big for the available blood delivered from the heart, and within a very short time there is insufficient fluid entering the arteries to keep them distended and hyperemic. To preserve an overfilling of the arteries of one region, there must be an extensive contraction of the arteries of other regions. The very convergence of the veins, so that all from relatively large districts come together and pour their blood into a common trunk, necessitates that any obstruction in this common trunk, or even in the heart itself, results in a heaping up of blood behind the point of obstruction; the blood becomes dammed in the main trunk or trunks and in the organs from which these trunks pass. In this way obstructive disease of the left heart leads to passive congestion of the whole pulmonary area; obstructive disease of the lungs or of the right heart causes cyanosis and congestion of the face, neck, liver, and other abdominal organs; obstructive disease of the liver or portal vein causes passive congestion of the intestines, spleen, etc. Paradoxically it may, and often does, happen that even complete blockage of a *small* vein leads to little or no passive congestion, and this because in most of the organs of the body the smaller veins present abundant anastomoses, as a result of which, if one vein becomes overloaded, the blood which should pass along it finds easy outlet along collateral channels. It is where these anastomoses do not exist, or are inadequate—in what is known as absolute or relative terminal veins—that we encounter the most extreme results of localized passive congestion.

The *causes* of arrested onflow of the blood in the veins are manifold. In the more widespread cases of passive congestion it is not essential that there should be actual narrowing of the vascular channel; mere weakening of the heart muscle, as from fatty degeneration without valvular disease, may result in lack of propulsive power, whereby the blood becomes heaped up in the venous system. Again, it has to be remembered that the normal advance of the blood along the veins is not dependent only on the *vis a tergo* of the ventricular pump acting through the arteries and capillaries. Every muscular contraction presses on certain veins, and through the agency of the frequent valves present in them drives the blood forward; every beat of the arteries must have a like influence on its venæ committentes.[1] The adjuvant action of the negative pressure on the thorax during inspiration and the negative pressure in the ventricles during diastole (see later[2]) need no comment. We mention these things in order to emphasize the fact that (1) cardiac weakness, (2) hindrances to perfect inspiration (paralysis of the diaphragm, or obstruction to the proper action of the same, accumulation of fluid, or new-growth in the pleural cavity, etc.), (3) lowered blood pressure and weakened pulsation, and (4) lack of muscular activity, all play a part in lessening the onflow of the venous blood, and all to a greater or less degree favor venous congestion.

Such congestion, it may be added, tends to show itself more especially in those regions in which the veins receive least support or compression from the surrounding tissues, and when at the same time these adjuvant factors are least brought into play. Thus, other things being equal, it is in those taking little exercise that piles or hemorrhoids are more particularly apt to show themselves; in those standing much on their feet, rather than in those indulging in much walking exercise, that varicose veins of the leg are to be encountered. Naturally, however, it is where there is narrowing, blocking, or obliteration of the venous channels that the passive hyperemia below the point of obstruction is most marked. To cite all the means whereby these conditions are brought about in the heart and veins would demand a very lengthy list; we must content ourselves with briefly classifying the main order of events into (1) conditions acting from within the blood channel (development of parietal thrombi, Chapter II), of intravascular new-growths, retrograde emboli (Chapter II); (2) conditions affecting the vessel walls, leading to stenosis or narrowing (endocarditis of heart valves, syphilitic, and other forms of phlebitis, new-growths involving the walls, etc.); and (3) conditions acting from without, compressing the vessel (tumors, fluid accumulations,

[1] Sir Lauder Brunton, Therapeutics of the Circulation, 1908: 5.
[2] Chapters VI and XI.

inflammatory cicatrices, granulomas, pressure of enlarged organs, *e. g.*, of the pregnant uterus, etc.). These conditions, to repeat, may affect the heart or larger veins, or, again, individual veins within an organ or tissue.

Results.—An organ or part which is the seat of passive hyperemia (1) is enlarged, primarily in consequence of the increased amount of contained blood, secondarily as a result of increased transudation from the distended capillaries; (2) is of a dark, purplish color, owing to the distension of its vessels with blood, which, owing to long continuance in the vessels, has become intensely venous; (3) is (when superficial) cooler than the surrounding parts, owing to the slowed circulation.

A few words are necessary regarding the significance of these different changes upon the blood, the vessels, and the tissues.

The Blood.—Relative or active arrest of the blood within the capillaries leads to greater giving up of oxygen and increased diffusion into it of carbon dioxide. It thus becomes intensely venous. Thus, Lépine found as much as 64 per cent. of CO_2 in the venous blood of a case of obstructive heart disease. It is this that explains the **cyanosis** (or "blue" state) of sufferers from passive congestion. One exception has to be noted: the brain and spinal cord, when congested, do not exhibit cyanosis; at most, multiple blood points (distended capillaries) stand out against the pale background of the cut surface of the white matter. Complete stasis or arrest may be followed by coagulation and thrombosis.

The Vessel Walls.—Continued passive congestion is constantly followed by indications of injury to the venous and capillary endothelium; in the first place, it is abnormally stretched and thinned; in the second, it exhibits fatty degeneration, presumably as a result of carbon dioxide intoxication.

The Tissues.—As a result there is increased transudation, and, it may be, modified (exudation), with some heaping of fluid in the interstitial tissue (œdema). This may not be marked in individual organs provided with a limiting capsule, but where there is general venous congestion of large areas, as from heart disease, it is one of the most striking features, with great accumulation of fluid in the body cavities (**ascites, hydrothorax**) and in the subcutaneous tissues (**anasarca**). The most rapid accumulation of fluid occurs in cases of sudden blockage or obliteration of the portal vein; here, apparently, in consequence of the portal blood with its material absorbed from the intestines being more toxic than systemic blood in general. Where the congestion is extreme and the capillaries ill-supported, there may be in addition repeated and multiple small capillary hemorrhages (Chapter III), and as a result of the breaking down of the hemoglobin the tissue may assume a brownish color. In addition, through malnutrition and through pressure, the specific cells of a tissue are apt to exhibit degeneration and atrophy. This is particularly well seen in the liver, where, through passive congestion, the cells of the centre of the lobule first undergo diminution in size with pigmentation, and eventually become completely atrophied and disappear, their place being taken by greatly dilated capillaries (Chapter **XXI**).

There is still some debate as to whether passive congestion of any order can lead to increased tissue growth. This we have already discussed (vol. i, p. 451). We would repeat that just as the Polish Jew or Chinaman can live and even thrive under conditions in which the Anglo-Saxon would starve, so when the congestion is of a moderate grade, the simpler and hardier white and yellow connective tissues may exhibit growth and proliferation at the same time that the more highly organized specific cells of a tissue manifest progressive atrophy. In addition to relative fibrosis due to this atrophy of the nobler elements, in the liver, for example, we have to recognize definite cases of productive fibrosis, not, we would emphasize, when the congestion is extreme, but when it has been of a moderate grade and long continued. Thus there is developed a true **cyanotic fibrosis** or **induration.** Where the congestion is extreme, where, that is, there is complete obliteration of the vein or veins of a part, with inadequate means of developing a collateral circulation, there the stasis of the blood is inevitably followed by necrosis or death of the whole area, resulting in the production of **gangrene** if the area of distribution be large, *e. g.*, the foot or leg (vol. i, p. 987), or of **hemorrhagic infarct** if the terminal vein of one portion only of an organ be involved.

Local Anemia.—Local anemia may be but part of a *general* bloodlessness—as after a profound hemorrhage; it may also be *collateral*, due to determination or drainage of blood to other regions, as in the anemia of the brain in syncopal attacks following upon dilatation of the splanchnic vessels (vol. i, p. 580). More often, however, we have to take into account the results of local disturbances of the blood supply through particular arteries, leading to deficient circulation in the areas served by those arteries. The causes of such local anemia are of the same order as are those of local passive hyperemia, though here it is the artery passing to a part that is affected, instead of the vein passing from it, and the results are widely contrasted. Disturbances may be brought about (1) by nervous influences acting upon the arteries, (2) by pressure upon it from without, (3) by disease affecting its walls, and (4) by obstruction or plugging of the arterial lumen by foreign or abnormal matter.

1. **Neurotic Anemia.**—With Lubarsch we can (perhaps somewhat insecurely) divide the cases in which individual arteries become contracted through nervous influences into the *direct* and the *reflex.* Thus, foremost among the direct he places the local anemias due to the action of cold. We admit freely with him that it is in females and those of a high-strung nervous temperament that such local contractions of the arteries most easily and most frequently show themselves. But in the first place, we are inclined to believe that cold, like heat, acts directly on the muscles of the arteries, and in the second, to doubt whether here, as indicated by the greater sensitiveness to, and perception of, cold by the affected individuals, there is not also a reflex element present. The case does not seem to be a pure one. More probably **Raynaud's disease** or symmetrical local asphyxia comes into this category. Here we deal

with a remarkable condition, at first spasmodic, later persistent, of contraction of certain arteries, usually symmetrical, most commonly of certain fingers and toes, although the whole hand or the pinnæ of the ears may be affected. The affected parts become first anemic and feel dead or tingle ("pins and needles"); if the condition continues for some hours, they gradually become blue (through lack of propulsion of the blood which slowly accumulates in the capillaries). After some time the condition may pass off and the affected area resume its normal appearance and warmth. The tendency is for the condition to last longer and longer until the prolonged anemia leads to death of the part and gangrene. Recent observations favor the view that in these cases we deal, if not at first, certainly later, with definite sclerotic changes in the arteries. It is, indeed, difficult to grasp the condition of prolonged tonic spasm of the arterial muscle. The cases thus may come into line with those of senescent or so-called spontaneous gangrene.

The type *reflex anemia* is seen in the pallor of fright or strong emotion; it is noteworthy that an emotion which in the one individual will stimulate the vasodilators and produce blushing, in another stimulates the vasoconstrictors and produces pallor.

2. Exogenous or Pressure Anemia.—Exogenous or pressure anemia may be produced by the compression exerted upon the artery running to an organ, by tumors, granulomas, cicatricial tissue, parasitic and other cysts, ligatures, etc. It deserves note that in many instances this form is preceded by passive congestion; when the pressure is of gradual development there is a first stage in which the accompanying vein with its lower blood pressure becomes first obstructed and then occluded, with the result that blood continues to be pumped into the organ or part through the still functional artery, and escapes with difficulty; only with increased pressure does the artery undergo obliteration.

3. Endogenous Local Anemia.—Endogenous local anemia is induced through changes in the arterial wall itself, *e. g.*, sarcomatous and other growths, or, the most frequent cause, endarteritis obliterans (see Chapter VIII).

4. Hematogenous Anemia.—Hematogenous anemia is brought about by coagulation of blood within an artery—thrombosis (see Chapter II), or by obstruction of the artery by foreign matter borne along the blood stream—embolism. The various substances which can act as emboli will be discussed more fully later (see Chapter II).

The *results* of defective blood supply to a part, and local anemia, are primarily: (1) pallor; (2) some reduction in size owing to lessened filling of the vessels; (3) firmer consistency; (4) lowered temperature of the part; (5) arrested function. With these there may or may not be secondary disturbances, either a dead feeling, or sometimes intense pain, *e. g.*, intense cardiac pain when a branch of the coronary artery becomes blocked, or agonizing cramps when there is anemia of the muscles of a lower limb.

The ultimate effects may or may not be of a more serious type, all depending upon the distribution of the vessels in the affected part.

(*a*) When through abundant arterial anastomoses a collateral circulation is rapidly developed, the disturbance may be but transient. (*b*) Where arterial anastomoses are present, but the area supplied by the blocked artery is large relative to the size of the collateral vessels, it is obvious that, at first, the region thus deprived of its normal blood supply obtains inadequate nourishment, and its functional activity is gravely depressed. Such conditions we find obtaining characteristically in the lungs, in which every region has a double arterial supply, in the main from the branches of the pulmonary artery, but in addition from the (smaller) branches of the bronchial arteries. (*c*) When the artery is truly terminal. We shall discuss the results in the following chapter.

CHAPTER II.

THE BLOOD—THE EFFECTS OF CLOSURE OF VESSELS.

It has been customary to discuss the effects of arrest of circulation through a vessel in connection with the treatment of ligation (in surgical works), or of embolism and thrombosis. The consequence has been not a little repetition, and a tendency to regard the results as due to one or other particular cause, and not as the natural outcome of the simple process of occlusion. It seems to us better to take up the broader subject of occlusion first, and later to deal with special modes.

It is obvious, in the first place, that arrest of the blood flow through a particular vessel, the general circulation continuing, may be brought about in three main ways: (1) By pressure acting from without; (2) by overgrowth of, or growth within, the vessel walls, either concentric and diffuse, or localized, so that the lumen becomes more and more reduced until it is wholly obliterated; or (3) by blockage from within. The pressure from without may be very variously produced—mechanically, as by ligature, or from general compression exerted over a part or over a particular vessel (e. g., by a tourniquet), by the growth of a tumor or cyst, enlarged glands, cicatricial bands, etc. The great cause of diminution of the vascular lumen by overgrowth of the vessel wall is arteriosclerosis (endarteritis obliterans). The corresponding condition, phlebosclerosis, does occur, but rarely proceeds so far as to obliterate the lumen of veins. The infiltration of the intima by new-growth may lead to like results. Blockage from within is due to either one of two causes, or a combination of the two, namely *thrombosis,* the intravital and intravascular "clotting" of the blood, and *embolism,* the arrest of matter foreign to the normal blood at some point where the size and configuration of the vessel prevents further progress along the lumen. Such foreign matter, if of irregular shape, may not at first cause complete occlusion, but upon it there may be deposit of platelets and clotting of the blood, so that the blockage tends to become complete.

The result depends upon whether we deal with occlusion of an artery or of a vein.

ARTERIAL OCCLUSION.

Many factors determine the result, namely, (1) the rate of narrowing or occlusion of the vessel, (2) the presence or absence of anastomosing arteries, (3) the size of the artery as compared with the collateral vessels, (4) the extent of the area supplied by the artery, (5) the condition of the heart and arterial blood pressure, (6) the venous blood pressure,

(7) the rate of flow, or perhaps more accurately, the difference between the arterial and venous pressure of a part.

We have placed in the first place what at first thought would seem to be a minor factor; further consideration shows that there is no factor that so materially modifies the result. The slow occlusion of an artery extending over days before it is complete permits the development of an adequate collateral circulation, so that when occlusion becomes complete the region supplied by the blocked artery may exhibit not a sign of disturbed nutrition; the sudden occlusion of an artery, as by an embolus, may be productive of grave disturbances, even of necrosis in the area of supply, and this notwithstanding the presence of collateral anastomosing vessels. Before these vessels become sufficiently dilated to afford an adequate blood supply, the imperfect aëration may have led to tissue death.

The presence or absence of anastomosing arteries is a very important factor. As Cohnheim pointed out, the arteries of the body are of two types, the *anastomosing* and the *terminal*, as indicated in the accompanying diagrams.

FIG. 1

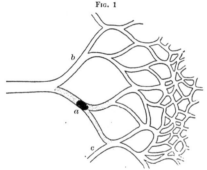

Schema of an anastomosing circulation. If a branch be ligatured or blocked as at *a*, the region supplied by that branch receives abundant blood through the anastomoses between it and other arteries, *b* and *c*. At most there is an arrested circulation in the artery itself as far as the nearest points of branching or anastomosis above and below.

ANASTOMOSING ARTERIES.—COLLATERAL CIRCULATION.—It is obvious that in those of the former order, ligature or blockage, say at *a*, will have very little effect upon the circulation of the area beyond; blood can so easily pass into the area from the arteries *b* and *c*. The case presents no difficulties under the simple conditions exhibited in the diagram. The conditions, however, are not always so simple. A large and important artery, such as one of the iliacs, may become obliterated. The dorsal aorta, even, through imperfect development, as in the condition known as coarctation, may be either excessively narrowed or completely blocked just above the region of entrance of the ductus Botalli. And notwithstanding the arrest of blood flow through such important channels, instead of the parts supplied becoming necrosed, we find that they receive sufficient nutrition to remain alive, nay, more, after a time the circulation through them may become wholly sufficient for the demands made upon the region in the course of every-day existence. In these cases we deal, it is true, with the same phenomenon, but with this difference, that the anastomosing or collateral vessels are often vessels which normally are inconspicuous, that it is not merely the branches immediately above and below the obliteration that carry the necessary blood, that vessels over a singularly wide area may be involved, and the collateral channels may be curiously round about. An extraordinary and widespread series of arterial anastomoses and enlarged collateral channels is to be made out in the cases of congenital coarctation of the aorta. Apart from persistence of the ductus arteriosus, what are

FIG. 2

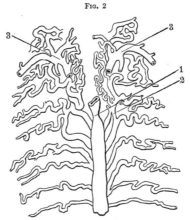

The main trunks of a collateral circulation established by means of the intercostals and neck vessels between the arch of the aorta and the dorsal aorta in a case of coarctation or congenital obstruction of the aorta in the region of the ductus Botalli. 1, region of coarctation; 2, anastomotic branches between the intercostal arteries; 3, subclavian arteries. From a man, aged thirty-five years. (After J. F. Meckel and Thoma.)

ordinarily unrecognizable anastomoses between the intercostal arteries become developed into arteries of the first rank, and a series of large anastomoses is to be made out between the arteries of the root of the neck and the upper intercostals, through which blood is conveyed into the aorta below the obstruction.

What, it may be asked, is the process whereby these small anastomosing vessels become enlarged, with hypertrophy of their walls, so as to function as main channels? It cannot be said that we wholly understand the process. Thoma, who has especially studied the subject, has laid down certain principles, but these do not explain; they only state the facts as we find them. With Thoma, we are forced to see that it is not primarily an active distension of the collateral vessels through increased pressure. It is true that where a large vessel becomes suddenly occluded, that occlusion induces increased pressure in the vessel (and its branches) behind the region of obliteration, but this is only a temporary state; within a very short time the blood becomes redistributed and the pressure falls to the normal. As von Recklinghausen pointed out, the important factor is the rate of blood flow. And here it must be noted that that rate is determined primarily by *relative pressure, i. e.,* by the difference in pressure in the vessels above the obstruction and those in the area whose supply has been cut off; the greater the difference between these two pressures, the more rapid the flow of blood into the part through vessels that are still open. Thoma lays down as his first principle that the distension of the vessels is dependent upon the rate of flow through them. This, however, does not carry us very much farther. Immediately after ligature or other obstruction, the pressure in the artery beyond the obstruction sinks to zero. Blood then pours into the artery from anastomosing vessels; the greater the pressure in the artery above the obstruction, the greater the rate of the flow through those vessels. But circulation cannot be reëstablished through the capillaries of the area supplied by the blocked artery until the pressure in those capillaries becomes higher than that in the veins. Or otherwise the time must come—and that relatively soon, unless the area of supply is to die from stagnation of the contained blood—when in the vessels forming the anastomoses there is no marked departure from the normal pressure difference between artery and vein, and when, therefore, the rate of flow must tend toward the normal and the dilatation of these collateral vessels, according to Thoma's principle, must be brought to an end and should give place to contraction.

We would suggest that another principle has to be taken into account, not considered by Thoma—the principle akin to that of Harris' "functional inertia," noted in our first volume (page 105), the principle of "overadaptation," which time and again we observe in vital phenomena. We would thus suggest that when collateral vessels expand, owing to increased rate of blood flow through them, the expansion is in greater ratio than the increase in rate of flow, with the result that the capillary pressure in the area of supply, instead of being lower, tends to become even higher than that in the surrounding tissues, whereby, in place of stagnation of the blood, an active circulation is favored, *i. e.,* a greater "fall" into the efferent veins. We fully accept Thoma's second mechanical principle, that with dilatation of a vessel the added strain of the larger stream of blood passing through it leads to growth of the walls—provided that the strain be not excessive (vol. i, p. 593). Thus it is that what had been little more than arterioles may become developed into relatively large, thick-walled arteries.

In other words, a collateral circulation can be maintained only in those cases in which the anastomosing vessels are sufficiently large or sufficiently numerous to preserve, when dilated, the circulation in the area beyond the obliteration. Where they are inadequate, there they pour blood into the area, and in the absence of a sufficient *vis a tergo*, the blood stagnates in the part, and by its stagnation the flow through the collateral vessels, instead of continuing, becomes arrested, and infarct formation or gangrene is the necessary consequence.

ANASTOMOSING VEINS.—In the case of the veins, we have, it is true, a somewhat different condition of affairs; the blood passing through the collateral vessels has not to supply later a capillary area; it has merely to find its way into another vein nearer the heart. The danger here is not one of stagnation in front, but of stagnation in the capillary area behind.

Venous anastomoses are freer and more widespread than are arterial, and, as a result, the extent of the collateral circulation set up is at times very extraordinary. Thus, when the portal vein becomes seriously obstructed, the blood from the portal area may find its way through a very wide series of tortuous collateral channels—through the coronary veins of the stomach into the œsophageal veins, through those of the gastro-epiploic omentum to the diaphragm and so into the vena azygos, through anastomoses between the inferior mesenteric and the hemorrhoidal veins, and through the retroperitoneal veins of Retzius joining the radicles of the portal veins in the mesenteries with branches of the inferior vena cava, as also through the veins of the round and suspensory ligaments of the liver to the epigastric and mammary veins. When the common iliac veins are occluded, or the lower end of the inferior vena cava, we similarly find the blood from the lower extremities conveyed through the epigastrics and veins of the anterior abdominal wall up to the mammary veins, with the formation of a pronounced **caput medusæ**, or congeries of tortuous distended veins in the region of the navel.

The obliteration of a large vein coming from a part must undoubtedly be followed by a marked rise of pressure behind the obstruction, and that rise and the accompanying dilatation of the capillaries of the area is frequently accompanied by œdema and accumulation of fluid in the tissues and spaces. Where it occurs, this indicates that adequate collateral circulation is not immediately developed, and that for some period, at least, the circulation through the affected part is impeded. The rise of pressure must materially increase the rate of flow through the collateral veins. Certainly the impression given is that the combined crosssection of these collaterals comes in many cases to exceed that of the obliterated vessel, and that the occlusion gains more than compensation. On the other hand, the great tortuosity of these vessels and their long and often roundabout course has to be taken into consideration, as counteracting the free discharge of blood from the affected area. On the whole, we see no reason to imagine that the same principles are not at work in the case of the development of a venous collateral circulation as in that of an arterial, and we think that for there to be free drainage, the dilatation of the anastomosing vessels must be more than proportional to the increased rate of flow through them.

TERMINAL ARTERIES.—The case is very different in cases of the latter order. Here ligature at *a* wholly cuts off the arterial supply to the region beyond. The only supply that can reach it is either by back flow through the vein of the part, or through the abundant capillary anastomoses at the periphery of the area. Not to enter into what has been quite an active discussion, we may say that the first of these methods is now generally discredited. Such back flow would not create a circulation, whereas microscopic examination of the peripheral capillaries shows that they become greatly dilated and distended with blood. Whatever circulation or entrance of blood occurs into the part we now attribute to those capillaries. But these may be inadequate to nourish the part, save, perhaps, at the very edge of the area of arterial supply, and as a result, the main bulk of the tissue undergoes a rapidly developing necrosis, and an **infarct** is produced.

FIG. 3

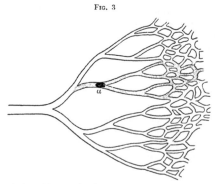

Schema of a terminal arterial system in which the anastomoses are only between the capillary loops. It will be seen that a ligature or obstruction at the point *a* may cut off the whole blood supply of the region supplied by the obstructed artery and its branches, unless the capillary circulation provided by neighboring arteries be so abundant as to afford nourishment to the blocked area.

The terminal arteries of the body as usually given are: those of the kidney, brain and spinal cord, spleen, the branches of the pulmonary arteries, the coronary arteries, arteria centralis retinæ, and superior mesenteric artery. More accurately, these are the arteries in connection with which infarct formation is encountered. Further investigation shows that these are not necessarily terminal arteries in the strict sense, so that Cohnheim himself was forced to modify his views, and speak of *functional* end arteries. The branches of the superior mesenteric notoriously have free arterial communication with those above and below, and yet true and often very extensive infarction of the small intestine is encountered. The same is true of the coronary arteries; these are not devoid of definite, if small, anastomoses, and the same may be said of the brain, and even of the kidney. In the lung, as again in the liver, while the pulmonary and hepatic arteries are of the terminal type, they do not afford the sole blood supply to individual areas; in the one case branches of the bronchial artery open into the same capillary network, in the other the portal vein supplies abundant blood. We come back then to this: *that it is not the absence of anastomoses or of other arteries supplying the same area that is essential to infarct formation, but the absence of arterial anastomoses sufficiently large to insure the proper nutrition of a part once the main nutrient vessel to that part becomes suddenly occluded.*

FIG. 4

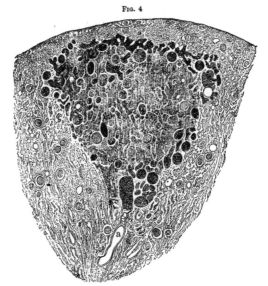

Anemic infarct of cortex of kidney to show coagulation necrosis, with surrounding zone of congestion: *a*, artery. (Orth.)

Infarct Formation.—What then is the nature of infarct formation? When such a main nutrient artery becomes occluded, collateral arterial supply is inadequate to cause a sufficient circulation through the associated capillary area, and, owing to the cutting off of the main *vis a tergo*, the blood pressure in the area sinks either to nil or, when there exist small collateral arterial supplies to the area, to a point which is below even the venous pressure of the surrounding tissue. As a consequence, the specific tissue cells of the part no longer gain sufficient oxygen; anabolism is arrested, although catabolism and disintegration of these substances may continue and result in the diffusion of carbon dioxide, and other end-products into the lymph and blood. We may compare the process with the continued discharge of carbon dioxide by the frog placed in an oxygen-free atmosphere, or the liberation of carbon dioxide from the removed kidney through which is perfused an oxygen-free salt solution. The result would seem to be a poisoning of the tissue with the products of its own disintegration. While this is proceeding, blood tends to pour into the capillaries of the part from the surrounding capillaries with their higher blood pressure. The extent of this passage we shall discuss later, but with it, following Weigert's conception of the process, there would appear to be some increased transudation of fluid from the capillaries, and absorption of the same by the tissue cells. The nuclei of those cells lose their chromatin. Whether this diffuses out, or is converted into non-stainable matter, must be left an open question. And now, through the formation or liberation of a thrombin or fibrin-ferment, the whole area, cells, lymph, and blood, undergoes a process of coagulation; it passes into a condition of coagulation necrosis. The whole affected area—usually wedge-shaped in consequence of the fan-like distribution of the branches of the affected artery—assumes a more solid consistence than the surrounding tissue, is swollen, so that if it abuts upon the surface of an organ it projects somewhat, and on section it cuts firmly, and is sharply defined. It may be either of a pale, grayish-yellow color—*white* or *anemic* infarct, or of a deep blood-red—*red* or *hemorrhagic* infarct.

White Infarct.—The white infarct is encountered almost constantly in the kidney, frequently in the brain, heart, and liver, less frequently in the spleen, rarely in the skin and intestine, practically never in the lung.[1] Where recent, the finer histology manifests a peripheral notably congested zone, in which the capillaries are greatly distended with blood, and within this, an almost hyaline mass, in which the outlines of the constituent tissues can be faintly distinguished, the constituent cells appearing to run into each other; the nuclei are invisible, and the whole area has a homogeneous, unstained appearance.

Red Infarct.—This, as regards incidence, is the converse of the white; is practically always the form present in the lung, is the commonest form met with in the intestine, is rarely present in the kidney, etc. We would add that the so-called red infarcts of the liver, due to obstruction of branches of the portal vein, cannot be considered as genuine infarcts; they exhibit, it is true, enormous congestion of the capillaries, but the liver cells and vessel walls are not necrotic. There is still in them a collateral circulation sufficient to prevent cell death.

Where recent, microscopic examination shows that not only are the capillaries throughout the red infarct greatly distended with coagulated blood, but in addition there is abundant evidence of hemorrhage; the tissue spaces are filled with extravasated blood cells. There is no evidence of actual rupture of the capillaries, the hemorrhage has been *per diapedesin.*

---

[1] We have on two occasions encountered soft, gray infarcts in the lung, but these were obviously late stages in the resolution of a red infarct, with breaking down of the erythrocytes, and diffusion out of the hemoglobin, and in one of the two cases, beginning organization.

The tissue cells of the affected area show necrosis and absence of staining of the same order as that seen in the white infarct. Here, one partial exception must be made: in most red infarcts of the lung we have been able to recognize still the nuclei of the capillary endothelium, staining, it is true, more feebly than normal, but standing out with some prominence in contrast with the surrounding non-staining tissues. This is, we hold, correlated with the existence of a second arterial blood supply to the part through the bronchial arteries. Such tissue is not absolutely necrotic, and through it the circulation can eventually become restored; considerations which explain the singular rareness of indications of old cicatrized infarcts in the lungs. It is, indeed, remarkable how rare it is to encounter anything that may be regarded as the cicatrix of a previous infarct in the lung, and yet infarction at a previous period must be common, especially in cases of long-standing cardiac disease. Where, as in the lung, there is this double circulation, we must conclude that in a certain, it may be a large, proportion of cases the vitality of the tissues is not entirely lost, and that subsequent resolution and regeneration of the alveolar epithelium, etc., is possible, the part returning to the *status quo ante*. We thus recognize a series of transitional cases, through the "red infarct" of the liver, with little or no necrosis, these red infarcts of the lung, with necrosis of some, but not of all the component tissues, up to the infarct proper, with complete coagulation necrosis.

Here, also, in passing, it must be emphasized that the red infarct is due not only to arterial obliteration, but may equally be produced by blocking of the efferent vein of an organ or part of an organ. Provided that there be no adequate venous anastomoses, the continued pouring of blood into the part by the artery leads to overdistension of the capillaries, stagnation of the blood, tissue necrosis, and hemorrhage. The picture is to all intents and purposes identical with that of arterial red infarct, save that the congestion and hemorrhage tend to be extreme. What is perhaps the best example of this form is occasionally encountered in infants in the hemorrhagic infarct of the adrenal, a rare cause of relatively sudden death. The primary disturbance would seem to be thrombosis of the adrenal vein. The organ is converted into a firm, swollen, intensely hemorrhagic mass of dead tissue. It is still a matter of controversy whether some, at least, of the red infarcts of the lung are not similarly due, not to embolism of branches of the pulmonary artery, but to thrombosis of branches of the pulmonary vein. It is quite possible that this may be the case; but, on the other hand, the more carefully these pulmonary infarcts are studied, the greater is the number in which arterial embolism is encountered. We must thus conclude that pulmonary infarct of venous origin is the exception and not the rule.

The Mode of Production of Red and White Infarcts.—Why under certain circumstances and in certain organs we obtain white infarcts, and in others red, has been angrily debated for now more than a generation. Intimately associated with this has been the whole study of the mechanism of infarct formation, and many of the positions taken have truly had more bearing upon this latter problem than upon the former. It is generally accepted that when the arterial supply to a part—or the venous discharge—is slowly obliterated, infarct formation does not occur. Time is then given for the establishment of collateral circulation. For infarct formation there must be relatively sudden arrest of the circulation in a part. It is accepted also that infarct formation may occur even when—as in the lungs, for example, and the intestines—a collateral arterial supply is present, *but is inadequate to provide, of a sudden, sufficient nourishment to the area.* Again, it is generally admitted that the blood that pours into an infarctous area does not enter by means of back pressure through the veins, but through the capillary anastomoses; there is a higher blood pressure in the surrounding capillaries than in the veins. But reviewing the ancient controversy, it is abundantly evident that considerations of general blood pressure, or capillary and relative arterial and venous blood pressure, give no satisfying explanation why, in some cases, the area becomes overfilled with capillary blood until hemorrhage occurs, and in others the coagulation necrosis occurs without those phenomena showing themselves. We have passed over the controversy very rapidly because we believe that these discussions upon relative blood supply, and the conditions affecting it, are, at the most, of but secondary importance. The explanation is to be sought along wholly different lines, and has been afforded by the more recent studies upon autolysis and tissue survival. It is, we hold, a fact of high significance that white infarcts involve just those tissues which either have been recognized as most rapidly succumbing to circulatory arrest, or, on the other hand, are those which after death afford the most abundant proteolytic and other ferments, and undergo autolysis most rapidly. Thus, for example, it is the heart muscle that of all the muscles in the body first shows rigor mortis, and first, through autolysis, passes out of that state; the nervous tissue that first shows lack of response (*i. e.*, dies) when its blood supply is cut off; the cortical tissue of the kidney that has empirically been selected to demonstrate the necrotic effects of temporary arterial ligature (Litten's experiment, vol. i, p. 929); the liver, kidney, spleen, and heart muscle that most rapidly exhibit autolysis. Or, otherwise, it is just those organs that either are most susceptible to arrest of blood supply, and whose cells die with relative ease, or again, those which, dying, discharge abundant autolytic enzymes, that may exhibit white infarct formation. Thus, we must assume that the essential cause of the white infarct is the relatively rapid death of the constituent cells of the affected area, with liberation of thrombin—or prothrombin—and that coagulation ensues, or rigor (for the two processes would seem to be of the same order), *before the capillary anastomoses have widened sufficiently to induce hemorrhage.* That in some organs we encounter now white, now red, infarcts would seem to gain its simplest explanation, not primarily in variations in blood pressure and in the rapidity with which blood finds its way into the vessels of the infarctous area, but, as Lubarsch points out, in the state of the cells at the moment when the circulation is cut off. He gives an excellent example in proof. In the healthy rabbit it is only after ligature of the renal artery for about an hour and a half that necrobiosis of the kidney is induced.   If, however, the animal be inoculated with diphtheria toxins, or better, if acute nephritis be set up by intravenous injections of ammonium chromate, and in the course of the next day the renal artery be ligated, now closure for only three-quarters to an hour is needed to induce complete infarction of the whole kidney, recognizable, not immediately, but eight hours or so after the temporary ligature.   He points out that by repeated closure of the artery for half-hour periods, eventually the kidney cells become so susceptible that half-hour closure is followed by infarction.   We may recall the parallel observations upon the great variation in the onset of rigor in muscles.   Where the muscle has been overexercised, as in the hunted animal, this may follow immediately upon death; in other cases putrefaction may ensue before it can show itself.   And so it has to be kept in mind that *infarct* formation does not necessarily follow upon closure of a terminal or functionally terminal artery.   The state of the tissues determines whether coagulation necrosis does or does not become developed.   This is particularly noticeable in the lung.   We have already pointed out that here infarction is often incomplete, but in addition it has to be noted that a large proportion of cases of embolism of branches of the pulmonary artery fail to show any sign of infarct formation This is more especially the case where large branches, such as those supplying a whole lobe, become blocked.   In these the most we obtain is congestion.   It is quite possible that another factor comes into operation here.   Weigert's postulate has to be kept in mind, namely, that for coagulation necrosis to ensue, there must not only be, as we may express it, the liberation of a prothrombin from the dying tissues, but a something supplied to the affected tissues by serous infiltration from the bloodvessels before coagulation can ensue.   Where a large tissue area has its blood supply suddenly cut off, the pressure in the capillaries of that area may never reach a sufficient height to permit this exudation, or only permits it at a period when further autolytic changes have already manifested themselves, and coagulation is impossible.   Here may be the explanation why infarct formation affects only relatively small areas, and why, when the blood supply is cut off from larger areas—a limb, for example—then, in place of infarct formation, we obtain a liquefactive necrosis or gangrene.

Here, farther, it must be pointed out, as shown by the researches of Greenfield and Beattie,[1] that it is not the mere presence or absence of blood in the vessels of the obstructed area that determines the existence of red or white infarct respectively.   These observers state that in experimental infarct formation *in all cases* examination during the first few hours shows the distension of the capillaries with blood.   It is evident that what determines whether the red or white infarct becomes developed is the rate of onset of the coagulation necrosis—whether this occurs after or before the distension has led to hemorrhage.

[1] Beattie and Dixon, A Text-book of Pathology, Lippincott, 1908.

The Results of Infarction.—1. *Complete Resolution.*—This, as already indicated, would seem to occur where the infarction has been imperfect, as in the lung. We have evidence of the existence of fibrinolytic ferments derived from both polynuclear and mononuclear leukocytes, as again of proteolytic ferments, broadly of a tryptic nature, liberated in autolysis. It is possible thus that capillary thrombi undergo complete absorption—that the hemorrhagic products in the lung alveoli become likewise absorbed, that with the reëstablishment of an adequate circulation the vascular endothelium regains complete vitality, as again, that the alveolar epithelium becomes regenerated from the periphery.

2. *Organization and Cicatrization.*—This is the more typical event. From the peripheral zone of congested capillaries abundant leukocytes pass into the necrosed area. Partly through the heterolytic enzymes, partly, it may be, through the autolytic, the necrosed area undergoes a process of solution, and as this proceeds, new capillary loops pass in from the periphery, and we have the familiar picture of the development of granulation tissue and of subsequent cicatrization of the same. It is a frequent experience to find the depressed cicatrix of old infarcts in the kidney and in the spleen.

3. *Cyst Formation.*—In the brain more particularly, in place of organization, cyst formation may show itself (vol. i, p. 864).

4. *Putrefaction.*—Where pyogenic organisms are in the affected area, or where the embolus causing the infarct is infective, there, according to the size of the infarct, we may encounter either a putrefactive softening of the infarct, with liquefaction of necrotic area through the proteolytic bacterial enzymes, and without the formation of true pus, or—

5. *Suppuration.*—In small infarcts, true abscess formation, with abundant leukocytes attracted into the area from the surrounding capillaries, may be developed.

6. *Calcification.*—The conditions favoring calcification of a necrosed area have already been discussed (vol. i, p. 927).

Mortification.—To recapitulate: where (1) there is inadequate anastomosis, and where (2) the area whose blood supply is cut off is extensive, there, in place of coagulation and infarct formation, we encounter mortification. We employ this term rather than what is usually regarded as its synonym, gangrene, because, to most minds, the latter carries with it the implied conception of putrefaction and decomposition of bacterial origin. More recent research shows that, at least in the first stages of cases of this order, there is an aseptic softening of the tissues due to autolysis.

We feel some hesitation in drawing this sharp distinction between infarction and mortification. It may well be that in the majority of cases in which tissue death occurs from the cutting off of the blood supply of a part there is at least a preliminary stage of rigor and coagulation necrosis. But if so, this may be imperfect, involving certain tissue constituents more than others, and passing off with relative rapidity as autolytic processes manifest themselves. We approach here a problem that has not yet to our knowledge been made the subject of investigation, namely, to what extent, if any, does the development of coagulation necrosis proper inhibit autolysis within the living body. It is not a little striking that in organs such as the kidney, which out of the body exhibit rapid autolysis, we encounter white infarcts which evidently are many days old, but which have remained firm with no signs of autolytic softening, or, at most, what has been termed heterolytic softening at the periphery through the agency of invading leukocytes; whereas, in other organs, in which infarct formation is not so noticeable, softening may ensue with relative rapidity. Our knowledge of the whole subject, in fact, of coagulation of the blood and of the tissues is in so chaotic a condition that it is impossible to lay down with any clearness why, when small areas are involved, we are more likely to get infarct formation; when larger areas, the process of mortification with softening. We see obscurely that for coagulation necrosis to ensue, there must be some liberation of kinase from the dying cells, which, interacting with bodies afforded by the surrounding lymph, favors the formation of a thrombin or ferment, which in its turn leads bodies of the nature of fibrinogen, both intracellular and extracellular, to undergo solidification, or coagulation. We cannot lay down with any clearness what it is, for example, that brings it about that where a small branch of the pulmonary artery becomes blocked, an infarct is produced; where a large branch, such as that supplying a whole lobe of the lung, no infarction ensues, but only mortification. Presumably the capillary pressure in the two cases and the extent of exudation play a part—but this is only a presumption.

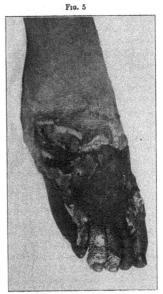

Fig. 5

Gangrene of the foot. (Montreal General Hospital.)

Gangrene.—Under conditions in which, either from coincident closure of the various anastomosing arteries of a relatively large area, or absence of anastomosing arteries in the same, it may happen that little blood passes into the dead area, and in that case in parts that are exposed and subject to evaporation, there is gradual desiccation and the development of *dry gangrene*. Where bacteria gain entrance, putrefaction ensues, and thus a form of *moist gangrene*—a form, it may be added, not so extreme as regards distension of the vessels, exudation, and hemorrhagic infiltration, as is seen where the efferent veins are blocked, the arteries still conveying blood to the part (see farther, vol. i, p. 988).

VENOUS OCCLUSION.

The causes of closure of veins are of the same order as those of arteries, although certain exceptions are to be noted. Thus neurotic or spastic occlusion is unknown; the condition also of endophlebitis obliterans, or proliferative overgrowth of the intima sufficient to induce obliteration, is almost unknown; at most, rare cases have been reported.[1] So also in regard to hematogenous occlusion, while thrombosis is common, embolism, from the nature of the case, is singularly rare, and can only be due to a retrograde passage or falling of foreign matter into a vein. This retrograde embolism will be discussed later. And obviously, by itself this can scarce induce complete occlusion; by inducing a surrounding thrombosis or, where of the nature of liberated portions of new-growth, by subsequent proliferation, it may bring about not an immediate, but a gradual complete closure.

Just as the primary effect of closure of an artery is to produce local anemia of the region of supply, the extent of the anemia depending upon the width of anastomosing vessels, so the primary effect of venous occlusion is the production of congestion, the corresponding artery or arteries pouring blood into the part which must become heaped up in the area, unless there be adequate anastomoses. In general, venous anastomoses are more abundant and larger than are arterial, and thus, in general, where we deal with the occlusion of a single venous branch in an organ the effects are little noticeable. It is thus more especially when all the veins coming from a part become occluded (as in the case of an incarcerated hernia), or where the occlusion affects the main vein coming from an organ after it has received all its subsidiary branches, that serious results ensue (as, for example, when the common iliac, the main portal trunk, or a main renal vein becomes blocked by a thrombus). Even in these cases the results are apt to be temporary rather than permanent. Anastomosing vessels of minute size undergo a progressive dilatation, and an abundant collateral circulation becomes developed. How abundant may be the paths of such collateral circulation may be indicated from a study of those cases in which there is obstruction to the main portal vein, such as occurs in cirrhosis of the liver. To those various collateral channels we have already referred (Chapter I).

It is noticeable that, despite these abundant anastomoses, it may be long before the collateral circulation is adequate. Thus, when the femoral vein becomes thrombosed, it may be long months before the congestion and œdema of a lower extremity completely disappear, and longer months, or even years, before any increased exercise with increased pouring of arterial blood into the part is not followed by indications that the circulation is still imperfect and only able to do little more than deal with the usual amount of blood—evidence in the shape of swelling of the limb and muscular exhaustion. And in portal

[1] See Meigs, Jour. of Anat. and Physiol., 34:1900:458

cirrhosis of the liver, even after providing additional anastomoses by causing adhesions between the omentum and the liver and the anterior abdominal wall, the congestion and accompanying ascites are still apt to continue, despite all the paths present or provided for the drawing away of the portal blood.

Where the main venous trunk coming from an isolated, encapsulated organ is suddenly blocked, there the opportunity for the carriage of the venous blood is at a minimum. The organ becomes hugely swollen and tense; there is complete stasis of the blood within it; interstitial hemorrhages occur, and the organ undergoes either infarction or mortification. We have already indicated (page 41), and here repeat, that hemorrhagic infarction may result from venous obstruction. Such mortification may give place to gangrene in those cases in which opportunity is present for the entrance and growth of bacteria, as in a strangulated hernia of the intestine or thrombosis of the veins of the leg.

Hence, to recapitulate, the results of occlusion of a vein may be:

1. Practically nil, when the vein is small and one of a series of abundantly anastomosing vessels.

2. Intense passive congestion, with exudation of fluid from the vessels, œdema, etc., and gradual development of a collateral circulation, the congestion and dropsy disappearing as the collateral circulation becomes more and more adequate.

3. Intense passive congestion with exudation, etc., giving place to stasis and hemorrhages in those cases in which a collateral circulation cannot be developed with sufficient rapidity. This stasis results in:

4. Hemorrhagic infarction.

5. Mortification.

6. Gangrene.

EMBOLISM.

Intimately associated with the subject of vascular closure is that of embolism. Literally, an embolus is something "thrown in;" actually, it is any body which, carried along in the blood stream, reaches some point at which the narrowing of the vessel causes its arrest, so that it either wholly or partially blocks the vessel. We are apt to conceive the embolus as always completely blocking a vessel. This is not essential; the shape of many solid foreign particles must be such that they permit some passage of blood around them. But undoubtedly their very presence favors a secondary deposit of thrombus material upon them, so that sooner or later the obstruction becomes complete. According to the size and the source of the foreign body forming the embolus, so may we encounter them in all parts of the circulating system—in the heart, aorta and arteries, capillaries, and veins.

Cardiac Embolism.—Cardiac embolism is very rare; occasionally a long thrombus of the femoral or iliac veins may become detached and be carried to the right heart, and there, becoming rolled upon itself, may form a plug sufficiently large to become arrested in the conus arteriosus, blocking the entrance to the pulmonary artery. We have encountered one such case. The ball thrombus of the left auricle referred to later (page 71) is not strictly an embolus, *i. e.*, it does not become firmly lodged in the stenosed mitral orifice; there are, however, one or two cases on record in which large, irregular, softened thrombi from the left auricle have become loosened and wedged in the stenosed mitral orifice, and thus have acted as true emboli. It is scarcely necessary to state that the result in these cases is sudden death.

Aortic embolism is also uncommon. While the aorta becomes very perceptibly narrowed in its lower portion after the renal arteries have been given off, it is rare to have a detached thrombus from the left heart, or of parietal nature from the upper part of the aorta, so large that it blocks this portion of the vessel. Along with others, we have, however, encountered a "riding embolus" poised upon the sharp angle of bifurcation of the common iliacs, which, itself loose and easily detached, had led to an obliterating thrombus filling the last portion of the aorta and there adherent.

Arterial embolism is the most common condition. As Professor Welch points out, it is difficult, if not impossible, to state with any degree of accuracy the frequency with which the different arteries are involved, and that because by no means all emboli give rise to symptoms, and as a result they are not sought after at autopsy. As indicated in the previous chapter, unless the embolism occurs in a functional end artery, the results are apt to be negligible. But observers are generally agreed that the most common site is in branches of the pulmonary artery, and the most common cause there is detachment of thrombus matter from one of the systemic veins or from the right heart. Sometimes—and this is most common during the puerperium—the detached thrombus liberated from some of the pelvic vessels is of such size that folded upon itself it fills the main pulmonary artery of one or other side at the point where it divides into its main branches. Here again the result is sudden death. Where it is of smaller size, there may be recovery after a period of intense respiratory distress and dyspnœa. It is possible, further, that a parietal thrombus in the proximal portion of a pulmonary artery may become detached and act as an embolus. Next most frequent, Welch is inclined to believe, on general principles, are emboli lodging in the arteries of the lower extremities, although these are apt to afford no symptoms; a detached cardiac thrombus of small size, or loosened cardiac vegetations, is more apt to be carried in the centre of the arterial blood stream —is more likely thus to be conveyed along the axial current into the common iliac of either side and its more direct continuation, the external iliac, than to be directed into a side branch of the main trunk. Nevertheless, it is in these side branches that the effects of embolism are most marked; they are most frequently detected, therefore, in the renal, splenic, cerebral, iliac and other arteries of the lower extremities, axillary and other arteries of the upper extremity, cœliac axis with its hepatic and gastric branches, central artery of the retina, superior mesenteric, inferior mesenteric, abdominal aorta, and coronary arteries of the heart.

This, according to Welch, is the order of relative frequency of emboli, that is, leading to observable symptoms and gross disturbances. These arterial emboli are, in the main, portions of detached cardiac thrombi from the left side of the heart or from the heart valves (vegetations), more rarely portions of parietal aortic thrombi or calcareous and necrotic matter from aortic atheromatous ulcers. It is possible also that detached thrombi from the pulmonary veins give occasional origin to emboli. Some few cases are on record of what is known as **paradoxical** or **crossed embolism**, in which matter originating in the systemic venous system or right auricle has been found plugging the systemic arteries. In such cases there is a relatively large patent foramen ovale. Patency of this communication between the two auricles is very common; in almost one out of every three hearts some communication exists, but usually very small, oblique, and valve-like, so that increased pressure in one or other auricle only serves to close the passage. In a certain number of cases the passage is wider and direct, and in these any increase in the right auricular blood pressure over that of the left auricle must be accompanied by flow of blood from the right into the left heart. As a matter of fact thrombotic material has been found forming an arterial embolus in the foramen ovale; one such case was encountered by Dr. John McCrae in our postmortem service at the Royal Victoria Hospital. Yet another form of crossed embolism can occur, though here the embolic masses are very minute. The capillaries of the lungs are relatively large and distensible, so large that it is possible for particles the size of tissue cells to pass through certain of these without being arrested. Thus, we have scraped the cut surface of a freshly excised rabbit's liver, made an emulsion of the scrapings, injected this into a systemic vein of another rabbit, and killing this after a few minutes, and making sections of the different organs, have encountered isolated liver cells and minute masses of the same in the arterioles of the kidney, determining at the same time that the foramen ovale was closed, or, more accurately, was non-existent.

Capillary Emboli.—Such minute masses, it is clear, are too small to be arrested in the arteries; at most, they can block the capillaries, and doing this, so abundant are the capillary anastomoses, that in the majority of instances they must cause no recognizable disturbance. Only when (1) these capillary emboli are extraordinarily abundant, or (2) have the capacity to propagate themselves, do they become manifest. It has been noticed, in the first place, that the pigmented remains of malarial parasites after sporulation are peculiarly apt to be arrested and accumulate in the fine capillaries of the brain and kidney, so that large numbers of the vessels become blocked, resulting in functional disturbance of these organs; in the second place, we encounter both microbic and neoplastic cell emboli. The former, by their continued growth, set up an inflammatory reaction, and thus induce the formation of multiple metastatic abscesses, hematogenous miliary tubercles, etc.; the latter form the centres for the development of metastatic new-growths. We are doubtful whether primarily the majority of so-called microbic emboli should strictly be regarded as such. When an infected thrombus breaks down, then undoubtedly the particles of softened matter form true capillary emboli; they block the small vessels, and the contained bacteria continue to grow until they form a dense mass filling and extending along the capillary; but in many cases of pyemia, what we deal with is the transport of individual microbes which, becoming taken up by the capillary endothelium without any circulatory arrest, multiply within the

Fig. 6

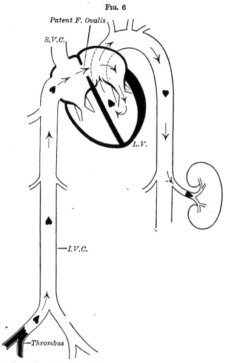

Schema of crossed embolism, to indicate the passage of thrombotic material from the veins to form emboli in the systemic arteries by passage through the fenestra ovalis.

endothelial cells, and only after distending and breaking these down grow into and along the lumen, obliterating the capillary. The chain of events is more akin to capillary thrombosis than to embolism or, otherwise, the embolism is secondary, not primary.

Venous Emboli.—We have to distinguish two orders of venous embolism: that occurring in the portal vessels of the liver, and that affecting the systemic veins proper. The portal vein in its branching and division into smaller and smaller vessels is strictly comparable with an artery, and the general principles governing arterial embolism govern it also. There may be extensive embolism in the liver through the liberation of thrombi from the splenic, the mesenteric, and other contributory veins of the portal system; the forms most frequently encountered are infective and multiple, secondary to suppurative thrombophlebitis, this in itself most frequently secondary to acute appendicitis. The liberation of the broken-down, infectious material may induce both venous and capillary emboli. Somewhat less frequently we encounter malignant emboli due to extension of malignant disease from the stomach, pancreas, and other abdominal organs into branches of the portal system, and detachment either of individual cells, or cell masses.

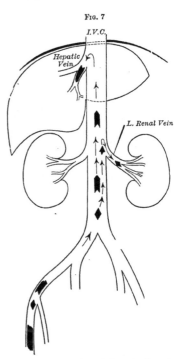

Fig. 7

In the ordinary veins which collect into larger and larger trunks, it is immediately evident that masses originating in and becoming detached from a smaller trunk cannot, under normal conditions, form an embolus, the lumen of the vessels through which it passes becoming progressively larger. The only possible conditions under which embolism can occur are when either the current of the venous blood becomes reversed, so that foreign bodies are carried by the stream into smaller and smaller veins until they become arrested, or when the very weight of the foreign body is such that under the action of gravity it falls

Schema of retrograde embolism, showing retrograde passage of thrombotic material to form emboli in the hepatic and renal veins, respectively.

against the blood stream into some more dependent vessel. It may be thought that these are scarcely possible conditions; that if momentarily the blood current were reversed or became slow enough for gravity to exert its effects upon contained larger masses, with the arrest of a mass at a point where two or more smaller veins joined to form a larger one, within a very short time the pressure of the venous blood behind the obstruction would liberate it and carry it forward toward the heart. But, as a matter of fact, several cases are on record which can only be explained as examples of the retrograde embolism. Only those examples can be taken as indubitable in which all possibility of crossed embolism is excluded; we can deal, therefore, only with cases in which the embolism is too large to have passed through the pulmonary capillaries, and in which there has been no patent foramen ovale. But when, to quote Lubarsch's case, there is encountered a primary ossifying chondrosarcoma of the right tibia, with a sarcomatous mass forming a riding embolus of the hepatic vein, and no other secondary growths in the liver; or, to instance one of von Recklinghausen's cases, where along with a primary myxochondrosarcoma of the tibia invading the veins of the leg there was found a similar myxochondrosarcomatous mass in the main renal vein extending by growth along the branches of the same, confined to this vessel and its branches with no other malignant involvement of the organ; then the only conclusion must be that there has been retrograde embolism.

And, as a matter of fact, Arnold, Lubarsch, and others have experimentally demonstrated the possibility of such retrograde embolism by the slow injections of thick emulsions of coarse meal into the neck veins, etc. More particularly when death occurred with severe dyspnœa, it was found that the coarse grains had made their way into the coronary veins of the heart, the renal and hepatic veins, the cerebral sinuses, etc. There has been considerable debate as to the exact mode by which the particles make their way against the normal course of the circulation, but this seems to be evident that both experimentally and in the cases in man so far recorded, there has been evidence of impeded respiration. This suggests that, as laid down by Heller, and von Recklinghausen, one essential for the retrograde transport is a temporary or continued removal of the negative intrathoracic pressure—a condition favoring the existence of positive pressure in the veins, with its accompanying obstruction to the onward flow of the venous blood, damming of the same in the large veins, and development of reversed current in the venæ cavæ at each contraction of the right heart. Both Arnold and Lubarsch have directly observed the regurgitation of foreign bodies from the inferior vena cava into the exposed renal vein upon the onset of respiratory convulsions in animals of the laboratory.

Following Ribbert's observations, we are, however, inclined to presume that the force with which foreign particles are driven back into the veins cannot be very great, and that what is necessary for the preservation of the foreign body *in situ* is a relatively rapid adhesion of the embolus by conglutination or the production of fibrin.

Lymphatic Emboli.—It is appropriate to note at this point that what applies to the systemic veins applies also to the lymphatic vessels. In them also retrograde embolism is apt to occur, apparently with fair frequency. More particularly does this explain the development of certain of the malignant metastases in the lymphatic system. The main cause of the retrograde current would seem to be closure of the main lymphatic channels of a part, with, as a consequence, reversal of flow in the branches, that the lymph may find an outlet by anastomosing vessels into other lymph channels that are not impeded. Such retrograde embolism is best fitted to explain the appearance of cancerous growth in the head of the humerus in cases of mammary cancer with involvement of the axillary lymph glands.

The Constitution of Emboli.—Any body which, free in the blood, may be carried forward until it blocks a vessel is capable of acting as an embolus. Emboli are thus of very varying nature:

1. By far the commonest causes of embolism are detached masses of **thrombotic material**, and this being so, it is evident that when, for example, we find recent cruor thrombus filling a vessel, it is at times impossible to determine whether we deal with embolism or local thrombosis. So, too, when the condition is of long standing, it is at times scarce possible to determine whether the whole occluding mass is thrombotic, or whether there has been a primary embolus with subsequent thrombosis developing upon it. In general, however, a difference in color can be made out between the primary mass that has acted as an embolus, and the secondary thrombus that has formed upon it; so also the embolus can be detached from the vessel wall and the secondary thrombus, and at times it is possible to straighten out the coiled-up embolic mass and detect the surface of detachment from the thrombus of origin; as also that thrombus of origin may be discovered elsewhere in the vascular system, and its broken surface may be seen and compared. It must be again recalled that detached vegetations from the cardiac valves form an important series of emboli of this order. Of other bodies found less frequently constituting emboli we may make a division into the endogenous and the exogenous, or, otherwise, into substances originating in and from the tissues and those of extraneous origin. Of the former we may have:

2. **Calcareous and atheromatous matter** from atheromatous ulcers.

3. **Tumor masses and cells** detached from new-growths which have penetrated into the vessels; these, forming emboli, may continue to proliferate, thus giving rise to secondary or metastatic new-growths.

4. **Detached tissue cells** or collections of the same. Of such, more particularly, there have been encountered *placental* cell (Schmorl) and *liver* cell emboli (Turner). The natural growth of the chorionic villi of the fœtus is into the uterine blood sinuses; conditions thus favor the detachment of certain of the cells or villous processes, which then may form pulmonary or other emboli. Ordinarily such cells undergo disintegration; rarely they proliferate, and so give rise to the chorioepithelioma malignum (vol. i, p. 665). The size of the liver, its abundant and large vessels, and the intimate relationship of the liver cells to the vessels, favor local dislocation of liver cells into the blood stream following blows upon the liver region, or disease in which congestion of the organ and degenerative disturbances of its cells are combined, as in eclampsia. The liver cells may be found in the heart, pulmonary vessels, and even in those of the systemic arterial system. They are to be recognized by their shape, the size of the nucleus, and the diagnosis becomes con-

vincing in those cases in which the cells contain bile pigment. A third
type of cell is occasionally encountered in the small vessels of the lung,
namely, the giant cells or megacaryocytes of the bone marrow (Aschoff),
often in a state of characteristic degeneration, with fusion of the multiple
nuclei into a single, large, irregular mass. The observations of Aschoff,
Fox, Lubarsch, and Langemann throw light upon this unexpected
process; wherever there is produced, either naturally or experimentally,
a condition of pronounced leukocytosis, with pouring of leukocytes out
of the blood-marrow, there along with the leukocytes a certain number
of these giant cells become liberated into the delicate capillaries with
which they are in intimate association, and, passing thus into the circulation, become arrested in the first series of other capillaries into which
they become carried. Very rarely, and in cases of either traumatic or
operative injury of bone, osteoclasts and fat cells from the marrow have
been noted in the lung capillaries.

5. **Leukocytes.**—In cases of myeloid leukemia, the capillaries of the
liver, kidneys, and other organs may be found so densely packed with
leukocytes that the condition must be regarded as embolic.

6. **Fat Embolism.**—Fat may be present in the circulating blood in
one of two forms, either a fine emulsion, as in lipemia, or coarse
droplets, as after rupture of fat cells and discharge of their contents
either directly into the bloodvessels or into lymph channels or spaces.
There is doubt whether the first of these conditions induces true capillary
embolism. It is true that in those dead of diabetic coma solid masses of
fatty matter have not been infrequently observed in the lung capillaries,
forming moulds of the same, but (1) these have not been detected in
autopsies performed within two or three hours after death; (2) they
are apt to have a granular, non-homogeneous appearance, as though
formed from the imperfect fusion of minute droplets; and (3) there is
a characteristic absence of surrounding hemorrhage or infiltration. All
these signs indicate a postmortem accumulation or "creaming" of the
fine fatty particles rather than an antemortem fusion into large drops
capable of acting as emboli.

There is now abundant evidence that these large drops or masses of
fat, liberated from fat-containing cells, cause capillary embolism in the
lungs with fair frequency, and in more extreme cases plug the capillaries
of the heart, the kidney (here more particularly the glomerular loops),
the brain, and other organs, setting up severe and often fatal functional
disturbance. The main cause would seem to be trauma, accidental or
operative, such as fracture of the long bones with accompanying rupture
of the fatty marrow cells, forcible breaking down of immobilized joints,
section, operative handling, and ligature through a large panniculus
adiposus, operative handling of the fatty omentum and mesenteries or
of other accumulations of fat in the patient, rupture or contusion of the
fatty liver. When there is no actual fracture of the bones, sudden
extensive concussion of the bony skeleton, such as follows falls from
some considerable height, has been observed to lead to fat embolism in
the lungs. It would seem that here the fatty cells and fine capillaries of

PLATE I

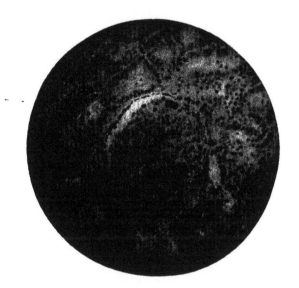

Fat-embolism of the Kidney.

The globules of fat are impacted within a glomerular tuft and are stained
red with Sudan III Reichert obj. No. 7, without ocular.

(From the Pathological Department, Montreal General Hospital.)

the bone marrow become jarred against or violently torn away from the more rigid bony framework. The fat embolism that has been noted after epileptic fits, eclamptic convulsions, etc., would seem best explained as due to a similar liberation from the bone marrow (Lubarsch). With Ribbert, then, we may regard violent shaking or concussion of bones as an important factor in producing the condition.

An obstruction of a few capillaries in the lung by fatty globules leads to no obvious disturbance, or at most to minute areas of congestion and hemorrhage; minute infarcts may be induced of no serious import. Occasionally these capillary emboli are present in great abundance, so abundant as to seriously obstruct the circulation through the lung, setting up grave and sometimes fatal dyspnœa. It is remarkable that symptoms of disturbance either manifest themselves within a few minutes to six hours after trauma, or only after four or more days. In the first case we see the direct effect of, more particularly, pulmonary embolism; in the second we are inclined to the view that through saponification the original fatty plugs in the capillaries at the site of injury, and again the emboli in the lungs, have become diminished and loosened. The contracted pupils, convulsions, and Cheyne-Stokes respiration suggest that now the fat has passed to the left heart and become lodged in the capillaries of the brain. For the fat forming these emboli tends to undergo absorption, and that in more than one way. Lipolytic enzymes exist in the blood, and gradually the droplets become saponified and dissolved. The fatty state of the endothelium of the affected capillaries indicates that these cells absorb it to some extent, and very possibly pass it on to underlying tissue cells, for these also may stain deeply with Sudan III. Add to this that there may be some accumulation of leukocytes around the fatty masses, suggesting a phagocytic activity on the part of these cells.

Emboli due to extraneous matter:

7. *Air Embolism.*—Occasionally during the course of operations upon the neck a suspicious sucking sound is heard, due to the entrance of air into a severed vein. If the vein be immediately closed before any large amount of air has been inspired no ill results may ensue, but at times death occurs with absolute suddenness, at others it is preceded by extreme dyspnœa, churning action of the heart, cyanosis, and convulsions. The nearer the heart and the larger the vein, the greater the danger of this event, but cases are on record in which sudden death of this order has followed operation upon the head, upper extremities, and uterus. The condition has been recognized for now more than a century, although, with Welch, we must ascribe many of the earlier cases of supposed uterine and intestinal origin not to air embolism, but to gas production by the Bacillus aërogenes capsulatus (Bacillus Welchii) or other gas-producing organisms.

As regards the cause of the sudden death, there are two main theories: (1) That it is essentially cardiac, due to the churning action in the right heart, so that a relatively small amount of air, as it becomes warmed up, expands to make a very considerable foam, which, accumulating behind the tricuspid valves, effectively arrests their activity; (2) that the essential cause is multiple air emboli in the pulmonary capillaries. That bubbles of air do not pass through the lung capillaries, but become blocked there has been proved by experiments on dogs; in experimental air embolism the left heart is found practically free from air, and the lungs show multiple hemorrhages, suggesting most significantly that the obstruction of a large number of capillaries has led to profound congestion and rupture of some. The more recent experiments of P. Wolf[1] are generally accepted as establishing this second theory, although the wide difference between the amount of air that can experimentally be injected into the veins of a healthy dog without fatal results (under 200 c.c.), and the much smaller amounts that have been estimated as causing sudden death in the human patient,[2] suggest that the right heart is a factor; that a vigorously contracting organ may be able to propel the air out into and through the lungs, distributing it thus to parts where it may become absorbed.

8. *Gas Emboli.*—Apparently of like order are the cases recorded by Janeway and Hun, in which grave cerebral symptoms followed the injection of peroxide of hydrogen into the abdominal and thoracic cavities.

A more common cause of gas embolism may lead to fatal results in divers and those working in compressed air; such gas embolism, in fact, would appear to be the essential causative agent in the so-called **caisson disease.** Workers in compressed air, who have for considerable periods been subjected to pressure of more than two atmospheres, if they emerge suddenly into the ordinary air, are liable either to show symptoms of dyspnœa and asphyxia, or to become victims of a series of intractable nervous disturbances, often fatal after a few days or weeks. These are of the nature of various paralyses, hemiplegia, etc. Examination of sections of the spinal cords from these cases shows the presence of multiple areas of necrosis in the posterior and lateral columns, without hemorrhages, but with ascending and descending degenerations. Von Schrötter and others have produced and studied these lesions in dogs and other animals subjected to compressed air. The partial pressure of the gases in the blood is dependent upon the atmospheric pressure; increase this last, and the blood passively absorbs air from the lungs; the greater the pressure the more the amount absorbed and held in solution. The oxygen of that air becomes fixed by the tissues, which also passively absorb some of the nitrogen. If the atmospheric pressure be reduced suddenly the blood now—and the tissues—can no longer hold the free nitrogen in solution. As a consequence, the gas separates in the form of bubbles, which grow in size and, carried in the blood stream, set up gas emboli in the various tissues, the results being most serious in the terminal arteries of the brain and spinal cord, leading to anemia and necrosis of the areas of supply.

The other form of gas embolism we have already indicated, that, namely, due to the products of activity of gas-producing organisms.

---

[1] Virchow's Archiv, 174:1903.; 454.
[2] See *Greene*, Amer. Jour. Med. Sci., 128; 1904: 1028.

While in the majority of cases the emphysema and gas in the vessels is a postmortem development, there are cases in which it is recognizable during life, and gaseous embolism may be claimed as a cause leading to the fatal event.

9. **Pigment emboli** (see p. 49).

10. **Bacterial emboli** (see p. 49).

11. **Animal Parasites.**—The symptoms of sleeping sickness are ascribed to the accumulation of trypanosomes in the cerebral capillaries, with blocking of the same, although it has to be admitted that the gradual development of these symptoms scarce suggests true embolism. Nevertheless, in trypanosomiasis the capillaries of more than one organ have been found completely blocked by dense accumulations of the parasites, herein corresponding with what has occasionally been observed with that other widespread protozoan parasite, the organism of malaria. Metazoan parasites may also induce embolism, notably the abundant larvæ of various strongyles. The classical example is afforded by the *Strongylus armatus* of the horse, whose larvæ, becoming arrested in branches of the abdominal aorta and other vessels, may with their growth and the irritation thereby induced cause thinning and giving way of the arterial wall, with the production of **verminous aneurisms.** Rare cases are also on record of the rupture of echinococcus cysts into a vein, with, as a result, embolism of the vessels of the lung by means of the daughter cysts or their membranes.

12. **Projectiles.**—Some three undoubted cases are on record in which bullets entering the heart or larger vessels have been carried in the blood stream until they have blocked and become fixed in some smaller artery.

The Results of Embolism.—These have already been discussed in the chapter on the effects of arterial closure and infarct function, and incidentally in the pages here preceding. One aspect of the subject was not touched upon, namely, the effects of embolism upon the vessel wall. Briefly, when embolism does not cause sudden death, and is not associated with rapidly fatal disease, the embolus, acting as a foreign body, produces a local irritation of the vessel with signs of inflammation, of the chronic or of the acute type, according as to whether the embolus is of the bland or of the infectious type. There may thus at the one extreme be developed a chronic thickening of the wall with accompanying organization of the embolus and permanent obliteration of the vessel, or in the other an embolic abscess. A less severe termination, also due to infection, is the production of the embolic **mycotic aneurism;** softening of the arterial wall, more particularly in arteries not well supplied by surrounding tissue, such as the cerebral, and branches of the mesenteric vessels, may lead to giving way of the same, with aneurism production. A form of embolic aneurism of the second degree may be brought about by embolic abscesses of the vasa vasorum of the aorta and large arteries, with weakening of the wall of the main artery and formation of a saccular pouch upon it.

THROMBOSIS.

When performing autopsies, it is a familiar experience to encounter clotted blood, either in the cavities of the heart or in the vessels, veins, or arteries, and immediately it becomes essential to determine whether the clotting has occurred before or after death, whether, that is, we deal with a condition which must have very materially affected the onward flow of the blood, and have been a factor in the production of symptoms of various orders, or whether with one which at most throws light upon the amount of coagulable material present in the blood. The latter condition differs in no important feature from the coagulation in blood escaping from the vessels during life; the former presents many departures, both in mode of development and arrangement of constituent elements. To it we give the name of *thrombosis*. To be exact, we should never speak of a "P. m. thrombus;" that expression involves a contradiction 'n terms.

A thrombus, therefore, is a solid body or mass situated in the cavity of the heart or vessels, formed during life of constituents derived from the blood. Some authorities would add to this definition, "formed *in situ.*" This we regard as a non-essential. The product of intravital and intravascular clotting of the blood is no less the result of thrombosis, and still remains a thrombus, even if detached and carried to a distance. Here at the most it is necessary to distinguish clearly between a thrombus and an embolus. An embolus is any free matter which, conveyed along the blood stream, becomes arrested at some point where the diminished diameter of a vessel becomes less than its own diameter. Anything which is capable of occluding a vessel constitutes an embolus; in simple English, it is a plug. A free, solid mass of clotted blood may thus be carried along a vessel until it blocks it, and so acts as an embolus. A thrombus may thus form one order of embolus, and that a very frequent one, but by no means all emboli are thrombi. What, however, is of importance is that thrombosis is, as we shall point out later, associated always with local disturbance of the vascular wall; it is doubtful whether a thrombus ever originates as a process of free precipitation out of the circulating blood; it develops in connection with an endothelial surface, the seat of some abnormal change.

Postmortem Clotting.—Before entering into the description of the process of thrombosis, it will be well to have a perfectly clear understanding of the appearance and characters of the postmortem clot, so that it may be differentiated and then set on one side. Briefly, such postmortem clot differs in no essential respect from the clot that forms in blood removed from the vessels during life.

I. It shows no stratification, *i. e.*, the blood has coagulated *en masse*. At most it may show two layers—a paler upper, and a dark red under layer. This is an indication that the clotting has not occurred immediately after the circulation has ceased, but some little time later. As can be seen so well after removal from the body of a slowly coagulating blood, like that of a horse, the lighter, white corpuscles rise to the surface and form a "buffy coat," and upon coagulation there develops a firmer pale upper layer and a dark red under layer, so here the upper layer is composed of a fibrin meshwork enclosing leukocytes. According, therefore, to (1) the rate of coagulation, (2) the number of contained leukocytes, and it may be, (3) the more or less hydremic condition of the blood, so may we distinguish three forms of postmortem clot, which pass one into the other: (1) The soft, homogeneous, red clot; (2) the clot with the firm, rather dry, adherent upper coat; and (3) the "chicken-fat" clot, with abundant moist, soft, glistening, and semitranslucent, buffy coat. This last form is found more particularly in leukemia and other states in which, along with increase in the circulating leukocytes, there is reduction in the erythrocytes and some hydremia.

II. Under the microscope the appearance is the same as that of extravascular blood clot. There is an abundant network of fibrin enclosing the corpuscles in no special order, save that the white cells become more and more abundant toward the upper surface, that the fibrin is more abundant and closer set in the upper buffy coat, being most abundant in the thin, upper layer of the second type. Blood platelets are characteristically few and far between, save it may be on the very surface.

III. The clot is loose and easily removed from the cavity in which it has developed. At most it may encircle the chordæ tendineæ and free columns of the musculi pectinati in the heart; it encircles these loosely, without being attached.

IV. The clot is of a moister consistency and not nearly so friable as the thrombus.

While laying down these differences so sharply, and while emphasizing the fact that these considerations in the majority of cases make it easy to distinguish between postmortem clot and antemortem thrombus, we have to admit that we occasionally encounter conditions in which we are at a loss to decide whether the clot has been formed immediately before or after death. We are still, that is, not wholly decided regarding the existence and frequency of **agonal thrombosis,** of a thrombosis occurring during the death agony which may, indeed, be the immediate cause of death. We know that very often in the last hours of life there is a pronounced terminal leukocytosis. If, as we believe, the leukocytes play a part in liberating the certain bodies essential to fibrin formation, it is conceivable that a rapid liberation of these bodies might induce a widespread coagulation of the blood. There are still those, for example, who hold that the extensive blood clots in those dying from acute lobar pneumonia, which fill the cardiac chambers and extend thence into the large vessels, are of this agonal nature. The abundant leukocytosis in this disease is certainly significant; but the absence of any lamination must, we think, negative the view that these are of antemortem or moritural development.

Considerations of space prevent us from treating this important process at length; for full details the student is referred to the "locus classicus" in our language, Professor Welch's article in Allbutt's *System of Medicine*.[1] We shall but call attention to the main data necessary for a sound understanding of the subject.

The thrombus differs from the postmortem clot in the following particulars: (1) It is firmly adherent on one surface to the heart or vessel wall, or, if not adherent, a study of the vessels will reveal the site at which it originated and had previously been attached. (2) It is of drier, more friable nature. (3) Under the microscope it shows an arrangement of its constituents which, even when fibrin is present, differs from that seen in the ordinary blood clot.

This last statement may seem somewhat vague; we make this broad statement because next it must be pointed out that there are thrombi of various orders and of different constitution. Thus we recognize:

1. **Hyaline Thrombi**.—These in general are small: they are characterized by a homogeneous, colorless appearance. In general they do not afford the staining reactions for fibrin, although at their edges there may be some development of fibrin threads. It is impossible at the present time to make a positive statement regarding the mode of formation of every thrombus of this order: this, however, may be said, that opinion is more and more swaying to the belief that they are due largely to a process of agglutination or conglutination rather than to coagulation. It would seem that we may distinguish at least two if not three forms.

(a) *The Pure Blood Platelet Thrombus*.—As first shown by Eberth and Schimmelbusch, if a needle or other fine foreign body be introduced through the walls of a vessel into its lumen, a thrombus becomes formed. Microscopic examination shows such a thrombus to be finely granular in appearance: higher powers resolve the granules into massed blood platelets, which in general take on the eosin stain somewhat deeply. Here and there a leukocyte may be included, but the mass is composed essentially of blood platelets. Almost imperceptibly the more granular portions of such a thrombus may pass into a completely fused hyaline mass.

There can be no doubt that the majority of white parietal thrombi in the heart and larger vessels originate thus by an accumulation of blood platelets. Those blood platelets, we may recall, are normally present in the healthy blood, and Wright has shown that some of them at least, and these perfectly typical, are derived from the megacaryocytes of the bone-marrow.

(b) *Hyaline Thrombi due to Conglutination of Erythrocytes*.—But more particularly in the smaller veins of various organs, in those of the liver and kidney for example, we encounter frequently translucent hyaline thrombi, sometimes filling up the whole lumen, more often partly occluding the vessel. and careful study of a series demonstrates, more particularly along the free side, that these, as Klebs was the first to point out,

---

[1] In German the fullest recent article on the subject is contained in Lubarsch's *Allgemeine Pathologie*, vol. i, Part 1. In both these places the allied subject of embolism is treated with equal thoroughness.

are composed of the colorless shadows of red blood corpuscles. The appearance suggests strongly a preliminary hemolysis and diffusion of the hemoglobin followed by agglutination into a hyaline mass. Flexner, Pearce, and others, by employing hemolytic agents, have experimentally produced thrombi of this type in the smaller vessels. Leo Loeb has demonstrated the wide extent of this agglutination process throughout the animal world. It is of interest to note that in man thrombi of this order are more particularly encountered in (*a*) infectious disorders,

FIG. 8

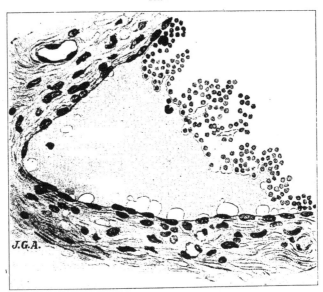

Hyaline thrombus in dilated venule of a hemorrhoid. This was perfectly homogeneous.
Reichert, obj. 7a, ocular 4. Camera lucida, reduced one-third.

suggesting that the bacterial toxins have been responsible for the hemolysis, and (*b*) in states characterized by destruction of the erythrocytes, in carbolic acid poisoning, for example, and eclampsia, and experimentally by the exhibition of ricin, diphtheria toxin, etc.

(*c*) *Hyaline Thrombi Associated with Plasmoschisis.*—But occasionally in the examination of these small thrombi we meet with appearances which it is difficult to translate, save on the assumption of an intermediate process. One portion may be completely hyaline and colorless: bordering upon this may be a granular area composed of masses of hyaline granules of the appearance of blood platelets, among these may at times be seen, now the transparent shadows of red corpuscles, now granulated red corpuscles, and these pass directly into a third layer of closely packed red corpuscles of which all, save it may be an isolated corpuscle here and there, are faded and have lost much if not all of their hemoglobin. The appearances strongly suggest the phenomenon, described by Arnold, of *plasmoschisis*, of the disintegration of the erythrocytes into particles of the size and appearance of blood platelets. We have observed this not a few times and are strongly of the opinion that Arnold is correct, and that prior to conglutination the corpuscles may undergo this dissociation into bodies curiously like blood platelets. Such appearances are capable of interpretation in two ways: either we must assume that not all blood platelets are derived from the megacaryocytes, but some gain origin from dissociation of erythrocytes, or that not all appearances of blood platelets in thrombi are truly of this nature.

2. **Fibrin Thrombi.**—Thrombi formed apparently from the onset of typical fibrin and of this alone are rare and small. They have been described as occurring in the vessels of the pneumonic lung, and Herzog has encountered them in the vessels of the renal glomeruli in cases of bubonic plague.

From these smaller thrombi we pass now to the larger forms present in the larger vessels and easily recognizable by the naked eye, and here we find a series of transitional forms leading up to a condition which, unless we examine carefully, we find difficult to distinguish from the product of ordinary postmortem intravascular coagulation.

3. **The "White Thrombus."**—In the chambers of the heart or adherent to the parietes of the larger vessels we may encounter sessile or subpedunculate thrombi. In the heart the surface of these polyp-like masses is not smooth, but irregular and ridged, with intervening depressions; in the large vessels, where the masses are more plaque-like, the surface is apt to be smooth. Sections of these thrombi show a surface layer composed mainly of white corpuscles lying upon and intermingled with a fibrinous layer. The interior of the mass, when it has not undergone the autolysis to be presently noted, exhibits a characteristic structure. Stained sections show areas which under the low power appear to be homogeneous, under the high power are seen to be composed of closely packed blood platelets. Among these may be relatively rare leukocytes. These areas are seen to be coral-like bands or strands cut in various directions; they may be separated from each other by a close network of fibrin, or by fibrin and leukocytes, or again, by accumulation of red corpuscles, leukocytes, and fibrin. We thus encounter various grades of the white thrombus, from (a) that composed in the main of blood platelets with occasional strands of fibrin, through (b) that in which leukocytes in clusters alternating with masses of blood platelets are the characteristic feature, to (c) that in which the admixture of red and white corpuscles is very noticeable, where, in fact, we have "*the mixed thrombus.*" More particularly, it would seem, where there is any extensive admixture of leukocytes, the central area of the thrombus is apt to undergo autolysis or heterolysis (vol. i, p. 371), and so to exhibit solution, the thrombus

becoming reduced to a thin shell of still solid fibrinous matter with inter_ mingled leukocytes, which is very friable, breaking very easily under the fingers, and then discharging a dirty creamy fluid, the result of self-digestion and solution.

4. **The Red Thrombus.**—From the above we pass on to states of more rapid and, in general, more extensive thrombosis, characterized by a more abundant imprisonment of red corpuscles between the strands

FIG. 9

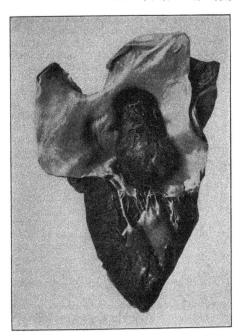

Thrombus originating in the left auricular appendix and increasing in size until it has largely occluded the mitral orifice. If its pedicle of attachment in the appendix became broken across the liberated main mass would form a ball thrombus. (Pathological Museum, McGill University.)

or layers of fibrin, so that the mass is of redder color, and with this the blood platelets become less and less evident. We approach nearer, that is, to the picture with which we are familiar in extravascular clotting. We recognize two forms of the red thrombus:

(a) *The Laminated Red Thrombus.*—This we find in aneurismal sacs that have undergone progressive filling up with thrombus, as again in the larger veins, such as the femoral and its branches, that have undergone eventual occlusion. What has happened in these cases is that over some one area necrosis has taken place, or removal of the endothelial lining. Here it would seem that at first the blood platelets have collected and undergone conglutination, next a fibrin layer with imprisoned leukocytes has formed over this, and as some of these have broken down and liberated their fibrin ferment more fibrin has been formed, enmeshing red corpuscles; more leukocytes, and it may be, blood platelets, have become arrested on the surface of the clotted mass, and in this way layer after layer is laid down, each layer consisting of a denser, more fibrinous, deeper portion representing the zone of earlier deposit of leukocytes, and a looser fibrinous meshwork enclosing abundant erythrocytes. The breadth of these layers is determined largely by the rate of the blood stream; where this is rapid, as over a parietal thrombus in the aorta, the layers are very thin and close packed. We have placed on record[1] a case of dissecting aneurism of the aorta in which through rupture of the intima in the lower thoracic region the blood dissected a channel between the layers of the media until it gained reëntry into the original channel through the femoral on the one side, the iliacs on the other. This channel was lined by a relatively thin layer of dense, mainly fibrinous, thrombus, which had become covered by a coat of endothelium. Once, that is, the channel had become patent and communicating, with rapid flow through it, the very rapidity of that flow, we must presume, prevented the arrest of leukocytes and platelets on the exposed surface of the thrombus, and with this arrest of fibrinous deposit the endothelium had spread over the surface. There had been some dissection also from the original rupture in an upward direction, but here no second communication had been established; no current had become developed. As a result, this upper cul-de-sac was completely filled with a red thrombus of the type now to be mentioned.

(b) *The Acute Red Thrombus.*—Where there is complete arrest of blood current, as in the above-mentioned case, or as occurs when a vessel is ligatured with injury to the endothelial lining, then the column of stagnant blood undergoes clotting throughout its whole mass, and if it be examined soon after the occurrence, before secondary changes have taken place, no distinction is to be made between the mass and a post-mortem or extravascular clot, save perhaps this, that at the region of origin and attachment of the thrombus, a collection of blood platelets, or more hyaline deposit with some accumulation of leukocytes, is to be made out. The origin, that is, is of the same order as in other forms of thrombosis, but in the absence of blood current there has been no arrest to the process of fibrin formation, which thus has extended through the whole mass of stagnant blood. The thrombus in an artery extends upward to the next branch of any size; once again its growth is arrested by the actively moving blood stream; in a vein it extends downward along the branches until a region or regions of anastomosis and collateral circulation is reached (see Fig. 11, p. 70).

[1] Adami, Montreal Med. Jour., 24: 1895-96: 945 and 25: 1896-97: 23.

We have here described the different forms of thrombus in the reverse
order of that usually employed, and have done this in order to lay
emphasis upon the divergencies between the main forms of thrombosis
and extravascular coagulation. It is obvious that although the end
result is the same, namely, the production of solid matter in the place of
fluid blood, that result is attained in more than one way. As to the
relative frequency and importance of these different modes of formation,
namely, by the conglutination of blood platelets, by the conglutination

Fig. 10

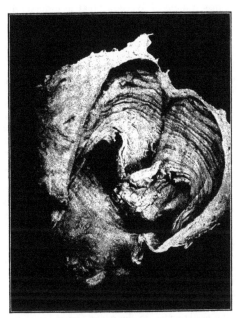

Sacculated aneurism of the ascending aorta, largely filled by firm laminated red thrombus.
(McGill Medical Museum.)

of red corpuscles, and by the development of a fibrinous network enmeshing the corpuscular elements we are still undecided; at most it can
be stated that the conglutinative forms are being more and more recognized as the more usual. For ourselves, judging from the specific
staining reactions, we believe that fibrin and the hyaline matter of white
thrombi are chemically closely allied and of the same order, and so are
developed as the result of similar reactions. The constant attachment
of the beginning thrombus to an area of the vascular wall, which in most

cases can be seen to have undergone injury or degeneration, indicates that either the damaged endothelium or the underlying cells supply something—probably of the nature of fibrin ferment—which initiates the conversion of the substance of the blood platelets or erythrocytes into fibrin-like material, and that once started, the process would seem apt to continue into the plasma outside and beyond as true fibrin formation. What part the blood platelets play in the ordinary process of coagulation is as yet undetermined; at most it is significant that in conditions in which their number is diminished, as in purpura, the coagulative power of the blood is likewise seen to be diminished. But unless we accept the observations of Wlassow,[1] that in ordinary fibrin formation in shed blood the conglutination of blood platelets is the first stage, it is difficult to bring into line with the prevalent theories of coagulation these observations upon thrombus formation, observations, be it noted, not of one isolated observer, but of a long series of trained pathologists, from Eberth and Schimmelbusch in 1888 onward.

It deserves note that Wooldridge derived his A fibrinogen from the blood platelets, and he held that fibrin is formed (without intervention of fibrin ferment) by a junction between this and other fibrinogens present in the plasma. His views have never gained general acceptance, and practically all modern physiologists recognize the part played by a fibrin ferment, even if most regard this as not liberated direct into the plasma, but require a *prothrombin*, present in, and capable of liberation from, leukocytes and most body cells, which, under the action of a zymoplastic substance, liberated from red corpuscles and other cells proper, gives origin to *thrombin*, or fibrin ferment proper. This thrombin in its turn is regarded as acting upon the paraglobulin of the plasma, converting it into fibrinogen, or metaglobulin, and eventually into soluble fibrin, and this in the presence of calcium salts becomes converted into the more solid fibrin. So many and so diverse are the theories of coagulation, that we do not in the least believe that the process here indicated is what actually occurs. No one appears to be satisfied that we have as yet gained a sure knowledge of the process. We have a certain satisfaction in leaving to the physiologists the teaching of a subject which they have for long years made peculiarly their own.[2] At most, we would urge that evidently something is involved which is common to the blood platelets, to the erythrocytes, to the white corpuscles (for it is where these are accumulated in greatest numbers that the fibrin is laid down most densely), and it may be also to the plasma (for in rapidly developing thrombi the fibrin threads extend into the plasma between the cells), and this something would seem to be of the nature of a globulin or globulins, for such are common to both cells and plasma, and there would appear to be an agreement among the physiological chemists that fibrinogen, the precursor of fibrin, is a metaglobulin.

[1] Ziegler's Beiträge, 15:1894:543.
[2] A very full review of the data and theories of coagulation is given by Buckmaster in Science Progress, 2:1907:51

The fact that the normal circulating blood does not coagulate, and that the ordinary thrombus is seen to develop in connection with the vessel wall at a region of disease or injury or loss of the endothelium, would suggest that something not ordinarily present in the circulating blood is given off at such an area, and initiates the conversion of the dissolved protein into its more solid modification, fibrin. The whole process points to the liberation of an enzyme. We do not pretend to say that the blood platelets are absolutely essential for the process; but the way in which, once the process has started in stagnating blood, the strands of fibrin spread rapidly through a relatively large mass, and the abundance of dense fibrin in immediate relationship to clusters of white corpuscles on the surface of ordinary white thrombi and elsewhere, prepare us to see that other cells besides those of the vessel walls may liberate the enzyme or initiator of the conversion of soluble protein into fibrin. Nay, more, although this is contrary to the generally received doctrine, just as, experimentally, by the injection of certain tissue extracts, it is possible to induce an almost universal thrombosis throughout the vascular system, so is it possible to imagine the existence of conditions, such as extensive disintegration of the circulating leukocytes, which would lead to a process of thrombosis independent of any disturbance of the vessel wall, conditions in which the multiple thrombi or masses of clotted blood would have no primary attachment. Admitting this, it has also to be admitted that the more we study actual cases of thrombosis the more we become impressed by the co-existence of lesions of the vascular wall.

The Factors Favoring Thrombosis.—The analyses made thus far of the incidence of thrombosis in man in various conditions of disease, and the experiments made upon the lower animals, indicate that very diverse orders of disturbance favor the development of thrombi—so diverse, in fact, that it is a matter of extraordinary difficulty to arrive at any sure conclusion, and as a result we find that different observers arrive at very different conclusions regarding their relative importance. We will here record these factors, giving the more important data and the conclusions that have been drawn, and then proceed to weigh the evidence in the light of what has already been laid down concerning the actual process.

1. **Slowing and Stagnation of the Blood.**—Thrombosis is more common in the venous system than in the arterial—according to Lubarsch, in the proportion of more than 4 : 1—as also it is peculiarly apt to occur in regions of dilatation of the channel where the current necessarily becomes slow, *e. g.*, in the auricular appendages, in the sinuses or depressions between the muscular bands of the heart chambers, in varicose veins, and in aneurisms. Where the blood stream is rapid, despite the existence of other favoring factors, thrombosis does not necessarily show itself, *e. g.*, there may be an extensive atheromatous ulceration of the aortic wall, with loss of endothelium, and no sign of thrombosis. This led Virchow to regard slowing of the blood stream as the prime factor.

2. Eddying of the Blood.—A factor upon which von Récklinghausen would lay great stress is the formation of eddies rather than the existence of simple stagnation in regions in which the vascular channel undergoes expansion. There is not, he urged, absolute stagnation in the pockets of the valves of the veins; nevertheless, these are peculiarly favorable seats for the origin of venous thrombi. If we conceive an eddy as a whirl, our first idea is that in it the blood flow is faster, and that, therefore, the conditions are unfavorable rather than favorable for the deposit of blood platelets and other cells. This, however, is not a complete conception; while at the edge of an eddy there is relatively rapid flow, at its centre there may be relative stagnation. What is more, the very whirling nature of the flow does away with any peripheral cell-free layer of the plasma, so that once cells become arrested in the quiescent area, the conditions distinctly favor the adhesion and accumulation of other platelets or cells.

3. Hemolysis and Destruction of Corpuscles.—It is those agents, exogenous and endogenous, that lead to corpuscular disintegration, which characteristically, when exhibited, bring about extensive thrombosis. There is a long list of exogenous poisons having such properties—salts of mercury, lead, arsenic, etc., potassium chlorate, sulphates and sulphites, nitrobenzole, toluylenediamin, and other toluylene compounds, various aniline derivatives, phenylhydrazin, etc., carbolic and salicylic acids, various compounds of vegetable origin, ricin, extracts of amanita and other poisonous mushrooms; others of animal origin, *e. g.*, snake venom and sundry enzymes, pepsin, etc. Of the endogenous poisons, the diffusible products from extensive burns, the (unknown) toxic agents in eclampsia and possibly toxic substances present in the blood in severe secondary anemias (*e. g.*, that accompanying cancer) may be mentioned. In all these conditions there is a marked tendency to thrombosis, either multiple and small in the capillaries, or sometimes of larger size in the larger veins. Stress is laid upon these data more particularly by those upholding conglutination as a main factor.

4. Bacteria and Their Products.—But it has to be admitted that intoxications pure and simple, whether endogenous or exogenous, are relatively infrequent compared with infectious and bacterial intoxication. Most people die from terminal infections, and attention is being increasingly drawn to the fact that even in what are recognized as bland thrombi bacteria are to be detected, or cultures gained, while conversely, as shown by Welch and Lubarsch, if known cases of infection be carefully studied—suppurative cases, lobar pneumonia, typhoid, appendicitis, diphtheria, acute rheumatism, measles, influenza, etc.—capillary thrombi in the brain, lungs, kidneys, and intestinal walls are found to be remarkably frequent.

There are different views as to how the bacteria act. Thus, certain observers have dwelt upon the hemolytic action, and have pointed out that the pyococcus aureus is most actively hemolytic, and is found associated with thrombi very frequently. But thrombi are frequent in acute tuberculosis and in typhoid, and the microbes of neither of these diseases have pronounced hemolytic powers. It is true that, as Professor Welch points out, in many of these cases examination reveals not the microbes of the main disease, but those of some secondary infection, streptococci, bacillus coli, etc. There is diversity of opinion, again, regarding the actual presence of the bacteria in the blood stream; some observers point out that the filtered culture fluids of forms like Bacillus typhosus, Bacillus coli, and Bacillus diphtheriæ, when injected into the veins, have little effect in inducing thrombosis (Jakowski); others, like Talke, demonstrate that parenchymatous inoculation of pyococci leads in the majority of cases to thrombosis of the vessels in the immediate neighborhood, and this without of necessity any bacteria being present in the thrombi. In our laboratory Leo Loeb demonstrated that the addition of cultures of certain organisms accelerated the rate of coagulation of extravascular blood, while cultures of other species had no effect. But accepting his data, his results bear little apparent relationship to the data of disease; thus, for example, the feebly pathogenic Micrococcus prodigiosus was found to have a greater accelerating power than the typhoid bacillus, and the streptococcus was without effect. Nor, so far as we can see, did his results tally with the hemolytic powers of the species tested.

5. **Disease and Injury of the Vascular Wall.**—We have already laid stress upon this as, in our opinion, a most important factor, but must again impress upon the reader that it is not everything. It is quite true that when we mechanically injure or destroy the endothelium of the living vessel, there we surely gain thrombus formation over the region of injury. But the extent depends very largely upon the *rate of blood flow* over the injured area; the more rapid the rate, the less the resulting thrombosis. Nevertheless, we can recall no observations in which destruction or grave injury to the previously intact endothelium has not been followed by some grade of thrombosis. Here a fine, but what must be considered an important, distinction must be made. We do not—because we cannot—hold that the thrombosis follows the exposure of what is dead or foreign material to the circulating blood. We know, for example, that the exhibition of foreign matter in the blood is not necessarily followed by coagulation. It is possible to place balls of perfectly smooth glass in the larger vessels or heart cavity without any clot forming around them. Guthrie, of St. Louis, has afforded the most remarkable instance to the point. Taking a length of the vena cava of the rabbit, he has hardened this in formalin solution for several days, washed out the formalin and dehydrated with strong alcohol, and then impregnated the piece with liquid paraffin, following upon which he has implanted the segment in the course of the rabbit's carotid artery. And notwithstanding the piece of dead vein has apparently functioned perfectly for twenty-two days with no sign of thrombosis. It is true that foreign bodies with rough surface introduced into the blood stream become covered with a layer of fibrin; blood platelets and leukocytes adhere to the surface irregularities, and their disintegration leads, we suggest, to the liberation of the substance which initiates coagulation and

fibrin formation. If the circumstances are such that this substance is not given off, or, being given off, is carried too rapidly by the blood stream, then thrombosis cannot ensue. It is in this way that we would account for the absence of thrombosis over exposed (dead) calcareous plaques and ulcers of the aortic wall. But admitting this, we have to acknowledge that there is a group of cases, more especially of capillary thrombosis, in which microscopic examinations reveal no recognizable departure of the endothelium from the normal, or, at most, a grade of fatty degeneration which is common in infectious processes, and most often found unaccompanied by thrombosis. Here we again revert to the same order of phenomena noted in connection with the coagulation occurring around foreign bodies; it is in the slighter cases of this order that we occasionally encounter vessels in which either desquamated endothelial cells, or leukocytes, or what are apparently clumps of blood platelets lying isolated in the blood, away from the vessel wall, are surrounded by a coarse radiation of fibrin filaments. Evidently all these orders of cell substance can give off the body—ferment or pro-ferment—which, interacting on substances in the plasma, gives origin to fibrin.

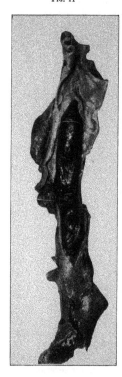

Fig. 11

Acute red thrombus of iliac vein.
(McGill Medical Museum.)

Localization of Thrombi. — They may occur in any portion of the blood system. Here we distinguish:

1. **Cardiac Thrombi.**—(*a*) Of these, the commonest form—although we are apt not to regard them as such—are the *vegetations* upon the valves in acute endocarditis. (*b*) The more typical thrombi, globular, sessile, or pedunculate, are found more particularly in the auricular appendices and at the apices of the ventricles—found in obstructive heart disease leading to cardiac insufficiency with retardation of the blood flow, and chronic diseases of the lungs, arteries, and kidneys, as again in cachectic states. We deal in these cases with retardation rather than with actual stasis of the blood, and this retardation is most manifest in the "pockets" of the heart. Along with this, microscopic examination reveals degeneration of the endocardium. (*c*) Another group of more flattened *mural* thrombi may be found in various positions either in the auricles or ventricles. These are situated over localized areas of necrosis or ulceration of the endocardium, due either to infection, infarction of the wall, or partial aneurism. (*d*) A form

apart is the *ball-thrombus*, found loose in the left auricle; some score of cases of this condition have been described. The condition is that of a relatively firm, globular mass, varying in size from that of a walnut to that of a hen's egg, lying loose in the cavity, and eventually causing sudden death by acting as a ball valve over the stenosed mitral orifice. Some examples have shown a rough area, indicating the recent detachment of a globular thrombus from the auricular endocardium, upon which a thrombotic area of origin has been detected; others have been smooth or homogeneous over the whole surface, indicating that the thrombus has been free for some considerable time before the fatal event, and that by the deposit of successive laminæ of fibrin it has increased in size while rotating in the auricle. Von Recklinghausen has doubted whether these necessarily cause sudden death, and much is to be said in favor of his arguments; we may conclude that they do not necessarily bring about sudden death, but that at the same time they must be regarded as producing it in the majority of cases. In only one other region do we know of the existence of similar ball-thrombi, and this is an individual observation of our own. In a case of sudden death we encountered a firm, oval, free mass occupying the cavity of the left coronary cusp of the aortic valve, and occluding the left coronary orifice. We have recently encountered an almost identical case of sudden death, but in this the globular mass was still attached by a delicate pedicle to the eroded aortic wall immediately above the left coronary orifice.

2. **Arterial Thrombi.**—Such may be found, either parietal or occluding, in the aorta or any of its branches, and then in general as the result of either mechanical injury (*i. e.*, ligature) or of arteriosclerotic changes, or lastly, as secondary to embolism. Most frequently, however, they are encountered in the arteries of the extremities, and more especially of the lower extremities. An important group occurs in connection with atheromatous degeneration of the cerebral arteries; another group, often but not always of embolic origin, in the pulmonary arteries.

3. **Venous Thrombi.**—These are in many respects of the greatest medical interest and the most widespread. Indeed, many factors combine to make the veins the seat of election for thrombosis—the poorer quality of the blood, its slower flow, the absence of pulsation, the presence of pockets behind the valves, the thinness of the walls, and low blood pressure, leading easily to local arrest of the blood flow in consequence of pressure from without. As Welch points out, thrombosis most often begins in vessels where these conditions are together most operative, namely, in the middle-sized veins rather than in the smaller, or those unprovided with valves. Thus, characteristically, thrombosis shows itself first in the femorals, and not in the smaller veins of the lower extremity, or in the vena cava, in the cerebral sinuses more often than in the cerebral veins. Once they originate, they are apt to extend progressively in both directions, although the smallest veins of a part usually do not become involved. It is the left common iliac vein that has the larger and more obstructed course, the left innominate vein that

is the larger and the more oblique channel for return flow; therefore, we find thrombi more common in the veins of the left leg and arm.

4. **Capillary Thrombi.**—We have already referred to the frequency of small hyaline thrombi in the smaller vessels, evidently of local origin; it is interesting in this relationship to call attention to what has been stated above, namely, that the ordinary retrograde thrombus does not in general extend back into the small veins and capillaries. Thrombosis of the ordinary type can, however, show itself in capillaries, and that in inflammations, and more particularly in infectious conditions, as in the zone surrounding a focal infectious condition, an abscess, or even a granuloma.

Effects of Thrombosis.—To discuss the effects of thrombosis of the arteries, veins, and capillaries is to pass in review the results of closure of all the vessels of the body, as that affects the different individual parts and organs. That is impossible; at most here it may be stated in the broadest way that there are certain main factors that determine those effects, namely, first and foremost, the extent to which the obliteration of a given vessel affects the nutrition of a part; and secondly, and of yet greater importance for the organism, the amount of tissue thrown out of gear relative to the importance of that tissue. Thus, for example, a very small vessel supplying just one small collection of nerve cells in the brain, if thrombosed, by leading to the destruction of an important centre, may have very profound if not rapidly fatal effects, whereas thrombosis of one renal vein, although leading to almost complete destruction of the whole kidney, through the compensating activity of the other kidney may be followed by very little general disturbance. Remembering that here we deal with phenomena that are the common end-results not only of thrombosis, but also of embolism, and in addition, of obliteration of vessels by very many means, it has seemed wise to discuss the broad general results of closure of vessels in an earlier chapter.

The Changes that Occur in the Thrombus.—Whatever the cause—whether the greater relative amount of fibrin entering into its composition, or its very architecture, whereby the contraction of the fibrin is more effective in driving out the serum—the thrombus is, even when recent, of a drier nature than the ordinary blood clot. If of long continuance, various changes may occur, some leading to greater firmness, others to softening, which, however, is quite distinctive. These changes are of the following orders:

1. **Absorption.**—When a thrombus is of moderate size, we have evidence that it may wholly disappear, the vascular channel becoming restored. The main agent at work in such cases is apparently leukocytic activity, with solution and absorption of the fibrin.

2. **Central Autolysis.**—This would seem to be closely allied to the previous change. It is most commonly encountered in old globular and mural cardiac thrombi. The thrombus apparently solid, with characteristic netted surface, is found to be a mere brittle shell filled with a discolored, puriform fluid. But this fluid is in no sense pus. It contains

granular debris, fatty globules, red corpuscles, and occasional fat-containing leukocytes, and is the result of self-digestion of the thrombus, or, perhaps more accurately, of heterolysis, by the agency of leukocytes, both those originally present and those wandering in from the surface.

3. **Organization.**—This is yet another natural process. The presence of foreign matter in the lumen of the vessel acts as a chemiotactic irritant, so that, in the first place, leukocytes are attracted into the substance of the thrombus from the vessel wall, not so much where the lining endothelium is intact, as where it is damaged and wanting, at the site of adhesion; and here also, following the leukocytic invasion, there would seem to be a similar chemiotactic entrance of capillary processes and loops. In this way, the leukocytes first digesting the fibrin, there is an entrance of granulation tissue into the thrombus, and this may advance and progress until the whole thrombus undergoes in part a slow heterolysis and absorption, in part replacement by well-formed and vascularized connective tissue. Through the absorption, or, again, through the contraction of the "cicatricial" tissue, what had been a large, obliterating thrombus comes to be represented by a small contracted mass of fibrous tissue.

4. **Canalization.**—Nor does this necessarily completely occlude the vessel. On the contrary, an old thrombus may come to be represented by one or more bands or bridles crossing the almost completely restored lumen of a vessel. Or the vessel may be narrowed and contracted at the site of the old thrombus, presenting one or more narrow channels through which communication is regained between the proximal and distal portions of the hitherto obstructed vessel. This process of "canalization" presents not a few points of interest. The channels, large or small, are lined with endothelium which is in direct continuity with that lining the normal vessel above and below. How have they come to be formed? It is easy to understand that a parietal non-obliterating thrombus should become covered in process of time by an extension of the endothelium lining the vessel immediately beyond the site of adhesion. This would explain the formation of a lateral channel; it does not explain the presence of central channels. For these the only adequate explanation would seem to be the establishment of free communications between certain of the capillaries of the replacement granulation tissue and the lumen of the obliterated vessel above and below. Once such communication is established, and the blood finds its way from the lumen above to the lumen below, then along the lines of Thoma's principles, the difference in blood pressure between the two parts and the rate of flow through the new channel would lead to its progressive dilatation, until from a mere capillary a wide channel becomes developed.

5. **Putrefactive Softening.**—We have already noted that even in what are of the nature of bland thrombi, bacteria have been detected; it is not, therefore, all bacteria that lead to disintegration of thrombi. More particularly when we isolate the pyogenic bacteria, more particularly again in the condition of thrombophlebitis, do we meet with a true

suppurative softening of a thrombus and replacement by true pus. It is not merely that these bacteria multiplying in the thrombus cause softening of the same through the action of their proteolytic enzymes, but in addition, through the diseased walls of the vein, leukocytes are attracted

Fig. 12

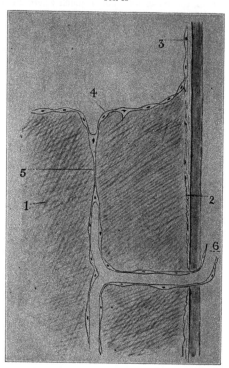

Schema of mode of canalization of a thrombus: 1, thrombus occluding a vessel; 2, diseased intima of vessel to which the thrombus is adherent; 3, endothelium of vessel above the thrombus, growing over the thrombus and at 4 passing downward into depression on its surface, one of its cells at 5 sending downward a process to join with similar endothelial process from one of the capillaries entering the thrombus at 6 in the process of organization of the same. The process at 5 will ultimately form a capillary channel of communication, which will undergo progressive enlargement.

in great numbers. Streptococci and Bacillus coli are most frequently found in these conditions, although the latter, with others of the group of intestinal bacteria, may also be found in conditions in which there is not so much an attraction of leukocytes as pure putrefactive disintegration.

6. Loosening of Thrombi and its Effects.—Such softening of thrombi, more particularly in the heart (endocardial vegetations) and in the veins, leads to liberation of the whole or portions of the same, and so to the formation of *emboli*. But embolism may be due also to portions of bland thrombi—cardiac vegetations, and polypoid thrombi of the heart, and mural thrombi of the aorta; these may become dislodged mechanically by the force of the blood stream or unusual movements either in the blood or the containing vessel. Similarly, the cases are fairly frequent in which, through some forced or unusual movement, relatively long thrombi in the systemic veins become broken across. The supervention of pulmonary embolism and sudden death is the gravest danger in these cases. The effects of embolism have been considered in another chapter.

7. Calcification.—In certain regions of the body, notably in the prostatic and uterine plexuses, and to a less extent in the spleen, thrombi of moderate dimensions become the seat of calcareous deposits, and so form phleboliths. This change has already been discussed (vol. i, p. 936).

CHAPTER III.

THE BLOOD—HEMORRHAGE.

STRICTLY speaking, hemorrhage[1] is a "blood burst," or is the process of escape of the blood out of the vessels in which normally it is confined; in practice the term covers not only the act of escape, but also the state of blood out of place, and thus in discussing hemorrhage we take into account not merely the means of escape and the results to the organism at large of such escape, but also the changes that occur in the extravasated fluid and the particular region involved.

Causes.—We recognize two orders of escape: (1) That brought about by gross breach of continuity of the vessel walls—hemorrhage *per rhexin*—and (2) that occurring in capillary vessels without gross breach of continuity, through interstices of the wall—hemorrhage *per diapedesin*. The causes of the first of these, of rupture, (*a*) may act from without, through injury, through inflammation, through atrophy secondary to pressure from tumors in apposition, etc., and through removal of the normal pressure upon and the support exerted by surrounding tissues; (*b*) may be due to disease and weakening of the vessel wall; and (*c*) may act from within through increased blood pressure. Two of these may be in action at the same time, as when in an artery sudden rupture occurs when the wall has become weakened through disease, the immediate cause being a sudden increase in blood pressure, through exertion or other cause; or again, the first and third may be involved, as in the multiple hemorrhages of high elevations, when there may co-exist heightened pressure within the vessels of certain areas, together with great lowering of the external pressure upon the vessels. Mere increase of blood pressure will not cause rupture of the healthy arteries, or larger veins, nor again of the heart, but only of the capillaries and smaller veins; sudden increase in pressure has been known to lead to rupture of the heart when the muscle is diseased. Thus, our museum at McGill contains a specimen contributed by Dr. Osler of a heart exhibiting advanced fatty degeneration, in which rupture occurred when the late owner was walking up a hilly Montreal street.

Hemorrhage per diapedesin occurs in the capillaries and venules as a result of dilatation of the same in conditions of hyperemia, either active or passive. The nature of this has been studied more particularly by Arnold, who first taught the existence of special spaces—stigmata and stomata—occurring here and there between the pavement endothelial cells. From this view he has withdrawn, and following his studies it is generally held that the passage occurs, between the endothelial cells, it

---

[1] From αἷμα, blood, and the stem, ῥαγ, from ῥήγνυμι, to burst or break.

is true, but as a result of stretching and enlargement of the spaces between the normally existing bridges joining the endothelial cells (see vol. i, p. 36), or, more probably, with distension of the vessels some of these bridges break down, and larger openings are thus provided, through which, under the blood pressure, the fluid and corpuscles of the blood are forced through between the cells. When the endothelium is already in a state of lowered nutrition, as happens in passive hyperemia, the hemorrhage is still more apt to occur. So, also, a favoring factor is lack of adequate support to the capillaries. Thus, hemorrhages of this nature are peculiarly apt to occur under conditions of great vascular dilatation in regions where capillary networks exist immediately beneath a delicate pavement endothelium, *e. g.*, into the alveoli of the lungs, in conditions of pronounced passive congestion, or pneumonic conditions; from the mucous membrane of the nostrils; from the pleural, pericardial, and peritoneal surfaces.

Capillary Hemorrhage.—Studying the different forms of capillary hemorrhage, it has to be admitted that time and again it is difficult if not impossible to differentiate clearly between cases due to rhexis and those due to diapedesis; there appears, indeed, to be evidence that in the same area and under the same circumstances both may occur. It is more satisfactory, therefore, remembering that both processes may occur, to consider these capillary hemorrhages in the light of their causation. Doing this we can distinguish several groups, according as we deal with increased internal pressure and no previous disease of the capillary endothelium; a combination of increased internal pressure with morbid state of the endothelium; and disease of the endothelium without increased internal pressure. Examples strictly of the first order are rare. Perhaps the commonest example is met with in the hemorrhages of the scalp and membranes of the brain which accompany prolonged labor, and due to the intense congestion involving the head when this is free and the rest of the infant still tightly compressed. Occasionally the small vessels rupture as the result of some vigorous effort, with consequent great rise of blood pressure, but this more often in the elderly than in the young, so that in general the existence of some previous weakness or disease of the walls may be suspected. Very closely allied are the petechial hemorrhages of serous surfaces seen when death has been due to asphyxia; these must almost certainly be attributed in the main to intense capillary congestion, although the accompanying extreme venous state of the blood and its effects upon the capillary endothelium cannot be wholly left out of account. Of the second order are the capillary hemorrhages of chronic passive congestion, in which we have well-marked indications of malnutrition of the capillary walls. Here are to be included the hemorrhages of the lungs, kidney, and other organs in obstructive heart disease, hemorrhagic infarcts, and the multiple minute hemorrhages which result from multiple capillary emboli (p. 49). Hemorrhages of a similar character found in many of the acute infections are found to be associated with the presence of hyaline thrombi in the capillaries, which obviously have the same obstructive effect, arresting the blood stream, leading to local stasis at either side of the block, and producing, in fact, minute hemorrhagic infarcts. In many of the cases of idiopathic purpura similar thrombi—or emboli—have been detected, and this in the absence of any bacteria; in cases of burns and frostbite (here in the kidneys and stomach; such are a possible explanation of the ulcers of the duodenum sometimes encountered in the former of these conditions); in certain cases of embolism, by body cells, placental cells, liver cells, etc.; in leukemia by leukocytes. In many infections, however, we have to deal with events of the third order, namely, with direct toxic injury to the capillary endothelium and with nothing else. To such must be ascribed the multiple capillary hemorrhages of the acutest types of the acute exanthemata—of hemorrhagic smallpox, scarlet fever, etc. The course of events in these cases may be of one of two orders—either *toxic*, due to the specific action of toxic substances upon the capillary endothelium, with giving way of the same, or *infectious*, due to actual growth of the bacteria or infectious agents within the endothelial cells and lumen of the capillaries, destruction of the cells, and escape of the blood. We meet with both events—the latter more particularly in cases of bacteriemia, in streptococcal and other terminal infections. As regards the former, it is, indeed, doubtful whether many of the hemorrhages of infectious cases accompanied by hyaline capillary thrombi are not of this nature—whether, that is, the localized coagulation of the blood is not secondary to epithelial degeneration. Similar toxic capillary hemorrhages may accompany certain exogenous intoxications (phosphorus, mercury, etc.), and these also must be attributed to direct action of the agents upon the endothelium, and lastly, the purpura and hemorrhages of those remarkable conditions, scurvy and Barlow's disease (or infantile scurvy), would seem to be due to endogenous intoxications—either to the presence in the blood of toxic albuminous bodies, the product of malnutrition, or, on the other hand, to the absence from the blood of certain elements necessary for the due nutrition of the capillary endothelium. Both conditions, it may be noted, are seen to be due to qualitative deficiencies of the food, and that deficiency is of the same order in the two cases, scurvy being due to a continued diet of what may be termed preserved or dead foods, Barlow's disease to a long-continued feeding of infants upon sterilized milk and prepared milk products. Both are recovered from by giving fresh food—in the adult, more particularly fresh vegetables; in the infant, unsterilized milk, and both may be warded off by the administration of small amounts of vegetable acids, lemon juice, etc.

It is the custom to refer to hemorrhages in different regions by different names. Thus, punctate capillary hemorrhages are known as **petechiæ**; more diffuse subcutaneous or interstitial hemorrhages as **suggillations** or **ecchymoses**; cerebral hemorrhage as **apoplexy**;[1] escape of blood from

---

[1] This term more accurately denotes the clinical symptoms that follow such hemorrhage, the stroke or loss of consciousness and power (ἀποπλήσσω, *active*, to strike to earth; *passive*, to be struck or to lose one's senses). It is thus utterly incorrect to **refer to** pulmonary hemorrhage as pulmonary apoplexy

the stomach as **hematemesis,** from the lungs as **hemoptysis,** from the nose as **epistaxis,** from the urinary channels as **hematuria,** from the uterus as **menorrhagia** and **metrorrhagia,** from the sweat glands as **hematidrosis.** Accumulation of blood in the various spaces of the body is known as **hematopericardium, hematothorax, hematocele.** This last term is by prescription more accurately confined to accumulation in the tunica vaginalis testis, but is also employed for limited accumulations of extravasated blood elsewhere. When the blood forms a cyst-like accumulation in the subcutaneous tissues, the term **hematoma** is not infrequently employed. **Purpura** is the name given to relatively small multiple cutaneous hemorrhages not due to injury, but to various diseased states; **melena,**[1] to blood which, escaping into the stomach or intestines, is so changed by the action of the digestive juices as to be discharged in a black condition. The localized infiltration of tissue with blood forming a **hemorrhagic infarct** we have already noted.

Local Effects.—As the result of rupture close to one of the surfaces of the body, or of trauma, whereby deeper lying vessels are exposed to the surface, the main effect is escape of blood and complete loss of the same to the economy. According to (1) the nature of the ruptured vessel, (2) the extent of the rupture, and (3) the duration of the escape of blood, so does this escape tell (a) upon the nutrition of the region supplied by or supplying blood to the ruptured vessel, and (b) upon the system at large. Very similar results follow rupture of vessels into one of the body cavities, though here, in addition, the changes taking place in the extravasated blood become a feature. Even in the first order of events, the blood coming into contact with tissues other than the normal endothelial lining of the vessels tends to undergo coagulation. This coagulation, with the progressive lowering of the blood pressure and diminution of rate of flow, with the contraction of the ruptured vessels as the internal pressure is removed, and in the case of arteries cut transversely, with the retraction and curling up of the middle coat, all together tend to bring the hemorrhage to a natural termination. Whether this natural arrest is accomplished or not, depends upon several factors—the nature of the ruptured vessel or vessels; the direction of the rupture (e. g., in arteries, rupture in the direction of the longitudinal axis cannot undergo closure by retraction, whereas this can take place when the rupture is transverse); the force of the heart beat (i. e., where the circulation is powerful there may be so rapid a loss of blood that death ensues before the natural arrest can come into play); and again the state of the blood, since, as will be discovered later (p. 85), the coagulating power of the blood varies considerably. Blood extravasated into the cavities of the body, into the pericardial or pleural cavities, for instance, if not discharged in sufficient quantities to lead to death, may remain fluid for some little time, and in this fluid state may undergo some reabsorption through the lymphatics, as regards both its fluid and its corpuscles. The tendency, however, is to undergo coagulation, and, following upon this, a slower

---

[1] From μέλας, fem., μέλαινα, black.

process of absorption under the combined action of autolysis (vol. i, p. 371) and leukocytic action.

Where we deal with suffusion, infiltration of the tissues, or hematoma formation, there we have to recognize both local changes in the tissue involved, and changes in the extravasated blood. Not only does the diversion of the blood from the normal channels bring about malnutrition of the area involved, but the presence of the blood under pressure in that area compresses the capillaries of the same, and arrests the circulation within them; while, thirdly, the force with which the blood escapes may lead to extensive laceration and destruction of the tissue. This last is particularly well seen in organs of a soft consistence, in cases, for example, of cerebral hemorrhage. Where the infiltrations are general and local, as in petechiæ, purpura, etc., and due to diapedesis rather than rupture, the local effects may be of the slightest order; there may be relatively rapid absorption with little tissue injury (although even here there is local deposit of pigment from disintegration of the escaped erythrocytes, which pigment undergoes slow removal, so that for long, cutaneous petechiæ leave behind them small brownish flecks). Where more extensive, we recognize a series of changes, of which the more important are: (1) Escape of hemoglobin from the extravasated erythrocytes, causing a hemoglobin **imbibition** which is accompanied by increased venosity and darkening of the suffused blood; (2) disintegration of the escaped hemoglobin, with production of **hemosiderin**, and, it may be, in more central parts of the infiltrated area, of **hematoidin** also (vol. i, p. 960). The successive stages in the disintegration of the hemoglobin cause the succession of vivid tints seen in the not unfamiliar "black eye." (3) Progressive absorption of the extravasated blood and its modified constituents. Again, it has to be observed that the extent of this absorption depends upon the extent and nature of the extravasation. In cases of even extensive subcutaneous suffusion it may be complete; in cases of hematoma-like accumulations it may be incomplete and accompanied by formation of granulation tissue replacing the destroyed tissue. The result may be either the formation of a firm fibrous cicatrix, or of a cyst with fibrous wall and fluid contents (vol. i, p. 863), whose contents at an early stage are deeply pigmented, but eventually through diffusion and leukocytic action become a clear colorless serum.

General Effects.—According to the extent and rate of the hemorrhage so may we observe:

1. Sudden death within a minute or two, as after rupture of the heart or bursting of a thoracic aneurism into the pleural cavity, trachea, or œsophagus.

2. Death preceded by collapse and all the symptoms of grave cerebral anemia.

3. Collapse followed by hydremia and eventual recovery.

4. Syncope, or temporary cerebral anemia with rapid recovery.

5. No disturbances due to cerebral anemia, but (in cases of internal extravasation) the development of a febrile state due to diffusion of disintegration products from the extravasated blood (vol. i, p. 484).

6. In cases of multiple repeated hemorrhages of moderate grade there may be eventual exhaustion of the hematopoietic tissues, and the development of a condition of the blood resembling that seen in true pernicious anemia, with poikilocytosis, presence of normoblasts, etc., but, unlike that condition, showing in the liver and other organs no indications of the results of excessive disintegration of the erythrocytes.

We have in our first book and in other chapters of this discussed most of these conditions. Here, therefore, they need but be called to mind. At most, it is necessary to add, as giving the basis of a scale for determining the incidence of sundry of these sequelæ, that according to the generally accepted estimate, the organism can withstand the loss of about 3 per cent. of the body weight without death ensuing, and that when "bleeding" was in vogue it was not unusual to remove thirty ounces from healthy adults without the supervention of any grave effects.

Hemophilia.—In this relationship, reference must be made to the very remarkable condition of the hemorrhagic diathesis known as hemophilia, a condition conveyed from one generation to another in a very striking manner (see the genealogical table given in our first volume, facing p. 164), and one in which the slightest trauma, *e. g.*, slight bruising or contusion, or some insignificant surgical operation, such as the removal of a tooth, is apt to be followed by almost intractable bleeding, lasting for days. It is still undetermined what is the essential cause of this condition. Virchow, it is true, observed a characteristic smallness and thinness of the walls of the aorta in these cases, and supposed an incomplete development or abnormal thinness of the vessels, but that has never been absolutely proved. What would seem more definite is a lowered power of coagulation of the blood. Just as in Barlow's disease and in scurvy, we see nowadays an explanation of the multiple hemorrhages in the presence in or absence from the blood of some element, owing to defective nutrition, so the tendency favored by the recent abundant studies upon immunity and cytolysis is to regard hemophilia as due to some inherited deficient reaction between the blood and the endothelium of the smaller vessels, leading, it may be, either to a state of weakness of that endothelium or to excessive development of bodies of the nature of antithrombin. The injection of horse serum has recently been noted to be followed by arrest of hemorrhage in these cases.

There is yet another form of capillary hemorrhage that must not be overlooked; we refer to the **nervous**. Examples of this are seen in certain cases of hysteria in which apparently almost, at will, the individual develops hemorrhagic suffusion of the skin or mucous membranes. Closely allied to this would seem to be the "stigmata" produced upon the hands and feet in cases of extreme religious exaltation or ecstasy, and other cases of bloody sweat or hematidrosis. Lubarsch would include here the hemorrhage of menstruation, pointing out that it is associated with definite nervous phenomena. It is a matter of present debate whether the menstrual flow is or is not intimately associated with the development of an internal secretion from the ovary, or again is preceded by degenerative changes in the endothelium of the submucous

vessels of the endometrium.   While admitting the very possible pres
of a nervous factor, we are inclined to doubt whether this be the con
ling agent. In the other uncomplicated cases the course of event
problematical; the suddenness with which the hemorrhages may be
duced by hysterical patients would seem to militate against local tro
changes; on the other hand, it is difficult to ascribe the escape of bl
purely to local action of the arterial vasodilators.

CHAPTER IV.

THE BLOOD—QUALITATIVE BLOOD CHANGES.

THE study of the qualitative changes in the blood has now become so special and so specialized a branch of pathology, with text-books and journals devoted to it, that to enter into the subject in all its modern detail would in itself demand a volume of fair size. Under the circumstances, the sense of proportion demands that we lay down at most the main outlines, at the same time emphasizing the fact that these are but the outlines, and that for a fuller knowledge the student must master such works as Ewing's *Clinical Pathology of the Blood* or Cabot's *Clinical Examination of the Blood,* and for the latest developments must consult that excellent journal, the *Folia Hematologica.*

In such a rapid survey we have to take into account, first, modifications in the different constituents—in the constitution of the plasma, and in the relative proportions of the corpuscular elements, erythrocytes, leukocytes, and blood platelets; and then pass in review certain of the more important blood dyscrasias as separate entities (chlorosis, secondary anemias, pernicious anemia, etc.).

THE PLASMA.

It is no false humility to state that despite the amount of research that has been devoted to the blood during late years, we are but at the beginning of a knowledge of its pathology. We have gained some knowledge regarding the red corpuscles and their function, and the significance of disturbances affecting the same; our knowledge of the white corpuscles, their mode of origin, relationships, functions, and morbid states has been materially widened, though much has yet to be determined; but as regards the plasma, the main medium of nourishment and interchange, the data we possess are painfully deficient. That plasma is the great medium of interchange; from it are constantly being abstracted materials needed for the elaboration of the different tissues; into it are poured many products of cell activities, internal secretions, enzymes, hormones, etc. The evidence is very clear that despite this constant change, the composition remains in health remarkably uniform. We are apt to attribute to the liver and kidneys the main function of removing the deleterious substances that would otherwise tend to accumulate—and here, it may be, we are correct, although we must take into account how other organs, like the ductless glands, evidently play a part in neutralizing certain bodies of a toxic type circulating within it.

But the study of immunity has revealed the existence of substances
in the plasma in minute amounts—enzymes and proteins—possessing
properties obviously of extraordinary importance for the general well-
being of the organism as a whole; we cannot isolate these, we can only
conclude that they are of proteid nature; we cannot surely state what
is their origin—we repeat glibly that the solid matters of the blood serum
constitute 9.2 per cent., and of this 7.6 per cent. is protein, in the main
serum albumin and serum globulin.   But having said this, we are ignorant of the exact source of these obviously most important constituents,
of the respective parts played by the two in nutrition, and consequently
of the significance of disturbances in their relative proportions.   We are
only slowly realizing that those names, serum albumin and serum globulin, cover not single entities, but groups of substances.   And if this is
true of the most abundant as well as the most sparse constituents of the
plasma, the poverty of our real knowledge stands revealed.

Briefly we may divide the constituents of the plasma into water,
proteins, and salts. The proportion of water maintains in health a
remarkable constancy, so that the specific gravity varies but slightly.
In disease greater variations show themselves, and the condition of
hydremia is not infrequent.   But here it has to be noted that a hydremic
condition of the blood may be brought about (1) by actual increase in
the amount of blood by increase in its watery content (true hydremic
plethora), as in obstructive heart disease; (2) by no increase in the total
amount of blood, but actual deficiency of proteins of the plasma, as after
severe hemorrhage; and (3) by increase in the salts of the blood, attracting more fluid out of the tissues in order to preserve the normal "tone"
of the plasma.   As already pointed out, this retention of salts is by some
held to explain the hydremia of nephritis.   Not until we possess a fuller
series of simultaneous observations on the total amount of blood (by
Haldane and Smith's or other method) and of the proportions of the
different main constituents of the blood shall we be able to speak with
decision about these matters.   In short, with our present lack of knowledge, it is difficult to do other than consider together those three possible
variants, water, proteins, and salts. A more watery condition of the
blood, however brought about, is encountered in obstructive heart and
lung and in kidney diseases, in severe infections and malignancy, and
after extensive hemorrhages.   It must not be thought that in every case
manifesting these particular morbid states, the condition of hydremia
necessarily manifests itself.   In by no means all cases of cancer or
sarcoma is there reduction of the circulating proteins, and as Grawitz[1]
has shown, in the different stages of tuberculosis marked variations are
to be made out in the composition of the blood serum; not infrequently
instead of being hydremic, the blood is found more concentrated and
viscid.   In conditions of nephritis it is more particularly the acute parenchymatous cases that exhibit hydremia (which it is to be noted is associated with extensive loss of albumin through the kidneys); it may be

[1] Deutsch. med. Woch., 19:1893:1347.

wholly absent in cases of chronic interstitial nephritis, and is not necessarily present in those of chronic parenchymatous nephritis.[1] And as regards obstructive heart and lung disease, a word of caution needs to be given. Where there is passive congestion there is coincidently an increased passage of fluid from the blood into the lymphatics, with, as a result, a marked concentration of the erythrocytes in the capillaries from which the exudation takes place. In these cases, as, indeed, in all, it is wrong to make any conclusions as to the quantity or quality of the plasma from an estimation of the number of erythrocytes per cubic millimeter. So also in this same series of cases the fact of this escape of fluid into the tissues has to be taken into account. By the ordinary means of piqure to gain capillary blood, that blood may be gained extensively diluted with œdema fluid. This, however, has been definitely determined, that the blood serum deprived of corpuscles obtained from those cases of cardiac insufficiency in the stage of imperfect compensation presents a recognizable reduction in its solids.

Of the proteins of the plasma as contrasted with the serum, **fibrinogen** must not be overlooked. To the modern views regarding this protein and its relationship to the coagulation process we have already referred (p. 66). Here it has to be noted that the amount exhibits very considerable variation, as evidenced by the varying quantity of fibrin obtained from different bloods. From the normal amount of 0.1 to 0.4 per cent. by weight there may be a rise to 1 per cent. and higher. Such **hyperinosis** is met with more particularly in certain infections, notably in acute lobar pneumonia, in acute rheumatism, and in some cases of acute pleurisy. In other infections, notably typhoid, there is found a condition of **hypinosis**, or reduction of the fibrin. The fact that hyperinosis and hypinosis in these febrile states show a remarkable parallelism with the presence or absence of leukocytosis suggests that it is not so much the fibrinogen as the fibrin ferment that undergoes variation. This, however, would not seem to be the case. The fibrinogen itself undergoes variations independently of the leukocytosis in leukemia[2] and in phosphorus poisoning,[3] where it may be completely absent. Variations in the amount of the ferment affect the *coagulation* time of the blood rather than (so long as any fibrin ferment is present) the amount of fibrin produced.

As regards the salts of the plasma, again it has to be noted that we possess scattered data[4] rather than a full knowledge of their variation in different morbid states. These salts consist in the main of sodium salts, of chlorides and phosphates. They evidently bear an intimate relationship to the state of solution of the proteins. Their nature is

[1] Hammerschlag, Ztsch. f. klin. Med., 21: 1892: 475.

[2] Pfeiffer, Th. Zentrbl. f. innere Med., 25: 1904: 809.

[3] Jakoby, Zeitschr. f. phys. Chemie, 30: 1900: 174.

[4] These data will be found collected and discussed in Hamburger, Osmotische Druck und Ionenlehre, 1906, and Limbeck, Pathologie des Blutes, 2d edition, Jena, 1896

such that the normal blood is definitely alkaline, and, as already pointed out in discussing acidosis (vol. i, p. 381), reduction in this alkalinity is associated with the gravest metabolic disturbances.

Lipemia.—One other constituent of the blood plasma deserves notice. There is always to be isolated from the fluid of normal blood a minute quantity of fat. As to the exact state in which this is present there is still debate, the evidence on the whole favoring the view that some at least is in the form of the more soluble salts of the fatty acids or soaps. What we have already said regarding the absorption of fats from the intestine (vol. i, p. 94) prepares us to find that after meals rich in fats the amount is definitely increased. Occasionally there is encountered a condition of **lipemia**—of extraordinary increase in this fat. In some cases of diabetes there may be as high a content as 20 per cent., the blood taking on a milky appearance, and the fat being present in an emulsified state in the form of fine globules. Once more it has to be acknowledged that we know little or nothing about the conditions leading to this lipemia—whether we deal with the absence of a lipolytic ferment either from the blood or from the tissue cells which normally absorb the fat, or again, of some constituent which converts the absorbed fat into a soluble salt, thereby preparing it to be taken up by the cells, or lastly the presence of acids splitting up the soluble soaps present in the blood and liberating thus the fatty acids and fats. In addition to diabetes, lipemia has been observed in conditions characterized by defective oxidation (and increased carbon dioxide content of the blood), such as pneumonia, phosphorus poisoning, and anemias.

THE ERYTHROCYTES.

Of the physiology of the red corpuscles, much may be said; regarding their pathology, we must be comparatively brief.

Variations in Number.—We have emphasized already that moderate increase or decrease in the number of erythrocytes per cubic millimeter in itself tells us little without, at the same time, there be present indications of either increased production or excessive destruction of the corpuscles, rather than variation in the amount of the fluid of the blood. Where there is great departure from the normal it is difficult to believe that in all cases the concentration or dilution of the blood alone is at fault. That it may be, is shown by the great apparent increase in the number of red corpuscles seen in cases of cholera nostras, cholera asiatica, and other conditions in which there is great drain of fluid from the intestinal canal. But in such cases there is abundant clinical evidence of loss of fluid, as, for example, the difficulty in obtaining blood from the finger or pinna of the ear, the feeble heart action, the tarry condition of the blood itself—all indicating reduction in the quantity of the blood and concentration of the more solid constituents of the same.

Polycythemia.—The polycythemia of high altitudes has been studied by a large number of observers (Paul Bert, Miescher, Mosso, Abderhalden, and others), and is very striking. It affects all vertebrates. Thus, in the South American Cordilleras, at a height of more than 12,000 feet, Viault[1] found that the count in the llama was as high as 16,000,000. There has been great debate as to its meaning, but this seems to be established: (1) That the total amount of blood remains unaltered, and thus the increase is not due to concentration; (2) that the arterial blood shows the increase, and thus we do not deal with concentration in the superficial capillaries; (3) that it supervenes with relative rapidity (Gaule records increase to 8,500,000 in a balloon ascension); (4) that it soon disappears upon descent toward the sea level.

Making due allowance for variations in individual reaction, it is difficult to regard the increase as other than adaptive, than a reaction to the need for more oxygen carriers in an atmosphere in which the amount of oxygen is diminished. A similar increase, it may be noted, has been observed by Nasmith and Graham[2] in animals made to breathe air containing carbon monoxide. That carbon monoxide is useless to the economy, but has a far greater affinity for hemoglobin than has oxygen; the organism evidently produces more hemoglobin and hemoglobin holders to counteract the using up of part of the circulating hemoglobin. We do not pretend that there are not facts in connection with the phenomenon that are difficult to explain. When the condition supervenes rapidly we have to postulate a rapid production of hemoglobin and rapid discharge of young erythrocytes from the bone-marrow, and so far only one observer, Gaule, has recorded the presence of (immature) nucleated red corpuscles in the circulating blood; others have failed to find them. So also what becomes of the excess of erythrocytes upon return to lower levels remains unsolved. These are matters regarding which we have incomplete knowledge, rather than facts absolutely opposed to the view here taken.[3] This may be spoken of as physiological polycythemia; pathological polycythemia is a condition which has come into recognition only during the last few years,[4] some fifty cases being on record. In these cases counts of 8,000,000 are common, and those of 10,000,000, 13,000,000, and even 14,000,000 corpuscles have been determined. There is an accompanying duskiness or cyanotic appearance of the skin, and frequent (though not constant) pronounced enlargement of the spleen. Cases have been reported of all ages, most frequently in advancing life. The presence of normoblasts and megaloblasts shows clearly that there is an active production of erythrocytes, and some of the few postmortems have demonstrated increase of the marrow, and one at least has confirmed Widal's view that the splenic

[1] Compt. rend. de l'Acad. des Sci., 112: 1891: 295.

[2] Journ. of Physiol., 35: 1906: 32.

[3] A thoughtful study of this problem is afforded by Krehl, Pathol. Physiologie, 5th German edition, Leipzig, 1907: 193. See also A. W. Hewlett's translation, Lippincott, 1907.

[4] The first case was recorded by Rendu and Widal in 1892. For bibliography, see Engelbach and Brown, Jour. of Amer. Med. Assoc., 47: 1906: 1265, and for a general description, see Cabot, Osler and McCrae's System of Medicine, 4: 1908: 678.

enlargement is due to resumption by the spleen of its fœtal properties of production of erythroblasts. With this there is in some cases a moderate grade of neutrophilic leukocytosis. The cause of the condition is wholly undetermined.

Variations in Size and Shape.—The normal erythrocyte is from 5 to 8.5 μ in diameter. In conditions of anemia and disturbed erythrocyte production, notably in pernicious anemia, cells 10 to 20 μ in diameter are encountered (**megalocytes**) along with others which may be but 2 to 3 μ in diameter (**microcytes**). In these cases of extreme anemia cells of very irregular form are also encountered—**poikilocytes,** pear-shaped, elongated, and sausage-shaped, etc.

Alterations in Structure and Staining Reactions.—The normal erythrocyte is homogeneous, its hemoglobin scattered evenly through it, and granules are absent when the ordinary processes of staining are employed. In a mixture of acid and basic aniline dyes (as in Romanowsky's stain and its many modifications) it takes up the acid dye.

If, however, the development be followed in the red marrow, a succession of stages may be made out, from the large erythroblast, with large, loosely skeined nucleus and without hemoglobin in its cytoplasm, through forms with scattered granules and masses of hemoglobin and small, condensed nucleus, the hemoglobin in these younger cells taking up the basic stain with more or less intensity and appearing purplish or even blue, to forms which have lost their nucleus and have the hemoglobin diffused evenly throughout them, but still tend to take a purplish rather than a reddish or orange color. These various immature forms of red corpuscles may be encountered in disease, and then indicate a pouring into the blood from marrow or spleen of imperfectly developed erythrocytes; indicate, that is, a condition of such stimulation of the hematopoietic system that with active proliferation of the erythroblasts the immature cells are discharged into the blood.

Polychromatophilia and the presence of **nucleated red corpuscles,** of megaloblasts (as the large, paler forms are termed), and of normoblasts (hemoglobin-holding cells of the normal size but nucleated) must then be regarded as evidence of excessive demand made upon the blood-producing tissues. Such conditions are most frequently seen in grave anemias. At the same time it has to be recognized that basic and irregular staining of the erythrocytes in another but widely different series of conditions is evidence not of regeneration, but of degeneration; in areas of interstitial hemorrhage, as again in areas of fresh thrombosis, such polychromatophilia is to be distinguished.

In the latter case it is associated with indications of disintegration. Of this, two forms have been distinguished by Arnold, namely, **Plasmorrhexis** and **Plasmoschisis.** The former is the condition often observed when erythrocytes are studied in film under the microscope, namely, the development of crenation and of a mulberry-like appearance with formation of peripheral globules of varying size, some very minute (resembling Müller's "dust bodies"), others it may be as large as blood platelets; and these become liberated, with progressive diminution in size of the parent corpuscle. In plasmoschisis what is observed is a rapid breaking up of the whole body of the corpuscle into small globules, which as they separate are seen to be free from hemoglobin and to be indistinguishable from blood platelets. Another modification of which the significance is not understood is seen in certain cases of lead poisoning in which ring-like accumulations of matter taking on the basic stain are seen within occasional erythrocytes. Since in this condition we are apt to meet with "stippling" or free granules of basic staining matter within the red corpuscles, with normoblasts and megaloblasts, the indications are that we deal with an anemia and accompanying overstimulation of the red marrow; and the suggestion is that here we deal with cells in which the conversion of the prehemoglobinic matter is not complete.

Variation in Amount of Hemoglobin; Hemolysis.—By the use of the hemoglobinometer we can determine the amount of hemoglobin in a given quantity of blood by comparing its color with that of a sample of normal blood of known dilution (or its colored equivalent). By the hemocytometer we can determine the number of erythrocytes per cubic millimeter of the same blood. Utilizing these two enumerations, we can arrive at the *color index, e. g.,* at the ratio of hemoglobin per corpuscle, taking the normal corpuscle with normal hemoglobin content as 1. A blood, for example, containing the normal 5,000,000 corpuscles, but only 75 per cent. of the normal hemoglobin, would have a color index of 0.75; having only 2,500,000, with a hemoglobin content of 75 per cent., would, on the other hand, have a color index of 1.5, *i. e.,* each corpuscle would possess half as much hemoglobin again as does the normal corpuscle. And, as a matter of fact, we find very considerable variations in this color index. In chlorosis, for example, it is reduced; in pernicious anemia markedly increased. And these findings tally with the clinical observation that in chlorosis very slight exertion brings on breathlessness—through lack of adequate oxygenation—whereas, in pernicious anemia the patient in general only consults his doctor for weakness when the number of red corpuscles has fallen to 2,000,000 or less.

Reduction of the color index may either indicate (as in chlorosis) a primary inadequate production of the hemoglobin, or, on the other hand, a diffusion of the same out of the corpuscles into the plasma. Such *hemolysis* occurs under a variety of conditions. Our attention has been drawn to it of late years more particularly by the studies upon cytolytic action, and the remarkable effects produced both by foreign sera from normal animals, and by the sera of animals of the same or other species which have received injections of cells of various orders. Such sera come to contain bodies which, both in the removed blood and when injected into the vessels, cause a marked "laking" of the blood, so that the corpuscles become represented by colorless shadows. There are many other agencies which have a like effect—cold, as in paroxysmal hemoglobinuria; heat, as in burns; and many chemical agents—potassium chlorate, ricin, toluylenediamin, glycerin, pyrogallic acid, etc. What is of particular interest as possibly explaining some at least of the secondary anemias, is the hemolytic action of not a few of the pathogenic microörganisms—Streptococcus, Pyococcus aureus, Bacillus pyocyaneus,

Bacillus coli, Pneumococcus, etc. These organisms may be grown in defibrinated blood solutions, when the laking can be readily observed by the change in the appearance of the medium, or laking may be directly induced by the addition of the fluids of culture.

In all these cases it would seem that we deal with more than the mere diffusion out of the hemoglobin. Some changes must occur in the physical state of the corpuscles before the pigment becomes liberated, and once it is liberated the corpuscle is rendered useless. We possess no evidence that the erythrocyte has the power to regenerate hemoglobin after loss. The fate of the affected corpuscles is to be removed from the circulation by the agency of the spleen. Any condition, therefore, bringing about severe or continued hemolysis causes with it a condition of (so-called) anemia, *i. e.*, a reduction in the number of circulating erythrocytes. The anemia so produced has been studied in our laboratory by Charlton, who injected over long periods into rabbits non-lethal doses of a relatively non-virulent colon bacillus isolated from the intestine of a normal rabbit. Bunting employed similarly repeated small doses of ricin. Charlton was able in several instances to bring down the number of erythrocytes to 1,000,000, and found that so soon as the number reached 2,500,000, poikilocytosis with occasional megaloblasts became developed; he found, however, little obvious change in the bone-marrow. In Bunting's cases the evidence of increased activity of the bone-marrow was well marked, the marrow closely resembling that seen in pernicious anemia. Other observers, like Hunter with his researches upon the effects of toluylenediamin, have studied the more immediate effects of hemolytic agents, as shown by the excretion of the liberated hemoglobin through the liver and kidneys, in the former case as bile pigment.

Chlorosis.[1]—Here it will be well to pass in review certain of the more important disorders characterized by altered states of the red corpuscles. And first we may consider chlorosis, a condition formerly very common, but now, according to Cabot, becoming relatively uncommon, at least in North America. It affects young women (94 per cent. of Cabot's cases were between the ages of fifteen and thirty years); rare cases have been recorded in young males, so rare that many writers doubt their existence. Save that the onset suggests some disturbance of the recently established menstrual function, and that the majority of cases are of girls in household service, who have exchanged the freer life in the country for one spent largely indoors under not the best hygienic conditions, we have practically no indications suggesting the causation of the disease—which in itself is not fatal, although it may predispose to tuberculosis and other more fatal conditions.

The characteristic features are the cachexia, the bloodless, pale complexion ("green sickness"), with pallor of the lips, the weakness and lassitude following upon slight exertion, the dyspepsia, capricious

[1] The fullest recent study of this condition is by Cabot, in Osler and McCrae's Modern Medicine, 4: 1908: 639, based on the study of 497 cases.

appetite, with gastric acidity, constipation, and palpitation, and the state of the blood. There is a slight but definite reduction of the number of erythrocytes, a marked reduction in the amount of hemoglobin per corpuscle; the color index averages about 0.5, but may be as low as 0.1. With this, as clearly demonstrated by Haldane and Lorrain Smith, there is pronounced increase in the amount of blood plasma, an increase more than sufficient to explain the reduction in the number of erythrocytes per cubic millimeter. There is a true serous plethora. Save that more might have been said regarding the symptoms, there is little to add that is definite in our knowledge of the disease, with the exception that the rapid general improvement which follows the proper administration of iron, accompanied by improved hygienic conditions, suggests that we deal very largely with a deficient building up of iron into the iron containing hemoglobin of the developing erythrocytes; that, in short, the reduction of the color index is the central feature of chlorosis. Several observers have called attention to the accompanying constipation and the improvement that follows when this is overcome; thus possibly an intestinal toxemia may play some part in the production of the condition.

Secondary Anemias.—With the exception of the above condition, when we can determine what appears to be a satisfactory cause for the diminution in the number of erythrocytes, we speak of a secondary anemia, and doing so, we leave as a class apart one condition of unknown causation, namely, idiopathic or primary pernicious anemia. Such secondary anemia may be acute, as after profound loss of blood. In these cases what has already been said will have prepared the reader to find a blood greatly diluted, owing to passage into it of lymph and tissue fluids, in order to preserve the amount of circulating fluid. The erythrocytes at first are normal in appearance and hemoglobin content, but eventually, if the loss of blood has been great and the pouring of new cells out of the bone-marrow excessive, there may appear a few immature erythrocytes and cells of the megaloblastic type. With this there may be a temporary actual increase in the number of circulating leukocytes (mainly neutrophile) and a lowering of the color index, due to the fact that the immature erythrocytes do not contain the normal amount of hemoglobin. Extensive hemolysis may also bring about an acute anemia; this may be induced by severe infections, and cases are on record in which, without the supervention of hemorrhage, the blood count has dropped to 1,500,000 within a few days of high fever. Certain drugs taken accidentally (*e. g.*, acetanilide) may induce active hemolysis and give a similar picture.

Chronic Secondary Anemias.—In these acute cases we have in the main the picture of great reduction in the number of erythrocytes, followed by stages of an imperfect hematopoiesis. In the chronic forms imperfect hematopoiesis may be said to hold the field. The main features are an abundance of cells smaller than normal, and a low color index. Much, however, depends, both as regards the erythrocytes and the leukocytes, upon the grade of the anemia, as again upon the cause. Thus, in the anemias due to intestinal parasites the milder cases show at most microcytosis with a characteristic eosinophilia, but grave cases, notably those due to the Dibothriocephalus latus, the fish tapeworm, present a picture indistinguishable from pernicious anemia. Lead poisoning, again, presents an undue proportion of nucleated reds with "stippling," *i. e.*, with basic granulation of the erythrocytes. In splenic anemia, the leukocytes are characteristically diminished in number, and the color index is very low. In infancy, the anemias present aberrant characters. In accordance with the other tissues, the regeneration of the blood cells is very active, with the result that abundant cells of erythroblastic type gain entrance into the blood, and the color index, instead of being low, is, as a rule, high.

As a general principle, it may be laid down for these secondary anemias that the more severe and the more long continued the causative conditions, the greater are the signs of exhaustion and using up of the erythroblastic mother tissues, until, in the advanced cases, we obtain pictures very similar to, and in fact at times indistinguishable from, those of pernicious anemia, to be presently noted.

Pernicious Anemia.—The picture presented by the sufferer from pernicious anemia is striking: the peculiar yellow cachexia, the absence of emaciation, and in its place the laying on of flabby fat, the weak heart action and pulse, and striking general weakness. At autopsy, the bright yellow color of the fat, the bloodlessness and anemia of all the organs, the pale color of what blood there is, the pronounced fatty degeneration of the heart, the presence of increased iron, more particularly in the liver, shown by either Quincke's or Perl's test, the increased red marrow of the bones, and the frequent presence of evidence of a chronic gastritis, all combine to form a combination that cannot be mistaken.

The most striking of these disturbances is the blood condition. That blood is both diminished in amount and characterized by a marked diminution in the number of erythrocytes. The number may fall to below 500,000. We have at the same time evidence of active disintegration of the red corpuscles (indicated by the increased storage of iron in the liver) and of active regeneration (indicated by the hyperplasia of the red marrow and the relatively abundant nucleated red corpuscles of different orders in the circulating blood). But the regeneration does not proceed at a rate sufficient to compensate for the destruction. What is characteristic is that the individual erythrocytes are many of them larger than normal, and they contain increased hemoglobin; so that a main feature is the very high color index. That the corpuscles are not healthy is indicated by the marked *poikilocytosis;*[1] they are flabby and assume various shapes. But despite the high index, owing to the great reduction in the number of corpuscles and reduction in the amount of blood, the total amount of hemoglobin is greatly lowered. To this lowered oxygen-carrying capacity of the blood must be ascribed the diminished metabolism and the storage of fat (a similar tendency to lay on fat is often observable in chlorosis), and possibly the continued malnutrition in itself is responsible for the fatty degeneration of the heart

---

[1] ποικίλος, varied or various (referring to shape).

PLATE II

FIG. 1

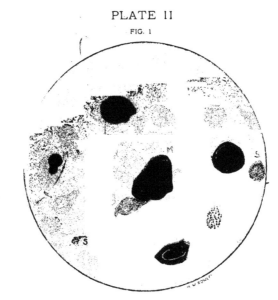

Pernicious Anemia. (Cabot.)

The field shows marked anisocytosis and poikilocytosis: M^1, young megaloblast (early generation); M^2 M^3 M^4, later generations of the megaloblast series; S S S, "stippled" red cells; R, ring body (nuclear remnant?); L, lymphocyte.

FIG. 2

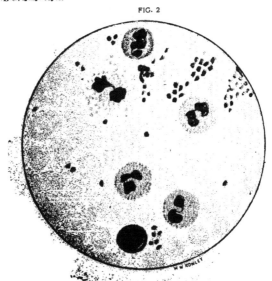

Eosinophilia (Trichiniasis). (Cabot.)

Copy of an actual field containing three normal polynuclear eosinophiles, one broken eosinophile, one polynuclear neutrophile, and one lymphocyte.

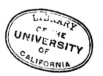

and other organs, although this may also be ascribed to the unknown toxic agent causing the hemolysis and continued blood destruction.

What this toxic agent is we still are in ignorance; obviously it is of hemolytic nature, and acts over long periods. One striking feature of the disease is that it is already far advanced, as a rule, before the patient feels himself ill enough to consult a physician; another, that apparently, despite the varied nature of the treatment afforded—save that the common basis of all forms of treatment is rest and simple diet—there occurs in the majority of cases a distinct remission; the number of erythrocytes increases, the general condition improves, until the blood returns practically to the normal and the patient is apparently restored to health. This may persist for but a month or two, as long as four years—only rarely is the improvement permanent. Then, without obvious cause, a relapse occurs. Cabot, from an analysis of several hundred cases, states that the average time of remission is for one year, and quotes cases in which the relapse has occurred at the same season in successive years; our impression is that too great stress must not be laid upon this regularity. The only suggestion that can be made to explain these remissions is that the enforced rest and dieting gives the system the opportunity to counteract the intoxication. More and more Hunter's conclusion that we deal with some alimentary intoxication is gaining ground. The frequency of a septic condition of the mouth, or of evidences of a chronic atrophic gastritis, the very frequent absence of hydrochloric acid from the gastric juice, the gastric distress, and the frequent condition of diarrhœa, all call attention to the digestive tract. And here three possibilities exist—either that we deal with (1) the absorption of hemolytic products of abnormal digestion, (2) the absorption of similar hemolytic products of abnormal bacterial fermentation, or (3) the presence and growth in the digestive tract of organisms of a low pathogenic type, and, as a consequence, the development of a state of subinfection (vol. i, p. 462), the increased carriage of organisms into the splanchnic blood stream being favored by inflammatory states of the alimentary mucosa.

Certain considerations favor either of the latter two theories, namely, (1) the known power of acid reaction of the stomach contents to arrest bacterial proliferation, and the converse, that absence of hydrochloric acid from the upper intestinal tract favors bacterial growth and abnormal fermentation; (2) the observed anemia that accompanies foul-smelling putrefactive states of the contents of the lower intestines.

Here at the present time the study of pernicious anemia may be said to rest. We are coming, that is, to the conclusion that pernicious anemia is not idiopathic; that the typical forms have associated with them bacterial overgrowth in the alimentary canal of such an order that hemolytic agents are developed in undue quantities, but still have to determine what particular order of bacteria are concerned, and how they act. In conclusion, we would repeat that it has to be kept in mind that a similar syndrome and extreme alteration of the blood may be produced by known agencies, by hemolytic substances, such as repeated small doses of ricin (Bunting), by the presence of the Dibothriocephalus latus in the intestines (whatever be its mode of action), and, rarely, in the latter stages of malignant disease. In this, Crile and others have determined the existence of hemolytic substances in the blood. We have seen the condition develop also in a patient the subject of repeated small hemorrhages extending over two years, from a villous papilloma of the bladder. In that case the picture was complete, save for the absence of excess of iron in the liver, *i. e.*, there had been no intravascular destruction of red corpuscles, but a steady loss of the same from the system. So also there was no recognizable disturbance of the gastro-intestinal tract.

Aplastic Anemia.—Rare cases are on record of a yet further stage in what appears to be the same process. In this it would seem that the overgrowth of the red marrow and excessive production of erythrocytes is followed by a stage of exhaustion, so that upon examining the medulla of the sternum or femur, etc., instead of finding an overabundance of red marrow, that red marrow is reduced in amount, and replaced, it may be wholly, by yellow fat; instead of hyperplasia there is aplasia; or, judging from the rapid course of many of the cases, it may be urged that from some congenital weakness or other cause the agent setting up the hemolysis does not excite an adequate hyperplasia from the first, and the erythroblasts are quickly used up. As indications of this exhaustion are to be noted the absence of normoblasts and megaloblasts, and the low color index. Poikilocytosis and anisocytosis[1] are found largely wanting, as are also the leukocytes proper, causing a relative abundance of lymphocytes. Hemorrhages are frequent. Cabot has collected twenty-two cases of this nature from the literature.

THE LEUKOCYTES.

With the present continued doubt regarding the relationship of the different forms of leukocytes in the circulating blood, it is essential that before discussing variations in the relative numbers of the different forms appearing in the blood, we should at least place upon record our opinions regarding that relationship; not that we consider our views so well founded that they are unlikely to undergo change, but because the whole of our treatment of leukocytosis is influenced by these views. We have discussed them elsewhere.[2]

Here, as regards the blood as distinct from the inflamed tissues, we recognize two well-defined groups: (1) The granular leukocytes, and (2) the lymphocytes, and these we hold are of separate origin. The different forms of the first group would seem all to originate from myeloblasts, large, non-granulated cells, which, in the adult, are present throughout life as "mother cells" in the bone-marrow. These originate, as do also

---

[1] ἄνισος, unequal (referring to size).

[2] Inflammation. London, Macmillan & Co., 4th edition, 1909

the erythroblasts, in intimate connection with the capillary endothelium,[1] whereas the lymphocytes are derived from the mother cells or lymphoblasts of lymphoid tissue. The myelocytes give origin to cells which exhibit granulations of different orders—either acidophilic, staining with the acid aniline dyes, or basophilic—while occasionally we may encounter cells which morphologically are of intermediate type. Despite the abundant studies that have been made, we still lack sure evidence that the fully developed cell, with, for example, coarse acidophile granules (eosinophile), undergoes conversion into one with finely granular basophile (neutrophile) granulations, or *vice versa*. All the evidence indicates that the neutrophile or ordinary polynuclear leukocyte, once it reaches this stage, remains a neutrophile and is incapable of conversion into other form. Still less do we have any indication of intermediate stages between the lymphocyte and the group of granular leukocytes. It is true that, contrary to general teaching, by special methods of staining the lymphocyte can be seen to exhibit extremely fine granulations, but these are of a special order, and are not demonstrable by the ordinary methods whereby the leukocytic granulations are brought out.

As to the functions of these cells under normal conditions in the circulating blood, while we have many indications, we know little that is absolute. We know much more concerning that function when they have made their way out of the vessels either into the lymph spaces or on to the surface of the body. These latter functions we have already discussed in our chapters upon Inflammation (vol. i, p. 413). It is quite possible that in the blood stream they act as scavengers, although normally, judging from the great rarity of any signs of inclusion,[2] this property is little called into play.

There are observations favoring the view that in the intestinal villi the circulating leukocytes may actively take up fatty globules, but it may be questioned whether such leukocytes have not actively taken up these globules outside, and then migrated into the veins. Again, according to Metchnikoff's views, it is the leukocytes that are the great manufacturers and storehouses both of immune bodies and complements. At the same time he holds strongly that where this is the case, the healthy leukocyte does not liberate these bodies into the blood plasma. On the whole, it would seem more probable that in the normal blood the leukocytes exert little functional activity, that the blood in the main acts as carrier for those cells, that their carriage throughout the body is to subserve their function of acting as patrols, so that, conveyed to any capillary region, they may make their way out into the tissues through chemiotactic attraction. Their activity, that is, would seem to be more extravascular than intravascular. In saying this we do not deny that circulating toxins have an influence upon the number of leukocytes in the circulating blood; this influence, however, would

[1] Vide Schridde, Centralbl. f. Pathol., 19:1908; 865.

[2] One of us once encountered a definite bacillus in a polynuclear leukocyte of his own blood, he being at the time in good health

seem to be exerted primarily upon the bone-marrow and lymph-glandular tissue, determining a greater or less discharge of the different orders of cells. It is to this, and not to any proliferation of the leukocytes in the blood that any leukocytosis or the reverse condition of leukopenia must be ascribed.

Leukocytosis.—The presence of any increase in the total number of white corpuscles in the peripheral blood above the normal constitutes leukocytosis. Usually one or other form is in relatively greater abundance; as subgroups we distinguish (a) a *polynuclear leukocytosis;* (b) *eosinophilia;* and (c) *lymphocytosis,* together with other conditions of the appearance of aberrant or immature forms constituting (d) *leukemia.* Strictly speaking, we do not consider that we deal with leukemia until the number of these aberrant leukocytes in the blood exceeds 15,000. Therefore, we may have a myelocytic leukocytosis, for example, that is not a leukemia.

Using the term in its broader sense, we distinguish next between *physiological* and *pathological* leukocytosis.

Physiological leukocytosis shows itself in a variety of conditions. In the first place, there is in the young a well-marked relative leukocytosis. During the first week of life the number of leukocytes varies between 15,000 and 30,000; during the first ten years of life it varies between 10,000 and 12,000. In the female toward the end of pregnancy there is a well-marked rise, reaching to 15,000 to 20,000 at the time of parturition. A distinct rise is to be noted after violent exercise, massage, cold baths, and the application of electricity; so also, full protein diet favors what is known as alimentary leukocytosis. Lastly, a *terminal* leukocytosis in the last hours of life is so common that it may be regarded as physiological.

Pathological Leukocytosis.—(a) **Polynuclear** or **neutrophilic leukocytosis.** It is in *inflammatory* and *infectious* conditions that we more particularly find this form of leukocytosis. We can produce it experimentally by the inoculation of many pathogenic organisms, *e. g.*, by inoculating non-lethal doses of the Pyococcus aureus into the peritoneal cavity, when for the first few hours there is a leukopenia, followed next day by a pronounced polynuclear leukocytosis. This is by no means a universal reaction to infection; notably it is wanting in typhoid, malaria, tuberculosis of the more chronic type, and, when without secondary infection, leprosy, measles, mumps, and most cases of influenza. But where there is localized or generalized suppuration, it becomes most pronounced; in pneumonia, again, there may be a leukocytosis of 100,000, with 95 per cent. of polynuclears. Our contention that these, the most actively phagocytic leukocytes, do not so much function in the blood as appear there to be utilized later in the tissues, is borne out by the fact that in malaria, trypanosomiasis, and other conditions in which animal microparasites multiply in the blood rather than in the tissues, a polynuclear leukocytosis is characteristically wanting; whereas in pneumonia and the suppurative diseases in which the irritants multiply outside the bloodvessels, there this form of leukocytosis is most extreme.

There is another group of conditions in which we encounter this type of leukocytosis—the toxic. Here are to be included posthemorrhagic leukocytosis, the later stages of hepatic cirrhosis, and other states characterized by grave disturbance of the liver cells (uremia, etc.), gout, the later stages of malignant disease, ptomaine poisoning, coal-gas poisoning, and the effects of certain drugs, antipyretics, salicylates, pilocarpine, etc. The presence, that is, of certain products of abnormal metabolism and cell disintegration on the one hand, and of certain exogenous chemical bodies on the other, set up an increased discharge of polymorphonuclear cells from the bone-marrow into the blood.

(b) **Eosinophilia.**—A distinct relative increase in the eosinophiles of the circulating blood is seen (1) in the majority of cases of helminthiasis, *i. e.*, of the existence of parasitic worms in the economy (vol. i, p. 349); (2) in a group of irritative skin diseases (pemphigus, dermatitis herpetiformis, etc.); (3) accompanying myelogenic leukemia; (4) in bronchial asthma, and to a slight extent in a variety of conditions which it is difficult to correlate: certain malignant cases of neoplasia, ovarian disease (where non-malignant and non-suppurative), and postfebrile conditions.

We know little regarding the significance of the eosinophiles. The larger oxyphile granules recall strikingly the granules of gland cells, but the observations of Kanthack and Hardy, to the effect that these may be actively excreted, are strongly contested by most hematologists, although we personally are prepared to accept the statements of these most accurate workers. They certainly play a part in the early stages of acute inflammation, being the first cells to be attracted; they accumulate in the omental vessels in cases of peritoneal inflammation; and very possibly the eosinophilia of diffuse cutaneous irritative lesions is of the same local type, *i. e.*, a determination of eosinophiles into the vessels of the inflamed areas.

(c) **Lymphocytosis.**—Actual or relative increase in the lymphocytes of the blood is seen:

1. In many diseases of young children, notably those affecting the gastro-intestinal tract. It will be recalled that the infant shows a marked relative and absolute lymphocytosis. This is doubtless associated with the greater relative amount of lymphoid tissue in the young individual, which continues into childhood, and is especially marked in the intestinal and mesenteric lymph-glands, so that irritation of this group of glands more especially is accompanied by a greater discharge of lymphocytes into the blood

2. In septic and other conditions in the adult, characterized by excessive enlargement of more than one group of lymph glands.

3. In whooping cough. Here the lymphocytosis is almost pathognomonic. A lymphocytosis of 20,000 and more is very frequent, and cases are on record of counts in the neighborhood of 100,000 (Steven Cabot).

4· In debilitating disease—scurvy, rickets, chlorosis, and various cachexias. Here the lymphocytosis is generally of a moderate grade.

In all the above cases we deal with the normal small lymphocytes.

(*d*) **Leukemia.**—We have in our first volume given our views regarding the relationship of the leukemias to simple hyperplasia on the one hand and neoplasia on the other. Here, we must briefly indicate the main features of the leukemic state, and the effects upon the organism. By leukemia, as distinct from leukocytosis, we signify not merely the excess of leukocytes in the blood, but the sum total of the disturbances which accompany the *continued* presence of a great excess of such lenkocytes. We do not employ the term when the number is below 15,000; indeed, when the excess is below that figure the syndrome of disturbances is scarcely recognizable. That it must have a beginning at an earlier period is obvious, but in general it is either progressive weakness, or the detection by the patient himself of a greatly enlarged spleen that first leads to an examination of the blood and recognition of an already advanced condition. And then one of two orders of disturbance is to be made out; either a great excess of myelocytes or of lymphocytes in the blood.

Myelogenic Leukemia.—Myelogenic leukemia is a disease affecting the male more often than the female, most often in early adult life, and showing itself especially by disturbances of the blood-forming organs and the results of the same. Those blood-forming organs, to repeat, are the bone-marrow, and, under pathological conditions, the spleen, liver, and lymph-glands, and all these may be involved, although the extent of involvement varies in different individuals. The bone marrow would seem always to be affected, exhibiting a replacement of the fat by hyperplastic gray marrow, in which cells of the myelocyte type preponderate, with transitional stages from myeloblast through myelocyte to the neutrophile leukocyte. Eosinophile cells may also be encountered, erythrocytes and nucleated red corpuscles, along with a distinct increase in the number of giant cells (megacaryocytes). Lymphocytic elements are relatively rare. Normally, the spleen after birth shows little evidence of myelocyte formation, but now it is pronounced, so that this organ takes on very much the appearance of the lymphoid Malpighian bodies. All the orders of cells seen in the leukemic marrow are encountered in this organ, which undergoes an enormous overgrowth, so that at times it may extend down to the pubes, still, however, retaining its shape and general proportions. In the more chronic cases there is in addition an extensive fibrosis of the organ. Like the spleen, the liver is actively involved in blood formation during antenatal life, and now it may revert to its fœtal activities. Regarding this there is still debate; many authorities hold that the great size of the organ and the appearances seen on section are due entirely to accumulation in the capillaries of cells conveyed from the spleen, and that the atrophy of the liver cells (which may be so extreme that considerable areas are encountered showing nothing but myelocytes) is due to the engorgement of and pressure exerted by the distended capillaries. Others see an activity on the part of the vascular endothelium, leading, as in the embryo, to a production of myelocytes and megacaryocytes both inward into the vessels and outward to form an extravascular accumulation. To

PLATE III

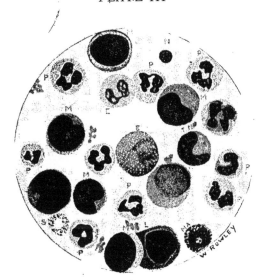

Myelogenic Leukemia. (Cabot.)

Copied from an actual field : P, polynuclear neutrophilic leukocytes ; M, neutrophilic myelocytes ; N, transitional neutrophile; M A, mast cell; L, "marrow lymphocyte;" E E, polynuclear eosinophiles; "stippled" erythrocyte; N, normoblast.

PLATE IV

FIG. 1

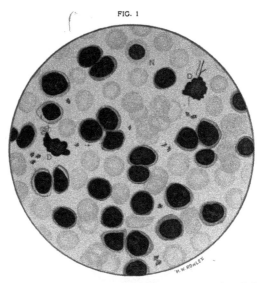

Chronic Lymphatic Leukemia (Actual Field). (Cabot.)

Twenty-nine typical small lymphocytes; *D D*, degenerating lymphocytes; *N*, normoblast.

FIG. 2

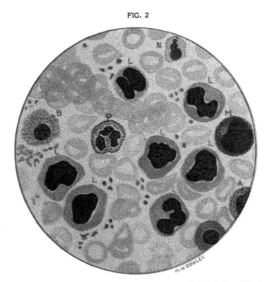

Acute Lymphatic Leukemia (Actual Field). (Cabot.)

atypical "lymphocytes" (Naegeli's myeloblasts); *M*, neutrophilic myelocyte; *P*, polynuclear neutrophile; *A*, "large lymphocyte," with "azur" granules; *B*, megaloblast (stippled); *N*, normoblast.

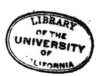

explain this divergence it must be recalled that not all parts of the hematopoietic system are necessarily involved at the same time and to the same extent, and thus it happens that in many cases the liver takes no active part. This organ also may attain great size. The lymph-glands are, as a rule, only moderately involved. Often, save for some accumulation of myelocytes in their vessels, they are normal; but occasionally some undergo the changes which make them closely resemble the modified bone-marrow and spleen. Accumulations of the modified leukocytes may fill the capillaries in the lungs, kidneys, myocardium, and other organs.

The diagnostic feature is, however, the blood. Here the average number of white corpuscles is between 400,000 and 500,000 (Cabot), varying from 60,000 to as much as 1,500,000 per c.mm. The increase involves all the orders of white corpuscles, the most striking increase being in the myelocytes, which may constitute about one-half the total, and the polynuclears, constituting almost the other half. There is a well-marked eosinophilia (but this relatively slight as compared with the increases above noted); an increase in the number of *mast cells* (coarsely granular basophiles), and though proportionately they are greatly diminished, the number of lymphocytes is actually greater than that found in normal blood.

As regards the red cells, until the final stages, there is usually only a slight diminution to not less than 3,000,000. Toward the end the diminution becomes much greater, and with this there may be poikilocytosis with presence of nucleated reds. We have indications, in short, of a profound hyperplasia, affecting especially those myeloblasts which give origin to the polynuclears, and in their proliferation are discharged as immature myelocytes. Simultaneously the other elements of the marrow tend to proliferate; hence, the eosinophilia, the nucleated reds, and somewhat increased discharge of lymphocytes.

This great increase in the large myelocytes leads to accumulation of the same in the organs possessing finer capillaries, and brings about both local malnutrition, through clogging of their channels, and general slowing of the circulation. Actual emboli may thus be formed. The accompanying reduction in the erythrocytes also favors malnutrition. These alone or combined may explain the dyspnœa, weakness, and moderate wasting characteristic of the disease, as again the epistaxis, retinal and other hemorrhages, and the persistent priapism occasionally encountered. But if there be increased production of leukocytes, there are also well-marked indications of increased destruction, foremost among which we to-day place the excessive discharge of uric acid through the kidneys due to the disintegration of the nuclei of the destroyed cells. We know of no microbic or other cause of the disease, and to the liberation of the products of cell disintegration may possibly be ascribed the fever present in practically every case. The course of the disease is distinctly chronic, lasting for from six months to several years.

LYMPHATIC LEUKEMIA.—This condition, again, is more frequent in the male than in the female, and in young adult life, though cases occur more widely distributed from infancy to old age. Unlike the myelogenic form, this may exhibit an acute onset and course, and we may broadly distinguish the two types: of *acute*, occurring more frequently in the first thirty years of life, and of *chronic*, in the latter half. Whereas it is the enlarged spleen that is the commonest physical sign of the former condition, here enlargement of the lymph-glands is the marked feature; weakness, dyspnœa, emaciation, .hemorrhages, are common to the two conditions.

The blood in the chronic cases shows an extraordinary preponderance of typical lymphocytes—typical, that is, in form, with large, deep-staining nucleus and small rim of cytoplasm, as again in size. In a large proportion of the acute cases we meet with cells so atypical, large, with abundant cytoplasm, and nuclei of irregular shape, and not so deeply stained, that while in many cases we distinguish transitional forms between these and the small lymphocyte, in others, doubts arise as to whether we deal truly with cells of the lymphocyte group—whether we have not to deal with myeloblasts, the non-granular forerunners of the myelocyte. It is worthy of note that it may be laid down that the more acute the case, the greater the tendency for the lymph-glands to be but slightly enlarged, and for the brunt of the hyperplasia to be found in the bone-marrow. We are inclined to the belief that up to the present, adequate means of distinguishing between the most immature forms of lymphoblast and myeloblast have not been elaborated, and that in this class we include the most acute forms of both lymphatic and myelogenic leukemia.

There is in most cases, both acute and chronic, some enlargement of the spleen, though this in general is not so marked as in the myelogenic form; the same is true regarding the liver. A condition peculiar to this disease is overgrowth of the multiple minute lymphoid collections in the skin, causing the appearance of multiple small nodules. The number of circulating leukocytes is, as a rule, not so great as in myelogenic leukemia; the average is in the neighborhood of 200,000. Counts between 400,000 and 1,000,000 are not common. What is characteristic is the infrequency of forms other than those above described; the polynuclears are few in number; eosïnophiles and mast cells may be wholly wanting; the basophile myelocytes are either absent or not abundant.

Lastly, these cases are characterized by a more continuous and sometimes high fever (102° to 104° F.) with severe sweats, so that without blood examination it is easy to mistake the condition for typhoid, acute tuberculosis, hepatic abscess, etc. The condition is most fatal.

What has been said regarding the relationship of the symptoms to the blood changes in myelogenic leukemia applies to this condition also.

Before leaving the subject it is necessary to call to mind that similar hyperplasia of the lymph-glandular system may present itself without excessive discharge of lymphocytes into the blood ("pseudoleukemia"), or, again, that the blood in the last stages of pernicious anemia may simulate that of leukemia, while similarly the last stages of myelogenic leukemia may be accompanied by so great a destruction or lack of production of erythrocytes as to bring about a condition much resembling pernicious anemia. With Cabot, we regard one or other of these conditions as explaining the condition of *leukanemia* of Leube[1] and other recent writers.

Regarding pseudoleukemia, Hodgkin's disease, chloroma, and lymphosarcomatosis, the reader is referred to our first volume (pp. 737–743).

THE BLOOD PLATELETS.

If only because they play so important a part in the process of thrombosis, it is necessary to have a clear understanding regarding the blood platelets, or, more accurately, regarding what is known concerning their origin. Apart from this, with the advent of the Romanowsky stain and its modifications, they have of late years come in for increasing recognition. There is no longer any disposition to regard them as artefacts, but there is still dispute as to their exact significance and as to their unity or duality.

They are small bodies of varying size, in general about $2\,\mu$ in diameter, oval or pear-shaped, evidently labile, and varying in shape with slight compression by neighboring cells or platelets, tending to be present in smears in small groups (possibly as the result of rapid agglutination in the shed blood). They are non-nucleated, although containing often fine, central granules, which assume a redder tint with the Romanowsky stain in contrast to the bluer groundwork. Pratt's careful studies show that they are present in the normal blood in greater numbers than the leukocytes, although the number shows wider variation—from 200,000 to 700,000 per c.mm. Since their discovery and the early papers by Hayem, Bizzozero, and Mrs. Ernest Hart, there have been very various views regarding their nature and mode of origin: (1) That they are precipitated globulin (Löwit, Wooldridge); (2) that they are products of disintegration of white corpuscles (Lilienfeld, Zenker, and others); (3) that they are given off from disintegrating red corpuscles (Mosso, Klebs, Arnold, etc.). The exquisite preparations made by J. H. Wright, of Boston,[2] demonstrate without possibility of doubt that some at least of the platelets, and those most typical, are normally derived from a particular order of cell, namely, from the giant cells (megacaryocytes) of the bone-marrow. These cells give off processes projecting into the lumina of the capillaries, and it is the distal portions of these which become liberated into the blood as platelets. As such they may, as Schimmelbusch was the first to demonstrate, retain some power of amœboid movement, but the mode of their development sets at rest the debate as to the nature of the central staining granules; they in no sense represent a nucleus.

The important question still to be determined is whether all the

---

[1] Deutsche Klinik, 1902, No. 42.

[2] Unfortunately, the photographs which illustrate his paper are not worthy of the preparations, and do not carry conviction.

blood platelets have this one mode of origin; and this is far from settled. That the leukocytes play any part in their production must, we think, be put on one side, although certain of the smaller "dust bodies" to be presently referred to would seem to have this origin. Their origin from erythrocytes cannot be so easily dismissed. Some would urge that there exist blood platelets proper, and other bodies, derived, it may be, from red corpuscles which are not platelets. But this cannot be seriously defended. The blood platelets, it has to be admitted, are very variable —variable in size from $1\,\mu$ up to half the diameter of a leukocyte; some have the central granules above described, others show more, and where granules are present they vary in amount and in position; most contain no hemoglobin, others have a hemoglobin tint. Now, it has been shown, more particularly by Arnold, that under conditions of intravascular and extravascular clotting the disintegration of the erythrocytes leads to the appearance of bodies which by no criterion can be distinguished from the platelets of ordinary blood. They may originate as discharged endoglobular bodies, which by diffusion soon lose their hemoglobin, by plasmorrhexis (detachment of peripheral nodular projections), or by plasmoschisis (whereby the whole body of the corpuscle breaks up into oval bodies which become separate platelets). Appearances which in our opinion can only be attributable to this breaking down of the erythrocytes are frequently to be noted in connection with thrombi of the smaller vessels (*e. g.*, of the liver), and if we do not accept these products of erythrocytic disintegration as platelets, then we are placed in the dilemma of regarding the process of thrombosis as due in a notable proportion of cases not to blood platelets proper, but to a conglutination of bodies which are not blood platelets, but simulate them in shape and properties. In short, we come perilously near occupying the position of the student who held that the *Iliad* was not written by Homer, but by another man of the same name. It is simpler to admit that the products of disintegration *en masse* of more than one order of cell afford bodies having the nature of blood platelets.

We must admit that in pernicious anemia the platelets are frequently (though not always) diminished in number, and that here there has been observed a lack of giant cells in the bone-marrow. In purpura they have at times been found completely absent. We know of no observations on the marrow giant cells in these cases. They are diminished also in typhoid—but increased in myelogenic leukemia, and in pneumonia.

DUST BODIES—HEMOCONIA.

Still smaller bodies or particles are to be recognized in the normal blood —$1\,\mu$ and less in diameter. To these H. F. Müller has given the name of dust bodies, or hemoconia. The observations of Nicholls[1] and others indicate that these also are the products of disintegration, more particularly of the erythrocytes.

[1] Trans Royal Soc. of Canada, 2d series, 11, 1905, sec 4:1

CHAPTER V.

RECENT observations have very materially altered our conception of the finer anatomy of the lymphatic system, and, with this, have, of necessity, modified the conditions which have to be taken into consideration in formulating our views regarding both lymph formation and the disturbances in the amount of lymph present in the tissues of the body. So recent are these observations that time has not yet been afforded for experimental review of the older hypotheses in the light of this newer knowledge. It is impossible, therefore, to write in other than a very tentative manner about what, from a pathological point of view, is the most important morbid state directly dependent upon alteration in lymph production and lymph discharge, the state, namely, of œdema.

The older, long-accepted view was that the lymphatic system had its origin in the intercellular spaces of the various tissues, and that these "lymph spaces" opened freely into an arborization of lymph channels, which differed from the spaces in being of a definitely tubular nature, and, like the blood capillaries, lined by an endothelium. The careful studies of, more particularly, W. G. MacCallum and Florence Sabin seem to demonstrate conclusively that the system of lymph vessels has arisen by a process of budding from the veins, and that it remains distinct from the system of intercellular lymph spaces—as distinct, that is, as are the blood capillaries. It follows, therefore, that in discussing lymph formation in, and lymph discharge from, any region, we have constantly to keep in mind not merely the mechanisms whereby fluid passes out of the bloodvessels into the tissues, but, in addition, those controlling the passage of fluid from the intercellular lymph spaces into the lymph vessels. We have to recognize thus (1) blood plasma, (2) intercellular lymph, (3) lymphatic lymph.

Doing this, we immediately find ourselves in an *impasse* so far as regards the establishment of hypotheses on the basis of exact data; the ultimate lymphatic vessels and the lymph spaces are of microscopic dimensions; in other words, no sure method has as yet been devised whereby to collect intercellular lymph; we cannot introduce the finest cannula into the tissues without breaking into lymphatic vessels; and so cannot compare lymphatic lymph and unmixed intercellular lymph formed at the same time. This has been abundantly determined, that the fluid obtained from a larger lymph vessel, from the thoracic duct, or one of the vessels of the extremity of the neck, differs materially in the relative amounts of its component constituents from the blood plasma. There is variation, even if slight, in the percentage amount of the most soluble inorganic salts. We have not, therefore, to deal with the simple leakage of fluid from one set of vessels into the other. But what is the nature of the process or processes of lymph formation is still a matter of keen debate. On the one hand, we have the upholders of the purely mechanical theory, first clearly formulated by Ludwig; those who hold that the laws of filtration, diffusion, and osmosis are adequate to explain the variation in the amount and composition of the lymph discharged from a part under varying conditions; on the other, those who, with Heidenhain, urge that while the known physical laws in part determine the production and constitution of lymph, there are alterations in amount and constitution which cannot be brought into harmony with the working of those laws. These workers demand a certain selective capacity and activity on the part of the capillary endothelium, determining to some extent the amount of at least some of the constituents of the blood plasma which is allowed to escape from the capillaries. The most prominent supporters of the mechanical theory at the present time are Starling[1] and Cohnstein; of the opposed view, are Asher, Hamburger, Lazarus, Barlow, Meltzer, and Carlson. These observers, it is true, differ among themselves as to cells mainly involved in the process of lymph formation, but are members of the "vitalistic" school to this extent, that they are unable to explain lymph formation by simple physical principles, and are compelled to fall back upon more elaborate processes occurring within the cell as introducing modification in the fluid during its passage from the interior of the blood capillaries to the interior of the lymphatics.

Here a word is necessary regarding the meaning of "vitalism." There are those who, with Haldane and B. Moore, see evidence of the existence of "biotic energy," of energy associated with and determining the activities of living matter, distinct from other forms of energy. This view necessitates the fatalistic attitude that vital phenomena are, beyond a certain point, incapable of explanation by the ordinary laws governing matter in general. With this view we have absolutely no sympathy. All that Heidenhain meant, and laid down with precision in his opposition to Ludwig, was that processes are undergone in the living cell which, while governed by the ordinary laws of physics and chemistry, are nevertheless so complicated that hitherto we have been unable to follow the successive forces acting upon the assimilated molecule in its passage through the cell; that the simpler processes of diffusion, osmosis, and filtration are at work, but are not everything. According to this view, it is quite possible that further research will throw light upon the nature of the intracellular forces. To this extent, and this extent only, with Heidenhain and Meltzer, we class ourselves with the vitalists.

---

[1] The clearest statement of the mechanical theory is afforded by Starling (Arris and Gale Lectures, Lancet, London: May 9, 16, and 23, 1906); a thorough and impartial criticism of all the theories up to date is given by Meltzer in the Harrington Lectures on Œdema, American Medicine, 8: 1904: Nos. 1, 2, 4, and 5. This latter is the fullest recent study on the subject, and is provided with a rich bibliography.

For ourselves we cannot accept the simpler mechanical theory, and this for the following broad, but we think obvious, reasons, namely, that this view presupposes that lymph is merely the outcome of the discharge through a single endothelial membrane, the blood capillary, into the lymph channels, takes no adequate account of the influence of the tissue cells in its composition, and, lastly, fails to explain how the interstitial lymph makes its way into the lymph vessels. The problem of lymph formation in reality consists of three parts: (1) What is the mechanism by which certain constituents of the blood plasma pass through the capillary wall? (2) How and to what extent is the interstitial lymph thus produced acted upon by the tissue cells which it bathes? (3) By what mechanism does the interstitial lymph gain entrance into the lymphatic vessels? If for the moment we admit, with Starling, that the first of these steps is purely a mechanical process determined by the interaction of two factors, the intracapillary blood pressure and the permeability of the capillary wall, we still have the other two problems to answer. Now, as regards the one of these, we are altogether too apt to repeat, parrot-like, that the tissues are nourished by the blood. As a matter of fact, save for the vascular endothelial cells, and one or two rare exceptions, like the Kupfer cells in the liver, in which tissue cells impinge directly upon the blood stream, the tissue cells are not nourished directly by the blood, but by the interstitial lymph; the nutritive fluid has to pass out of the capillaries into the lymph spaces surrounding the individual tissue cells before those cells can abstract from it the particular foodstuffs needed by them. This demands that the different orders of cells abstract from the interstitial lymph different orders of substances, as also that they excrete or discharge into it very varying products of metabolism; in short, demands conditions of give and take of so complex a nature that even if broadly, under certain conditions of experiment, thoracic duct lymph has the character of a filtrate through a semipermeable membrane, it cannot, in its finer analysis, conform to a fluid of that nature, and under normal conditions of moderate flow, must inevitably depart widely from this type of fluid.

And as regards the last of these problems, there are again, it seems to us, insuperable difficulties in regarding the eventual lymph of the lymph vessels as a filtrate or product of diffusion. The ultimate lymph vessels are so delicate that we fail to recognize their existence in ordinary sections, even under high powers. We utterly fail to conceive how the result of increased accumulation of lymph in the tissue spaces can result in an increased filtration of that lymph into these delicate vessels. On the contrary, the greater the interstitial pressure, the greater the tendency for these delicate channels to become collapsed and obliterated. And, as a matter of fact, the extreme tension of the tissues in cases of advanced anasarca of the lower limbs, for example—a tension so great that the lymph is apt to ooze through the deeper layers of the cutis and form "blebs"—indicates that this actually happens. But in other cases, as, for example, in inflammatory œdema, we obtain a marked increase in the discharge of lymph through the lymph vessels coming from the inflamed area. The simplest and most rational conclusion to reach is, that ordinarily the lymphatic endothelium actively absorbs and secretes the interstitial lymph into the vessels, and that under certain conditions this secretion is increased. Only in this way can we imagine an active flow becoming set up within them. And if we are forced to predicate such powers for the lymphatic endothelium, then, by analogy we must suppose that the capillary endothelium has powers of a like order, and, with Heidenhain, must endow this with a certain grade of selective secretory activity. Indeed, the conception of the tissue cells as nourished not directly by the blood, but by the lymph, would seem to demand that the capillary endothelium of the various tissues abstracts particular substances from the circulating blood necessary for the specific metabolism of these tissues, and passes these into the interstitial lymph. We cannot, for example, comprehend the extraordinary passage of fats into the milk, unless the capillaries of the mammary gland in the first place possess a selective power.

Under the term œdema we include all abnormal accumulations of fluid approximating in its constitution to that of lymph, and occurring in the tissue spaces and serous cavities of the body. To these accumulations in different regions special names have been given, and with this newer knowledge we can divide them into distinct classes:

1. **Anasarca,** or interstitial œdema, as of the limbs and body wall. **Chemosis** is the name given to serous infiltration of the subconjunctival tissue. **Œdema glottidis,** to anasarca of the upper portion of the larynx.

2. Accumulations in serous cavities, including **ascites,** involving the peritoneal cavity; **hydrothorax** (the pleural); **hydrocele** (the tunica vaginalis); **hydrocephalus,** internal and external, involving the ventricles of the brain and the pia-arachnoid spaces.

3. Accumulations of albuminous fluids which, strictly speaking, are outside the body, *i. e.*, affect surfaces in direct communication with the exterior. The important example of this form is pulmonary œdema.

A little consideration shows that in these three classes we have three different orders of accumulations:

ANASARCA.

The essential feature of the anasarcous state is the excessive accumulation of intercellular lymph. In other words, the discharge of this lymph into the lymphatic vessels has not kept pace with the formation of lymph by passage of fluid through the capillary walls. Examination of dropsical tissues under the microscope shows the individual cells composing the tissue widely separated, in consequence of the intercellular accumulation. What is characteristic is that the lymphatic vessels are not obvious. On the contrary, the absence of distended lymph vessels suggests that the interstitial pressure due to fluid accumulation has brought about a relative, or, it may be, a complete occlusion of the delicate lymphatic channels, and that one of the factors in the continuous and progressive intensity of anasarca is this local obliteration of these vessels. A comparison between sections from simple anasarca and those from elephantiasis or macroglossia, due to acquired or inherited obstruction of the lymph vessels of a part, shows that we have to deal with two distinct conditions, namely, of (1) interstitial tissue accumulation of lymph, and (2) lymphangiectasis, or distension of the lymph vessels. Even prior to a knowledge of the barrier separating the lymph spaces from the lymph vessels, it had become recognized that this latter condition was a separate entity, although it had been in general neglected in the discussion of œdema. In the existence of these two pathological states we possess the confirmation of the conclusion reached by MacCallum and the anatomists.

ASCITES AND ALLIED CONDITIONS.

The serous cavities are lined throughout by an endothelium. It follows thus that serous fluid accumulations within them have passed through not one but two endothelial layers in the process of production. To this extent they correspond with lymph-vascular lymph. Here again we note that there may be pronounced (interstitial) œdema of the intestines, with little or no ascites, and *vice versa*. As to how the ascitic and pleural fluid gain entrance into the efferent lymph vessels proper is still a matter of debate. The more recent teaching is, that under normal conditions the peritoneal cavity is closed off from the underlying efferent lymphatic channels, and that an endothelial layer covers over the apparent ostia. We find it difficult to harmonize this teaching with the abundant injection of the diaphragmatic lymph channels with red blood corpuscles which rapidly follows the introduction of blood into the peritoneal cavity. Such abundant passage can only, we hold, be due to the existence of actual stomata, or channels of direct communication, and we have explained the curious minute hemispherical pits occasionally observable in plastic exudates covering the dome of the liver as caused by eddies opposite to those stomata in the diaphragm. While saying this, we cannot pass over the evidence adduced by MacCallum and others that sections through the diaphragm demonstrate the presence of a distinct membrane separating the diaphragmatic lymphatics from the peritoneal cavity. The only satisfactory compromise would seem to consist either in concluding that under certain conditions, by retraction or contraction of the endothelial cells constituting or affording the membrane, what had been an intact membrane becomes provided with a central stoma or passage of direct communication, or that there exists normally a combination of intact membranes and occasional scattered stomata. We confess that the latter view does not appeal to us; the existence of lining membranes would seem to predicate a certain selective function and control of the composition of the efferent lymph; that of course pores or stomata would be diametrically opposed to any such selective action. On the other hand, the existence of potential stomata, which act as weirs, closed under normal conditions, but permitting the free passage of fluid and free particles when the intraperitoneal pressure becomes excessive, would seem not irrational. We bring these matters forward at this point in order to indicate that, according to the one view, accumulations in serous cavities are distinct from lymph-vascular lymph; according to the other, the normal existence of a dividing membrane would indicate that under more natural conditions there may be essential differences in the composition of the two fluids, although, under abnormal conditions, the contents of the serous cavities may pass unchanged into the efferent lymphatics. We regret that in the present state of our knowledge it is impossible to afford dogmatic teaching on this point. The fact that in a hydrocele, or in a case of ascites, the fluid may accumulate until there is very high pressure is not to be brought forward on one side or the other; there might be abundant stomata, and nevertheless the pressure be such as to obliterate the underlying network of delicate lymph channels, and thereby arrest the outflow. There is, however, one striking feature in connection with simple transudates (as distinct from inflammatory exudates) into the serous cavities, namely, that they contain much less solids than either serum or ordinary lymph, the reduction being especially marked in albuminous matter. This in itself may justify us in considering them as constituting a class apart.

PULMONARY ŒDEMA.

There can, however, be no doubt as to the necessity of regarding pulmonary œdema as belonging to a distinct class. That fluid is always pouring from the pulmonary capillaries into the alveoli is clearly shown by the abundant moisture contained in the expired air; the accumulation of serous fluid in the alveoli is, therefore, only to be regarded as an exaggeration of a normal process. What is distinctive is that here the accumulation of fluid is not interstitial, but is, strictly speaking, external to the body; the discharge is onto surfaces communicating with the exterior. It is not, therefore, determined by any force acting on the capillaries from without; neither diffusion nor osmosis can be called into play to determine the discharge. What is more, the delicate alveolar epithelium is so directly applied over the capillary network that we appear to have a relationship similar to that seen in the glomeruli of the kidneys, with a practical absence of intervening lymph space between vessel and epithelium. Here, then, again, we have a different order of conditions.

Briefly, while it is impossible not to be impressed by Professor Starling's valiant support of Ludwig's mechanical hypothesis, a study more particularly, of actual clinical cases of œdema cannot but convince us that this hypothesis does not satisfy. Pressure plus variation in permeability alone will not explain the great varieties of cases in which we encounter the œdematous state, nor the variations in the constitution of the œdema fluid. It will not, for example, explain Leber's experiment,[1] in which he showed that the cornea with intact epithelium of the membrane of Descemet will stand a pressure of 200 mm. of mercury, whereas, once that epithelium is removed, solutions readily filter through; or the observations of Tigerstedt and Santesson that the freshly removed lung of a frog filled with 0.6 per cent. NaCl solution will stand a pressure of 14 mm. of mercury for several hours without any escape of the contained fluid, whereas the same lung killed by slight heat, or by pouring in distilled water or (frog's) bile, at once allows filtration.

Something is necessary to explain the sudden change in the porosity of these membranes over and above the ordinary physical laws determining the rate of filtration through dead membranes.

We are apt to regard the endothelial cells of the vessels and capillaries as of an extraordinarily low type, as flattened plates of cytoplasm and little more; on the other hand, we admit freely that bacteria, organisms much more minute, and of a much lower type of structure, possess selective assimilative powers. The position is irrational. These endothelial cells are nucleated; they are actively phagocytic; can proliferate actively; and, as observed in inflammatory states, are acutely sensitive to changes in their environment. While admitting that, other things being equal, they permit a more active passage of plasma under a higher pressure, and conform in many respects to the laws governing filtration, diffusion, and osmosis, it must, we think, be concluded that certain substances are taken up by them selectively, while at times other substances of equal solubility are not taken up. We feel some compunction in dealing thus so largely in generalities. The subject is most complicated, and to analyze conscientiously the data at our disposal would consume more space than we can afford. At most, keeping these views in mind, we believe that the different forms of œdema, and the variations seen in these, become more comprehensible. These forms are:

1. **Congestive Œdema.**—This is the commonest clinical type, and is met with in cases of obstruction to the venous onflow, either local or general. The most extensive cases are seen in obstructive heart disease. In such cases there is (a) increased venous pressure, (b) increase in the total amount of blood within the vessels, (c) dilatation of the capillaries and increased capillary pressure, (d) slowing of the blood stream, (e) increased venosity of the capillary blood. The increased capillary pressure is here not the sole factor. Thus, œdema does not ensue if the main vein of a limb be ligatured in a healthy animal. Again, the variation in albuminous contents is too great to be ascribed to mere difference in the permeability of the capillary wall. As shown by Reuss, pleural transudations on the average contain four times as much albumin as do those from the subcutaneous tissues, and twice as much as does ascitic fluid. We are forced to the conclusion that the cells in these different regions have a varying sensibility, and are affected differently

[1] *Leber*, Archiv f. Ophthalm., 19: 1873: 125. Tigerstedt and Santesson, Bijhang till K. Svensk. vet. Akad. Stockholm, 11; 1886; No 2.

by the increased venosity of the blood. It may further be noted that
there are pronounced individual differences in the reaction to one and
the same lesion.   Thus, long-continued mitral stenosis commonly
results in pulmonary œdema; we have, nevertheless, encountered two
cases of this disease in which, with extreme anasarca and ascites, there
has been inconsiderable hydrothorax, and the lungs have been devoid
of serous effusion.   Cases of advanced anasarca with little or no ascites,
and of the converse condition, are far from infrequent.

2. **Lymphatic Obstruction.**—The accumulation of fluid in the spaces
of the body is dependent on the interaction of two factors—the rate
of discharge of fluid from the bloodvessels and the rate of removal.
If the latter be less than the former, then an œdematous condition must
develop. We should then expect a *priori* to find that lymphatic obstruction is a potent cause of œdema.   But this is not the case.   The main
lymphatics of a part may be ligatured or compressed, and yet, as a rule,
no œdema occurs.   Even when the thoracic duct is ligatured, ascites
may develop, though slowly, yet, as Cohnheim showed, œdema does
not result.   Two factors are responsible, namely, the existence, in many
cases, of abundant collateral channels, and the reabsorption of the
tissue lymph into the bloodvessels.   And the latter would seem the more
important—so important, in fact, that we seem justified in regarding
the lymph channels not as the prime, but as an accessory factor in tissue
drainage, with the additional function of removing selectively certain
products of metabolism.   Even during the process of bleeding an animal
to death, the last portions of blood are much more watery than the first,
a fact which can only be explained by the passage of tissue fluid into the
circulation through the capillary walls.   And as shown by Roy and Lloyd
Jones, after less extreme hemorrhage, the specific gravity of the tissues
becomes rapidly raised, that of the blood diminished.   The exchange
of fluid between the surrounding tissues and the blood may, nay, must,
be most considerable.   This, first demonstrated by Magendie, has been
convincingly shown by Starling and Tubby.[1]   Methylene blue or indigo
carmine injected into the pleural cavity appeared in the urine within
five minutes, whereas the lymph presented no trace of coloration for
another twenty minutes, or it might be two hours.   Lymphatic obstruction alone is thus little likely to cause œdema.   It is true that occasionally
we meet with this condition following obstruction; thus, secondary cancer
of the axillary glands, with the not infrequent extension of the malignant
growth along the lymph channels, or extensive removal of the axillary
lymphatic chain, may be followed by œdema of the arm.   But this is
not a necessary outcome, and where it occurs we must conclude that
hydremia, or a toxic condition of the blood, with altered state of the
capillary endothelium, is superadded.

As already noted, where there is lymphatic obstruction there the
vessels behind the obstruction are apt to become dilated; and from these
dilated vessels it is evident that fluid may escape into the tissues and

[1] Jour. of Physiol., 16: 1894: 140.

spaces of the body. This is often to be determined where there has been cancerous or tuberculous growth involving the region of the receptaculum chyli. Radiating from the affected area are distended lymph vessels, or white streaks, filled with semisolid inspissated lymph, consisting of fat droplets and cell debris. This, it may be noted, only in the upper abdominal area; to our knowledge, this inspissation is never encountered in cases of lymphangiectasis of the limbs or face—a further evidence of the selective activity of the lymph-vascular endothelium.

Chylous Ascites.—Did the lymph vessels communicate freely with the tissue spaces, we should expect ascitic fluid to approximate in composition to the chyle in the abdominal lymphatics; but this is notoriously not the case under ordinary circumstances. Under abnormal conditions we obtain this approximation. A condition of true chylous ascites is found in cases of rupture of the receptaculum chyli, the fluid affording, upon analysis, a relatively high percentage of proteins and fat, the latter, though small in amount, giving it a milky appearance. Rupture of the thoracic duct may similarly lead to **chylous hydrothorax** (of the renal or bladder lymphatics in filariasis and other states, to **chyluria**). The thoracic and pleural accumulations may occur not only through trauma, but through inflammatory erosion, or sometimes as the result of obstruction and dilatation.

Chyliform Ascites.—The above condition is with some difficulty to be distinguished from one seen occasionally in low forms of serous peritonitis, most frequently due to abdominal carcinoma or tuberculosis, in which the fluid becomes milky from fat liberated by the breaking down of leukocytes and endothelial cells which have undergone fatty degeneration. The percentage of fat is in general high (as high as 6 per cent. in some cases, compared with 0.5 per cent. and less in true chylous ascites). Sugar and diastatic enzymes, frequently to be detected in the former condition, are absent in this.

Pseudochylous Ascites.—More frequent than either of these states is that termed pseudochylous ascites, in which the milky fluid simulating chyle is found to be free from fats. There has been much obscurity as to the cause of the turbidity; in some cases it is apparently due to the presence of mucoid substances;[1] in others, it would seem, to partly dissolved proteins.[2] Joachim ascribes it to a combination of lecithin and pseudoglobulin.[3]

3. **Inflammatory Œdema.**—In this group of œdemas either we can recognize under the microscope changes in the endothelial lining of the capillaries, to which we ascribe largely the increased transudate (exudate), or by analogy we hold that changes of like order must obtain. The type example is to be seen in acute inflammation. In this, in addition to arterial and capillary dilatation, the capillary endothelium is swollen and more prominent, and there are other indications of alteration in the

---

[1] Gourand and Corset, Compt. Rend. Soc. Biol., 60:1906:23.
[2] Poljakoff, Fortschr. d. Med., 21:1903:1081.
[3] Joachim, Biochem. Centralbl., 1:1903:437.

state of these cells, such as adhesion of the leukocytes (suggesting, as Wells has pointed out, an altered surface tension), and nuclear enlargement and proliferation. Associated with these various changes we find increased pouring of fluid from the tissues along the lymphatics, higher protein content of the discharged lymph, and increased cell contents, both leukocytes and, it may be, red corpuscles. Such modified transudate is termed an exudate. In constitution it approaches more nearly to the blood plasma than does congestive œdema fluid. It has, however, to be admitted that in different inflammations we find every transition from fluid of the one type to the other, and that in practice it is at times practically impossible to state with precision whether we deal with a hydrothorax, for example, or a mild form of serous pleurisy.

There can be little doubt regarding physical changes in the capillaries being responsible, to a very large extent, for the increased transudate: the increased intracapillary pressure, the dilatation and thinning of the capillary walls, the dilatation of the stigmata of the vessels, or formation of stomata or passages where the leukocytes and red corpuscles pass out. Such gross openings in the capillary wall, when present, must necessarily cause the exudate to approximate in composition to the blood plasma. At the same time, the indications of reactive change in the endothelial cells at least suggest the co-existence of some amount of selective activity on the part of the endothelial membrane, while, at the same time, the enlargement, nuclear and cytoplasmic changes in the tissue cells of the inflamed area suggest an altered interchange between them and the tissue lymph, and that the resultant lymph-vascular lymph is much more than the result of mere filtration, diffusion, and osmosis.

4. **Toxic Œdema.**—Intimately allied to this last is the group of toxic œdemas. As Heidenhain demonstrated, there is a class of substances which act as lymphagogues, *i. e.*, circulating in the blood, set up increased lymph formation in sundry areas. Some of these set up alterations in blood pressure, which may be an important factor but others (curare, extract of mussels, crab, etc.) induce lymph flow in the absence of noticeable change in the circulation. The logical conclusion is that they act directly on the vascular endothelium of certain areas, modifying its properties. It is the custom to describe these bodies as having a toxic action; the difficulty is where to draw the line between stimulation and irritation. Thus, it may be laid down as a rule that increased glandular activity is accompanied by marked increase in lymph flow. This is notably the case in the liver. It is scarcely to be imagined that when in the course of its normal function the liver removes deleterious agents from the portal blood, we are dealing with a diseased, toxic state of the capillary endothelium. Rather we must conclude that that possesses a selective capacty; that certain substances contained in the portal blood stimulate it, and that only when these are in excess is there an overstimulation and toxic state of the cells induced. While saying this, we have also to recognize that lowered vitality of the endothelium is accompanied by increased passage out of fluid. We need only recall the difference in transudation between living and dead membranes.

A well-marked example of this order of toxic œdema is seen in the so-called ischemic œdema supervening after prolonged lowering of the blood supply of a part after ligature, compression (as by Esmarch's bandage), or frostbite. In these cases, clearly, the inadequate blood supply has deleteriously affected the endothelium, and now, upon the circulation being resumed, the escape of fluid into the tissues is extreme. But, admittedly, it is difficult to determine in every case which of these two conditions we have to deal with. Thus, we are still undetermined where to place one of the most common examples of widespread œdema and anasarca, namely, the œdema of acute parenchymatous nephritis. This differs from the œdema of heart disease in its relatively rapid onset and in its primary distribution. Thus, a favorite seat for its early appearance is in the loose tissue of the orbit, resulting in a puffiness around the eyes. Congestion and alteration in blood pressure cannot explain its development, and the experiments of Cohnheim and others prove definitely that mere hydremia will not reproduce the condition. We can only conclude that in consequence of the renal incompetence certain toxic substances circulating in the blood have a more or less specific action upon the vascular endothelium of certain areas. But what is the nature of this action we do not know—whether depressant, lowering the vitality, or, on the contrary, stimulant, leading to the active absorption and removal of fluid plus toxic substances from the blood stream. The matter has to be left *sub judice*.

5. **Neuropathic Œdema.**—Here, in connection with œdema, as with inflammation and so many other processes, we find that nervous influences alone can set up disturbances of the same type as those due to local irritation. We may encounter (1), as we have already pointed out (vol. i, p. 449), a collateral or sympathetic œdema in the areas innervated from the same region of the brain or cord as that controlling a focus of acute inflammation; or (2), in association with definite nerve lesions, may find œdema of particular fields of nerve supply, as in herpes zoster. But in addition to these, and unassociated with any apparent inflammatory disturbance, we meet with a remarkable series of **angioneurotic œdemas** exhibiting sudden and acute pouring out of fluid into particular areas, for which we can ascribe no cause other than nervous influence upon the vessels of the part. It is true that the line distinguishing these from the *urticarias* of cases of idiosyncrasy is not always easy to draw. In the latter the exhibition of certain foods, even in minute amounts, leads to local vascular disturbances with infiltration and subcutaneous or submucous swelling. Underlying this there would seem to be a neurotic influence, though the suggestion has of late received credence that, as in serum sickness, some substance present in the circulating blood in minute quantities has a specific lymphagogue action upon the endothelium of the vessels of particular regions. But as in hay fever, and in those severely affected by the mere presence of a cat in their neighborhood, acute local œdematous conditions may be induced by influences acting through the respiratory system which it is difficult to attribute to any but pure reflex nervous

influence, with vascular instability of particular regions. An important group of spasmodic asthmas would seem to come into this category, at least in part due, not merely to constriction of the bronchial musculature, but also to sudden congestion and œdema of the bronchial mucous membrane. It would thus seem necessary to distinguish a class of pure angioneurotic œdemas from that of the idiosyncratic œdemas of what, failing a better term, we must still refer to as toxic in origin.

FIG. 13

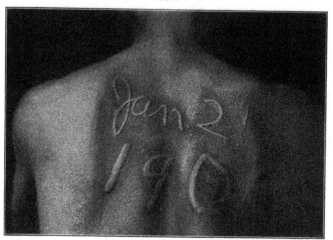

Urticaria factitia (angioneurosis). (Hyde and Ormsby.)

6. **Hydrops ex Vacuo.**—Lastly, reference must be made to the condition in which, with atrophy of tissues, there is replacement by lymphatic fluid. Practically the only region in which this is recognizable is in the brain case and vertebral canal following upon shrinkage of the brain and cord. Here clearly the lack of pressure must be the main reason why the extravasated cerebrospinal fluid fails to be discharged into the lymph vessels, and as a consequence accumulates. Allied to this is what we may term the *replacement hydrops*, seen in the development of necrotic and hemorrhagic cysts (vol. i, p. 864).

From the above recital it is obvious that (1) the time has not yet arrived to lay down any broadly simple laws regarding the nature of œdema, and that (2) we must recognize a varying interaction of several factors—blood pressure and filtration, diffusion, osmosis, the selective activity of the vascular endothelium, the tissue cells, and, it may well be, the endothelium of the lymph vessels. Much has still to be done before we can speak with precision of the relative value of these different agencies.

CHAPTER VI.

CARDIAC FUNCTION AND ITS DISTURBANCES.

Embryological Considerations.—The more important congenital abnormalities of the heart and bloodvessels will be discussed more fully later (see pp. 118 and 142). At most, we can here refer to only a few general points.

It will not be unscientific, in view of the close relationship existing between the heart and vessels, on the one hand, and the blood, on the other, to conceive of these elements as forming integral portions of one functional entity—the blood-vascular system, the more so that the vessels and the contained fluid are derivatives alike of the mesoblastic layer. Structural defects in the heart and vessels cannot, therefore, fail to affect the blood and through it the nutrition of the body as a whole. Conversely, abnormalities in the quantity and quality of the blood immediately and ultimately profoundly modify the structure and function of the containing structures. As an illustration in point, we may cite the opinion of certain eminent authorities that chlorosis is due to a congenital stunting of the cardiovascular system. Besides this, however, we think we must lay some stress on an inadequate blood formation. As a more remote result of the imperfect nutrition thereby induced we sometimes get hypoplasia of other parts, the hair and the genitalia, for example, or even the body as a whole. A moderate grade of dwarfing has been observed by Gilbert and Rathery[1] in some cases of congenital mitral stenosis. The partial or complete congenital occlusion of the vessels springing from the heart and the defects of the septum, all of which are not particularly uncommon, have a general effect on function comparable to inefficiency of the cardiac valves, that is to say, hypertrophy and dilatation of the chambers with other more remote results, and can profitably be included under our discussion of the latter conditions later.

Anatomy.—We must take for granted a knowledge of the gross anatomy of the heart, here merely recalling (1) that the weak muscular tissue of the auricles is independent of the strong musculature of the ventricles save for a small connecting bundle first noted by Stanley Kent, and later by the younger His. As we shall see, this bundle plays an important part in the regulation of the heart beat; (2) that the musculature of the ventricles is not entirely independent, there being an extensive crossing of, more particularly, the outer bundles from the one ventricle to the other, whereby it comes to pass that the work of the two ventricles must

---

[1] Presse Médicale, May 7: 1900.

be largely synchronous, and (3) that we have evidence of the existence of both motor and sensory nerves in association with this organ. Fibers pass to the root of the heart from both vagi, others again from the upper dorsal sympathetic ganglia; and by physiological methods we have determined the existence and some of the functions of nerve bundles of different orders.

As bearing upon disturbed function, certain considerations regarding the physiology of the heart demand somewhat fuller treatment. As a mechanism for the propulsion of the blood, we observe in that mechanism (1) chambers for the collection of the blood; (2) the motor apparatus proper for the propulsion of the blood; (3) valves to determine that the blood is discharged in a particular direction, so that the heart being interpolated in a system of closed vessels, a circulation, and not merely a flow and ebb of the blood, is assured.

1. THE CARDIAC CHAMBERS.

Applied Physiology.—The heart is a double pump, each moiety consisting of two chambers, or more accurately, of an auricular antechamber leading into the ventricular chamber, or pump proper. Undoubtedly, the **auricles**, through the muscle in their walls, do act as pumps propelling the blood; nay, more, we possess ample evidence that the normal cardiac contraction originates at the venous ostia, where the venæ cavæ open into the right ventricle, and that the auricular muscle is essential for the due conveyance of the wave of contraction from this region to the ventricles. Further, there is evidence that in certain states the auricular pulse wave is demonstrable in the arterial pulse, or, otherwise, the effect of the contraction of the auricular muscle is then sufficiently powerful to be conveyed through the ventricular blood into the column of aortic blood. But admitting this, it has also to be admitted that the muscular contraction of the auricular walls is not the dominant force leading to the filling of the ventricles. It is but necessary to observe the auricles of the exposed mammalian heart to note that their contraction is incomplete; that it does not empty the auricles at each beat. What is more, we have accumulated increasing evidence (see p. 124) that the ventricular expansion is active, and that a large proportion of the blood filling the ventricles enters it before the auricular systole occurs; in other words, that systole is not absolutely essential for the onward passage of the blood; at most, when through the progressive filling and expansion of the ventricle the active diastole is becoming weak, the auricular contraction acts as a final but auxiliary force whereby the intraventricular blood pressure is raised, and thereby (we would hold) the automatic or idiomuscular contraction of the ventricular muscle is stimulated, or perhaps, more accurately, the muscle fibers are placed in that tense state which favors contraction following upon a minimal stimulus. There are, indeed, cases in which obviously the auricles are incapable of exciting any propulsive action, and, nevertheless, the circulation continues.

Thus we have seen the left auricle completely filled and distended with blood clot save for two passages leading from the right and left pulmonary veins respectively to the ventral orifice. In this case, judging from the appearance of the thrombus, the auricle must have been out of action for days rather than hours; nevertheless, the circulation was not noticeably impeded. And, as Hoover points out, there are not a few cases recorded by veterinarians in which the auricles in the horse have been found completely rigid from universal calcification. Thus we are

FIG. 14

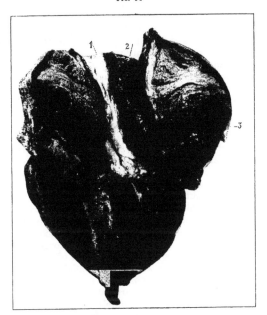

Thrombus completely filling the left auricle except for two passages; 1 and 3 represent the channels from the right and left pulmonary veins.

inclined to regard the auricles as essentially antechambers for the gradual collection of blood from the veins prior to the active diastole of the ventricles. Did these antechambers not exist; did the thin-walled and collapsible veins open directly into the actively expanding ventricles, then the suction force exerted by the ventricles would tend to approximate the venous walls, and arrest the circulation into the ventricles. These collecting chambers prevent any such catastrophe.

Use of the Ventricles.—These are essentially the pumping apparatus of the circulating system, and as such their functions are best considered under the next heading. Here we would only note that their walls are far from rigid, but elastic, and that, just as if we attach a weight to a resting band of muscle, such as the gastrocnemius of a frog, we find that the band undergoes progressive elongation, so, similarly, if through positive pressure increasing volumes of fluid seek to gain unimpeded entrance into the ventricles, or, to express it otherwise, if a column of blood of increasing length becomes connected with the ventricular cavity, this has the same result—the resting muscle expands and the chamber undergoes distension. We shall have more to say regarding this when we come to consider the subjects of hypertrophy and dilatation.

Abnormalities.—The most serious disturbances of the heart, considered as a series of chambers, occur in connection with certain congenital vices of development. Although the heart develops into the two distinct pumping systems, right and left, already noted, it must be recalled that at an early stage it exists in the embryo as a two-chambered organ with a single auricle and a single ventricle. By a very complicated series of outgrowths there develop septa dividing each of those primary chambers into two; so that the normal state after birth is that the right heart is completely closed off from the left. Up to the time of birth the separation between the two auricles is wanting to this extent, that there exists a passage or foramen (the foramen ovale) whereby the blood from the inferior vena cava (more particularly) crosses the right auricle and enters the left. In quite a large proportion of cases this undergoes incomplete postnatal closure; in a few cases it remains widely open; or there may be yet more incomplete formation of the interauricular septum. In all these cases there is the possibility of mingling of the venous blood entering the right heart, with the oxygenated blood entering the left. The same is liable to happen when the interventricular septum is imperfect. Yet graver disturbances ensue when, through abnormalities in the division of the originally single vessel of discharge, we gain a long series of anomalies, from mere narrowing—congenital stenosis—of either pulmonary artery or aorta to conditions of complete "Rechtslage," in which the systemic arteries are supplied with blood from the right heart, the pulmonary arteries with blood from the left. These abnormalities in the growth of the arterial septum downward are very frequently associated with incomplete development of the interventricular septum upward, so that there is combined free communication between the two ventricles, with consequent admixture of venous and arterial blood.

2. THE MOTOR APPARATUS.

Here we deal essentially with the ventricles, and of these, the left ventricle more particularly concerns us.

Arrangement of the Muscle Fibers.—In the first place, it must be noted that the ventricle does not contract as a sphere and thus become narrowed in every direction. The successive layers of muscle fibers are so arranged that, with contraction, the length of the left ventricle is practically unaltered. The form of this ventricle and mode of contraction are such that in systole singularly little internal pressure is exerted upon the apex. It is a fact which we think is not generally known that the total thickness of the ventricular wall at the apex of the heart is little more than one-eighth of an inch. The arrangement of the fibers and the mode of their contraction is such that the walls of the apical half are brought together and the blood propelled upward, *i. e.*, toward the aorta. Another fact not generally recognized is that the left ventricle never becomes completely emptied; there is always left some of what Roy and Adami have termed residual blood. As may be determined by inserting the little finger through a small slit in the apex of a large animal that has been curarized, the lower half of the ventricle contracts tightly round it in systole, but above the level of the apices of the papillary muscles there is a persistent chamber.

Two accessory muscle systems are to be noted, the papillary (Albrecht), whose function is to keep taut the mitral valve and prevent this from becoming everted into the auricle; the fibers from this pass downward, then laterally and forward and to the surface of the septum; and the ring musculature (Krehl), controlling the upper orifice of the ventricle.

The contraction of the right ventricle is not so complete; the shape on transverse section is that of a crescent applied to the more circular left ventricle. The result of contraction is that the outer wall becomes approximated to the inner, a process aided by the bands of muscle which pass across the cavity.

Nature of the Cardiac Contraction: Systole.—Our conception of muscular contraction is naturally based upon what we know regarding the contraction of the skeletal muscles. In them we know that a nervous stimulus is, under ordinary conditions, the originator of the contraction, and we are apt to neglect Sherrington's observation on the nature of the patellar and other reflexes, that these occur so rapidly after the blow that induces them that they can only be explained as the direct response of the muscle fibers to a sudden strain, and cannot be of nervous origin. Thus it is that the early view of the cardiac contraction was that each systole was the result of a nervous impulse.

The Myogenic Theory.—We owe more particularly to Gaskell (1883)[1] the view which prevails to-day—that the cardiac contraction is automatic, or, more accurately, is myogenic rather than neurogenic, the muscle directly responding to stimuli, the contraction stimulus travelling not by the nerves, but along the muscle cells. Thus, in the embryo, the primitive heart is the earliest organ to present active function, and that long before there is any sign of the development of the peripheral nerves. We see it there as a tube bent upon itself, and undergoing rhythmical contraction, contractions which begin at the one end, and continue as a peristaltic wave to the other. And still, in the fully developed higher

---

[1] German writers are apt to give the credit to Engelmann, whose work was later, as also, it may here be noted, they credit His, Jr., rather than the earlier English observer Kent, with the discovery of the auriculoventricular bundle.

animal, it is seen that the wave of contraction begins at the region corresponding with the sinus venosus, or first portion of the more tubular heart of the embryo and of lower forms of life.   The earlier difficulty in understanding the conveyance of the wave from one chamber to the other in the apparent absence of any muscular band of connection between auricles and ventricles has been solved by the important discoveries of late years with which one associates the names of Stanley Kent,[1] the younger His,[2] Aschoff and Tawara,[3] Erlanger,[4] and Keith and Flack.[5] Such band of connection does exist, and is of a very remarkable character. Thus, in 1893 the first two of these observers demonstrated the existence of a peculiar band of fibers of muscular type, which, beginning apparently in a small node in the wall of the right auricle near the coronary sinus, continues downward into the ventricles.   The course of these fibers has been very thoroughly studied by Tawara, working under Aschoff, who has found that forming a node above the auriculoventricular junction,

FIG. 15

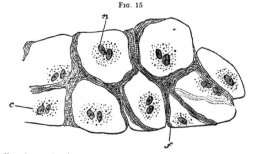

Purkinje's fibers from a sheep's heart: *n*, nuclei; *c*, protoplasm; *f*, striated muscular substance.
(After Ranvier, Leçons d'Anatomie Générale sur le Système Musculaire, Paris, 1880, p. 300.)

the band divides into two main branches, one for each ventricle, and each, becoming superficial, ramifies in the subendothelia tissue, important branches passing to each papillary muscle.   The cells forming these subendothelial fibers had hitherto been known as Purkinje cells, and had been regarded as a layer of vegetative muscle cells (Fig. 15).   Whether there exist two orders of cells in this position, those of the conducting system, and myoblasts, has still to be determined.   The cells of this system, it may be added, are not ordinary muscle cells—they are relatively large and clear, with only occasional sarcous elements; they recall, in fact, cells of a more embryonic type.   More recently Keith and Flack have demonstrated a sino-auricular ring or node of cells of similar order

[1] Journal of Physiology, 14: 1893: 229.
[2] Arbeiten a. d. med. Klinik zu Leipzig, 1883:21.
[3] Das Reizleitung system der Säugethiere, Jena, Fischer, 1906.
[4] Jour. of Exp. Med., 7:1905: 676; see also Erlanger and Blackman, Amer. Jour. of Physiology, 19:1907: 125.
[5] Journ. Anat. and Physiol. (Proc. Anat. Soc. Great Britain), 37: 1903.

situated at the opening of the superior vena cava into the right auricle. The connection of these with the auriculoventricular node has still to be worked out.

The significance of these observations is shown by experiments in which (a) the sinus region is by pressure cut off from the auricle, or (b) the auricles separated from the ventricles. The result in either case is, at first, arrest of the heart wave beyond the point of stricture. After a certain period, in the first experiment, the auricles begin to beat again, but at a rate slower than that of the sinus; and in the second, the ventricles begin contracting, but at a rate slower than that of the auricles, or otherwise the individual parts of the heart are capable of exhibiting automatic contraction, but ordinarily the stimulus to contraction, originating in the sino-auricular node, is conducted to the auricular walls, thence to the auriculo-ventricular node, and thence to the ventricular muscles.

Before considering the significance of these observations, other characteristics of the cardiac contraction have to be briefly referred to. In the first place the heart muscle differs from the skeletal in this, that whereas the latter can be tetanized, the former cannot. That is to say, with ordinary muscle the state of contraction does not prevent a nervous electric stimulus still influencing the fibers, so that if stimuli be repeated with sufficient frequency, the muscle passes into a state of persistent contraction. The heart muscle, on the other hand, exhibits a **refractory stage** (Marey), whereby we mean that when once in the state of contraction it is refractory to, or uninfluenced by, stimuli, and this state persists for a certain period. Associated evidently with this is the further characteristic known as the **law of maximal contraction,** that *the weakest stimulus adequate to produce a contraction evokes as powerful a contraction as the strongest* (Bowditch). This, we would emphasize, is not the same as saying that every contraction of, say, the left ventricle, is of equal force. There are, as we shall point out, conditions under which the refractory period may be prolonged—in which, therefore, the amount of "contractile material" becomes increased, and the subsequent contraction is therefore more powerful. It only signifies that this subsequent contraction will be equally powerful, whether incited by a minimal or a maximal stimulation; that the explosion of the keg of gunpowder will be equally forceful, whether caused by the scarce glowing stump of a match or a 2000 volt electric current; the amount of gunpowder in the keg will, however, modify matters. According, therefore, to the myogenic theory, the "explosion" of the cells of the sino-auricular node —and of the heart muscle fibers in succession—is followed by a period of resuscitation of the contractile matter, and with this accumulation the cells become more and more excitable until some stimulus, not nervous—it may be the strain put upon the cells by the accumulation and presence of the blood in the auricle—induces another explosion. Or, again, it may be that the very excitability of the elements which go to form the contractile material, leads, as they become stored up, to an active rearrangement of these elements. This is still undetermined.

The Neurogenic Theory.—What part, then, is played by the nervous mechanism of the heart, for this, as we have pointed out, definitely exists, both nerves coming from without, and intrinsic ganglion cells in the auricular septum and elsewhere. The vagus fibers, we know, can completely arrest the heart, but with more moderate power of stimulation they slow the heart beat, increase the refractory period, so that the individual contractions are fewer in number, but each individual beat more powerful, although in a given period the main result is that the work done by the heart is lessened. The accelerator fibers, on the other hand, reduce the refractory period, so that the beats succeed each other with greater rapidity. At the same time they appear to stimulate the increased formation of the contractile material, as shown by the fact that the work accomplished by the heart in a given time is increased. For this reason they have also been described as augmentor fibers.[1]

The more recent work of Engelmann[2] indicates that those nerves may control the heart work by various means. Thus, he distinguishes between *inotrope* influences (causing change in the force of the heart beats), *chronotrope* (causing change in the rate), *dromotrope* (causing changes in the rate with which the wave of contraction is conveyed from one segment of the heart to the other), and *bathmotrope* (causing modifications in excitability). We would add that changes other than nervous may also affect the heart in one or other of these directions.

As already indicated, the myogenic theory here put forward is still strongly opposed by not a few physiologists; more particularly Kronecker and his school have brought forward data which are difficult to reconcile completely with the theory of muscular conveyance of the cardiac wave. Thus, Kronecker and Imchanitzky have shown that the bundle of His can be ligatured without disturbing coordination between the auricles and ventricles, and Paukul has demonstrated the existence of nerve plexuses accompanying the bundle,[3] and has found that if these be injured, incoördination is induced. It is not, therefore, according to this school, the muscle bundle itself, but the accompanying nerves that constitute the coördinating mechanism.

There is a remarkable condition of irregular, independent contraction of the heart muscle fibers which may be brought about in various ways in animals of the laboratory. This is known as **fibrillation**. If, for example, the anterior coronary artery of the dog's heart be ligatured, or puncture made into a particular spot in the interventricular septum (Kronecker), the heart passes into this state, and from regular contractions takes on the appearance of a thin bag filled with actively wriggling worms. In general this state is not recovered from, and from arrest of circulation, death ensues. If, now, the heart be treated by a strong fixative agent

[1] Roy and Adami, Phil. Trans. Roy. Soc., Lond., 183 B; 1892:199.

[2] Arch. f. Anat. Physiol (Physiol. Abth.), 1900: 315, and Deutsche Klinik, 4: 1903: 215.

[3] It deserves note that Tawara had described the co-existence of nerve fibers in the bundles.

when in this state of fibrillation, Imchanitzky[1] has shown that the state of striation in adjoining cells may be sharply contrasted; at one side of the dividing line between two cells the striæ may be widely apart, at the other close together; the one cell in a state of expansion, the other of tense contraction. The appearances are certainly not those we would expect to find were there the conduction of the contractile wave from one cell to the next in series. This argument, however, does not strike us as absolutely convincing, for she admits that there may be the same sudden change of striation in the course of a single cell.[2] On the other hand, the earlier observations point strongly in the direction of the fine plexus of nerves interspersed through the heart musculature serving as the main coördinating mechanism.

To reconcile these divergent views, we would again have recourse to the parable of the coach and its horses and the driver (vol. i, p. 489). We cannot but think that under normal conditions the fibers contract under the influence of the "strain" to which they are subjected, although constantly under the controlling influence of the nerve plexus, which are to the cells what the reins and bit are to the horses.

Meltzer[3] points out a possible means of reconciling the myogenic and neurogenic theories. Tawara has described in the atrioventricular bundle the existence of a peculiar mass of net-like structure containing both nerve cells and nerve fibers (Tawara's node), while Keith and Flack have discovered a similar body at the junction of the superior vena cava and auricle (Keith's node). We may suppose that the normal wave of cardiac contractions originates in Keith's node, and that under exceptional circumstances Tawara's node can automatically set up the ventricular contractions independent of the more proximal sino-auricular node, or otherwise the contractions originate usually in the heart itself, but through the agency of these nerve-containing centres.

Parenthetically, in this connection, it must be recalled that the heart possesses also efferent nerves. These are not sensory nerves proper, in the sense that we normally *perceive* the effects of their stimulation. Normally, that is, like other visceral nerves, stimuli do not extend beyond the cord, or at most the medulla, there setting up reflexes. Only in cases of more severe stimulation of certain orders do we in lower degree obtain a vague sense of discomfort that cannot be accurately localized, in the higher degree acute pain, which, again, is not sharply localized, but is recognized more definitely to be in the cardiac region. What is more marked in these cases—in angina pectoris, for example—is the "referred pain;" pain referred to the areas innervated by the first and second dorsal nerves, to the skin over the upper part of the thorax, down the inner side of the left arm as far as the elbow, more rarely down

---

[1] Arch. Internat. de Physiol., 4: 1906: 1. This article gives a *resumé* of the literature on this subject.

[2] The same phenomenon has been observed in human hearts exhibiting fragmentation; it may be the indication that in these cases death has been due to the heart assuming the state of fibrillation.

[3] Medical Record, 75: 1909: 873. An excellent *resumé* of recent studies.

both arms, or to the little finger or fingers.   As pointed out by Sir Lauder Brunton, Harvey knew that the outer wall of the heart is insensitive to touch.   It is either anemia of the ventricular muscle, or distension from within that induces cardiac pain.   The referred pain is an irradiation effect.   Stimulation of the specific ganglion cells in the first dorsal region, if extreme, causes an overflow to neighboring cells, those associated with tactile and other cutaneous sensations of the first dorsal area; and as these have cerebral connections, stimuli proceeding along them to the brain are referred to the regions they innervate.   At most, efferent cardiac stimuli reach normally the medulla.   It may be questioned whether in cases of severe stimulation we here again deal with irradiation effects, or whether there is thence a normal direct path to the cerebrum, which, being little used, does not, when stimuli pass along it, convey to us an accurate sense of the locality of the primary stimulation.   The majority of patients, for example, cannot surely determine whether they experience cardiac or gastric pain.   These considerations apply not only to cardiac pain, but to visceral pain in general.

Diastole.—Although, as we have pointed out, the properties of the cardiac muscle fibers differ in important particulars from those of ordinary striated muscle, it is, nevertheless, natural that our conceptions of their mode of action are based upon our knowledge of that of voluntary muscle. Hence, as it is firmly fixed in our minds that muscular contraction alone is an active process, relaxation being passive, for long the tendency has been to regard diastole as passive, as a mere act of relaxation.   For long there have been observations known opposing this view, such as the evidently forcible rounding of the ventricles in diastole, when the living and beating heart of an animal is held between finger and thumb, an expansion too forcible to be explained by the internal blood pressure or by elastic recoil.   So long ago as 1885 Pawlow demonstrated that in the fresh water mussel there exists a muscle which expands on stimulation, contracting when that stimulation is removed.   It has, however, been difficult if not impossible to demonstrate the active nature of muscular expansion in warm-blooded animals.   And so it follows that the negative pressure which can often be determined in the ventricular cavities of the mammalian heart under experimental conditions has been ascribed to the elasticity of the heart wall, the general negative pressure of the thoracic cavity during inspiration acting as an adjuvant.

Under ordinary conditions of experiment—*e. g.*, in Rolleston's valuable studies upon the intraventricular pressure—it is difficult to demonstrate this negative pressure as constantly existing during the diastolic phase, and that because, coincident with the expansion of the ventricles, the blood pours into the ventricles under definite positive pressure; it is only when this flow becomes slowed that, prior to systole, a brief period of negative pressure shows itself on the curves.   Recently, Stefani,[1] working under Luciani, has placed the existence of active diastole beyond reasonable doubt.   Enclosing the dog's heart in a cardiometer or box,

---

[1] Luciani, Physiologie der Menschen, 1: 1905.

such as that employed by Roy and Adami, he found that the heart was still able to propel the blood into the aorta when the pericardial pressure (*i. e.*, the pressure of the fluid within the box enclosing the heart) was 25 cm. H_2O higher than within the cava, *i. e.*, within the right ventriele. Further, when the pressure acting upon the heart from without was so increased that no blood entered the heart, and none, therefore, passed into the aorta, stimulation of the peripheral end of the cut vagus led to the appearance of an aortic wave. Evidently, therefore, vagus stimulation increased the active expansion of the ventricles, permitting blood to enter their cavities, which blood became expelled in systole. The heart, therefore, is not merely a force pump, but is also a suction pump, and in both ways brings about the circulation of the blood. From a pathological point of view these observations are of importance as throwing light upon its action in cases of circulatory obstruction. The hypertrophy that occurs in these cases, it is suggested, is not only due to increased work in propulsion, but also to increased suction in diastole. We thus gain an explanation, hitherto wanting, for the not infrequent cases in which uncomplicated stenosis of the mitral valve is accompanied by hypertrophy of the left ventricle. If systolic effort alone induced overgrowth, then, less blood reaching it through the narrow valve, that chamber should remain small, but as above noted, that frequently is not the case.

Here must be called to mind the similar indication of active dilatation of the muscles of the arterial wall. The well ascertained existence of vasodilator nerves, which on stimulation cause enlargement of the arterial lumen, in contrast to the vasoconstrictor fibers, can only mean that dilatation of the muscle fibers is an active process. Here, it is true, we deal with non-striated muscle fibers, but in their relationships these are strictly homologous with the cardiac muscle, which we must regard as a highly differentiated development of the muscle layer of one part of the hemal tube. With Sir Lauder Brunton[1] we may assume the existence of two orders of contraction on the part of these muscles, (*a*) longitudinal contraction, leading to a shortening of the long diameter, and (*b*) transverse, leading to a lengthening of the same.

Arrhythmia.—For us the main significance of these recent developments of the myogenic theory is the light they throw upon various orders of cardiac irregularity. It cannot be said that we as yet have fully solved by any means all the problems which these cardiac irregularities present. There are still those inclined to uphold the pure neurogenic or the pure myogenic theory of origin of many of these states. But if what has been laid down in the previous volume be kept steadily in mind, namely, that analogous series of reactive phenomena may present themselves, set up by the direct action of noxæ upon the tissues and by nervous influences respectively, as demonstrated by the existence of neurogenic and "referred" inflammatory disturbances, and of neurogenic hyperpyrexia, then, applying the same consideration to the heart

[1] Therapeutics of the Circulation, London, J. Murray, 1908: 43.

action, we can harmonize what appear to be absolutely contradictory findings. Of these arrhythmias six types are to be recognized:

(1) **Respiratory.**—It is a very old observation that the rate of the pulse is accelerated with inspiration, slowed with expiration. At times, in neurasthenia, those recovering from acute infections, etc., this difference in rate is greatly exaggerated, the pulse during inspiration becoming so rapid and the heart beats so small as to be scarcely recognizable. Mackenzie[1] ascribes this to pressure influences acting upon the sinus, or as we may express it, to excitability of Keith's node.

(2) **"Extrasystolic."**—Experimentally upon the hearts of animals of the laboratory, working regularly, it is possible to interpolate extra contractions or systoles, and where this is done by ventricular stimulation it is found that (1) this interpolated beat is smaller than normal; (2) that it is followed by a longer diastole, and this (3) by a systole more powerful than usual in such a way that the diastole before the extra beat and the comparatively lengthened post-systolic period together equal in length two diastoles, while it may be suggested that the small extra systole and the following delayed systole together in effectiveness correspond to two ordinary beats. In the conditions of pulsus bigeminus, pulsus trigeminus, etc., we have indications in man of the existence of this extra systole, and this is the most common type of cardiac irregularity. What is the meaning or the cause of this extra systole is still an open question. For ourselves, studying a large series of tracings, we cannot but be impressed with their resemblance to interference curves, namely, to the interference between two series of waves of different length and rate.

The character of the pulse tracings in this series of cases is, we would emphasize, that of "interference curves;" it corresponds, that is, with the orders of tracings that can be obtained by the interference of two sets of periodic waves of differing wave lengths, with these distinctions (1) that owing to the law of maximal contraction, where the waves augment each other, *i. e.*, when the upstrokes of the two coincide there is no summation; and (2) that the existence of a refractory period following the wave of the one order prevents the appearance of waves of the other order timed to show themselves during that refractory period. We have in the previous paragraphs suggested that these two orders of waves are the nervous stimuli and the automatic contractions respectively. There are, however, difficulties in accepting this view. If the assumption of the physiologists be correct, that the law of maximal contraction demands that each contraction of the heart muscle necessitates the explosion or using up of all the contractile material accumulated during the previous refractory period, it must follow that where stimuli of two rates of periodic incidence act on the ventricular muscle, the waves of greater frequency alone will be effective, the other order of waves will make no impression upon the curves. The very existence, however, of these irregular curves of heart beat, in which it by no means necessarily

---

[1] Diseases of the Heart, London, 1908: the fullest study upon this and allied phenomena that has yet been published.

follows that the longer the interval between the beats the greater the size of the subsequent wave, shows that our ordinary conception of the significance of the refractory phase is not wholly satisfactory. It is at least worthy of suggestion that the refractory phase corresponds with the stage of active expansion of the heart fibers, already noted (P. 124).

If we assume that active contraction and active expansion are under the control of different nerves (*e. g.*, the accelerators and the vagi, respectively), then were the stimuli to pass down these nerves to the ventricular muscle at different rates, we would, it may be suggested, obtain interference curves of the nature of those observed in this order of cases.

(3) **Due to Disturbance in Conduction.**—Great interest has of late been manifested in cases of what is termed the Stokes-Adams syndrome, or "heart-block." In this there is a striking bradycardia, or slowing of the pulse. By fluoroscopic examination, or by simultaneous register of arterial and venous (jugular) pulses, it is found that the ventricular beat occurs only with every other auricular contraction, or, it may be, with every third or fourth. Along with this there may be Cheyne-Stokes breathing, attacks of syncope or of epilepsy, or even apoplectiform seizures. Since the publication of Tawara's paper autopsies upon quite a series of sufferers from this syndrome have recorded the existence of disease affecting the region of the atrioventricular node, degeneration of the myocardium and necrosis involving the region, fibrosis and gummas, leading to partial or complete destruction of the same: conditions, that is, which evidently have obstructed or completely destroyed the band of communication between auricle and ventricle. They amply explain the lack of coördination between the two sets of chambers.

(4) **Of Central Origin.**—But there are other cases on record in which anemia of the medulla or vagus irritation can alone be invoked. Bradycardia, or abnormal slowing of the heart beat, and tachycardia, or abnormal rapidity, may both experimentally be produced by nervous influences alone. It is possible that efferent impulses alone may so depress the excitability of ventricular muscle that, instead of there being (as in some cases) simple bradycardia, auricle and ventricle becoming equally slowed, arrhythmia may be produced of such a nature that only every other, or it may be only every third or fourth, auricular contraction may be followed by a ventricular systole. With Erlanger[1] we may explain this as due not to absence of stimulus conveyed from auricle to ventricle, along the "bundle of His," but as due to the fact that, following a ventricular beat, the contractile material is so slowly accumulated (or the muscular excitability so depressed) that the next stimulus passing from the auricles fails to arouse a contraction. Only with further accumulation of the contractile material will a second or later stimulus, of like strength, become effective.

Here, the opposite condition must also be noted. Of this we know only one instance, observed in our laboratory at the Royal Victoria

[1] Journ. of Exp. Medicine, 7: 1905: 676: and Bull. of the Johns Hopkins Hosp., 16: 1905: 234.

Hospital by Dr. Klotz in the heart of a late patient of Dr. C. F. Martin
—the condition of complete interruption of the bundle of His or conducting system, with, nevertheless, no sign of cardiac irregularity or heart-
block.   In this case there was complete replacement of all the tissues
in the region of the auriculo-ventricular node by a very extensive sarcomatous infiltration.   At most, some scattered and greatly degenerated
fibers were to be detected, which might possibly represent isolated cells
of the system.   The patient had for long been bedridden, and as the
Stokes-Adams syndrome is peculiarly apt to manifest itself after some
act of exertion, it may well be that in this case the ventricles were beating
automatically, *i. e.*, had assumed their own independent rhythm of contraction—just as happens experimentally and eventually after compression or destruction of the bundle of His, and, doing this, were able to
fulfil all the needs of the organism.

While everything indicates that the heart automatically may take up
an independent rhythm which results in irregular action, *i. e.*, that
direct stimuli acting on the ventricular muscle may stimulate the
production of independent contractions, nevertheless, the indications
are that very often vagus action is responsible for cardiac arrhythmia.
The many years of study of the mammalian heart by Roy and one of us[1]
led to the conclusion that the main function of the vagus is to protect the
heart, even, if need be, at the expense of the body in general.   Moderate
vagus stimulation slows the heart beat, the individual beats becoming
stronger, but undoubtedly the work accomplished by the heart is lessened
—the output of the ventricles in a given time is reduced.   Stronger vagus
stimulation actually stops the auricles, and experimentally we can produce the various grades of (1) temporary complete stoppage of the
ventricles, and so of the pulse; (2) assumption by the ventricles of an
independent rhythm, the auricles still being arrested; and (3) various
grades of arrhythmia.   It is not that the vagus directly stimulates the
ventricle or auricle to contract; on the contrary, we have evidence that
this wave lowers the excitability of both the auricular and the ventricular
muscle.   Rather along the lines suggested above, we may regard the
vagus as the anabolic nerve, or, at least, as the nerve favoring the
active expansion of the heart muscle.   Thus, if stimuli conveyed down
this nerve be sufficiently powerful they may neutralize and overcome
those passing down the atrioventricular bundle and favoring contraction.   And now, when through the action of vagus stimuli there has
been increased accumulation of the contractile or expansive material
either a minimal nervous stimulus to contraction may result in a
maximal contraction, or other stimuli, not of nervous origin, may be
directly effective in causing contraction.   In other words, according to
the conditions acting upon the heart, so may there be either nervous or
automatic contraction of the ventricles manifesting itself.   We may thus
lay down that when the ventricles are overworked, as is the case in

[1] Roy and Adami, Contributions to the Physiology and Pathology of the Mammalian Heart, Phil. Trans. Roy. Soc., London, 183 B: 1892· 199 to 298.

beginning failure of compensation, then for self-protection, afferent impulses from the heart call the vagus heart centres into activity. It is under these conditions that arrhythmia shows itself. Or otherwise, arrhythmia is frequently an indication that the ventricles are working at the limit of their reserve force, and need vagus assistance in order to prevent complete cardiac exhaustion. Further, other reflex arcs may stimulate the vagus centres. These centres may be acted upon by emotional and psychic influences, or influences reaching them from the gastric or splanchnic areas and from sensory surfaces. The analysis and determination of the cause in any particular case of cardiac arrhythmia demands, therefore, a wide survey of conditions throughout the organism.

(5) **Pulsus Alternans.**—Of this and the next form of irregularity of heart beat less has been determined. In the pulsus alternans a strong ventricular beat alternates with a weak, *with equal intervals between the beats.* It occurs with indications of great cardiac weakness. We have already indicated that in "extra systole" the lengthened diastole is associated with ventricular disturbance. The want of such lengthening in these cases suggests that the disturbance originates in the auricle or at Keith's node.

(6) **Aperiodic Irregularity** (*pulsus irregularis perpetuus*).—Markedly irregular irregularity is encountered in cases of advanced mitral and tricuspid stenosis and incompetence. Mackenzie assumes that there is some break in continuity of the conducting paths between the sino-auricular and the atrioventricular mode. It cannot, however, be said that we have adequate anatomical or other data upon which to base a conclusion.

The Filling of the Ventricles, and its Effect on the Muscle Fibers.—Distension, Hypertrophy, and Dilatation.—The work accomplished by the heart in a given time is determined by the amount of blood propelled in that time, and the external (arterial) pressure against which it is discharged. And the amount propelled—or expelled—is the product of the amount discharged per heart beat into the number of heart beats. The pressure remaining the same, the like amount of work is accomplished by a rapidly beating heart discharging a small quantity of blood at each systole, as by a heart beating at half the rate, discharging each time twice the quantity. It will be realized that in those two cases the conditions within the ventricles may be very different, to the extent that the diastolic expansion in the latter case will, in the normally acting heart, be roughly twice that seen in the former, or otherwise, the muscle fibers in the latter case have to contract against twice the load, and, in diastole, expand to a greater extent under this increased load.

The physics connected with this aspect of cardiac work are not a little interesting, inasmuch as they give a clearer understanding of what happens in the not infrequent cases of obstruction to the outflow of blood from the heart. Here we may, we think, employ safely our knowledge of the laws of contraction of voluntary muscle. The ventricle, that is, under its load of blood to be expelled, may be compared with the familiar gastrocnemius muscle of the frog. If a series of weights be attached to such a muscle hanging at rest, it is to be noted that some weights are so small that the length of the muscle is not altered; the natural tonus of the muscle is greater than the expanding force exerted by those weights. With progressively increasing weights, however, the resting muscle becomes more and more stretched, at first with relatively rapid increases in length, later as the limit of elasticity is reached, with lessened increment in length. The application of these facts to the ventricle is that, with increase in load, even within normal limits, the ventricles show distension, and that increase in work per individual systole is accompanied by a *natural distension* of the ventricle. In other words, within normal limits increased work of the heart is followed by increased size of the organ in diastole. There is a natural distension as distinguishable from a pathological dilatation.

On the other hand, still considering the gastrocnemius, if we record the excursion of this muscle when stimulated with the like strength of electric current, but when bearing a succession of increasing loads, we find that the work accomplished by the muscle, i. e., the weight raised multiplied by the distance to which it is raised, is far from being at its maximum with the smallest weight. The work done when progressively increasing weights are attached undergoes increase up to a certain point, or, otherwise, there is an optimum load which with a given muscle and given strength of stimulus leads to the accomplishment of the greatest amount of work. Here the application is that the heart accomplishes most work not when the arterial pressure is lowest, but under a certain mean arterial pressure, which of necessity varies with different individuals and different states of nutrition of the ventricular muscle. So also it would seem that a certain amount of diastolic stretch of the muscle fibers, or distension of the ventricles, results in more effective contractions, i. e., in the expulsion of the greater amount of blood as the result of individual contraction.

Or we can approach this subject from another point of view. If, as shown by Roy and Adami,[1] two points be taken upon the surface of the left ventricle of a dog, and by a proper instrument the distance between these points under various conditions be recorded, it is found that upon increasing the intraventricular pressure, as by narrowing the aortic arch by means of a ligature, the heart becomes more filled in diastole, and the two points become farther apart, while in systole, the points do not approximate to nearly the same extent as when there is less resistance. Similar results are obtainable if, instead of primarily increasing the pressure in the arterial system, the heart is given more work to do by increasing the amount of blood supplied to it. This can be accomplished, temporarily, by pressure upon the abdomen, or over longer periods, by injecting into the venous circulation some few hundred cubic centimeters of defibrinated blood. Again, there is the same filling in diastole, and relatively slighter approximation of the points in systole. With increased work of the heart accompanying the dis-

[1] Practitioner, 52: 1894: 81.

tension in diastole, there is a dilatation in systole also; the fibers do not shorten to the same extent. There is of necessity *residual blood* in the ventricular chambers. The significance of this is grasped if we consider the ventricular chambers as a sphere.[1] There is this to be noted concerning the relationship between the circumference of a sphere and its contents, namely, that as a sphere expands, its cubic contents increase

Fig. 16

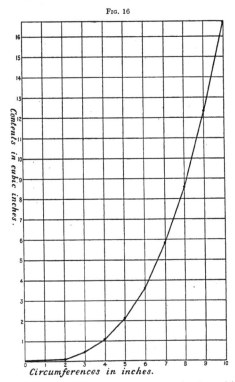

Curve representing the relationship between the circumference of a sphere and its volume, with successive unit increments of circumference. Ordinate—volume in cubic inches. Abscissæ—circumference in inches.

out of all proportion to its increase in circumference, or, more accurately, the ratio of increase is not an arithmetical ratio, but is such that if the circumference be taken as abscissæ, the corresponding volumes as ordinates, the curve of successive values is what is known as a cubical parabola (Fig. 16). From this it follows that a degree of shortening

[1] This is the nearest geometrical figure that we can employ here for purposes of illustration.

of the fibers of the heart wall sufficient, let us say, to reduce the circumference of the ventricle an inch, will cause a greater diminution in volume (or greater output) the more distended or dilated the ventricle is at the beginning of its contraction. For example, a diminution of the circumference by an inch of a sphere of ten inches' circumference causes a diminution of volume, or an output, equal to 4.5 cubic inches, when a diminution by one inch in the circumference of a sphere five inches round causes an output of only 1.027 cubic inches, although in the first case the circumference was reduced only one-tenth, in the second one-fifth. That is to say, with moderate distension or dilatation of the heart, the fibers will need to contract a very small amount in order to expel a given amount of blood compared with the amount of their contraction in a normal undilated heart. It is thus very possible that, in a hard-working heart, a certain grade of distension is economical, and that the presence of residual blood by diminishing the extent to which each fiber is called upon to contract, may be a saving to the heart and to the organism as a whole.

From these considerations and observations it follows that *hypertrophy is never primary;* distension (or, as it is usually termed, dilatation) always precedes hypertrophy. The only distinction—and perhaps it is a necessary distinction—that we can recognize between these two terms—distension and dilatation—is that the former is a temporary state which disappears as soon as the heart is relieved, the latter is a more permanent condition, brought about by disease, and still persisting when the cause ceases to be effective. Possibly, we may add that dilatation proper should only be regarded as present when there is actual incompetence of the heart muscle and incapacity to contract to an extent commensurate with the load borne by the muscle. If we deal simply with distension, and the heart muscle be well nourished, we have the inevitable sequel that continuance of increased work within reasonable limits leads to hypertrophy—either hypertrophy proper, or hyperplasia, or often a combination of the two (vol. i, p. 591). Such hypertrophy or hyperplasia will either relatively or absolutely lessen the load of each individual muscle fiber. As a result, with lessened load, each fiber will contract more completely, and the dilatation will tend to disappear. In such cases we deal with **simple hypertrophy.**

There can be no doubt that where there is ample reserve force and good compensation, this simple hypertrophy exists and may persist for years, though it is the exception rather than the rule upon the postmortem table. Where there is persistent cause for increased heart work (as in aortic stenosis or incompetence), then more often we find that the reserve force of the ventricular muscle becomes diminished or exhausted, and **eccentric hypertrophy** supervenes; that is to say, we have combined a pathological dilatation with hypertrophy. Not a few authorities still describe a **concentric hypertrophy.** In our opinion this is non-existent. It is true that now and again we encounter an apparent, a false concentric hypertrophy upon the postmortem table, in which what is striking is the tensely knit ventricular muscle, greatly increased in amount, with practically no lumen to the ventricle. All the cases we have seen of this condition have been from cases examined within the first six hours or so after death. They represent rigor mortis, the heart muscle passing into this state in one hour after death. Seen next day, such hearts present well-marked hypertrophy with dilatation. There is no such thing as true concentric hypertrophy; it implies that the ventricle, in contracting, expends a large part of its energy in compressing the more internal fibers, a most unnatural lack of economy in the work of the organ. The causes of hypertrophy and dilatation will be dealt with seriatim on pp. 155 and 156.

3. THE HEART VALVES.

The mechanism of the action of the heart valves is, or should be, so well known that little need be said regarding their physiology, although in discussing their pathology certain less known aspects of their normal mode of function will have to be dwelt upon. We have to consider the results of their imperfect closure and imperfect opening: of *incompetence* and *stenosis*. Practically all the. disturbances we have to consider, whether congenital or of postnatal origin, come under these two headings.

Incompetence.—This ·may be relative, due to no disease of the valves themselves, but to a giving way and expansion of the ring of tissue to which the valves are attached, so that their cusps do not meet and close the aperture; or actual, due to disease or injury to the cusps, producing the like result. As a consequence, at the period of the cardiac cycle, when the valves should be closed, there is **regurgitation** of blood, and passage back of the same into chambers from which it had previously been discharged. The blood thus regurgitated constitutes an additional load for these chambers to propel at their next systole in addition to the normal load reaching them from the normal source or sources. To accommodate this additional blood the affected chambers undergo distension (or physiological dilatation); to cope with the increased work they are called upon to perform, they exhibit hypertrophy.

The study of the heart post mortem suggests that incompetence is a more frequent condition than is recognized clinically; or otherwise, that frequently regurgitation exists without the existence of murmurs calling attention to its presence. Notably is this the case in connection with the tricuspid; the shape and the relative weakness of the right ventricle may almost be said to favor incompetence and regurgitation with even a moderate grade of distension of the ventricle. Such distension is the outcome of either (1) incompetence or stenosis of the pulmonary valve, (2) obstructive disease of the lungs and pulmonary circulation, or (3) obstruction to outflow of the blood through the left heart. The result is distension of the right auricle, and, as there are no adequate valves at the entrance of the venæ cavæ, with contraction of the ventricle a reverse wave of blood is propelled into the larger systemic veins, and these become distended at a period when normally the blood should be pouring from them into the right auricle. The result is a marked obstruction to the venous circulation. The greatly distended right auricle undergoes some hypertrophy, but very soon the compensation is incomplete, with the result that the blood accumulates or is dammed back on the venous side of the heart, passive congestion showing itself in the liver and other organs, and with the other consequences already discussed on p. 106 et seq.

A similar relative incompetence is not infrequent at the mitral valve, whether as the result of high blood pressure or obstructive aortic valve disease, or again through acute or terminal dilatation of the left ventricle; acute dilatation being brought on by the action of toxemia, alcohol and other drugs; terminal, being due to failure of compensation after long-continued hypertrophy or progressive malnutrition. Nor is this relative incompetence unknown in connection with the pulmonary and aortic orifices; the fact that in the last three years we have encountered at autopsy no less than three cases of the last condition, makes us think that it is more common than is generally suspected. In one of these three the regurgitation had evidently been of long continuance, for the corpora Arantii and free edge of those portions of the cusps which did not meet at the centre had been thickened and rounded. Such relative incompetence of the pulmonary and aortic valves would seem to be brought about in part by dilatation of the origins of the pulmonary artery and of the aorta; in part by a giving way of the muscular ring immediately beneath the valves.

Actual or organic incompetence of the heart valves will be discussed in the chapters devoted to the morbid anatomy of the heart. Here, it is only necessary to call attention to the fact that incompetence most frequently co-exists when there is stenosis. The narrowing of the cardiac orifices is rarely of such a nature as to permit complete apposition of the diseased components of the valve.

The results of incompetence, whether relative or actual, are of the same order, whichever valve is involved, namely: regurgitation, over-loading of the chambers into which the blood regurgitates, distension of the same, followed by compensatory hypertrophy. The overfilling of the chamber behind the incompetent valve sooner or later brings about further damming back of the blood toward the venous side of the heart, until eventually, in aortic incompetence, for example, we obtain mitral incompetence, pulmonary congestion, tricuspid incompetence, and general passive, venous congestion of the organs.

CHAPTER VII.

THE HEART: PATHOLOGICAL ANATOMY AND HISTOLOGY.

FOR purposes of description it is convenient to regard the heart as consisting of three portions: the pericardium, the myocardium, and the endocardium. It should be borne in mind, however, that no serious affection of any one of these structures can exist without involving the others to a greater or less extent.

Being a hollow viscus that contains a constantly moving fluid tissue, the bulk of which is constantly altering, and, moreover, being subject to various peripheral impressions, the heart is in a state of physiological unrest and is consequently proportionately liable to be affected by disease processes.

The average weight of the heart in the adult male is 300 grams; in the female, 250 grams.

THE PERICARDIUM.

The pericardium is a serous sac composed of an elastic connective-tissue membrane lined with endothelium. Unlike the other large lymph spaces of the body, it usually contains a relatively large amount of fluid, viz., from 30 to 50 to 100 c.cm., even in the absence of any pathological condition. No doubt, the presence of the larger quantities is to be regarded as an agonal manifestation. From the fact that the pericardial fluid contains considerable albumin, we must conclude that the vessels of the pericardium have a physiologically greater permeability to their fluid contents than have those of the other serous cavities. This will explain the greater susceptibility of the pericardium to exudative processes and the formation of large amounts of fibrin.

The close relationship of the pericardium to the heart, lungs, and pleural cavities renders it also especially liable to secondary invasion by infective agents, and the free movement of its two layers, one upon the other, explains the rapid propagation of the various inflammatory processes to which it is subject.

DEVELOPMENTAL ANOMALIES.

In acardiac monsters the pericardium is more or less imperfectly developed.

Complete or partial *defects* occur in rare cases, generally associated with other malformations. The sac may be quite absent or represented by a few fringes at the base of the heart. More commonly there is a partial loss of substance over the left ventricle, through which the heart may protrude into the pleural cavity.

Hernia of the endothelial membrane through the outer fibrous layer is very rare. *Diverticula* are also recorded (*Rohn*).

CIRCULATORY DISTURBANCES.

Anemia.—This may affect the pericardium in common with the rest of the body.

Hyperemia.—Active hyperemia is met with in cases of death from pressure on the base of the brain, and in commencing inflammation. Passive hyperemia occurs from the same causes as it does elsewhere, and in death from suffocation. It may lead to rupture of the vessels and the formation in their neighborhood of small *ecchymoses* or subserous hemorrhages, which are most commonly present about the base of the heart. *Petechial spots* are so common at autopsy that it is probable that they are frequently produced during the death agony.

Similar extravasations are the effect of poisons (*e. g.*, phosphorus), septicemia, morbus Werlhofii, pernicious anemia, leukemia, and the various infections.

Hematopericardium.—Hematopericardium is the condition in which blood is found in the pericardium. This is due to wounds of the heart; rupture of the heart wall, of an aortic aneurism of the aorta, pulmonary artery, or coronary vessels. More often it is a concomitant of inflammation, as in tuberculosis and carcinoma of the sac, or is an expression of some blood-dyscrasia, such as scurvy and leukemia.

Hydropericardium.—Hydropericardium, or *hydrops pericardii*, may be part of a general anasarca but is also met with in hydremia, cachectic states and chronic Bright's disease. Occasionally, it is seen as a compensatory process in cases of brown atrophy of the heart (*hydrops ex vacuo*). The amount of fluid sometimes reaches as high as one liter. The fluid is pale amber or greenish in color, clear, without flocculi, and poor in albumin (as compared with an inflammatory exudate). Stray leukocytes and endothelial cells, more or less hydropic and degenerated, are to be found. The condition is important, as it leads to stretching of the pericardium, pressure upon and even atrophy of the heart, and pressure upon neighboring structures.

PNEUMATOSIS.

Pneumopericardium.—Air in the pericardium may be due to fistulous communication between the hollow viscera, such as the œsophagus and stomach, and the pericardial sac; to subdiaphragmatic abscess, to the extension of a pyopneumothorax, or to fracture of the ribs and traumatic perforation; or, again, to the presence of certain bacteria like the Bacillus Welchii and the B. coli. In the last contingency the sac is often empty and the surface of the heart resembles meat dried in the sun. A very striking example is recorded by one of us,[1] where, in a case of perforative appendicitis, pneumopericardium developed during life, with a distinct musical sound over the precordium, which could be heard at a considerable distance. At the autopsy there was a subdiaphragmatic pus collection, but the continuity of the pericardium was intact. The B. Welchii was found in all the organs.

INFLAMMATIONS.

Pericarditis.—The most important disease of the pericardium is *inflammation*, which may present a variety of characteristics.

Primary idiopathic pericarditis, so called, probably does not exist, except in those cases due to wounds of the pericardium. The cases recorded in children, while they may be "idiopathic" clinically, almost certainly are due to some mediastinal lesion.

Secondary pericarditis is a term applied to those forms due to extension of disease from other parts. It is less misleading, however, to divide the cases into (1) *hematogenic*, in which the irritants reach the pericardium by way of the blood, as, for instance, miliary tuberculosis and those forms that complicate acute rheumatism, smallpox, influenza, nephritis, diabetes, septicemia, and cerebrospinal meningitis, and (2) those arising *per extensionem*. In the latter class the disease may arise from a great variety of causes, among which may be mentioned pneumonia, chronic pulmonary tuberculosis, acute pleurisy, empyema, aortic aneurisms, inflammation of mediastinal and peribronchial glands, acute and chronic endocarditis, and many abdominal conditions, such as peritonitis, appendicitis, abscess of the liver or pancreas, and ulcer of the stomach. In 91 cases of which we have notes, occurring in the postmortem practice of the Royal Victoria Hospital, 58 per cent. arose by extension, of which three-quarters were due to preëxisting disease of the lungs or pleura.

While it is true that in some cases cultures have failed to show the presence of microörganisms, it is almost certain that all exudative. as distinguished from transudative processes, are due to their action. The organisms which are usually found are Diplococcus lanceolatus, B. coli, Staphylococcus pyogenes, Streptococcus, B. tuberculosis, Friedländer's pneumobacillus, M. meningitidis intracellularis, and B. Welchii. One case has come under our notice where B. pyocyaneus was present. Mixed infections are not uncommon, and B. tuberculosis is at fault in more cases than are usually suspected.

The relative frequency with which pericarditis complicates endocarditis, particularly of the aortic valves, is readily explained when we remember the close anatomical relationship of the pericardial reflexion to the aortic ring. That the inflammation can extend through the vessel wall at this point is beyond a doubt, and not only acute, but chronic endocarditis may provide a starting point.

When pleurisy exists, it is very common for the outside of the peri-

[1] A. G. Nicholls, Brit. Med. Jour., 2: 1907: 1844.

cardial sac to be affected (*pericarditis externa*). Often in such cases
the pericardial fluid is increased in amount, but without flakes (*inflammatory hydrops*), while the superficial vessels of the pericardium are
congested and the surface of the heart may show a rosy flush. Though
the endothelium may, in general, be quite smooth, even at this early
stage bacteria may be present. The condition is sometimes called
pericarditis serosa. This form rapidly passes over into a serofibrinous
inflammation, in which the sac becomes distended with a fluid exudate of
a yellowish turbid appearance, sometimes stained with blood, in which
float flakes of fibrin. The amount of the exudate may be small or may
reach a liter or more. The character of the exudate varies considerably,
depending on the nature of the infection.

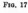

FIG. 17

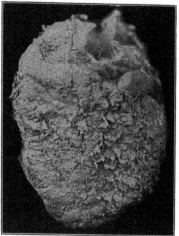

Fibrinous pericarditis.   (From the Pathological Museum of McGill University.)

The fibrin may take the form of a granular deposit, rendering the
fluid turbid, or it may exist in large flakes, or again may be gelatinous.
If pus-producing organisms be present, such as the staphylococcus and,
in certain cases, the pneumococcus, the exudate is purulent (*pyoperi-
cardium*). The amount of fluid may be so small that the fibrinous
deposit is quite thick and dry (*pericarditis fibrinosa sicca*). This condition
may alternate with the serous outpouring, or may be due to absorption
of the fluid during the later stages of the affection. The deposit
does not form a layer of even thickness upon the epicardium, but,
owing to the movements of the heart, tends to collect in little clumps.
The condition is aptly described by Laennec, who compared it to the
appearance produced by the rapid separation of two slices of bread and

butter. In some cases the fibrin over the left ventricle is arranged as a raised network, while over the right it takes the form of transverse parallel bands. When the deposit is thick and in the form of long tags, the condition is known as the *cor villosum*. The serous fluid may contain so much blood that a characteristic appearance is presented, known as *pericarditis hemorrhagica*. In such cases there may be relatively little fibrin. This form occurs in debilitated persons and alcoholics, or as a manifestation of a hemorrhagic diathesis, for example, in scurvy and morbus maculosus. Tuberculous and carcinomatous disease of the pericardium also at times produce this appearance. In the case of drunkards, the condition is analogous to pachymeningitis hemorrhagica interna. In cases of some standing one sees the process of organization

Fig 18

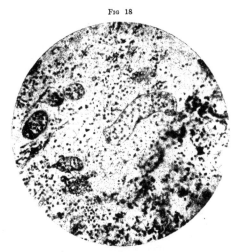

Organizing pericarditis. Section shows newly-formed capillaries in the pericardial exudate. Zeiss obj. DD., ocular No. 1. (From the Pathological Laboratory of McGill University.)

beginning. Small vessels are seen to be springing from the deeper layers of the pericardium and making their way into the exudate, which now shows signs of disintegration.

If the heart in a case of fibrinous pericarditis in the early stages be examined microscopically, it will be seen that the flattened endothelial cells lining the sac are swollen and desquamating, lying free in little masses upon the surface. The vessels of the pericardium are congested and there is beginning extravasation of leukocytes. The pericardial connective tissue and the superficial layers of the heart muscle are oedematous. In parts where the process is somewhat more advanced, there is upon the surface a distinct layer of fibrin, forming a meshwork mixed with leukocytes and containing numerous bacteria. This frequently stains rather badly, as if undergoing disorganization. In some instances the fibrin melts together and forms hyaline clumps. In severe cases the underlying heart muscle shows marked cloudy swelling and congestion.

When the exudation into the sac is marked it leads to pressure upon the heart and great vessels, causing more or less stasis of the circulation. The lung often becomes, to some extent, atelectatic. Acute pericarditis may extend to the pleura and peritoneum. When it heals, but few traces may be left of its occurrence.

Pericarditis Chronica.—Acute pericarditis may eventually become chronic, in that, owing to repeated relapses with partial absorption of the exudate, the process may extend over weeks and result in thickening of the pericardium and fibrous adhesion between the two leaves of the sac. Many cases which start clinically as acute are really chronic in their nature. Chronic pericarditis may also start insidiously. The disease is perhaps most common in young persons. In developing cases, where pericardial thickening is going on and more or less adhesion of the surfaces has taken place, one can see remains of the exudation in the form of disorganized, granular, rather inspissated, masses of fibrin. The adhesions are partial or complete, and in some cases calcification of the fibrinous material takes place.

An important type is the **indurative mediastinopericaːditis**, where not only are the pericardial layers fused, but the connective tissue of the mediastinum is thickened, so that the heart may be firmly united to the chest wall, the lungs, and the diaphragm. The etiology of this form is somewhat obscure. The most potent cause appears to be acute pericarditis, either rheumatic or following some of the infectious fevers. A peculiar form of chronic pericarditis is that in which the pericardial sac is obliterated and the two layers are converted into a thick hyaline membrane of gristly consistence. This form is nearly always seen in association with similar disease of the pleura and peritoneum, but Eichorst[1] has recorded a case in which the pericardium alone was affected.

The most important chronic conditions are tuberculosis and syphilis.

Tuberculous Pericarditis.—Tuberculous pericarditis may be hematogenous or extend from the mediastinal and peribronchial glands, or from the lungs and pleura. It begins with the formation of small grayish tubercles on the inner surface of the sac, which are surrounded by a hyperemic zone and often capped with granulation tissue. As the condition progresses, exudation takes place, the tubercles enlarge and coalesce, forming ultimately caseous nodules. The exudate may be serofibrinous, fibrinous, purulent, or hemorrhagic. It is usually moderate in amount, and much productive change is going on. The disease at times assumes the guise of a simple serofibrinous inflammation, or the two walls of the pericardium may be completely and firmly united by a thick layer of newly formed connective tissue containing caseous foci. This layer is often very thick and may have a semitranslucent, structureless appearance resembling partially solidified celloidin.

---

[1] Eichorst, Zuckergussherz, Deutsche med. Woch., 28:1902:293.

Syphilitic Pericarditis.—Syphilitic pericarditis is rare, generally depending upon syphilis of the heart wall. It leads to adhesions.

Actinomycosis.—Actinomycosis of the lungs, mediastinum, œsophagus, and peritoneal cavity occasionally extends to the pericardium.

The results of pericarditis, when healing takes place, may be that the exudate is absorbed and there is complete return to the normal condition. Or the fluid portion may be absorbed, leaving a granular, fatty, and caseous-looking detritus between the layers of an adherent pericardium. Such deposits may even calcify. **Milk spots** (maculæ tendineæ), which are so common[1] on the front of the right ventricle, are by some thought to be due to preëxisting pericarditis. Most often they would seem to be of the nature of "corns" of the serosa, the result of intermittent pressure. A more important sequel is the formation of fibrous adhesions between the two layers of the pericardium. These occur in about 3.5 per cent. of all postmortems. Fine fibrous bands near the aortic ring are very common, and are due to extension of inflammation from the valves. Local adhesions by veil-like processes may be present (*partial synechia*), or the two layers may everywhere be in such close and firm contact that it is impossible to separate them (*total synechia*). The latter form leads to dilatation of the heart chambers. On the other hand, great thickening of the pericardium may lead to atrophy of the heart. Such a condition is often spoken of under the term "chronic adhesive pericarditis," but since it is a result and not a process, it would be more correct to call it *pericarditis adhesiva obsolescens*.

Parasites.—*Trichinæ, Cysticerci*, and *Echinococci* have been found in the cavity.

Foreign Bodies.—Foreign bodies may enter from without or from ulcerative processes. It is peculiarly frequent in cattle to have needles, wire, etc., which have passed through the walls of the first stomach, find their way into the pericardium and lead to sudden death by puncture of the heart. Analogous cases occasionally occur in man.

RETROGRESSIVE METAMORPHOSES.

Serous Atrophy.—Serous atrophy of the pericardial fat occurs in cases of effusion and in individuals the subjects of senility, marasmus, and cachexia. The fat is grayish, gelatinous in appearance, and, microscopically, shows swelling and hydropic degeneration of the fat cells with reversion to the primitive connective-tissue type.

PROGRESSIVE METAMORPHOSES.

Tumors.—**Primary Tumors.**—Primary tumors are very rare. **Carcinoma** (?) and **endothelioma** are recorded, as are also a few instances of

---

[1] According to our Montreal statistics they are to be found in more than 14 per cent. of all autopsies.

primary sarcoma.[1] **Fibroma** (Kaufmann)[2] and **lipoma** (McKechnie)[3] are also described.

Secondary Tumors.—Secondary growths may be extensions from tumors of the mediastinum, bronchus, lung, œsophagus, and stomach, or may be metastatic. Of the first, carcinoma and lymphosarcoma may be mentioned, and of the second, carcinoma and melanotic sarcoma.

THE MYOCARDIUM.

CONGENITAL ANOMALIES.

Congenital peculiarities are said to be more frequent in the male than in the female sex. In general, they are due to a retardation or an actual vitium in the development of certain parts. More rarely, they are to be attributed to inflammatory processes occurring during fœtal life. Many of them are of great practical importance, inasmuch as their presence may prevent an independent existence on the part of the offspring, or if life be possible, grave circulatory disturbances may be the consequence, with abnormal susceptibility to disorders of related parts and all that this implies.

The number of the cardiac anomalies of this class is legion, and we cannot, for lack of space, do more here than indicate in a sketchy fashion the more important forms.

In a general way the developmental anomalies of the heart and its sinuses may be summarized as follows:

1. Numerical variations.
2. Displacements.
3. Anomalies of the heart as a whole.
4. Anomalies and defects of the various septa.
5. Anomalies of the lumina of the various ostia.
6. Anomalies of the semilunar cusps and auriculoventricular valves.
7. Patency and other anomalies of the ductus arteriosus.
8. Anomalies of the vessels in immediate relationship to the heart.

Under the category of numerical variations we note the condition of total **absence** of the heart, as, for example, in the monstrous birth known as acardiacus. This is associated with other grave anomalies of development. One case is on record, also, of a **double heart**. Verocay has described and figured a case of seven hearts in a series found in a chicken.

The heart may be displaced in various ways as a result of errors of development or acquired disease. Thus, it may be **rotated** upon its vertical or anteroposterior axis. Under the term **dextrocardia** are recognized two conditions: one, in which the heart occupies a position on the right side of the thorax; and the other, in which, while the heart

[1] J. C. Williams, New York Med. Jour., 71: 1900: 537.

[2] E. Kaufmann, Text-book of Special Pathological Anatomy, Reimer, Berlin, 5th edit., 1909, p. 12.

[3] McKechnie, British Medical Journal, 2: 1906: 76.

is found at its normal site, its various chambers and sinuses are simply reversed (true dextrocardia). The latter form is, as a rule, though not invariably, found associated with transposition of other viscera. **Ectopia cordis** is a condition in which the heart is situated outside the thoracic cavity. Should the organ remain high up in the neck, we have *ectopia cervicalis;* should it enter the abdomen through a slit in the diaphragm, it is called

Fig. 19

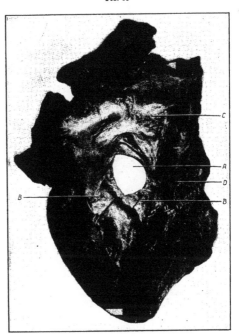

Heart showing (*A*) defect of interauricular septum below (persistent ostium primum), with (*B*) cleavage of right anterior segment of mitral valve. (*C*) Interauricular septum above, showing closed foramen ovale. (*D*) Left posterior mitral segment. From a woman, aged thirty-two years, without cardiac symptoms, dying of perforative appendicitis. (From a specimen in the Pathological Museum, McGill University.)

ectopia abdominalis; should it appear beneath the skin of the thorax through a defect of the sternum, it is known as *ectopia pectoralis.* In such cases the pericardium is sometimes wanting.

The chief anomalies of the heart as a whole are **bifid apex, diverticulum primary hypertrophy,** and **hypoplasia.** Hypoplasia is not uncommon, and is usually found in the vessels as well as the heart. The heart is either small at birth or the whole vascular system gradually lags behind in the general bodily development. In long-standing cases, cardiac insufficiency and dilatation come on. Rokitansky has noted the occasional association of the condition with defects of the external genitalia. Bamberger and, later, Virchow pointed out the relationship of cardiovascular hypoplasia to chlorosis. Ortner and others hold that the condition predisposes to infection. We, ourselves, have noticed, post mortem, the great frequency with which the condition is present in cases of tuberculosis, especially in young people. The vessels are thin-walled and show a tendency to fatty change.

The commonest defect of the septa is the **patent foramen ovale**. This is so frequent that it can hardly be called an anomaly, unless it is so widely open as to allow free communication between the auricles. In

Fig. 20

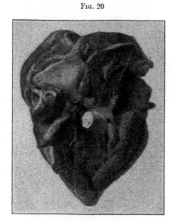

Defect of the interventricular septum at undefended space. Heart of infant. No other anomaly. (From a specimen in the McGill Pathological Museum.)

1500 autopsies at the Royal Victoria Hospital, the condition occurred 220 times, or in 14.7 per cent. When patent, the opening may be merely of pin-point size or may admit a finger. Defects of other parts of the auricular septum may also occur, These defects are often associated with other abnormalities, such as coloboma, or mental degradation.

The interventricular septum may be partially or totally wanting. Defect of this kind is usually associated with pulmonary stenosis and *rechtslage* of the aorta, and constitutes one of the commonest forms of congenital heart disease. When the septa are completely wanting, we have a two-chambered heart (**cor biloculare**). Absence of the ventricular septum, with presence of the auricular, constitutes a three-chambered heart (**cor biatriatum triloculare**). A remarkable instance of this latter form is to be found in the Pathological Museum of McGill University, the gift of Dr. A. F. Holmes, one of the original founders of the Medical Faculty.[1]

The aortic septum may be partially or completely defective.

Pulmonary stenosis is one of the commonest of cardiac anomalies. Both it and the severer grade of atresia are commonly associated with defects of the septum.

Aortic stenosis and atresia are rare.

The ductus arteriosus Botalli may be *absent, patent,* or *anomalous* in its course. Patency of the duct is sometimes associated with stenosis of the pulmonary artery, or of the aortic isthmus. It occurred 6 times in 1500 autopsies at the Royal Victoria Hospital.

The coronary arteries may be increased in number, may have an abnormal origin, or may take an abnormal course.

Aberrant chordæ tendineæ are not uncommon: a case, giving rise to a remarkable musical murmur, has been recorded by W. F. Hamilton.[2]

Those desiring more detailed information than that given here are referred to Dr. Maude Abbott's admirable article in Osler's *Modern Medicine* (vol. iv, 1908, p. 323), an article that will be for long the "last word" on this most important and interesting subject.

CIRCULATORY DISTURBANCES.

Anemia.—This may be part and parcel of a general anemic condition, or may be a local condition due to a narrowing or obliteration of the branches of the coronary arteries. A pericardial exudate or hydropericardium also produces a local anemia by pressure. The affected muscle has a pale grayish-brown or yellow color. As sudden death is frequent from acute anemia, the coronary vessels should always be examined for sclerosis, thrombi, or emboli.

Hyperemia.—Active Hyperemia.—Active hyperemia occurs in acute infections, in abnormal nervous conditions, and in death from respiratory failure.

Passive Hyperemia.—Passive hyperemia is found under the same conditions as elsewhere.

Hemorrhage.—Interstitial hemorrhage is often due to obliteration of the arteries, as in hemorrhagic infarction, or to spontaneous rupture of the venules in the state of passive congestion. Apart from these conditions it is not common, but is sometimes present in certain dyscrasias, as in the various infective diseases, the hemorrhagic diatheses, leukemia, pernicious anemia, and in poisoning with phosphorus, arsenic, and morphine. In some cases it is due to the death agony.

Leukemia.—In this affection we find either multiple isolated aggregations of leukocytes in the form of nodules, or a diffuse infiltration of the heart wall.

[1] Trans. Medico-Chir. Soc. of Edin., 1824. Reprinted by Abbott, Montreal Med. Jour., 30:1901: p. 524.

[2] Montreal Medical Journal, 28: 1899: 508.

Myomalacia Cordis.—By this is understood a degeneration of the heart muscle resulting from arterial anemia. Atheroma of the coronary vessels, with its attendant thrombosis, is the most common cause. Embolism in the coronaries is a less frequent one, inasmuch as these vessels are so placed that foreign bodies cannot readily enter. The essence of the process is that it is a rapid one, bringing about what is practically a white infarct, with subsequent softening and degeneration of the muscle.[1]

The affected area, according to its age and vascular relationship, varies in appearance at different times. At first, it is still firm and of a dull yellow color. Later, the patch becomes yellowish white and friable. If the neighboring capillaries rupture, a red infarct is the result, presenting a dull, reddish appearance. Later still, the color changes to a rusty brown and, as fibrosis occurs, to a dull gray. Microscopically, the affected muscle fibers appear to be swollen, hyaline, and have lost their characteristic structure. If they take the stain, it is with a diffuse glassy appearance. As in other infarctous conditions, an inflammatory reaction shows itself at the periphery of the necrobiotic area, when of any standing. The site of election for the process is in the wall of the left ventricle, at or below the junction of the lower and middle thirds, at the tip of the papillary muscles, sometimes in the right ventricle, more rarely in an auricle.

Such localized areas of degeneration may produce a rupture of the heart wall leading to hematopericardium and sudden death, or, if fibrosis has had time to develop, may result in the formation of a partial aneurism in the wall. This is most frequent in the anterior wall of the left ventricle, next, in the posterior, and occasionally in the septum. Such aneurisms may lead to an imperfect discharge of the heart's contents and to the formation of parietal thrombi with their attendant dangers. Lazarus-Barlow[2] has described a seemingly unique case of dissecting aneurism of the right heart wall.

Fibrosis of the Myocardium.—This condition has much in common with the last mentioned, but differs from it in that it is a fibrous degeneration of the heart muscle, which is very slowly produced. It is often called "chronic interstitial myocarditis," but incorrectly, since it is primarily a degenerative process. Owing to sclerosis of the coronary vessels, which leads to a narrowing of their caliber and consequently impoverished blood supply, the muscle bundles in the affected tract undergo starvation atrophy. Associated with this is proliferation of the preëxisting interstitial connective tissue which gradually invades the degenerating part—a true replacement fibrosis—and is reparative in its result. This is the pure type. It cannot be denied, however, that other cases exist in which, in addition to the "replacement fibrosis,"

---

[1] See R. Marie, L'infarctus du Myocarde et ses conséquences, Paris, 1897.

[2] Brit. Med. Jour., 2: 1899: 1344. For dissecting aneurisms, see also Vestberg, Om dissekerande hjärtaneurismer, Nordiskt Med. Arkiv., Ny Föjd, 7 : Nos. 26 and 30 : 1897.

there is the production of a cellular granulation tissue that may either develop into scar tissue or may, in its turn, participate in the degenerative change. Such inflammatory changes must, we think, be regarded as due to the irritation produced, and secondary in nature. It would consequently seem more rational to include this condition among the degenerations rather than the inflammations.

The scar tissue may be fairly diffused throughout the organ, giving it a tough feel like leather, Much more commonly, the change is localized to certain parts. On section, the muscle shows grayish streaks running parallel to the muscle bundles, particularly in the wall of the ·left ventricle and at the tip of the papillary muscles. If the condition be more extreme, one sees irregular areas of a semitranslucent appear-

Fɪɢ. 21

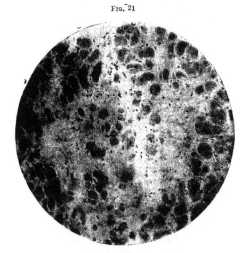

Myocardial fibrosi from disease of coronary arteries.   Leitz, obj. No. 7 without ocular.
(From the collection of Dr. A. G. Nicholls.)

ance, and of a grayish or grayish-white color, sharply defined from the healthy muscle, which are sunken below the general level of the cut surface. These have the appearance of tendon. Besides the favorite site in the wall of the left ventricle, similar areas may be found in the columnæ carneæ, the septum, or even in the right ventricle.

Microscopically, the condition is characterized by the presence among the muscle bundles of larger or smaller fibrous patches often presenting a stellate appearance. The muscle fibers about the margin show definite evidence of atrophy, and melt away into the fibrous mass. Sometimes in the centre of the patch can be seen a few isolated muscle bands, atrophied by compression. The scar tissue is generally very poor in nuclear elements, but toward the outer margin is more cellular. New-formed capillaries can be made out, with perhaps small areas of inflammatory infiltration. The more healthy muscle fibers usually show marked hypertrophy, as evidenced by the fact that the nuclei are relatively large, stain deeply, and are blunted at the ends.

INFLAMMATIONS.

Acute Inflammations.—Inflammation of the heart muscle, apart from the mild reactive form which sometimes accompanies ischemic necrosis, is mostly due to infection or intoxication. The various agents may reach the muscle from the contiguous pericardium or endocardium, or from more distant regions by means of the blood stream.

According to the anatomical distribution of the lesions some authorities recognize a *parenchymatous* and an *interstitial* myocarditis, but this distinction is largely academical. It is impossible for the inflammation to be confined to the muscle of the heart without the connective tissue being involved more or less, and *vice versa*. At most, we can say that the process is more in evidence in one or other constituent part. In general, the lesions in the parenchymatous form are degenerative in character, while those in the interstitial are exudative and productive. In both types of involvement the changes in question may be *localized* or *diffuse*.

A notable form of myocarditis occurs in the course of many infective fevers, such as typhoid, diphtheria, scarlatina, rheumatism, pneumonia, septicemia, pyemia, and other similar conditions. The first obvious change is cloudy swelling, and Virchow is probably correct in regarding this as the first stage in an inflammatory process. But besides this *myocarditis parenchymatosa*, in many cases there is evidence of an interstitial process as well, for we see collections of inflammatory leukocytes between the muscle fibers, together with connective-tissue proliferation. This form is called by Orth *myocarditis degenerativa*. The affected muscle is pale, soft, and friable, and often œdematous. Hemorrhagic points may frequently be seen through its substance. The cavities, particularly the left ventricle, are dilated.

Microscopically, the fibers are swollen, the striation faint, and the nuclei indistinct (cloudy swelling). Vacuolation is sometimes seen, and fragmentation. If the process continue, the nuclei swell and divide and the fibers show fatty or hyaline degeneration. The vessels are usually congested and may show proliferative changes. Collections of inflammatory leukocytes in many cases are seen between the muscle fibers, and in the later stages proliferation of the connective tissue, with the formation of fibroblasts. In this form, suppuration does not occur. If the patient survive, the inflammation, if slight, may entirely resolve. In other cases a diffuse fibrosis of the heart muscle is the result.

The interstitial form of myocarditis is usually purulent but not necessarily so. In this connection it might be mentioned that Aschoff and

Tawara[1] have lately drawn attention to a special form of acute myocarditis occurring in acute rheumatism with endocarditis, in which scattered foci of leukocytic infiltration are found along the course of the vessels, in type suggesting an infective origin, but not going on to suppuration. Local or diffuse fibrosis may result.

Purulent myocarditis can arise in various ways. Apart from those cases which are due to a direct extension from a purulent pericarditis or an ulcerative endocarditis, an embolic infection is the commonest cause. The so-called idiopathic heart abscess, where there is usually a single pus collection of some size, is distinctly rare. Formerly, many cases of myomalacia were erroneously classed under the term abscess. Most cases are simple expressions of a general pyemia.

The bacteria found in such cases are usually Staphylococci and Streptococci, occasionally Pneumococci, rarely Gonococci.

On examination, the affected heart is seen to be riddled with opaque grayish or grayish-yellow dots the size of a pin-head or larger. Many of these are surrounded by a hemorrhagic zone. Small hemorrhages are often seen, and all grades occur from this to true pus collections. The heart may be dilated, and show cloudy or fatty change.

Microscopically, these areas are seen to consist of pus cells with cell detritus. The vessels are often found to be plugged with microorganisms. In many cases the bacteria have penetrated the vessel walls and appear within the leukocytes or are lying free. The muscular fibers show cloudy swelling or fatty degeneration. The vessels in the neighborhood are greatly congested.

In the event of recovery, the detritus may be absorbed and a fibrous scar be produced, or the area may become calcified. More often the patient dies, but if he survive for a time the abscesses may coalesce, and rupture into the pericardium or into a cavity may occur. Thus communication can be opened up between two cavities, or a partial heart aneurism can result. Occasionally an abscess becomes encapsulated.

Acute Miliary Tuberculosis.—Acute miliary tuberculosis is somewhat rare, only one case having come under our observation. It is a part of a disseminated miliary process.

Chronic Inflammations.—Tuberculosis.[2]—Most frequently the tuberculous affection is an extension from a tuberculous endocardium or pericardium, especially from the chronic caseating form. It is rarer to find smaller or larger caseous foci in the heart wall. The differential diagnosis between this condition and syphilitic gumma is very difficult, and often can only be made after a general survey of the whole case, or from the discovery of the B. tuberculosis in the affected area. Gummas, however, are apt to be enclosed in a dense mass of hyperplastic connective tissue.

[1] Die heutige Lehre von den pathologischen-anatomischen Grundlage der Herzschwäche, Gustav Fischer, 1906.

[2] For a full description of Tuberculosis of the Myocardium, see Anders, Jour. Amer. Med. Assoc., 39: 1902: 1081.

Syphilis.—Syphilis is an infrequent cardiac affection. According to H. P. Loomis,[1] syphilis of the myocardium takes the form of (1) gummatous foci, almost invariably in the wall of the left ventricle; (2) fibroid induration, either localized or diffuse; (3) amyloid infiltration; (4) endarteritis obliterans, often causing infarctions. Indurative inflammation is perhaps the most common.

Solitary gummas may reach the size of a pigeon's egg. They are rare in inherited syphilis. Multiple miliary gummas are also described. Fatty degeneration of the muscle is a more frequent manifestation of the specific virus. Rupture of the wall or a partial heart aneurism may result.

Actinomycosis.—Actinomycosis is very rare, and is secondary to actinomycosis of the mediastinum, lungs, and pericardium. It takes the form of small granulomas of a grayish or yellowish-white color, often suppurative in character.

Trauma.—Solution of the continuity of the heart muscle arises in various ways. Wounds inflicted by instruments or bullets, either wholly or partially penetrating the wall from without, are not uncommon. An ulcer of the stomach has been known to penetrate the wall.

Foreign Bodies.—Foreign bodies are sometimes found in the heart wall. These may come not only from without, but from the œsophagus and stomach, and are usually needles, bullets, fish bones, knife blades and the like. The condition may be latent or, on the other hand, lead to sudden death.

Parasites.—Parasites are extremely rare. *Echinococci, Cysticerci,* and *Pentastoma* have been found. *Trichinæ* are said not to be found. Echinococcus cysts may burst into a cavity, causing a general infection or sudden death from pulmonary embolism.

RETROGRESSIVE METAMORPHOSES.

Atrophy.—**Simple Atrophy.**—Simple atrophy of the heart is characterized by a general diminution in the size and weight of the organ. The arteries do not partake so much in the process, consequently, owing to the shrinkage of the muscle, they become tortuous. The epicardium and the endocardium alike from the same cause present a rumpled appearance and often secondary thickening. The muscle is firm and tough, and may be of a dull, dark brown color—**brown atrophy.**

Microscopically, the fibers are thinner than normal. The outline of the cells is well marked, owing to an actual separation of the muscle bands. This is regarded as being due to a disintegration of the fibers in consequence of impaired nutrition of the cement substance. In brown atrophy, in addition, there is a great increase in the amount of the pigment which is usually situated about the poles of the nuclei, and the pigment takes a dark brown color. In severe cases brown granules are seen to be scattered throughout the cell.

[1] American Journal of the Medical Sciences, 110: 1895: 389.

Whether the affection can occur as a purely senile change has been doubted; nevertheless, routine examination of sections from the post-mortem room shows that after middle age some degree of brown atrophy is very common. More certain causes are marasmus, malignant disease, and tuberculosis of the lungs. Some cases are due to pressure, as from mediastinal lesions or from progressive relapsing pericarditis.

Local Atrophy.—Local atrophy is due to pressure or to sclerosis of small branches of the coronary arteries. Atrophy of the columnæ carneæ of the left ventricle, which is so common in valvular affections of the heart, may result from either of these causes.

Degenerations.—Cloudy or Albuminoid Degeneration.—This is a very common condition. The heart muscle has a grayish, cloudy, opaque appearance not unlike parboiled meat or raw fish and is some-what more friable than normal. Microscopically, the fibers are seen to be opaque from the deposit of numerous minute granules which obscure the nucleus and transverse striæ. The condition is best made out by making a thin section of the fresh muscle. The nature of the granules is not definitely settled, but they appear to be albuminoid in their character. On adding a drop of acetic acid to the section, the granules dissolve and the normal translucency of the fibers is restored.

Cloudy swelling is very common in severe anemias and in the course of the infectious fevers, and is due to the action of specific toxins with or without prolonged high temperature, or to disorders of metabolism.

Fatty Degeneration.—This common condition is characterized by the presence of minute globules of fat in the muscle fibers, which are de-posited in small droplets, generally in the line of the longitudinal fibrillæ of the cell. In the severer affections the whole muscle fiber may be full of fat. The change often begins with cloudy swelling, but while acetic acid and potassium hydrate have the power of restoring a cloudy cell to its normal appearance, these agents have no effect on fat globules. Osmic acid, however, stains the fat black, and Sudan III, a yellow or carmine red. At first, the transverse striation of the cells is readily made out, but tends to become obscured the more advanced the degeneration. The condition may affect the whole heart, one side of it, or one side of the wall of a cavity.

Macroscopically, the muscle is soft, friable, and of a pale color, the degenerated portion showing up as yellowish streaks or specks, by preference on the endocardium, the papillary muscles, and in the wall of the left ventricle. In well-marked cases the muscle has a mottled appearance—the so-called *"thrush-breast"* heart.

In advanced fatty change, when there is anemia as well, the heart muscle is very pale and of a yellowish white or clay color. In this state it is soft and cuts like cheese.

The main causes of fatty degeneration are general, that is to say, those acting through the circulation, and local.

The infectious fevers, particularly typhoid, and diphtheria; the anemias, as pernicious anemia, and leukemia; poisons, like phosphorus, arsenic, and sulphuric acid, are the common general causes. Whether we are to regard with Virchow the fatty degeneration occurring in the infections as a sequel of a parenchymatous myocarditis is perhaps doubtful. Many cases, however, are beyond a doubt pure degenerations.

The local causes are sclerosis of the coronaries and valvular lesions. Whenever hypertrophy, dilatation, and incompetence co-exist, fatty degeneration is almost certain to be present.

Fatty degeneration also accompanies inflammation, as in acute pericarditis and acute interstitial myocarditis.

Fig. 22

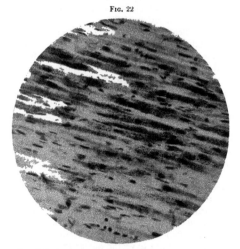

Fatty degeneration of the heart muscle. The fibers in the upper and lower portions of the field are normal. Those in the centre contain fat droplets, showing as black dots. Zeiss obj. DD, ocular No. 1. (From the Pathological Laboratory of McGill University.)

Fatty Infiltration.—Fatty infiltration is not to be confused with the last condition. In this the normal amount of fat which is present about the base of the heart and in the coronary sulci is greatly increased. The fat forces its way in between the muscle bundles and may even appear on the endocardium. While the heart may be much enlarged, it is at the same time greatly weakened, since the muscle fibers are markedly atrophic— a true pressure atrophy (*atrophia lipomatosa*). In advanced cases the front of the right ventricle and even the left may be permeated with fat, in addition to that which is present in the sulci and about the main vessels. Often the apex of the right ventricle in cross-section shows scarcely any muscle. Obesitas cordis is frequently a manifestation of general corpulency but may occur independently.

Microscopic sections show merely masses of fat lying between the muscle bundles, which are usually paler and more yellowish brown in color than healthy muscle. The fibers are atrophic, often granular, and may show signs of fatty degeneration.

Hyaline Degeneration.—Hyaline degeneration is a glassy or waxy condition of the muscle fibers, in which they gradually lose their striation and become homogeneous, presenting a hyaline, shiny appearance not unlike amyloid, but not giving the same chemical reactions. More often the hyaline change involves areas of fibrosis.

Vitreous Degeneration.—The vitreous degeneration, which von Zenker described in the muscles, especially the recti of the abdomen, and occurring in typhoid and other infectious diseases, is probably a localized necrotic change (vol. i, p. 979). The fibers of the heart, when affected, become brittle and break up into lengths, or we may see globules of hyaline material embedded in the fiber. In the later stages, the interstitial fibrous substance proliferates, and we may find it passing in between the various muscle fragments. The change is seen mainly in the acute infections or associated with parenchymatous inflammation.

FIG. 23

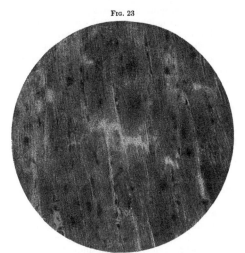

Fragmentation of the fibers of the heart. Leitz obj. No. 7, without ocular. (From the collection of Dr. A. G. Nicholls.)

Segmentation.—Segmentation of the fibers is seen in hearts that are dilated, relaxed, soft, and brittle. The individual fibers are separated and broken up into short lengths, the "myocardite segmentaire" of the French writers (Renaut, Landouzy). The parts usually affected are the septum and the papillary muscles. Many opinions have been advanced as to the nature of this condition. It occurs in cases of sudden death from acute dilatation of the heart, in prolonged muscular strain, in the various infections and intoxications, in Bright's disease, in hyaline degeneration, and, as Landry has shown at the Royal Victoria Hospital, in a large proportion of cases of aneurism of the aorta. Some think it is produced during the death agony. It can be produced **experi-**mentally by the action of digestive ferments upon the heart muscle.

Hektoen[1] recognizes two forms, true *fragmentation*, in which the muscle fiber is actually ruptured at some part of its course, and *segmentation*, in which the primitive segments of the fibers become simply dissociated. The first form is due to strain upon a weak and insufficiently acting muscle. J. B. MacCallum[2] concurs in this division and is disposed to regard segmentation as a form of "reversionary" degeneration. Both Hektoen and MacCallum regard it as of antemortem occurrence, but there are not wanting those who regard the condition as a simple artefact.

Amyloid Degeneration.—This never affects the muscle fibers, but the interstitial cement substance and the bloodvessels. It is part and parcel of a general amyloid degeneration. It is rare to find the process so extreme that it can be recognized macroscopically.

Calcification.—This is usually a terminal event in the course of myomalacia or of fibrosis, but may be part and parcel of a general lime metastasis. The deposit of lime salts which is seen so often in the thickened mitral ring in cases of mitral stenosis may encroach considerably upon the heart muscle, and we have seen one case in which a large calcareous mass in this situation all but penetrated the wall of the ventricle.

Degeneration of the Heart Ganglia.—This has been described. Putjatin found it in various chronic affections of the heart and aorta, and in syphilis. The changes were fatty and pigmentary degeneration of the ganglia, with hyperemia and productive inflammation in the neighborhood. No doubt some nutritional disturbance is at work, but the significance of the changes is not made out, farther than that serious interference with the power and function of the heart is the result.

Rupture of the Heart.—Spontaneous rupture is a rare event, and never occurs unless the heart has been weakened by disease. The most frequent causes are fatty degeneration or infiltration of the muscle and occlusion of the coronary arteries. Less commonly, myomalacia, abscess, gumma, echinococcus cyst, and new-growths are responsible. Rarely an aortic aneurism has ruptured into the auricle, as in cases reported by von Wunscheim[3] and A. McPhedran.[4] Death is usually instantaneous, but a few cases have been recorded where the patient has lived several hours or even days. Deposits of fibrin are usually found in the neighborhood of the tear, and more or less blood is effused into the pericardial sac.

PROGRESSIVE METAMORPHOSES.

Enlargement of the Heart.—This is due to *hypertrophy* or to *dilatation*, or both, affecting one or more cavities. In general hyper-

---

[1] Amer. Jour. Med. Sci., 114: 1897: 555.   [2] Jour. Exper. Med., 4: 1899: 409.
[3] Prager medizinische Wochenschrift, 18: 1893: 175.
[4] Canadian Practitioner, 21: 1896: 578.

trophy of the heart the organ has a more rounded appearance than normal, and its transverse breadth is greatly increased. The enlargement may be so great that the heart approaches that of the bullock in size—*cor bovinum.*

Fɪɢ. 24

B

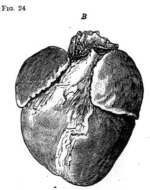

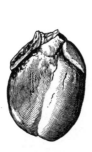

A, normal heart of rabbit; B, hypertrophied heart of rabbit due to repeated inoculations with small doses of adrenalin extending over several weeks. The adrenalin causes contraction of the arterioles, heightened blood pressure, and increased heart work. (From specimens of Dr Klotz in the McGill Pathological Museum. Natural size.)

Hypertrophy.—Hypertrophy is in most cases due to increased resistance to the heart's action, provided that the muscle is able to respond to the increased demand. Or otherwise, anything that increases the work of the heart, short of causing cardiac exhaustion, leads to hypertrophy. We may classify the causes as follows:

I. Obstruction to egress of blood.
    (*a*) Endocardial, from stenosis of one of the valves.
    (*b*) Arterial, from diminution of the arterial lumen, sclerosis, contraction of the smaller arteries, etc.
    (*c*) Pericardial, from complete synechia.

II. Increase in the volume of blood to be propelled.
    (*a*) Actual increase in the amount of circulating blood, plethora, Munich beer heart, etc.
    (*b*) From regurgitation, as in mitral and aortic incompetence.

III. Increase in rate of blood flow.
    (*a*) From tachycardia, as in exophthalmic goitre.
    (*c*) As a response to systemic needs, as in the athlete.

The chamber to be first affected is that one which first experiences the unusual strain. Thus, in arterial sclerosis, Bright's disease, and aortic endocarditis the left ventricle is the first to suffer. In pulmonary endocarditis and many lung affections (fibroid tuberculosis, emphysema, and pleuritic adhesions) where there is obstruction in the lesser circulation, it is the right.

General hypertrophy will, in time, supervene upon partial hypertrophy. It may occur from overexertion, as in excessive muscular work, hysteria, neurasthenia, prolonged mental strain, exophthalmic goitre, in pericardial synechiæ, and, very commonly, from overeating and drinking. The Munich "beer-heart" is a good example of general hypertrophy due to the prolonged overdistension of the vessels with fluid.

Fɪɢ. 25

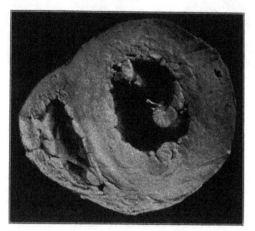

Cross-section of the heart, to show hypertrophy of the walls. The cause; increased peripheral tension. (Pathological Museum, McGill University.)

Dilatation.—Reference has been made in the preceding chapter to the distinction between (physiological) distension and (pathological) dilatation. As the hypertrophied heart becomes weaker the latter becomes manifested. Most of the causes that produce hypertrophy are competent to cause dilatation in time. It is a frequent result of sudden strain, as in prolonged races. The most frequent cause of simple dilatation is degeneration of the muscle, usually fatty, such as occurs in typhoid fever, pneumonia, and other infective fevers, and also in pernicious anemia. Acute dilatation may also be induced by alcoholic excess, and experimentally by chloroform and other agents. Local dilatation (aneurism) has already been referred to.

In dilatation the heart wall is generally thin, flabby, softer than normal, and pale in color from fatty change. The papillary muscles are thin, elongated, and the columnæ carneæ are flattened and atrophic.

The determination of the presence of **hypertrophy** is best made by consideration of the volume and weight of the heart. The organ may

FIG. 26

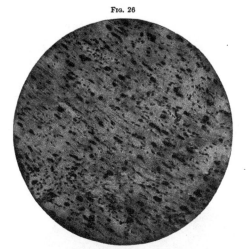

Simple hypertrophy of the heart. Leitz No. 7, without ocular. Shows large blunt-ended nuclei, occasionally dividing. (Dr. A. G. Nicholls.)

FIG. 27

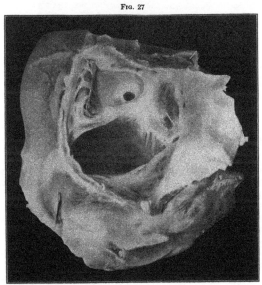

Relative dilatation of the left ventricle of the heart. Patent foramen ovale. (From the Pathological Museum of McGill University.)

weigh from 600 to 800 grams. Stokes records one of 1980 grams. The average normal thickness of the left ventricular muscle is from 15 to 20 mm., but reference to this standard only gives imperfect information, since other factors may intervene to prevent a correct conclusion being formed.

Should the right ventricle be mainly involved, the heart becomes as it were rotated on its long axis, the right side coming more to the front and the left receding from view. The heart as a whole is plumper and squarer, and the axis is broadened.

In hypertrophy of the left side rotation occurs in the opposite direction and the apex is formed mainly of the left ventricle. The heart is elongated and more conical. The papillary muscles and columnæ are correspondingly enlarged.

FIG. 28

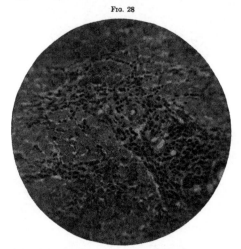

Heart muscle invaded by round-celled sarcoma.   Reichert obj. No. 7a, without ocular.
(Collection of the Royal Victoria Hospital.)

The hypertrophied muscle is of a marked brownish-red color, with often the sheen of raw ham. Its consistency is increased so that when cut it does not collapse, but remains firmly in position.

Microscopically, the muscle fibers are increased in thickness and probably in number (hyperplasia). The nuclei are very large, deeply staining, with bluntly rounded ends. Sometimes they appear to be increased in numbers. Often fatty changes in the bands can be made out.

Tumors.—Tumors of the heart can be either primary or secondary. By far the majority are due to the extension of malignant growths from neighboring parts, as the pericardium, mediastinum, lung, œsophagus, and stomach, or to metastasis.

Primary neoplasms are excessively rare. This is probably to be attributed to the fact that the heart above all organs is constantly in a state of great efficiency, well nourished, well innervated, and functionally always active, so that it is less likely to take on aberrant growth. The usual growths are **fibroma, myxoma,** and **lipoma,** the relative frequency being in the order named. These are generally subendocardial in situation, and form nodular or polypoid outgrowths, which project into the heart cavity.

Fibromas have been found in various parts of the heart. Age has nothing to do with their occurrence. One case is recorded in a child aged three months. Many of the cases are congenital, and to this class also belongs the interesting **rhabdomyoma,** of which twelve examples have been recorded.[1] These are hyperplastic growths, with stellate transversely striated muscle cells. One of them was also telangiectatic, and is, no doubt, similar to a recorded case of cavernous angioma, which probably was originally a myoma.

The secondary tumors are **carcinoma, sarcoma, lymphosarcoma, melanosarcoma,** and **osteoid sarcoma.** Metastatic growths may be found in any position, subpericardial, subendocardial, or intramural. Metastatic carcinoma is recorded, but is rarer than secondary sarcoma: of the latter, the melanomas present the most abundant metastases throughout the organ.

The results of such growths are various. When they project into a cavity, thrombosis and its attendant embolism may occur; fragmentation of the tumor, causing disseminated metastases; sudden death from pulmonary embolism; or, lastly, rupture of the heart.

THE ENDOCARDIUM.

The endocardium, or lining membrane of the heart, consists of a thin layer of connective tissue, containing elastic fibrillæ arranged after the fashion of a fenestrated membrane. The inner surface is covered with a single layer of flattened endothelial plates similar to those lining bloodvessels everywhere. Further, the endothelial lining of the heart is in direct continuity with that of the bloodvessels.

The valves are formed by a reduplication of this membrane in which the fibrous tissue has become somewhat thickened. In the case of the tricuspid and mitral valves, a few muscle fibers from the myocardium, together with a few small bloodvessels, pass in to the base of the valve, but the aortic and pulmonary valves are devoid of even these.

The endocardium is richly supplied with lymphatics, and the nerve-supply is from a plexus situated in the connective tissue beneath the endocardial layer.

The anatomical structure of the membrane has an important bearing upon the character of the pathological processes affecting it. Since that portion of the lining usually affected by disease is devoid or relatively devoid of bloodvessels, we get in inflammation a good example

[1] Wolbach, Jour. of Med. Research, 16:1907: 495; also, Abricossoff, Ziegler's Beiträge, 49: 1909.

of the process as it affects a non-vascular structure, and for the same reason infective processes of embolic origin are of the rarest occurrence.

Further, when erosion of the endothelium takes place, we find a deposit of blood platelets and fibrin, with resulting thrombosis.

Lastly the endocardial cells possess a marked phagocytic power.

CONGENITAL ANOMALIES.

Apart from those conditions due to intra-uterine inflammation, several malformations must be mentioned. **Fenestration** of the aortic and pulmonary similunar valves is so common that it need only be referred to. An **abnormal shape** of the valves, owing to a loss of substance on the free margin, is occasionally met with. The **number** of the cusps of the aortic and pulmonary valves may be diminished, or increased to four or even five. The pulmonary valve is the more apt to be affected. A perfect additional cusp may be inserted, or there may be merely a septum attaching the free border of the cusp to the ring, thus dividing it into two portions. When an extra cusp is inserted it may be only one-half the height of the others. Such reduplication is not excessively rare Three instances have been met with by us in 1500 autopsies, and two more are recorded by Powell White.[1] Three instances of reduplication of the aortic valves was also met with in our series. Complete doubling of the left atrioventricular ostium with doubled mitral orifice is much rarer. Dr. M. E. Abbott figures an example from the McGill collection.[2]

Mitral stenosis and **atresia** and **bicuspid stenosis** and **atresia** are recorded.

Hematoma of Valves.—These are small bodies, the color of raspberry jelly and of pin-head size, seen most frequently along the closing edge of the mitral segments, more rarely near the edge of the aorta cusps. They are seen only in infants, disappearing in childhood. According to Kaufmann, they represent unused remains of the (vascular) nodes or eminences from which the valves are developed. Wegelin,[3] in a quite recent publication, points out that in the course of development small pockets lined with endothelium are formed on the ventricular aspect of the auriculoventricular valves and on the distal side of the semilunar valves. These cavities eventually become covered in by the proliferation of the endothelium to form closed sacs. Valvular hematomas are always found to be covered by endothelium, and Wegelin holds that they are formed by the extravasation of blood into the aforesaid pockets. They are not vascular ectases, as some have thought.

[1] Lancet, Lond., 2: 1898: 1194. See also Osler, Montreal General Hospital Reports, 1880.

[2] Osler and McCrae's Modern Medicine, 4:1908:394.

[3] Frankfürter Ztschrft. f. Pathol , 2: 1909: 411

CIRCULATORY DISTURBANCES.

Œdema.—Marked œdema does not occur, but a slight grade may be evidenced by a shiny gelatinous appearance of the endocardium.

Hemorrhages.—Subendocardial hemorrhages occur from blood dyscrasias, such as scurvy, morbus maculosus Werlhofii, pernicious anemia, leukemia, and in the infections, like scarlatina and smallpox. Venous hyperemia or increased arterial pressure may lead to rupture and hemorrhage. When, in consequence of inflammation, newly formed capillaries are present in the valves, plugging of these may lead to hemorrhagic infarction of the segments.

Blood Imbibition.—A reddish staining due to blood imbibition is often met with. It is most probably a postmortem change and is specially common in septicemia and in infection with the B. Welchii.

Thrombi.—When atheromatous ulceration of the endocardium exists, or stenosis of any of the ostia, thrombi are apt to form in the cavities. These may form a dense layer over the atheromatous plaques, or may form polypoid excrescences. Occasionally a ball thrombus may be produced. This form is fairly frequently seen in the left auricle in cases of mitral stenosis. A ball thrombus may soften in the centre and form a bladder-like mass containing puriform or grumous fluid. Thrombi also occasionally calcify.

Among other causes of thrombosis may be mentioned dilatation of the heart, slowing of the blood stream, and changes in the composition of the blood. Thrombi are usually found in the right side of the heart, particularly in the appendix and near the apex, but are not uncommonly present in the left auricle. A distinction should be made between true thrombosis and the clotting of the blood that is so commonly produced at the time of death or subsequent to it (see p. 58). Postmortem clots are soft, moist, translucent, and elastic, and are of a yellowish-red, or mixed color. Extensive oily looking yellow clots are common in those diseases where leukocytosis is a marked feature, notably pneumonia. Real thrombi, however, are reddish gray, dry, friable, and opaque. They are generally firmly adherent to the endocardium, which often shows some pathological change.

The thrombi produced *intra vitam* are of grave significance, as they may lead to obstruction of the valvular orifices or to emboli in distant parts. Ewart and Rolleston[1] have reported a case where a thrombus arising from the fossa ovalis passed through the mitral orifice and gave rise to signs of mitral stenosis.

INFLAMMATIONS.

Endocarditis.—Inflammatory changes in the endocardium may affect any portion of it, the valves, the tendinous cords, the papillary

[1] Clinical Society's Transactions, 30: 1897: 190.

muscles, or the mural lining. The valvular form is by far the commonest, and is often associated with inflammation of the neighboring heart wall. For the mural endocardium to be alone affected is one of the greatest rarities.

Acute Endocarditis.—Primary endocarditis is said to occur, and does no doubt from a clinical point of view, but careful search post mortem often reveals an external cause for the condition, so that from pathological experience we must believe that every case is secondary to some other condition, such as intoxication or infection. Indeed, it may even be doubted whether intoxication has any influence except as a predisposing cause, and whether all acute cases are not due to bacterial invasion.

Repeated studies have proved that the cases usually classed as "simple" are due to microörganisms. Consequently, the old division of endocarditis into "simple" and "ulcerative" no longer holds good except for convenience of description, for these terms merely represent grades in the one process.

Etiologically, the condition cannot be regarded as a distinct entity, for a great variety of microörganisms enter into its causation. Strictly speaking, it is more correct to speak of a pneumococcus or streptococcus infection, etc., with endocarditis.

Acute endocarditis may occur as a secondary manifestation in the following diseases: chorea, inflammatory rheumatism, septicemia, pneumonia, scarlatina, tonsillitis, erythema nodosum, peliosis rheumatica, Bright's disease, diabetes, pyelonephritis, tuberculosis, smallpox, typhoid, gonorrhœa, and malignant growths. That overstrain is a possible cause is to some extent supported by experimental evidence.[1]

The bacteria at work are numerous and the infection may be mixed. The chief organisms are Diplococcus pneumoniæ, Streptococcus parvus, Streptococcus pyogenes, and Staphylococcus pyogenes aureus; but B. coli, B. diphtheriæ, B. influenzæ, B. pyocyaneus, gonococcus, B. tuberculosis, Micrococcus endocarditidis rugatus, Micrococcus endocarditidis capsulatus, and B. endocarditidis griseus, have been met with.

Endocarditis due to the Gonococcus is now well recognized, although many cases occurring in gonorrhœa are the result of secondary infection with pus organisms. Thayer and Lazear[2] have analyzed sixteen cases. The lesions usually are ulcerative with large vegetations, and the aortic valve may be affected.

A peculiarity of endocarditis that deserves mention is its tendency to relapse. Atheromatous valves are also liable to become inflamed. Statistics show that acute inflammation supervenes on chronically sclerosed valves in from 60 to 90 per cent.

With regard to the frequency with which the various valves are involved, Washbourn[3] refers to 309 cases of infective endocarditis; the

[1] Roy and Adami, Brit. Med. Jour., 2:1888:1325.
[2] Johns Hopkins Hospital Bulletin, 7: 1896: 57.
[3] The Pathology of Infectious Endocarditis, British Medical Journal, 2:1899: 1269.

mitral was alone affected in 115, the aortic and mitral together in 73, the aortic in 69, the tricuspid in 28, the pulmonary in 19.

Acute Granulating Endocarditis.—Acute granulating endocarditis, sometimes called simple or rheumatic endocarditis, is produced by the invasion of the endothelial and subendothelial cells by bacteria reaching these tissues from the blood stream. The germs are, no doubt, taken up by the phagocytic action of the endothelial cells and soon spread to the deeper parts, where they produce swelling and coagulation necrosis of

FIG. 29

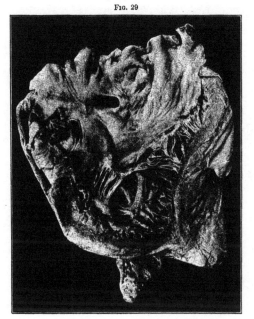

Acute verrucose endocarditis affecting the mitral valve. The efflorescence of granulation tissue is seen as a dark band along the closing surface of the mitral cusps. (From the Pathological Museum of McGill University.)

the affected region. This process begins on the closing surface of the valve, and at first leads to a grayish, condensed appearance. The endothelium is soon shed, and as a result a thrombus, formed at first of blood platelets, but ultimately of leukocytes and fibrin, is produced. This results in the formation of warty excrescences or granulations (**endocarditis verrucosa**), either as small nodules, or villous or polypoid outgrowths (**vegetative endocarditis**) that may reach the size of a plum. These are particularly large in pneumococcus and gonorrhœal cases. Subsequently, the intimal cells proliferate and there is an exudation of leukocytes. This is a late event in the case of the aortic and pulmonary valves, as they do nót contain bloodvessels, but may be a marked feature in the mitral and tricuspid forms from an early stage. New bloodvessels may be formed and grow into the exudation, so that typical granulation tissue is produced.

That the infection may take place through infective emboli in the bloodvessels of a valve is said by some to occur, but Orth, in a wide experience, has never met with an instance of it, although it is certainly

FIG. 30

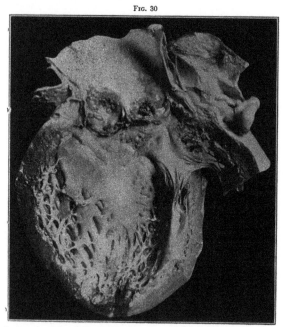

Acute ulcerative endocarditis, affecting the aortic valve and the wall of the left ventricle.
(From the Pathological Museum of McGill University.)

possible in relapsing cases, when new vessels have been formed in the cusps.· Welch has pointed out the striking similarity between the endocarditic process and venous thrombosis.

In very severe cases the necrotic process is in excess of the reparative. When this is the case, if the granulations be broken off, we often see little areas of suppuration in the affected valve (**endocarditis pustulosa**). This leads to actual ulceration with necrosis, rupture, or perforation of the valve, and the formation of an acute valvular aneurism.

The characteristics of **endocarditis ulcerosa acuta** are that a part of the valve is destroyed while the remainder shows signs of a fresh inflammatory process. The process reminds one of pharyngeal diphtheria, and in its earlier stages might easily be overlooked. The first stage is a small, somewhat opaque, yellow patch, with a slightly uneven surface. In other parts such a patch may show a distinct loss of substance. Upon these shallow ulcers reddish-gray thrombotic masses are deposited, which may attain considerable size. If the clot be carefully removed, the tissue beneath is seen to be swollen, ulcerated, and of a yellowish color.

Microscopically, such a section would reveal in the fibrinous deposit countless bacteria. The tissue about the microörganisms shows coagulation necrosis with loss of the nuclei. Later on in the process there is a definite leukocytic infiltration of the necrosing parts. In relapsing cases we often see newly formed capillaries distended with blood, and frequently hemorrhage into the inflamed area. True suppuration in this form is decidedly rare.

The affection may spread to the base of the valve, to the tendinous cords, or to the endocardium of the ventricular and even of the auricular wall.

An unbroken continuity of the inflammatory process is not necessary, as the inflamed areas may be sporadic in their distribution. This is due to the vegetations on the valve coming in contact with the heart wall during the movements of the heart, thus bringing about a direct infection. In the milder forms, healing may take place with fibroblastic change and calcification. Generally, however, the condition leads sooner or later to death.

One of the results of acute endocarditis may be that small portions of the thrombi may break loose and cause infarction in the brain, spleen, or kidneys. These are the more dangerous if they contain microorganisms, for in this way miliary metastatic abscesses are produced. Besides the production of incompetence or stenosis of a valve, already referred to, the inflammation may spread to the myocardium or even the pericardium, and sometimes leads to abscess of the heart and rupture.

Chronic Endocarditis.—There are, etiologically, two conditions which, since their end results are very similar, have until the last few years been regarded as one process under the common heading of Chronic Endocarditis. These are chronic endocarditis proper or secondary sclerosis, and primary or work sclerosis.

Secondary Sclerosis.—It is the outer non-vascular portions of the valves, along the proximal margin of the line of apposition of the cusps, that, with rare exceptions, become the primary seat of acute inflammation. And, to repeat, the succession of events occurring in the inflamed areas is identical with that seen in the cornea and other non-vascular areas, with, in addition, a marked liability to the formation of thrombotic vegetations upon the ulcerated surfaces. Thus, save when the process assumes a rapid, progressively destructive type, there occurs a vascularization of the cusps, and later a new-growth of fibrous cicatricial tissue in the region of the previous ulcer; this, in part through proliferation of the connective tissue of the deep layers of the cusps in part through organization of the thrombi. The result, therefore. of a single localized focus of ulcerative inflammation is a local fibrosis with some contraction of the involved area of the cusp.

Thus, localized cicatricial areas may surely be ascribed to previous inflammation. The cusp so affected, becoming deformed, is relatively weakened, and at the same time subject to increased strain in the performance of normal function. Hence, in the first place, as a *locus minoris resistentiæ*, it is more liable to succumb to a second infection if pathogenic agents again appear in the circulation, and hence, more particularly in acute rheumatism, in which recurrent infection is peculiarly liable to occur, we are apt to find indications, clinical and anatomical, that the

Fig. 31

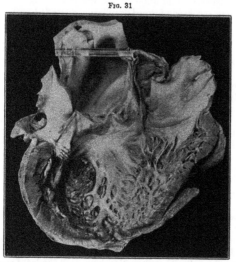

Calcareous infiltration of the aortic valves, with regurgitation. Dilatation of the left ventricle: atrophy of the columnæ carneæ. (From the Pathological Museum of McGill University.)

same valve (most often the mitral) has been the seat of repeated attacks of inflammation, and, as a consequence, exhibits extensive fibrosis and deformity. In the second place the deformed valve cannot function normally: the new tissue is not the equivalent of the old: now under what for a normal valve are normal conditions it is subjected to strain, and the result is that complicating the inflammatory sclerosis, there is a marked liability for adaptive or work sclerosis to show itself of the type to be described immediately. It is this frequent combination in the same cusp of the two types that renders it difficult in case after case to distinguish the sequence of events.

Primary Sclerosis.—In discussing the nature of arteriosclerosis in Chapter VIII. it will be demonstrated that the pronounced fibroid thickening of the intima of the arteries seen in this condition is the direct result of increased strain to which this layer may become subjected: that, in brief, increased work within physiological limits leads to increased growth of connective tissue, as of other cells of the organism. That strain, we shall show, may be brought about by either actual or relative increase in the blood pressure. Now, accompanying this condition of arteriosclerosis we encounter time and again an identical condition of, more particularly, the aortic valves, although in succession all the valves may come to show the same changes. (These valves, it must be remembered, are merely folds of the vascular intima.) Namely, we find that the cusps are the seat of a diffuse fibrosis. The new tissue is laid down in orderly layers, the most superficial being the most récent; it is non-vascular; there is the greatest development in those parts of the cusps that are subjected to the greatest strain—at the bases and along the margins of apposition of the aortic cusps; along the areas of apposition of the mitral cusps; the deeper layers like those of the sclerosed intima are apt to exhibit hyaline degeneration necrobiosis or atheroma, calcification and ulceration. The process is identical with what we find in arteriosclerosis, and just as in that condition we conclude that the intimal changes are non-inflammatory, so we cannot but conclude that this type of valve thickening is equally non-inflammatory.

But now, just as in the inflammatory type, a strain sclerosis is apt to supervene, so it has to be recognized that in this there may be secondary inflammatory disturbances. The valves are abnormal and so more liable to irritation. Thus, it is not uncommon to find the aortic cusps undergoing fusion along their opposed angles.

In both forms of sclerosis we find certain common features. The new connective tissue manifests the characteristic tendency of new connective tissue in general to undergo contraction, hence the aortic and pulmonary cusps undergo shortening along their free edges, with resulting incompetence. It is usual to state that the mitral cusps undergo fusion. This is a false conception. The mitral and the tricuspid do not possess distinct cusps: they form a veil or tube hanging into the ventricular cavity, which veil is now longer, now shorter, but continuous around its whole circumference. The length of the different portions varies considerably in different individuals. When there is fibrosis and contraction, it depends upon the relative proportions of the different sections whether there develops a funnel-shaped or a button-hole stenosis, the latter occurring when the short areas joining the longer so-called cusps are of small dimensions.

In both forms also, degenerative changes, calcification and atheromatous ulceration, may show themselves, as also the chordæ tendineæ may undergo thickening and contraction, the latter at times so extreme that the cusps appear to be inserted upon the apices of the papillary muscles.

Tuberculosis.—The occurrence of simple (so-called) endocarditis in connection with tuberculosis elsewhere is not uncommon in our experience. True tuberculous lesions of the valves are, however, rare.

Miliary tubercles have been seen on the valves in cases of general miliary affection, but such are more common on the mural endocardium about the conus arteriosus pulmonalis. The specific bacilli have been detected in the lesions. The experimental work of Michaelis and Blum has demonstrated the possibility of this form.

Syphilis is also rare.

Traumatism.—Rupture of one of the cusps of the healthy aortic valve is recorded, but, as would be expected, is more often found in a diseased valve. It is due to excessive muscular strain. The tendinous cords may give way from the same cause.

ALTERATIONS IN THE SIZE OF THE OSTIA.

Tricuspid Valve.—**Stenosis.**—Stenosis of the tricuspid valve may be congenital or acquired. The congenital form is due either to a defect

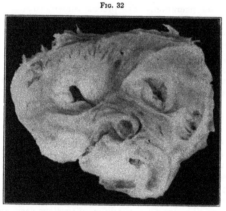

Heart viewed from above, showing stenosis of aortic, mitral, and pulmonary ostia. (From the Pathological Museum of McGill University.)

of development or to fœtal endocarditis. It is rare for the tricuspid to be alone affected. Usually mitral stenosis exists as well; less frequently both mitral and aortic stenosis are present. Rarely, an adherent thrombus may obstruct the passage.

Insufficiency.—Insufficiency is usually caused by relative dilatation of the right ventricle owing secondarily to mitral lesions and to affections that increase the vascular tension within the lung, such as emphysema and fibroid induration. Primary insufficiency due to endocarditis is not common.

Pulmonary Valve.—**Stenosis.**—Stenosis of the pulmonary ostium is almost invariably congenital, and is generally associated with grave defects of development, such as patent ductus Botalli or imperfect septum. Rarely, in endocarditis, a thrombus may more or less completely occlude the opening.

Insufficiency.—Insufficiency is excessively rare. It may occur from rupture of an acute aneurism of the valve, or from other manifestations of endocarditis.

Mitral Valve.—Stenosis.—Stenosis is nearly always caused by endocarditis, and is usually combined with insufficiency. As a rule, the obstruction is brought about by the fusion of the valve segments, together with calcification, so that a narrow orifice is produced. An adherent thrombus upon one of the cusps may produce a similar effect. Not only does the thickening and fusion of the cusps lead to obstruction, but, owing to the impossibility of closure, leakage is a common result. The relationship between the stenosis and regurgitation varies considerably in different cases.

Insufficiency.—Insufficiency may be due to loss of substance of the cusps, retraction, or dilatation of the ventricle (*relative insufficiency*).

Aortic Valve.—Stenosis.—Pure aortic stenosis is rare. It is due in part to the fusion of the semilunar valves or to narrowing of the aortic ring, but the most important element is the deposit of lime salts in the cusps and ring. This prevents the proper collapse of the cusps during systole. Aortic stenosis is commonly associated with insufficiency.

Aortic Insufficiency.—Insufficiency may be due to ulceration and loss of substance of the valve or to the contraction that results from chronic endocarditis. Rarely, it is due to rupture of a cusp. Relative insufficiency is not very uncommon, and is usually secondary to dilatation of the left ventricle, or to dilatation of the first part of the aorta from atheroma or aneurism.

The Lesions Associated with Valvular Disease.—In acute endocarditis the heart muscle is invariably affected to some extent, owing to the action of the same toxic cause. We find not only cloudy and fatty degeneration of the fibers, but also in some cases acute interstitial myocarditis, and hyaline thrombi in the smaller vessels. Again, acute pericarditis may be set up. This is more frequent in children, and is most likely to occur in aortic endocarditis, for the reason that there is but a small distance between the valve and the pericardial sac, viz. the thickness of the aortic wall. It is fairly common at autopsy to find in cases of endocarditis fine adhesions at the upper cul-de-sac of the pericardium. Small portions of the vegetations may break off and give rise to embolism in remote organs, or, if infective, to multiple abscesses.

In the case of chronic endocarditis, changes in the heart wall are often marked. In the degenerative and sclerotic form, the coronaries are apt to be affected from the same cause, leading to myodegeneration In aortic insufficiency, owing to the imperfect filling of the aorta, the blood pressure within the coronaries is diminished, and, in consequence the heart becomes atrophic. Banti has also pointed out that venous stasis within the heart causes degeneration of the muscle bands and interstitial fibrosis, a condition that he terms venous cirrhosis. A most important result of valvular affections is hypertrophy and dilatation of the heart muscle and cavities. The mechanics of this, however, has been discussed fully in another place (see p. 129).

RETROGRESSIVE METAMORPHOSES.

Degenerations.—**Fatty Degeneration.**—Fatty degeneration appears in the form of slightly elevated scattered patches of a yellowish-white color upon the valves, less frequently on the mural endocardium. These are due to the transformation of the protoplasm of the connective tissue and endothelial cells into fat. In advanced cases, fat droplets may be seen in the spaces between the connective-tissue cells. The condition is met with usually in elderly people, but is not very uncommon younger individuals, in cases of marasmus, anemia, valvular disease, intoxications, and infections. The first stage of atheroma is fatty change.

Mucoid Degeneration.—Mucoid degeneration occurs particularly in advanced life and almost without exception upon the valves. Circumscribed nodules of gelatinous appearance at the closing edge of the valve are of this nature. They may contain true myxoma cells or may be merely masses of gelatinous substance. The condition is often associated with fatty degeneration.

Hyaline Degeneration.—This is met with in the valve segments or mural endocardium as a late transformation of connective tissue.

Calcification.—A deposit of lime salts is not infrequent in atheromatous processes in the valves, or as a result of chronic valvular endocarditis. The formation of *cartilage* or *bone* in a valve is rare.

Amyloid Disease.—Amyloid disease not infrequently affects the subendocardial connective tissue under the same conditions as elsewhere. It is often combined with hyaline degeneration.

PROGRESSIVE METAMORPHOSES.

Tumors have already been dealt with under the heading "Myocardium." Kanthack and Pigg[1] have recorded a unique case in which a carcinoma of the testis, or, more accurately, a teratogenous blastoma (see vol. i, p. 660), formed secondary growths lying free in the right heart and inferior vena cava.

[1] Trans. Path. Soc., London, 48:1897:1391.

CHAPTER VIII.

THE VESSELS. VASCULAR FUNCTION AND ITS DISTURBANCES.

WE are apt to repeat glibly that the arteries are composed of three coats—intima, media, and adventitia—and with this to regard the whole arterial tree as uniform throughout, save that the constituents of the different coats become progressively reduced as we pass from the aorta to the arterioles. Undoubtedly there is a certain amount of truth in this general conception, but undoubtedly, also, we have thus far allowed the view to prevail too fully, to a neglect of the study of the histology of individual arteries. We still need, for example, more exact information regarding the extent and variations in the deeper musculo-elastic layer of the intima, to which Jores has called attention, and, as Meigs points out, until we study the arteries of different regions not under various degrees of contraction as we encounter them in the usual run of post-mortem tissue, but uniformly expanded (and this has not been done), we obtain wholly false ideas as to the relative development of the different layers.

Failing such exact study, we have to content ourselves with laying down that the arteries may be divided into the two broad groups of those of the elastic type, and of the muscular, respectively. The presence of abundant layers of yellow elastic tissue such as we find characteristically in the aorta and its main branches connotes two things: (1) That the vessel is capable of undergoing passive dilatation up to a certain point, and of returning passively to the normal when the distending force is removed; and (2) that only with difficulty can it be contracted beyond a certain mean, the very elasticity of the tissue acting as a counteracting force against obliteration or collapse of the vessel. Here it may be noted that the wrinkled, wavy appearance of the internal elastic lamina, the "plicated" membrane, or, as the French term it, the "bandelette," of medium-sized arteries is a postmortem appearance, due to rigor and contraction of the muscle coat. This appearance, of course, must be reproduced when the arterial muscle is contracted, but be absent in the uncontracted vessel. As we shall have to note later, even in arteries of the elastic type, there is fairly abundant muscle in the form of layers between the elastic sheaths which must play a part in modifying the caliber. It is generally accepted that this musculature, from the beginning of the aorta down to the smallest arterioles, has the property of automatic contraction similar to that possessed by the heart muscle. It is at the other extreme, in the arterioles, that the muscular sheath is most prominent, the elastic least.[1]

Very slight changes in the tonus of the small arteries of the body must induce great changes in the stream bed, and must materially alter the volume of the blood passing through the vessels and the presence of the same.

So far as we can see, capillary contraction must be left out of account as a primary factor in causing rise of blood pressure. With Meltzer and Leonard Hill we are prepared to admit that the capillaries possess some power of contraction; we doubt, however, whether this is sufficiently great to be of any effect when the arterioles are uncontracted and supply blood to the capillary area at relatively high pressure; only when the arterioles are contracted and the blood supply low does it appear possible that the contraction can be effective. It is by capillary contraction under those conditions that we would explain the rather striking pallor of the ordinary arteriosclerotic individual.[2] The size of the capillaries, that is, depends in the main upon the amount of arterial blood supply on the one hand, the venous pressure on the other. At the same time, the capacity of the capillary system is so much greater than that of the arterioles, that were the latter generally dilated, the free passage of blood into the wider capillary channels would almost immediately empty the arterial tree and bring the circulation to a stop by the individual bleeding into his own capillaries. We know that this may happen when dilatation occurs merely of the arteries of the splanchnic area. The muscular arterioles, then, as guarding the gateway into the capillaries, are, with the heart, the main agents in maintaining the circulation; and, as a rule, through the marvellously developed vasomotor apparatus, they act in absolute harmony with the heart on the one hand, with the needs of individual organs on the other. Now one, now another organ may demand a larger blood supply, and presumably in the main, through reflex stimulation, the arteries to that organ undergo dilatation, but with this, presumably also in the main under the control of the vasomotor centres, other arteries contract, and thus a mean arterial blood pressure of about 120 mm. Hg is preserved with great regularity.

[1] It may well be that the size of a plain muscle fiber relative to the caliber of a vessel determines to some extent the need or lack of need of an elastic-tissue framework; that in an arteriole, for example, the range of contraction of a muscle fiber relative to the load that fiber has to bear (namely, to the blood pressure) may be such that there is little danger of overextension of the muscle; that, in short the presence of elastic tissue in the aorta and larger arteries is a factor of safety, preventing excessive strain on the muscular elements of the wall. In a small artery a very slight expansion or contraction of the circular fibers will induce a relatively great alteration in the size of the lumen, altogether out of proportion to the change in size of the large aorta produced by the same extent of contraction of its musculature.

[2] With prolonged reduction of blood supply to a part we should expect to obtain a venous congestion owing to the lack of *vis a tergo;* this, characteristically, is wanting in the arteriosclerotic as contrasted with the sufferer from Raynaud's disease.

Everyone is familiar with the existence of vasoconstrictor and vaso-dilator nerves; we need not here enter into a description of their action; what is important is to determine whether these alone determine the contraction and expansion of the arteries. The indications are that we have the identical problem before us that we had in connection with the heart. There is evidence, that is, that besides the central nervous control exerted from centres in the bulb, there exists a system of nerve cells with processes tending to form a plexus in the arterial wall, and further, that the muscle fibers of the media are capable of direct stimulation. Cut through the nerve supply of a limb, and immediately the arteries lose their tone and dilate, but eventually, although still unconnected with the central nervous system, they regain their tone. There is one very important series of arteries in which no one has yet been able to discover any proper vasomotor system—namely, the cerebral arteries. At most, individual nerve cells are to be made out in the arterial walls, provided with processes; from which it would appear that these cerebral vessels possess a self-regulating apparatus—that the condition of the brain matter and the nature of the circulating blood determine the blood flow through them. The indications are that the brain is superior to all other organs, and that it governs its own blood supply untrammelled by vasomotor interference from other parts.

The above conditions might be determined through the local nerve mechanism. On the other hand, we know how rapidly nerve cells die when cut off from their blood supply or when removed from the living body. Now, as MacWilliam has shown, the larger arteries removed from the body after death respond to direct stimuli, and are capable of a strong contraction many hours after death. More precise data to the same effect have been supplied by Brodie and Dixon,[1] who have shown that the vasoconstrictor nerves to the limbs are no longer irritable three hours after death, while six hours after death the arteries still contract under the influence of adrenalin. This indicates independent contractibility of the arterial muscle fibers in response to direct stimuli. We will not here discuss the finer points brought out by those observers, Ellicott[2] and H. H. Dale, as to the existence of modes of stimulation through the neuromuscular junction and through the muscle substance proper. Adrenalin, pituitary extract, and ergot have all been shown to act directly upon the arterial muscle, and judging from the similarity of their effects, the same is true of a large number of other bodies, barium chloride, nicotine, etc. We must accept, therefore, all three modes of stimulation as inducing contraction of the arterial muscle, giving the place of honor, in normal conditions, to control from the vasomotor centres. It is this that determines the dilatation with profound lowering of the blood pressure seen in syncope and shock. Whether it is the essential cause of general relaxation of the arteries, with lowering of the blood pressure seen in the acute fevers, is still a matter of some debate.

[1] Jour. of Physiol., 30: 1904: 494.
[2] Ibid., 32: 1905: 401

That relaxation may show itself early in a fever is evidenced by the dicrotic pulse, and then it may be accompanied by no weakening of the heart action, but, if anything, by the very reverse. It has to be admitted from the experiments of Roger and others that different bacterial toxins act in different degrees upon the different segments of the coördinating apparatus; some, like the diphtheria toxin, appear to act directly upon the heart, others directly upon the arterial wall. But the general trend at he present time, strongly supported by the experiments of Romberg and his pupils, is to lay the greatest stress upon the direct action of the bacterial toxins upon the vasomotor centres in the medulla. The opposite condition of vasocontraction has, of late years, attracted not a little notice, and that from a clinical point of view. The indications are that arterial spasm—prolonged extreme contraction of the arteries of individual areas—is a not uncommon condition. To this condition and its results we have referred in discussing Raynaud's disease. Pal[1] more particularly has studied the vascular crises affecting the splanchnic vessels; Osler and others, the contracture of arteries of the lower extremities leading to **intermittent claudication** or limping, due to the sudden cutting off of blood supply and muscular anemia. As Sir Lauder Brunton indicates, arterial contraction probably plays an important part in a very common form of migraine known at times as "bilious headache." In this form, with the development of premonitory symptoms, the blood pressure is found distinctly raised well above the normal, and it continues to rise. Such rise can only be due to arterial or arteriolar contraction, and, as a matter of fact, superficial arteries, like the temporals, can be seen firm, contracted, and whipcord-like. When the condition has become almost unendurable, and the patient finds himself thoroughly exhausted, the attack passes off, the headache disappears, the pulse becomes soft, the circulation resumes its normal condition. In such cases there would seem to have been not merely a local, but a general vascular crisis; it is difficult to explain the raised blood pressure otherwise. How this is brought about we cannot positively say; those liable to the condition know full well that certain errors in diet surely invoke this Nemesis. It is possible, on the one hand, that certain products of imperfect metabolism or other poisons act generally on the arteries, but the direct action of the same on the vasoconstrictor centres would equally explain.

Here, leading up to the consideration of arteriosclerosis and its causation, a phenomenon must be noted which has been emphasized by Leonard Hill—namely, the paradox that arteries tend not to expand but to contract under heightened internal pressure, and this so immediately that the contraction must be a local reaction, not reflex. When in conjunction with this we realize that the smaller the circumference of the artery the greater is the effect of the contraction of the muscle cells upon the reduction of the arterial lumen and the diminution of the blood stream, we are led to see that this phenomenon leads to the establishment

[1] Pal, Gefässkrisen, Leipz., 1905. S. Hirzel.

of a vicious cycle. The higher the blood pressure, the greater becomes the contraction of the arterioles; the less, therefore, the blood supply to the tissues and the greater the call upon the central nervous system for more blood. Whether from reflex stimulation of the heart to increased activity in order to supply the tissues, or from direct automatic action of the increased aortic pressure in raising the intraventricular pressure, and so stimulating the ventricles to more forcible contraction, the blood pressure becomes yet higher, and, as a result, the arteries still further contracted. It is along these lines that we would explain the progressive rise of blood pressure and contraction of the smaller arteries in migraine. In this order of cases we must suppose that the eventual result is a veritable spasm of the arteries, which continues until the muscle fibers become exhausted, dilate, and cause lowering of the blood pressure and return to the normal. That exhaustion is the only means whereby, in general, the blood pressure, once raised, becomes reduced, we do not for a moment mean to suggest. These vascular crises are the exception and not the rule; there must be other reflexes; must, for example, be the means of pouring into the blood substances which neutralize the agents causing arterial contraction and high blood pressure in the first place. But in this class of cases these opposing agencies must be either inadequate or temporarily inhibited. The studies on the ductless glands have demonstrated that the system produces both internal secretions, which raise the blood pressure (*e. g.*, products of the activity of the adrenal and pituitary bodies), and others which, on the contrary, reduce it (*e. g.*, the thyroid extract). At most, what we desire to emphasize here is that *arterial contraction, and particularly a generalized arteriolar contraction, is the primary cause of heightened blood pressure.* It would require a very much greater increase in force and frequency of the cardiac contractions to raise and maintain the blood pressure that we ordinarily encounter if, with rise of blood pressure, the arteries underwent a corresponding dilatation. The drugs which characteristically cause heightened blood pressure of any duration act by contracting the arterioles.

Clinically, what is a more common event than arterial spasm is a persistent rise of blood pressure, or state of "hyperpiesis," as Sir Clifford Allbutt has termed it. In this, for long periods the blood pressure, instead of being in the neighborhood of 120 mm. Hg, is raised to 180, 200, or 250 mm. Hg., or even higher. It is this continued rise of blood pressure, due as we have said to increased contraction of the arterioles, that is the commonest precursor of arteriosclerosis.

ARTERIOSCLEROSIS.

Strange to say, for that which, in civilized lands among those attaining adult life, is the commonest of all morbid states, we possess no adequate and comprehensive name. It is a condition in which evidently the arteries are primarily involved, and what is the most obvious lesion is a fibrotic thickening of the intima, whence the term arterio-sclerosis has obtained wide acceptance. It is, however, doubtful whether sclerosis (hardening) is the essential change, and certainly the later stages in the larger vessels are of the nature of a softening and degeneration; whence Marchand has suggested the name *atherosis*, and this is being widely taken up by German workers. But here again the "ἀθήρη," or porridgy state of intimal degeneration, only affects the larger arteries, and is a secondary and not a primary condition. The name given thirty years ago by Gull and Sutton of "arteriocapillary fibrosis" is quite as defensible, and that because a fibrosis of the arterioles characterizes the most important group of cases, and has a very clear relationship to the development of the changes seen in the larger vessels. We shall speak of general arteriosclerosis, waiting for some thoroughly satisfactory name to be proposed in the future.

More accurately there are two main causes of arteriosclerosis, either (1) increased strain thrown upon the arterial wall by heightened blood pressure, or (2) a weakened state of the wall, either from congenital causes or from disease of the same. If the pressure be normal but the walls weakened, the results are of the same order as when the pressure is heightened but the walls of normal resisting power. It is the lack of recognition of this central fact that is at the bottom of the confusion that has reigned all these years regarding the etiology of arteriosclerosis. It is not high pressure alone that causes arteriosclerosis; that condition may show itself without rise of blood pressure above the normal; but it is *the ratio between the resisting powers of the vessel wall and the pressure to which they are subjected from within*. If this be accepted, then, secondly, we are forced to realize that *the arterial tree is by no means necessarily equally resistant in all its parts*. In some individuals, whether from hereditary or acquired conditions, the aortic wall is relatively weak compared with the walls of the smaller vessels; in them the aorta may become affected when there is little or no change in the smaller arteries or arterioles. In others the aorta is resistant and the smaller arteries weak and apt to show arteriosclerotic change. In others the change is universal—although in these the series of alterations seen in the smaller vessels are from a histological point of view wholly different from those seen in the aorta.

Before going farther and adducing the observations upon which these statements are based, it becomes essential to describe briefly the changes seen in arteriosclerosis of arteries of different size, that the series of changes to which we must refer may be clearly understood.

Aortic Arteriosclerosis.—The slightest change observable in the aorta is the appearance of small streaks in the intima, opaque, white, fatty looking, and tending in general to a longitudinal arrangement. They are most common in those dying from infection and acute intoxication. Microscopic examination shows that they are not, as usually considered, confined to the endothelium, but represent a fatty degeneration of the deepest layer of the intima, the musculo-elastic layer. Their arrangement and position makes us doubt whether these "fatty streaks" bear any relationship to the series of changes to be presently noted constituting arteriosclerosis proper.

Besides these, as demonstrated by Klotz and confirmed by Saltykow, certain bacteria and their toxins lead to a definite proliferation of the aortic endothelium and intima—a true proliferative intimitis. Again, we are doubtful whether this should be regarded as a true arteriosclerosis, or, more accurately, we lack evidence that this intimal thickening proceeds onward to afford the familiar picture of the atheromatous aorta. The typical arteriosclerotic aorta shows changes which, to the naked eye, characteristically affect the intima. That undergoes a notable thickening, not uniform but nodose, although in advanced cases the thickened plaques may be so close that they fuse into large areas. In these plaques we observe a succession of stages. The slightest cases are those of either proliferation of the superficial layers of the intima, forming a layer of dense fibrous tissue, the fibers running parallel to the surface, or of a somewhat similar proliferation of the deeper, musculo-elastic layer of the intima, not so purely fibrous, but exhibiting

Fig. 33

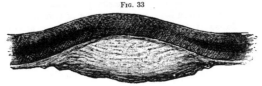

Section of the aorta from a case of nodose arteriosclerosis, to show the bulging and thinning of the media, prepared by Dr. Mathewson. × 8 diameters. The section shows also the hyaline degeneration of the deeper layers of the overgrown intima, and the persistence of a fine layer of less altered intima tissue immediately beneath the media. The media in this case showed evidences of calcareous degeneration in patches with some hyaline change.

also a proliferation of yellow elastic tissue. In either case we deal with simple hyperplasia of the intima, with no sign of leukocytic infiltration, of new vessel formation, or of inflammation as usually accepted. More often we encounter degenerative changes in these plaques. The layers nearest to the intimal surface may show little or no change, but deeper down (1) the layers become swollen and hyaline, or (2) as a more advanced change, exhibit fatty degeneration, loss of nuclear staining, disintegration of the tissue, with presence of tablets of cholesterin; in short, evidence of necrosis and autolysis; this is the typical atheromatous material. (3) Suitably stained, as by von Kossa's method, such softened areas show also the presence of calcareous matter, and this may accumulate, becoming more and more abundant, until gritty masses and extensive brittle plates of calcification become developed. In either of these later stages the superficial, thin, but hitherto intact layer of the intima may give way and be torn off, an **atheromatous ulcer** becoming formed, shallow, and with rough necrotic floor.

These in brief are the changes undergone by the intima. Normally that intima possesses no vessels; its nutrition—and that also, we may add of the inner portion of the media—is gained in part from the aortic lumen by infiltration of the blood plasma. Obviously, with the progressive laying down of layers of dense fibrous tissue, the nourishment of the older, deeper layers becomes cut off and necrosis results. Save in syphilitic cases, it is only exceptionally that we encounter a secondary granulation process occurring in the atheromatous plaque, with entry of capillary loops from the vasa vasorum of the media, and when this is the case we meet with a distinct reparative process, absorption of the atheromatous material, and laying down of new fibrous tissue to replace that which has undergone necrosis. Where this is the case, the plaques, instead of remaining flattened, become puckered, often with an obscurely stellate depression. This puckering is, we may add, the main naked eye indication of syphilitic aortitis.

But while thus, macroscopically, the intima is the site of the most marked change in aortic arteriosclerosis, microscopic examination with the employment of suitable stains demonstrates that the media is also involved—nay, *is the seat of the primary change.* This change, so far as we have at present determined, may be of one of two orders.

Syphilitic Mesaortitis.—A frequent source of aortic arteriosclerosis in those of early middle age is syphilis. The researches of Heller and his pupils and of Chiari (which since have been abundantly confirmed in other laboratories) have proved that the primary lesion here is a small-celled or granulomatous infiltration of the media, along the course

Fig. 34

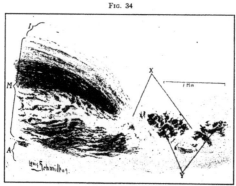

Section from aorta of syphilitic mesaortitis to show extreme degeneration of media and absorption of elastic tissue: *I*, thickened intima; *M*, media, the darkest parts being the elastic tissue. At *X* this has disappeared. At *Y*, round-celled infiltration.

of individual vasa vasorum. Klotz, Bruns,[1] and Wiesner[2] have pointed out that a similar change may be encountered in congenital syphilis. Accompanying the infiltration there is a well-marked localized atrophy

[1] Berl. klin. Woch., 8: 1906: 217.
[2] Centralb. f. allg. Path., 16: 1905: 822.

and disappearance of both elements of the medial coat, of the muscular and elastic-tissue layers, the absorption of the latter being very striking (Klotz). *This is the primary change.* The process does not extend beyond the media into the intima, but, as a secondary process, that intima undergoes proliferative thickening. It is only at a later period, when the fibrosis has given place to atheroma, that the vessels above noted extend into the necrotic area. We see here a syphilitic mesaortitis followed by intimal sclerosis and its sequelæ. As to the relationship of the syphilitic lesion to aneurism production, we shall speak later. This form of arteriosclerosis is frequently, but not necessarily, accompanied by high pressure and peripheral arterial sclerosis—frequently because your syphilitic is apt to indulge his various appetites, and if, according to Cabot, alcoholism, contrary to the general opinion, is not a cause of arteriosclerosis, all are agreed that overeating is.

Senile Degeneration of the Media and Arteriosclerosis.— Another well-marked type of aortic arteriosclerosis is the *senile*. This also is not necessarily accompanied by high pressure, and that in spite of well-marked signs of peripheral sclerosis. With advancing age the force of the heart beat becomes progressively weaker, and the blood pressure tends normally to diminish; and thus, what for a middle-aged adult would be a normal blood pressure is relatively a high pressure in an old man. The main feature is the widespread alteration in the media of the aorta and larger vessels with dilatation and tortuosity. In these cases the internal thickening of the aorta is apt to be not nodular, but more diffuse, without puckering, and whereas the syphilitic lesion has as its site of election the first part of the aorta, here we not

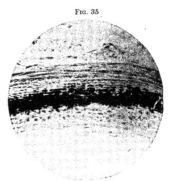

Fig. 35

Section of human aorta of elderly individual, treated by von Kossa's method, to demonstrate calcification of media, and more particularly of the muscular bands. (Klotz.)

infrequently find comparatively little intimal change in the arch, which, on the contrary, may show thinning of its wall and some diffuse enlargement; where the condition is not generalized it is the lower part of the abdominal aorta that is most involved. Working in our laboratory at the Royal Victoria Hospital, Klotz has called attention to the fact that if the aortas of those thirty-five and upward be examined—aortas not necessarily showing any sign whatever of intimal sclerosis—and if these be treated to demonstrate the existence of calcareous deposits, it is rare to encounter a section which does not show some degeneration of the media. The earliest change is in the middle layers of this coat, and then in connection with the muscle cells. These show first some fatty change, later a fine powdering with calcareous granules; later the muscle cells, as such, become indistinguishable, much shrunken, so that the elastic bands on either side become approximated, separated by a collection of the fine calcareous granules; later the elastic lamellæ exhibit also calcareous degeneration.   It is at times remarkable what extreme degencration of the media may be found in a comparatively thin and not particularly rigid aorta exhibiting none of the ordinary signs of arteriosclerosis.   These observations are in complete harmony with earlier observations upon the progressive loss of elasticity of the aorta with advancing life.   Whereas strips of the aortas of young individuals have great elasticity, there is little stretching power in strips taken from elderly individuals.   These observations of Klotz show that not only the elastica but also the muscle cells participate in the progressive degeneration.

Moenckeberg's Sclerosis.—Moenckeberg was the first to direct attention to the widespread degeneration of the media.   He was of the opinion that it was a condition quite distinct from intimal sclerosis. Now, it is quite true, as we have pointed out, that it may occur in a diffuse form without accompanying thickening of the intima; indeed, with some thinning of the same.   Indeed, it can immediately be diagnosticated in the lower abdominal aorta and the common iliacs and their branches by the development of a succession of what are truly shallow aneurismal pouches lying with their long axes transverse, with intervening ridges. But here we have, only on a somewhat larger scale, the phenomenon noted in connection with syphilis, namely, that one and the same cause now leads to intimal thickening, now to aneurism.   Why this is we shall explain later.   We would only note here that all arteriosclerosis of the senile type presents this underlying medial degeneration; that this is very common; that it involves also the middle-sized arteries in which medial calcification may be extreme; and that the "pipe-stem radial," for example, is not an example of intimal, but of medial calcification.

Nodose Aortic Sclerosis: Hyperpiesis.—It is clear that the unceasing recurrent strain of the pulse wave seventy times a minute or thereabouts, through the whole twenty-four hours, day after day, year after year, eventually wears out the elastic tissue of the aorta. The rate at which it does so varies, and undoubtedly there enters an hereditary factor, so that in some families this senile change appears at a comparatively early period, in others is long delayed; but in all, sooner or later, this loss of elasticity shows itself.   Where, in addition, there are causes leading to marked continued contraction of the arterioles, there the prolonged rise of blood pressure materially hastens the giving way of the media.   It is, we admit, difficult to draw a sharp line between the senile arteriosclerosis and the arteriosclerosis accompanying this state of hyperpiesis.   The two merge one into the other; but when clinically we encounter high blood pressure in those without syphilitic taint, there anatomically we find not so much a diffuse intimal thickening as a nodose arteriosclerosis.   And here, as Thoma was the first to lay down with precision, we find evidence of local and restricted giving way of the media.   As he showed, the first localities to give way are those of natural

weakness. Thus, the earliest regions to show the arteriosclerotic change
are at and around the mouths of the intercostal and other arteries, where
the regular order of the muscle and elastic bands of the media becomes
interrupted or pushed to one side to allow the exit of the lateral arteries.
Here, we find the intima presenting the same proliferation and fibroid
change noted in the other conditions, passing on to necrotic, and later
calcareous change in the lower layers. With this, other scattered or
sporadic, plaque-like foci of fibrosis show themselves along the length
of the aorta, and these may eventually show atheromatous change and
ulceration. That the media gives way in these cases was demonstrated
in a striking manner by Thoma. Post mortem, when the aorta is opened,

FIG. 36

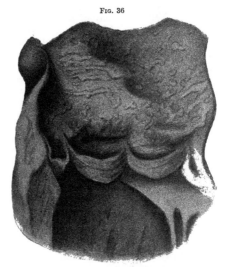

Atheromatous plaques on the lining of the aorta. (Graupner and Zimmermann.)

these nodes of intimal thickening project well above the general surface;
Thoma showed that if the recently removed aorta be filled with warm
tallow at blood pressure, and it be cooled and the aorta cut away
from the solid core of tallow, this is found perfectly cylindrical with no
depressions corresponding to the plaques; or otherwise, in life these
intimal thickenings evidently fill little bays in the media, the intimal
proliferation compensating for the giving way of the middle coat, and
the aortic lumen being thus kept of even diameter. This experiment
of Thoma's does not always succeed; there are even cases in which the
intimal thickening is in excess of the medial giving way—cases of over-
compensation; and there are those who deny that in every case the media
shows thinning at the regions corresponding to the intimal plaques.

But if in certain cases this thinning is not very obvious, appropriate staining shows often that the media at these areas is degenerated; that the thickening is only apparent, due to the elastic contraction which causes the intimal mass to be projected post mortem into the aortic lumen.

It should be added regarding the extent of necrosis and calcification that this may involve the most internal layers of the media. As already noted, the nutrition of these inner layers is, in part, at least, from the lumen of the aorta, and consequently suffers when there is this deposit of impermeable fibrous tissue in the intima. So as not to confuse the reader by the introduction of minute details, we have purposely neglected to lay stress upon the minute anatomy of the arteriosclerotic change. Many recent workers, notably Jores and Marchand and Aschoff and their schools, have paid attention to the histology of the changes here described; they have more particularly called attention to the increase in yellow elastic, as well as white connective tissue in the intima, and there has been not a little divergence regarding the respective parts played by muscular and elastic tissue degeneration in the media, the existence or non-existence of spontaneous rupture of the elastic tissue lamellæ, etc. But these matters do not modify our conception of the broad nature of the main process. To epitomize so far as concerns aortic sclerosis we have determined:

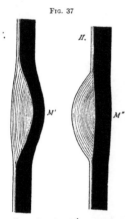

Fig. 37

I, media weakened at *M'* with overgrowth of intima filling in the depression; *II*, with postmortem rigor and contraction of the muscle of the media and removal of the blood pressure from within, the stretched media at *M''* contracts, the intimal thickening thus projecting into the arterial lumen.

1. In the vast majority of cases, if not in all, a weakness and giving way of the media is the primary anatomical lesion.

2. There is the possibility that, as the result of a subacute proliferative intimitis, due to bacteria and their toxins, the thickening of the intima, by cutting off the nutrition of the inner layers of the media, may weaken that coat, and so cause a local dilatation of the aortic lumen, followed by a secondary and further thickening of the intima; but it is also possible that the infective endaortitis which undoubtedly exists has no direct association with the general process here described, and that when, after typhoid and other infections, there develops a premature arteriosclerosis, here, again, we deal with a primary sporadic degeneration of the media, set up by the bacterial toxins.

3. The affection of the media may be either a primary degeneration without signs of preceding inflammation, or may be of inflammatory origin (as in syphilis).

4. The intimal change secondary to the medial degeneration has none of the features of an extension of the morbid process from the media, but is of a wholly different nature. It is primarily of hyperplastic type —a simple connective-tissue hyperplasia unaccompanied by the phenomena which we associate with inflammation.

Sclerosis of Arteries of the Second and Third Degree.—These same changes—syphilitic, senile, and ordinary nodose—affect also the branches of the aorta and their ramifications, but with this main difference, that only in the larger branches do we encounter anything like extensive necrosis and atheroma of the intimal thickening. These thickenings, compared with the size of the artery, may be extreme, but in absolute size they do not compare with what may be found in the aorta. The absence of necrosis is to be ascribed to the fact that in general their size is not such as to inhibit the percolation of lymph through them;

Fig. 38

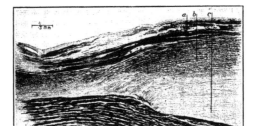

From a syphilitic aorta, showing a moderate grade of medial degeneration and giving way, to demonstrate the simple connective-tissue hyperplasia of the intima, in regular layers. The outer layers at *a* exhibited diffuse fatty degeneration, at *c* they were more hyaline. (From Dr. Klotz's collection.)

all parts are able to gain some nourishment. Saying this, it must not be thought that these arteries do not present calcification; on the contrary, that may be extreme. Long stretches of such arteries as the radials, the circle of Willis and its branches, the splenic, etc., may be found converted into rigid tubes. But this deposit is in the media, and at most involves the internal elastic lamina and the deepest portion of the thickened intima. It may be added that it is the smaller arteries that demonstrate most strikingly the thinning and giving way of the media beneath the overlying great thickening of the intima.

Sclerosis of the Smaller Arteries and Arterioles.—There is great variation in the appearance of the arterioles in different cases, and, indeed, in different organs from the same case—differences which, nevertheless, we believe represent different stages in the same process, modified, it may be, by variations in the reactive powers of the different tissues, intimal and medial, to like noxæ. In this way two broad groups of cases may be distinguished: (1) That in which pronounced thickening and hypertrophy of the muscularis is the most marked feature, and (2) that in which a generalized proliferation of the intima dominates the field. We are inclined, on general principles, to believe that the first represents the earlier condition; that the first effect of substances circulating in the blood, stimulating the smaller arteries to increased contraction, must, of necessity, be to bring about an hypertrophy of the muscle cells; it has already been noted that to this generalized contraction of the smaller arteries and arterioles must be ascribed the continued elevation of the blood pressure.

But just as in the heart hypertrophy beyond a certain point is succeeded by incompetency and degeneration, so here eventually the muscle fibers degenerate and fail to maintain the narrowed lumen; and where this is a progressive process, and the artery as a whole tends to give way under the internal pressure, there is developed a compensatory fibrosis and thickening of the intima, with simultaneous evidence of atrophy and fibrosis of the media, so that now we encounter vessels with greatly increased intima, a media which approximates now, it may be, to the normal width, or if thickened is fibroid and hyaline, presenting a replacement fibrosis. The indications are that in some individuals and tissues the muscular elements are incapable of pronounced hypertrophy, and give way at an early stage in the process, so that in them the intimal change is the more pronounced; in others the muscular hypertrophy is exceptionally well marked, the intimal change slight. This pronounced muscular hypertrophy, we should add, is by no means confined to the arterioles; it is to be observed in arteries of much larger size, in the radials, for example; and then, as Savill and Russel both point out, it may be present either with or without intimal thickening.

What is a characteristic feature in connection with the arterioles is the very frequent surrounding fibrosis, or, as it is termed, chronic periarteritis. We know little or nothing regarding its causation—whether it is irritative, due to seepage of irritative substances out of the vessels, or whether it is of compensatory nature, or of the same order as the intimal fibrosis. That it is due to malnutrition from the lessened circulation, the fibrous tissue replacing nobler tissue elements, is scarce likely; the histology does not suggest this, while, further, any such malnutrition should show itself at the periphery of the capillary area supplied by a given arteriole, rather than at the centre. As Huchard has pointed out, we occasionally encounter examples of this *dystrophic* peripheral fibrosis. They clearly are of another order.

In the arterioles, as in the aorta, we encounter a very definite infective or toxic endarteritis that causes confusion from its similarity to certain phases of arteriosclerosis. More particularly in connection with secondary subacute syphilitic disturbances, in the neighborhood of tuberculous foci, and, as our former colleague, Duval,[1] has shown in connection with subacute glanders, the same is to be met with. His very full study shows that this is primarily a proliferation of the endothelium of the arterioles; the cells attain great size, exhibit mitoses, and soon com-

[1] Journal of Exp. Medicine, 9:1908:241.

pletely fill the lumen. At times they form giant cells. More often their overgrowth results in the production of several layers of a flattened type of cell. According to him, degeneration of the media is secondary to this proliferation. His figure, however, shows the familiar picture of localized giving way of the media with overlying intimal proliferation, and as he expressly notes that the internal elastic lamina at the region of this giving way loses its plicated, wavy appearance and becomes even and without curves, the alternative explanation seems to us possible that where this occurs, the giving way of the media is primary, the intimal overgrowth a secondary phenomenon. We admit, freely, that is, the endothelial proliferation due to bacterial toxins; we doubt whether the medial degeneration is truly secondary to this, believing it to be equally primary, and due to the action of the toxins.

Experimental Arteriosclerosis.—What, then, is the exact meaning of all these changes? The answer is supplied by the abundant experiments of the last few years upon artificially produced arteriosclerosis. There had been many attempts to reproduce the condition by setting up internal and external injury to the arteries, and by causing localized infection. None of these were surely successful until Jores reported his results with adrenalin. It is now one of the most familiar facts of physiology that intravenous injections of adrenalin induce a most pronounced rise of blood pressure. As Langley has shown, these injections reproduce exactly the effects of sympathetic stimulation; or otherwise, adrenalin directly acts upon the muscle of the smaller arteries and causes these to contract. The effect is temporary, but if the injections be repeated in the rabbit, eventually there is developed a profound alteration in the aorta. There have been doubts as to whether the changes produced correspond accurately with those of human arteriosclerosis. Certainly they do not correspond with those of the ordinary nodose sclerosis. They are, however, indistinguishable from the changes seen in Moenckeberg's type of medial degeneration. There is the same atrophy and giving way of the media, with the production of pouchings which at times become so extreme as to become definite, small saccular aneurisms. And, as Klotz has shown, what happens is a fatty, followed by a calcareous, degeneration of the muscular layers, with subsequently a similar calcareous degeneration of the elastic-tissue elements of the coat. Identical changes have been produced by other observers, using barium chloride, nicotine, and other drugs which cause pronounced rise of blood pressure.

There has been great debate as to what precisely is the action of these drugs; do they act directly as poisons of the muscular coat, or of the elastica; do they contract the vasa vasorum, and so bring about malnutrition, or is the degeneration due not to the drugs but to the high pressure they induce? This last has been shown to be correct by Harvey[1] (of Toronto), working in Professor Dixon's laboratory at Cambridge, and independently by Klotz[2] in our laboratory. Harvey employed

[1] Jour. of Med. Research, 17:1907:25; Virchow's Archiv, 196: 1909: 303.
[2] Centralbl. f. allgem. Pathol., 19:1908:535

temporary digital compression of the abdominal aorta of a rabbit for many successive days; Klotz, taking healthy, young rabbits, suspended them head downward for three minutes daily for one hundred and twenty days or more. In both cases the only disturbance induced was rise of blood pressure in the thoracic aorta and its branches; no drug was introduced; but changes were gained of the same order as those obtained with adrenalin. Klotz's results were especially valuable. The heart was found distinctly hypertrophied; the thoracic aorta showed a diffuse, almost aneurismal enlargement compared with the abdominal aorta. There was little sign of intimal sclerosis, but sections showed well-marked medial degeneration of the Moenckeberg type. But now upon examination the main vessels of the neck, which, if anything, had through gravity experienced the daily rise of blood pressure to an even greater degree than the aorta, exhibited most exquisitely a sporadic intimal sclerosis of the nodose type. The condition was indistinguishable from that seen in man.

FIG. 39

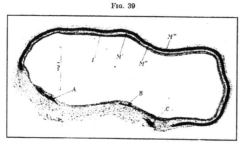

Transverse section of thoracic aorta of rabbit that had been suspended by the hind legs for three minutes daily for 130 days: *I*, intima; *M′*, unaffected inner layer of media; *M″*, degenerated middle layer of media with calcareous degeneration; *M‴*, outer layer of media. The portion of the artery between *A* and *C* has not undergone extreme distension; at *C* there is beginning degeneration of the media; at *A* and *B*, slight patches of intimal overgrowth. (Dr. Klotz.)

Let us put these facts together. Raised blood pressure may induce (1) localized giving way of the media, or (2) diffuse giving way of the same with no accompanying overgrowth, in the first place causing a saccular, in the second a diffuse fusiform aneurism; or (3) it may cause a slighter degeneration and giving way of the media, which now is accompanied by pronounced proliferation of the intima. How are we to reconcile these apparently contradictory results?

The reconciliation is simple and straightforward once we accept the existence of what one of us has termed "strain hypertrophy" (vol. i, p. 451) and of "overstrain atrophy." It is a matter of common teaching that, provided the nutrition be adequate, muscle fibers, whether striated or plain, subjected to strain slightly above the normal, undergo both hypertrophy and hyperplasia; such moderate extra work is a stimulus to increased growth. Subjected to greater strain, they, on the contrary, become exhausted and tend to atrophy. Now, this same law holds for the tissues in general (vol. i, pp. 593 and 871). If the media gives way only slightly and gradually at the region where it bulges, the overlying endothelium and intima, being pressed outward, become stretched, subjected, that is, to increased strain; and the strain not being excessive, the cells proceed to multiply until the concavity is filled up and the strain is removed. The explanation of the difference in the results in Dr. Klotz's experiments between the aorta and the carotids is that the artery of smaller lumen and relatively more powerful media can stand a greater dilating force than the artery of large lumen and relatively weaker walls. Regarded thus, the sclerotic thickening of the intima is in no sense an inflammatory process, any more than is cardiac hypertrophy. At the most, it is compensatory to the weakening of the media. When, on the other hand, the giving way of the media is more extreme and more rapid in its progress, there the strain to which the intima and endothelium are subjected becomes excessive, and proliferation of the cells is inhibited, so that aneurism formation takes the place of compensatory intimal fibrosis or sclerosis. These views were enunciated by one of us[1] in 1896, but then gained little acceptance; the results of this experimental production of arteriosclerosis have demonstrated their

Fig. 40

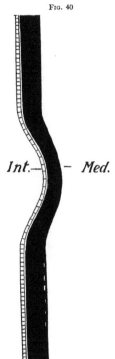

Int.— *— Med.*

Schematic representation of the increased strain brought to bear upon the cells of the intima, *Int.*, when the media undergoes a localized expansion, through relative weakness.

Fig. 41

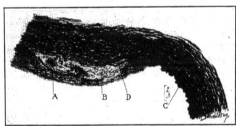

To show nodose sclerosis of intima of carotid of same rabbit: *A*, outer layers of new fibrous tissue showing little degeneration; *B*, atheromatous degeneration of deeper layers, apparently of musculo-elastic layer; *C*, unaffected intima.

[1] Adami, Middleton Goldsmith Lectures, New York Med. Record, 1896:469 and 505.

accuracy. The final and complete proof has been afforded by Carrel's remarkable observation,[1] that if a length of vein be transplanted into the course of an artery, that vein in the course of a few months is found to present an extraordinary fibroid hypertrophy. It is unnecessary, with Thoma, to invoke the difficultly comprehensible local changes in rate of blood flow and nutrition to account for the intimal hyperplasia.

Throughout the whole of this arteriosclerotic process we see, therefore, relatively simple forces at work. In one important series of cases, direct stimuli acting upon the media of the smaller arteries cause increased tonic contraction, or, as Russel terms it, *hypertonus* of the same, and this, raising the blood pressure, affects secondarily the media of the aorta. The musculature of the media, becoming overworked, undergoes atrophy and degeneration, and, gradually giving way, induces a local compensatory fibrosis of the intima. Similarly, the musculature of the smaller arteries giving way induces in them also fibrosis of the intima. In the other series of cases, without, of necessity, any contraction of the peripheral arteries and rise of blood pressure, weakness of the media of the aorta and larger vessels, whether inherited or acquired, makes the media give way under the normal blood pressure, and again the dilatation may be followed by compensating fibrosis of the intima, with the successive stages leading up to atheroma. In either series of cases, if the giving way be widely diffused or sudden and extreme, in place of this compensatory sclerosis aneurism formation results.

In these cases of hyperpiesis and hypertonus of the more peripheral arteries with the increase in blood pressure there is also increased strain thrown first upon the cusps of the aortic valve, and next upon those of the mitral. The arteriosclerotic thickening and fibrosis of the cardiac valves in these cases is of exactly the same nature as the intimal thickening of the arteries; the cusps, indeed, are but infoldings of the intima, or its homologue, the endocardium. These also afford examples of strain hypertrophy and fibrosis, and, as already noted, are apt to present identical degenerative processes, atheroma, calcification, and atheromatous ulceration.

Sclerosis (Functional) and Regeneration of the Uterine and Ovarian Arteries.—A remarkable condition to which attention was first directed by Westphalen[2] in 1886, that has come in for renewed attention during the last few years by Pankow,[3] Sohma,[4] Szasz-Schwarz,[5] Goodall, and others, deserves mention here. The increased blood supply to the uterus during pregnancy is accompanied by great dilatation of the uterine arteries, so great and so long continued, that after childbirth they would seem unable to contract to their previous dimensions. And now there may be the development of a complete new artery (as regards adventitia, media, and intima), within the old, which exhibits fibrosis, hyaline and other degenerative changes. Failing this,

---

[1] Jour. of Exp. Medicine, 10:1908:630.   [2] Virch. Arch., 106:1886:420.
[3] Arch. f. Gynäk., 80:1907:pt. 2.   [4] Ibid., 84:1908:pt. 2.
[5] Révue de Gynec., 7:1903:593.

there is extensive intimal overgrowth. Our colleague, Dr. Goodall, has followed the succession of changes, and concludes that there is an intermediate stage of active proliferation and wandering inward of cells from the various coats resulting in these new cells assuming orderly relationships with the production of a new arterial wall.

The factors determining this remarkable process have not been fully worked out. It may be suggested that with the contraction of the uterine muscle, and it may be the contraction also of the terminal arterioles, there is pronounced obstruction to the outflow of the arterial blood and the production of increased strain: that the condition is identical with the intimal thickening which Thoma noted as affecting the proximal part of an artery after ligature. But this is not sufficient to explain the development of a well-formed new artery within the old. Aschoff[1] places this in a special class as functional sclerosis.

The process affecting the ovarian arteries after menstruation and ovulation is of the same order.

ANEURISM.

We shall, in the next chapter, pass in review the various forms of aneurism, or localized expansion of the arterial wall. We would, in this connection, merely emphasize here that the factors which are productive of arteriosclerosis are the same as those producing aneurism —only that in the case of aneurism we have a severer disturbance of the equilibrium between the pressure within the vessels and the strength of its walls. The studies of the last thirty years have amply confirmed Scarpa's observation (1804) that the strength of arteries depends upon the middle coat, and that either localized degeneration or localized inflammation of the media, particularly syphilitic mesaortitis,[2] is the main cause of the condition (Köster, Eppinger, Thoma, Heller, Chiari, Benda). · The distension induced is so marked that characteristically in the aneurism there is no compensatory hyperplasia of the intima. On the contrary, the strain thrown upon this and the other coats is so great that the tendency is to atrophy, and with this a gradual absorption of the thinned coats may become followed by a complete disappearance of the same and the production of a "false" aneurism, the walls of which are formed of the condensed tissue of surrounding parts and organs. There is but one possible factor for the production of aneurisms which, so far, has not been recognizable as inducing arteriosclerosis, namely, trauma; sudden mechanical injury to the arterial coats is most apt to be followed by sudden giving way of the vessel, and such sudden distension of the intima certainly does not favor hypertrophic changes.

[1] Beihefte zur med. Klinik., 4:1908:pt. 1.
[2] The majority of statistics give from 60 to 85 per cent. of aneurisms as of syphilitic origin. Of recent workers, Hausmann is the only one who depreciates this cause, ascribing only 18.75 per cent. of cases thereto.

CHAPTER IX.

As will be readily understood, the various portions of the vascular system stand in such close functional and anatomical relationship to each other that the pathological processes involving them, while possessing some few characteristics and peculiarities, on the whole present much similarity

ARTERIES.

The walls of the arteries are composed of three layers, the tunica intima, the tunica media, and the tunica adventitia. The first is avascular, deriving its nourishment from the circulating blood within the vessel, while the adventitia derives its blood supply from small arterial twigs, the vasa vasorum. In the case of the media the condition varies in different places, the media of the aorta having vascular twigs which reach to the intima. The intima is an endothelial lining directly continuous with the endocardium and the wall of the finest capillaries.

The thickness of the arterial walls and the caliber of the vessels varies at different periods of life and with different individuals. According to Orth, the thickness of the aortic wall from the age of twenty-five to seventy-five is, on the average, 1.5 to 2 mm. The circumference of the aorta just above the valves is 6.1 to 8.3 cm.; of the thoracic aorta, 4.4 to 5.95 cm.; of the abdominal aorta, 3.2 to 4.33 cm. The circumference of the pulmonary artery just above the valves is from 6.4 to 7.5 cm. In early life the pulmonary artery is somewhat larger than the aorta; in middle life they are the same size; and in old age the aorta is the larger. This last condition is due to the fact that degenerative processes in the aorta are so common after middle life.

CONGENITAL AND DEVELOPMENTAL ANOMALIES.

Defects of development have a close relationship to those of the heart, and have already been touched upon. Abnormalities in the course or number of the arteries have no pathological interest.

The aorta may participate in the condition of transposition of the viscera, or may be duplicated, either in whole or in part.

More important is general hypoplasia of the arterial system, which may exist alone or in combination with a similar defect in the heart. The condition is found in both sexes, but is most common in chlorotic girls about the age of puberty. We have found it with striking frequency in young people who have died of tuberculosis. The aorta is narrowed and the circumference may be only 2 cm. At the same time the wall is thinned and the elasticity is decreased. Other physical defects may be associated, particularly hypoplasia of the genital system. Arterial hypoplasia has also been met with in cases of hemophilia.

CIRCULATORY DISTURBANCES.

Blood Imbibition.—Owing to the avascular character of the intima, circulatory disturbances in this portion do not occur. At most, we may find a diffuse rosiness due to **blood imbibition**, which is most likely a postmortem change. This is found in septicemia, passive congestion, and infection with the B. Welchii.

In the adventitia and media, and even in the intima, where newly formed vessels have invaded this coat, small **hemorrhages** are found in passive congestion and in inflammation. Of special interest to the medicolegal expert are hemorrhages into the wall of the carotid in those who have been hanged or throttled.

INFLAMMATIONS.

Arteritis.—Arteritis may be hematogenic, may arise from trauma from direct extension of inflammatory processes, or complicate degenerative changes. Traumatic causes are, rupture, wounds, or ligature of a vessel. Apart from injury, the most important factors are infections and intoxications, due to microörganisms, tubercle bacilli, and the syphilitic virus. A very common occurrence is the inflammation of a vessel from the presence of a thrombus, either infective or simple.

According to the chief localization of the process we may recognize an *endo-*, *meso-*, or *peri-arteritis*. When all the coats are uniformly involved we have a *panarteritis*. The acute forms are *simple* and *suppurative*. The chronic are always *proliferative*.

Thrombo-arteritis.—Thrombo-arteritis is the form associated with the presence of an autochthonous thrombus or an embolus. Examples of the former are found in traumatism to the vessel wall and in the infections. As a rule, inflammation of the artery is primary and the thrombus is secondary, but undoubtedly the reverse can occur. The character of the inflammation, whether suppurative or proliferative, depends upon the nature of the obstruction.

Suppuration results when the thrombus or embolus contains pus organisms. The affected spot is of a yellowish-white color, swollen, and more friable than usual. The intima is first swollen, and later there is rapid infiltration of all the coats from within outward, with inflammatory aneurism or a local abscess.

Thrombo-arteritis proliferans occurs when the thrombus or embolus is not infective. According to the degree of proliferation, localized patches of thickening or thread-like projections are formed upon the vessel wall. If the process be extensive enough to obliterate the artery, we can speak of an *endarteritis obliterans*.

The proliferative change consists in the substitution of the thrombus by connective tissue. The arterial wall is infiltrated with leukocytes, and many fibroblasts can be seen, which invade the intima and penetrate the substance of the thrombus, eventually bringing about complete organization. Newly-formed capillaries can be made out within the fibrous mass. If the intima be preserved, it may also show changes of a proliferative character. The thrombus may thus be converted into a solid mass of tissue or may be tunnelled through (*canalization*), the various channels being ultimately lined with endothelium and the blood flow thus restored (see p. 73). In some cases a calcareous deposit takes place, and an *arteriolith* is the result.

Proliferative arteritis, leading to gradual thickening of the vessel and even to obliteration, is also found in the arteries of a tissue which is chronically inflamed. It is well seen in cases of chronic interstitial nephritis, tuberculosis, and syphilis, and is very common in almost every form of tumor, as in soft sarcomata and carcinomata, but particularly often in those forms which contain much connective tissue, such as elephantiasis, fibroma, and scirrhous carcinoma.

Arteritis also arises by the extension to the vessel of a neighboring inflammatory process, such as an abscess, ulceration, infected wound, tuberculous cavity, and the like. In these cases the inflammation begins first in the adventitia, and subsequently invades the other coats. It may lead to thrombosis of the vessel or to rupture.

Periarteritis Nodosa.—This is a curious condition, first fully described by Kussmaul and Maier,[1] in which small nodules are formed in the walls of the smaller arteries of the muscles, serous membranes, spleen, abdominal glands, uterus, and mucous glands. According to Freund, who has published a careful research, the changes are sometimes most marked in the adventitia, sometimes in the intima, but usually the process affects chiefly the media.

The adventitia shows cellular infiltration, chiefly of the mononuclear variety, together with spindle cells. The intima is often thickened and hyaline. The hyaline change also extends into the media. In the earlier stages round cells from the adventitia penetrate the media. From this description of the lesion it will be seen that the term "periarteritis is not strictly applicable. The character and the multiplicity of the affection render it probable that infective agents or circulating toxins are the cause of the condition (H. Morley Fletcher[2]). Thrombosis and acute aneurismal dilatation often accompany the process.

Tuberculous Arteritis.—Tuberculous arteritis may arise from infection through the blood or from the extension of a tuberculous process outside the vessel. The latter event is the more common. In the arterial wall typical tubercles can be seen, or a more diffuse inflammatory infiltration. The tubercles sometimes caseate, and rupture of the vessel takes place; the vessel may become thrombosed, or the infective substance may be discharged into the lumen. Under favorable conditions, fibrous hyperplasia takes place. Most frequently the adventitia is affected; but the

[1] Deutsch. Arch. f. klin. Med., 1: 1866:484.
[2] Ueber die sogenannte Periarteritis nodosa, Ziegler's Beiträge, 11:1891:323.

intima may be considerably thickened as well. In the case of the smaller vessels the lumen may be entirely occluded. Tuberculosis of the large arteries is rare. Blumer[1] has recorded two cases.

Syphilitic Arteritis.—Syphilitic arteritis occurs as a distinct entity or as an extension of a local syphilitic infection. The arteries of the brain and heart, and the aorta are the vessels chiefly affected. In the first form a thickening of the intima and adventitia occurs either as circumscribed gray or grayish-white, semitranslucent masses (gummata), or a section of a vessel may be transformed into a firm, grayish-white cord. Or, again, the vessel wall is infiltrated with gummatous masses or is enclosed in dense, fibrous tissue. In the aorta the disease affects primarily the adventitia and media with secondary fibrosis of the intima (see p. 178). Reuter,[2] Wright, and others have detected Treponema pallidum in cases of specific aortitis.

Actinomycotic Arteritis.—This is rare.

RETROGRESSIVE METAMORPHOSES.

Atrophy.—Atrophy of the arterial system occurs in general marasmus and severe anemias, or a particular organ may be affected. Stenosis of the aortic ring and extreme atrophy of the heart may also result in this condition. In amputated limbs the vessels of the stump become smaller. Increased blood pressure leads to atrophy of the tunica media.

Degeneration.—**Fatty Degeneration.**—This is a very common condition found at autopsy, and while it usually affects the intima, is also met with occasionally in the media and adventitia. It is due to anemia, to circulating toxins, or again to increased blood pressure. The last form is often seen in the pulmonary artery, for instance, in pulmonary tuberculosis, and in prolonged congestion of the lesser circulation. The toxic form is well illustrated in the case of typhoid fever and pulmonary tuberculosis. The fatty patches appear in small streaks or flecks of a whitish or yellowish-white color, which may or may not be slightly elevated above the general surface. Microscopically, the stellate cells of the deeper layers of the intima are filled with fat droplets. The condition can result in a small local loss of substance, which, in the capillaries of the brain and lungs, may even lead to rupture of the vessel. In the larger vessels a *locus resistentiæ minoris* may be thus produced, which may very possibly prepare the way for sclerotic changes.

Necrosis and Calcification.—These are also frequent sequels. The media is the chief seat of calcareous deposit, and the intima may at the same time exhibit productive change. The thickened vessels of the aged are no doubt of this type. Such arteries are a frequent cause of thrombosis and anemic necrosis, as well as glandular atrophies.

Hyaline Degeneration.—Hyaline degeneration affects chiefly the intima of the larger vessels or the wall of aneurismal sacs, but is frequently found in the finest capillaries. It is a common accompaniment of arteriosclerotic change. It is often present in the glomerular tufts of the kidney

---

[1] Amer. Jour. Med. Sci., 117:1899:19.   [2] Zeitschr. f. Hygiene, 54:1906:49.

in chronic nephritis, in the choroid plexus of the brain, and in the capillaries of atrophic lymph-glands. The change consists in the formation of a homogeneous hyaline substance, resembling amyloid, but not giving the same chemical reactions, in the cell protoplasm. It is due to mechanical, chemical, or dyscrasic causes. In certain tumors, hence called "cylindromata," the vessels are found converted into thick tubes of this material.

Amyloid Infiltration.—Amyloid infiltration attacks by preference the smaller arterioles of the various organs, though in very severe cases of the affection the large trunks do not altogether escape. The deposit is seen first in the media, following the course of the circular muscle fibers. The condition may spread to the adventitia and, in large vessels, to the intima.

Arteriosclerosis.—Arteriosclerosis is an affection of the arteries most frequently found in the aorta, but often also in the arteries of the brain, heart, extremities, the kidneys, and the spleen. It is somewhat rare in the mesenteric and pulmonary arteries. The lesions vary much in their distribution; at one time the major trunks, at another the medium-sized vessels, or, again, the finer arterioles show the most advanced changes. Even the capillaries may be involved in a widespread process, the arteriocapillary fibrosis of Gull and Sutton (angiosclerosis of Thoma). If the lesions are extensive and widespread, we recognize an *arteriosclerosis diffusa*; if scattered and localized, an *arteriosclerosis nodosa*. According to Rokitansky, the following is the order of frequency with which the vessels are affected: Ascending aorta, the arch, the thoracic aorta, the abdominal aorta, iliacs, crurals, coronaries of the heart, cerebrals, vertebrals, uterine arteries, spermatics, hypogastrics.

At an early stage of the process, gray, semitranslucent patches, sometimes of a gelatinous appearance, are found in the intima (*plaques gélatiniformes*). They have, in part, the structure of mucoid tissue, the cells of which are either well preserved or more often fattily degenerated or necrosed. Later, the patches are harder, of a cartilaginous appearance and gray-white color, forming round, oval, or irregular areas more or less raised above the general surface. These are composed of newly-formed connective tissue which already begins to show retrogressive changes. The tissue has lost its stratification, the cells are swollen and stain poorly, the whole eventually forming a structureless, hyaline mass. Associated with this may be fatty degeneration of the cells and the production of a granular, shreddy detritus (*atheroma*). A true necrosis is thus the result, and in the advanced stages we frequently find a deposit of lime salts in the areas of degeneration (*calcified plaques*). Very frequently the necrobiotic tissue breaks down into a shallow ulcer (*atheromatous ulcer*), the base of which is formed of cholesterin and granular debris. On such ulcers thrombi may form, although more often they are characteristically not produced. If the destructive process goes on in the deeper layers, leaving the necrotic area still covered by the thickened intima and endothelium, an abscess-like cavity is the result. The degenerative changes just described are by no means re-

stricted to the intima, but may extend quite deeply into the media. The
muscle fibers are atrophic and show hyaline, fatty, and calcareous change.
The elastic fibrillæ are usually degenerated, and often torn. New
formation of elastic tissue takes place, especially in the intima. In
addition to the appearances mentioned in the class of case just described,
there are others of an inflammatory nature which have led many pathologists to regard the whole process as inflammatory. Both in the media
and the adventitia small collections of leukocytes are found, situated
around the vasa vasorum, which also seem to proliferate, for we find
newly-formed capillaries developing in the media and even pushing their
way into the intima, indications of a reparative process. Where this is
notably the case we deal with **syphilitic mesaortitis** (see p. 178). With the
vessels a certain number of fibroblasts are carried in which go to form
scar tissue, thus assisting repair. When the vessels come in contact with
calcareous deposits these may be absorbed, and in the aorta, at least,
a formation of bone may take place. All stages of the affection are
found in the vessels at the same time.

The recent studies upon experimental arteriosclerosis have demonstrated that at least three forms of sclerotic disease of the arteries must
be recognized: (1) Mönckeberg's type of medial degeneration followed
by medial calcification; this is the form present in the radials of
clinical arteriosclerosis, and may be reproduced by adrenalin injections.
(2) Productive endarteritis; this may be reproduced experimentally,
even in the aorta, by injections of pyococcus toxins (Klotz[1] and
Saltykow[2]); and (3) inflammatory periarteritis extending into the media
by injury to the outer walls. The syphilitic virus, it may be noted,
more particularly invades the arteries through the vasa. The relationship of the common nodose type of arteriosclerosis of the aorta to
these, whether in the main compensatory to medial giving way, or
productive, is still a matter of dispute.

As would naturally be expected, such grave disturbances bring in
their train further secondary manifestations. The larger vessels become
elongated and dilated in whole or in part. In the smaller vessels, such as
those of the brain and heart, owing to the thickening of the intima, the
lumen is greatly obstructed or even obliterated. Such vessels on cross-
section show a characteristic signet-ring appearance.

Among the consequences of arteriosclerosis may be mentioned, thrombosis, embolism, rupture of the vessel wall, aneurism, necrosis from
ischemia, contracted kidney, and enlargement of the heart.

Aneurisms.—As to what constitutes an aneurism authorities differ.
The subject is still further confused by a multiplicity of terms. It is
perhaps simplest to define "aneurism," with Orth, as any circumscribed
dilatation of the lumen of an artery.

If the aneurismal sac be constituted of all or any of the coats of the
arterial wall, it is called a "true" aneurism. If, on the other hand,

---

[1] British Med. Jour., 2: 1906: 1767.
[2] Saltykow, Cent. f. Path. Anat., 19: 1808: 321. Ziegler's Beiträge, 42: 1908: 147.

a portion of the sac be composed of the surrounding tissues or a newly-formed fibrous investment, we speak of a "false" aneurism. In advanced cases, however, it may not be possible to draw this distinction.

In the immense majority of cases aneurisms are due to the action of a normal or increased pressure of the blood upon an arterial wall weakened from disease; syphilis is the most potent cause; tobacco, alcoholism (?), gout, and lead poisoning are also effective in some instances. Some cases are due to muscular strain, direct injury, inflammatory processes in the vessel, or rarely to defective development of the arteries.

The following classification is offered as a convenient and comprehensive one:

I. **Aneurism from dilatation.**
   (a) Arteriectasis.
   (b) Cirsoid or racemose aneurism.
   (c) Serpentine aneurism.
   (d) Cylindrical aneurism.
   (e) Fusiform aneurism.
   (f) Sacculated aneurism.
II. **Aneurism from rupture.**
   (a) Dissecting aneurism.
   (b) Sacculated aneurism.
   (c) Anastomotic aneurism $\begin{cases} \text{Varicose aneurism.} \\ \text{Aneurismal varix.} \end{cases}$
III. **Aneurism from external erosion.**
IV. **Aneurism from embolism.**
   (a) Tearing of the intima.
   (b) Mycotic.
V. **Aneurism from trauma.**
VI. **Aneurism from traction.**

The forms in the first group are differentiated according to the form which the dilatation takes.

Arteriectasis is a tubular, spindle-formed, or nodular dilatation of an artery affecting a more or less considerable extent of the vascular tree. Such is commonest in the aorta or some portion of it, as the thoracic aorta and the arch.

When, in addition to the dilatation of the vessels, there is great tortuosity with free anastomosis, we speak of **cirsoid aneurism.** These are found in the large vessels of the pelvis, and on the scalp. Some of them should possibly be classified with the angiomas. A sub-variety is the **serpentine,** characterized as its name implies.

Cylindrical and **fusiform** aneurisms are found commonly in the thoracic aorta and in the great vessels springing from the arch.

A very important form is the **sacculated,** in which, springing from the side of the affected vessel, is a saccular diverticulum, often of large size, and communicating with the lumen of the vessel by a comparatively narrow opening. Such are the aneurisms which especially give rise to pressure symptoms, erosion, rupture, and the like.

Sometimes the various forms may be combined. An aneurismal sac usually shows some variation in thickness in its various parts, inasmuch as the wall is generally extensively diseased; some parts showing advanced atheromatous degeneration, while in others the wall of the sac may be quite thin, one or more coats being absent. Within the sac one often sees local deposits of fibrin or possibly organized clot adherent to the atheromatous plaques. Any considerable amount of clot or reparative

Fig. 42

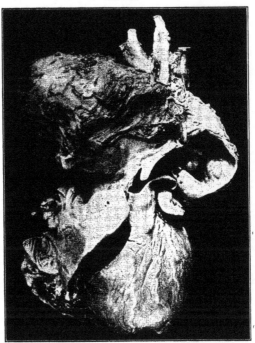

Sacculated aneurism of the ascending and transverse arch of the aorta. (From the Patho-logical Laboratory of the Royal Victoria Hospital.)

change is distinctly rare; in one specimen, however, in the museum of McGill University, where complete cure took place, the sac was quite obliterated by the organization of clot.

As will be readily understood, in a diseased and weakened arterial wall rupture very readily takes place.

If the rupture be through the intima into the media, the blood finds its way along the vessel between the layers of media, and a **dissecting** aneurism is the result. These are found frequently in the aorta and the vessels of the brain. Usually swiftly fatal, they have been known to undergo repair.[1] The exciting cause is usually some strain or injury. If all the coats be ruptured, there is naturally hemorrhage about the vessel, with the formation of a hematoma, or hemorrhage into some cavity. In some cases, where the intima and media are torn through,

FIG. 43

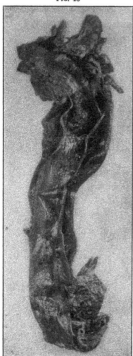
Dissecting aneurism of the aorta.
(From the Pathological Museum of McGill University.)

a local or sacculated dilatation is formed, owing to the distension of the weak adventitia. Such may be quite large, or, again, small and multiple in distribution. They sometimes heal up, leaving few traces.

In the outer wall of the sac secondary inflammatory change is common, leading to a development of fibrous tissue.

When rupture takes place into a vein, in the cases where the artery and vein have become closely united, we get an **aneurismal varix** produced. In other instances a false aneurism is the result, which later breaks into a vein, so that there is an indirect communication between vein and artery. This is a **varicose aneurism.**

Aneurisms from **erosion** are found chiefly in suppurating wounds and in tuberculous cavities. They are due to the extension of the necrotic process to the wall of the vessel, thus rendering it weak and unsupported. In tuberculous cavities one frequently sees the vessels stretching across with small aneurismal dilatations upon them (see Fig. 72). The hemorrhage so common in cases of ulcerative tuberculosis of the lungs is frequently due to the rupture of one of these minute aneurisms. In most cases, however, the vessel is thrombosed and the lumen obliterated before the tubercle begins to soften.

Embolic aneurisms are of two forms. In the first, sharp calcareous particles break loose from an ulcerated valve of the heart or an atheromatous patch, and are carried along in the blood stream to some small vessel, where they tear the intima, producing hemorrhage or an aneurism from rupture. In the second form, the mycotic, infective emboli set up degeneration and inflammation of the arterial wall and thus bring

[1] Adami, On Arrested or Repaired Dissecting Aneurisms, Montreal Med. Jour., 24: 1895–96; 945, and 25: 1896: 23.

about weakening and rupture. Osler has drawn attention to multiple aneurisms of this type occurring in ulcerative endocarditis. J. McCrae has also recorded a case.[1] In the horse similar aneurisms are produced by parasites, such as Strongylus armatus.

Traumatic aneurisms are formed by the rupture of one or all of the arterial coats due to external violence, particularly penetrating wounds. Many of the false aneurisms, as well as the anastomotic, come under this head.

FIG. 44

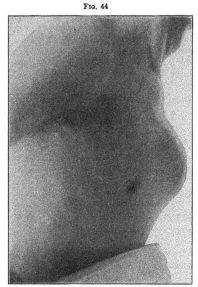

Aneurism of the aorta. Here the sternum and costal cartilages were extensively eroded, a large false aneurism pulsating under the skin and eventually undergoing external rupture. (From the Medical Clinic of the Royal Victoria Hospital, under the late Dr. J. Stewart.)

The commonest sites for aneurisms are the aorta, chiefly the arch, the abdominal aorta, the popliteal, femoral, subclavian, carotid, innominate, and iliac arteries, in the order named. Aneurisms are not uncommonly multiple in distribution. Multiple miliary aneurisms are often found in the arteries of the brain, particularly those supplying the lenticulostriate region, and are a fertile cause of cerebral hemorrhage. Aneurisms of the aorta, according to their size and position, produce a variety of effects. If large, they dislocate various organs and produce collapse of the lung, necrosis, or form adhesions. Aneurisms of the middle part of the arch press upon the left recurrent laryngeal nerve and the œsophagus. The ribs or the vertebral column may be eroded and the vertebral canal

[1] J. McCrae, Jour. Path. and Bact., 10:1905:373.

may be opened. Rupture can take place into a right auricle of the heart, as in a case recorded by McPhedran,[1] the bronchi, the œsophagus, the trachea, the pleural cavity, or externally.

PROGRESSIVE METAMORPHOSES.

Hypertrophy.—The cause of general arterial hypertrophy is increased function—due to excessive intravascular pressure, overwork, or nervous influences.

True hypertrophy is found in tumors and in organs or portions of an organ which are the sites of compensatory hypertrophy. The enlargement affects both the thickness and the length of the vessel, so that it frequently becomes tortuous. All coats may be affected, but particularly the media, the latter condition being marked in that form of arterial hypertrophy found in chronic Bright's disease.

Cirsoid aneurism, or the angioma arteriale, is by some classed under this head.

Physiological hypertrophy is found in the uterus as a change incident to pregnancy.

Tumors.—Primary tumors of the arteries are very rare. Brodowski has recorded a case of primary **sarcoma** of the thoracic aorta. A very interesting form of tumor is the **perithelioma**, which may be either benign or malignant. This is found in the suprarenals, the prostate, the thyroid, and in the brain. It is a vascular tumor, really a spindle-celled sarcoma, which originates in the perithelium of the vessels.

Myomas are also said to occur.

Secondary tumors arising by direct extension or from embolism are not uncommon.

Cysts.—Freedman has described an apparently unique case of a **lymphangiectatic cyst** of the carotid artery.[2]

THE CAPILLARIES.

Thrombosis of the capillaries is probably not so rare as has been taught, and **embolism** is not uncommon.

Capillary **aneurisms** are met with frequently, due to active or passive congestion. These are seen particularly well in the lung, where in such a condition the capillaries of the alveolar wall assume a tortuous or varicose appearance.

In exudative inflammations the capillaries play an important part. The component cells show swelling of the nucleus and cell body, with some granulation of the protoplasm.

In proliferative inflammation the appearances are similar, but are of a more progressive character. Owing to local collections of granular

---

[1] Canadian Practitioner, 21: 1896: 578.
[2] Montreal Med. Jour., 38: 1909; 583.

protoplasmic substance, small buds are produced which ultimately develop into new capillaries. The same process is seen in many tumors.

Like the arteries, the capillaries are frequently affected by **fatty degeneration, calcareous deposit, hyaline** or **colloid degeneration.** Perhaps the most important of these is **amyloid disease.** In the case of the lymph-glands, the liver, spleen, and the kidneys, amyloid disease is amyloid disease of the capillaries.

Capillary **angiomas (teleangiectases)** are generally congenital, but may appear or increase in size after birth. They form usually flat tumor-like masses in the subcutaneous tissues of soft consistency, and of bright red color. They may be combined with true tumor formation, as sarcoma, carcinoma, or lipoma.

THE VEINS.

The pathological changes in the veins are very similar to those of the arteries, except that inflammation is distinctly more common, and there is greater tendency to neoplasia.

DILATATION OF THE LUMEN.

Phlebectasia.—This is a dilatation of a vein due to a mechanical hindrance to the free return flow of the blood, to local or general stasis, to compression of the veins, thrombosis, and heart weakness. Disease of the venous wall is a predisposing cause. The vessel may be dilated cylindrically, or become sacculated (**varicosity**), or, again, complicated loops may be formed. Adjacent loops may fuse so that anastomosing venous sinuses are produced. The walls are often thinned, but in time become thickened (*phlebosclerosis*) or even calcified, and the vessel is usually both tortuous and elongated. Varices are found most frequently in the lower extremities, pelvic veins, the broad ligaments, spermatic veins, prostate, bladder, scrotum, labia, and the rectum (**hemorrhoids**). In cases of cirrhosis of the liver, the veins of the œsophagus, the portal vein, the veins of the abdominal wall and hepatic ligaments are often greatly dilated.

Varices are a frequent cause of hemorrhage, œdema, inflammation, ulceration, thrombosis, calcification, and pachydermia.

Phlebitis.—Simple and Suppurative Phlebitis.—This frequently occurs, and the histological changes are similar to those in the case of the arteries. The causes also are similar.

Thrombophlebitis.—Acute phlebitis, particularly the infective variety, is very commonly combined with thrombosis. The well of the vein is infiltrated with inflammatory products and the cavity occluded by a degenerating clot. Suppuration at the site of the process is not uncommon, and general septicemia is an ever-present danger. *Prolifera-tive thrombophlebitis* is frequent in the veins of the lower extremities, the pelvis, and the sinuses of the brain. As in the case of the arteries, it can lead to partial or complete obliteration of the lumen. The thrombus may calcify, forming a *phlebolith.*

Tuberculous Phlebitis.—Tuberculous phlebitis and periphlebitis is analogous to tuberculous arteritis and peri-arteritis.

FIG. 45

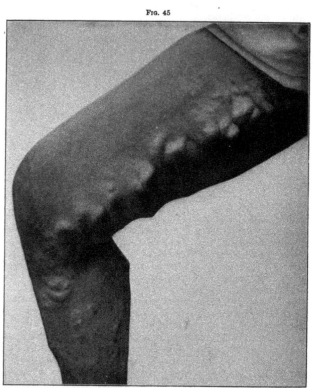

Varicose veins of the leg. (From the Surgical Clinic of the Montreal General Hospital.)

Syphilitic Phlebitis.[1]—Syphilitic phlebitis is most frequent in the district of the portal vein and in the umbilical vein of the newborn.

Phlebosclerosis.—A condition of fibroid thickening of the intima and media of veins closely resembling that seen in arteriosclerosis is much more common than is usually imagined. Such phlebosclerosis affects more particularly veins that are poorly supported, and this even in

[1] For literature see Thorel, Lubarsch and Ostertag's Ergebnisse, 9: 1904.

young adults: it is unassociated with any signs of progressive inflammation, and as our colleague Dr. C. F. Martin[1] concludes, must be placed in the group of "strain fibroses."

THE LYMPHATIC VESSELS.

Affections of the smaller lymphatics are almost invariably associated with disease of the tissue in which they lie. Pathological conditions of the larger trunks, in the main, concern us here. When we remember, however, that the pleura, the peritoneum, and other serous sacs are large spaces in close relationship with the lymph-channels, the subject attains notable proportions.

The lymphatics derive their importance from the fact that they afford a ready means for the invasion of the organism or particular regions by inflammatory processes, and for the dissemination of malignant growths. Further, by their obstruction they give rise to several remarkable conditions.

Lymphangitis.—A frequent disorder of the lymphatics is **lymphangitis** and **perilymphangitis**. It is almost invariably due to the presence of an infective inflammation in some part drained by the affected vessels. Infective organisms pass rapidly up the channels from the wound, and may ultimately reach the lymph-glands, where they often set up hyperplastic and even suppurative changes. Thus, infection from a wound of the foot may reach the inguinal glands. The affected lymphatics are seen as reddish lines extending up the limb, and are somewhat painful. In the mildest form, the endothelial cells are swollen and show nuclear division. In more advanced cases, they are desquamated and the lumen of the vessel is filled with debris, lymphoid cells, and fibrin. In the suppurative form the channels may be dilated, owing to collection of the pus, and may thus resemble a rosary. The inflammation spreads to the surrounding tissues, which are œdematous, hyperemic, and infiltrated with leukocytes. Lymphangitis may heal completely with regeneration of the destroyed cells, abscesses may form, or induration from fibrous hyperplasia may result.

Chronic lymphangitis, as it affects the smaller lymph capillaries, gives rise to a notable proliferation of the lining endothelial cells, whereby the vessel is converted into a solid band of cells, devoid of lumen, recalling somewhat the appearance of a glandular carcinoma (*lymphangitis productiva: endolymphangitis proliferans*). The larger vessels are gradually converted into thick fibrous cords (*lymphangitis fibrosa obliterans*).

Of much importance are the specific inflammations, especially the tuberculous.

Tuberculosis.—Tuberculosis attacks the various organs with great avidity through the lymphatics. Tuberculosis of the thoracic duct is

[1] Transactions Assoc. of Amer. Phys., 20: 1905: 525. See also Fischer, Ziegler's Beitr., 27:1900:494.

a frequent cause of miliary tuberculosis in children, and tuberculous lymphangitis is a common method of infection in the lungs. In tuberculous ulceration of the intestines, one can frequently see subserous tubercles situated along the course of the lymphatic vessels.

Syphilis.—In syphilis, in addition to a proliferative lymphangitis, gummatous infiltration of the wall is seen. The lymphatics are also affected in **leprosy** and **glanders.**

Fig. 46

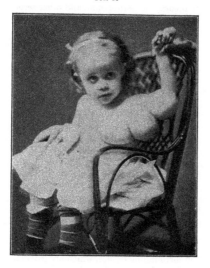

Cavernous lymphangioma of the axilla of congenital origin.   (Warren.)

Dilatation (Lymphangiectasis).—Dilatation is the result of some obstruction to the free outflow of lymph. This may be due to pressure of external tumors, aneurisms, enlarged glands, metastatic growths in the wall, chronic inflammation, impaction of filaria, thrombosis of the left innominate vein or of the duct itself, backward pressure in the subclavian vein from tricuspid insufficiency. The condition is often seen very prettily on the serosa of the intestine in the neighborhood of tuberculous and typhoid ulcers, where the chyle vessels are found as delicate transparent tubes filled with clear fluid. As a consequence of overdistension, or in the course of operations, the vessel wall may be ruptured and a condition of **lymphorrhagia** may be the result. The interesting condition of **chylous ascites** is due to the rupture of the lymph channels from traumatism, erosion, or to rupture of the thoracic duct itself (see p. 111). Similarly **chylous hydrothorax** may be produced. The allied conditions of chyliform and pseudochylous ascites have already been described (p. 111).

Where dilatation is combined with chronic lymphangitis and perilymphangitis, as it may be in the case of the skin in the neighborhood of ulcers, especially where the regional lymph nodes are destroyed or have been removed by operation, a brawny induration of the part results (*pachydermia lymphangiectatica*).

Parasites.—Among parasites found in the lymph-vessels may be noted *Echinococcus* and *Filaria sanguinis*. The latter is associated with certain cases of elephantiasis found in the tropics and the condition known as **chyluria.**

FIG. 47

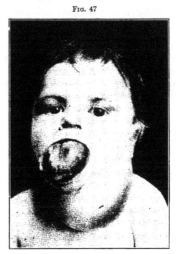

Macroglossia.   (Dr. Shepherd's case, Montreal General Hospital.)

The retrograde changes are of little importance. **Fatty degeneration** of the endothelium is common; and **calcification** of the thoracic duct as a result of productive inflammation has been observed.

Hypertrophy of the walls of the lymph channels has been noted in cases of obstruction.

More important are the **tumors. Carcinomata** have a special tendency to spread by means of the lymphatics, and often considerable portions of a vessel may be blocked by cancer cells. This occurs not merely in the neighborhood of the original growth (local metastasis), but affects even distant parts, as, for example, when we get metastases in the supraclavicular glands in cases of carcinoma of the stomach. Besides carcinomas, chondromas seem to have a tendency to grow into the lymphatics. The most important and interesting primary tumor is the **endothelioma,** a growth which has some resemblances both to carcinoma and sarcoma, and hence has been called by some, ill-advisedly, sarcocarcinoma. This tumor is found particularly in connection with the larger serous sacs, but also originates in the vessels. It develops, consequently, in the pleura, the peritoneum, the dura mater, and the various organs. The growth forms either multiple small nodules on the serous membrane, only slightly elevated above the general level and often so minute as to be easily overlooked, or extensive sheet-like masses. Microscopically, it consists in masses of cells, not unlike epithelial cells, having an alveolar arrangement, which are really only lymphatic channels with thickened and proliferated endothelium. The growth is malignant.

A second primary tumor is the **lymphangioma**, which presents itself either as a diffuse enlargement of the part with preservation of its outward contour, or as a definite tumor mass. It occurs chiefly in the connective and submucous tissues in the throat, neck, tongue, and lips (*macroglossia, macrocheilia*), the extremities, mesentery, and kidneys. Most of these are more accurately conditions of congenital lymphangiectasis (vol. i, p. 818), although the true lymphangioma does occur.

Allied to this is the condition known as **elephantiasis lymphangiectatica,** which is seen most frequently in the extremities, the scrotum, and the vulva.

CHAPTER X.

THE BLOOD-FORMING ORGANS.

THE LYMPHATIC GLANDS.[1]

LYMPHADENOID tissue is widely distributed throughout the body, being found in almost all the organs in the form of follicles or scattered lymphoid cells. More important than this, it is aggregated in certain regions into definite glands, which form an integral part of the lymph-vascular system. The structure of a lymph-node is fairly simple. It is composed of a fibrous capsule sending in trabeculæ, which break up into innumerable fine ramifications, so as to form a reticulated stroma. On the walls of the spaces thus produced are situated large mononuclear cells with clear protoplasm—the endothelioid plates. The remaining portion of the cavities is filled up with small, round cells, which contain a single, relatively large, and deeply staining nucleus, in all respects resembling the lymphocyte of the blood. In the outer zone the lymphoid elements are grouped into follicles to form the cortex of the node. In the central portion, or medulla, wavy strands of connective tissue, lined with endothelioid cells, are found, constituting the sinuses, which are directly continuous with the lymphatic vessels. The cells of the medulla are larger and stain more feebly than those of the cortex, and the nuclei frequently show evidences of mitosis, proving that this portion is the germinal centre of the node. A striking point in connection with the lymphatic glands is that they possess the embryonal characteristic of active growth, so that the cells, under the influence of a very slight stimulus, rapidly undergo nuclear division and proliferation. This is the feature that dominates the picture in all the important pathological processes affecting these structures.

Lymph-nodes are of two kinds—ordinary lymph-nodes and hemo-lymph-nodes. The latter were first discovered by Gibbes,[2] and more fully described by Robertson[3] and Swale Vincent.[4] They have been found in the sheep, ox, pig, horse, and man. The most recent and comprehensive study of these structures is that of Warthin,[5] who divides

---

[1] While strongly objecting to this designation, on the ground that, speaking of these as glands, the student becomes confused in his conception of glandular activity, we realize that the term is so firmly established that it would be pedantic to change it.

[2] Quart. Jour. Micr. Sciences, 24:1884:186; and Amer. Jour. of the Med. Sci., 24:1893:316.

[3] Lancet, London, 2:1890:1152.   [4] Jour Anat. and Physiol., 31:1897:176.

[5] A Contribution to the Normal Histology and Pathology of the Hemolymph Glands, Jour. of Medical Research, 6:1901:3.

them into two varieties, splenolymph-nodes and marrow lymph-nodes, with numerous transitional forms.   He has shown that there is a close relationship between the lymph-nodes, the spleen, and bone-marrow, and that the hemolymph-nodes can take on more or less completely the structure and function of the spleen or marrow when either of these is incapacitated through disease.   Under normal conditions the hemolymph-nodes are concerned chiefly in hemolysis and leukocyte production.   The spleno-lymph-nodes are found chiefly in the neighborhood of the solar plexus, adrenal and renal vessels, omentum, mesentery, epiploica, thymus and thyroid glands.   The marrow lymph-nodes are found only in the retro-peritoneal tissues, near the great vessels, particularly the vena cava, aorta, and common iliacs.   Unlike the ordinary lymph-nodes, the hemo-lymph-nodes, except the transitional forms, contain blood-sinuses but no lymph-sinuses.   Hemolymph-nodes are dark red or bluish in color, possess a hilus into which a large vessel enters, and are usually surrounded by a plexus of veins.   On section they resemble spleen pulp.   They have a particular importance in connection with the various forms of anemia.

The function of the lymphatic glands is to act as a sort of filter for the lymph, which enters the sinuses in the medulla and gradually percolates into the cortex,.where it is taken up by the efferent lymphatics. In this way, should the lymph contain any foreign substance or toxic material, these tend to be stopped within the gland, and thus, not only on account of the anatomical peculiarities of the structure, but also of the cellular hyperplasia that results from the irritation, this barrier action is a very effective one.   It is most effective, naturally, in the case of the grosser foreign particles which reach the part, such as, for example, broken-down blood corpuscles, tissue detritus, and tumor cells.   Bacteria are more likely to pass through.   Yet, even in the latter case the retardation is by no means slight, for the endothelioid plates before referred to are actively phagocytic and do much to minimize the activity of the invaders, not only by engulfing them, but by opposing a physical obstruction to their onward course, an obstruction that may be very considerable where the sinuses are blocked by proliferating cells. Possibly, too, farther protection is afforded by extracellular substances derived from the lymphatic cells themselves or from leukocytes which are attracted to the region.   The lymphatic glands are, therefore, set like sentinels to guard all the orifices and channels of the body, and frequently prevent systemic infection.   This function has been clearly demonstrated by the researches of Bizzozero, Ruffer, and Ribbert, who have shown that the glands in the pharynx, neck, root of the lungs, and mesentery in healthy animals contain bacteria.

A further important function is said to be the formation of leukocytes, which is especially active under most conditions of infection.

As will readily be inferred, the most important affections of the lymph-nodes are the inflammatory, and this from a clinical as well as a pathological point of view.   They are, however, rarely affected as a system, except in the possible case of leukemia and lymphosarcoma.   As a rule, only the glands belonging to a certain anatomical district are involved, though in some affections like syphilis, the lesions are rather widespread. The glands nearest the primary focus of infection are the most markedly involved, but the process often spreads by way of the lymphatic channels to more distant glands, the more rapidly the more virulent the nature of the offending microörganisms. In septic cases we get not only inflammation of the various lymphatics and glands but of the adjacent tissues as well. Abscesses and general systemic infection may finally result. In more chronic cases where there is time for reactive hyperplasia of tissue, we may get obstruction and serious interference with the lymph circulation of the part.

A word or two should be said in regard to the role played by the lymphatic glands in the dissemination of malignant new-growths. Carcinomas are preëminently the ones which spread in this manner. Usually the nodes nearest to the site of the tumor are those that show the greatest involvement, in fact they may become enlarged to such a degree as to overshadow the original growth. Not infrequently, however, emboli of cancer cells are carried farther on and may invade other lymph districts. Occasionally the involvement is more diffuse affecting not merely nodes and lymphatics but the surrounding tissues, giving rise to a sort of brawny induration. This is seen well in the so-called "cancer en cuirasse" of the skin secondary to cancer of the breast. A very pretty example of the widespread diffusion of the cancerous process is that seen occasionally in the pleura, where the affected lymphatics stand out as a pearly network of the surface of the lung. From obstruction of the lymphatics or pressure on important veins, œdema of a part may result. Thus extensive œdema of the legs and lower part of the trunk may indicate the pressure upon the inferior vena cava of cancerous masses in the retroperitoneal tissues. A knowledge of the line of transmission of metastasis is useful in determining the site of the primary growth when this is concealed.

CONGENITAL ANOMALIES.

These are not important, with the exception of that excessive production of lymphoid tissue throughout the body characteristic of the so-called "status lymphaticus." It may, perhaps, be noted here that in infancy and childhood the lymph-glandular system is very prominent, and as puberty is reached it becomes relatively less important.

CIRCULATORY DISTURBANCES.

Anemia.—The circulatory disturbances are also of no special interest. The lymph-glands normally contain but little blood, and in general anemia even this may disappear.

Hyperemia.—Hyperemia is almost inseparably associated with inflammation. The glands are reddened, enlarged, and succulent.

Hemorrhages.—Hemorrhages in such cases readily occur, which may also be due to minute **emboli** in the cortical vessels leading to rupture.

Œdema.—Œdema may be inflammatory or part of a general anasarca.

Varices.—A curious occurrence is the formation of varices or **cysts** in the centre of the nodes owing to obstruction of the efferent lymphatics, which is generally brought about by inflammation.   In severe cases the dilated and tortuous sinuses may coalesce and the node-substance be distended into a large cystic space (*adenolymphocele*),[1] varying in size from that of a nut to that of one's head.   The inguinal glands are those usually involved, and young people are particularly liable to be affected. The disease is endemic in some tropical countries.

INFLAMMATIONS.

Lymphadenitis.—Inflammation of the lymph- glands—lymphadenitis—is one of the commonest of conditions.   It is usually brought about by infective agents or toxins reaching them through the afferent lymphatics· Not infrequently, also, the process arises by extension of inflammation from the adjacent structures; more rarely the affection is hematogenic.   Lymphadenitis is invariably secondary to infection elsewhere.   The glands nearest the point of entrance of the offending bacteria are chiefly affected, but those at some distance are quite commonly involved, owing to the· action of diffusible toxins.   In many diseases, such as diphtheria and variola, lymphadenitis is a marked feature, and in one—plague—it may give the character to the clinical type (bubonic plague).   In certain other diseases, such as leukemia and Hodgkin's disease, the involvement of the glands is striking.   The relationship of chronic inflammatory change to the latter condition has been discussed in our first volume (P. 739).

Acute Lymphadenitis.—Acute lymphadenitis is *simple* or *suppurative.* Both forms have much in common, for the suppurative variety generally supervenes upon the other.   Suppurative lymphadenitis is due to infection with pyogenic microörganisms, and may result from septic wounds, puerperal metritis and endometritis, gonorrhœa, chancroid, diphtheria, and scarlatina.   When inflamed, the glands are enlarged, hyperemic, and soft (*bubo*).   On section, they vary in color from gray or grayish-white·to pink, and are succulent, so that a milky juice can be scraped from the surface.   In the early stages the congestion is confined to the cortex, but sooner or later it becomes impossible to differentiate between the cortex and medulla.   In some cases, as of diphtheria and typhoid, one can make out dull, opaque, necrotic areas, and, in the most severe forms, softening, with the formation of thick, greenish-yellow pus. In many instances the fibrous capsule of the glands and the neighboring tissues are œdematous, infiltrated, and congested (*perilymphadenitis*).

[1] Auger,· Des Tumeurs érectiles lymphatiques (adenolymphocèles), Thèse de Paris, 1867.

Microscopically, the enlargement of the glands is found, in the main, to consist of a hyperplasia of the cellular elements, as evidenced by nuclear division and increase in the number of cells. Not only are the lymph elements affected in this way, but the endothelial plates proliferate and are found in great numbers, often with several nuclei, more particularly in the lymph-channels. This "catarrh" of the plates, as has been shown by Mallory,[1] is a prominent feature in the mesenteric glands and, to some extent, in others, in typhoid fever, where in many cases they fuse into giant cells having phagocytic properties. The trabeculæ and the capsule may be œdematous and infiltrated with cells. Not infrequently the lymph-sinuses are dilated with an exudate con-

FIG. 48

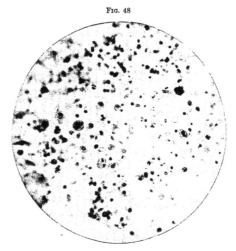

Section of mesenteric gland in typhoid fever, showing the enlarged endothelial and giant cells. Zeiss obj. $\frac{1}{12}$, oil immersion, without ocular. (From the Pathological Laboratory of McGill University.)

taining but few cells. In the severer forms of inflammation the exudate may be fibrinous or hemorrhagic, or both. Fibrinous deposit is seen chiefly in the sinuses, and is especially prominent in lobar pneumonia and diphtheria. Occasionally spots of necrosis may be seen where the lymphoid cells and those of the stroma lose their staining power, become granular, and finally disintegrate. This change is brought about by the direct action of the toxin, but also, no doubt, by the obstruction to the circulation caused by the cellular proliferation and accumulation of debris. Should suppuration occur, there is an abundant aggregation of polymorphonuclear leukocytes in the lymph-

[1] Jour. Exper. Med., 3:1898:611.

spaces, together with necrosis and, ultimately, liquefaction. When this event does not occur, it is possible for the inflammation to resolve. The redundant cells and fibrin undergo fatty degeneration, and finally disintegrate and dissolve, the debris being carried off in the lymph-stream or taken up by the phagocytes. In cases where hyperemia has been marked, or where hemorrhage has taken place, it is common for pigment to be deposited. In the severer forms it is usual for the gland to remain somewhat enlarged and firm, owing to fibrous hyperplasia. Where necrosis or suppuration has occurred, a definite scar may be the result, or, if the necrosed substance be not absorbed, the gland may undergo calcification. In some cases, where the gland has burst externally, a sinus discharging lymph has persisted for some time.

Chronic Lymphadenitis.—Chronic lymphadenitis occurs as a sequel to the acute form, but may arise independently. In the latter case it is due to the action of mild or repeated irritation. Apart from syphilis or tuberculosis, the most common cause is the presence of dust or other foreign material. The process is seen most commonly in the peribronchial glands, where large amounts of coal, stone, steel, or other dust may be deposited, and in the axillary glands after tattooing.

The affected nodes are enlarged, firm, and variously pigmented, according to the nature of the offending material. In the earlier stages the enlargement is due to simple cellular hyperplasia, but soon the capsule and stroma become noticeably thickened, encroaching gradually upon the lymphoid cells, until, eventually, there is atrophy of the lymphoid elements, and the node is converted into a fibrous nodule or encapsulated mass of pigment. In other cases the necrosis is so rapid that the node softens and its contents may be discharged into the nearest hollow viscus.

Tuberculosis.—Tuberculosis of the lymph-glands, in most cases, is brought about by bacilli that reach them through the afferent lymph-vessels; more rarely from the blood-stream. The glands chiefly affected are the cervical, peribronchial, and mesenteric.

In exceptional cases the disease is widespread, involving the axillary, inguinal, and retroperitoneal regions as well. Often the organs from which the infected lymph is derived show evidences of tuberculosis, but this is by no means necessary. In the case of the lungs, for instance, while affection of the peribronchial glands is attributable in some cases to a primary pulmonary lesion, yet, as Ribbert and Baumgarten have shown, the reverse process is frequently at work, and, in tuberculosis of the cervical glands, where infection takes place through the tonsils, gums, and nasopharynx, it is rare for the latter structures to show the lesions of the disease. Similarly, in tuberculosis of the mesenteric glands, the mucous membrane of the intestines may entirely escape.

The affected glands are noticeably, and in some cases enormously, enlarged, presenting all the signs of a more or less intense inflammation. In the earlier stages section reveals a homogeneous, translucent infiltration of grayish color, affecting either the greater portion of the gland or merely scattered areas. Later, this becomes opaque, granular looking, and may finally caseate, so that the mass becomes yellowish-white in color, granular, and friable. In some cases, possibly from secondary infection, the glands suppurate and may discharge their contents into the nearest cavity. Rupture into a vein or into the thoracic duct is the most potent cause of systemic miliary infection with tuberculosis. Rupture may also take place into the pericardium, mediastinum, œsophagus, and intestinal tract. In long-standing cases the glands become shrunken, more or less fibrosed, and destroyed, and may contain calcareous spicules.

Microscopically, there is an increase in the number of round cells, partly from the proliferation of the lymphoid elements and partly from the diapedesis from the vessels. With this, there is more or less hyperplasia of the endothelioid cells. In the more advanced stages the centre is occupied by isolated or confluent areas of caseation, the tissue in the neighborhood showing evidences of cellular disintegration and nuclear destruction. In chronic cases giant cells make their appearance about the periphery of the tubercle, and in still more chronic forms there is an attempt at walling off the dead material with fibrous tissue. Calcification may also be noted. True bone has occasionally been observed.[1]

A peculiar form, which deserves special mention on account of its resemblance to Hodgkin's disease,[2] is **chronic hyperplastic tuberculosis.** This disease has been described in connection with the intestinal tract, the serous membranes, and the lymphatic glands. The glands are considerably enlarged, and are hard, showing no striking evidence of acute inflammatory action. On section, they are firm, grayish, and translucent in appearance, or present small grayish dots. Caseation is absent, or at least reduced to a minimum.

Microscopically, the chief feature is a proliferation of the endothelial plates, with little or no leukocytosis. The endothelial cells at first form small masses, which ultimately coalesce and encroach upon the lymphoid structure of the gland, so that the hyperplastic tissue is made up of large mononuclear cells, either round, stellate, or spindle-shaped, with pale nuclei and relatively abundant protoplasm. Very often these cell collections undergo hyaline change and are converted into translucent, structureless masses. Caseation is seen only in very long-standing cases. This affection is apparently the benign form of tuberculosis. Duval[3] has reproduced it in the rabbit by injections of attenuated tubercle bacilli.

Syphilis.—The initial lesion of syphilis is followed by a slow, painless enlargement of the nearest lymph-glands (*indolent bubo*). The inguinal, axillary, and epitrochlear, cervical and prevertebral glands have been found affected. The glands are moderately enlarged and firm. Microscopically, the condition is found to be due to thickening of the capsule and septa, with hyperplasia both of the lymphoid and endothelial cells.

[1] Lubarsch, Virch. Arch., 177·1904:371.
[2] See Fagge, Path. Trans., Lond., 25:1874:235; and Bonnet, Jour. de Phys. and Path. gén., 10:827:1899.
[3] Jour. of Exp. Med., 11:1909:403.

The endothelial plates lining the lymph-spaces are the ones chiefly involved. The Spirochæta pallida may often be detected by appropriate staining.[1] The condition may persist for months or even years. When healing takes place, the cells undergo fatty degeneration, the swelling subsides, and the glands become more or less indurated. Gumma formation occurs in tertiary syphilis, and affects usually the inguinal, submaxillary, and cervical glands. As a rule, only one or two are affected.

Plague.—In one form of plague, "pestis bubonica," the involvement of the lymph-glands is striking. In about one-half of the cases the inguinal glands are those first attacked, and in about 25 per cent. the axillary. While the chain of glands next the site of the inoculation is chiefly involved, those elsewhere, notably of the pharynx, the root of the lungs, and the mesentery, are usually quickly attacked. The nodes first infected are greatly enlarged, reddened, and hemorrhagic, and the tissues in the neighborhood show hemorrhagic œdema. In the early stages, or if the infection be not very virulent, they are quite firm, but in other cases they are softened and even liquefied. On section, the nodes are of a grayish-red color, with areas of hemorrhage, or the entire substance may be densely infiltrated with blood. In the severest form they undergo colliquative necrosis and contain a semifluid gummy material, or a substance not unlike lard. The distinction between cortex and medulla is usually lost. In the more remote nodes hemorrhage does not occur except in cases of relapse.

Microscopically, the bloodvessels and the lymphatics are engorged with cells and contain abundant pest bacilli. There is proliferation both of the lymphoid and the endothelial cells, and the latter contain large numbers of bacilli within their protoplasm. An unusual number of "Mast-zellen" is also noticeable. Almost the whole gland may be converted into finely granular material, consisting of a few cells with abundant cellular debris and hosts of bacteria. A few plasma cells may also be seen, but polymorphonuclear cells are quite scarce. It is incorrect, however, to call the softening "suppuration," as is so often done. Bacterial thrombi may be found in the bloodvessels and lymphatics, which are greatly distended and show proliferation and degeneration of their endothelium. Fairly numerous and well-preserved red cells can usually be seen within the necrotic areas. The tissues surrounding the infected glands show inflammatory œdema, the bloodvessels are dilated, and there is an exudate of lymphoid cells and erythrocytes into the lymph-spaces. The bloodvessels contain numerous bacilli. The lymph-glands at some distance from the main lesions are somewhat enlarged and of a darker color than normal, but show merely congestion and hyperplasia.

Leprosy.—In leprosy, changes in the axillary, inguinal, and mesenteric glands are sometimes met with. The affected structures are enlarged, soft, and of yellow color.

---

[1] Tchlenhoff, Roussky Vratch, June 18, 1905, confirming Hoffmann.

Microscopically, all the signs of hyperplastic inflammation may be seen. Fatty changes in the lymphoid cells and reticulum have also been observed, as well as phagocytes containing pigment and blood cells. The specific bacilli may be demonstrated within the nodes.

Parasites.—*Filaria, Trichina, Echinococcus, Cysticercus*, and *Pentastomum* have been met with.

RETROGRESSIVE METAMORPHOSES.

Simple Atrophy.—Simple atrophy occurs as an involution process in old age. The condition affects chiefly the lymphoid elements, although the stroma is relatively or even absolutely increased. The glands are small, increased in consistency, and contain but little juice. An interesting variety is the so-called "lipomatous" atrophy. Here the lymphoid cells of the medulla gradually disappear and the fibrous stroma undergoes fatty metamorphosis. The process gradually extends to the cortical portion and the original follicular structure may in time be utterly destroyed. The affection is said to occur chiefly in the glands of the mesentery, especially in cases of obesity and chronic alcoholism.

Amyloid Disease.—The lymph-glands, particularly those of the abdomen, may be affected in cases of widespread amyloid change. Occasionally, especially where there is chronic bone disease, they may be early or alone involved. In advanced cases the nodes are enlarged, hard, and of a grayish-white semitranslucent appearance. The disease begins in the walls of the arteries and capillaries of the cortex and in the fibrous septa, where it leads to the production of small flattened nodules that gradually encroach upon the lymphoid cells, and in time bring about complete atrophy. In rarer cases the walls of the lymph-sinuses in the medulla are chiefly or alone affected.

Hyaline Degeneration.—This is found particularly as a secondary manifestation in tuberculous nodes. Generally, the reticulum and the lymphoid cells are swollen, hemorrhagic, and transparent, and are fused into irregular masses. Such hyaline degeneration is apt to be the precursor of necrosis, though it is not invariably associated with tuberculosis, being met with also in cancerous glands. Less frequently the degeneration affects the walls of the smaller vessels.

Calcification.—Calcification is usually met with in connection with chronic tuberculosis and certain forms of carcinoma of the glands, but may be found in previously healthy glands, as in osteomalacia.

Pigmentation.—The pigments found in the lymph-glands are either derived from disintegrating red blood corpuscles, present in the nodes themselves or in areas drained by the affected lymph system, or from foreign matter, of the nature of dust, reaching the nodes from extrinsic sources.

The most common type is that known as **anthracosis**, in which coal dust inhaled into the upper respiratory passages is carried by the lymph stream to the nodes, particularly those at the bifurcation of the trachea.

Stone, iron, and other mineral substances sometimes produce an analogous condition. The affected nodes are enlarged and become fibrosed, occasionally calcified. Now and then they are softened.

In cases of **tattooing** the regional lymph-nodes show small deposits of whatever pigment is employed, gunpowder, cinnabar, or other substance.

Necrosis.—Necrosis is fairly common in cases of inflammation, occurring, for instance, in diphtheria, typhoid, tuberculosis, bubonic plague, and septicemia. It is usually due to blocking of vessels, owing to hyperplasia of their endothelial lining. Extensive glandular necroses have been described in connection with severe burns of the skin. J. McCrae has produced a careful study of this form.[1]

PROGRESSIVE METAMORPHOSES.

In the present transitional state of our ideas it is impossible to give a thoroughly scientific description of the progressive changes affecting the lymph-glands.

Hyperplasia.—Hyperplasia is one of the commonest of these changes, and arises from a number of different causes. It is frequently impossible to draw a hard and fast line between what are merely compensatory or inflammatory hyperplasias and true tumor formation. The whole subject of overgrowth of the lymphatic glands at the present time is in such almost hopeless confusion that at this point we have thought it better to deal chiefly, and that in a very sketchy way, with the anatomical conditions of the glands, leaving the fuller consideration of the subject to another place (see vol. i, p. 737).

Many observers, notably Winogradow, Pio Foa, and Mosler, have noted *compensatory hyperplasia* of the lymph-glands after experimental extirpation of the spleen in the lower animals. A similar condition has been observed occasionally in man. The compensation, however, appears to be temporary.

Lymphadenia.—Under the term lymphadenia, or "progressive hyperplasia of the lymph-glands," we may include a number of allied conditions in which there is an increase in the lymphoid and other elements of the glands, whereby they become notably enlarged.

Under this caption we may conveniently deal with the conditions known as **chronic hyperplasia, Hodgkin's disease, leukemia, typical** or **benign lymphoma, atypical** or **malignant lymphoma (lymphosarcoma).**

The distinctions between these various affections have not in the past been by any means clearly defined, nor even yet is their pathogeny fully understood. The confusion that has existed in this regard is to be seen, to take a single example, in the numerous synonyms that have been proposed for Hodgkin's disease, namely, simple adenia (Trousseau), lymphosarcoma (Virchow), malignant lymphoma (Billroth), and pseudo-

[1] The Nature of Internal Lesions in Death from Superficial Burns, American Medicine, 2:1901:735.

leukemia (Cohnheim). More recent studies have done something to bring order out of chaos. To begin with, it is now beyond question that we can get a relatively enormous enlargement of the regional lymph-nodes as a result of inflammation. The majority of such cases are probably due to tuberculosis, which gives rise to two types of lesions, the ordinary granuloma with caseation, and a more chronic hyperplastic form without caseation. In the latter the fibrous tissue is increased, large endothelial cells are numerous, and the lymphoid elements are diminished. Caseation is

FIG. 49

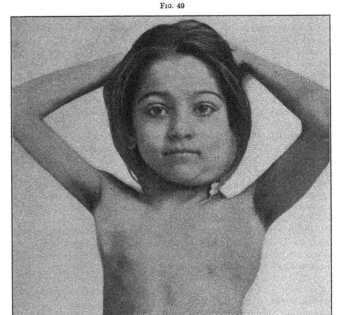

Hodgkin's disease in a young girl. (From Dr. F. G. Finley's clinic, Montreal General Hospital.)

not present here, and the specific bacilli can be detected with difficulty. These are the cases which, as Hilton Fagge was the first to point out,[1] simulate Hodgkin's disease very closely, and no doubt the two affections have been frequently confused. In **Hodgkin's disease** the cervical nodes are the first to be noticeably involved, becoming gradually greatly enlarged and consolidating into dense masses. Subsequently, the axillary, inguinal, retroperitoneal, peribronchial, mediastinal, and

[1] Path. Trans., London, 25: 1874: 235.

mesenteric glands present a similar change, and finally the spleen and liver become enlarged.

Histologically, the process apparently begins with the proliferation of the endothelial plates of the lymph-sinuses and the large cells in the germinal centres. Later, the lymph-sinuses and reticular spaces are filled with proliferating lymphoid and endothelial cells. Numerous giant cells and plasma cells are also to be seen. Goldmann and Kanter[1] pointed out the great abundance of the eosinophile cells in the nodes in this disease, a fact that has been emphasized by some, though, in our judgment, erroneously, as a diagnostic point between Hodgkin's disease and tuberculous adenitis (Dietrich, Fischer, Reed[2]). As the disease advances, the fibrous septa of the nodes increase in size, dividing them into coarse lobules, and gradually bring about a degeneration of the lymphoid and other cellular elements. This connective tissue may show hyaline metamorphosis, and large areas resembling ischemic necrosis are frequently seen. The histological appearances in Hodgkin's disease suggest undoubtedly an inflammatory and probably an infectious origin.

In **leukemia** (of the lymphatic type) the lymph-nodes all over the body are enlarged. Lymphoid tissue everywhere is increased, and the spleen reaches truly colossal proportions. Histologically, all the elements of the nodes are increased, and, unlike Hodgkin's disease, there is no special increase of fibrous tissue. A striking and characteristic feature is the alteration in the blood (excessive lymphocytosis).

Benign lymphoma is extremely rare, but its occurrence is recognized by Le Count[3] and Kundrat.

Lymphosarcoma, histologically speaking, is a small round-celled sarcoma, originating in the proliferation of the lymphoid elements of the lymph-nodes. The nodes enlarge, fuse together, and infiltrate locally, so that enormous solid masses of new-growth are produced. It is found commonly in the thorax, involving the mediastinum and the structures in that region; and has also been noted as beginning in the submucosa of the intestine. It does not form distant metastases. The relationship of this condition to diffuse lymphomatosis has already been discussed (vol. i, p. 737 et seq.).

Tumors.—The only primary growths are **lymphoma, sarcoma, fibrosarcoma, enchondroma,** and **carcinoma.**

According to histological structure, the sarcomas may be divided into round-celled, spindle-celled, and alveolar. The growth may originate in the perithelium of the vessels (*angiosarcoma*), the endothelial lining of the lymph-sinuses (*endothelioma*), from the lymphoid cells (*lymphosarcoma*), and from the connective-tissue stroma (*sarcoma*). The true round-celled sarcoma is hard to distinguish from the lymphosarcoma previously

---

[1] Centralbl. f. allg. Path., 5: 1894: 299.

[2] See Dorothy M. Reed, On the Pathological Changes in Hodgkin's Disease, with Special Reference to its Relationship to Tuberculosis, Johns Hopkins Hospital Reports, 10· 1902 :133.

[3] Jour. of Exper. Med., 4: 1899: 559.

FIG. 50

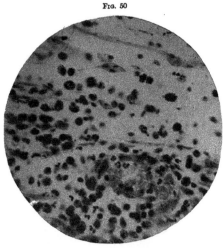

Lymph-node in Hodgkin's disease. The section shows a portion of the cortex of a node with the capsule. The warty-looking cells are eosinophiles, which were numerous in this region. Zeiss obj. $\frac{1}{12}$, oil immersion, ocular No. 1. (From the Pathological Laboratory of the Montreal General Hospital.)

FIG. 51

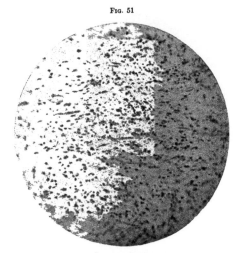

Lymph-node in Hodgkin's disease, showing the extensive fibrosis occurring in the later stage Reichert obj. 7a, without ocular. (From the collection of the Montreal General Hospital.)

FIG. 52

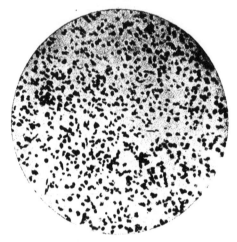

Lymphosarcoma. Leitz obj. No. 7, without ocular. (From the collection of Dr. A. G. Nicholls.)

FIG. 53

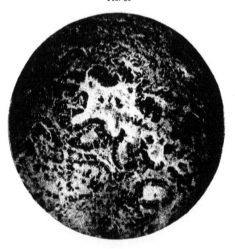

Secondary columnar-celled carcinoma of lymph-node. Zeiss obj. DD, without ocular. (From the collection of the Royal Victoria Hospital.)

referred to. It, however, originates in a single gland and does not tend to involve the neighboring glands. It rather invades the capsule and other tissuès, and produces distant foci of metastatic deposit.

Primary carcinoma has been described.[1] (This should probably be designated alveolar endothelioma).

The secondary growths are carcinoma, sarcoma, chondroma, and myxoma. In secondary sarcoma the glands nearest the primary growth become first involved. They are enlarged and infiltrated with a new-formation more or less perfectly resembling the primary growth. The cells of the secondary growth are formed into clusters or bands surrounded by connective tissue derived from the proliferation of the stroma.

THE SPLEEN.

The exact function of the spleen is still in doubt, but, from the anatomical structure of the organ and from experiment, we can deduce certain conclusions 'that are important, so far as they go. In general terms, the spleen may be described as an organ composed of numerous bloodvessels which discharge their contents into a peculiarly arranged lymphadenoid tissue. The organ, which weighs on an average 170 grams, is bounded by a capsule of fibrous and elastic tissue that sends prolongations or trabeculæ into the substance of the gland. In the central portion these trabeculæ break up into finer ramifications, so as to form a spongy matrix. From the hilus passes in the artery, whose branches follow the connective-tissue septa. The Malpighian corpuscles are seen on section as whitish dots that contrast with the red of the spleen pulp. They consist in small collections of lymphoid cells, either encircling or situated to one side of the afferent arterioles, together with reticulated tissue derived from the adventitia of the vessels. They generally, though not invariably, contain capillaries that empty into the spleen pulp. The circulation is very free. The blood enters at the hilus by the splenic artery, whence it diffuses through to the cortex. There is no doubt now that the arterioles ending in small dilatations, the ampullæ of Thoma, discharge directly into the pulp, while at the same time they communicate closely with the veins.

The pulp is composed of a reticulated fibrous-tissue stroma in which lie numerous lymphoid cells. The walls of the spaces are lined by large mononucleated cells, or endothelial elements, similar to those lining the bloodvessels of the lymph-sinuses. Besides this we may see red blood cells in various stages of degeneration, blood pigment, and phagocytes containing cellular debris and pigment. From this it may be inferred that there is a close relationship between the spleen and the vascular system. The lymphoid character of the pulp cells suggests that one of its functions is to produce lymphocytes, and this is possibly correct. It used to be taught that the large mononuclear and transitional cells of the blood were formed in the spleen, hence they were called "spleno-

[1] V. Willmann, Inaug. Diss. Münch., 1904.

cytes." But we know now that the spleen is not at least the only source of origin, for the splenocytes may still be found in the blood after experimental extirpation of the organ. The main function of the spleen, therefore, seems to be the destruction of the red blood-cells which are found in all stages of disintegration in the pulp. For it has been found that when red blood-corpuscles in excess are introduced into the circulation, there is a great increase in the amount of the erythrocytes and pigment in the spleen. It is now practically settled that the spleen is not normally concerned in the formation of red cells, except during fœtal life and in the first year after birth. In cases of destruction of bone-marrow, it may resume this function.[1] The hyperplasia of the spleen, which is so common a feature in many infective fevers, suggests also that this organ may play a part in the neutralization of toxins. As demonstrated by Roy, the organ exhibits a periodic contraction and expansion (through the agency of the plain muscle fibers present in its capsule). By this means the contents of the sinuses undergo renewal. Owing to this and the close connection with the vascular system, which has suggested the name "abdominal heart" for the spleen, we can understand readily how it is that the spleen is especially liable to be involved in changes in the blood, either from foreign substances reaching it, from the action of soluble toxins, or from alterations in blood pressure. Again, as the splenic vein forms part of the portal system, the pathological conditions in the liver react upon the spleen, and *vice versa*.

CONGENITAL ANOMALIES.

The rarest anomaly is complete **absence** of the spleen. This is most often found in association with other grave defects of development. The splenic artery is usually wanting in such cases. About thirteen cases are on record,[2] but only one, that of Birch-Hirschfeld,[3] is beyond cavil.

More often the place of the spleen is taken by scattered nodules of splenic tissue in various parts (*splenunculi*). H. Albrecht[4] has recorded a remarkable case in which nearly 400 of these splenunculi were found scattered throughout the abdominal cavity. Probably the most common anomaly is the occurrence of **accessory spleens.** These occur in our experience in 11 per cent. of all autopsies. They vary in number from one to twenty, and may be scarcely recognizable or as large as a walnut. Care should be taken not to mistake hemolymph-nodes for accessory spleens. The latter are found usually on the under side of the gastrosplenic omentum, the mesentery, the wall of the intestine, and

[1] Meyer u. Heineke, Verhandl. d. deut. Path. Gesellschaft, 9 : 1905 : 224; Morris, Johns Hopkins Hospital Bull., 18: 1907: 200.
[2] See Hodenpyl, Med. Record, 54:1898:695.
[3] Defect der Milz bei einem Neugeborenen, Arch. f. Heilk., Leipzig, 12: 1871: 190.
[4] Ziegler's Beiträge, 20:1896:513.

in the tail of the pancreas. Irregularities in shape and position are rather common. Rolleston has recorded a remarkable case in which there was a tongue-like process extending into the scrotum.

Congenital dislocation of the spleen has been observed in cases of umbilical and diaphragmatic hernia. The so-called *"wandering spleen"* is in part due to congenital laxity of the tissues at the hilus, but perhaps more important is increased weight of the spleen, such as may be brought about by malaria. In these cases the spleen may be found in the pelvis. In *transposition* of the viscera, the spleen may be found on the right side.

Alterations in Position.—The spleen may be found in almost any part of the abdominal cavity. This may be due in part to congenital laxness of its attachments, but increase in the weight of the organ is the chief cause. In other cases the organ may be dragged down, as in gastroptosis and enteroptosis. Occasionally, inflammatory adhesions fix it in the abnormal position.

CIRCULATORY DISTURBANCES.

Anemia.—Anemia of the spleen is found in all forms of generalized anemia and in compression of the organ from any cause. The organ is small, the capsule somewhat wrinkled, and on section the tissue is pale, grayish-red, and less pulpy than usual, while the trabeculæ stand out prominently.

Hyperemia.—**Active or congestive hyperemia** is found in cases of infection or intoxication, and is closely allied to acute inflammation, of which it forms the first stage. It leads to rapid swelling of the organ, with distension of the bloodvessels, so that the part contains more blood than normal. The spleen is usually greatly enlarged, the capsule is tense and thin, and through it can be seen the congested pulp. The swelling may be so great that spontaneous rupture of the organ may occur. On section, it is soft, pulpy, and intensely reddened, so that the corpuscles and trabeculæ are quite indistinct.

Passive Hyperemia.—Passive hyperemia is a common condition and is brought about by obstruction to the free exit of blood from the spleen such as may result from valvular disease of the heart, defective pulmonary circulation, cirrhosis of the liver, and thrombosis of the splenic vein The affected organ is somewhat enlarged, the capsule tense, opaque and sometimes thickened. The consistency is also increased. On section, the tissue is, as a rule, dark purple-red in color, firm and dry, and the trabeculæ and bloodvessels are thickened.

Microscopically, the veins are congested, even cavernous, and the pulp is greatly suffused with blood, and may contain blood pigment. The trabeculæ and reticulum generally are thickened, and the vessels may show endarteritis. This condition is called *cyanotic induration*

Infarction.—This is a fairly common event in the spleen, owing to the fact that the splenic artery is a large vessel that breaks up quickly

into branches forming relatively small end-arteries.   The usual cause of
embolism is the dislodgment of fine particles from the heart-valves or
aorta.   An occasional cause is thrombosis of the splenic artery, more
rarely of the splenic vein.   Osler has recorded infarction in a movable
spleen due to twisting of the pedicle.   Embolic infarcts are single or
multiple, and are of small size, or, again, may involve the whole thickness of the organ.   The smaller infarcts are more or less wedge-shaped,
with the apex toward the hilus.   Recent infarcts form a firm prominence

Fig. 54

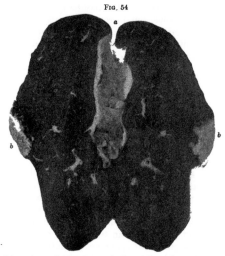

White infarct of the spleen.   Section was made through the infarct, the organ being thereby
laid open.   (From the Pathological Laboratory of McGill University.)

on the surface of the organ.   On section, the affected area is ivory-white
in color, less commonly somewhat hemorrhagic, and sharply defined
from the rest of the splenic tissue.   Mixed forms also occur, where the
centre is pale and the periphery infiltrated with blood.   According to
Orth, all infarcts at first are white, but later some may become hemorrhagic.   Beattie and Dixon claim on the other hand that all infarcts
exhibit a preliminary congestive stage, which may pass on either to the
white or the hemorrhagic stage.
    Microscopically, the anemic region shows coagulation-necrosis, the
cells are swollen and granular and their nuclei indistinct.   In advanced
conditions, the nuclei have disappeared and the tissue is converted into
a granular, slightly refractile, fibrinoid material.   In parts, especially
about the periphery, the cells show a certain amount of fatty degeneration.   As a rule, surrounding the infarct there is a zone of reactive
inflammation.   As the infarct ages, the necrotic material is gradually

-softened and absorbed, while vascular granulation tissue develops at the periphery and gradually substitutes the damaged area, until finally only a pigmented scar remains. In the red infarct the vessels are greatly distended and the pulp 'is densely infiltrated with blood. When the emboli are infective the infarcts rapidly soften and are converted into abscesses. Rarely, these heal and may cause local adhesive perisplenitis. Or, again, they may burst into the peritoneal cavity and set up a fatal peritonitis.

Hemorrhage.—Hemorrhage into the spleen is of frequent occurrence, but it is often difficult to be sure of the condition, since the spleen pulp normally contains such great numbers of red cells. Apart from traumatism and infarction, the usual causes are malaria, typhoid, variola, leukemia, and purpura hæmorrhagica; in fact, any condition that may set up acute splenitis. The hemorrhages are recognized as dark red spots or streaks in the parenchyma.

INFLAMMATIONS.

Splenitis.—**Acute Splenitis.**—Acute splenitis is closely associated with congestive hyperemia, and, indeed, can hardly be considered apart from it. The condition arises in the course of a variety of infective fevers, such as typhoid, pneumonia, scarlatina, diphtheria, septicemia, malaria, and relapsing fever, and is characterized in the main by hyperplasia. The spleen is enlarged, sometimes to several times its usual size, soft, and the capsule is tense. On section, the organ in the earlier stages is intensely hyperemic and firm. Later, it becomes pulpy, almost diffluent, and of a grayish-red color. The follicles are usually not prominent, but may be noticeably enlarged in scarlatina. Not infrequently on the capsule is a fibrinous or fibrinopurulent exudation (*perisplenitis*).

Microscopically, there is a numerical increase chiefly of the lymphoid cells, many of which show fatty change, while large multinucleated cells are to be seen containing pigment, broken-down blood-corpuscles, and lymphoid cells. The vascular sinuses and lymphatics are dilated and their endothelium shows signs of proliferation and fatty degeneration. Small hemorrhages into the splenic substance are common. In certain cases the follicles also participate in the acute hyperplasia. . In connection with scarlatina, Klein[1] has described hyaline degeneration of the smaller vessels.

Besides the appearances just described, there are certain others that deserve mention. Rarely, the follicles are found to be of a yellow color in the centre and softened, having undergone, not suppurative, but rather colliquative, necrosis. This has been described particularly in connection with typhus exanthematicus and relapsing fever. More common are areas of necrosis which may be merely of microscopic size, but which occasionally reach that of a cherry. These are found chiefly in typhoid, diphtheria, scarlatina, and relapsing fever, either in the pulp

---

[1] Trans. Path. Soc. Lond., 28:1877:430.

or follicles. The affected cells are found in all stages of disintegration, so that in the affected area we find fragments of nuclei and cellular debris. About the periphery is an extravasation of leukocytes. The condition is due, in part, to the direct action of bacterial toxins, but chiefly to anemia brought about by the obstruction of the bloodvessels and lymphatics through cell proliferation and the accumulation of debris. The larger necrotic foci may soften or suppurate and may burst through the capsule, thus setting up purulent peritonitis.

The results of acute splenitis are various. Commonly, the process subsides, the hyperemia gradually disappears, the hyperplastic cells are disintegrated and absorbed, and complete resolution takes place. Rarely, the simple splenitis may become suppurative, or the process may become chronic.

Suppurative Splenitis.—In this form the whole spleen may be diffusely infiltrated with pus, but it is more common to find multiple abscesses. The condition is usually due to a hematogenic infection with pyogenic microörganisms, such as occurs in ulcerative endocarditis and septicemia. Here the process is frequently combined with hemorrhagic infarction. In other cases the inflammation may extend from neighboring parts, as, for instance, in ulcerating carcinoma of the stomach, abscess of the pancreas, perinephritic abscess, and purulent peritonitis. The abscesses may rupture into the peritoneal cavity, the left pleura, left lung, stomach, or intestines. Should the patient live, the abscesses, when small, may be absorbed and become fibroid; the larger ones finally become enclosed in a fibrous capsule, while the contents become inspissated or calcareous. Calling to mind the relative frequency of pyemic and bacteriemic states, the rarity of suppurative disturbances in the spleen is very remarkable. It can only be explained on the assumption of strong bactericidal properties on the part of this organ.

Chronic Indurative Splenitis.—This may be the result of acute splenitis or may be an insidious process from the first. It is found chiefly in malaria, cirrhosis of the liver, rickets, kala-azar, and late syphilis, and leads to considerable increase in the size of the organ (splenomegaly).

In malaria the process may, for a time, run an acute course, just as in other infective fevers, but, as a rule, the spleen, in addition to the signs of active inflammation, contains yellow, brownish, or black pigment in the pulp and in the centre of the follicles. In relapsing cases and chronic malarial cachexia the spleen becomes permanently enlarged and firm in consistence, owing to the overgrowth of fibrous connective tissue (ague cake). The capsule is usually thickened and the organ is more or less firmly attached to the diaphragm. The enlargement may be so great that the spleen may become dislocated, or grow until it reaches the pelvis. It is not uncommon, also, to find amyloid change. The overgrowth of fibrous tissue is permanent, but the organ may occasionally diminish in size, owing to the destruction of the lymphoid elements.

Another form of splenomegaly that has been confounded with malaria, associated with febrile disturbance, is found in kala-azar. Here the parasites are enclosed in the smaller endothelial cells. The spleen is enlarged and firm, but friable and not sclerotic.

A very puzzling form of enlargement of the spleen that should be referred to here is **Banti's Disease**,[1] which is believed to be a primary splenomegaly characterized by a progressive hyperplasia of the connective tissue of the organ and a moderate grade of systemic anemia. After some months the liver becomes enlarged and a slight grade of jaundice becomes manifest. Later, the liver contracts, ascites sets in and we get the usual picture of Laennec's cirrhosis. The disease differs from the latter affection in that the spleen is more enlarged, and in the order in which the various symptoms become developed. The relationship to Laennec's cirrhosis and to so-called anemia splenica is still disputed. Banti himself regards the affection as a manifestation of an infectious or toxic influence brought to the spleen through the blood, where it produces a fibrosis beginning in the centre of the follicles that spreads to the pulp and eventually produces a sclerosing phlebitis extending to the portal vein. Good results in early cases have followed removal of the enlarged spleen.

It may be remarked in this connection that the term "anemia splenica" is not a very illuminating one, for anemia associated with splenomegaly is met with in more than one affection, notably, for example, in malaria, tuberculosis, leukemia, pseudoleukemia, and hereditary syphilis.

A still more obscure affection is the so-called **Idiopathic Splenomegaly** (Gaucher[2]). Here there is enlargement of the spleen and liver (but without ascites), anemia, melanosis of the skin, and a tendency to purpura. Histologically, in the spleen one sees an accumulation of large hyaline-looking cells, either diffused throughout the organ or arranged in clumps and strands. Similar cells are found in the liver, lymph-glands, and bone-marrow. They are probably of endothelial origin and the affection appears to be one of the entire lymphatic and hematopoietic systems.

In cirrhosis of the liver the spleen is often noticeably enlarged and this both in the portal and the biliary forms (Hanot's type), the enlargement being more marked in the former. It used to be thought that this was due to stasis in the portal circulation, but this is undoubtedly not the whole explanation, for the spleen may be enlarged and hyperplastic in cases where portal obstruction is not present, while its substance may be pale red and soft, quite unlike the hard cyanotic spleen of passive congestion. It is more probable that infective microörganisms, or circulating toxins, are at work here as well. The hyperplasia affects the pulp, which contains numerous red and white cells without any special change in structure. Later, the arrangement of the pulp becomes confused and there is a cellular transformation of the reticular connective tissue.[3]

---

[1] Banti, Lo Sperimentale, 1894, and Zeigler's Beiträge, 24: 1898.

[2] Thése de Paris, 1882.

[3] A good resumé of the subject of splenomegaly, apart from leukemic conditions, is given by Osler, British Medical Journal, 2: 1908: 1151.

Tuberculosis.—This is rarely primary in the spleen. *Acute miliary tuberculosis* occurs in systemic dissemination of the tuberculous infection. The spleen is enlarged, the parenchyma on section is soft, swollen, and dark red in color, and is universally scattered over with minute round grayish tubercles.

Microscopically the miliary nodules may be purely lymphoid in type, but more commonly endothelioid, and giant cells are present as well. Slight caseation is often observed.

In another form the tubercles may be fewer, rarer, and caseous These are found in the Malpighian bodies and about the bloodvessels There is apt to be more or less adhesive perisplenitis.

FIG. 55

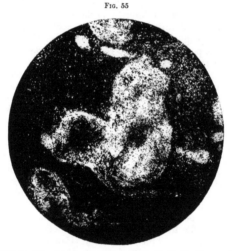

Caseous tuberculosis of the spleen (miliary type).   Leitz obj. No. 7, without ocular.   (From the collection of Dr. A G. Nicholls.)

Syphilis.—*Miliary gummas* are rare, but are met with in **both** inherited and acquired syphilis. Large gummas, varying in size **from** that of a pea to that of an egg, have been described.

Diffuse hyperplasia is by far the most common and important syphilitic manifestation. The condition may be acute, affecting the lymphoid cells, or may lead to chronic thickening of the reticulum and trabeculæ. In long-standing disease amyloid change is also met with. In some cases of old lues the spleen contains abundant pigment.

Leprosy.—The spleen is enlarged and presents numerous granulomas, which contain the specific bacillus.

Glanders.—The organ is enlarged, soft, greatly reddened, and studded with multiple abscesses, containing thick yellow, rather viscid pus, in which the specific bacillus may be demonstrated. In chronic cases amyloid deposit may also be observed.

Actinomycosis.—This is rare in the spleen and generally a secondary manifestation. It leads to the formation of isolated abscesses filled with glairy pus, in which can be recognized the actinomycosis "grains."

Parasites.—*Echinococcus, Cysticercus,* and *Pentastomum denticulatum* have been met with.

RETROGRESSIVE METAMORPHOSES.

Atrophy.—Atrophy of the spleen is found in old people and in those suffering from long-standing disease. It may follow acute splenitis and may be produced by general anemia or by any obstruction of the splenic artery leading to local anemia. The spleen is small, firm, and the capsule wrinkled. On section, the pulp is noticeably diminished, the trabeculæ are prominent, and the organ contains but little blood.

Hyaline Degeneration.—Hyaline degeneration has been observed in the vessels and reticulum. It is sometimes superadded to amyloid disease.

Amyloid Infiltration.—This is a fairly common occurrence. There are two main types, the "sago" spleen and the diffuse amyloid or "bacony" spleen, but these forms are frequently combined. In the first type, the spleen is not enlarged to any extent and its consistency is but little altered. On section, the pulp is red and thickly studded with firm, translucent, gelatinous-looking bodies, varying in size from a millet seed to a pin's head or somewhat larger. These are the amyloid Malpighian bodies, and they bear a close resemblance to grains of boiled sago, whence the name. Microscopically, the amyloid material is laid down in the walls of the smaller arterioles and capillaries, chiefly in the intermediate zone of the Malpighian bodies, so that the appearance presented is that of a ring of amyloid material. In more advanced conditions, the whole corpuscle may be thus transformed. The vessels are of course thickened and the lymphoid elements tend to atrophy. It may happen, however, that the vessels are not particularly involved.

In the diffuse form, which is less common, the organ is moderately enlarged, the capsule distended, and the edges rounded. The tissue is firm like rubber and is translucent when a thin section is held up to the light. On section, by reflected light, the surface is of a peculiar semitransparent, reddish color, as if covered with a thin coating of gelatin, whence it has been compared to ham or bacon (Speckmilz).

Microscopically, the amyloid change affects the walls of the venous radicles and the reticulum of the pulp. The endothelial lining of the vessels is unaffected and the lymphoid cells show merely the effects of pressure. The Malpighian bodies, as a rule, escape in this form.

The causes of amyloid disease are the usual ones, chronic wasting affections and cachexias, osteomyelitis, suppuration, septicemia, tuberculosis, syphilis, intermittent fever, chronic glanders, carcinoma, and the like. Associated with the disease, and depending equally upon the initial cause, are pigmentation, infarction, and fibrous hyperplasia.

Pigmentary Infiltration.—This is met with in cases of passive congestion, the cachexias, leukemia, and all diseases associated with blood destruction.   It is well marked in malaria and in hemochromatosis; rarely, particles of coal dust may reach the spleen.   According to its nature, the pigment is golden, reddish, reddish-brown, through all shades of brown to black.   It is laid down chiefly about the bloodvessels in the trabeculæ, but may lie free or within phagocytic cells.

Necrosis.—Necrosis may involve the spleen in cases in which the blood supply is suddenly cut off.

PROGRESSIVE METAMORPHOSES.

Regenerative Hyperplasia.—Regenerative hyperplasia has been observed in cases where a portion of the spleen has been destroyed. Both the Malpighian bodies and the pulp participate in the process.

FIG. 56

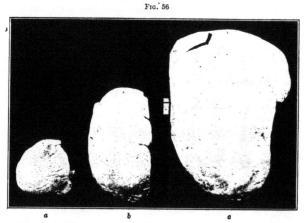

a   *b*   *c*

The spleen in three different conditions, to illustrate variations in size.   From left to right. *a*, normal spleen; *b*, typhoidal spleen; *c*, leukemic spleen.   (From the Pathological Museum of McGill University.)

Nodular hyperplasia, the so-called "splenadenoma," which perhaps ought to be classed with the tumors, is met with in dogs and has occasionally been seen in man.   It forms a nodular mass the size of a cherry or less, of a bright grayish-red color, fairly well defined from the rest of the spleen.   It is occasionally surrounded by a fibrous capsule.

Microscopically, there is hyperplasia not only of the lymphoid cells, but also of the fibrous stroma.

As in the case of the lymph-nodes, it is difficult to draw the line between inflammatory hyperplasia of the spleen and tumor formation, and there are certain enlargements of the organ, notably in leukemia, pseudo-leukemia, and Hodgkin's disease, which belong to this debatable ground.

The changes found in the spleen in leukemia and pseudoleukemia are practically identical. The organ may be greatly enlarged, so that it reaches even into the pelvis, and may weigh as much as 3 kg. or more. The capsule is thickened in places and covered with numerous shaggy adhesions, binding it to the diaphragm and the neighboring structures. Two main forms are recognizable: the first in which the hyperplasia is confined to the spleen pulp, and the second where the Malpighian corpuscles are involved. In the first, the parenchyma is soft and bright red or reddish-gray, while the corpuscles show little or no change. Hemorrhagic infarcts of considerable size are not uncommon. Microscopically, one sees hyperemia with hyperplasia both of the lymphoid cells and the connective-tissue stroma. In the second variety, the Malpighian bodies are greatly enlarged, forming whitish, tumor-like masses arranged in nodules or bands. They vary in size from that of a pea to that of a walnut. In long-standing cases, owing to the overgrowth of fibrous tissue, the organ becomes firm and the color gray, often streaked with brown or brownish-black pigment. In these diseases the spleen may be the first and only organ to be affected, but, as a rule, analogous changes are to be found in the lymph-nodes and bone-marrow.

Tumors.—Tumors do not commonly involve the spleen. Among the primary benign growths may be mentioned **fibroma, chondroma, osteoma,** and **lymphangioma.** Langhans[1] has recorded a curious case of **angioma cavernosum** (angiosarcoma?) in which small secondary masses were present in the liver. **Dermoid cysts** are rare. **Simple cysts,** containing clear or blood-stained fluid, may arise from degeneration of the parenchyma, the dilatation of the lymph-spaces (Fink and Aschoff), or from the inclusion of peritoneal endothelium (Renggli[2]).

Sarcoma.[3]—Sarcoma occurs occasionally as a primary growth, but is usually secondary. A form arising from the endothelial plates has been described.[4] **Melanotic sarcoma** not uncommonly leads to metastases in the spleen, which, however, are not necessarily pigmented.

Carcinoma.—Carcinoma is invariably secondary and arises either by metastasis or direct extension from the stomach. It is rarer even than secondary sarcoma.

THE BONE-MARROW.

Anatomically speaking, the marrow forms an integral portion of the bones, so that it is difficult to conceive of it as detached from this association. Nevertheless, the marrow can hardly be regarded as forming a

[1] Virch. Archiv, 85: 1879· 273; see also Thiele, Virch. Arch., 178: 1904.
[2] Inaug. Diss Zurich, 1894.
[3] See Jepson and Albert, Annals of Surgery, 40:1904:80.
[4] Bunting, Univ. of Penna. Med. Bull., 16:1903:188.

part of the supporting structure of the body, except in so far as it contributes to the nourishment of bone. Histologically, its structure is closely akin to that of the spleen and lymph-nodes, and as its main function undoubtedly is to produce certain types of blood-cells, it seems more logical to consider it in its physiological rather than its anatomical relationships.

The bone-marrow is in its young state soft, cellular, and well supplied with bloodvessels. The stroma is composed of branching connective-tissue cells forming a fine reticulum, in the meshes of which lie a great variety of cells, namely, red blood-cells, hematoblasts, lymphocytes, eosinophiles, pigmented cells, and multinucleated giant cells (myeloplaxes; megacaryocytes). The bloodvessels are wide, thin-walled, and arranged so that collapse cannot occur. On account of its appearance and structure, this form is called the red or lymphoid bone-marrow. Red bone-marrow is present in all the bones at birth, but gradually changes its character, the cells of the supporting stroma being transformed into fat (*lipoid atrophy*). The color thus changes from red to yellow, hence the term "yellow" bone-marrow. At about the age of puberty all the long bones contain this yellow marrow. The red marrow, however, persists into advanced life in the sternum, ribs, vertebræ, and skull. With old age the yellow fatty marrow exhibits serous atrophy.

The function of the bone-marrow is to produce blood-corpuscles and to absorb or otherwise render harmless foreign substances in the blood. The giant cells just referred to can also on occasion act as osteoclasts.

CIRCULATORY DISTURBANCES.

Anemia.—Anemia occurs, but is so closely associated with regeneration of the medulla that it is better dealt with under the Progressive Metamorphoses.

Hyperemia.—In hyperemia the yellow marrow assumes a reddish-yellow color.

Hemorrhage.—Hemorrhage into the medulla occurs from traumatism and from obstruction to the free exit of blood from the part.

INFLAMMATIONS.

Inflammatory infections so commonly involve the bone as well, that they are better considered under affections of the bones. The usual forms are **osteomyelitis, metastatic abscesses, tuberculosis, syphilis,** and **leprosy.** Litten and Orth[1] have pointed out that in many infectious diseases associated with acute splenic tumors, such as sepsis, typhoid fever, fibrinous pneumonia, an analogous hyperplasia is present in the bone-marrow. This has been confirmed for acute endocarditis

[1] Ueber Veränderungen des Marks in Röhrenknochen unter verschiedenen pathologischen Verhältnissen, Berl. klin. Woch., 14:1877:743.

by Ponfick, and for variola by Golgi. In addition to hyperplasia, fatty degeneration of the vessels has been noted, as well as the presence of numerous-cells containing broken-down blood-corpuscles and pigment.

Metastatic Abscesses.—Metastatic abscesses are found in the marrow not uncommonly in septicemia and certain other infectious fevers, notably variola.

Tuberculosis.—Tuberculosis arises as a hematogenic infection in most cases, and usually begins in the cancellous part of the bone. It occurs also in the miliary form, in general systemic tuberculous infection.

Syphilis.—Syphilis takes the form of gummas. It is rare in the marrow.

Leprosy.—Granulomas containing the characteristic bacillus have been found.

RETROGRESSIVE METAMORPHOSES.

Atrophy.—Atrophy of the bone-marrow occurs in old age, in chronic pulmonary emphysema, chronic pulmonary tuberculosis, chronic nephritis, and in death from starvation. The fat cells are gradually absorbed and the tissue shrinks. Its place is taken by a mucinous fluid, so that the marrow becomes gelatinous, translucent, and somewhat brownish (Gallertmark). The condition is identical with the *serous atrophy* of fat that occurs elsewhere.

Fatty Degeneration.—Fatty degeneration of the capillaries and medullary cells is met with in certain of the infectious fevers, notably typhoid, typhus, and relapsing fever.

Focal Necroses.—Focal necroses may occur under similar circumstances.

PROGRESSIVE METAMORPHOSES.

Hyperplasia.—Hyperplasia of the fatty tissue of the marrow is met with in the generalized atrophy of the skeleton that occurs in old age. Not only are the medullary canals enlarged, but the bone itself becomes rarefied, cancellous, and infiltrated with fat. Not infrequently the fat gradually disappears and there is a hyperplasia of the marrow, so that it reverts to the more primitive form of red or lymphoid marrow. This occurs in anemia, leukemia, chronic pulmonary tuberculosis, suppurative bone disease, and cancerous cachexia. It has also been found in many of the infectious diseases, such as typhoid, pneumonia, septicemia, acute endocarditis, and variola, also in cases where death has occurred after prolonged illness. The process begins first in the long bones and involves the epiphyses of the upper part of the bones, gradually spreading to the whole medulla. The fatty tissue is gradually reduced and replaced by lymphoid cells until the medulla assumes a reddish-gray or dark red color and, in severe cases, the appearance of raspberry jelly.

Microscopically, there is a great increase in the number of all the marrow cells, but particularly the nucleated red corpuscles, suggesting that the process is a regenerative one. The lymphoid cells are often fatty, and there are numerous phagocytic and pigment-bearing cells. Besides these, there may be seen numbers of small octahedral crystals, the so-called Charcot-Neumann crystals.

Neumann[1] was the first to draw attention to that form of leukemia in which the bone-marrow was first and chiefly affected, hence called **medullary** or **myelogenic leukemia.** The changes in the marrow have been regarded as the cause of the altered blood condition. Pure myelogenic leukemia, that is, leukemia apart from marked changes in the spleen and lymph-glands, is certainly rare, but one instance has come under our notice at the Royal Victoria Hospital. This occurred in a man, aged sixty-eight years. The bone-marrow presented a marked raspberry-jelly appearance, while the spleen was small. The retroperitoneal glands were somewhat enlarged, but not more so than in many cases of other forms of disease. The bone-marrow is not always soft, juicy, and gelatinous in myelogenic leukemia, but, as Ponfick[2] pointed out, may assume a grayish-yellow or even green color, owing to the great increase in the numbers of the colorless cells (*pyoid marrow*). Not only this, but the marrow is anemic from compression of the vessels and inflammation of their walls. Red blood-cells normal and nucleated, fattily degenerated leukocytes, and Charcot-Neumann crystals are here found in varying amounts. The two forms, therefore, seem to be but variations of the same condition.

In **pseudoleukemia** the changes in the bone-marrow are also variable. At one time there is hyperplasia such as is found in anemias, at another lymphomatous nodules.

Tumors.—Tumors of the medulla may arise from the cellular elements or from the fibrous stroma. Many of these lead to rarefaction of the bone through pressure or the action of osteoclasts. With this there is frequently a new formation of bone from the periosteum. This is particularly well seen in the giant-celled or "myeloid" sarcoma, or more accurately myeloma (see vol. i, 733), which may start from the medulla and form a large tumor. On the surface of the growth can be felt thin plates of bone that give on pressure a peculiar sensation resembling the crackling of an egg shell. There is in tumors of this kind a tendency to develop bone in their interior. Among the malignant growths, besides the sarcomas, **carcinomas** are sometimes met with.

Among benign growths may be mentioned **fibroma, chondroma, myxoma,** and **fibromyxoma.** Virchow has described a myelogenous **angioma** of the vertebræ.

Of these various tumors, **sarcomas** are by far the most common. Several forms are described. The most usual site for their development is in the maxillæ and the epiphyses of the long bones, especially the humerus and tibia. They may, however, start in the diaphysis. In the early stages they produce a gradual caries of the bone, so that spontaneous

[1] Berl. klin. Woch., 14:1877·685.　　　　[2] Virch. Arch., 56:1872:550.

fractures are not rare, and eventually lead to great expansion and rarefaction of the bone. The softer growths are round-celled, while the
firmer are spindle-celled, but mixed forms occur. Of the mixed type
the most interesting is the **giant-celled myeloma** (*tumeur à myeloplaxes*
of Nélaton). Here in the ground substance are round, spindle, or
mixed cells, with a varying amount of connective tissue and numerous
large, multinucleated cells. These tumors are often very vascular,
owing to the presence of wide vessels. These may give way, so that

FIG. 57

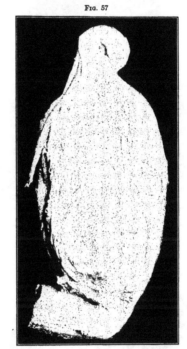

Sarcoma of the shaft of the humerus. (From the Pathological Museum of McGill University.)

hemorrhage and degeneration are not infrequent occurrences. The
presence of so much blood gives them a bright red appearance that is
somewhat characteristic. They are relatively less malignant than other
forms of sarcomas in that they do not tend to form metastases. Not
infrequently, masses and bands of osteoid tissue or even true bone are
formed (osteoid sarcoma, osteosarcoma). Retrogressive changes are
not uncommon in this form of tumor, and we meet with fatty degeneration
hemorrhage, pigmentation, liquefaction, and cyst formation. Occasion-

ally, the greater portion of the tumor may be destroyed. Another form is the **alveolar sarcoma,** in which the stroma is arranged in alveoli containing nests of relatively large cells, so that an appearance not unlike

FIG. 58

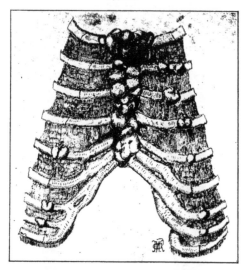

The sternum and ribs, showing the location of myelomatous growths. (Herrick and Hektoen's case.)

FIG. 59

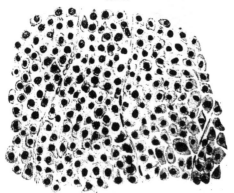

Section of myeloma of vertebra. X 600. (S. Saltykow.)

carcinoma is produced. An **alveolar endothelioma** has been described by Billroth,[1] Hildebrand,[2] and Driessen.[3] Some, at least, of these and of the alveolar sarcomas of bone would seem to be secondary adrenal growths.

An interesting form to which much attention has been paid recently is one resembling a small round-celled or lymphosarcoma, the so-called **myeloma.** The exact etiology of this growth is yet a matter of doubt, as is proved by the great number of names that have been proposed for it, namely, angiosarcoma, lymphosarcoma, lymphadenia ossium (Nothnagel[4]), general lymphadenomatosis of bone (Weber), myeloma (v. Rustizky, Klebs, Herrick and Hektoen[5]), and plasmoma.

The peculiarities of this growth are that it develops usually in old persons, forms multiple apparently individual growths in different portions of the bony skeleton, and takes the shape of nodules or diffuse infiltrations of soft consistency. The skull, vertebral column, and ribs are the sites of election. Multiple spontaneous fractures of the bone frequently result. As a rule, but little new bone is formed, yet exceptions to this statement occur. Microscopically, there is a delicate connective-tissue stroma inclosing masses of small round cells and presenting numerous large and imperfectly defined bloodvessels. Wright[6] has pointed out that most of the cells closely resemble "plasma" cells. A curious point associated with this growth is the excretion of albumose in the urine.[7] As we have pointed out in the first volume, the multiple nature and characteristics of this form of growth place it among the blastomatoid formations, as a **myelomatosis** rather than a **myeloma.**

Carcinoma of the bone-marrow is invariably secondary and arises by direct infection or by metastasis. Nodular and diffuse forms are met with.

It may be remarked in this connection that carcinomas of the thyroid gland, prostate, and breast, as well as hypernephromas, exhibit a special tendency to involve the bone-marrow in their metastases.

[1] *Langenbeck's Archiv.*, 11:1869:244.

[2] *Deutsche Zeitschr. f. Chir.*, 31:1891:263.

[3] *Ziegler's Beitr.*, 12:1893:65.

[4] *Internat. Beitr. Festschr. f. Virchow*, 1891.

[5] *Medical News*, 65:1894:239.

[6] *Boston Soc. of Med. Sci.*, 4:1900:195.

[7] See Bence-Jones, *Phil. Trans. Royal Soc.*, 1848 : Part I : 55.

SECTION II.

THE RESPIRATORY SYSTEM.

CHAPTER XI.

THE RESPIRATORY FUNCTION AND ITS DISTURBANCES.

Embryological Considerations.—We need not detain ourselves long over the consideration of the practical bearing of questions of development of the respiratory system. Few of the anomalies are of much clinical importance, though many are of scientific interest. The formation of the upper respiratory passages is closely connected with that of the cephalic bones and cerebrum and will be dealt with more fully elsewhere. Of some surgical importance are **branchial fistulæ cysts**, due to imperfectly closed bronchial clefts which may, among other situations, be found in close proximity to the larynx. (See Vol. I, p. 852.)

.The trachea, bronchi, and lungs develop as a diverticulum from the primitive alimentary tract. This relationship is shown in the occasional persistence of fistulæ between the trachea and œsophagus, and the occurrence of cysts on the posterior wall of the trachea or in the wall of the œsophagus.

Anatomy.—There are a great many points in connection with the anatomical structure of the respiratory organs which call for remark. Many of these, however, are more conveniently and usefully dealt with when we come to speak of questions of function, so that at this point we will confine ourselves to the more general considerations.

The first thing that strikes one is that the lungs are so constructed that the maximum amount of blood is brought into close proximity to the maximum amount of air, thus facilitating the interchange of gaseous and other substances. Next, the presence of abundant elastic fibrils in the alveolar walls assists in the recoil of the lung and.directly promotes the elimination of the unused residue of the air and the circulation of blood and lymph. This movement of the lung tissue, which is, of course, absolutely necessary for the maintenance of life and health, may, under certain circumstances, as, for example, when there is a local area of infection, prove an actual menace in that it tends to disseminate the causal agents of the disease. The trachea and bronchi, with the exception of the terminal ramifications, are practically rigid tubes which, therefore, do not become occluded without the existence of some very gross condition. In this connection it may be mentioned, as a practical point, that the orifice of the right bronchus is wider than that of the left and its direction is more vertical, so that foreign bodies accidentally inhaled almost invariably pass into the right lung.

The lungs possess a double blood supply, from the right ventricle through the pulmonary artery, and from the aorta through the bronchial arteries. While many of the arteries of the lung are end-arteries, we can, nevertheless, readily understand how it is that obstruction in one set of vessels does not entirely cut off the blood supply of the affected part. The nourishment of the lung is good. Consequently, anemic infarcts are almost unknown, and necrosis (as a result of circulatory disturbances alone) is practically impossible, unless both sets of vessels are interfered with at the same time. On the other hand, congestion and hemorrhage are quite common. This is due to the fact that the capillaries, which possess a most tenuous structure, are but badly supported by the scanty connective and elastic tissue of the alveolar walls. The capillaries, therefore, can readily become overdistended and can equally readily give way. As will easily be understood from what has just been said, in such a delicate organ as the lung circulatory disturbances may make their appearance very quickly and usually produce marked effects.

Finally, the free communication of the lungs with the external air renders them the more liable to irritation and infection from extrinsic causes.

Applied Physiology.—In discussing the broad pathology, as distinct from the pathological histology, of the respiratory system, we have to keep constantly before us the primary function of that system, namely, the intake of oxygen and the discharge of carbon dioxide for the benefit of the economy. All other functions are in comparison of minor importance. Strictly speaking, respiration is concerned with the whole problem of gaseous interchange, not merely between the system and the external medium, but also between the blood, the internal vehicle, and the tissue cells.

Internal Respiration.—This latter, the internal respiration, we can but glance at incidentally, although it is the process to which the other is subservient. The data regarding the conditions in which oxygen exists in the blood, the avidity for it exhibited by the hemoglobin of the erythrocytes, its entrance into combination with the same, are known to every first year student of medicine. But of the processes occurring in the capillaries governing the discharge of the oxygen, of its entrance into the tissues and into the cells, and of the changes undergone in these cells we know singularly little.

The arterial blood, we know, is almost saturated, but not quite, with oxygen, nor is this wholly used up in the circulation through the tissues; even in the last stages of asphyxia some oxygen can still be gained from the blood. In other words, the blood carries more oxygen than is needed by the tissues. Some of this oxygen, but only a small portion, would seem to undergo direct reduction in the red corpuscles, with production of carbon dioxide. This, however, is but an inconsiderable fraction of the gaseous interchange. We possess abundant evidence that the active interchange occurs in the tissue cells. These have an intense avidity for oxygen, and take it up from the surrounding blood and lymph— nay, more, are capable of storing it to some extent, for it has been shown that muscle and other tissues are capable of active metabolism for some little period, in an atmosphere deprived of oxygen, or when transfused with oxygen-free saline solution, and during this metabolism they discharge abundant CO_2. The appearance of glucose, lactic acid, etc., in the urine of animals kept upon an insufficient oxygen supply, indicates that the oxygen thus taken into the cell in excess enters there into loose chemical combinations, and that when this store of oxygen is needed, and there is continued discharge of CO_2, these bodies also become discharged from the cells. Ultimately the amount of oxygen removed from, and of CO_2 afforded to the capillary blood, depends upon the relative tension of the two gases in the blood and tissue cells respectively; but of the stages whereby the combined oxygen of the erythrocytes becomes liberated into the surrounding plasma, and thence passes to the lymph, and thence to the tissue cells, our knowledge is minimal.[1]

External Respiration.—In connection with this we have to pass in review: (1) Disturbances in the mechanism whereby air gains entrance into the lungs, and their effects. (2) Disturbances in the air sacs of the lungs, the medium of gaseous interchange between the air and the blood, and their effects. (3) Disturbances in the composition of the air entering the lungs.

THE RESPIRATORY MECHANISM.

This may be discussed under four heads: (*a*) The air passages; (*b*) the muscles of respiration; (*c*) the pleural cavities; and (*d*) the nervous mechanism.

The Air Passages.—Under these are to be included the whole tract from the external nares to the terminal bronchioles. These, it will be recognized, are of considerable length, and their effect upon the air passing down them is that with normal respiration it enters the air sacs (1) at the body temperature instead of at that of the external air; (2) impregnated, if not saturated, with moisture; and (3) devoid of dust and foreign particles, and, as a consequence, sterile.

A multiplicity of mechanisms bring about these results, and disturbances of any one of them tends to modify the quality of the air gaining entrance to the air sacs. The nasal passages are factors of high importance; the wide surfaces of the turbinated bones being of peculiar service, both in warming the inspired air after the manner of radiators, and in imparting moisture to the same. To a considerable extent, also, these moistened, somewhat glairy surfaces detain foreign particles present in

---

[1] For the main data bearing upon the internal respiration, see Pembrey's article on Respiration, in Schäfer's Physiology, vol. 1: p. 780.

the air passing over them. It cannot be too strongly emphasized that persistent mouth-breathing is harmful in that it favors the air entering the air sacs being deficient in each of these respects. Hence, it favors irritation of the lower air passages and of the lungs, with resultant inflammation. Such mouth-breathing results from nasal obstruction of several orders—congenital narrowness of the nares, acquired stenosis of these passages, from trauma, chronic syphilitic and other inflammations, acute and subacute catarrh with excretion of abundant thick mucus, the presence of overgrowths and tumors within the nasal passages, most commonly of mucous polyps in the posterior nares and of adenoids in the nasopharynx. These last, occurring in childhood, and arresting the function of the nose, arrest also its due development, so that even after removal it may happen that the passages remain abnormally small, and nasal respiration is not as free as it should be. The result in all these cases is a peculiar liability to inflammation of the throat and lower respiratory passages, increased susceptibility to infection, and in children a distinct delay in bodily and even in mental development. Your mouth-breathing child not only looks, but actually is, more stupid than the average of normal-breathing children.

The condition of the inspired air may also affect the nasal passages, and, influencing their function, adversely affects the lower respiratory passages and the lungs. The nasal mucosa is distinctly sensitive, with abundant vascular supply and rich supply of mucous glands. Extremes of temperature of the air, the presence of irritant gases and particles, induce congestion and inflammation with relative facility, an inflammation characterized by abundant mucous discharge. That discharge would appear to have several functions; it protects the underlying epithelium; washes off and dilutes irritant substances, and is to some extent bactericidal, in addition to which, by its physical constitution, it arrests the passage and spread of bacteria.

If chronic and long-continued, catarrh is apt to be followed by atrophy of the nasal mucosa. Such *atrophic rhinitis* being accompanied by reduction of discharge and direct lodgement of irritant particles on the nasal mucosa, favors ulceration and deep inflammation, and as regards the lower respiratory passages, from presence of irritant bodies in the inhaled air, and from relative lack of moistening of that air, tends to produce results similar to those brought about by mouth-breathing.

The Pharynx.—The moist surface of the pharynx, together with the sudden bend in the direction of the stream of inhaled air, converts this more particularly into an adjuvant apparatus for removal of dust and other particles. It can be demonstrated experimentally that if a current of air impinges upon a moist surface at an angle of 45° or thereabout, it delivers up to that surface the majority of its contained solid particles. The mucous glands of the pharyngeal mucosa provide a mechanism whereby this surface is kept continually moistened, and the abundant lymph-glands of the tonsils and pharyngeal roof constitute a further protective mechanism. That they function in arresting pathogenic bacteria is indicated by the acute tonsillitis which is the first active symptom in so many diseases which we regard as air-borne, notably the acute exanthemata. Although the diphtherial membrane may show itself primarily in the nasal passages, or upon the back of the pharynx, it is over the tonsils that it most often makes its first appearance. Adenoids and other growths of the upper part of the pharynx, inflammatory and neoplastic growth of the tonsils, of necessity obstruct the passage of air to a greater or less extent.

Stertor.—Yet another form of obstructed breathing is brought about by loss of tone or actual paralysis of the muscles of the soft palate—that form of stertor known as *snoring*. As the reader may determine for himself, three factors are necessary to produce this, namely, a flaccid, soft palate, a combination of mouth- and nose-breathing, and relatively deep inspirations.

The other forms of stertor may here be noted in passing. They are: (2) *Nasal* stertor, seen in apoplexy, with paralysis of the muscles of the alæ nasi, the inhaled air, as in sniffing, drawing the alæ against the septum. (3) *Buccal* stertor, or puffing out and flapping of the cheeks. This may occur in cases of paralysis of the facial nerves, or again, as in the snoring sleeper, from flaccidity of the muscles with partial closure of the mouth. (4) *Pharyngeal* stertor, due to falling back of the base of the tongue with obstruction to the laryngeal entrance. (5) *Laryngeal* stertor, heard most commonly, according to Lister, during chloroform inhalation, and also in paralysis of some of the muscles influencing the vocal cords; and lastly, (6) *Mucous* stertor, due to the bubbling of air through mucoid fluid in the larger air tubes. Of this nature is the "death rattle." As pointed out by Bowles, most of these can be prevented by altering the posture of the individual.

The Larynx.—Two main functions are to be ascribed to the larynx— phonation, and the provision of a firm base for attachment of the epiglottis and control of its movements in the act of swallowing. As regards the former, it has to be admitted that the physiology and pathology of voice production lead us so far from the main object of this chapter —that of discussing the disturbances of respiration and their nature— and constitute in themselves so large a subject, that here we can at most call attention to them parenthetically. We would recall that the larynx, essential for the singing voice, is not essential for speech; that speech is possible after the complete extirpation of the larynx, although then it is hollow, and little more than a whisper; that variation in the "note" of the voice is determined by the tension and consequent rate of vibration of the vocal cords and communication of the waves thus set up to the issuing air; that thus to this extent the voice is affected by pathological conditions of the vocal cords; that these pathological conditions range themselves into two groups: (1) The nervous, excessive stimuli leading to spasmodic contraction of the intrinsic laryngeal muscles, with closure of the laryngeal aperture; defective or arrested stimuli, leading to flaccidity and paralysis of the vocal cords with lack of the finer vibrations; and (2) intrinsic disturbances of the cords, either diffuse or localized inflammatory thickening of the same, or the development of tumors upon them;

by each of these disturbances the cords become "muted;" that the "timbre" of the voice depends upon the various resonating cavities communicating with the main air stream, upon their size and the freedom of communication, upon the lungs and thoracic cavity, the laryngeal sacculi, the sphenoidal, frontal, ethmoidal, and antral sinuses, etc., as also upon the extent of development of the palatal arch; that variation in the development of these, obstruction of their orifices, inflammatory and other conditions leading to the accumulation of liquid or solid matter within the cavities, materially affect the resonance of the voice; that *articulation* is dependent upon the lips, teeth, palate, and tongue, and this is materially affected either by congenital or acquired defects in these organs, or by paralysis of the muscles of the lips, tongue, and lower jaw.

We are apt, on first thought, to cite the crossing of the respiratory and alimentary tracts as an example of evolutionary imperfection. Undoubtedly it has its disadvantages. With imperfect action of the larynx or disease of the epiglottis, foodstuffs may gain entrance into the trachea and lungs; with paralysis of the soft palate, such as is apt to occur after diphtheria, fluids, instead of being swallowed, may pour into and through the nares; the infant suffering from obstructive nasal catarrh cannot suckle. But this same infant, under the same conditions, were there no alternative respiratory channel through the mouth, could not breathe; and when we come to consider the secondary employment of the organs of mastication, of the mouth and mouth parts for articulation and speech, it may be regarded as at least doubtful whether man, as a communicative animal, does not to a very great extent owe his position in nature to the utilization of this apparent imperfection.

The more recent studies upon deglutition indicate that the epiglottis is to be regarded as an adjuvant rather than the essential organ in preventing the entrance of foodstuffs into the larynx during the act of swallowing. This view is supported by the fact that in tertiary syphilis more particularly, as again after extensive tuberculous ulceration, there may be most extensive erosion and destruction of the epiglottis, and this evidently of long-standing, without observed suffocative attacks. During swallowing, that is, the laryngeal entrance is raised under the backward projecting root of the tongue, so that the bolus of food or stream of fluid passes well behind it.

Lastly, it has to be noted that the passage through the vocal cords constitutes the region of greatest narrowing of the main respiratory passage. Here, therefore, the slightest grade of narrowing by any cause —spasmodic contraction, inflammatory deposits, new-growth, etc.— produces relatively the most obstruction to the respiratory act. But the larynx as a whole is a region of narrowing of the passage, and thus affections of the glottis in general are liable to induce grave obstruction. More especially the loose attachment of the mucosa (save over the vocal cords) renders congestion and œdema a not uncommon event, either as the result of trauma or other irritation, of infection, or rarely of angioneurotic type, as one manifestation of the tendency to local œdema of sudden development and unknown causation which may attack individual portions of the digestive and respiratory tracts. In all these cases, the upper opening of the larynx, the epiglottic and aryteno-epiglottic folds are most involved, and may by their swelling cause such narrowing of the passage that, unless intubation or tracheotomy be performed, death may ensue from asphyxia.

The Trachea and Bronchi.—Beyond the larynx the respiratory passage widens again into the trachea, which, it may be noted, is not of uniform diameter, but according to the measurements of Braune and Stahel[1] is at its broadest about half-way between the larynx and the point of bifurcation, slowly narrowing below this. The transverse section of the larger bronchi is again greater than that of the lower end of the trachea, and greater than that of the combined smaller bronchi. The result of these variations, both in the shape and the transverse section volume of the respiratory passages, must necessarily be to intermingle the different portions of the inspired air-stream, and so favor all portions of that stream coming into contact at one or other point with the walls of the channel. There are, indeed, indications that the stream eventually acquires a spiral instead of a direct motion. The moist ciliated surface which extends from the larynx to the terminal bronchioles thus tends to arrest such solid particles as have managed to pass the upper respiratory passages, and through the action of the cilia these are passed upward to be expelled through the larynx by an act of coughing. An adjuvant in the removal of matter are leukocytes which migrate on to the free surface, and either become expectorated or wander back into the lymph-glands, notably into the group below the bifurcation of the trachea.

Despite the mechanism of cartilaginous bars, by means of which the trachea and bronchi are kept patent and at the same time mobile, there may be hindrance to passage of air through them either from (1) the entrance of foreign bodies, (2) inflammatory deposits or contraction, (3) new-growths, or (4) pressure from without. The last may be variously produced by aneurism, goitre, mediastinal tumors, enlarged tuberculous lymph-glands, and, very possibly, by the enlarged thymus, Regarding the capacity of the enlarged thymus to produce direct compression of the trachea in the striking and fatal condition known as **thymic asthma**, there is still debate. The sudden onset of the dyspnœa and the stridor suggest spasm of the glottis, and although in these cases postmortem examination reveals an enlarged thymus, there is no sign of narrowing or distortion of the trachea. Nevertheless, it may be urged that the thymus of young children is a very vascular organ; that a sudden congestion may greatly increase its size and the pressure that it exerts upon the trachea where this passes through the narrow orifice of the chest; and that such sudden compression cannot be expected to show permanent effects upon the tracheal tube. Certain it is that recent cases are on record in which the operative removal of the thymus during paroxysms of this form of spasmodic dyspnœa has been followed by marked disappearance of symptoms. We have encountered similar paroxysmal attacks of dyspnœa in cases of goitrous enlargement of the

[1] Berichte d. K. Sächs. Gesell. d. Wiss., Math. Phys. Cl., 1885: 326.

middle lobe of the thyroid which could only be ascribed to congestion and accompanying increase in size and pressure of the goitrous mass.

Of peculiar interest are those forms of obstruction, whether of the larynx, trachea, or bronchi, which assume a valvular nature permitting free inspiration or expiration, but not both. Thus, œdema of the glottis or a polypoid tumor in the glottis will obstruct inspiration, as will also a growth of the walls projecting from a smaller into a larger bronchus. On the other hand, a diphtheritic membrane, or a polyp attached below the vocal cords, will permit inspiration, but act as a valvular plug preventing expiration, as may also an enlarged and partly detached tuberculous gland or other tumor in this region projecting into one of the larger bronchi at the root of the lungs.

Yet another form of obstruction is associated with bronchial narrowing, namely, **asthma**. The symptoms here point very definitely to a spasmodic narrowing of the bronchi; the extreme grade of distension of the lungs developed during the attack indicate that through the active inspiratory efforts air is sucked into the alveoli, but with expiration cannot be expelled to the same extent. Evidently, also, the whole bronchial tree is simultaneously involved, for all the lobes of both lungs are simultaneously expanded. The sudden onset of the condition, and sudden departure, indicate a nervous origin, that the condition is a neurosis; and, as a matter of fact, it has been observed that in many susceptible subjects particular odors and surroundings induce the condition, while there is in some a small area of the posterior and upper portion of the nasal septum, irritation of which induces an asthmatic attack. Various theories have been adduced to explain the development of the condition— that it is due to spasm of the bronchial muscle sheath; that it is due to hyperemia and swelling of the bronchial mucous membrane (Traube, Weber, Clark); that in many cases it is a special form of inflammation of the bronchioles, **bronchiolitis exudativa** (Curschmann); that it is due to a reflex spasm of the respiratory muscles. This last may be dismissed; it does not explain the overfilling of the lungs. Curschmann's theory also is untenable; the onset is too sudden for any known inflammation. Brodie and Dixon[1] have brought forward strong evidence in favor of the bronchial spastic theory. It had already been shown (MacGillavry, Einthoven, Beer) that the vagus contains motor fibers for the bronchial muscles. By oncometric records of the lobe of the dog's lung under artificial respiration, they proved that vagus stimulation could produce rapid arrest both of entry into and of exit of air from the air sacs, as again, the state of overdistension of the organ. They point out that those drugs which are of service in asthma are just those which by experiment they determined cause paralysis of the nerve endings, and point out that ether, which is of material benefit in asthma, notoriously causes hyperemia of the mucous membrane and increased secretion from the bronchial glands. In our first volume we had called attention to Auer's observations upon the anaphylactic spasm of the bronchial muscles in the guinea-pig. In this way, as Meltzer points out,

---

[1] Trans. Path. Soc. London, 54: 1903:17.

we can experimentally produce the asthmatic condition. Nevertheless, it does not seem to us that Brodie and Dixon have adequately explained all the symptoms of all cases. They pass too slightingly over the discharge which, while not primary, nevertheless soon makes its appearance in a larger proportion of cases, and this even when there has been no attack for a long period. As is well known, this discharge is characterized by the presence of Charcot-Leyden crystals and Curschmann's spirals (p. 280). And they depreciate the vascularity of the bronchial mucous membrane. But, as every one knows who has studied sections of the lungs in acute bronchitis, that mucous membrane is highly vascular. Admitting freely that the condition is brought about by reflex nervous stimulation, as also the value of Brodie and Dixon's observations, we still cannot but consider that, in one order of cases at least, the abundant exudate, and the similarity of the causative factors to those seen operating in hay-fever suggest the presence of a similar angioneurotic œdema.

The General Effects of Obstruction to the Air Passages.—It is scarce necessary to state that complete obstruction of the air passages for more than a few minutes ends in death by asphyxia. If the obstruction be incomplete, then according to its nature do we find either inspiratory or expiratory dyspnœa, or both, and according to its degree do we have either death by progressive slow suffocation, or a remarkable adaptation of the respiration and of the bodily activities in general to the lessened supply of oxygen. With obstruction to inspiration, the respiratory acts become slow and labored, and not only are the diaphragmatic contractions deeper, but also the accessory muscles of respiration are called into play, so as to secure the greatest extent of thoracic enlargement. In marked contrast, the expirations are short and not labored. The swift passage of the air through a narrowed passage leads to inspiratory stridor. The reverse is the case in expiratory obstruction. Here it is the expiration that is slow and labored; the accessory muscles called into play are those which most reduce the thoracic capacity, notably the abdominal muscles and those bending the vertebral column, bringing the ribs closer to each other.

Where only one main bronchus is obstructed the results are different; a period of rapid, not to say tumultuous, respiration is followed by indications of adaptation, the one lung being capable of performing the functions of both. The rapid irregular respiration may be ascribed to the different periods at which the vagus inspiratory and expiratory stimuli are initiated in the two lungs (see p. 251 et seq.).

THE MUSCLES OF RESPIRATION.

In ordinary quiet breathing the expansion of the lungs in inspiration is an active process, expiration being largely, if not entirely, passive, due to relaxation of the diaphragm, and pressure upward of the abdominal viscera under the normal abdominal tension, and to the elastic reaction of the distended lungs and of the thoracic musculature. In children of both sexes, and in the adult male, the distension of the lungs in inspiration is in the main brought about by contraction of the diaphragm. The use of corsets, and that only, would seem to reduce the diaphragmatic activity and cause inspiration of the costal type. Women who do not employ corsets are found to exhibit the diaphragmatic type of inspiration indistinguishable from that of men.

But while the contraction of the diaphragmatic muscle, by separating the circumferential portion of this septum from the costal wall, is the main factor in increasing the thoracic cavity, it must be kept in mind that in inspiration the thorax increases in every direction—in lateral and fore and aft diameters, as well as in the vertical. It is thus obvious that the costal musculature is a factor even in pronounced cases of diaphragmatic breathing. According to Mosso, during natural sleep this thoracic breathing is the normal condition. Of the muscles causing elevation of the ribs and lateral and anterior expansion of the thoracic cage, the external intercostals are the most important. In forced inspiration a large number of other muscles are called into play; the head, shoulder, and arm are all called upon to form fixed supports for muscles which, passing from them to the thorax, elevate and rotate the ribs forward and outward, that the thoracic cage may attain its greatest capacity; as again, that the increase in the negative pressure within the thorax may cause most forcible inhalation. The more important of these muscles are the sternomastoids, the pectoralis minor, the lower part of the pectoralis major, and the lower segments of the serratus magnus. In normal inspiration also the central tendon of the diaphragm does not alter its position; with forced inspiration, with more vigorous contraction of the diaphragmatic muscle, it is pulled downward, thus raising very materially the negative intrathoracic pressure. Yet other accessory muscles must be noted. Even in ordinary respiration, the larynx moves downward during inspiration through the contraction of the sternohyoid and sternothyroid muscles, the upward movement in expiration being aided by the thyrohyoid muscles. In forced inspiration the larynx is to some extent pulled downward by the descent of the lungs and trachea. In forced inspiration, also, and where there is nasal obstruction (and in the quiet breathing of children, also, with their smaller nasal passages), the dilator naris comes into play, widening the nostrils.

Expiration.—Normal expiration is wholly, or almost wholly, a passive process. As Starling expresses it, the inspiratory enlargement of the lungs not only acts against gravity in raising the ribs, but also stores up potential energy in consequence of a stretching of the rib cartilages and of the elastic lungs. Thus it follows that as the muscles relax, gravity and the elasticity of the cartilage and lungs come into play, and restore the thorax to its resting state and original size. Where, however, there is obstruction and forced expiration, there muscular aid is given to lessening of the thoracic cavity, more particularly by contraction of the abdominal wall, whereby the abdominal contents force the diaphragm upward, while at the same time the ribs and sternum are pulled downward. The lower ribs are further pulled downward by the serratus posticus inferior and the sacrolumbalis.

THE PLEURAL CAVITIES.

Intimately associated with the muscular apparatus of the thorax in bringing about the distension of the lungs we have to consider the pleuræ. These form closed cavities around each lung. Were the lungs directly attached to the parietes (as happens in cases of universal pleural adhesions), expansion and contraction could occur, but the extent would vary greatly in different regions. With diaphragmatic contraction there would be great expansion of the lower lobes, whereas the apices would be scarcely influenced, and, as a consequence, there would be little interchange of air occurring in them. The pleural cavity, with the free movement of the visceral over the parietal pleura, insures that with inspiration the lungs undergo uniform expansion; if the excursion of the lower parts of the lower lobes is the greatest, this at the same time causes the expansion of the whole organ and of its individual air sacs.

According to Donders, the elastic pull of the lungs in expiration—and this is equivalent to the negative pressure in the pleural cavities—is 7.5 mm. Hg. in the expiratory phase; it is increased to about 9 mm. in ordinary inspiration, and to 30 mm. in the deepest inspiration.

Pneumothorax.—This negative may be converted into a positive pressure in either or both cavities by the entrance of air or gas into them. Contrary to the general teaching, we would point out that a small opening into the healthy pleural cavity is not necessarily followed by pneumothorax. We have made such an opening in the dog (without artificial respiration) and seen the visceral pleura move across it with each breath without the lung undergoing collapse, the viscous adhesion of the two layers of the pleura surrounding the opening being sufficient to neutralize the positive pressure upon the exposed surface. This, it must be added, is exceptional; ordinarily, air rushes into the cavity, and the pressure it exerts upon the lung causes collapse of the same. Nay, more, where the orifice, either in the thoracic wall or in the lung, is of a valvular nature, the air drawn into the pleural cavity during inspiration, and unable to escape during expiration, may accumulate and come to exert a pressure upon the lung in excess of the atmospheric pressure, causing an extreme filling of the side of the chest, even to the extent of displacing the heart and compressing largely the other lung, thus rendering adequate respiration and continued existence impossible.

Two main forms of pneumothorax may, therefore, be distinguished, the *open* and the *closed*. In the former there is free communication with the external air, either through the thoracic wall, or an abdominal viscus, or most often through the lung; here of necessity the pressure within the cavity is positive, and the lung undergoes complete collapse, unless there be pleural adhesions which keep portions of the organ distended. In closed pneumothorax the communication has become occluded, or, as in gaseous pneumothorax, may never have existed. In such cases, according to the amount of contained air or gas, we may have merely diminution of the negative pressure or low positive pressure; and here respiration is not wholly arrested in the affected lung. There is considerable divergence of opinion regarding the effect of these two forms upon respiration. In general it would seem that in both there is a tendency to deeper respiration, with increased rapidity in the open form and some slowing in the closed.[1]

Pleural Effusions.—The mechanics and the effects upon respiration of the accumulation of fluid in a pleural cavity form an interesting study. Upon first consideration we would imagine that the effect of accumulation of fluid in a closed cavity is to diminish the space that can be occupied by the lung; that the lung in consequence cannot fully expand, and that thus the results are similar to those of a positive pressure exerted upon the lung, which, as a matter of fact, in extreme cases becomes completely collapsed, lying against the vertebral column. Garland, however, urges (1) that a pleuritic exudation does not compress the lung as universally taught, but, on the contrary, by virtue of its weight exerts a negative pressure; (2) that the lung does not swim upon the effusion, but by virtue of its retractility it supports the entire body of the effusion, together with the diaphragm, until the weight of the fluid exceeds the lifting force of the lung; (3) that the diaphragm does not bag down until the weight of the fluid exceeds the lifting force of the lung, and (4) that the heart is not pushed out of place by an effusion, whether of air or fluid, but that those parts are drawn over by the negative pressure in the other pleural cavity. Enormous effusions increase this displacement.

While there is much that we must accept in these conclusions of Garland, it is difficult to accept them in their entirety. Let us begin by considering the normal lung at the end of expiration. That organ is still in a state of distension—of distension so considerable that its elasticity, or the force necessary to keep it distended, is, as already stated, equivalent to a negative pressure of about 7 mm. Hg. With ordinary inspiration that force is only increased by about 2 mm. Hg. Suppose that now the pleural cavity became filled in the expiratory phase either with fluid or with a solid growth. The lung would thereby become collapsed and airless, and with ordinary inspiration, instead of expanding to the extent of bringing about a negative pressure of 9 mm., the total amount that it could exert would be only 2 mm. (*i. e.,* 9–7 mm.). In other words, the elasticity of the lung which causes the negative pressure to come into play is exerted to a very slight extent when the organ is collapsed; just as a rubber band exerts very little pull when it is flaccid compared to the pull exerted when it is taut. This progressive reduction of the pull exerted by the lung, due to the elasticity of the same, would seem to have been largely neglected by Garland. Nor is it merely the intrathoracic negative pressure that keeps the diaphragm bowed upward in spite of extensive fluid in the pleural cavity A more important factor is the upward pressure of the abdominal

[1] For a full study of the mechanics of pneumothorax, see Emerson, Johns Hopkins Hospital Reports, 11:1903:1.

viscera under the influence of the muscles of the abdominal wall. It is very rarely that we find the diaphragm bulging actually downward, and then in conditions of marked abdominal flaccidity. When this occurs it is to be noted that each contraction of the diaphragm, instead of producing a negative, must materially increase the positive pressure in the pleural cavity.

Thus, our opinion is that Garland's conclusions are only valid for conditions where there is but relatively small accumulation of fluid in either cavity; any considerable quantity so hinders the expansion of the lung that its elasticity cannot be effective, while the very weight of the fluid, if it does not materially lower the diaphragm, and so lessen its excursion and with that the distension of the lung, must at least interfere with the excursion of the thorax by increasing the load which the costal muscles of inspiration have to carry. Whether the diaphragm or the costal muscles bear the brunt of the increased load will depend materially upon the position of the patient. Here we would add that the accumulation of fluid below the lung in the lower part of the thorax can only exert a negative pressure upon the lung when its weight has become sufficient to neutralize the upward pressure of the abdominal organs upon the diaphragm. As a matter of fact, the singular freedom with which, in general, fluid escapes from the chest in thoracocentesis, and this during both the inspiratory and the expiratory act, and the absence of suction of air into the chest, demonstrate that this fluid is under a positive, and not under a negative pressure. It is only when the amount of fluid is, or has become, small that there is danger to be anticipated of suction, or, more accurately, of forcible entrance of air into the cavity.

THE NERVOUS MECHANISM OF RESPIRATION.

The acts of inspiration and expiration being determined by muscular activity, and the skeletal muscles not acting automatically but contracting under nervous stimuli, it is clear that we have in the first place to look to the nervous system for the initiation of active breathing, and, secondly, that disturbances affecting the centres controlling the work accomplished by the muscles concerned must materially affect those acts.

There must, in the first place, be as many centres as there are individual muscles. We know, indeed, that the intercostal muscles have their innervation through the series of dorsal motor roots, and conclude that the neurons that cause these muscles to contract originate in the anterior horns of the dorsal cord. The diaphragm is innervated by the phrenic nerves, and these have their origin from the fourth and fifth cervicals; the alæ nasi are innervated by the seventh cranial; the muscles of the vocal cords by the recurrent laryngeal branches of the vagus. It follows from this that the performance of normal acts of respiration depends upon the coördinated stimulation of a series of centres situated in the medulla and cervical and dorsal cord, as also that destruction of particular centres or of the nerves passing from them to particular muscles, must modify the respiratory act in particular directions; that section of one phrenic, for example, must arrest diaphragmatic respiration upon one side. But if these centres are coördinated, there must be some supreme or coördinating centre. The striking fact is that after all these years we still are unable to state exactly what particular group of cells forms this centre. We know that if the brain be separated from the cord by section through the upper part of the medulla oblongata respiration is unaltered; that, therefore, the centre is not in the brain. The observations of Flourens and several others indicate that it is bilateral and situated in the medulla; but the experiments of Gad and Marinesco show that the localization given by Flourens, Gierke, and Mislawsky is either incorrect or too limited; while the very extent of the area which they, in their turn, lay down, namely, the cells of the *formatio reticularis* upon either side of the median line, would seem too vague and widespread to constitute what is generally considered a spinal or cranial centre. Granted that there be such a coördinative respiratory centre—which some still deny—how does it work? Does it send down automatic and rhythmic impulses, or, on the contrary, is it only stimulated by afferent impulses, or, thirdly, is its activity rhythmic, but capable of material modification by afferent impulses reaching it from other regions of the organism, as again by nutritional influences due to alteration in the gaseous contents of the blood circulating through it? These questions also cannot be said to have gained an absolutely certain answer. This much is clear: (1) That stimulation of several regions of the brain, as again of many peripheral nerves, modifies, at least temporarily, the respiratory act, and that thus the respiratory rhythm is influenced by afferent impulses; (2) that the pulmonary branches of the vagus nerves stand out preëminently in exerting an influence upon the respiratory rhythm; they are the foremost afferent nerves of respiration; and (3) that the activity of the centre is materially affected by the blood passing through the medulla, being stimulated by increased presence of CO_2, and depressed, not so much by over-oxygenation, as used to be taught, as by reduced CO_2 tension. The brilliant studies carried out by Head[1] in Hering's laboratory established firmly the second of these conclusions, studies in which he was able to observe the uncomplicated movements of the main muscle of respiration—the diaphragm—by recording the contractions of a small isolated band of the same, which, in the rabbit passes to the ensiform cartilage, and is capable of isolation along with its nerve and blood supply without disturbing the thorax or its contents. The extent of the contractions of this muscle and variation in the rate of its contraction can be recorded without being disturbed by passive movements of the thorax. By this means the observations of Hering and Breuer were confirmed, that the normal stimulus to both the inspiratory and the expiratory act is due to influence of the intrapulmonary conditions upon the nerve endings of the vagus. Collapse of the lung for example, induces a prolonged contraction of the diaphragm—as it were, an intense inspiratory effort on the part of this muscle; inflation of

[1] Jour. of Physiol., 10: 1889: 279.

the lung, on the contrary, relaxation of the diaphragm, such as accompanies the passive expiratory act in the rabbit. The immediate effect of section of both vagi is to produce inspiratory tone, or partial contraction of the diaphragm, and to lengthen individual inspiratory contractions of the same; the individual contractions are slower and more violent. What is the meaning of these phenomena is still a matter of debate—whether, for example, with relaxation of the lung, stimuli pass up the vagi which set in action the inspiratory muscles, or, on the contrary, inhibit the expiratory mechanism; or whether, again, the only impulses which pass up the nerve are expiratory in nature; or, lastly, whether, as Meltzer[1] has urged, the vagus contains both positive, inspiratory and inhibitive, expiratory fibers. Further, it is to be kept in mind that vagus stimulation is not necessary for respiration; after division of both vagi respiration gradually assumes a regular although slower rate, with long and powerful inspirations with intervening complete expirations. These may, it is true, be brought about by impulses reaching the coördinating centres through other afferent nerves. They, at the same time, raise the question whether the centre may not possess an automatic rhythm of its own, normally always in action, but modified by impulses proceeding from the lungs and other cerebral and spinal centres. The existence of this automatic rhythm is inferred from several considerations. Thus, more particularly, several observers have shown that if the medulla be separated from the brain above, and the lower cervical cord be cut across, along with all sensory nerves reaching the cord between these two sections, a rhythmical contraction of the diaphragm is still in evidence, slow but definite. It may, however, be objected that the trauma of the cut ends of the sensory nerves still acts as a sensory stimulus. The problem thus is one that it is practically impossible to solve by direct means. We can only repeat that the bulk of evidence is in favor of this automatic rhythmic action of the coördinating centre.

And further, we must imagine that the condition of the blood raises or depresses the activity of the main respiratory centre, thereby increasing or decreasing both the rate of the rhythm and the force of the individual respiration. Both Miescher and Head have shown that by over-ventilation of the lungs, and, therefore, of the blood, a condition of *apnœa* or arrest of the respiratory acts can be produced even when both vagi are cut; when, therefore, the arrest is not due to afferent impulses from the lungs, but presumably is due to the influence of the blood upon the respiratory centre. Similarly, *asphyxia* may be brought about by cutting off the blood supply to the medulla, or by bleeding an animal so as to produce universal anemia, and such asphyxia, as will be presently noted, is characterized in its earlier stages by the contrary stage of excessive force of the respiratory movements. The researches of Haldane and Priestley show that it is not want of oxygen but increased amount of carbon dioxide that is the influence exciting the respiratory centre to increased activity.

[1] Arch. f. Physiol., Leipzig, 1892: 340.

With this general and brief review of what is a most complicated sub. ject, we may now pass on to consider the more characteristic disturbances of the respiratory process.

Sneezing.—Sneezing is characteristically a reflex act; the usual cause is from nasal irritation, by stimulation of a branch or branches of the fifth nerve; it may be initiated, however, by exposure to intense light, by stimulation of the optic nerve. The act consists of a spasmodic, deep inspiration, followed by a strong expiratory effort. While this last is proceeding, the mouth passage is at first closed by approxima- tion of the dorsum of the tongue to the soft palate. The first portion of the expired air passes, therefore, with considerable force through the nostrils, tending to dislodge irritant particles if they be present. Almost immediately the tongue is slightly depressed, so that the remainder of the air is forced through a relatively narrow passage between the tongue and the upper jaw, producing a characteristic sound.

Coughing.—Coughing may be either a voluntary or a reflex act, the reflex originating either from irritation in the larynx (most common), in the lungs, or of the pleural surfaces. Here a deep inspiration is fol- lowed by closure of the glottis, which continues during the first part of the strong expiratory act, so that with sudden opening of the glottis, the air under considerable pressure in the main air passages is liberated, and escapes with much force, carrying with it mucus or other matter in the bronchi, trachea, or larynx.

Dyspnœa.—The term dyspnœa is used in two senses, to indicate both the sensation of air-hunger and, more commonly, and we think more correctly, the condition of labored respiration brought about by obstruction to the entrance of an adequate amount of air into the lungs, and broadly by all conditions of accumulation of increased amounts of CO_2 in the blood, with or without deficiency of oxygen. The condition may or may not be accompanied by cyanosis, according to the activity of gaseous.interchange possible in the lungs. Here we have to recognize the existence of a protective mechanism; whenever there is a tendency to deficient ventilation in the lungs, then constantly the general metabo- lism becomes lessened by all possible means; the individual indulges in the least possible muscular and other exercise, whereby both the call for oxygen is brought to a minimum, as is also the discharge of carbonic acid. Coincidently, even in the absence of sensation of air-hunger, there may be increase in the rate of the respiratory act, the more rapid if shallow inspirations leading to increased respiratory interchange, and favoring thus a better condition of the blood. When the venous condition of the blood becomes more aggravated, such rapid respiration is replaced by deeper inspirations and slow, labored breathing, correspond- ing to the first stage of asphyxia. But at the same time it is evident that prolonged relative venosity of the blood dulls the respiratory centre; in other words, the subject of respiratory obstruction may endure with little respiratory distress a state of venosity of the blood, which, sud- denly produced in a healthy person, would be accompanied by the gravest respiratory distress. This is equivalent to recognizing—as from other

considerations we must recognize—that the sensitiveness of the respiratory centre is capable of considerable variation; and, as a matter of fact,
there exists the opposite condition of hypersensitiveness of the centre.
Thus, we occasionally encounter a pronounced dyspnœic condition in
connection with hysteria and melancholia, in states, that is, in which
there is no evidence of any modification in the gaseous tension in the
blood.

Keeping these matters in mind, we may sum up the conditions under
which dyspnœa may manifest itself. They are:

1. Conditions of severe hindrance to entrance of normal amount of air:
(a) In the air passages, leading to diminished ingress and egress of
air (foreign bodies, inflammatory and other narrowings of the larynx,
trachea, or bronchi, compression from without). (b) In the lungs
themselves—collapse, diminution of the ventilating surface by exudates
into the alveoli, tuberculous and other growths in the lung substance,
destruction of the lung substance (gangrene, cavitation, etc.), fibroid
induration, atrophy, emphysema.

2. Conditions affecting the muscular mechanism of respiration:
(a) Diseased conditions, inflammation, etc., of the diaphragm or other
respiratory muscles, more particularly the former. (b) Pathological
conditions of the main and secondary respiratory centres and of the
nerves forming the respiratory arc, paralysis or irritation of the centres,
trauma or destruction of the afferent (vagus) nerves, as again of the
efferent nerves (more particularly the phrenics).

3. Conditions obstructing the circulation of blood: (a) Through the
lungs (obstructive heart disease, emphysema, chronic interstitial pneumonia, etc.); (b) through the medulla.

4. Conditions modifying the constitution of the inspired air—rarefaction of the air as at high altitudes, reduction of the amount of contained
oxygen, increased CO_2 content, presence of CO, which, uniting with
the hemoglobin, permits less oxygen to be taken up, and reduces thus
the gaseous interchange in the medulla and tissues generally.

Asphyxia.—Dyspnœa connotes the existence of at least the minimum
gaseous interchange necessary to maintain life, the obstruction to that
interchange being overcome either by increased rate or increased amplitude of the respiratory acts, and the calling into play of the accessory
muscles of the respiration. Asphyxia or suffocation, on the other hand,
connotes a condition in which that minimum cannot be attained, and
in which, as a consequence, the progressive accumulation of carbon
dioxide in the blood circulating through the medulla eventually arrests
the action of the respiratory centre, and brings about death unless the
obstruction to the gaseous interchange be rapidly removed. It is true
that the progressive exhaustion of the respiratory centre in dyspnœa
through overstimulation may usher in a quiet death with progressive
cyanosis, but little or no struggle. But more often in dyspnœa when the
venosity of the blood becomes excessive, and always when the hindrance
to respiration is of sudden development, we obtain that intense respiratory
struggle which forms the typical picture of asphyxia. In this acute

condition three stages may be recognized: a first, of increased amplitude, as well as rate of the respiratory movements; a second, with increase of the expiratory movements out of all proportion to the inspiratory, the expiration becoming prolonged, the inspirations short and convulsive. To produce these violent expirations the whole musculature of the body appears to be called into play. In the final stage these violent expirations cease almost suddenly, and now slow, deep inspirations manifest themselves. The mouth is widely open, the head is stretched back, so as to gain the fullest freedom for entrance of air into the trachea, the body stretched, the arms raised. There is now complete insensibility; the dilated pupils do not react, the inspiratory movements become farther and farther apart, become weaker and weaker, until, in the course of a few minutes (the time varying) the last gasp is taken.

These stages are accompanied by changes in the circulation, of which the most marked is rise in the blood pressure. It is evident that the venous blood stimulates the vagus and vasomotor centres in the medulla, so that there is both slowing of the heart beat and contraction of the arterioles. With the advent of the third stage, the heart poisoned with venous blood begins to fail; its beats become weaker and ineffective, and death occurs with all the chambers of both sides hugely distended, and with the blood pressure rapidly sinking. It may be noted in passing that during the second stage, if the blood pressure be taken, large secondary waves show themselves of progressive increase and decrease of the general blood pressure, embracing many pulse waves. These, the "Traube-Hering curves," indicate the existence of a rhythmic action of the vasomotor centres in the medulla. They are of no small interest, as being analogous to the phenomenon to be immediately discussed.

Cheyne-Stokes Respiration.—The first clear description of this type of respiration was given by Cheyne, of Dublin, in 1818; the first full study by Stokes of the same city in 1854. Both these physicians observed it in connection with cases of fatty degeneration of the heart. To quote Stokes: "It consists in the occurrence of a series of inspirations increasing to a maximum, and then declining in force and length until a state of apparent apnœa is established. In this condition the patient may remain for such a length of time as to make his attendants believe that he is dead, when a low inspiration, followed by one more decided, marks the commencement of a new ascending and then descending series of inspirations. This symptom, as occurring in its highest degree, I have only seen during a few weeks previous to the death of a patient." Herein fuller study has shown that although frequently seen in association with fatty degeneration of the heart, and although most frequently manifested in the last few days of life, periodic breathing of the same order may present itself in several morbid states, and not necessarily as a penultimate event. As Traube pointed out, there are two main groups of conditions in which these respirations make their appearance—circulatory disturbances with no obvious brain disease, and intracranial diseases without heart disease. Of the first group, the most common disorders are those associated with chronic interstitial nephritis and arteriosclerosis—cardiac degeneration, aortic and mitral stenosis and incompetence, etc.; of the second, cerebral hemorrhage and tumors, tuberculous meningitis, hydrocephalus, and other conditions leading to increased intracranial pressure, with (presumably) compression and lowered blood supply to the medulla. Yet a third group should be added, that of the intoxications, including (rare) cases of · infection (typhoid, diphtheria, smallpox, pneumonia), and the narcoses (morphine, ether, and chloroform in association with morphine, chloral). A mild form of the same type of ascending and descending periodic breathing, with brief apnœic pause, may not infrequently be heard during the afternoon siesta of the middle-aged who have many years of life still before them. According to Ede, the breathing of certain individuals during sleep is constantly periodic, and Gibson[1] suggests that this is a familial peculiarity. We encounter grades of the periodic breathing from those in which ascent follows descent with no absolute pause, to others in which the apnœa may persist for half a minute and more. There may or may not be associated changes in the general blood pressure, unconsciousness during the apnœic pause, contraction and dilatation of the pupil.

In attempting to elucidate this peculiar phenomenon, Gordon Douglas and Haldane,[2] as also Haldane and Poulton,[3] found they could produce it experimentally by breathing deeply and rapidly for about two minutes. Whenever any desire to breathe returned, the process was allowed to take its own course, with the result that the Cheyne-Stokes type of respiration was induced. The first-mentioned observers, in studying farther the intra-alveolar air in regard to oxygen and carbonic dioxide pressure, conclude: (1) that the periodic breathing is excited by the periodic occurrence and disappearance of the (indirect) stimulating effect of want of oxygen on the respiratory centre; (2) the want of oxygen may be due to an abnormal deficiency in the intra-alveolar oxygen pressure or to the effect on the circulation of changes in the breathing, or to both causes combined.

There have been abundant theories, and at times angry debate as to the meaning of this type of respiration; more particularly the studies and views of Traube, Filehne, Wellenbergh, Luciani, Rosenbach, Mosso, Murri, and Gibson stand out prominently. But notwithstanding all this work, it cannot be said that any consensus of opinion has been reached. Without attempting to lay down any full hypothesis, we could point out:

1. That the phenomena and the records taken of those phenomena have essentially the characters of what physicists term interference curves, i. e., of a series of waves of one rhythm modified by the super-position of waves of another rhythm, which at one period augment, at another neutralize, each other.

---

[1] Cheyne-Stokes Respiration, Edinburgh, Oliver and Boyd, 1892: 122. This work gives a full bibliography of the subject up to date, with discussion of the many theories.

[2] Journ. of Physiol., 38:1909:401. [3] Medico-Chir. Trans., 40:1907:49.

2. That there is a curious likeness between these Cheyne-Stokes curves and those of certain forms (the so-called "extra-systolic") of periodic cardiac irregularity; and that, if in the latter case we conclude that in addition to evidence of the manifestation of an automatic rhythm, there are manifested opposite phases of muscular contraction and dilatation, so in connection with the respiratory act we have similar indications.

3. To the existence of an automatic rhythm reference has already been made (p. 253). Whether this is truly automatic, or whether it represents the rhythmic resultant of stimuli other than those proceeding ·from the lungs must, for the present, be left an open question. What is of import is that in the absence of normal vagus stimuli the centre has been demonstrated to initiate rhythmic contractions.

4. The respiratory cycle is what may be termed a double-phase act: inspiration demands that expiratory stimuli be inhibited, and *vice versa*. The inspiratory contraction with the succeeding expiratory contraction may be compared with the cardiac muscular contraction with the succeeding refractory period, which, as we have pointed out, may be regarded as indicating active dilatation of the cardiac fibers.

5. As in connection with cardiac irregularity, so here, we may presume that want of coördination between these factors and the establishment of interfering rhythms is at the bottom of the production of these periodic alterations in rate and volume of the respiratory curves.

6. There are other forms of irregular breathing, not possessing, on the one hand, the marked periodic character of the Cheyne-Stokes type, and on the other hand, not manifesting the progressive ascent and descent in the amplitude of the contractions. Thus, some would separate what is termed "Biot's respiration." This is seen in meningitis and some other cases of brain disease, and is characterized by irregularly periodic periods of apnœa, lasting for many seconds up to half a minute. These may be encountered in uremia, diabetes, and sundry nervous states, as again under the action of certain drugs. Here presumably stimuli of another type act upon the main respiratory centre. Still less is known regarding the mode of development of these than of the Cheyne-Stokes type.

THE AIR SACS.

We shall in the next chapter describe in detail the various disorders which may affect the air sacs. Here we have to consider the broad effects of these disorders upon the work of the lung and upon the system in general. Speaking generally, these disorders range themselves into two classes: those in which more particularly the entrance into and egress from the air sacs of the proper amount of air is prevented, and those in which changes occurring in the walls of the air sacs prevent the air which has entered them from being properly utilized for purposes of gaseous interchange. There are not a few cases in which diseases of the first group lead to the development of disorders of the second; we might

thus constitute a third group of the combined disorders. It will, however, be simpler to consider the cases according as one or other of the
two main orders is primary. Leaving out of consideration those cases
in which obstruction occurs in the air passages, the entrance of a due
amount of air into the sacs may be prevented either by want of distension
of the sacs, as in **atelectasis** and **collapse**, or by the collection within
them of fluid or solid matter. By atelectasis is understood the condition
of primary imperfect expansion of the air sacs (ἀτελής, incomplete;
ἐκτάσις, expansion); by collapse, the closure of air sacs which have
previously been expanded, although—we are inclined to think incorrectly
—the term atelectasis is coming to be used for both conditions. If of
limited extent, neither condition produces any recognizable disturbance;
the surrounding unobstructed air sacs undergo a compensatory enlargement; nay, more, the whole of one lung may undergo collapse, and if the
other be healthy it is able to suffice for the needs of the organism. Only,
as already noted, if the one lung be put out of action suddenly, there is a
period of tumultuous breathing and dyspnœa before adaptation to the
changed circumstances becomes complete, while, further, the respiratory
system is working perilously near to the limit of its reserve force, so that
bronchial and other disturbances, of little import when both lungs are
functional, now assume a serious aspect.

The air sacs may become filled, and the air they should contain be
replaced,-(1) by serous fluid, as in cases of acute or chronic congestion,
(2) by blood, as in rupture of an aneurism of one of the branches of the
pulmonary artery in a tuberculous cavitation, or of an aortic aneurism
into the trachea, from an infarct, etc.; (3) by water or other fluid from
without, as in cases of drowning;. (4) by inflammatory exudates and
migrated cells, as in pneumonia. The effects upon respiration are of the
same order as in the former group of cases; whether there be no noticeable
results, or rapid respiration, dyspnœa, and eventual adaptation, or
the development of asphyxia and death, depends primarily upon the
extent of lung tissue involved, secondarily, upon the causative agent.
The diffusion of the products of coagulation and death of the erythrocytes
in cases of hemorrhage, and of toxins and cytolytic products in cases of
pneumonia, sets up a febrile state, and doing this, *inter alia*, directly
affects the respiratory centre, inducing an increased rate of breathing
out of proportion to the extent of lung substance involved. Further,
it must be remembered that *an acute lobar pneumonia is always a pleuropneumonia*, and that the painful irritation of the pleural surface inhibits
the excursion of the thorax; here, again, is a cause of the rapid and
shallow respirations present in this condition. But even in acute lobar
pneumonia the exudate may completely distend all the air sacs of a
whole lung, or the lower lobes of both lungs, and bring about complete
displacement of the air in the same without a fatal result; or, more
accurately, at autopsy we may encounter cases showing a distribution
of the pneumonic disturbance, which has evidently been of some days'
duration, and in which the lethal event is seen to be due to recent and
further extension of the process beyond these limits. Certain distinc-

tions of some practical importance must be drawn between fluid agents and those which, like blood and inflammatory exudates, are liable to coagulation and solidification. In the first place the site of accumulation of fluid depends upon the position of the individual; they naturally accumulate in the more dependent parts of the lungs, and, indeed, by turning the individual upon one or other side, they may drain from one side to the other, often with grave disturbance of the respiratory act in the process. Or, as in Sylvester and Schäfer's methods of resuscitation from drowning, the fluids can be drained out through the trachea. In the second place, when the air sacs become distended with solid contents, there is the greater interference with the circulation. In collapse and atelectasis the absence of the air pressure within the alveoli, as again the lack of distension of the same and of consequent flattening and elongation of the capillaries within their walls, induces a dilatation of the bloodvessels of the affected area, and consequent free flow of blood through the same. When serous fluid percolates into the air sacs, then also we find a congestion, either active or passive. When passive, it is not the lung condition, but obstruction to the onflow of blood from mitral or other obstructive disease in the left heart that is the cause of the great dilatation of the capillaries, and this dilatation continues, however advanced the serous accumulations within the alveoli. In pneumonia and hemorrhagic infarcts, with coagulation and progressive passage of more material into the air sacs, these become overdistended, and the result now is that eventually, from great congestion, we pass to a state of narrowing and compression of the interalveolar capillaries, and when the conditions affect any large portion of the lungs, the result is well-marked increase in the work of the right heart, with dilatation of the same, and some incompetence. It is remarkable how relatively rare are local necrosis and gangrene of the affected lung as the result of this induced anemia; nevertheless these conditions occasionally show themselves.

Changes in the Walls of the Air Sacs Hindering Due Aëration. —These changes may be of two orders, either atrophic, or of the nature of interstitial deposits in the alveolar walls. The first of these leads to or accompanies the not uncommon condition of either localized or generalized vesicular *emphysema*. As will be more fully described in the next chapter, we find in this state a great dilatation of the air sacs, with pronounced thinning of the interalveolar septa, leading to atrophy of the same, with fusion of contiguous air sacs into large chambers, a process inevitably accompanied, not only by reduction of the respiratory surface, but also by a harmful alteration in the relationship between the mass of air within the alveoli, and the surface of the same, and so hindrance of the gaseous interchange with the blood in the alveolar walls.

Emphysema.—To understand the ill effects of the emphysematous condition, it is necessary to realize the mechanics of its production. Let us take first the condition of *localized* emphysema, in which the change affects one small bronchial tree and its associated air sacs, the rest of the lung being in a normal state. It is obvious here that the primary condition has involved the bronchus. We can best explain the development by presuming a narrowing of the lumen of the bronchus, whether congenital or induced by inflammatory thickening, or by the presence of thick exudate within it. In such a case the forcible nature of the inspiratory act draws air into the associated air sacs; the passive nature of the expiratory act may prevent an equal amount of air becoming expired. The result will be that with successive acts of inspiration, the air sacs will become more and more distended, as demonstrated by Brodie and Dixon's experiments, already noted (p. 246). There is, it is true, an active force opposing overdistension, namely, the fairly abundant elastic tissue in the alveolar walls. This force is most effective when the air sacs are in a state of distension; it is of little effect when the alveoli are only moderately filled. Time and again at autopsy we notice that a very slight grade of bronchitis suffices to prevent the postmortem collapse of the lungs. Thus, under the condition postulated, both the expiratory

Fig. 60

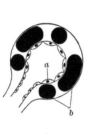 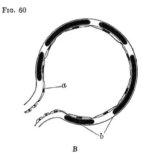

A   B

Diagram to demonstrate the effect of emphysematous dilatation of the air sac upon the epithelial lining of the air sac (a) and upon the capillary network of the alveolar walls (b). A, normal air sac; B, expanded air sac.

act and the elasticity of the alveolar walls are unable to reduce the air sacs to the collapsed expiratory state (Fig. 60). If the state of distension be kept up, it materially affects the abundant capillary network of the alveolar wall. When that wall is collapsed, the pressure from without upon the capillaries is reduced, they are circular in section, and there is a minimal obstruction to the onflow of blood. When, on the contrary, the air sac is distended, not only do the capillaries become stretched, but, in addition, they are subjected to increased pressure from the contained air. The result is that the individual capillaries become flattened and elliptical in section; not only can they contain less blood but that smaller amount of blood is exposed to a larger surface, and consequently to increased friction. Thus, if the distension be continued, the final result is continued malnutrition of the alveolar wall, reduced gaseous interchange, atrophy of the wall, diminished elastic tissue, and diminished elasticity; yet further dilatation, with fusion of the air sacs, until now, even if the obstruction be removed and the ingress and egress of air be restored, the atrophy of the tissue, and the want of proportion between the volume of the air in the greatly dilated system and the cross-section of the emergent bronchioles render the emphysematous condition permanent. Thus in an otherwise healthy lung we may encounter thin-walled translucent sacs with occasional thin septa crossing them which may attain to the size of a pigeon's egg or larger, and project prominently from the surface of the organ. A similar state may be brought about by somewhat different means in the condition of compensatory emphysema. Here, with collapse of the air sacs connected with certain bronchi, the force of the inspiratory negative pressure leads to an overdistension of air sacs connected with other bronchi, and especially of such air sacs —e. g., those at the edges of the lobes—as are not supported by mutual compression. Such extreme distension is apt to overstrain the elastic tissues of the alveolar walls and bring about atrophy.

Now these same conditions must be operative in causing generalized emphysema. In perhaps the majority of cases microscopic examination reveals the existence of a chronic bronchitis and peribronchitis, i. e., suggests that the main causative factor has been a diminution of the lumen of entrance and exit of air to and from the air sacs. But in other cases, as in children after prolonged whooping-cough, in glassblowers, players upon wind-instruments, the obstruction has been situated higher up in the respiratory passages. But in many of these cases also it is to be noted that the condition develops with advancing life; i. e., just as in the vessels, so in the lungs, there is a progressive diminution in the elasticity, and an atrophy of the elastic connective tissues, so that the lung-tissue does not sufficiently aid the thoracic wall in bringing about expiratory contraction of the lungs.

The effects of such generalized emphysema are thus: generalized expansion of the lungs, coincident enlargement of the thorax, which assumes a characteristic barrel shape (the "air hunger" demands constantly the entrance of more air into the already overfilled air sacs, and therewith increased inspiratory expansion of the thorax), prolonged expiration, diminished gaseous interchange, obstruction to the passage of blood through the lungs, hypertrophy and dilatation of the right heart, and eventually dyspnœa and cardiac failure.

How, it may be asked, does this conception agree with the various views that have been enunciated regarding the etiology of vesicular emphysema? Laennec was of opinion that mucus in the lumen of the bronchi exercised a ball-valve action admitting the entry, but preventing the discharge of air from the air sacs. This, it will be recognized, is a possible cause of one series of cases. Gairdner, in 1857, held that collapse, either complete or partial, of one portion of the lung was a necessary antecedent of emphysema in another part; that the condition was compensatory. This, again, can be applied to only one series of cases, and cannot explain diffuse emphysema. Of more importance are the views of Mendelssohn, followed by Jenner, that obstructed expiration is the essential cause. They showed clearly that the emphysematous condition followed violent expiratory effort, and pointed out that the increased pressure in the alveoli must tend to affect most those portions of the lung which have least support from their surroundings, and that so, as a matter of fact, emphysema shows itself most extensively along the edges. This view, however, leaves out of account the nature of the lung substance as a factor in the development of the condition. J. Jackson, Jr., of Boston, was the first to direct attention to an inherited liability to emphysema, and to the fact that it is more common in the young than is usually supposed. This seemed to point to some developmental defect in the lung tissue as a factor. Cohnheim concluded that the explanation was to be sought in a congenital imperfect formation of the elastic tissue, basing the view upon experiments which demonstrated the singular loss of elasticity of the lung in advanced emphysema. Eppinger, admitting this loss of elasticity, held that in the majority of cases it was a secondarily induced, and not a primary condition. Lastly, Isaaksohn regarded the disease as essentially due to vascular disturbance. As we have pointed out, the vascular disturbance naturally follows persistent distension of the alveoli. It will be seen that our conception of the nature of the process takes into account both the factors which may be regarded as clearly established, namely, (1) increased difficulty of expiration, leading to raised intra-alveolar pressure, and (2) diminished elasticity of the alveolar wall. It must be freely admitted that these interact, and that one or the other may be the more prominent in the early stage. Thus a congenital deficiency in elasticity will render a relatively slight obstruction to expiration the more effective, while, contrariwise, in the lung possessing well-marked elasticity, prolonged distension of the alveoli eventually brings about atrophy of the elastic tissue. Further, it has to be noted that the elastic tissues of the body are liable to lose their elasticity with advancing age, and that so, conditions which have little effect in early life favor the development of emphysema at a later period; this loss of elasticity is a characteristic feature of arteriosclerosis; we are thus prepared to find that emphysema and arteriosclerosis are very commonly associated conditions.

Bronchiectasis.—Here, in passing, may be noted the contrasted condition of bronchiectasis, in which, through atrophy of their walls or, again, through tension exerted upon them from without by the contraction of interstitial fibrous tissue, the bronchi and bronchioles undergo dilatation. Whether, as in the latter category of cases, the alveoli have undergone a coincident compression by the interstitial tissue or not, the dilated bronchi take the space that should be occupied by functionating air sacs. Here also the result is a diminished aëration of the blood. The different forms will be found described on p. 283.

Interstitial Deposits.—New tissue, whether fibrous, as in chronic interstitial pneumonia; granulomatous, as in tuberculosis. syphilis actinomycosis; or neoplastic, leads to compression and diminution, if not absolute occlusion of the air sacs, and in addition affords a mechanical resistance to their expansion during inspiration. According, therefore, to the extent of the development of these interstitial deposits within the lung substance, so do we obtain greater or less reduction in the functional capacity of the lungs. Nor has the amount only of the new tissue to be taken into consideration, and the lessened amount of air which in consequence can be inspired. Such interstitial deposits gravely obstruct also the pulmonary circulation; interstitial fibrous tissue, as it contracts, obliterates largely the capillaries of the alveolar walls; the granulomas and tumors, as they grow, obliterate the surrounding air sacs, and if situated within the lung substance rather than at the surface, obstruct the blood supply of the tissue lying between them and that surface.

Modifications in the Constitution of the Inspired Air.—This is a subject so fully treated in the larger text-books of physiology that here it is only necessary to recall the main facts that have been ascertained.

Oxygen is the essential constituent of the inhaled air. In the normal animal this may be materially increased in amount without modification of the respiratory exchange; nay, if the animal breathe pure oxygen instead of air, there is little immediate effect, metabolism being regulated by the needs of the tissues, and not by the amount of oxygen presented. When, however, the blood comes to contain one-third more oxygen than normal, metabolism is arrested and the animal dies. Such increase may be brought about by inhalation of the gas under pressure, and, as shown by Paul Bert, if this pressure be increased to six atmospheres, the animal dies in violent convulsions. The same effects may be induced by breathing air under pressure, although here the pressure has to be raised to a much greater extent in order to attain a partial pressure of the contained oxygen of the same value. As shown recently by Leonard Hill, where the individual through muscular exercise —as in runners and those engaged in football matches—is in need of oxygen, the effects of inhaling pure oxygen are immediate, relieving the hyperpnœa (*i. e.*, rapid, labored breathing) and fatigue. The same is true when the respiratory surface is diminished, as in pneumonia. The opposite condition of diminished atmospheric pressure produces its results by diminution of the partial pressure of the oxygen, and so of the amount of this gas which can diffuse or otherwise gain entrance into the blood. When the atmospheric pressure is reduced to half an atmosphere, marked discomfort is felt, with dyspnœa and rapid breathing; with reduction to 250 mm., the symptoms become violent, with profound diminution of the oxygen in the arterial blood, convulsions, insensibility, and death. Similar results are produced by maintaining the normal atmospheric pressure, while reducing the amount of contained oxygen, *i. e.*, reducing the partial pressure of the oxygen. An air, for example, that contains only 5 per cent. of oxygen produces insensibility in man within a minute.

The **nitrogen** of the air is wholly inert, and variations in its amount are without effect so long as the partial pressure of the oxygen is maintained. Though here, again, as in **caisson disease**, with increase in atmospheric pressure, an increased amount is taken up by the blood, and if the pressure be suddenly removed, the liberation of the gas in the capillaries in gaseous form leads to profound and often fatal results.

Hydrogen is similarly inert; animals can breathe without apparent ill effects a mixture of equal parts of oxygen and hydrogen. **Argon** is also stated to be inactive.

Carbon Dioxide.—Excess of this gas in the air produces effects more rapidly than does deficiency in oxygen; or otherwise, to this gas more particularly are due the deleterious effects of air vitiated by being breathed over again in a confined space without ventilation. The figures given by different observers for the maximum amount of this gas which can be inspired without discomfort vary somewhat widely. The most accurate appear to be those of Haldane and Lorrain Smith. They found that the presence of 18.6 per cent. induced in them hyperpnœa and distress, with flushing, cyanosis, and mental confusion, and this within a minute or two, and that when the carbon dioxide in vitiated air rose to from 3 to 4 per cent., symptoms of hyperpnœa and distressed breathing gradually developed. On the other hand, hyperpnœa from defect of oxygen only showed itself when the oxygen was reduced to 12 per cent. in one individual, to 6 per cent. in another. The volatile substances exhaled or given off from the skin, whose presence is so pronounced in the air of crowded and ill-ventilated rooms, are doubtfully toxic, but undoubtedly they cause discomfort in breathing. Pure carbon dioxide is irrespirable; it causes an immediate spasm of the glottis. The cyanosis and toxic effects of the gas are due to its accumulation in the blood; where the amount in the inspired air is excessive, there, instead of being discharged from the blood, it is absorbed from the pulmonary air. Speck found abundant absorption when the air contained 11.51 per cent. CO_2.

Other gases, like **ammonia** and **nitric oxide**, are irrespirable even in small amounts, in consequence of the spasm of the glottis induced by them. Yet others, like **nitrous oxide, carbon monoxide**, and **hydrogen sulphide,** can be breathed and undergo absorption, producing specific effects. Of these, the most important is **carbon monoxide**, and this because the hemoglobin of the corpuscles has an intense avidity for the same, combining with it to the exclusion of oxygen. As shown by Haldane, symptoms manifest themselves when the corpuscles become about one-third saturated, and become urgent when they are half saturated. These symptoms are identical with the effects of reducing the amount of oxygen in the respired air. With the presence of 0.05 per cent. of this gas in the air, symptoms show themselves; when the percentage rises to 0.2 they become severe. It is this carbon monoxide poisoning that is the cause of the frequent deaths from inhalation of coal gas, from the fumes of charcoal and coke fires, kilns, and noxious gases in coal mines, more especially after explosions.

CHAPTER XII.

THE NOSE.

CONGENITAL ANOMALIES.

THE most common anomaly is an asymmetrical position, generally due to deviation of the bony septum, a condition which is present in more than 50 per cent. of individuals. Malformations of high grade, however, are almost invariably associated with other defects of the face and often of the cerebrum. For example, in the condition known as cyclops the nose may be absent or rudimentary. One or more of the turbinated bones may be absent, the anterior or posterior nares may be occluded, or there may be defect in the alæ or the floor of the nasal cavity. The last-mentioned condition may be found associated with harelip or cleft-palate.

CIRCULATORY DISTURBANCES.

Owing to its excessive vascularity, the nasal mucosa, particularly the erectile portion of it in the neighborhood of the lowest turbinal, is specially liable to sudden and extreme disorders of circulation.

Hyperemia.—**Passive Congestion.**—Passive congestion is found in heart and lung diseases, and in consequence of the presence of tumors in the nasal cavity.

Active Hyperemia.—Active hyperemia is common at the commencement of inflammatory processes and in some infective fevers, such as measles, typhoid, and influenza. It very readily leads to rupture and hemorrhage (epistaxis).

Hemorrhages.—Hemorrhages are also common in ulceration, hemophilia, leukemia, scurvy, death from suffocation, and as a result of trauma. Of more than ordinary interest are the cases of vicarious hemorrhage taking the place of ordinary menstruation. In fact, there seems to be some sympathetic relationship between the nasal mucosa and the sexual organs, for during sexual excitement the membrane becomes turgescent.

Œdema.—Œdema is a frequent result of inflammation.

INFLAMMATIONS.

Acute Catarrh or Coryza (Acute Rhinitis).—Acute rhinitis occurs as a primary affection which is usually attributed to the effects of exposure to cold and wet, and to bacterial influences. It is probable that individual peculiarities are also operative. Chemical irritants, such as ammonia, formalin, nitric and osmic acids, can induce severe rhinitis. Some people are very susceptible to the influence of volatile substances, like ipecacuanha, the scent of certain flowers or animals, pollen, etc. To this group belongs **hay fever**, which seems to be due to personal idiosyncrasy of this kind. This affection, like the nasal catarrh (*rhinorrhœa*) that is due to sexual excess, is not a true rhinitis or inflammation, but rather a reflex vasomotor effect. Coryza is met with also as a complication of many infections, as measles, scarlatina, erysipelas, variola, typhus fever, and influenza.

In acute coryza the mucosa is swollen, hyperemic, of a deepened color, with often considerable thickening, and feels dry and irritable. After this first stage there is an abundant secretion of a clear, watery, very slightly viscid or mucoid irritating fluid, which contains leukocytes and ciliated epithelium. Erosion of the edges of the nose and upper lip is frequently the result of its irritating qualities.

The condition is often important, as the inflammation may spread to the accessory cavities and sinuses, to the throat, to the Eustachian tubes, and middle ear.

Purulent Rhinitis.—This form may develop into a purulent rhinitis. It is characterized by greater inflammatory reddening and swelling of the mucosa, with an abundant purulent exudate, often mixed with blood, and having a foul odor. It may lead to collections of pus in the various accessory cavities (*e. g.*, empyema of the antrum of Highmore), and may even infect the meninges. The suppurative process may extend into the deeper parts, leading to the formation of local abscesses and erosion of bone or cartilage. Suppurative rhinitis may occur also as a primary infection, as from the gonococcus and glanders bacillus, or may be a complication of infectious diseases, such as scarlatina, variola, and diphtheria.

Croupous and Phlegmonous Inflammation.—Croupous and phlegmonous inflammation are also described. In the former the diphtheria bacillus is an important factor in the etiology.

Chronic Rhinitis.—Chronic rhinitis occurs frequently in those of a phthisical or syphilitic habit, but sometimes in healthy individuals.

In the productive forms there is a generalized cellular infiltration of the mucosa, particularly that covering the lowest turbinals, together with proliferation which lead to a more or less extensive thickening of the membrane (*rhinitis hypertrophica*). The process may be most marked on the middle or lower turbinals and result in the formation of polyps. This form gradually gives way to a contracting fibrous tissue, relatively poor in cellular elements, in which the glands are atrophic, that ultimately leads to atrophy of the bony parts (*rhinitis atrophica*). In these later stages the mucosa is covered with a thick yellowish or yellowish-green purulent secretion, together with thick scabs. These have a very characteristic and offensive odor (*ozæna*).

Tuberculosis.—Tuberculosis takes the form of milia, tuberculous granulations or actual ulceration. It is, on the whole, not frequent, except when there is most advanced tuberculous disease of the respiratory passages, the palate, or the pharynx. Lupus of the face frequently extends into the nose and causes widespread destruction.

Syphilis.—Syphilis may present the features of a purulent catarrh, which is very common in the eruptive stage of the disease, and in the congenital lues of the newborn. As with other mucous surfaces, the nasal mucosa can be the site of condylomata. More frequent is the gummatous form of the disease, which may begin either in the mucosa or in the bony and cartilaginous structures. This leads often to perforation of the septum and the hard palate, with the production of the characteristic saddle-shaped deformity. It is associated with a thick purulent secretion, which dries into hard scabs and has a very offensive odor (*ozæna syphilitica*). The primary sore is rare in this situation.

Glanders.—Glanders causes a purulent or a purulent-hemorrhagic discharge from the nose, and produces in the mucosa either a diffuse inflammation or multiple small abscesses. The process may lead to destruction of the bone.

Leprosy.—Leprosy is found in the form of nodular granulomas, which may form ulcers covered with thick crusts.

Rhinoscleroma.—Rhinoscleroma is a peculiar disease first studied fully by v. Frisch, Paltauf, v. Eiselsberg, and O. Chiari, which is characterized by the formation of nodular masses of almost ivory consistency, chiefly upon the nasal mucosa, but also upon the skin and the upper lip. Later, the masses coalesce and lobulated tumors are produced.

Microscopically, in the submucosa and subcutaneous tissues a round and spindle-celled infiltration is seen. The infiltration is perhaps more marked in the deeper layers where the cells are larger and often hyaline or show mucoid degeneration. The walls of the vessels are thickened, and all parts show a chronic productive inflammation. Numerous "mastzellen" are found in the infiltrated areas. The condition is due to a specific microörganism closely resembling Friedländer's bacillus, which is found abundantly in the swollen cells.[1]

Parasites.—A great variety of these have been described. Besides the *schizomycetes*, may be mentioned *Oïdium albicans*, *Scolopendra*, and the larvæ of various diptera (producing a condition of **myiasis**).

Foreign Bodies.—These are very frequently inserted into the nose by children. Many substances have been found, such as marbles, peas, beans, paper, and wood. H. S. Birkett[2] has recently recorded a curious case in which a thimble was embedded in the nose for eighteen years. It was found to be incrusted with salts, the surface being quite smooth.

RETROGRESSIVE METAMORPHOSES.

Calcification.—Calcification of the mucosa is recorded. It takes the form of scattered spicules of lime embedded in the membrane, or of actual plates.

---

[1] For bibliography, see Babes, Kolle-Wassermann, Handb. d. path. Mikroorganismen.

[2] Montreal Medical Journal, 28:1899:449.

Rhinoliths.—Rhinoliths, or concretions, may be formed in plugs of inspissated mucus, but more usually the salts are deposited about foreign bodies. Sometimes, instead of a calcareous coating, a caseous-looking mass composed of dead epithelium, leukocytes, and detritus may be deposited upon the offending substance.

Necrosis.—A perforating ulcer of the septum (apart from the syphilitic and tuberculous variety) is decidedly rare. According to Zuckerkandl, it does not necessarily follow inflammation, but may be a purely retrogressive phenomenon. It may perforate or, healing, leave a dense scar. The condition has been attributed to coagulation-necrosis, capillary thrombosis, the action of bacteria, and to a trophoneurosis.

PROGRESSIVE METAMORPHOSES.

The mucous membrane of the nose and of the accessory cavities often shows **hyperplastic growth** or actual **tumor** formation, which may be due to a preëxisting inflammation or may arise without discoverable cause.

Fig. 61

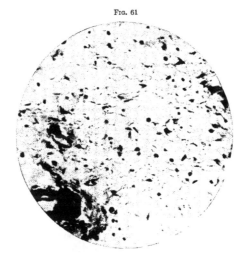

Myxomatous polyp from the nose. Winckel obj. No. 6, without ocular. (From the collection of Dr A. G. Nicholls.)

The lesion is diffuse or may result in the formation of local excrescences or *polyps*. A common form is the soft or **myxomatous polyp**, which is of a grayish semitranslucent appearance. Nasal polyps are frequently multiple and may attain a considerable size. They are composed of tissue identical with that of the mucous membrane, except that it is more cellular. Within this growth glands may become entangled, which sometimes become dilated, owing to the retention of secretion, so that cystic tumors are the result. In other cases the glandular elements proliferate, giving rise to **adenoma**. From the deeper fibrous structures, particularly from the bony parts, **fibromas** often develop. These often become oedematous, thus simulating the myxomatous polyp. They have a more yellow color, however. Owing to excessive development of the bloodvessels, **teleangiectatic** or **cavernous fibromas** are produced. Nasal polyps may undergo hyaline or calcareous degeneration. Strictly speaking, most of these polyps are not true tumors but should be classed with the hyperplastic formations resulting from a preëxisting inflammation.

Carcinoma.—Primary carcinoma takes the form of medullary cancer or of epitheliomatous growths of the order of Krompecher's "basal-celled" cancer (vol. i, p. 801).

Sarcoma.—Sarcoma, as a primary disease, is rare in the nose, but usually extends from sarcoma of the antrum or the neighboring parts. It occasionally forms polypoid excrescences.

More rarely, **chondroma** and **osteoma** are met with.[1]

THE PHARYNX.

This will be considered along with the Digestive Tract in Chapter **XVII**.

THE LARYNX AND TRACHEA.

The predominant etiological factor in the production of diseases of the larynx is the character of the respired air. The physical and chemical peculiarities of the air; affections of neighboring organs, particularly the pharynx, the thyroid gland, and the lungs; constitutional tendencies, all play their part. "Catching cold" is an important predisposing cause. It has been shown experimentally by Rossbach that anemic and hyperemic conditions of the larynx can be induced by the action of heat and cold upon the skin of the body at some distance from the larynx itself.

MALFORMATIONS.

Complete **absence** of the air passages, in common with absence of lungs, occurs only in connection with other grave defects, as in the condition of Acardiacus amorphus and A. acephalus. Particular cartilages or portions of them may be deficient or absent. **Hypoplasia** occurs in aplasia of the testicles or early castration. Partial or complete **fissuring** of the epiglottis has been observed. There may be sacculated diverticula of the sinuses of Morgagni, as again of the sacculi laryngis, recalling the pouches normally found in monkeys. The most important anom-

---

[1] The literature on the pathological disturbances of the nose is given in Suchannek's article in Lubarsch and Ostertag's *Ergebnisse* der allgemeinen Pathologie.

alies of the trachea are atresia or abnormal narrowing of the tube, fistulous communication with the œsophagus, or imperfect closure of the branchial clefts.

CIRCULATORY DISTURBANCES.

Owing to the loose tissue of the submucosa, circulatory disturbances can quickly arise and as quickly disappear. Thus it is, that when, for instance, marked œdema of the glottis has been present during life, at postmortem examination all traces of it may have passed off.

Anemia and Hyperemia.—Anemia and hyperemia may be local or a part of a general condition. Anemia of the larynx is well known to be an early manifestation in some cases of tuberculosis and chlorosis.

Active hyperemia may result from excessive use of the voice, the inhalation of dust and irritating gases, and from inflammation.

Prolonged **passive hyperemia** may lead to a permanent dilatation of the veins (*phlebectasia laryngea*).

Hemorrhages may occur from traumatism, acute inflammation, ulceration, the hemorrhagic diathesis, morbus maculosus, scorbutus, and phosphorus poisoning. They may amount to the formation of a hematoma which may lead to death from suffocation.

Œdema.—The most important condition, in that it may lead to rapid death by suffocation, is œdema, which leads to partial or complete obstruction of the rima glottidis. The swelling affects those parts in which loose submucous tissue abounds, the aryepiglottic folds, the epiglottis, the false cords, the arytenoid cartilages, and more rarely on the vocal cords. The condition is due to a variety of causes, among which may be mentioned cardiac and renal dropsy, pressure from cervical and mediastinal tumors, aneurisms. These forms are mostly chronic. The acute type is, as a rule, inflammatory in origin.

INFLAMMATIONS.

Acute Laryngitis.—According to the character and intensity of the causative agent, acute laryngitis may be classified as *catarrhal, herpetic, fibrinous (membranous), diphtheritic, phlegmonous,* and *ulcerative,* in addition to certain more specific forms found in *tuberculosis, syphilis, variola, rhinoscleroma, glanders,* and *leprosy.*

Acute Catarrhal Laryngitis.—Acute catarrhal laryngitis is a very common affection, but comes much more frequently under the observation of the laryngologist than of the pathologist.

The condition is usually brought about by mechanical, chemical, or thermic irritation, and occurs in one of those situations that is affected readily by climatic and atmospheric conditions. It occurs also in the course of the infective fevers, measles, scarlatina, variola, typhoid, while in certain others, such as influenza and whooping-cough, it is often the most prominent feature. The distribution and intensity of the process are affected mainly by the nature and virulence of the infecting agent. The epiglottis or the vocal cords may be chiefly affected, or else the intermediate portion. At first there is more or less redness and swelling of the parts. Sooner or later, a catarrhal secretion makes its appearance, which is at first viscid and glassy, but soon becomes more cloudy, grayish, or grayish-yellow from admixture with leukocytes. The secretion rarely forms hard crusts. From loss of the lining epithelium small superficial erosions are produced. From the irritation produced by coughing, small quantities of blood are often effused. The catarrh from influenza usually begins in the nose and spreads downward into the bronchi and the lungs. The secretion is viscid, mucopurulent, and glairy, and of a pale greenish color. Within the leukocytes, and lying free, the minute bacillus of Pfeiffer can be demonstrated. The process in whooping-cough usually begins below the vocal cords, and thence spreads into the bronchi.

Acute Catarrhal Tracheitis.—Acute catarrhal tracheitis does not differ materially in its etiology and progress from catarrhal laryngitis. Acute catarrh, if neglected, or if the cause be not removed, may ultimately assume a chronic course, particularly in those who suffer from some constitutional taint. Catarrh may also be chronic from the first in those who use the voice much or are addicted to the immoderate use of alcohol or tobacco.

Laryngitis Herpetica.—Laryngitis herpetica is characterized by the formation of vesicles on the edge of the epiglottis and on the vocal cords. Small erosions may be caused by the rupture of the vesicles. The condition is rare.

Membranous Laryngitis.—This form is characterized by the production of a fibrinous membrane of a gray or grayish-white color, somewhat elevated above the general level of the mucosa and varying in extent. The condition is usually not confined to the larynx, but extends upward to the epiglottis, throat, tonsils, and buccal cavity, and downward to the trachea and bronchi. The infection is usually a descending one, but not invariably so, for the larynx may be affected while the pharyngeal structures remain free. When the membrane is removed, which can often be accomplished without difficulty, the surface is found to be reddened and more or less swollen. The thicker the membrane is, the firmer and more elastic it appears to be. In the neighborhood of the patch the mucosa shows the usual changes of a simple or mucopurulent catarrh.

Microscopically, the membrane is seen to consist of fine threads of fibrin, or sometimes broader bands, which form a thick meshwork and in many instances have undergone hyaline change, so that it presents a superficial resemblance to cartilaginous tissue. In the meshes of this membrane are numerous cells, chiefly leukocytes and desquamated epithelium. These cells often show signs of necrosis. It is not always possible to differentiate macroscopically the true diphtherial from other forms of membranous inflammation. A distinction is drawn, pathologically, between a fibrinous or croupous, sometimes called pseudomembranous, exudate, which merely lies upon the top of an epithelial surface and which can readily be removed, from another form, of which true diphtheria is the type, where the mucosa and submucosa are the site of a fibrinous inflammation, and both the exudate and the deeper tissues have undergone a form of coagulation-necrosis, welding them into a united mass. It should, however, be mentioned that the adhesion or otherwise of the membrane depends largely on the nature of the underlying epithelium. Where columnar epithelium exists, the membrane is readily removed, but where the epithelium is absent or where the cells are of the squamous variety, the exudate becomes firmly attached. The term "croup" has unfortunately given rise to much misunderstanding in this connection. If we employ it in regard to those forms of laryngitis characterized by a stridorous respiration, we have to recognize with Virchow a catarrhal, a fibrinous, and a diphtheritic form. It is better, however, to discontinue the use of the word "croup" as misleading, and speak of a fibrinous laryngitis.

With regard to the etiology of laryngitis, a variety of factors may be at work. Any cause which destroys the lining epithelium of the larynx and irritates the underlying structures is sufficient. Children have a greater liability to the affection than have adults. Chemical and thermic irritants play a certain part, but by far the most important factors are the infectious diseases, such as variola, measles, typhoid, pyemia, and pneumonia. The most frequent causes are diphtheria and scarlatina. In both the last-named diseases, the condition is usually secondary to an affection of the pharynx, but in some few cases the larynx alone is attacked. It must be admitted that whatever the original cause of a laryngitis may be, bacteria sooner or later play an important role. The germs chiefly concerned are the diphtheria bacillus and the various pus-producing organisms, notably the streptococcus. It should not be forgotten that the pyogenic cocci are quite competent to produce an adherent membrane closely resembling that of diphtheria.

The forms due to the Klebs-Loeffler bacillus and pyogenic cocci are much more intense than are the others. Any case of membranous laryngitis that lasts longer than twenty-four hours should rouse the suspicion of diphtheria. The examination of swabs from the throat, or of the expectoration, for the specific germ is, however, the only sure way of making a differential diagnosis.

Phlegmonous Laryngitis.—Phlegmonous laryngitis is characterized by the formation of a purulent or fibrinopurulent infiltration in the mucosa and submucosa, and frequently is a late complication of inflammatory œdema of the larynx. The parts affected are the loose connective tissues, the epiglottis, the aryepiglottic folds, and the false cords, more rarely the under surface of the true cords. Local abscess formation with ulceration is not uncommon. It is a frequent complication of diphtheria, erysipelas of the face, and the other infectious diseases. It may spread to the cartilages, causing a perichondritis, that may lead to sequestration of the part and the formation of a fistula.

Chronic Catarrh.—Chronic catarrh of the larynx leads to hyperemia of the parts, with hypertrophy of the mucosa and submucosa, together with fibrous-tissue proliferation. Secretion is scanty and tenacious. Localized thickenings, either flat or warty, are found not infrequently upon the vocal cords, of a gray or whitish-gray color (*Pachydermia laryngis verrucosa*). They are often found in speakers and singers. In other cases the glands are enlarged, so that a granular condition is produced.

Tuberculous Laryngitis.—This is a very frequent complication of pulmonary tuberculosis. Rarely, the larynx is affected in general miliary tuberculosis, and more rarely still primary tuberculosis of the larynx

FIG. 62

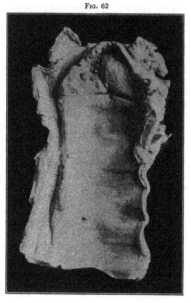

Chronic tuberculosis of the larynx and trachea. The thickening of the epiglottis is well shown, and numerous superficial erosions are also apparent. (From the Pathological Museum of McGill University.)

has been recorded (Orth). The infection is usually brought about through the sputa. The lesions generally take two forms, ulceration and diffuse infiltration.

Tuberculous ulcers vary a good deal in appearance. They may be shallow and lenticular, deep and crateriform, few or numerous. The lenticular form is seen most typically on the epiglottis with a pale, flat base and rounded margin. In other cases, on the contrary, hyperemia is marked. The process begins with small foci of cellular infiltration in the subepithelial tissue, which give rise to minute nodules projecting above the surface. These caseate and produce shallow ulcers. In other cases the infiltration is more extensive and severe, forming a subepithelial granulation tissue in which typical tubercles are found embedded. This gives rise to warty projections of the epithelial surface, so that a hypertrophic appearance is produced. Through caseation ulcers are produced in this form also.

On the primary infection can supervene a secondary development of tubercles in the neighborhood of the original lesion, which takes the form of small inflammatory foci in the mucosa, submucosa, and perichondrium, or in the mucous glands, or even between the muscle bundles. Microscopically, the appearances are those of a vascular granulation tissue, with epithelioid and giant cells and central caseation. The ulcers are found on the epiglottis, the anterior or posterior portions of the thyroid cartilage, the arytenoid cartilages, the false and true cords, but the greatest variety exists in the distribution of the lesions. In addition to the specific lesion, there is usually a marked simple catarrh. Supervening upon the condition, œdema of the glottis, phlegmon, and sequestration of cartilage may occur. In the most severe cases of tuberculous laryngitis scattered ulcers are to be found for some distance down the trachea.

Syphilitic Laryngitis.—Syphilis may produce a simple congestion or catarrh of the parts, but there is often a definite infiltration. Ulceration may take place, the base and edges of the erosions being greatly thickened. Owing to the prolonged irritation, the mucosa is often hyperplastic and thrown into polypoid or warty elevations, which later on may ulcerate and finally may become more or less normal from absorption of the exudate. The ulcers are found usually upon the epiglottis, the vocal cords, and the back part of the larynx.

A second variety is characterized by the formation of gummas, which are to be found usually in the submucosa of the epiglottis and on the vocal cords. From their size they may obstruct the lumen of the air passages. Perichondritis and necrosis of the cartilages and epiglottis are not uncommon. Small gummas may be absorbed, but when there is destruction of tissue, scars are the result. These are hard, whitish, and contracted, leading to great deformity of the organ with stenosis of the lumen. The mucosa between the contracted bands often shows warty or polypoid hyperplastic growth. The combination of recent ulceration, loss of tissue, and dense scarring is very characteristic of syphilis.

Typhoid Fever.—This may give rise to catarrh, which leads to desquamation of the epithelium, hemorrhagic infiltration, and superficial erosion. The lesions are usually to be found on the edges of the epiglottis. There is very little exudate, and the inflammation is apt to be desquamative in character. Often there is marked œdema of the parts, and perichondritis and erosion of the cartilages are not uncommon. In other cases there is a fibrinous or so-called "croupous" exudate. In this case the mucosa of the epiglottis, the anterior surface of the larynx, and the vocal cords are covered with a distinct membrane composed of desquamated and necrotic epithelium, leukocytes, fibrin, and bacteria.

A specific typhoid lesion, however, exists, in which there is swelling of the lymphoid follicles at the base of the epiglottis, the false cords, the inner side of the arytenoid cartilages, and the anterior commissure. Just as in the intestine, the swelling of the lymphoid tissue tends to the production of definite elevations upon the mucous membrane. These become necrotic and may develop into ulcers with swollen infiltrated margins. In severe cases the infiltration can extend beyond the limits of the lymphoid tissue to the neighboring parts. Ulcers analogous to those found in the intestine are thus produced.

Perichondritis without previous ulceration of the superficial parts has been met with, but is rare.

Ulceration of the larynx may also occur in glanders, leprosy, variola, actinomycosis, and rhinoscleroma.

Parasites.—In *trichinosis* the parasites are found early and in considerable numbers in the muscles of the larynx.

RETROGRESSIVE METAMORPHOSES.

Simple Atrophy.—Simple atrophy, leading to a thinning of the mucosa, diminution of secretion, atrophy of muscle and cartilage, fatty degeneration, and calcification of the various cartilages, is found in old age, premature senescence, and in certain cachexias.

Ossification.—Ossification of the cartilages has been recorded as a result of chronic inflammatory processes.

Rarely, a deposit of *uric acid salts* has been observed in the cartilages and ligaments in gouty cases.

Amyloid deposit, in the form of a diffuse infiltration or tumor-like masses, has been described. It is rare.[1]

PROGRESSIVE METAMORPHOSES.

Simple Hypertrophy.—Simple hypertrophy of the mucosa leads to the production of small local verrucose overgrowths, often taking the form of polypi. These are found by preference in those situations that are rich in glandular elements. Polypoid masses are also met with in the neighborhood of tumors and scars.

Tumors.[2]—The most common form of tumor is the **papilloma** or **papillary fibroma.** This forms a warty or papillomatous growth, often resembling the acuminate condyloma. It is usually situated on the vocal cords, and consists of a fibrous ground substance covered with stratified pavement epithelium. Round cells are often seen and the growth may contain numerous wide vessels. The diffuse variety is

[1] Herxheimer, Virchow's Archiv, 174: 1903; 130.
[2] For literature on tumors of the larynx, see Krieg, Beiträge z, klin. Chir., 58: 1908.

called by some **pachydermia laryngis**. These growths frequently return after removal, but only rarely develop into carcinoma.

Nodular fibromas are found also on the vocal cords, particularly in singers.

Enchondroma, lipoma, myxoma, angioma, lymphangioma, adenoma, and **lymphadenoma** have been found. **Cysts** are fairly rare, and are found in the epiglottis[1] and on the sinuses of Morgagni.

Aberrant masses of thyroid tissue may rarely be present in the larynx and trachea and give rise to tumors.[2]

Of malignant growths, the most frequent is the **carcinoma**. This is usually of the squamous variety, but a soft glandular carcinoma and even scirrhus have been recorded.

FIG. 63

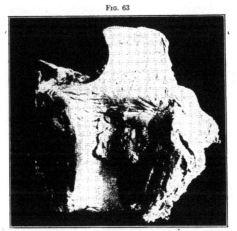

Carcinoma of the larynx.   (From the Pathological Museum of McGill University.)

Carcinoma of the larynx usually starts from the true or false vocal cords, the ventricles, or even lower down (*intrinsic laryngeal carcinoma*). Rarely, it extends from the epiglottis, pharynx, or adjacent parts (*extrinsic carcinoma*). It is apt to spread locally, but distant metastases may be formed, particularly in the liver.

Sarcoma, either round or spindle-celled, is rarer.

Secondary growth is rare.

ALTERATIONS IN SIZE AND SHAPE.

These affect mainly the trachea, but the lumen of the larynx may be obstructed either partially or completely by œdema, inflammatory

[1] See H. D. Hamilton, Montreal Med. Jour., 28:1899: 602.
[2] Meerwein, Deutsche Zeitschr. f. Chirurgie, 91: 1908: 334.

infiltration, tumors, or exostoses. **Atresia,** or narrowing of the lumen, may be due to structural defects or to contraction of scar tissue, but usually is the result of pressure exerted upon the tube from without. Such may be brought about by tumors of the thyroid glands, peritracheal abscesses, enlarged glands, and aneurisms. Pressure, if long continued, may lead to atrophy of the cartilages and give rise to the clinical symptoms of asthma, as in a case under our own observation at the Royal Victoria Hospital. Here obstruction was brought about by an enlarged middle lobe of the thyroid, which led to acute bronchitis and death from atelectasis of the lungs and secondary pneumonia.[1] Perforation of the trachea may be due to ulcerating tumors, peritracheal suppuration, and aneurisms.

Dilatation.—Dilatation, either complete or partial, in the latter case leading to the formation of saccular diverticula, is occasionally found.

THE BRONCHI.

The pathological changes that are apt to be met with in the bronchial tree are somewhat diverse, the details of the processes being considerably modified by the anatomical peculiarities of the parts affected. Thus, the larger bronchi, which have cartilaginous walls, bear a closer relation, pathologically speaking, to the larynx and trachea than to the lungs, while the terminal bronchioles are in such intimate connection with the lung substance that lesions of the one structure profoundly affect the other.

CONGENITAL ANOMALIES.

Supernumerary bronchi have been met with. Congenital **atresia** and **bronchiectasis** are more frequent, but still rare.

CIRCULATORY DISTURBANCES.

Passive Congestion.—Passive congestion is frequently met with, and is found typically in connection with valvular diseases of the heart. The mucous membrane is swollen and deep red in color. When catarrhal inflammation supervenes, as it frequently does, there is a slight sticky mucoid exudate. The congestion affects not only the mucosa, but the deeper structures as well. In some cases small ecchymoses are produced or even extravasation of blood into the lumen of the bronchi. Congestion is also a constant accompaniment of bronchitis.

Hemorrhage.—Hemorrhage into a bronchus does not often occur, unless from erosion a communication is made with some branch of the pulmonary artery, or when an aneurism ruptures into the tube. **Petechiæ** are seen in the hemorrhagic diatheses and in many of the infective fevers.

Vicarious menstruation from the bronchi is recorded.

---

[1] Adami, Canada Lancet, 35 : 1902 : 373.

INFLAMMATIONS.

Bronchitis.—Bronchitis is one of the most frequent pathological conditions that we meet with. The inflammation may be restricted to the bronchial structure, but it is frequently associated with other and more serious disturbances. The condition is usually bilateral, but not invariably co-extensive with the whole bronchial tree. Certain portions seem to be more often affected than others. Bronchitis affecting the larger bronchi is always associated with tracheitis and often with laryngitis. The same condition of the minuter bronchioles is apt to be associated with peribronchitis and bronchopneumonia.

Bronchitis arises from many causes and assumes various forms. It may result from the inhalation of irritating substances derived from the air or the nasopharyngeal cavity, and is a frequent accompaniment of the infective fevers, particularly typhoid, measles, diphtheria, tuberculosis, influenza, and variola. Bronchitis is a constant accompaniment of emphysema of the lungs, bronchiectasis, pneumonia, and abscess of the lung. In bronchiectasis it is very apt to assume the putrid type. Passive congestion of the lungs, especially when due to a valvular heart lesion, favors the development of bronchial inflammation.

The macroscopic appearances of the lungs in this condition vary somewhat according to the type of the affection present, but in the simple catarrhal form the mucous membrane is reddened, swollen, and covered with more or less sticky exudate. In the simpler forms, this is of a clear grayish appearance and largely mucoid in nature, but when the exudate is more cellular, and tends to approach the mucopurulent or purulent type, the secretion is thicker and more opaque. When a section is made through the lung, small drops of muco-pus may often be squeezed out of the openings of the bronchioles. Usually the lung substance is more or less reddened.

Acute Bronchitis.—Acute bronchitis may be divided into the following forms: *Simple catarrhal, purulent, membranous, putrid* or *gangrenous*, and *specific*.

In **catarrhal bronchitis** the character of the secretion may vary considerably. As a rule, desquamation of the epithelium is not such a prominent feature as the conversion of the epithelial into muciniparous cells, resulting in hypersecretion. Sometimes the secretion is only scanty, transparent, and adherent, the so-called "*dry catarrh.*" In other cases it is more abundant, mucoid, or even purulent. In still others, it is very abundant, thin, and watery (*serous catarrh*). The last form is apt to occur in passive congestion of the lungs. A few instances have been met with where several liters of fluid have been expectorated daily.

Purulent Bronchitis (Bronchoblennorrhœa).—This is a more serious affection and is apt to be found in the smaller bronchi associated with certain chronic pulmonary affections, such as bronchiectasis, tuberculosis, abscess, and the like. When the secretion is retained and becomes

decomposed from the action of putrefactive microörganisms, it becomes
altered in color and very fetid.   In such cases the wall of the bronchus   ·
may be destroyed.   This is putrid or gangrenous bronchitis.   It is often
the result of abscess of the lung, but may be primary.

Microscopically, sections through an affected bronchus show œdema,
congestion, and cellular infiltration in the mucosa, and in severe cases
in the submucosa.   There is also desquamation of the lining epithelium,
with an abundance of mucin-containing goblet cells.   On the free surface is a certain amount of exudate made up of mucin, fibrin, and
leukocytes.

FIG. 64

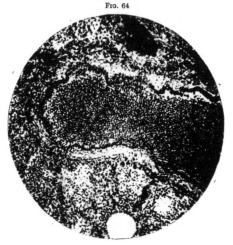

Acute purulent bronchitis with early bronchopneumonia.   Leitz obj. No. 7, without ocular.
(From the collection of Dr. A. G. Nicholls.)

Under the term "bronchiolitis exudativa," Curschmann[1] has described a form of bronchial catarrh that is by some regarded as the
main lesion of bronchial asthma.   In this form the exudate is scanty,
clear and glassy, and very viscid.   It is coughed up in small pearls that
are characteristic.   When these are spread out on a glass plate on a black
background a very peculiar appearance can be observed.   This consists in the arrangement of the sputum in a spiral form about a central
fine thread.   These are the so-called "Curschmann's spirals," and may
often be made out with the help of a hand-lens.   They are not absolutely
pathognomonic of asthma, as they have been described as present occasionally in lobar and lobular pneumonia.   In the secretion, octahedral
crystals, the so-called "Charcot-Leyden crystals," have been met with
in asthma, but are found in fibrinous bronchitis also.   A striking

[1] Deut. Archiv f. klin. Med., 32:1882:1.

feature of asthmatic sputum is the presence of considerable numbers of eosinophile cells. They are found in other conditions as well.

Membranous Bronchitis.—Membranous bronchitis is nearly always associated with a similar affection of the trachea. It is most often due to the diphtheria bacillus, but is occasionally due to the inhalation of septic microörganisms from the mouth. The mucosa is covered with a membrane of varying thickness, usually most extensive in the larger bronchi. The bronchioles may be blocked with leukocytes and fibrin intermingled.

Chronic Bronchitis.—Chronic bronchitis is practically always purulent, and while, in most particulars, it closely resembles the acute form, it differs from it in the presence of a more deeply penetrating inflammation and in the production of fibrous tissue. It is common in emphysema and bronchiectasis, in valvular heart disease, chronic nephritis, and as a result of the inhalation of dust. The mucous membrane is swollen, reddened, infiltrated, and covered with purulent secretion. Leukocytic infiltration can be made out in all the layers of the bronchi, the walls of which are also, according to Orth, hypertrophic. Not infrequently the mucosa is thrown into little polypoid excrescences, partly due to contraction and partly to fibrous proliferation. The walls of the bronchi become thickened and there is often a fibrous peribronchitis, which in time may lead to induration of the lung (*indurative pneumonia*). In very long-continued cases, however, the inflammatory products may be absorbed, the mucous glands, muscle bundles, and cartilages gradually disappear, and as a consequence the bronchial walls become thin and dilated.

Under the specific forms are included tuberculosis and syphilis.

Tuberculous Bronchitis.—Tuberculous bronchitis is a very frequent occurrence in the course of pulmonary tuberculosis, and may be found as a secondary affection in the aspiration form of the disease. In other cases the bronchus is involved by the extension of a caseous focus from without. In the first form little tubercles develop in the mucosa and submucosa and by degeneration lead to the formation of small ulcers. These may coalesce and in some cases the whole bronchial wall becomes caseous.

Primary tuberculosis of the trachea and bronchi has been observed.[1]

Syphilis.—Syphilis of the bronchi resembles the same affection of the larynx and trachea. From fibrous contraction, great distortion of the bronchi may occur. It is, however, a rare condition.

Foreign Bodies and Parasites.—Foreign bodies, such as corks, particles of bone, slate-pencils, etc., are occasionally inhaled into the bronchi. They are most frequently found in the right side, the right bronchus being wider and more vertically situated than the left. The symptoms produced depend largely on the nature of the substance inhaled. If this be septic, putrid bronchitis and abscess of the lung are the results. In other cases a mild bronchitis or pneumonia follows. When the obstruction of the branch of the bronchial tree is complete,

---

[1] See Hedinger, Verh. d. deutsch. path. Ges., 1904.

collapse of the corresponding portion of the lung occurs. Bronchiectasis and fibroid induration of the lung are occasional sequels.

Broncholiths.—Broncholiths formed of inspissated secretion in which lime salts have been deposited are occasionally met with, especially in cases of bronchiectasis.

Parasites.—Apart from the various schizomycetes, parasites are not commonly found in the human lung. In the lower animals a very common organism is the *Strongylus*, of which several varieties have been noted.

Mycosis Aspergillina.—A mycosis aspergillina, due to the growth of *Aspergillus fumigatus*, has been described in connection with bronchiectasis. Rarely *Echinococci* and *nematode worms* have been met with.

RETROGRESSIVE METAMORPHOSES.

These are not of much practical importance. Atrophy and degeneration of the muscle of the bronchi occur in chronic bronchitis, as well as fatty degeneration of the cartilaginous rings. More noteworthy are the cases of generalized calcareous degeneration of the bronchi, analogous to the changes in the cartilages elsewhere, that are met with in old people.

PROGRESSIVE METAMORPHOSES.

Hypertrophy.—Hypertrophy of the muscular tissue is frequently found in chronic bronchitis. A general hyperplasia of the bronchial wall has been described by Heller in cases of bronchitis, and this seems to form a starting point for many varieties of tumors, such as the chondroma, osteoma, myxoma, papilloma, lipoma, adenoma, and mixed growths, for it has long been known that these are relatively more frequent in connection with bronchiectasis than in affections of the lung proper.

Tumors.—The benign growths are exceedingly rare. Malignant growths, originating as primary tumors in the larger bronchi, are uncommon. Those beginning in the finer branches cannot be distinguished from those beginning in the lung itself. **Carcinomas** either originate from the lining columnar epithelium or from the peribronchial mucous glands. *Squamous epithelioma* of a bronchus has been reported.[1] This is probably due to metaplasia of the lining columnar epithelium of the mucosa. **Sarcoma** and **lymphosarcoma** are rare. Metastatic growths, however, are common enough.

ALTERATIONS IN THE CONDITION OF THE LUMEN.

Perforation.—Perforation of the bronchial wall may arise from a variety of causes. Tuberculous or purulent inflammation, parasites, or foreign bodies may erode through the bronchial wall into the lung

---

[1] P. Ernst, Ziegler's Beiträge, 20:1896:155.

substance. Caseous lymph-glands, cancer of the œsophagus, abscesses, and more rarely aneurisms, may burst in from without.

Bronchial Occlusion.—Bronchial occlusion may be brought about by foreign bodies, such as corks, slate-pencils, or bits of bone, that have been accidentally inhaled. Exudates and excretions sometimes also collect in the tubes, and, while they are often got rid of by coughing, they may, owing to inspissations or caseation, form a permanent obstruction. Such exudations may become calcified and form *broncholiths.* In rare instances, as in a case recorded by one of us,[1] the occlusion is brought about by intrabronchial tumors. Pressure from without is a not infrequent cause, and is usually due to inflammatory processes in the neighborhood of the bronchus, enlarged lymph-glands, tumors of the mediastinum, lung or œsophagus, and aortic aneurisms. By far the most potent cause is inflammation of the bronchial wall, which is often associated with inflammatory changes in the lung substance in the immediate neighborhood. In such cases secretion and exudation are usually present. When tuberculosis is the underlying condition, the bronchial wall is often caseous and the lumen plugged with a more or less dry, cheesy mass. In some forms of inflammation, notably the syphilitic, the process as it heals leaves a contracting scar-tissue, that gradually squeezes in the bronchial wall and thus produces distortion, or even complete occlusion. In those cases where the obstruction of the bronchus is complete, the corresponding lobule of the lung becomes in time quite collapsed, owing to the absorption of the contained air. When the obstruction is only partial, the alveoli become dilated and a form of emphysema is the result. Much depends, too, upon the nature of the obstructing substance. Tuberculosis is, of course, a progressive affection, and may lead to a local destruction of a bronchus and of the lung itself. Even when the offending substance is of a benign nature, secondary infection is apt to occur, so that septic pneumonia, abscess, and even gangrene are not infrequent results. In many instances the trouble is only temporary, for if the obstructing substance be coughed up, restoration to the normal condition is more or less complete.

Bronchiectasis.—Bronchiectasis is the condition in which the bronchi are dilated and often distorted. The factors concerned in its production are increased intrapulmonary pressure, disease of the bronchial walls, pressure of accumulated secretion within the bronchi, and certain chronic affections involving the parenchyma of the lung. Usually more than one cause is at work in any given case. A congenital form is recognized, but is rare.

According to the appearance of the dilatations, the following varieties have been recognized: the **saccular,** the **cylindrical,** the **fusiform,** and the **varicose.** The condition may be localized to one region of the lung or may be disseminated.

In the saccular form, the dilated portion is somewhat globular in shape and often more or less eccentrically situated; in the cylindrical, the whole

[1] Adami, Montreal Medical Journal, 24:1895–96:510.

tube is evenly dilated. The fusiform and the varicose are sufficiently described in their designations. The condition of the bronchial wall varies a good deal according to the etiological factor at work, being at one time dilated and thinned (*atrophic form*), at another dilated and thickened (*hypertrophic form*). When the bronchial wall is weakened, as, for instance, from long-continued inflammation, increased pressure of air within the tube will naturally produce dilatation and atrophy. In the atrophic form the dilatation is usually cylindrical, but if the pressure has been unevenly exerted, the sacculated form will be produced. Within the lumen the wall is seen to be encircled by a number of sharp ridges which represent the muscular and elastic constituents of the wall, while the more widely dilated portion is the connective tissue.

The hypertrophic form is most frequently found in those cases where the lung is fibroid and certain portions are, as a consequence, impermeable to air. The dilatation is not so much due to weakness of the walls as to irregular pressure. As can be readily understood, when a portion of the lung is cut off in any way from its air supply the bronchi of the unaffected portion are subjected to increased pressure and therefore dilate. In chronic indurative pneumonia bronchiectasis is not uncommon where there are pleural adhesions, owing to traction of the fibrous bands upon the bronchi. Great dilatation and deformity may thus result.

We may, further, recognize, with Orth, a **primary** and a **secondary** bronchiectasis.

Of the primary form, chronic catarrh and productive inflammation are the most potent causes. Owing to the cellular infiltration and the exudative and productive processes, the bronchial wall becomes less resistant, so that it gives way before any increased demand upon it, such as is made by prolonged coughing and difficult respiration.

The secondary variety is due to some cause apart from the condition of the bronchial wall. The forms described are the *compensatory*, the *atelectatic*, the *cirrhotic*, and the *paretic*.

The compensatory form is seen where a portion of the lung is compressed, collapsed, or indurated, so that the bronchioles in part, are obstructed; those in the more healthy portion may then become dilated. This affords the most typical example of atrophic bronchiectasis.

The atelectatic form is met with in cases where a lobe of the lung is collapsed but not compressed, as in pleural effusions and in congenital atelectasis. The bronchi of the affected portion may dilate and their walls become hypertrophic.

Cirrhotic dilatation is found in fibroid lungs. Here the condition is due not only to increased intrabronchial pressure, but also to traction upon the bronchial wall by the newly formed fibrous tissue.

In the paretic form, none of the ordinary causes are at work, but the most important factor is the pressure of secretion which has stagnated in some portion of the bronchial tree.

The appearance of the lung in bronchiectasis will, of course, vary according to the causes at work. The condition is usually recognized from the fact that the bronchi are dilated and consequently occupy more than they should of the pulmonary area. The dilated bronchioles can often be traced to the very periphery of the lung. The mucous membrane is reddened and there is some secretion. The parenchyma of the lung may present the appearance of compression, collapse, cavitation, or fibroid induration. Gangrene is an occasional sequel. In all forms of bronchiectasis the mucous membrane is more or less infiltrated with inflammatory products and may present evidences either of atrophy or proliferation according to circumstances. The cartilaginous plates are degenerated and often invaded by vascular newly formed fibrous tissue. The ducts of the mucous glands are dilated. The lining ciliated epithelium is sometimes intact, but more often desquamated or in a state of hypersecretion, goblet cells being quite numerous. Very rarely, polypoid outgrowths of the mucosa have been met with.

CHAPTER XIII.

CONGENITAL ANOMALIES.[1]

The anomalies of development are of little practical importance.

Complete absence of both lungs has been found in acephalic monsters, and is, of course, a condition quite incompatible with life. Complete absence (**agensia**) of one lung and imperfect development (**hypoplasia**) are occasionally met with, but still are rare. Again, a lobe may be rudimentary. With some of these defects bronchiectasis may be associated. More common is **abnormal lobation** of the lung, which is rather more frequent on the right side. In addition to the usual fissures, there may be several extra ones more or less perfect or, again, the right lung may consist of only two lobes. In 1500 autopsies at the Royal Victoria Hospital abnormal lobation was met with 71 times; on the right side, 54 times; and on the left 11; on both, 6.

An interesting condition is that in which the right apex is cleft by a fissure passing from above downward and inward. In the cleft is usually a fold of the parietal pleura, along the edge of which the azygos vein runs. It would seem probable that the explanation is to be found in an abnormal course of the azygos vein. In our series we have met this condition six times. **A supernumerary left lung** has been met with by Dürck.[2] Accessory lungs have recently been described as occurring within the abdominal cavity.[3]

Atelectasis or Apneumatosis.—Atelectasis or apneumatosis is a persistence of the fœtal type of the lung tissue. It is due to the failure of the alveoli to expand. This may be caused by any obstruction to the free entrance of air, to pressure on the lung, and to general feebleness. The presence of this condition is of much importance in medicolegal cases. Congenital atelectasis is also brought about by certain intrauterine affections, such as hydrothorax or pleurisy.

CIRCULATORY DISTURBANCES.

Anemia.—Anemia of the lungs may be part of a systemic oligemia, or may be partial and due to local causes. Thus, pressure of a pleuritic exudate or effusion, or of a mediastinal growth, may lead to this condition.

---

[1] The literature on this subject up to 1904 will be found in Eppinger's article in Lubarsch and Ostertag's Ergebnisse, 8: 1904.

[2] Münch. med. Woch., 42: 1895:456. [3] Seltsam, Virch. Archiv, 180: 1905: 549.

In emphysema, there is always a certain amount of anemia owing to the fact that the vessels are occluded from pressure, atrophy, and endarteritis. The anemia that is part of a systemic condition is most marked about the apex and the anterior border of the lung. The organs are pale, colorless, and on section very dry. By many it has been thought that anemia of the lungs, such as is brought about by congenital smallness of the pulmonary artery or hypoplasia of the cardiovascular system as a whole, is a potent predisposing cause of pulmonary tuberculosis. According to Rindfleisch, the fact that the apex of the lung is the first to suffer in anemia explains why tuberculosis so frequently starts in that situation.

Œdema.—This is of frequent occurrence, being found at almost every autopsy—*agonal œdema*. The condition may involve the whole lung or may be confined to one or more lobes.

The lungs are somewhat heavier and firmer than normal, pit on pressure, and on section the tissue generally is filled with a rather thin, watery fluid, which can readily be demonstrated by squeezing the lung between the hands. When the fluid is removed the lung regains its normal crepitant condition. The fluid is largely serous in character and may contain a few red cells and leukocytes, as well as swollen epithelial cells, loaded with coal or blood pigment, that have been desquamated from the alveolar walls. The most frequent cause is the relaxation of the vessels that takes place just at the time of death. This is probably assisted by the toxic condition so often associated with the last hours of life. It is rather curious that in this form the upper lobes of the lungs are frequently most affected, and often one more than another. Why this should be has never been adequately explained.

A second form—*congestive œdema*—is that seen in connection with passive hyperemia, in which case the posterior portions of the lungs are most affected. Here the fluid is often reddish or reddish-brown, from admixture with blood or blood pigment. In cases of long-standing, chronic œdema is not infrequently found. In this form the fluid is more viscid, and when the lung is squeezed the fluid does not readily flow away.

A third form is the *inflammatory œdema*, which is found in the early stages of pneumonia, at the periphery of pneumonic patches, and occasionally in cases of septicemia. This differs from the other varieties mentioned, in that the fluid is richer in albumin and apt to contain cellular elements in greater abundance. This form readily passes over into catarrhal inflammation.

A fourth form is the *acute fulminating œdema*. This comes on suddenly, sometimes in those who are apparently in perfect health. Usually, however, the persons attacked are the subjects of arteriosclerosis or chronic nephritis. Allbutt has observed it in connection with aortitis. Cases often run their course rapidly, and may end fatally in an hour. In one case coming under our knowledge pints of watery fluid poured out of the mouth for some hours before death, and at autopsy the lungs were completely waterlogged. The condition has been produced experimentally by the injection of adrenalin.

Microscopically, œdema of the lungs shows little worthy of note. The vessels of the alveolar wall are somewhat congested, and the alveoli contain a few large, round, mononuclear cells derived from the lining epithelium, with a few red and white blood cells. Should the œdematous fluid contain much albumin, although it usually does not, the albumin appears as a fine granular deposit or in the form of minute clear globules produced by the coagulation of the albumin in the process of hardening.

Hyperemia.—In the production of the various forms of congestion of the lungs, a number of factors, mechanical, physical, chemical, and thermic, are concerned, apart from the question of inflammation. Thus heat, cold, irritating gases, and other changes in the respired air are often responsible for the condition. Too great functional activity, such as sometimes arises from severe muscular strain, leads to marked hyperemia, which in some cases has been so severe as to cause death (*apoplexia pulmonum vascularis*).

Of those due to mechanical causes may be cited the hyperemia (active) of the lungs which is found so often in cases of death from respiratory failure, such as occurs from certain lesions producing pressure upon the base of the brain, and the compensatory forms, as, for instance, the hyperemia of one lung which is present when the other lung is collapsed or compressed. In another class the condition is due to reduced external pressure, for example, in aëronauts and after thoracentesis. One of the main types is that known as **hypostatic congestion.** This occurs whenever there is obstruction to the free outflow of blood from the lungs or deficiency in the driving power of the heart or arteries. As will readily be understood, the lower and posterior portions of the lungs are the parts first and chiefly affected. This form is seen in patients that have been confined to bed for a length of time, or where there is degeneration of the muscle of the heart, such as occurs in the severer forms of the infective fevers, for example, typhoid and pneumonia. Mechanical obstruction within the lung itself may be at the bottom of this, or the heart may have given way from cloudy and fatty changes and dilatation. It is also obvious that this condition will be aggravated whenever, as so frequently is the case in severe fevers, the respiratory movements are weak. Deficiency in the driving power of the right heart is a potent cause, as it allows the blood to remain in the lesser circulation longer than it should do normally. A weak left heart, by lessening the power of the general circulation, acts in a similar way, but to a less extent.

The most striking examples of the obstructive form are those due to insufficiency or stenosis of the mitral valve, or to other cause of increased pressure within the lesser circulation. In a marked case the lung is somewhat enlarged, its consistency increased, and its elasticity diminished. On section the tissue may not be œdematous, but is full of blood of venous appearance. The color is dark red, or purple red. Being a chronic condition, there is apt to be proliferation of the fibrous tissue in the septa of the lung, so that the tissue becomes firmer than ·normal, the so-called **cyanotic induration.** In cases of a longer standing still, more or less blood is effused by diapedesis, and the red cells are eventually broken down, liberating the blood pigment. In such cases the fibrosis is still more marked. This condition is called **brown induration,** from the fact that the cut surface of the lung is of a dark, rusty brown color. On squeezing such a lung, the fluid which is exuded is also of a brownish color, and if a little of it be examined under a microscope it is seen to contain large, clear, mononuclear cells loaded with brownish pigment. These are the so-called "heart-failure" cells.

Microscopically, the appearances in congestion of the lungs are characteristic. The vessels are found to be distended with blood. This is extremely well seen in the delicate capillaries of the alveolar walls, which can be made out to be filled with red blood· cells. They are over-distended, in fact, so that they assume a beaded or varicose appearance and project into the alveolar spaces. An occasional red cell may be seen lying free in ·the alveolar spaces. In the chronic cases, such as those due to a long-standing valvular lesion of the heart, there is in addition to the appearances just mentioned a fibrous hyperplasia of the septa of the lung, which are, in places, infiltrated with small, round cells, probably young fibroblasts. Besides this, in the alveolar spaces there are often considerable numbers of cells of the heart-failure type just mentioned. These have the appearance of large mononuclear cells, containing the shadows of red cells, or blood and coal pigment. They are derived either from the desquamated lining cells of the alveolar walls or are wandering cells. In the advanced cases the pigment is not confined to the desquamated cells, but is found in the connective tissue, lymphoid and epithelial cells as well.

Hemorrhage.—Effusions of blood within the lung substance may affect the parenchyma of the organ or may involve the various air spaces. The latter event is by far the more common. As a rule, the blood is derived from the pulmonary vessels, but occasionally it comes from outside the lung altogether, as, for instance, when an aneurism of the aorta bursts into a bronchus. Occasionally the blood is aspirated from the nose or mouth.

The effused blood may be small in amount, taking the form of petechial spots, varying in size from that of a pin-head to that of a bean, or large areas may be involved, even to the extent of a whole lobe. The smaller hemorrhages are usually but imperfectly defined from the unaffected lung tissue and more or less patchy in character. In the case of the larger areas, notably in infarcts, the line of demarcation is usually very distinct.

With regard to the ultimate causes of these effusions, it may be said in general that the extravasation is due to alterations in the vessel walls or to the obstruction of the lumen. Thus, in the early stages of lobar and lobular pneumonia, blood may be extravasated in large amounts, owing to diapedesis. In a few cases, as in vicarious menstruation, it would appear that the condition is due to some defect in the innervation of the vessel walls, for the lung is in such cases practically intact.

Any solution of continuity of a vessel wall is also a cause, such as may result from fatty and hyaline degeneration, ulceration, or traumatism. A similar condition of things is found in connection with lesions of the pons, medulla, and occasionally the cerebral cortex.

The traumatic form is seen in wounds of the lung produced by shooting or stabbing, or by a broken rib. In rare instances, rupture of the lung occurs from severe strain without any of these causes.

By far the most common cause of the larger hemorrhages is ulceration or degeneration of the vessel walls in the course of necrotic or tuberculous inflammation of the lung substance.

It occasionally happens that in gangrene of the lung a vessel is opened and free hemorrhage takes place into the cavity, which may eventually discharge into a bronchus. This is, however, a much more frequent event in chronic ulcerative tuberculosis.

In the course of the caseous and necrotizing inflammations which result in cavity formation, the fibrous septa and bloodvessels, which are the most resistant of the tissues, are laid bare. The bloodvessels are often found projecting in loops from the wall of the cavity or running in fibrous bands across the space, where they are badly supported. The vessels themselves do not escape, however, but are the seat of a pan-arteritis or endarteritis, which in some cases, but not invariably, lead to obliteration of the lumen. The vessel walls become thickened through a chronic productive inflammation, and from the inner layers a fibrinohyaline degeneration sets in, which gradually spreads to the periphery and may eventually involve the whole circumference. In this way, the tissues become soft and are no longer able to resist the pressure of the blood. Usually some part of the wall gives way and an aneurism is formed or rupture takes place. These aneurisms vary in size from that of a pin-head to that of a cherry, and may fill up the entire space of the cavity. Rupture readily takes place, and the resulting hemorrhage may be very severe or even fatal. Often, however, death is not brought about by a single hemorrhage, but by repeated attacks, leading to oligemia and cachexia. Post mortem, it is not always easy to find the aneurism or ruptured vessel, for when the bleeding has been repeated and prolonged, the vessel is often obliterated, owing to pressure and inflammation.

Perhaps the most striking form of hemorrhage into the lung is the hemorrhagic **infarct**. This is found most frequently in the right lung and in the lower lobe, but may be multiple and bilateral.

In a well-marked case, the infarct is cone-shaped and more or less sharply defined from the rest of the lung. It is usually situated near the pleural surface, the apex of the cone being innermost. The pleura over the affected part is elevated, of a dark, purplish-red color, and the lung is felt to be occupied by a firm mass. The pleura in the early stages is still quite smooth, but in a case of some standing is covered with a slight fibrinous deposit, due to reactive inflammation. On cutting through the mass, the affected area is found to be solid, friable, and of a dark, purplish-red or rusty-brown color. The edges may be quite sharply defined from the rest of the lung, or the infarct may be of a more patchy character. In an infarct of some standing, there may be slight softening and the apex and edges of the cone are somewhat grayish in color, due in part to a deposit of fibrin and a leukocytic infiltration. On scraping, the surface is at first dry and granular, subsequently more juicy.

Microscopically, the changes in the affected tissue are very plain. The alveolar spaces are filled with red blood cells so as to be quite airless. An occasional leukocyte or thread of fibrin may also be seen. The alveolar walls are thin and compressed, the nuclei staining badly or not at all. The various interlobular septa are free from any extravasation. About the margins of the infarct, where a certain amount of reactive inflammation is taking place, the leukocytes are more numerous in the alveolar spaces and the fibrin is more abundant. The lymph channels about the periphery of the infarct, in addition to the perivascular and peribronchial lymphatics, are filled with reabsorbed blood cells.

As the infarct ages, a characteristic series of changes takes place. The extravasated cells gradually break down and the pigment is set free in brownish granular masses. Gradually the circulation is restored through the bronchial arteries, the alveoli become emptied, and the part becomes functional. Rarely do we have necrosis and cicatrization as in infarcts elsewhere. A rare event is for the centre of the infarct to soften and then become absorbed, producing a form of cyst; or the infarcted area may become infiltrated with calcareous salts and a hard nodule be left. In those cases where the infarct is infected at the start, or becomes so later, a septic pneumonia may develop with the formation of a lung abscess or a patch of gangrene.

With regard to the etiology of infarct of the lung, much has been written. A variety of factors seems to enter into the causation. The most important and constant is the condition of the bloodvessels. As a majority of instances of lung infarct arise in connection of valvular lesions of the heart, emphysema, inflammations, senile and marantic conditions of the general system, we can look for a main contributory cause in the fatty and hyaline degeneration of the capillaries and smaller vessels which is so often present in such cases. A sudden disturbance of the blood pressure of the part or a loss of the normal vascular balance which should exist between the different portions of a lung area are powerful factors also, since such may lead not only to degenerative changes in the vessels themselves, but to actual rupture of their walls.

The most frequently found condition is a clot within the main vessels leading to the infarcted area. The pulmonary artery at the apex of the wedge-shaped mass is usually stopped by a thrombotic embolus. The pulmonary vein may be thrombosed, but it may not infrequently be free from clot, except in its terminal ramifications. The vessels affected may appear to be comparatively healthy, or they may show fatty and other endarteritic changes. Sometimes the clot, from its condition and appearance, can be clearly made out to be an embolus which has reached the lung from some other part. This is seen not infrequently in cases of endocarditis, and when thrombi in the larger vascular trunks have become dislodged. In the latter cases the emboli may be so large as to occlude the main trunk of the pulmonary vein and lead to instant or rapid death. The condition of thrombosis of the crural veins or of the uterine veins after childbirth is of much importance in this connection.

The various theories regarding the mode of formation of these infarcts have already been discussed on page 39 et seq.

In connection with infarction we have spoken so far only of emboli that are formed of blood clots, but on occasion other substances, such as fat, air, coal dust, cells from tumors, fragments of vessels, calcareous salts, and parasites enter the vessels, although they do not by any means always result in infarction.

Embolism.—Fat Embolism.—Fat embolism occurs whenever fat in any quantity gains entrance into the blood. Thus, in the case of fractures of the long bones, suppurative osteomyelitis, crushing injuries to the body wall or the liver, the lipemia of diabetes, in eclampsia, in extensive destruction of the brain substance, in fatty degeneration of thrombi, fat droplets can be found in the capillaries not only of the lungs, but of the other organs as well (see p. 54). A rapid method for demonstrating the condition is to cut a thin slice of tissue with a double-bladed knife, which can then be examined directly with the low power. The fat in the larger vessels looks like an elongated drop of some semifluid substance, clear and refractile. In the smaller capillaries the droplets have a more varicose appearance. If the tissue be treated with Sudan III or osmic acid, the fat takes either a red or brownish-black stain.

Air Embolism.—Air embolism is apt to occur when from any cause a large venous trunk is laid open to the air (see p. 55).

Emboli composed of portions of *tumors* are important, since it is in this way that metastases in the lungs are usually produced.

CONDITIONS DUE TO DISTURBANCE OF THE RESPIRATORY FUNCTION.

Atelectasis.—By this is commonly meant the condition in which the alveolar spaces are either partially or completely undistended by the air. The term "atelectasis" is, strictly speaking, only applicable to cases where the lung has undergone primary imperfect expansion. When complete airlessness exists, "apneumatosis" is the better term.

The condition is *congenital* or *acquired.* Before birth the lung is a solid organ, the alveolar walls lying in close contact. The lining epithelium of the alveoli is composed of small polyhedral cells and the smaller bronchioles are thrown into folds longitudinally. Thus, not actual but only potential air spaces exist. With the first inspirations the lung begins to expand, the alveolar walls are thrust apart, and the lining cells are converted into flattened plates. The bronchioles thereupon assume their permanent shape. The condition of the lungs in the newborn is of great importance from a medicolegal standpoint, to determine whether the infant has breathed or not.

A number of causes may contribute to the persistence of the fœtal condition.. Such are, general asthenia and muscular weakness commonly present in premature children; weakness, owing to a syphilitic or other constitutional taint; lesions of the central nervous system, like cerebral hemorrhage or similar lesions of the brain; defects of development, such as hypoplasia of the lung and diaphragmatic hernia; finally external causes, as compression of the thorax, obstruction of the bronchi by foreign bodies, meconium, or secretion.

The causes of the acquired form may be included under the general heads of (1) defective respiratory function within the lung itself, and (2) external mechanical pressure.

Fig. 65

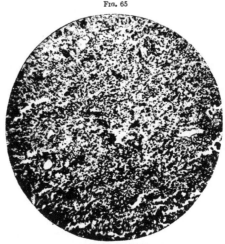

Compression collapse of the lung. Note the fact that the alveolar spaces are obliterated, the walls being in contact. Zeiss obj. DD, ocular No. 1. (From the Pathological Laboratory of McGill University.)

Of the first type the commonest form is that found in cachectic or moribund individuals. Owing to weak inspiratory movements the lung tissue is not perfectly distended. Consequently, small areas, chiefly at the margins of the lungs, become partially or wholly collapsed. This is among the commonest conditions found post mortem.

Another form is that where the bronchial tree in some portion becomes occluded (**obstructive atelectasis**), as from a foreign body, the accumulation of secretion in the lumen, and intrabronchial and intrapulmonary tumors. The collapse in these cases is brought about in part by the obstructing material acting as a kind of valve, whereby air does not readily enter the affected portion while it passes freely out. This mechanical action is, however, not entirely adequate to explain the condition, for the whole of the contained air could not be got rid of in that way. The residual air is absorbed into the blood (**absorption atelectasis**) and the collapse thus becomes complete.

External pressure upon the whole lung or any part of it is a very frequent cause of atelectasis (**compression atelectasis**). Pressure may be exerted by fluid or air within the pleural cavity, an elevated diaphragm, aneurisms or tumors in the mediastinum, kyphosis and scoliosis of the vertebral column, enlargement of the heart or pericardial cavity, thickening and contraction of the pleura. The effect is due not only to direct pressure, but also to the interference with the proper respiratory movements.

Atelectasis may affect one or both lungs, one lobe, or any portion thereof. When the lung as a whole is atelectatic, as, for instance, in hydrothorax, it lies close to the spinal column, somewhat high up in the thorax. Its volume is much diminished and the surface is thrown into fine wrinkles. The consistence is increased and the organ has a leathery feel, the normal crepitation of the healthy lung being absent. In color it is usually purplish or brownish-red. If, as sometimes happens, the tissue is ischemic from pressure, it assumes more of a grayish or slaty appearance. On section, the lung does not crepitate, and resembles flesh. The affected part sinks in water. If squeezed below the surface of the water a few air bubbles may sometimes be expressed. In most collapsed lungs there is a tendency to vascular stasis, so that the cut surface is congested. When only a portion of a lobe is collapsed, the affected part is of a dark purplish-red color, and somewhat sunken below the general level of the lung. The pleura is smooth and the tissue has all the characteristics already described.

Microscopically, the alveolar walls are found to be in more or less close contact, so that the alveolar spaces are obliterated. Occasionally, in the infundibula, groups of epithelial cells can be made out. The cells lining the alveoli have resumed, in fact, the embryonic type. The bronchioles are corrugated and the bloodvessels are everywhere congested. Sometimes small hemorrhages and masses of blood-pigment can be observed.

When of long standing, atelectasis is frequently complicated with other conditions. Thus, in infants, bronchiectasis has been observed. Again, from the fact that the atelectatic portion is usually congested while the cause of the condition is often an inflammatory one, infection readily takes place. Bronchopneumonia, therefore, is not an infrequent sequel. In other cases, the lung undergoes a chronic, indurative change, owing to proliferation of the fibrous tissue, fatty degeneration of the alveolar epithelium, and becomes permanently collapsed and carnified.

Emphysema.—Emphysema of the lungs is one of the commonest pathological conditions. The term "emphysema" was originally applied to a condition in which air is found in the tissues (**interstitial emphysema**), but is very appropriately applied to that affection of the lungs in which they are overdistended and contain more than the normal amount of air.

The condition may be generalized, affecting nearly the whole of both lungs, or may be restricted to certain parts. In an advanced and typical case of generalized emphysema the patient has a characteristic appearance. The neck is short and thick; the chest is enlarged in all its diameters, but particularly anteroposteriorly, so that it assumes a barrel shape; the abdomen is relatively sunken and the accessory muscles of respiration are well developed.

When the thorax is opened the lungs are more voluminous than normal, encroaching upon the cardiac area, and do not collapse. The costal cartilages are lengthened and sometimes calcified. While the lungs are considerably enlarged, their weight may be actually diminished. The tissue is inelastic and much less crepitant than normal, retaining the impress of the fingers and having the feel of a bag of feathers. The pleural surface is very pale, and the pigmentation of the lung is not so conspicuous as it usually is. With a hand lens, or even with the naked eye, small vesicles, the size of a pin-head or less, which represent the enlarged alveolar spaces, can be seen on the surface. In advanced cases these vesicles may attain the size of peas, or even larger, giving the lung a bullous appearance (*emphysema bullosa*). In the larger vesicles can often be traced the remains of what were originally the alveolar walls. On section, the lung is pale and dry and the larger vesicles collapse. These can, however, again be made manifest with water. Associated with the condition is usually a certain amount of chronic bronchitis, with some thickening of the bronchi and pulmonary septa. Bronchiectasis, however, is not often met with. In less extreme cases, the apices, the anterior borders, and the inner surface near the root are the parts affected. These areas are somewhat distended or inflated, as compared with the rest of the lung, and present the characters just mentioned.

Several classifications of emphysema have been proposed. The usual one of hypertrophic, atrophic, and compensatory forms, while a useful clinical division, is open to some criticism from the point of view of the pathologist. Perhaps the best general division is into *vesicular* and *interstitial* emphysema. In the first variety it is the alveolar spaces that are distended and contain a surplus of air. In the second, the air is present in the interstitial tissue of the lungs.

Vesicular emphysema may further be subdivided into (1) *essential* or *substantial* emphysema, and (2) *complementary*.

Essential Emphysema.—Various grades of essential emphysema exist, which pass imperceptibly one into the other. Orth recognizes three forms: (1) **Simple emphysema,** in which the lung is simply inflated with air to its full capacity, or, in other words, is in a permanent inspiratory position. This form is Traube's *Volumen Pulmonum Auctum,* and while, on anatomical grounds, it is correctly differentiated from the other forms of emphysema, it cannot be separated clinically from them by any definite signs. (2) **Ectatic emphysema.** This is a farther stage in which the limit of physiological dilatation of the alveoli is overstepped and the spaces become enlarged though without actual atrophy.

The structural changes present consist in dilatation of the alveolar spaces in connection with certain infundibula. The alveolar walls become gradually stretched and thinned, and the spaces tend to assume a globular form. Thus, the multiloculated structure of the lung becomes much simplified. (3) **Atrophic emphysema.** In this variety, the alveolar walls atrophy and the vessels gradually become obliterated. Rupture of the air spaces is here a striking feature. Several alveolar spaces are thrown into one, so that actual bullæ are the result.

In atrophic emphysema, the microscopic changes are well marked. The alveolar walls are thinned and in many cases broken. Thus, we see large spaces which are clearly due to the coalescence of several adjacent alveoli, for the remains of the ruptured walls can be seen projecting into the cavity. The bloodvessels are small and in many places obliterated. The atrophy affects first and chiefly the bloodvessels and

FIG. 66

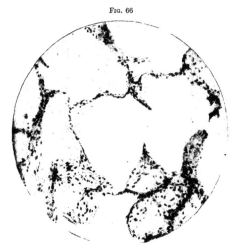

Emphysema of lung. Leitz obj. No. 7, without ocular. The atrophied alveolar walls and the rupture of several of them are well shown. (From the collection of Dr. A. G. Nicholls.)

elastic tissue, the connective tissue being more resistant. By special preparation, the lining epithelium can be recognized on the alveolar walls. The cells are, of course, forced apart by the process of distension, but isolated ones can be made out here and there on the walls, many of them fattily degenerated. In the infundibula small groups of these cells can be found. The bronchi usually show signs of chronic inflammation and the septa are infiltrated. This is not a feature of the emphysema, however, but is due to the inflammation and catarrh which is so frequent an accompaniment of the disease.

Complementary Emphysema.—Complementary emphysema is generally localized to one or more lobules, but may, under certain circumstances, affect a whole lung. Local emphysema is quite a common condition, and is frequently only a temporary state, due, not to structural changes in the lung, but, for the most part, to irregularity in the intra-alveolar pressure. Thus, in pneumonia, fibroid induration, and in tuberculosis, where a portion of the lung becomes impervious to air, the remaining air sacs are subjected to increased pressure and in consequence become distended. As soon as the cause is removed the affected air sacs return to their normal state, but in prolonged or repeated attacks the temporary may give place to a permanent condition. The distension of the alveoli is due to a compensatory process and is found in the neighborhood of the atelectatic or consolidated areas of the lung.

Interstitial Emphysema.—Interstitial emphysema is a relatively unimportant condition. Here air is present in small beads in the interstitial tissue. The air bubbles remind one of a string of beads and may clearly define the various lobules. The bubbles rarely attain any size and can be pushed along the septa with the finger. The condition is usually met with beneath the pleura, but may spread to the hilus of the lungs and even to the mediastinal tissues. A similar state of affairs may result from putrefaction. This form may be present in ordinary emphysema due to rupture of an alveolus, in injuries of the lung, and in those who have died of suffocation. The artificial inflation of the lungs of the asphyxiated newborn infant has been known to produce it.

A word should be said about the conditions due to and associated with pulmonary emphysema. In advanced cases there is nearly always chronic bronchitis and sometimes bronchiectasis. Owing to the increased intrapulmonary pressure the right side of the heart becomes hypertrophied, and eventually the whole heart may become hypertrophied and dilated with evidences of valvular incompetency. Arteriosclerosis is also a not infrequent accompaniment. The peculiar changes in the chest have already been referred to.

In **senile emphysema** of the lung, which is not properly emphysema at all, though classed with it by many writers, the thorax and indeed the whole body is small and shrunken, the ribs close together, and very obliquely situated, so that they approximate very closely to the crest of the ilium. The lungs in such cases are small, generally atrophied, and, as Jenner expressed it, feel like an inflated bag of wet paper.

INFLAMMATIONS.

Pneumonia.—Pneumonia is to be referred to the direct irritant action of microörganisms upon the lung substance. While, however, certain clinical types are recognized on the ground of the anatomical distribution of the lesions and a well-defined clinical course, it should be remembered that there are many intermediate and atypical forms, so much so that to the bacteriologist pneumonia is not a single disease entity, but rather a multiplicity of pathological manifestations dependent on a variety of causes.

Numerous inquiries into the etiology of acute pneumonia have been made in recent years, and almost all the known pathogenic microörganisms have been proved to be capable of producing pulmonary inflammation.[1] Among these may be mentioned the Fraenkel-Weichselbaum Diplococcus of pneumonia, Friedländer's pneumobacillus, Streptococcus pyogenes, Staphylococcus albus and aureus, B. tuberculosis, B. typhi abdominalis, B. coli communis, B. influenzæ, B. pestis, B. anthracis, B. diphtheriæ, B. enteritidis of Gaertner. Any one of these alone is able to cause the affection, but mixed infections are common. A curious and extremely fatal form that should be mentioned is that known as **psittacosis**, which is due to a typhoid-like organism. The infection has been traced to birds, particularly parrots.

To produce the disease it is necessary for the bacteria to invade the lung, and this they do, either through the bronchi (*inhalation* or *aërogenic pneumonia*) or through the blood and lymph-stream (*hematogenic, lymphogenic pneumonia*). Some of the germs above mentioned have been found in the buccal secretion of healthy people, so that it is not surprising that inhalation or bronchogenic pneumonia is a common affection.

Recent investigations go to prove that the lungs and peribronchial glands play an important role in the protection of the organism from infective agencies coming from without (see vol. i, p. 319). Barthel[2] found in the healthy lung both pathogenic and non-pathogenic bacteria in the trachea and larger bronchi, though the bronchioles and alveoli were free. The bacteria, of which the diplococcus was most frequently present, were more abundant in the lung than in the mouth, a condition of things due possibly to local growth or to the inhibiting and eliminating power of the saliva. The later researches of Beco,[3] on the whole, confirm this view.

It would appear, too, that bacteria may pass by means of the lymphatics through the lung without eliciting any manifestation of their presence. Whether pneumonia is produced or not must depend, therefore, upon some second cause, either increased virulence of the bacteria or diminished resisting power on the part of the organism. In the case of Diplococcus pneumoniæ, increased virulence is scarcely likely to be an important factor, for, as we know, this germ, when freely exposed to the air, rapidly loses its power, and is readily killed out by the presence of certain other microörganisms. Any diplococci, therefore, in the mouth or respiratory tract are likely to be so weakened that in many instances they are non-pathogenic. Susceptibility seems to vary also in different individuals and races. Thus, for man the Diplococcus pneumoniæ is comparatively mild, for the majority of cases, at least in healthy adults, get well. In the case of some of the lower animals, such as mice and rabbits, the infection is very severe, so much so that when infected they

[1] For a study of the bacteriology of pneumonia, see Curry, Jour. of Exper. Med., 4: 1899: 169.

[2] Centralbl. f. Bakt., 24: 1898: 11.

[3] Arch. de méd. expér. et d'anatom. path., May, 1899.

die from general bacteriemia rather than pneumonia. It may be remarked, moreover, in passing, that the oftener careful bacteriological studies are made, the more frequently do we find that pneumonia, even in man, is to be regarded as a generalized infection with a local manifestation, as is the case also with typhoid fever and some other infections. Any circumstance that leads to a lowered vitality of the organism may be a predisposing or contributory cause, such as previous attacks, wasting diseases, alcoholism, diabetes, Bright's disease, pulmonary lesions, traumatism to the lung, bodily injuries, chronic nervous disorders, and exhausting occupations. Climate, season, and age are of some importance, as affecting the resisting power of the system. "Catching cold" does not seem to have the importance that once was thought. The influence of traumatism is shown very prettily in a case cited by Lucatello,[1] where, in a patient in previously perfect health, pneumonia developed a few days subsequently to a severe contusion of the shoulder.

On account of the anatomical structure of the lungs, inflammatory processes occurring therein differ materially from those met with, for example, in the secreting glands. The chief characteristic is that the inflammatory products are poured out into the alveolar spaces, while the cells lining these spaces undergo degeneration and desquamation. The process may be more or less confined to the alveolar walls, but in many cases the interlobular septa are involved, so that an interstitial process is at work as well. The changes are exudative and desquamative rather than parenchymatous.

The anatomical picture in pneumonia varies greatly. Sometimes the whole or the greater part of a lobe is affected, hence the term **lobar** pneumonia. At other times the disease is confined to the lobules—**lobular** pneumonia—or to minute but numerous portions of the lobules—**miliary** pneumonia.

The infection is in many cases derived from the air passages, and to an important group of these, in which the process seems to begin in the smaller bronchioles and extends to the alveoli, the term **bronchopneumonia** has been given. The **miliary** form is due to infection through the blood stream. In certain other cases, inflammation begins in the neighboring tissues and spreads to the lung by means of the lymphatics. An important type of this form is the so-called **pleurogenetic pneumonia**, where the disease begins in the pleura and extends as a lymphangitis and perilymphangitis of the lung substance.

In most varieties of pneumonia the bronchi are more or less affected, either primarily or secondarily, and the peribronchial lymph-glands are enlarged, succulent, and inflamed.

Pneumonia may be *acute* or *chronic*, depending upon the nature of the offending microörganism and the resisting power of the tissue.

It is perhaps difficult to account satisfactorily for the variability in the distribution of the lesions. Certain germs like the Diplococcus pneumoniæ and the Pneumobacillus of Friedländer tend to produce the

[1] Centralbl. f. Bakt., 8: 1890: 239.

lobar variety, while others like the pus cocci, the Bacillus of influenza, and the B. coli, nearly always produce a lobular inflammation. The explanation probably is that the Diplococcus pneumoniæ, being relatively non-malignant in man, can only act in the event of a *locus resistentiæ minoris* being formed, and this in ordinary healthy people is apt to be present in only one portion of the lung. Lobular pneumonia, however, while it does occasionally develop as a primary affection, nearly always occurs in those previously weakened by disease. It is characteristically a "terminal" infection, and as in all chronic cases the lungs are uniformly weakened, not only from degenerative processes, but also from defective respiration, any infective agents present in the respiratory passages are likely to exert a disseminated activity. The hematogenic and lymphogenic forms are, of course, more easily understood.

Another important feature in the differentiation of the various pneumonias is the character of the exudate. From this, we are often enabled to decide as to the nature of the infecting microörganism. According to the acuteness of the case, the inflammatory products are exudative or productive, and either element may predominate over the other. In one common form, the so-called "fibrinous" or "croupous" pneumonia, due to the Diplococcus pneumoniæ, the alveoli are filled with a rather dry, granular exudate of a grayish color. When resolution is commencing, the alveolar contents can be expressed in the form of little plugs. In the form due to the Friedländer bacillus, the lung is congested-looking, juicy, and the cut surface has the appearance of being coated with gelatin. The exudate can be scraped off with the knife, and is so viscid that it depends in long, glairy strings from the knife.

Acute Lobar Pneumonia.—In acute lobar pneumonia (Fraenkel-Weichselbaum diplococcus) the lung is usually said to pass through four stages: (1) Engorgement, (2) red hepatization, (3) gray hepatization, and (4) resolution. This is a convenient division for purposes of description, but it is very doubtful how far it is warranted by the actual facts. The mode of development of the lesions is certainly quite varied and a uniform order is not always adhered to. It is not uncommon to find several of the above-mentioned stages present simultaneously in the lung. There can be no doubt, however, that the inflammation begins with congestion followed by consolidation. The first two stages are rarely ever seen except in persons dying by accident, or in limited areas at the edge of a creeping pneumonia, for, as might be supposed, the cases that come to autopsy are in the advanced stages.

In the period of *engorgement* the condition is that of a simple active or inflammatory hyperemia. The lung is redder than normal and possibly slightly edematous. Microscopically, the capillaries in the alveolar walls are congested and varicose, the epithelial cells are swollen and occasionally desquamated, and there may be an occasional red corpuscle in the alveolar spaces. In the *second stage* the affected portion of the lung is swollen, heavier, and firmer than normal, pitting on pressure, and somewhat friable. It is intensely red, and on section an abundant turbid, blood-stained fluid can be squeezed out. Although the exudate appears reddish

Fig. 67

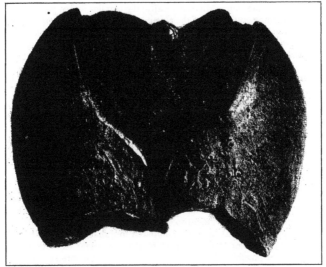

Acute lobar pneumonia (gray hepatization). The lower lobe is involved. (From the Pathological Laboratory of the Royal Victoria Hospital.)

Fig. 68

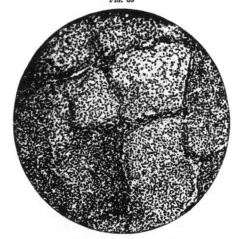

Acute lobar pneumonia. Leitz obj. No. 7, without ocular. The alveolar spaces are filled with leukocytes and fibrin. (From the collection of Dr. A. G. Nicholls.)

and contains a majority of red corpuscles, even at this early stage numerous leukocytes are present. Microscopically, the capillaries are greatly congested, the lining epithelium of the alveolar spaces is swollen, and the cells are found in all stages of proliferation and desquamation. The alveolar spaces are more or less filled with red blood cells, and desquamated epithelial cells—the so-called "catarrhal" cells—enmeshed in fibrin, but numerous leukocytes can be seen. A round-celled infiltration is also to be noted about the vessels of the interlobular septa. Owing to the solid appearance of the lung and its reddish color, it was compared by the older pathologists to the liver, whence the term "red hepatization." Imperceptibly the condition passes on into .the *third stage*, that of gray hepatization. Here the lung is still more swollen, so that it shows the impression of the ribs, is heavy and firm to the touch. The pleura has lost its glassy appearance, is granular and cloudy, and covered with a varying amount of fibrinous exudation. In fact, every acute lobar pneumonia is also a pleuropneumonia. The lung is quite airless, friable, and sinks in water. On section, the surface is granular, and, according to the age of the process, of a color varying from dark red through the different shades of reddish-gray to gray or yellow. This, with the deposit of coal pigment so often present, gives the lung a curious mottled appearance that has been compared to granite. The characteristic ashen-gray color is due in part to the leukocytic exudation and in part to the anemia of the tissue produced by the pressure of the alveolar contents upon the vessels. On scraping the surface, a small amount of granular material can be removed. The bronchioles of the affected area are usually blocked with fibrin. Microscopically, the alveolar walls are compressed and the capillary channels are obliterated. The exudate is made up almost entirely of leukocytes and fibrin, with an occasional erythrocyte and catarrhal cell. By Weigert's method the fibrin threads can be beautifully demonstrated, and may sometimes be seen passing through the stomata from one alveolar space to the other.

When the fibrin is beginning to break up and become granular, and the leukocytes show advanced fatty degeneration, the stage of *resolution* is being initiated. The lung begins to shrink, the pleura is relaxed and thrown into folds, and the organ has a boggy feel. On section, the tissue is grayish verging on yellow, and is moist, so that a fluid not unlike pus can be expressed. On scraping, little plugs of fibrin and leukocytes readily come away. Microscopically, the appearances are not unlike the last stage, except that the alveolar capillaries are again becoming permeable, the fibrin threads are broken up into a granular debris, and the leukocytes especially about the margin of the clot show signs of fatty degeneration and solution (autolysis). Later, regeneration of the alveolar epithelium takes place. The exudation is removed chiefly by the lymphatics but also to some extent through expectoration. The lymphatics are frequently found distended with leukocytic and fibrinous exudation. Indeed, a true lymphangitis and perilymphangits may occur, so that the framework of the lung is profoundly involved in the inflammatory process. Should the lymphatics be damaged by previous disease, as, for instance, from emphysema, absorption is rendered so much the more difficult.[1]

As has been remarked, it is by no means necessary for pneumonia to pass regularly through the stages described. Clinical experience teaches us that some cases attain their acme very rapidly and subside in two or three days instead of lasting ten or more, as is the rule. Some variation in the amount of exudation occurs also. In children, the aged, and the asthenic, the amount of fibrin produced may be small and the alveoli not greatly distended, so that the usual dry, granular appearance of the lung is not observed.

As to the site of the pneumonic process, according to Orth, 52 per cent. occur on the right side, 33 per cent. on the left, and 15 per cent. on both. When both lungs are involved it is common to find the process less advanced in one than in the other. One lung may be in the stage of gray hepatization, while the other shows merely engorgement or red hepatization. The portions of the lung uninvolved in the consolidation are not free from pathological change. They are usually much congested and there may be local emphysematous dilatation of the alveoli of a compensatory character.

With regard to the distribution of the lesions in the lung, the lower lobe of the right lung is the one most frequently affected, next to this the lower lobe of the left lung. The tendency is for a whole lobe to be involved. Atypical forms are, however, not infrequently met with, as, for instance, the "central" pneumonia, where the process begins about the hilus and is most in evidence in the centre of the lung. In other cases the disease may be localized to a small area in the apex of the lung—"apical" pneumonia. The presence of such a focus, by the way, should always raise the suspicion of tuberculosis. A curious form is the so-called "creeping" pneumonia, in which the consolidation presents various stages of development, at one part resolution being in progress, at another fresh pneumonic infiltration. This conforms to a well-known clinical type.

It is not very uncommon for pneumonia to be associated with or complicated by inflammatory processes elsewhere in the body. Chief among these should be mentioned pleurisy, pericarditis, endocarditis, peritonitis, nephritis, meningitis, and lesions of the bones and joints.

It is the rule in young and otherwise healthy persons for resolution to take place, but, apart from a lethal termination, certain other results may follow. Not infrequently, tuberculosis is superadded and the case progresses instead of resolving. Rarely, the exudate dries up within the alveoli into a granular caseous mass, so that the condition resembles massive tuberculosis. Again, secondary infection may take place, and if pyogenic or putrefactive microörganisms be present, abscess or gangrene may result. Further, there is a close relationship between abscess of the lung and gangrene, for the one may initiate the other.

[1] For a study of the histological appearances, see Pratt, Jour. Boston Soc. of the Med. Sci., 4: 1900: 183,

While it must be admitted that the pneumococcus is capable of producing a suppurative and necrosing process, it is probable that this is a rare event. No doubt, owing to the close resemblance between a pneumonic exudate when undergoing liquefaction and absorption and pus, two different conditions have been confused. Gangrene is said to be more frequent than abscess. Here, the lung is converted into a foul, pulpy mass of dark greenish color. When softening has taken place, irregular cavities with shaggy, necrotic walls are seen. A line of demarcation is not usually formed. Gangrene is specially apt to supervene in those cases where there is putrid bronchitis and bronchiectasis, where the circulation is poor, and in cases where a hemorrhagic exudate is a prominent feature. The most common sequel, however, is fibroid induration of the lung. Here, with the signs of delayed or absent resolution, the exudate becomes organized by a process similar to that occurring in a thrombus. The affected part is enlarged, very firm and heavy, cutting with some difficulty. The color is reddish or reddish gray, mixed with the black of the coal pigment, and the septa are prominent as bands of grayish-white appearance. Thus, a peculiar marbled appearance is the result. The pleura is also greatly thickened. If the patient live long enough, the exudate is absorbed and the lung shrinks into a hard, irregular, fibrous mass.

Acute Lobular Pneumonia (Catarrhal Pneumonia, Bronchopneumonia).— This form differs somewhat from lobar pneumonia in that the exudate tends to be catarrhal rather than fibrinous. The process is associated with bronchitis, and, indeed, almost always starts with inflammation of the smaller bronchioles, which spreads to the adjacent alveoli (bronchitis and peribronchitis). This is the "capillary bronchitis" of the older writers. The exudate is at first serous and contains a few erythrocytes, but more numerous white cells. A striking feature is the great abundance of the so-called "catarrhal" cells, large mononuclear cells with clear protoplasm. These are believed by many to be swollen and desquamated epithelial cells from the alveolar walls, and, while they are present in all forms of pneumonia, they are specially numerous in the lobular variety.

Only exceptionally does this disease occur as a primary affection. As a rule, it is a sequel of bronchitis or a complication of the infective fevers, such as measles, scarlatina, whooping-cough, diphtheria, influenza, typhoid, and variola. It is generally found in the young or aged, or in those debilitated from any cause. Particularly is it liable to attack the bedridden and those suffering from congestive conditions of the lungs (*hypostatic pneumonia*). A class of cases worthy of special note is that due to the inhalation of infective material from the mouth and upper air passages (*aspiration pneumonia*). This is met with after operations upon the nose and mouth and in certain nervous diseases with involvement of the vagus nerve (*vagus pneumonia*). The microorganisms at work here are the same as in the lobar form, but there is a greater tendency for the pyogenic cocci to be concerned.

The disease usually affects both lungs, but may involve only one, or even a single lobe or portion thereof. The affected organ is heavier than normal, somewhat congested, and in its substance can be felt areas of increased consistence. These are friable, of a reddish-gray, gray, or grayish-yellow color, contrasting somewhat with the rest of the lung. In other cases the whole or the greater part of a lobe is consolidated, but irregularly so, pointing to the origin of the condition in the coalescence of isolated foci. On pressure, a turbid blood-stained fluid can be expressed, in which may be seen small particles of a more gray, grayish-yellow, or purulent appearance. These often represent the contents of the bronchioles. From the sporadic distribution of the consolidated areas, the term "splenization" has been given to the condition. As in the lobar form, both red and gray stages are recognized. On section, the lung as a whole is markedly hyperemic. The smaller bronchi and bronchioles show inflammation and are filled with exudate. In the alveolar spaces the exudate consists mainly of serum, a few red cells, abundant leukocytes, and "catarrhal" cells. These catarrhal cells frequently contain pigment and bacteria. Fibrin is not a striking feature, and in this the lobular differs materially from the lobar form. At most, a few of the alveoli at the periphery of a consolidated patch may contain scattered threads of fibrin. Consequently, granulation of the lung is absent. It is worthy of note that pneumonic infiltration may supervene upon the previous collapse of a pulmonary lobule. The explanation is simple, since bronchitis and obstruction of the bronchial lumen lead alike to collapse and bronchopneumonia. In the form due to the presence of foreign bodies in the bronchi or to the inhalation of infective material, the exudation may become purulent. Such a condition usually leads to a diffuse purulent infiltration of the lung and eventually abscess.

Like lobar pneumonia, the lobular form presents several variations in its course and development. It is a serious affection, since it nearly always attacks those of low vitality, or complicates other grave disease. A fatal termination is therefore quite frequent. When resolution does occur, it takes place quickly, for a relatively small area of lung substance is involved, and the lymphatics are less interfered with. In certain cases, when the inflammatory process has originated in an area of old fibroid or caseous pneumonia, the secretion tends to become fatty and finally inspissated, so that the affected area remains consolidated and appears somewhat gelatinous with yellowish specks. This condition was called by Virchow "chronic catarrhal pneumonia." Occasionally abscess and gangrene of the lung may result. This is the case in aspiration pneumonias, in the weak, and those with general circulatory disturbance. In another class of cases local areas of induration result with bronchiectasis. An important sequel is secondary infection with the tubercle bacillus, so that a miliary or caseous bronchopneumonia results.

Septic or Purulent Pneumonia.—The characteristics of this form are its great intensity, a purulent exudation into the alveolar spaces and into the interstitial tissues, and a tendency to destruction of the lung. Expectoration in some cases is profuse, and the sputum may contain elastic tissue and other fragments of lung substance. The process is rarely primary, but usually occurs as a sequel or complication of some other condition. It is due to the action of pyogenic microbes that reach the lung through the air passages, the bloodvessels, and lymphatics. The type of the bronchogenic form is the so-called "aspiration" pneumonia. According to the virulence of the infecting agent a simple catarrhal pneumonia may be the first result, leading eventually to suppuration or rapid destruction with gangrene. One or both lungs may be affected and the lower lobes are the seat of election. According to the character and amount of the aspirated material, scattered foci of infiltration, separated one from the other by comparatively healthy lung tissue, may be seen, or a diffuse and confluent condition. The affected lung is usually congested and œdematous, and the abscesses can frequently be recognized on the surface as nodules of a reddish or reddish-yellow color, over which the pleura shows some cloudiness and injection. On section, the nodules referred to are seen to be due to a more or less complete consolidation. The centre is apt to be broken down and composed of thick, yellowish, or blood-stained pus. About the affected areas there is generally a zone of intense hyperemia. The tissue is very friable, and if the process be of some standing, cavitation may be observed. Sometimes gangrene supervenes and then the affected part is of a dirty, greenish color with a foul odor. The bronchioles are often plugged with exudate.

Microscopically, the parenchyma of the lung is intensely congested. The smaller abscesses are composed of an intense intra-alveolar and interstitial leukocytic infiltration, forming a local cellular focus, the centre of which stains badly and contains leukocytes in all stages of degeneration and debris. In the neighborhood, the capillaries of the alveolar walls are much congested, and there is a certain amount of œdema and desquamation of the lining cells, together with some diapedesis of the red and white cells. Frequently, little clumps of bacteria can be seen in the centre of the mass. Stained with hematoxylin, these are a purple-black color.

Metastatic or Septic Embolic Pneumonia.—Metastatic or septic embolic pneumonia is more common than the last form, and is the type of purulent pneumonia. It is hematogenic in origin and due to the lodging of multiple infecting agents in the vessels of the lung. It is commonly met with as a manifestation of general septicemia, and results from such conditions as osteomyelitis, thrombophlebitis, septic arthritis, septic endometritis, malignant endocarditis, erysipelas, and the like. In cases of infarction of the lung, when due to an embolus containing pyogenic microörganisms, suppuration will result. In other cases clusters of bacteria are found obstructing the capillaries, and thus bring about the condition. It is not likely that germs are ever in the blood in such quantities as to form emboli, but it is more probable that one or two become entangled in the lining cells of the vessels and, being strong enough to overcome the defensive power of the cells, proliferate there.

Both lungs are usually uniformly affected, but, exceptionally, only a few lobules, chiefly those of the lower lobes. The abscesses appear as multiple nodular swellings beneath the pleura, varying in size from that of a pin-head to a cherry or even larger. The areas are usually more or less spherical or, if the condition have originated in infarction, irregularly wedge-shaped. The overlying pleura is congested and cloudy and generally covered with fibrinopurulent exudation. On section, the lung is filled with inflammatory foci in all stages, from simple consolidation or purulent infiltration to actual abscess and excavation. The color varies from reddish-yellow to yellow. In the earlier stages there is not much destruction of tissue, but softening soon occurs and the lung has the appearance of a loose, spongy matrix filled with a thick, reddish-yellow purulent fluid. Sequestration of the tissue is not uncommon, and in advanced stages, on washing out the pus, the abscesses are revealed as cavities with dirty, necrotic walls, surrounded by a zone of intense inflammatory hyperemia. In cases which have lasted some time the cavities may be bounded by a rather dense layer of infiltration walling off the abscesses more or less completely, the so-called "pyogenic" membrane. In certain cases of intense infection gangrene supervenes.

Microscopically, the picture is much like that in other forms of suppurative pneumonia, with the exception that the process is more localized. The minuter abscesses show merely collections of small round cells, but the larger ones stain badly in the centre, owing to necrosis. Œdema, congestion, and hemorrhage in the neighborhood are marked features.

Besides the bronchogenic and hematogenic forms just described, local suppurative and gangrenous inflammation may occur in the lung as the result of traumatism.

Perhaps more frequently than in any other organ secondary suppuration is met with, complicating, for instance, fibrinous pneumonia, chronic ulcerative tuberculosis, actinomycosis, and echinococcus disease. Buhl has described a purulent peribronchitis that may lead to septic pneumonia.

Septic Pneumonia by Extension.—Another important form of septic pneumonia is that arising by extension. Abscesses of the liver, subphrenic abscess, and suppuration of the lymphatic glands may extend to the lung. Frequently, the infection is by way of the pleural cavity and lymphatics (_pleurogenic_). This gives rise to a suppurative interstitial lymphangitis (_peripneumonia_), and is said to be most common in children, especially in connection with empyema. In this case the subpleural lymphatics are dilated, varicose, and of a yellowish color. On section, the lobules are found to be separated from each other by broad succulent yellowish bands representing the connective-tissue septa. The process may go on to the extent that portions of the lung tissue are sequestrated and cast off (_pneumonia dissecans_ of Ziegler). The lung tissue, as a whole, except in the neighborhood of the affected lymphatics, departs but little from the normal. As a rule, if recovery take place, the affected tissue remains somewhat thickened.

Chronic Pneumonia.—This is characterized by the overgrowth of connective tissue in the lung, so that it becomes hard, traversed by fibrous bands, and more or less shrunken. The condition leads to destruction of the alveolar spaces, sometimes with bronchiectasis, and always to marked impairment of function. As already mentioned, it may be one of the methods of termination of ordinary lobar pneumonia,

and may also follow catarrhal, tuberculous, and syphilitic disease of the
lung, ulceration and gangrene, and frequently passive congestion or atelectasis. This may be called (1) the **secondary fibroid or indurative pneumonia;** (2) or it may follow the inhalation of various kinds of dust, and
is then termed **pneumonokoniosis;** (3) lastly, it may arise by the extension
of chronic pleurisy to the lung substance—**pleurogenetic fibroid pneumonia.**
    The induration following upon ordinary acute pneumonia, when of
the lobar type, takes the form of a generalized substitution of the spongy
tissue by compact fibrous bands, while the pleura and the interlobular
septa are thickened as well.   When due to lobular pneumonia, the fibrous
tissue production follows the course of the bronchial tree (peribronchial
fibroid pneumonia).   The lung is greatly increased in weight, has lost
its spongy feel, and is quite hard.   It cuts firmly and is of a grayish-
white color, mottled with black from the inhaled coal dust.   Sometimes

Fig. 69

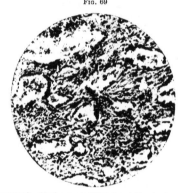

Chronic indurative pneumonia, showing great thickening of the alveolar walls and distortion of
the alveoli. Zeiss obj. DD, without ocular. (From the collection of Dr. A. G. Nicholls.)

small areas of necrosis not unlike caseation may be seen.   In advanced
cases the pleura is thickened and the lung is greatly distorted.   The
two layers of the pleura are usually matted together and the tissues of
the mediastinum may be indurated.   Not infrequently, contraction of
the fibrous tissue leads to deformity of the chest, drooping of the shoulder,
and scoliosis.   Microscopically, the condition is seen to be due to an
imperfect absorption of the exudate within the alveolar spaces and
the overgrowth of connective tissue, so that not only are the septa of the
lung thickened, but the newly formed fibrous tissue grows out into the
alveoli and thus tends to obliterate them.   The affected alveoli are small,
collapsed, or compressed, and often all that can be made out is an
irregular cavity containing a few catarrhal cells or a leukocytic exudation
in various phases of degeneration and absorption.   Small bands of
fibrous tissue project into the cavity of the alveolus and may even form

polypoid excrescences. The bronchi are either compressed so that they are thrown into longitudinal folds, or are dilated and irregular from traction. Here and there in the fibrous tissue are large masses of inflammatory leukocytes and young fibroblasts, pointing to a continuous proliferative process. Greatly contracted alveoli may be found almost devoid of lumina, and lined by an epithelium which is of cubical type.

In cases due to passive congestion the fibrosis is never so extreme, and there is considerable deposit of blood-pigment with dilatation of the veins, while the alveoli contain numerous catarrhal cells filled with pigment. The lung presents a brownish color (*brown induration*).

An important variety is that due to the inhalation of dust. But a small part of the dust that we commonly inhale reaches the lungs, and what finally gets there probably does not reach the termination of the bronchial tree, but is carried into the lung by means of the phagocytes. With regard to the events that follow, much depends upon the nature of the dust inhaled. All kinds lead to a certain amount of bronchial irritation and inflammation, and when carried along the peribronchial lymphatics into the substance of the lung, are deposited in the alveolar walls and the deeper layers of the pleura, where they lead to catarrhal inflammation and leukocytic infiltration. The more irritating kinds of dust, such as stone or iron, may lead to much more extensive lesions. The particles, being sharp, penetrate the walls of the bronchioles and the alveoli and lead to marked inflammation with proliferation of the connective tissue. Thus, it is common to see in the neighborhood of the bronchi and in the alveolar walls more or less rounded nodules of considerable hardness that are composed of connective tissue enclosing a granular detritus with clumps of pigment. In advanced cases the peribronchial glands are greatly enlarged and full of gritty material. Occasionally, the pigment may pass the lung and be deposited in the glands about the lesser curvature of the stomach and the hilus of the liver, and may even reach the liver and general circulation.

Among the forms of dust that are inhaled may be mentioned coal dust, stone dust, kaolin, iron, wool, flour, tobacco, iron oxide, and ultramarine blue. When coal dust is present, the condition is called *anthracosis*. This condition is found in the lungs of all those past the age of infancy, and is more marked in those living in the cities. Coal dust is relatively innocuous, and all we see is scattered patches of black pigment with comparatively little fibrosis. Sometimes small, rounded nodules with a black centre are met with, the so-called "anthracotic tubercles." It is the rule for the peribronchial glands to be enlarged and contain coal pigment. In coal miners the lung is uniformly infiltrated with coal, is heavy, and has a gritty feel on cutting. In such cases the expectoration may be black. In cases of pneumonokoniosis due to stone dust or particles of steel, fibrosis may be very marked. In the stonemason's lung (*chalicosis*) the lung is heavy and filled with a grayish, gritty material. *Siderosis* is the name applied to those cases due to the inhalation of iron or steel, such as is seen among needle grinders, file makers, and founders. The results of pneumonokoniosis are not unlike those of the secondary fibroid pneumonias. There is the same induration and contraction of the lung, together with deformity of the thorax and dislocation of the mediastinal tissues. Calcification has been observed, and true bone formation. In rare cases, suppuration and cavitation has been met with. It should be noted that the presence of dust within the lung predisposes to tuberculosis.

Pleurogenetic Fibroid Pneumonia.—Pleurogenetic fibroid pneumonia is due to an extension of pleuritic inflammation, whereby both the pleura and the septa leading from it are infiltrated with inflammatory products and show fibrous hyperplasia. This condition is also frequently complicated with collapse of the lung.

Tuberculosis.—This disease may present both acute and chronic manifestations, and, as its name implies, is characterized by the formation of tubercles or specific granulomata in the lungs. The disease is caused by the B. tuberculosis, first described by Koch in 1882. This microörganism is constantly present, and conforms to all the requirements of Koch's law as to specificity. The search for the bacillus in the sputum is now one of the routine practices of clinical research. Some difficulty has been imported into the subject, owing to the discovery of several forms of acid-resisting bacilli that morphologically and tinctorially are similar to the tubercle bacillus, some of which are met with under similar circumstances. Such are the smegma bacillus found in cases of gangrene of the lung by Pappenheim and Fraenkel,[1] the butter bacillus of Möller, the timothy-grass bacillus, the bacillus of Lydia Rabinovitch, and certain streptothrix forms described by Flexner.[2] Some of these can produce granulomata in the tissues, so that the resemblance to the true B. tuberculosis is close. Careful culture experiments alone will differentiate. We have to recognize now that, as there is a colon group of bacilli including a great number of allied forms, so there is a tuberculosis or acid-fast group, containing several forms differing in virulence and in minor cultural peculiarities.

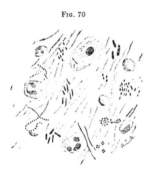

Tuberculous sputum stained by Gabbett's method. Tubercle bacilli are seen as red rods; all else is stained blue. (Abbott.)

With regard to the modes of infection, it may be said at once that tuberculosis is practically never inherited. Some few authenticated cases are on record of the transmission of the specific bacillus from mother to offspring through the placental blood, but such cases are so rare that direct inheritance may be dismissed as an unimportant factor. At most, we can say that there is an inheritance of the soil, in that in certain individuals there is a weak resisting power of the tissues toward the tubercle bacillus, so that when invasion takes place there is growth of the bacillus within the body with all its couse-quences.·

The *primæ viæ* of infection are various. It used to be, and in many quarters still is, accepted by clinicians and pathologists that tuberculosis of the lungs is bronchogenic as a rule. It should be mentioned, however, that by certain observers, notably Ribbert, Aufrecht, and Baumgarten, a more or less successful attempt has been made to disprove this. Ribbert,[1] while not denying absolutely that infection may take place by inhalation, believes that pulmonary tuberculosis is usually hematogenic, in the sense that the peribronchial glands are infected through aerial trans-mission by way of the buccal mucosa and cervical glands, and that when they break down the products of the destructive inflammation are discharged into the blood and so reach the lung. Baumgarten[2] goes still farther, and holds that the glands also are invaded hematogeneously. The experiments of Aufrecht[3] would seem to prove that it is impos-sible for bacilli to reach the terminal bronchioles and alveoli through inhalation (save in the possible case of forced inspiration), and post-mortem evidence also supports this contention. It would seem probable that we will have to give up the view that the bronchi are the first structures to be attacked, and adopt a modified inhalation theory, somewhat similar to Ribbert's, admitting an infection through the blood or lymph-stream from the mouth and nose and the upper respiratory passages. The possibility of a tuberculous lymph-gland bursting into a bronchus and so causing an inhalation infection is obvious.

Ravenel,[4] further, has shown recently that tuberculous material, when ingested, frequently reaches the tonsils and peribronchial glands. In some cases the lungs have become secondarily affected from tuberculous disease of the intestinal tract. This is rare, at least in this country, although apparently more common in Great Britain. In 1200 autopsies at the Royal Victoria Hospital, Montreal, active tuberculous lesions of one kind or another were found 295 times; in only three of these was the disease obviously primary in the intestine,[5] although this source of origin seemed probable in six more.

In rare instances the lungs have been infected in cases of primary tuberculosis of the skin. The skin is, however, a relatively unfavorable medium for the growth of the tubercle bacillus, probably owing to local temperature conditions and the nature of the epithelium, so that the disease does not often become general. The bovine strain of the organ-ism, however, when invading the human subject in this way, is apt to rise to widespread and virulent infection.

After a careful consideration of the modes of infection of the lung we are reduced to three: (1) the aërogenic, (2) the hematogenic,

[1] Deut. med. Woch., 17: 1902: 17: 301.

[2] Wien. med. Woch., November 2, 1901.

[3] Pathologie und Therapie der Lungenschwindsucht, Wien, 1908.

[4] Amer. Jour. Med. Sci., 134: 1907: 469.

[5] Nicholls, Montreal Med. Jour., 31: 1902: 327

and (3) the lymphogenic.   Frequently two or even all three may be combined.[1]

The first method, if tuberculosis of the bronchi be an essential lesion, would appear to be rare, except in those cases where a lobe of the lung is secondarily involved by the inhalation of infective excretions from some other part of the respiratory tract.   Such cases, however, do not represent the frequency of infection through the air, as it is possible for bacilli to pass through an intact bronchial mucosa and lodge in the deeper structures, and, moreover, as may be inferred from what has been said above, we must distinguish between aërogenic and bronchogenic tuberculosis.   The disease usually arises from the inhalation of dried sputum, but infective material from tuberculous cavities or caseous peribronchial glands may be aspirated into the air passages.

When the bacilli are inspired into the lung they become entangled in the mucus at certain parts of the bronchial tree, where they set up irritation.   Judging from clinical experience, bronchitis is a frequent result, but postmortem studies suggest that this is simple and not caseous, for primary caseous bronchitis is rare.   As a rule, the bacilli are picked up by the phagocytes and carried through the lymphatics to the recesses of the lung.   Thus, a lymphogenic distribution of the infection is quite common.

In another set of cases infection is through the blood, as, for instance when a caseous gland discharges its contents into the pulmonary artery, or when the receptaculum chyli or the thoracic duct are invaded.

Aërogenic Tuberculosis.—Wherever the bacilli become lodged is a focus for the development of a tuberculous lesion, and the number of these will, of course, depend very much on the amount of infective material reaching the lung, and the character of the phagocytes and lymph currents. The anatomical picture frequently produced is that of a localized bronchopneumonia.   In adults the site of predilection is just below the apices, probably because the excursion of the lung is slighter at these points and the movements of fluids and gases are consequently slower.   At first, the patch of infiltration is small, somewhat gelatinous in appearance, and imperfectly defined from the healthy tissue.   At this stage the vessels of the alveolar walls are congested and a cellular exudate is thrown out into the alveoli.   The vessels gradually become blocked, owing to proliferation of the endothelium, and the picture speedily changes as the centre of the area breaks down and becomes caseous.   A sharply defined nodule thus results.   This may heal, being finally represented by a fibrous scar with some puckering of the apex, or a fibrous nodule containing caseous or calcareous matter.   Should, however, the process continue,

---

[1] For a very good consideration of the modes of infection in tuberculosis, see D. E. Salmon's report on the Relation of Bovine Tuberculosis to the Public Health, U. S. Dept. Agric. Bureau of Animal Industry, Bull. No. 33: 1901: Washington; also A. D. Blackader, Montreal Med. Jour., 30: 1901: 905; Baumgarten, Berliner klin. Woch., 42: 1905: 1329; Raw, Tuberculosis, 1906; Beitzke, Tuberculosis, 1906; Tendeloo, Münchener medizinische Wochenschrift, 3: 1907; Orth, 6 inter. Tub. Konferenz, Wien, 1907; Escherich, Wiener klin. Woch., 15: 1909.

as frequently happens, the bacilli are carried along the lymphatics of the neighboring septa, and secondary foci are the result. The original lesion gradually increases in size through continued infiltration and proliferation, until coalescence takes place between it and the surrounding nodules. The disease may spread rapidly, especially in children, so that the most distant parts of the lung become involved. Where the lesions reach the surface the pleura is inflamed. The peribronchial glands are commonly infected.

The lung-substance between the tubercles may show little or no change, but in their immediate vicinity there are always congestion, inflammatory infiltration, and cell-proliferation. The tubercles are commonly sur-

Fig. 71

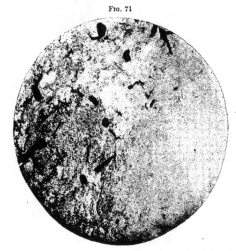

Caseation (tuberculous) in the lung. Area of caseation to the right; the bloodvessels injected to show the avascularity of the necrotic part. Leitz obj. No. 3. (From Dr. A. G. Nicholls' collection.)

rounded by a zone of simple pneumonia, which, in turn, rapidly becomes caseous. In the progressive form the original focus may attain considerable size, and, owing to the interference with the circulation and the toxic action of the bacilli, undergoes caseation and colliquative necrosis. A ragged cavity is the result. Even in the more chronic cases, where there is much fibrous tissue, this, in turn, may become caseous. The cavities are usually circumscribed and filled with soft, puriform material containing granular and calcareous particles, with shreds of tissue. In many cases the cavity becomes lined with pyogenic membrane or bounded by a fibrous wall. Bands of tissue are not infrequently found traversing these cavities, and represent the original interlobular septa of the lung. In the strands, bloodvessels, sometimes showing aneurismal dilatations,

may be found, the rupture of which leads at times to fatal hemorrhage.
Small cavities may gradually shrink and their contents become inspissated, so that a cheesy and calcareous nodule surrounded by dense fibrous
tissue results. The larger ones may contract, but seldom become
obliterated.

Fig. 72

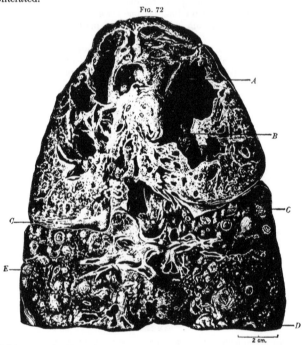

Left lung, superior lobe, and upper part of lower lobe, the former containing a number of
communicating caverns, brought about by tuberculous infiltration, caseation, and evacuation of
the contents through the bronchi. *A*, aneurismal dilatation of an artery spanning one margin of a
large cavity; *B*, communication with another cavity; *C, C*, thickened and adherent pleura
between the two involved lobes. The pleura over both lobes is thickened, and at the autopsy
the cavity had been obliterated by universal adhesion; *D*, the pointer from the letter *D* leads to
a small group of tubercles in which caseation is just beginning; *E*, a fused group of tubercles,
farther advanced than at *D*. (Hare.)

When free communication exists between a cavity and a bronchus it is a common thing to find a condition of **tuberculous broncho-**
pneumonia in the other lobes or in the opposite lung. This is due to
aspiration of the infective products, a process that is rendered easy
by cough, forced inspiration, or bodily activity. Here, in the earlier
stages of the process, small isolated tubercles form along one or more
branches of the bronchial tree, which eventually coalesce and produce
large and perfectly defined caseous masses surrounded by a zone of

simple pneumonia. The course of the disease depends on the nature of the infection. Many cases are examples of mixed infection with the bacillus tuberculosis and pyogenic microörganisms. This aspect of the subject has received considerable attention, notably from Ortner[1] and Sprengler.[2]

In a moderately severe form of secondary tuberculous bronchopneumonia, a local cellular exudation and proliferation take place, followed shortly by the formation of a caseous nodule. When such an area is examined microscopically, one sees at the periphery of the caseous mass an exudation of fluid into the alveolar spaces, diapedesis of leukocytes, swelling and desquamation of the lining epithelium, and occa-

FIG. 73

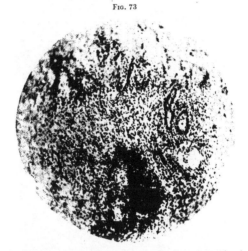

Fibroid induration of the lung in tuberculosis. The alveoli are destroyed and replaced by fibrous tissue. Round-celled infiltration is marked at the lower part. Zeiss obj. DD, without ocular. (From the collection of the Royal Victoria Hospital.)

sionally threads of fibrin. The alveolar walls show round-celled infiltration, and the lymphatics, not only the perivascular and peribronchial, but also the interalveolar and interlobular, are more or less blocked with inflammatory products. As the process extends, all the manifestations seen in the original focus are repeated. The degree of involvement of the bloodvessels in the neighborhood of the tubercles is a matter of some importance. Generally, owing to proliferation of the lining endothelium, they become more or less occluded. Thus, the tubercle is avascular. It sometimes happens, however, that erosion of the vessel

[1] Die Lungentuberculose als Mischinfection, Wien, 1893.
[2] Lungentuberculose u. Mischinfection, Zeitschr. f. Hyg., 18: 1894: 343.

walls takes place and hemorrhage results. Again, a caseous focus may erode into a vessel and lead to a miliary dissemination of the bacilli in other parts of the lung or throughout the body.

As we meet with this form of tuberculosis post mortem, the lung is more or less adherent to the thoracic wall, is increased in weight, the upper lobe largely caseous with multiple cavities, while tuberculous nodules are scattered here and there throughout the rest of the lung. The bronchi are usually inflamed. The cavities that are so frequently found in this form of tuberculosis are produced by the softening and subsequent evacuation of the contents of a caseous focus, or at times by the enlarge-

Fig. 74

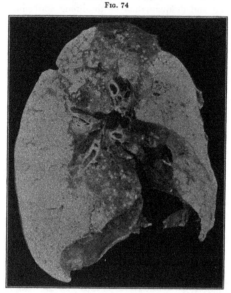

Tuberculous pneumonia (acute pneumonic phthisis). (From the Pathological Laboratory of McGill University.)

ment of a bronchiectatic cavity through necrosis of its walls. Their numbers and size vary considerably. Sometimes a single cavity, the size of a walnut, is found near the apex, or, again, a whole lobe may be converted into a thin shell. It is not uncommon to find the upper part of the upper lobe riddled with caverns of varying size, communicating more or less freely one with the other. Depending upon the chronicity of the process, the walls are either rough and shaggy, lined by a pyogenic membrane, or smooth and fibrous. The walls are often irregular from the presence of the fibrous septa of the lung, which are more resistant than the rest of the lung, so that an imperfectly loculated cavity is the result. The cavities contain, besides air, a mixture of serum, pus cells, caseous matter, and detritus, occasionally blood. One or more of them may communicate with the bronchi, which show ulceration and other inflammatory change. In the older regions of the disease considerable fibroid induration may be met with.

Besides the common form of tuberculous involvement just described, which may be correctly termed the **caseofibroid** variety, or **chronic ulcerative tuberculosis,** there are several others arising in the same way that are worthy of attention. Not infrequently, a fibroid or calcareous focus in the lung, or a partially healed cavity, for a long time giving rise to no symptoms, will suddenly start into activity and rapidly invade the rest of the lung. In one form, minute miliary tubercles

FIG. 75

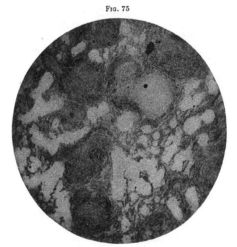

Miliary tuberculosis of the lung.   Zeiss obj. DD, without ocular.   (From Dr. A G. Nicholls' collection.)

are produced along the course of the bronchi, and a picture not unlike the hematogenic miliary tuberculosis is the result. This has been termed **disseminated miliary tuberculous bronchopneumonia.** In other cases the foci become rapidly larger and coalesce, showing little or no tendency to fibrosis, so that caseation and softening proceed apace. This is the **caseous nodular** or **lobular bronchopneumonia.** Again, a whole lobe, or, indeed, a whole lung, may become rapidly and uniformly involved, owing to the coalescence of the various foci, and we get the **caseous lobar pneumonia** or **acute pneumonic phthisis.** This is the form that has been called by clinicians "florid" phthisis or "galloping consumption." Here the affected lobe or lung is uniformly consolidated, very heavy, with a thickened and adherent pleura. On section, it is dry, granular, and caseous, and in it may be small areas of cavitation near the apex. The condition is not unlike lobar pneumonia, except that the infiltration is denser and the exudate white and caseous, rather than gray and fibrinous.

Another type is the **chronic fibroid tuberculosis**, a disease that often lasts for years. Here tissue proliferation is in excess and leads to induration, contraction, and deformity of the lung. The organ is traversed by numerous bands of fibrous tissue, with some caseation and old contracting cavities. The parenchyma of the lung is greatly damaged, being substituted in great part by compact fibrous tissue. In the parts less affected the alveoli are emphysematous. This form may affect the upper lobe, which may appear a very small appendage to the rest of the lung, and may contain partially contracted cavities and calcareous nodules. The bronchi are often dilated. The pleura is also greatly thickened and is adherent. After a time, owing to contraction, deformity of the chest wall sets in with, sometimes, dislocation of the heart. This form frequently arises from old apical disease, but is occasionally pleurogenic.

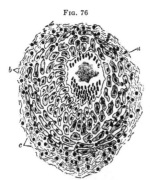

Fig. 76

Schematic representation of a tubercle: *a*, giant cell with necrotic centre and multiple nuclei peripherally arranged; *b*, epithelioid cells; *c*, lymphocytes.

Hematogenic Tuberculosis.—Hematogenic tuberculosis may be part and parcel of a generalized systemic dissemination of the infection, or may be confined to the lungs alone. The specific bacilli are conveyed to the lungs by the blood stream. The condition often arises from the discharge of a caseating lymph-gland into a vein or from tuberculosis in the neighborhood of the receptaculum chyli and thoracic duct. As a rule, the tubercles are numerous but minute (**miliary tuberculosis**).

A lung affected in this way is dark red from hyperemia and somewhat heavier than normal. In the earlier stages the tubercles can be felt rather than seen as minute shotty granules. Later, they are noticeable as small pin-point dots of a grayish color, becoming in time caseous. In the generalized systemic infection the tubercles are numerous and uniformly scattered throughout the lungs and on the pleuræ. In other cases they are confined to one lung or to one lobe. The lung is less crepitant than normal and the bronchi are reddened and inflamed.

Owing to the small size of the lesions, they are a convenient form for the study of the development and minuter structure of the typical tubercle. The bacilli usually lodge in the capillaries of the alveolar walls. Here they become entangled in the endothelial cells lining the vessels, which possess phagocytic powers, and proliferate there. The irritation produced leads to inflammatory hyperemia and the out-pouring of leukocytes, chiefly lymphocytes, not only into the interstices of the alveolar septa, but also into the alveolar spaces. Accompanying this there is œdema, exudation of fluid, and desquamation and prolifera-ation of the cells lining the alveoli. The cells lining the capillaries also proliferate, so that sooner or later obstruction of the lumina takes place. As the disease progresses, another type of cell makes its appearance, somewhat larger than the leukocyte, with a single pale nucleus—the so-called "epithelioid" cell. The exact origin of these is not settled, but they are probably derived from the proliferation of the fixed mesoder-mic connective-tissue elements. Thus, a typical tubercle consists in a localized collection of lymphocytes with, toward the centre, a num-ber of epithelioid cells, accompanied by the usual signs of inflam-mation, viz., hyperemia, exudation of fluid sometimes containing fibrin, and catarrh of the cells lining the alveoli. As the condition progresses, the central portion of the tubercle breaks down or caseates. In the more chronic forms, large, multinucleated cells—giant cells—make their appearance at the periphery. Any that may have been present in the central portion are usually destroyed in the caseating process. The tubercle increases by the gradual involvement of the peripheral cells in the caseating process. It used to be thought that giant cells were characteristic of tuberculosis, but we know now that they are present in many forms of chronic inflammation and wherever foreign matter is being absorbed. In fact, there is nothing character-istic in the structure of the tubercle as a whole, except in the prepon-derance of lymphocytes, the caseation, and the presence of the specific bacilli. Both plasma cells and "Mast-zellen" are met with in tubercles, but are equally non-specific.

In the more chronic forms, or where the resisting power of the individual is strong, there is a new formation of connective tissue which tends to wall in the focus. This may be so well marked that firm shotty masses, the size of hemp seeds, with relatively little central caseation may be produced. This is the *chronic miliary tuberculosis*, or the *chronic granular tuberculosis* of the Vienna school.

Lymphogenic Tuberculosis.—Infection of the lungs by way of the lymph-paths may occur in cases of tuberculous caries of the ribs or vertebral column. Where, again, as so commonly happens, the peri-bronchial lymph-glands are softened and caseous, the disease process may spread to the lungs either by retrograde embolism or by direct continuous extension. By far the most frequent examples of this mode of infection, however, are seen as a secondary process within the lungs themselves, where it forms the usual mode of extension of the disease from the original main focus.

Pseudotuberculosis.—This term has been employed to designate a con-dition closely resembling tuberculosis, but due to microörganisms other than the bacillus of Koch. The lesions found, like those of tuberculosis proper, may be caseous granulomata or abscesses. The etiology of the condition is, curiously, most diverse. Perhaps most of the cases recorded have been due to bacterial microörganisms allied to the streptothrices or to certain hypomycetes, but some have been due to animal parasites, and even to foreign bodies.

One form, the pseudotuberculosis of rodents (*tuberculose zoogléique*), is found in guinea-pigs, rabbits, hares, and mice, but occasionally, also, in chickens. An organism has been isolated, which seems to belong to the same class as the bacillus of hemorrhagic septicemia. Two cases are reported where this form of the disease has been transmitted to man. The evidence is, however, somewhat inconclusive.[1] Some few cases, also, have been described in which pseudotuberculosis in man, though not of the lungs, has been caused by germs not identical with Bacillus pseudotuberculosis rodentium, but only differing from it in minor points.[2] Preisz[3] and Kutscher[4] have met with instances due to organisms resembling the bacillus of diphtheria. Eppinger[5] has reported a case of pseudotuberculosis due to a cladothrix, and Flexner,[6] one apparently due to a form of streptothrix.

An interesting form of the affection, found in pigeons and transmissible to man, has been described by Chantemesse.[7] A number of cases affecting the lung in man have been reported. The organism at work here is usually Aspergillus fumigatus. We have found this also common in quite young chickens.

An organism, producing a rare and curious disease of the skin, found in South America and California, and allied to blastomycetic dermatitis, has been known to invade the internal organs, including the lungs, producing lesions resembling those of tuberculosis.[8]

Among the animal parasites that may cause pseudotuberculosis, we may mention the eggs of the strongylus, found by Marsden[9] in the lungs of hogs, sheep, and goats.

Small, dead, foreign bodies can also produce nodules if they enter the lung, as has been shown by Cruveilhier[10] and Waldenburg.[11] Tubercles of this order, due to coal dust, are quite common.

Syphilis.—Syphilis of the lung, apart from the congenital form, is rare, and does not always manifest itself in a characteristic way. It is at times difficult to differentiate it from other forms of inflammation. No doubt, many of the cases of bronchitis and pneumonia attributed to syphilis are more correctly to be regarded as complications or examples of mixed infection. The disease is met with in the form of **gummas** and **diffuse interstitial fibrosis**.

Gummas are rare in acquired syphilis and are not common even in the lungs of newborn syphilitic children. The gummas, which are usually

[1] Massa and Mensi, Rev. Baumg. Jahresb., 1895.
[2] Wrede, Ziegler's Beit., 32: 1902: 526.
[3] Lubarsch u. Ostertag's Ergebnisse, 1: 1896: 733.
[4] Centralbl. f. Bact., 17: 1895: 835.　　　[5] Ziegler's Beit., 9: 1890: 287.
[6] Jour. of Exper. Med., 3: 1898: 435.　　　[7] Rev. Centralbl. f. Path., 1: 1890: 581.
[8] Ophüls and Moffitt, Phila. Med. Jour., 5: 1900: 1471.
[9] Münch. med. Woch., 35: 1898: 1100.　　　[10] Traité d'Anat. path. gén., 4: 1862.
[11] Tuberculosis, Pulmonary Phthisis, and Scrofulosis, Berlin, 1869.

quite numerous, when present, are in the earlier stages grayish-red or grayish-white, somewhat translucent, and form nodules of all sizes up to that of a hen's egg, surrounded by an area of congestion. Later, they undergo a process allied to caseation and become opaque white and more or less walled off by connective tissue. The contents of the granuloma may liquefy and be discharged into a bronchus, or again may become inspissated and calcareous. Healed gummas are to be distinguished from old tubercles and abscesses only with the greatest difficulty. They may lead to marked fissuring of the lung (*pulmo lobatus*). Gummas are more common near the hilus of the lung than elsewhere. Microscopically, they only can be distinguished from tubercles by the absence of the tubercle bacilli.

In the second type the lung becomes the site of a more or less diffused and extensive cellular infiltration, together with hyperplasia of the connective tissue and proliferation and desquamation of the alveolar epithelium. To any one who has seen the extraordinary number of spirochetes present in these cases, this marked inflammation is not surprising. The alveolar walls become greatly thickened, and large areas are converted into a somewhat fibrous mass, in which compressed-air spaces and groups of cells, representing the proliferated and desquamated epithelium, can be recognized. The bloodvessels are thickened so that the lung is pale and anemic, an appearance that has given to the condition the name of "white pneumonia." Diffuse pneumonia of this type may be combined with gummas. Virchow, followed by Pankritius,[1] has described a form of induration starting from the hilus of the lung as of syphilitic origin. Others mention a form starting from the pleura and interlobular septa. Reuter[2] has demonstrated the presence of Spirochæta pallida in the lung of a child dying of hereditary syphilis with "white" pneumonia.[3]

Actinomycosis.—This disease may affect the lung primarily, but it is more common for it to originate from inhalation in actinomycosis of the mouth or pharynx, or by extension from the anterior mediastinum or œsophagus. Occasionally the disease is metastatic, as in a case we saw in which the primary lesion was in the liver.

Multiple nodules of a miliary type are met with, or there may be large areas of infiltration formed by the fusion of several granulomas. Not infrequently, the affection conforms to the type of a bronchopneumonia. Clinically, the disease may resemble bronchitis, there being a discharge of fetid mucopus, containing at times the characteristic "sulphur grains." Under the microscope these are found to be the specific ray-fungus. In more chronic cases, signs of consolidation and cavitation of the lung may be met with, so that the disease is not unlike chronic tuberculosis.

In the metastatic form, the lungs are riddled with small abscesses

---

[1] Ueber Lungensyphilis, Berlin, 1881.   [2] Zeit. f. Hyg. u. Infect., 54: 1906· 49.
[3] For literature, see Herxheimer, Lubarsch und Ostertag's Ergebnisse, 1: 1907, and 12: 1908.

containing creamy pus and surrounded by an inflammatory areola. When young, the granulomas are grayish or grayish red in color and surrounded by a pneumonic zone, or what amounts to a vascular granulation tissue.

In long-standing cases the nodules are more or less completely walled off by fibrous tissue, the interlobular septa are thickened, and there are all the signs of a diffuse fibrous hyperplasia with alveolar catarrh and inflammatory exudation. The lung may eventually be converted into a contracted nodular mass full of cavities and riddled with sinuses. The disease occasionally spreads through the thoracic wall and invades the pectoral muscles, or, again, may spread through the diaphragm to the abdominal viscera. The mediastinum and pericardium are liable to be involved.[1]

Glanders.[2]—This is rare in man, and is almost invariably contracted from animals suffering from the disease. The affection takes the form of multiple cellular nodules of a grayish or yellowish-white color, varying in size from a millet-seed to a pea. In other cases there is lobar or lobular pneumonia, or a diffuse purulent infiltration, with abscess formation. The affection can only be recognized by the presence of the mallein reaction during life, or the detection of the B. mallei in the excretion.

Parasites.—Apart from the bacterial forms already mentioned, such as B. tuberculosis, Diplococcus pneumoniæ, pyogenic cocci, B. mallei, B. anthracis, and Actinomyces, vegetable parasites are rare and few of them are of importance.

Various forms of moulds, such as *Aspergilli, Mucor, Eurotium,* and the *thrush-fungus,* have been described. They are liable to be found wherever destruction of the lung substance is going on or where there is stagnation and decomposition of secretion. Some are accidental, while others must be regarded as pathogenic. A *Pneumonomycosis aspergillina,* as it has been termed by Saxer,[3] has been described by Virchow, Dieulafoy, Chantemesse and Widal, and later by Risel.[4] Cases also have been reported in England by Boyce, Arkel, and Hinds, and by Pearson and Ravenel[5] in America.[6]

The disease is met with in birds, horses, and cattle, but occasionally attacks man. The lesions produced resemble those of tuberculosis (see above).

Of the animal parasites, the most important is *Echinococcus.* Echinococcus disease may be primary or secondary. ·The lung may be invaded from the liver. Rarely, infection takes place through the hepatic vein, the inferior vena cava, and the right heart. The cyst may be

---

[1] For literature see Schlagenhaufer, Virch. Archiv, 184: 1906; also Karewski, Arch. f. Chirurgie, 84: 1907: 403.

[2] For a histological study see MacCallum, Ziegler's Beiträge, 31: 1902: 440.

[3] Pneumonomycosis Aspergillina, Jena, 1900.

[4] Etude sur l'aspergillose chez les animaux et chez l'homme, 1897.

[5] Proc. Path. Soc. Phila., new series: 111: 1900: 10.

[6] See also Rolleston, Article on Pulmonary Aspergillosis, Allbutt and Rolleston's System of Medicine, 5: 1909: 440.

single or multiple, and may reach the size of a man's head. The cavities are filled with clear fluid containing the characteristic hooklets, or again may suppurate. When healing takes place, the fluid is to some extent absorbed, and calcareous deposit may take place. Occasionally the cysts may rupture into a bronchus, the pleural cavity, or the abdomen. Dislocation of the neighboring organs is likely to occur.

Cysticercus cellulosæ is rare. *Strongylus longivaginatus, Monas lens, Cercomonas, coccidia, Pentastomum denticulatum,* and *psorosperms* have been met with.

A rare but important affection is that called by Stiles[1] "*Paragonimiasis.*" This is due to a trematode worm, the "lung fluke" or Paragonimus Westermannii. It is most common in Asia and Africa, although some few cases have been met with in America. The disease affects the tiger, cat, dog, and swine, and sixty-six cases in man have been collected by Stiles. The infection is probably through drinking-water.

The most striking symptom is hemoptysis. The parasites, which look not unlike small almonds, fix themselves by their suckers to the mucosa of the bronchi and burrow their way through the lung, so that a series of intercommunicating cavities are produced. These may open into a bronchus. The bronchi are much inflamed and the lung tissue near the cavities is much congested. The cavities contain broken-down lung tissue, ova, hematoidin, and the parasites. The disease tends to run a chronic course. Recovery is the rule.[2]

RETROGRESSIVE METAMORPHOSES.

Atrophy of the Lungs.—This is a comparatively unimportant condition.

The senile form, sometimes called "atrophic emphysema," has already been referred to. It is to be regarded as a physiological involution rather than a pathological process. Emphysema may, however, be associated with it, and is generally due to a concomitant chronic bronchitis which is found in so many old persons.

Besides this, a certain amount of local atrophy is found in a variety of conditions, such as emphysema, atelectasis, and indurative pneumonia.

Rokitansky[3] also recognized a form of atrophy due to inactivity of the lung in cases where the pleura presents marked thickening.

Degenerations.—Fatty Degeneration.—This affects chiefly the alveolar endothelium and the walls of the bloodvessels. It is found in poisoning by arsenic and phosphorus, and as a secondary manifestation in a great variety of inflammations and new-growths. The change is best seen in the epithelial cells lining the air spaces, which are swollen and desquamated.

[1] Proc. Path. Soc. Phila., February, 1901.
[2] For details of pathological anatomy, see Katsurada, Ziegler's Beitr., 28: 1900: 506.
[3] Lehrb., 3: 1861: 47.

Hyaline Degeneration.—This also affects the alveolar epithelium and the walls of the bloodvessels. It is found chiefly in tuberculous and syphilitic affections of the lung. The so-called *corpora amylacea* have been referred to elsewhere (vol. i, p. 901).

Amyloid Disease.—This is singularly rare in the lungs. Only in the most extensive condition of disseminated amyloid disease do we find the vessels of the lungs affected. Occasionally, in cases of syphilis, with induration of the lungs and marked amyloid degeneration of the organs, the condition is met with.

Calcareous Degeneration.—This is seen usually in the form of concretions, old tuberculous foci, and in tumors. A rare condition is a deposit of lime salts in the alveolar walls, bloodvessels, or septa of the lung. This has been attributed to a lime metastasis, where the blood is loaded with salts derived from the skeleton (see vol. i, p. 926).

Pneumonomalacia.—Apart from that form of gangrene of the lungs due to inflammation or to the germs of putrefaction, there is a form analogous to myomalacia of the heart and encephalomalacia. Small areas are seen which are softened, shaggy, and necrotic looking. The patches have a reddish-brown color and are devoid of any putrid odor. The condition seems to be a simple necrosis. It is, of course, rare, as will readily be understood when we consider how easy it is for any diseased portion of the lung to become infected by germs. Some cases are due to pulmonary embolism; others are met with in diabetes.

PROGRESSIVE METAMORPHOSES.

Hypertrophy.—We must be careful not to conclude that because a lung is enlarged it is hypertrophic, for, unlike other organs which belong to the group of epithelial glands, the lungs do not tend to undergo hypertrophy. Owing to its anatomical structure, when from any cause a portion of the lung is rendered functionless, the rest becomes enlarged, it is true, yet not from hypertrophy but from emphysematous dilatation of the air spaces. Still the lung does seem to have a certain amount of regenerative power, for cases are on record where, in the event of complete atrophy of one lung, the other enlarged so much as to fill not only one pleural cavity but to encroach upon the other, and this in the absence of sufficient emphysema to account for the enlargement.

Besides this form, which is rare, hypertrophy of the muscle fibers about the smaller bronchioles has been observed in cases of brown induration of the lungs. This is probably to be attributed to the catarrh of the bronchi, which is usually present in such cases and should be classed with the hypertrophies due to increased work.

Tumors.—Primary tumors of the lung are comparatively rare. Among the benign growths, fibromas, lipomas, chondromas, and osteomas have been observed. Not all the cases reported as "osteomas," however, are to be regarded as true tumors. Many are examples of ossification developing in hyperplastic connective tissue arising from chronic inflammation (metaplasia). Ribbert has described ossification in caseous areas, and we have met with the same condition ourselves. Care should also be taken not to confuse the calcification that takes place in old tuberculous and other inflammatory foci with tumor formation. Chondroma is also rare and arises from the bronchial cartilages, and, possibly, from embryonic "rests."

Teratoids.—*Dermoids* are occasionally met with. Albers has described a case in which there was a cystic tumor communicating with a bronchus. For years hairs were discharged in the sputum. *Adenorhabdomyoma* has been observed (Helbing, Zipkin[1]).

Adenoma.—Adenomas derived from the peribronchial mucous glands have been described by Chiari,[2] but are very rare.

Sarcoma.—Primary sarcoma is also rare. Ranglaret[3] has recorded a case of spindle-celled sarcoma of the left lung, and Reymond[4] one of the round-celled variety. *Lymphosarcoma* is not so uncommon. Less frequent are the cases that arise in the mediastinal tissues and the lymphglands at the root of the lung. It is interesting in this connection to note that chronic irritation from certain kinds of dust seems to be an exciting cause, for Ancke[5] has pointed out how frequent sarcoma of the lung is among the miners of the Schneeberg district. Very interesting and important are those new-growths—the *endotheliomas*—that are intermediate in structure between the sarcomas and the carcinomas. They develop superficially in the pleura, or at the hilus of the lung in the lymph-channels. The aberrant growth, however, soon passes beyond the lymphatic vessels and invades the adjacent tissues, forming larger or smaller nodules, arranged, in some cases, about the bronchial tree like a string of beads.

A very rare form of primary growth is the simple **melanotic tumor** (tumeur melanique simple) described by Cornil and Ranvier,[6] which may take on malignant action.

Carcinoma.—Primary carcinoma of the lung generally affects by preference the right side, and is either nodular or diffuse. There are three main types, in which the new-growth starts from the bronchi, the alveolar epithelium, or the peribronchial mucous glands. The first form is composed of columnar cells, while the second is made up of flattened plates in which cell-nests may sometimes be seen. It is characteristic of carcinomas in this situation that they readily soften or become hemorrhagic, so that they are not unlike caseous tuberculous masses. In such cases, when the contents are discharged through a bronchus, cavities are the result. Metastases appear to be relatively infrequent.

Secondary growths are much more common, and are generally due to

---

[1] Virch. Archiv, 187: 1907.
[2] Verschiedene Tumoren, Prager med. Woch., 1883.
[3] Bull. de la soc. anat. de Paris, Ser. V: Tom. VII: Fasc. 22: p. 591.
[4] Ibid., p. 256.
[5] Dissert. Munich, 1884.
[6] Tumeurs melaniques simples, Manuel d'histol. path., 2: 1882: 140.

malignant emboli that get into the venous circulation, an event t
easily occurs.   The first to be mentioned is the *chondroma,* whi
when found in the lungs, is nearly always secondary.   *Osteoïd chondro
myxomas, lipomyxomas,* have also been met with.   Besides these
the *sarcomas,* including pigmented forms, and all varieties of *carcinom*
In the case of the latter the primary seat is nearly always in the stoma
or mamma.   An interesting and not uncommon form, in our experien
of secondary carcinoma is that in which small cancerous nodules
formed along the course of the pleural lymphatics, so that a disti
network is produced.   *Chorioepithelioma malignum uteri* may fo
metastases in the lungs.

CHAPTER XIV.

THE PLEURÆ.

THE pleuræ are sacs composed of a thin, rather loose, connective-tissue membrane, containing numerous bloodvessels and elastic fibrillæ. They are covered by a single layer of flattened mononuclear cells—the endothelium. The pleuræ are not very liable to be affected by primary disease, but owing to their close association with the lungs are frequently involved by contiguity or extension. Not only so, but inasmuch as the pleural sacs are lymph-spaces having communication more or less closely with the pericardial and peritoneal cavities, inflammatory processes originating in either of these regions readily extend to the pleuræ. Disease, therefore, of the lungs, peribronchial and mediastinal glands, œsophagus, aorta, thoracic duct, stomach, liver, and thoracic wall may rapidly involve the pleuræ. Conversely, lesions of the pleuræ may extend to the contiguous parts. In the dissemination of disease the great power of absorption of the membrane and the movements incident to respiration play an important part.

ANOMALIES OF DEVELOPMENT.

Perhaps the most common anomaly is an **infolding** of the membrane at the upper part of the cavity associated with the apical fissure of the lung before referred to. Along the free border an abnormal azygos vein frequently runs. Partial **defects** of the pleuræ are found associated with congenital diaphragmatic hernia. In monstrous births the pleura may be **absent** altogether or **redundant**. In the rare congenital atrophy of the lung, the pleural cavity may be filled with fat mixed with a mucoid connective-tissue substance.

CIRCULATORY DISTURBANCES.

Hyperemia.—*Active Hyperemia.*—Active hyperemia occurs as an accompaniment of congestion of the lung proper, and also from a sudden relaxation of tension, such as takes place during the operation of thoracentesis. In the latter event the vessels not infrequently give way and hemorrhage results.

Passive Hyperemia.—Passive hyperemia is found in all forms of obstruction to the greater or lesser circulation.

Hemorrhages.—Multiple hemorrhages, ecchymoses, and petechiæ are common. They are found especially in cases where there has been marked interference with respiration, as in death by suffocation. Similar manifestations are met with in kidney and heart affections, in the infections and intoxications, in nervous diseases, and in the hemorrhagic diatheses.

Œdema.—Œdema of the pleura is indistinguishably associated with œdema of the lungs.

ABNORMAL STATES OF THE PLEURAL CAVITIES.

Hematothorax.—When blood is effused into the pleural cavity, the condition is called hematothorax. It is somewhat rare for the sac to contain pure blood, for the fluid is generally mixed with transudation or the products of inflammation. The affection is brought about by tearing of the vessels, and is not infrequently met with in rupture of tuberculous and gangrenous cavities, in certain forms of inflammation, and in carcinoma. Other causes that should be mentioned are the bursting of an aneurism into the cavity, fracture or caries of the ribs, and bullet and stab wounds of the chest.

Hydrothorax.—Hydrothorax is a collection of transuded fluid in the pleural cavity. This occurs by preference on the right side, although it may be bilateral. The reason for this is said to be that most people lie upon the right side, or else that there is pressure of a distended right heart on the veins of that side. When pleural adhesions are present, the effusion may be sacculated.

The fluid is usually pale, straw-colored, alkaline, the specific gravity varying between 1009 and 1012, or a little higher, and contains no flakes. The amount of albumin varies from 2.78 per cent. (Hoppe-Seyler) to 4.97 per cent. (Scherer). Microscopically, there are a few leukocytes and desquamated cells from the pleural endothelium. The pleural surface is still smooth, but may be slightly sodden, and in long-standing cases the membrane becomes turbid, pearly, and somewhat thickened, owing to overgrowth of the connective tissue.

Small quantities of fluid may be poured out into the cavity during the death agony, but the larger collections are found in nephritis, uncompensated heart lesions, nodular cirrhosis of the liver, hydremia, pulmonary œdema, and poisoning with carbon monoxide.

Chylous and Pseudochylous Hydrothorax.—Chylous and pseudochylous hydrothorax are due to rupture or obstruction respectively of the thoracic duct above its point of entrance into the pleural cavity. The fluid is opaque, milk-white, and contains granules and lymph cells. In chylous fluid fat globules are also present.

Small collections of fluid in the thorax are of no significance, but the larger ones lead to compression and collapse of the lung and dislocation of the neighboring structures, such as the heart and diaphragm.

Pneumothorax.—When the pleural cavity contains air, the condition is termed pneumothorax. Owing to the nature of the exciting causes, the affection is accompanied, in the vast majority of cases, by inflammation, so that the cavity contains serum or pus as well as air (*hydropneumo-thorax, pyopneumothorax*). Pneumothorax is rare as a primary disease, and is usually due to a lesion of the lung or pleura. The most frequent cause is the rupture of a tuberculous focus in the lung during cough or other strain. Occasionally, it follows the rupture of a gangrenous or suppurating area. It is said that it may also be caused by the giving way of an emphysematous bulla. It may be regarded as certain that it never occurs from the rupture of a healthy lung. Air may also enter the pleura as the result of penetrating wounds of the chest, fractured ribs, thoracentesis, or from the stomach, œsophagus, and bowel. In the last case the usual condition found is a malignant growth in the viscus, which attaches it to the diaphragm. An empyema may also erode its way into the lung and discharge into a bronchus.

Pneumothorax due to perforation has been divided by Weil into three varieties: (1) **Open pneumothorax**, in which air passes freely in and out. (2) **Ventilated pneumothorax**, in which there is an oblique or valve-like opening, so that air enters readily but cannot escape. (3) **Closed pneumothorax**, where the opening has become occluded. In many cases the fistula becomes closed, and at autopsy it is frequently impossible to find the point of rupture.

Laennec was perhaps the first to describe pneumothorax without perforation. Although for some time doubted, it is now abundantly demonstrated that there is such a thing as non-perforative or **essential** pneumothorax, caused by the growth of gas-producing microörganisms in the pleura. Cases due to the B. coli have been recorded by R. May and Adolf Gebhart,[1] and in other cases the B. Welchii has been found.[2]

The result of pneumothorax will depend very much on the cause and on the persistence or otherwise of the communication with the outer air. So long as the fistula remains, the lung is completely collapsed unless this result be prevented by the presence of adhesions. In cases where a valvular opening is present, the pleural cavity becomes gradually inflated with air, so that the lung is compressed, the heart pushed over to the opposite side, the diaphragm depressed, and the whole side of the thorax distended. In cases of pneumothorax without infection, the wound may close and the air is then gradually absorbed, so that the lung resumes its normal condition. A *false* pneumothorax is met with post mortem owing to self-digestion of the walls of the stomach and the diaphragm and a consequent discharge of gas into the pleural cavity. Cases with serofibrinous inflammation or empyema, provided they are cured at all, generally leave traces in the shape of pleural thickening and adhesions.

INFLAMMATIONS.

Pleurisy.—Inflammation of the pleura (**pleurisy** or **pleuritis**) is only occasionally a primary affection, and usually originates in disease of

[1] Deuts. Archiv f. klin. Med., 61 : 1898 : 323.

[2] Nicholls, Brit. Med. Jour., 2 : 1897 : 1844.

the lung, mediastinum, or the neighboring cavities. Not a few cases are metastatic, being dependent on or associated with infections elsewhere, or affecting the body as a whole. This form is met with in cases of septicemia, acute inflammatory rheumatism, typhoid, the exanthemata, and nephritis.

The type of disease varies considerably according to the nature of the infecting agents. These are almost invariably bacterial, since the lung, owing to its association with the outer air, always contains bacteria. Pleurisy may be partial or complete, the exudate free or sacculated. Frequently, pleurisy, particularly when left-sided, is combined with pericarditis. It is not uncommon also for several serous membranes to be progressively involved, a condition for which certain Italian observers have proposed the term "polyorrhomenitis." According to Taylor,[1] the course of involvement of the various serosæ is as follows: (1) Peritoneum involved first with extension to the pleura, usually the right; (2) the pleura, then the peritoneum; (3) the pleura of one side and then of the other; and (4) one pleura, then the peritoneum, and finally the other pleura. According to the course of the inflammation, we may recognize *exudative* and *productive* pleurisy. These forms may exist independently, but it is not uncommon for exudative pleurisy to develop into the productive variety.

Exudative Pleurisy.—Exudative pleurisy is met with occasionally in persons of low vitality or as a manifestation of the rheumatic infection. It is very common in pneumonia, tuberculosis, infarction, and in newgrowths.

The exudation may be fibrinous (plastic), serofibrinous, fibrinopurulent, purulent, or hemorrhagic.

Fibrinous Pleurisy.—In the fibrinous form, or what is sometimes called "dry" pleurisy, the pleura is opaque, slightly turbid, and upon it lies a delicate layer of fibrin which can readily be scraped off. Microscopically, the tissues are œdematous; the vessels of the pleura, both blood and lymphatic, and the subjacent portions of the lung are congested, with some perivascular leukocytosis; not infrequently meshes of fibrin can be made out within the layers of the connective tissue of the pleura. Upon the surface the exudate is seen to consist of delicate interlacing fibrillæ of fibrin with some leukocytes. Occasionally, the fibrin is fused together into hyaline masses. By appropriate methods of staining, bacteria may be demonstrated in the exudate. In the early stages it is not always easy to detect the presence of pleurisy, since there may be merely a trifling cloudiness and turbidity of the membrane, but in more advanced cases the fibrin forms a definite layer, even amounting to a membrane.

Serofibrinous Pleurisy.—Very few pleurisies remain dry for long and 'there is usually a more or less abundant outpouring of fluid into the cavity (*serofibrinous pleurisy*). The serum exuded is of a yellowish color, clear, or, if mixed with cells, somewhat turbid. The fibrin is usually abundant in the fissures of the lung and in the dependent or posterior

[1] British Medical Journal, 2 :.1900 : 1693.

portions of the pleural cavity. It is often curdy, whitish-yellow, and forms shaggy masses adhering to the lung and thoracic walls. In many cases, loose, friable, rather gelatinous-looking clots are produced. The amount of exudation varies from a few cubic centimeters to several liters. The specific gravity is almost always above 1025. The fluid coagulates readily on the application of heat, and often spontaneously when removed from the body. The exudation differs from the fluid of hydrothorax in being of higher specific gravity, containing more albumin, and also more uric acid, cholesterin, and sugar. Microscopically, it contains leukocytes and blood cells, bacteria, somewhat swollen endothelial cells, and shreds of fibrin.

FIG. 77

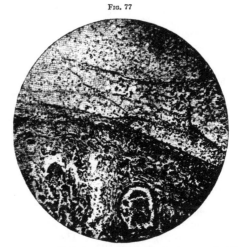

Acute serofibrinous pleurisy. Zeiss obj. DD, ocular No. 1. Long strands of fibrin, between which inflammatory leukocytes are enmeshed, are well seen on the surface of the lung. (From the Pathological Laboratory of McGill University.)

When the effusion is large, the lung is more or less completely compressed and atelectatic, lying in the upper part of the pleural cavity close to the spine, unless previously existing adhesions limit its movements. When free, the fluid moves on posturing the patient. The airless portion of the lung is tough, lacks crepitation, and is of a dull gray, grayish-brown, or blue-black color. The heart may be dislocated to the side and the large thoracic vessels compressed. The diaphragm is depressed and the intercostal spaces may bulge. In large right-sided effusions the liver is pushed down. When healing takes place, the fluid portions are absorbed by the lymphatics, the fibrin breaks down, becomes granular, and in its turn is carried off. Thus, few signs of trouble may remain, except possibly a slight thickening

of the pleura. Not infrequently, the connective tissue, however, proliferates, grows into the fibrinous layer, and leads to adhesion of those
parts which are in contact. The union is at first intimate, but, as
the lung regains its function, the adhesions are pulled upon so that
velamentous strands are produced. These are very commonly found
between the lobes and about the upper lobe posteriorly. The adhesions
may be partial or lead to complete obliteration of the pleural space.

Purulent Pleurisy.—Serofibrinous pleurisy occasionally develops into
a *purulent* or *fibrinopurulent* one (*empyema*). Here the exudate is
more cloudy, yellowish, and contains abundant leukocytes. There is
often more or less fibrin, but it tends to diminish both absolutely and
relatively, as both less is produced and what is present is gradually
digested by the action of the pus corpuscles. Empyema is rarely a
primary affection, except in children. It sometimes is met with in pneumonia, especially that form due to influenza, but occurs perhaps most
commonly from the rupture of a tuberculous cavity in the pleura or
follows abscess and gangrene of the lung. A subdiaphragmatic abscess
may perforate into the pleura as well as cancerous or other ulcers
of the œsophagus, stomach, or bowel. When putrefactive germs are
present, the pus is often dark colored, decomposed, and very foul
smelling (**putrid pleurisy**). Some of the bacteria, notably Diplococcus pneumoniæ and B. typhi, which usually produce a simple
inflammation, are competent to produce pus, either from an increase in
their virulence or a diminution in the resisting power of the patient. As
a rule, however, when a simple pleurisy becomes purulent, it is due to
secondary infection with pus-producing organisms.

Unless relieved by surgical interference, the consequences of empyema
are apt to be serious. The patient may die of exhaustion, amyloid disease,
or septicemia, or the pus may burrow through the lung and discharge into
a bronchus, with the formation of pyopneumothorax. The pus may also
dissect its way beneath the parietal pleura and point externally, thus
finally discharging (*empyema necessitatis*). The usual site for this is
near the lower end of the sternum. The pus may also discharge into
the œsophagus, stomach, peritoneum, pericardium, or mediastinum. Empyema, as a rule, unless recognized and treated early, usually leads to
great thickening of the pleura and, in protracted cases, to deformity of
the chest. In some cases the pleura becomes so infiltrated with lime salts
that it is converted into a dense calcareous cuirass.

Hemorrhagic Pleurisy.—Hemorrhagic pleurisy is not rare as a secondary
complication. It is found in debilitated persons or those suffering from
scurvy, icterus, and the hemorrhagic diathesis. It is common in tuberculosis and carcinoma of the pleura. In one variety, which is strictly
comparable to pachymeningitis hæmorrhagica, there is a formation of
a vascular granulation tissue upon the surface of the pleura.

Chronic or Productive Pleurisy.—Chronic or productive pleurisy is
common. It may exist as a late manifestation of an acute simple or
purulent inflammation, or may begin insidiously as a primary affection
without exudation. The condition leads to great thickening of the pleura

with more or less extensive adhesions. The lung is coated with a firm whitish or whitish-gray membrane which may be one or more centimeters thick. Microscopically, it is composed of somewhat interlacing fibrils of connective tissue with areas of coagulation necrosis, and in the deeper layers newly-formed capillaries and perivascular leukocytic infiltration. In some cases, the membrane is very thick, pearly white, and of a firm cartilaginous consistence (*Zuckerguss*). This form is rare as a primary disease of the pleura, but usually is due to a chronic inflammation extending from the peritoneum or from the pericardium. Rosenbach[1] has pointed out that chronic pleurisy may extend to the liver capsule causing contraction of the organ and to the pericardial sac, which, in time becomes obliterated. The cartilaginous appearance is due to extensive hyaline degeneration of the connective tissue. In such cases the lung usually shows some atrophy, but when adhesions have not taken place it may be considerably contracted and deformed. In other cases, particularly those connected with pneumonia, the lung itself participates in the proliferation and becomes indurated. In long-standing cases, calcareous masses, and even plates of cartilage and bone, are formed in the pleura. The disease has been known to follow simple pleurisy and tuberculosis.

Tuberculosis.—Exceptionally, tuberculosis of the pleura is met with as a primary manifestation without discoverable disease elsewhere. Such cases are difficult of explanation, but the bacilli probably reach the sac through the blood-stream or the lymphatic system. A common form is that in which the pleura is affected as a part of a general miliary dissemination of the disease. Here the membrane is studded with pinpoint tubercles, with possibly slight surrounding congestion, but without exudation or adhesion, so that the inflammatory manifestations are of the slightest. Most frequently, tuberculosis of the pleura is an extension from the lung or peribronchial glands, and it has been found to be occasioned by tuberculosis of the peritoneum, the ribs, and the spinal column. In tuberculous bronchopneumonia it is not uncommon to find clusters of tubercles upon the pleura, somewhat elevated above the general surface, and covered with a delicate layer of fibrin. In other cases, a more abundant exudation takes place, frequently of a serofibrinous character, and with some admixture of blood. The surface of the lung is covered with a layer of blood-stained fibrin that may be readily removed. On scraping it off, one can make out tubercles on the under surface. When the disease is of long standing, several layers of caseating tubercles are formed in the exudation which is converted into a thick, cheesy, and brittle membrane. Another common form, sometimes combined with the last, is that where a more or less extensive adhesion of the pleural surfaces takes place. In the adhesions, which are due to the organization of the exudate, isolated or confluent caseous tubercles are produced, leading to marked thickening.

A purulent tuberculous pleurisy also exists and is due commonly to the rupture of a cavity into the pleural space. Here, no doubt, a mixed infection is at work.

---

[1] Die Erkrankungen des Brustfells, Nothnagel, 14: 1894: 1: 18.

A word should be said here about a peculiar form that is common
in cattle and has been met with, though rarely, in man—the so-called
"grape disease" or "Perlsucht." In cattle, the disease is frequently
found not only in the pleura, but in the lungs, lymph-glands, pericardium,
peritoneum, and liver. As it affects the pleura, the disease presents a
very striking and characteristic appearance. The tubercles vary somewhat in size and take the form of warts and polypoid excrescences, often
bound one to the other by fibrous bands, so that they have been been compared to pearls on a string. At first they are of a gray or grayish-red
color but sooner or later degenerate at the centres, becoming opaque,
yellow, and brittle. They may finally calcify. Hodenpyl regards the
minute, lenticular, pearly dots sometimes found on the pleura as of
tuberculous nature.

Syphilis.—Syphilitic induration of the lung, already referred to,
commonly leads to thickening of the pleura. Lancereaux[1] has described
a *pleuritis gummosa*. It is excessively rare.

Leprosy.—This is found in the form of granulomas of varying size
upon the pleura.

Foreign Bodies.—These are rare, except blood and pus, as already
mentioned. Foreign bodies may be introduced from without, or may
gain entrance from the stomach and œsophagus. Rarely, detached
portions of tumors may be found, or sequestra from the lung.

Parasites.—*Echinococcus cysts* are found both primarily and secondarily. *Psorosperms* have also been met with. *Amœba coli* is found
in cases where an amœbic abscess of the liver has ruptured into the
pleura.

PROGRESSIVE METAMORPHOSES.

Hypertrophy.—Hypertrophy, if it can be regarded as occurring
at all, is possibly that form of enlargement of the pleura that occurs
when the volume of the lung is increased.

Tumors.—Tumors are primary and secondary. The primary
benign growths are **fibroma, lipoma, chondroma, osteoma, neuroma,** and
angioma. Lipomas originate in the subserous fatty tissue of the intercostal spaces, but Rokitansky has described a branching lipoma (*lipoma
arborescens*), starting at the free edge of the base of the lung.

The most important malignant growth is the **endothelioma,** which is
found in the pleura more frequently than elsewhere, save the dura mater.
This may occur, as in a case coming under our own observation, in the
form of minute flattened nodules of miliary type, but more frequently large
scattered or coalescing nodules of whitish color, occasionally connected by
fibrous bands, are produced. The growth leads to considerable infiltration
and thickening of the pleura, and is usually accompanied by a serous or
hemorrhagic pleurisy. Sometimes large, soft, solitary tumors are produced, but generally the tumor has more the characteristics of a **hard**

[1] Traité de la Syphilis, 1873: 326.

cancer. ·Microscopically, it consists of a dense, fibrous stroma, in which are nests of cells of an endothelial type. When, however, the tumor is soft and rapidly growing, the resemblance to sarcoma is somewhat close. The growth originates in an overgrowth of the lining cells of the pleura and may gradually extend to the lung and lymphatic glands.

Primary **sarcoma** is usually of the spindle-celled variety and begins in the subpleural connective tissue. It is said to be common in children. It may extend to the lung and lead to pressure upon the brachial plexus and axillary vessels, as in a case examined by one of us.[1] Other forms met with are *angiosarcoma, fibrosarcoma, chondromyxosarcoma,* and *neurofibrosarcoma.*

Secondary tumors invade the lung by metastasis or by direct extension The most common are those due to carcinoma of the thyroid, mamma, stomach, and œsophagus.

[1] Stewart and Adami, Montreal Med. Jour., 22: 1893–94: 909.

CHAPTER XV.

THE MEDIASTINUM.

THE mediastinum is that portion of the thorax which lies between the two pleuræ, bounded in front by the sternum and behind by the vertebral column. The anatomists generally divide it into two parts—the superior mediastinum, lying above the pericardium; and the inferior mediastinum, which is further subdivided into three, the anterior, median, and posterior mediastina. The anterior mediastinum is bounded in front by the sternum, laterally by the pleura, and behind by the pericardium. The posterior is bounded in front by the pericardium and roots of the lungs, laterally by the pleuræ, and posteriorly by the spinal column from the lower border of the fourth dorsal vertebra downward. The middle mediastinum is the remaining space.

Pathologically, the mediastinum interests us on account of the great number of important organs which it contains and its intimate relationships with other parts. All the viscera of the thorax with the exception of the lungs and pleuræ are to be found within it.

The superior mediastinum contains the origins of the sternohyoid and sternothyroid muscles and the lower ends of the longus colli; the transverse part of the aortic arch; the innominate, left carotid, and subclavian arteries; the vena cava superior, the innominate veins, and the left superior intercostal vein; the pneumogastric, cardiac, phrenic, and left recurrent laryngeal nerves; the trachea, œsophagus, and thoracic duct; the thymus gland and lymphatics.

The anterior mediastinum contains the origins of the triangularis sterni muscles, the internal mammary vessels, some areolar tissue, and some lymphatic channels and nodes.

The middle mediastinum contains the heart and pericardium, the ascending aorta, the superior vena cava, the bifurcation of the trachea, the pulmonary arteries and veins, and the phrenic nerves.

The posterior mediastinum contains the descending limb of the aortic arch, the descending thoracic aorta, the greater and lesser azygos veins, the pneumogastric and splanchnic nerves, the œsophagus, thoracic duct, and some lymph-nodes.

In the consideration of disorders of this part of the body, we need deal with only a few, but they are of not a little importance. The affections of the trachea, bronchi, œsophagus, heart, pericardium, vessels, and nerves are more conveniently described elsewhere, though it must not be forgotten that the mediastinum is often secondarily involved in disease of these structures. In this place, therefore, we shall confine our remarks chiefly to the areolar connective tissue, the lymph-nodes, the thymus gland, and the various ailments affecting them.

CONGENITAL ANOMALIES.

The mediastina will, of course, be modified in their shape, extent, and boundaries by anomalies of development of the heart, lung, vertebral column, and sternum.

ACQUIRED ANOMALIES OF SIZE, SHAPE, AND POSITION.

Transudations, inflammatory effusions, extravasations of blood; infiltrations, inflammatory or neoplastic, whether of the mediastinal space itself of the neighboring viscera and serous cavities; and aneurisms will alter the size, shape, and position of the mediastina. In cases of extensive pleural effusion the heart and mediastinum may be dislocated considerably to one side; or the mediastinum may be dragged out of its normal position by induration and retraction of the lung.

CIRCULATORY DISTURBANCES.

Hyperemia.—Active Congestion.—Active congestion occurs in the first stages of acute inflammation.

Passive Congestion.—Passive congestion is found in general venous stasis, and in local conditions which lead to obstruction in the veins leaving the mediastinum, such as enlarged glands, and tumors. Hemorrhage into the mediastinum may arise from traumatism, the erosion of vessels, or the rupture of an aortic aneurism.

INFLAMMATIONS.

Mediastinitis.—Inflammation of the mediastinum—mediastinitis—is not uncommon, and is to be attributed to trauma, the extension of disease from neighboring parts, and to hematogenic infection.

Traumatic Mediastinitis.—The traumatic form is due to external injuries, such as stab wounds or gunshot wounds. Occasionally, too, foreign bodies within the œsophagus may be the cause.

Mediastinitis by Extension.—Mediastinitis arising *per extensionem* is much the most common form. It may be secondary to pleurisy, pericarditis, or peritonitis; it may extend from the neck along the vessels, from the retropharyngeal glands, the larynx, trachea, or œsophagus; from the thymus, lungs, or bronchial glands; or from the vertebræ. According to the type, we may recognize *simple, suppurative,* and *specific mediastinitis;* these may, again, be *acute* or *chronic.*

Hematogenic or Metastatic Mediastinitis.—Hematogenic or metastatic mediastinitis has been met with in connection with typhoid fever, erysipelas, acute rheumatism, pneumonia, and variola.

Simple mediastinitis usually is a complication of acute pleurisy or pericarditis. It is almost certain, too, that there is an inflammatory hyperplasia of the mediastinal glands in cases of bronchitis, pneumonia, and many of the infectious fevers. No doubt most of these cases heal without leaving any untoward results, but occasionally the process ends in suppuration, or the glands become chronically enlarged and indurated. Subsequently, should contraction of the inflamed structures occur, we may get traction or pressure upon important structures, such as the vessels, trachea, bronchi, or œsophagus. One form of diverticulum of the œsophagus is due to the traction of a contracting gland which has become adherent to this organ. Mediastinal abscesses may extend and rupture externally, but have been known to discharge into the trachea, œsophagus, pleural cavity, pericardial sac, left ventricle, and aorta. A common sequel of mediastinal inflammation is the formation of bands of adhesion between the external surface of the pericardium and the pleuræ, or between the pericardium and the chest wall (*mediastino-pericarditis*). In the latter event systolic retraction of the thoracic wall in the neighborhood of the apex of the heart may be produced (provided that there is concretion of the apex of the heart with the parietal pericardium), a fact that is of some diagnostic import in connection with pericarditis. In some cases adhesions may be so widespread that the mediastinal space is practically obliterated.

Apart from the adhesion and induration of the tissues just referred to, which are to be regarded rather as relics of an inflammation past and gone than as evidences of a presently active process, there is a form of chronic mediastinal inflammation which is of a steadily progressive character. In this case the process begins either as a perihepatitis, which extends to the mediastinum by the lymphatics, involving in its course the right pleura, or as a pericarditis. The mediastinal space is obliterated and the various serous sacs are eventually more or less completely involved (multiple progressive hyaloserositis,[1] chronic multiserositis, polyorrho-menitis, Concato's disease). The adhesions produced are very numerous and dense and the newly-formed fibrous tissue may undergo hyaline degeneration, so that a peculiar substance, of pearly white color and cartilaginous appearance, is produced. This material may form thick sheets on the surface of the different viscera, liver, lungs, or heart (*Zuckerguss*).

Tuberculosis.—Tuberculosis of the mediastinum arises by extension from the vertebral column or from the lymph-nodes. It is frequently suppurative in type.

Syphilis.—Syphilis of the mediastinum appears to be as rare as tuberculosis is common. The few recorded cases appear to have been secondary to gummata of the sternum or ribs. In one there was enlargement of the mediastinal glands as well.

No consideration of inflammation of the mediastinal structures would be complete without a more detailed reference to the important role played by the mediastinal lymph-nodes. Repeated observations have proved beyond question that the tracheobronchial lymph-nodes, both in man and the lower animals, not infrequently contain living bacteria,

---

[1] Nicholls, Studies from the Royal Victoria Hospital, 1: 1902: No. 3.

even in the absence of local disturbance or disease elsewhere. The presence of pneumococci, staphylococci, or tubercle bacilli has been determined in these cases. Pizzini, for instance, found the bacilli of tuberculosis in the peribronchial nodes of non-tuberculous adults, dying from accident, suicide, or acute infectious disease, in 42 per cent. of cases. This being the fact, the potency for evil of the mediastinal lymph apparatus must be admitted. Moreover, in probably every case of bronchitis and pneumonia the tracheobronchial and peribronchial lymph-nodes are involved, as are the anterior mediastinal nodes in acute peritonitis. A simple inflammatory hyperplasia may result, either acute or chronic, which may lead to enlargement and often, finally, induration of the structures; or, again, a suppurative process may be initiated. Among the commonest forms of disease of the mediastinal lymph-nodes is tuberculosis, which may be of the acute miliary or the caseating type. It was for a long time thought that this affection was secondary to pulmonary tuberculosis. Considerable evidence has now accumulated to show that this view is incorrect, however. Weigert has demonstrated that the dissemination of tubercle bacilli in the lung follows the same path as the absorption of coal dust or other pigments, and the work of Aufrecht proves that it is next to impossible for foreign particles to reach the alveoli of the lung by inhalation, save in the possible case of forced inspiration. The observations of Ribbert, Baumgarten, and others, referred to above, strongly support the view that tubercle bacilli do not reach the lungs directly, but, entering by way of the nasopharyngeal mucosa, pass into the cervical chain of lymph-nodes and thence into the tracheobronchial and peribronchial group. The exact method by which the lungs eventually become infected is less certain, but it is probable that it is either by retrograde metastasis in some cases, or, in others, by the rupture of a caseous focus into one of the pulmonary arteries. The presence, then, of infected lymph-nodes opens up several possibilities. Inflammation may spread throughout the mediastinum and eventually involve important structures. Enlarged masses of nodes may press upon the trachea, bronchi, œsophagus, or large vessels. Cicatricial contraction of the chronically inflamed groups may lead to traction upon the same structures. In this way diverticula of the hollow viscera are not uncommonly produced. Caseous or suppurating foci may discharge into the mediastinal space or into the trachea, bronchi, arteries, or veins. Further, abscesses have been known to rupture externally, or into various cavities and viscera. The results are often, therefore, far-reaching.

Parasites.—*Echinococcus* cysts of the mediastinum have been describd.

PROGRESSIVE METAMORPHOSES.

Tumors.—Tumors of the mediastinum are relatively rare and may be primary or secondary. The secondary growths originate in the bronchi, lungs, or œsophagus, and involve the region by direct extension, or, again, are metastatic. The primary neoplasms begin in the lymph-nodes, connective tissue, thymus, in the thyroid or an accessory thyroid.

The primary benign growths reported are **lipoma, fibroma, adenoma, lymphoma, chondroma,** and **teratoma.** In some cases, however, it is impossible to determine whether such tumors have developed primarily in the mediastinum or not.

Among the more common of the benign tumors are the **teratomas** (dermoid cysts), of which Christian[1] has made the most recent study. They are usually benign, but occasionally show evidences of malignancy. They originate, according to Marchand, Koster, and Pinders, from the thymus gland, but have also been explained as due to inclusion of epiblast in the course of the closure of the thoracic wall, and again to fœtal inclusion. Waldeyer describes one which contained thyroid tissue. They may also contain cartilage, bone, and mucous membrane.

Dermoid cysts are usually soft, fluctuating, occasionally pulsating, and are situated under one clavicle or on both sides of the sternum. The pulsation, which may be due to their own vascularity or to transmitted impulse from the aorta, has led to their being mistaken for aortic aneurism. The contents of the cyst are similar to those of dermoids elsewhere. These cysts are dangerous, inasmuch as they may ruture into some important structure, such as the pericardium, pleura, left lung, the bronchus, or aorta. In about 20 per cent. of cases they have been diagnosticated by the presence of hair in the sputum.

Tumors of the mediastinum may arise from thyroid tissue. Occasionally, the thyroid gland is situated much lower down than usual, lying behind the sternum between the trachea and œsophagus. Accessory thyroids may also at times be found in the superior mediastinum. Wuhrmann has recorded 91 tumors of thyroid origin in the mediastinum, 75 benign and 16 malignant. Such tumors may assume the type of an adenoma, carcinoma, or sarcoma. They may attain a large size. Dittrich mentions a substernal "endothoracic struma," the size of a man's head, which had compressed the right lung.

Altogether, the most common primary new-growths of the mediastinum are those originating in the thymus or the lymph-nodes. These are by far the most frequently malignant and sarcomatous in type, but **benign lymphoma** has been described.

Benign lymphomas are to be distinguished from malignant lymphomas or lymphosarcomas, on the one hand, by their localized non-infiltrating character, and from leukemia and pseudoleukemia, on the other, by the absence of the peculiar blood changes and of enlargement of the spleen and liver.

The most frequent primary tumor of the mediastinum is the **sarcoma,** which may assume the form of *lymphosarcoma, fibrosarcoma, round* or *spindle-celled,* and *alveolar sarcoma.* **Endothelioma** is also met with.

---

[1] Dermoid Cysts, Jour. of Med. Research, 2 (N. S.):1902:541.

These growths originate either in the mediastinal lymph-nodes or in the areolar connective tissue; it is not always possible to determine which.

Lymphosarcomas of the mediastinum are soft, yellowish-white in color, with thin-walled vessels. They usually infiltrate somewhat rapidly, but occasionally are of slow growth. The newgrowth begins in the lymph-nodes, bursts through the fibrous investiture of these structures, eventually invading all the tissues of the mediastinum and fusing them into a more or less homogeneous mass. The resulting tumor is often of enormous size and extent, and may involve the heart, lungs, bronchi, œsophagus, the sternum, and vertebral column. It has been known to reach even the meninges by way of the intervertebral foramina. Unlike other forms of sarcoma, the mediastinal lymphosarcoma gives rise to metastases by preference in the intestinal tract, less often in the parenchymatous organs, such as the liver, spleen, and kidneys. On the whole, however, mediastinal sarcoma tends to spread by local diffusion, and distant metastases are not common.

Histologically, we find an aggregation of small round-cells, held together by a variable amount of fibrous reticulum, and, if small, presenting evidence of a capsule. Multinucleated and spindle-shaped cells are not often seen.

According to Hare,[1] the most frequent malignant newgrowth of the mediastinum is the **carcinoma**. This, however, is almost always secondary in character, the few exceptions being those forms derived from thyroid tissue above referred to. Some of the cases reported by the older pathologists as carcinomas probably would now be placed in the category of endotheliomas.

Cysts, lined with ciliated epithelium, are occasionally met with, due to partial persistence of the original communication between the œsophagus and trachea, or to dilatations of rudimentary accessory bronchi.

The secondary tumors of the mediastinum are carcinomatous or sarcomatous, and are confined to the lymph-nodes. In the case of carcinoma, the primary growth is usually to be found in the breast or lung, less often in gall-bladder, kidney, pancreas, or stomach.

Secondary sarcoma is not very frequent, but has been observed in cases of sarcoma of the upper extremity.

The symptoms resulting from the presence of mediastinal tumors of all kinds depend largely on their size and position, and, in general, are those of pressure and irritation, together with, in some instances, the ordinary features of malignancy. At first, there is usually a subjective sensation of fulness and pressure, generally referred to the neck, with some palpitation of the heart, but with at first no pain. Later, actual dyspnœa sets in, due to pressure upon one or more of the important structures within the thorax, trachea, bronchi, the veins of the heart, nerves, or lungs. Irritation of the vagus possibly accounts for the cough, vomiting, palpitation, regurgitation of food, and the girdle

---

[1] Affections of the Mediastinum, Philadelphia, 1889.

sensation complained of in some cases. Irritation of the sympath
leads to dilatation of the pupil on the affected side; destruction of
nerve, to contraction of the pupil. Pressure on the aorta will prod
a difference in the volume of the radial or carotid pulse of the two si
Irritation of the phrenic nerve, which is rare, produces severe pain
singultus.   Compression of the œsophagus and the thoracic vein
common.   Where there is much obstruction to the venous return,
nosis of the head, chest, and arm, dilatation of the superficial veins,
later, local œdema, are met with.   Pulsation may be detected and l
to the suspicion of an aneurism.

SECTION III.

THE ALIMENTARY SYSTEM.

CHAPTER XVI.

THE DIGESTIVE FUNCTIONS AND THEIR DISTURBANCES.

Developmental Considerations.—Before we can acquire an adequate conception of the great diversity of disease processes that occur in the alimentary tract, we must be conversant with certain features of the development and anatomical structure of this system. Furthermore, it is necessary to have a working knowledge of its normal functions, inasmuch as it is from the physiological side alone that we can attack many of the problems that confront us as a result of disordered activity. We can in this way, and in this way only, become competent to recognize and to appreciate not only the structural evidences of morbidity, but also the internal and external manifestations of abnormal function to which they give rise. A very cursory examination, indeed, would be all that is necessary to convince us of the wide range and importance of this part of our subject, for its complexity is evident at once.

The alimentary tract is derived from the invagination of the endodermal layer of the embryo, supported by the visceral portion of the mesoderm. The former provides the lining epithelium of the entire digestive tube, as well as its accessory structures, the lungs, liver, and pancreas. The latter forms the muscular and serous coatings, together with the mesentery and great omentum. We will not take up space in describing the complete chronological sequence of events, for that would be beside our immediate purpose, but will confine ourselves to indicating those features that will be of importance in our subsequent consideration of our subject. The invagination of the two tissue layers just mentioned continues until a complete tube is formed, the primitive gut or archenteron. This is at an early period of embryonic existence a simple straight tube, recalling the condition of things found in certain adult fishes and amphibians, terminating blindly at each end without external communication. The central portion, or mid-gut, as it is called, is connected with the yolk-sac by a wide passage, which ultimately becomes contracted to form the *omphalomesenteric* or *vitelline duct*. From the posterior part, or hind-gut, a diverticulum grows out, forming a thick-walled stem, the *allantoic stalk*. These two structures eventually become approximated, and, together with the umbilical arteries and vein, form the umbilical cord. As development proceeds, the primitive gut increases in length, but the body cavity enlarges disproportionately, so that the tissues uniting the dorsal and ventral aspects of the gut to the body wall become elongated and form ultimately two ligaments, each composed of two serous layers united by connective tissue. These are the dorsal and the ventral mesenteries. During the fourth week of fœtal life the various parts of the alimentary tract begin to be differentiated. The dorsal aspect of the tube toward the head gradually bulges

Fig. 78

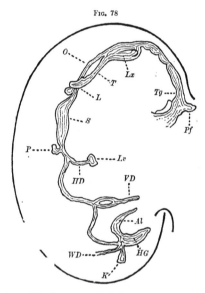

Diagrammatic schema of the alimentary canal of a human embryo, twenty-eight days old: *Pf,* pituitary fossa; *Tg,* tongue; *Lx,* larynx; *T,* trachea; *O,* Œsophagus; *L,* lung; *S,* stomach; *P,* pancreas; *HD,* hepatic duct; *Lv,* liver; *VD,* vitelline duct; *Al,* allantois; *HG,* hind-gut; *K,* kidney; *WD,* Wolffian duct.

backward to form the primitive stomach. The liver begins as a diverticulum, which arises on the ventral aspect of the archenteron just below a point corresponding to the future duodenum. Sometime later, a similar pouching of the dorsal side of the same portion gives rise to the pancreas. The accompanying diagram shows very clearly the position of things at this stage.

The mouth is at first indicated by a pit (stomodœum) on the under surface of the primitive head, which gradually deepens until it meets the blind end of the foregut. At first, a thin membrane, composed of ectoderm and endoderm, the pharyngeal membrane, separates the two, but this finally ruptures and communication is thus established. The anus is formed in a somewhat similar way. The tissues in a small area on the ventral aspect of the body, in front of the neurenteric canal, become thinned and again form a depression (proctodœum) which gradually approximates to the hind gut until it is separated from it by an anal membrane, which, in time, also disappears.

The intestine thus constituted soon loses its primitive simplicity. It becomes somewhat folded, and we can early distinguish four divisions: The first becomes the duodenum; the second, the small intestine; the third, the colon; and the fourth, the sigmoid and rectum. There is at first no ascending colon, for the cecum is situated high up under the liver. It gradually descends, however, and this portion of the gut elongates to form the ascending portion. Finally, the small intestine becomes extremely long and convoluted.

The stomach, which at first is vertical, its long diameter being parallel to the vertebral column, a condition that occasionally persists into adult life, alters its position considerably by rotation in two axes. The long axis becomes oblique and, later, almost transverse, owing to rotation on the dorsoventral axis. The pylorus, thus, comes to be on the right side and lies somewhat higher than the cardia. During the same period the stomach also rotates on its longitudinal axis, the left aspect becoming anterior and the right posterior. Thus, the greater curvature assumes the lower position, and the lesser the upper. This torsion, also, to some extent affects the lower part of the œsophagus.

A recollection of the facts just mentioned will suggest an explanation for many of the anomalies of development that are met with in later life; for example, atresia oris, imperforate anus, tracheo-œsophageal fistula, omphalomesenteric fistula, preperitoneal cyst, enterocystoma, aberrant pancreas and liver, certain regional hypoplasias, and the like.

Apart from the embryological considerations that we have just discussed, there are certain other points which have an important bearing on the etiology of disease of the alimentary tract and its accessories, to which a brief reference should be made. These have to do, on the one hand, with the anatomical structure and peculiarities of the tract itself, and, on the other, with the relationships which the tract bears to other systems and to the body at large.

Anatomical Features.—The first important fact is that the mucous membrane of the alimentary system is lined with cells that are of different types in various parts. Thus, in the mouth and œsophagus we have stratified squamous epithelium; in the stomach, columnar cells of certain specialized types; in the intestine, columnar cells, of a different character still, arranged in a characteristic and complicated way. The squamous cells have little to do with absorption or with secretion, and from their nature are adapted rather to a protective function. Therefore, they are but little likely to get out of gear and are relatively insusceptible to irritation and other forms of trauma. The more highly specialized and delicate cells of the stomach and intestine are much more easily deranged and are liable to disorder from a great variety of sources. Any disturbance, too, of these structures will be likely to be attended by far-reaching results.

Another point is, that there are several places at which the epithelium is transitional, for example, at the lip, the passage of the œsophagus into the stomach, the pyloric ring, and the anus. These are points of danger, because the lining cells at these points are more or less unstable. Consequently, we find that they are the favorite seats of carcinoma.

Again, at certain points, the lumen of the alimentary tube is narrowed, for instance, at the level of the cricoid cartilage, the pylorus, and the anus. Mechanical irritation and stasis are, therefore, more likely to occur at such places and set up inflammation and new-growth. A similar result is apt to occur at points where there is an abrupt turn in the direction of the tube, at the cardia of the stomach, the duodenum, the ileocecal valve, the hepatic and splenic flexures of the colon.

The extreme mobility of the gastro-intestinal tract is also an element of danger, in that dilatation and obstruction of the lumen, displacements, kinks, twists, and invaginations are comparatively easily brought about, any of which may be of most serious moment.

Moreover, the alimentary tube, being in direct communication with the external air, is a breeding place for bacteria, some harmless or possibly even beneficial; others potentially dangerous and at times working havoc, not only on the alimentary tract itself, but in the general bodily system.

The digestive tract, finally, is brought into touch with the body, as a whole, through the medium of the blood and lymph-circulatory systems and the nervous system. Toxic substances and infective agents may be carried to the tract or away from it, congestion may occur and lead to lowered vitality, catarrh, and impaired function. Disorders of the nervous mechanism may lead to impaired motility and secretion. The absorption of toxic matters, in turn, may affect the nerve trunks and centres. These relationships will be dealt with in more detail later.

Applied Physiology.—The functions of the alimentary system, stated briefly, are: (1) to ingest foodstuffs, and, by mechanical action, to render them more easily acted upon by the various digestive ferments; (2) to convert by the secretory activities of the mucous membranes lining the digestive tube, and of the parenchymatous cells of its accessory glands, substances largely insoluble into those that are largely soluble, thereby preparing them for incorporation into living cells and vital fluids; (3) to absorb and assimilate the substances thus transformed; and (4) to eliminate from the body those products that are unnecessary or even harmful to the economy. We may, therefore, consider this subject under the headings of mastication and propulsion, digestion, absorption and assimilation, and finally, excretion and elimination. Or, in other words, it may be discussed from a mechanical, a chemical, and a vitalistic point of view. While this method conduces to precise thought, it must not be imagined, however, that the subject in hand is so simple as, at first sight, it might appear. Even the normal processes connected with the function of alimentation are highly complicated, and this complexity and confusion become still more confounded when we come to deal with diseased conditions. While in the alimentary system we have particularly well exemplified the peculiar features of a division of labor, the factors above mentioned, while separate and distinct, are still in a large measure mutually complementary. A disorder of one function is liable to be followed by disorder of another, and may even lead to a derangement of the general system. Thus, an insufficiency in the motor power of the digestive tube leads to abnormal fermentation of its contents, impaired digestion, inflammation, and systemic intoxication. Defects in its secretory functions, again, may alter its motor functions. Not infrequently a "vicious circle" is thus produced. Or, again, a local condition of the tract will produce an effect for good or evil on a distant portion of it or on the economy at large. A correlation, more or less intimate, therefore, exists between its various functions and between its anatomical divisions.

THE MECHANICS OF DIGESTION.

The purely mechanical functions of the alimentary tract are concerned with the duties of ingestion, mastication, deglutition, admixture, propulsion, and defecation.

Food is taken into the mouth through the mutual coöperation of the lips, teeth, cheeks, and tongue. It is ground up by the teeth and jaws so as to provide a greater surface for the action of the digestive ferments. It is, by the tongue and cheeks, intermingled with saliva and mucus, and rolled into a bolus convenient for swallowing. The process of deglutition is somewhat intricate, for during the act the larynx must be shut off by becoming raised up under the back of the tongue and by the epiglottis; the nasal cavity, by the soft palate and the superior constrictors of the pharynx. This part of the mechanism is a reflex one, the centripetal impulses originating in the pharyngeal mucous membrane, being conveyed to the appropriate centre in the medulla, and from thence reflected to the muscles concerned by means of the trigeminal and vagus nerves.

When, by the contraction of the muscular wall of the œsophagus, the bolus is conveyed to the stomach, it is stored up in the fundal portion. There, after a brief period of rest, it is intimately mixed with the gastric secretion, owing to a quiet, rhythmical churning action of the cardia, and is then passed on. The antrum pyloricum seems to have the power of picking out the water and the finer particles of food from the rest before permitting it to enter the intestine. By this selective action the more delicate bowel is protected from possible injury by the larger masses of food. Only a small proportion of the total meal can be acted on in the duodenum, so that an important function of the stomach is to act as a receptacle for food. It is known that the action of the pyloric sphincter is intermittent, periods of relaxation alternating with periods of contraction, thus allowing only small amounts of food to pass at a time. How this is brought about is not yet well understood, and has led to considerable theorizing. The most we can say positively is that the act appears to be reflex and dependent on the amount and condition of the food in the pyloric antrum and its degree of acidity. Once in the duodenum, the acidity of the partially digested food is quickly neutralized by the alkaline contents of that portion of the bowel, and it is thus prepared for the action of the pancreatic secretion, the succus entericus, and the bile.

The semisolid and partially digested food, or chyme, as it is now called, is rapidly passed on through the small intestine by peristalsis. The movements connected with peristalsis appear to be threefold. There is, first, a simultaneous contraction of the circular and longitudinal fibers of the muscular wall, which has the effect of thoroughly mixing the chyme and bringing every part of it in contact with the mucous membrane; secondly, waves of contraction, affecting the circular layer of muscle, which tend to progress forward and, as a consequence, carry along with them the intestinal contents; thirdly, simultaneous contractions and relaxations of the muscle, producing a rhythmical segmentation of the bowel and its lumen.

The ileocecal valve is the boundary between the large and small intestine. It is slit-like in shape, and when the cecum becomes distended with food products, or is the site of muscular contraction, it is closed, thus preventing the return of the contained material into the small bowel. The movements of the large intestine are not unlike those of the small, but are slower and less vigorous. In the sacculated portion, they result largely in the transference of material through contraction from one sacculus to another, which dilates to receive it. The movements of the sigmoid and rectum are comparatively infrequent.

Defecation, or the expulsion of the unused residue of the food from the body, is, in infants, at all events, a purely reflex act. In adults it may be. The sphincter ani is usually kept in a state of tonic contraction through the action of a centre in the lumbar cord. The accumulation of feces in the large bowel leads to increased peristaltic action, and, therefore, increased pressure against the sphincter. The lumbar centre is then inhibited, and through the combined action of the intestinal and abdominal muscles and the levator ani, the contents of the bowel are ejected. It should be remarked, however, that in human beings, at all events, the act of defecation is largely controlled by the will. The power of the will to hasten or to delay defecation is too well known to require comment. The glottis is closed, the diaphragm is fixed, and with the chest thus splinted, as it were, the abdominal muscles can contract effectively, and drive the contents of the large bowel forward.

DISORDERS OF THE DIGESTIVE MECHANISM.

Serious results may follow the imperfect performance of any of the motor functions of the alimentary canal, results that are often far-reaching in their character.

1. **Mastication.**—Insufficient mastication may, for example, result from deficient or painful teeth, inflammation of or injury to the maxillæ or temporomaxillary joints, spasm of the muscles of the jaw, or paresis of the muscles concerned with the movement of the food within the mouth. Moreover, painful affections of the mouth, tonsils, or parotid glands will render patients averse to taking a sufficient amount of food. If such conditions be of some standing, malnutrition of the body, as a whole will inevitably result. When food is imperfectly chewed or insalivated, the burden of the stomach is greatly increased, and digestion may be greatly delayed. In aggravated cases even gastritis may be induced.

2. **Deglutition.**—Deglutition may be rendered difficult or impossible from defect in the palate, and through paralysis of the tongue, cheeks, or œsophagus. Thus, the motor nuclei in the medulla may be destroyed, as in bulbar paralysis and tumors of the medulla, or there may be a peripheral neuritis, such as is not infrequently met with in diphtheria. Similar results may follow diminished excitability of the centre or of the sensory nerves. Spasm of the necessary muscles, again, such as we meet with in tetanus, strychnine poisoning, hysteria, and hydrophobia, may prevent deglutition. The appropriate movements, not being properly coördinated, or being rendered impossible through disease or physical defect, may result in the food taking an abnormal course, for example, into the larynx, trachea, or bronchus, or, again, into the nasal cavity. Obstruction of the larynx leads rapidly to suffocation, if the condition be not promptly relieved, or, should the offending substance become lodged in the lung, an infective pneumonia, with not infrequently gangrene, is almost certain to result. The passage of food into the nasal cavity is attended with discomfort rather than danger, but may be so disagreeable that the person so affected refrains from eating. A large proportion of the food may be lost in this way. Pain in swallowing, like pain in chewing, may lead the patient to take insufficient nourishment and thus induce marasmus.

In the case of the œsophagus, difficulties in the matter of deglutition are usually to be referred to positive **obstruction.** This may be due, on the one hand, to inability of the muscle to force the food onward, or, on the other, to a narrowing of the lumen, which renders the onward passage of the bolus difficult or impossible. Not infrequently, both conditions are combined.

Muscular insufficiency of the œsophagus is always associated with dilatation of its lumen. Some of the acute cases are, beyond doubt, due to a primary paralysis of the musculature, for the condition has been produced experimentally in the dog by cutting both vagi in the neck. As a result, though the cardia remains open, the food does not pass into the stomach, but accumulates in the œsophagus, decomposes there, and eventually causes death. There are some cases, also, of so-called "idiopathic" dilatation that are apparently congenital and developmental.

Narrowing of the lumen of the œsophagus arises from a variety of causes. Some few cases, such as those found in hysteria and hypochondriasis, appear to be due to a functional disorder of the nature of a spasm of the lower end of the organ. The majority, however, result from some demonstrable physical condition, cicatricial contraction, the pressure or traction of inflammatory bands, the pressure of enlarged glands, tumors, aneurismal sacs, or diverticula. When the obstruction is gradual in its onset, the walls of the œsophagus above the stricture hypertrophy and for a time may be able to force the food onward. Sooner or later, however, disability becomes apparent, only the smaller particles of food being able to pass, and, finally, liquids alone. Hypertrophy is succeeded by dilatation and the inability may then become complete. Inflammation, and even ulceration, of the œsophagus may be induced, and death result from infection or from starvation.

The symptoms are those of obstruction to the passage of food, stasis and decomposition of the contents of the sac, and regurgitation. The regurgitation is quite different from vomiting, inasmuch as the food appears to return of itself; there is no nausea, and the abdominal muscles are not called into play. The symptoms occasionally resemble those of rumination. In the cases where there is only a partial anatomical obstruction or an intermittent functional stenosis, symptoms may occur irregularly, and the condition is compatible with prolonged periods of perfect health. A persistent close stricture, on the other hand, which cannot be relieved, results in death.

Apart from muscular weakness or stenosis, deglutition may be rendered impossible through a solution of the continuity of the œsophagus. **Rupture** of the organ from traumatism, cancerous infiltration, or peptic self-digestion and ulceration has occasionally been met with.

3. **Gastric Motility.**—The disturbances of the motor functions of the stomach take the form of overactivity and insufficiency.

Overactivity may be the result of excessive irritability of the nervous mechanism of the stomach, but is much more often due to some difficulty in discharging its contents. Any obstruction at the pyloric orifice may bring this about, whether it be from newgrowth, the pressure of enlarged glands, the traction of inflammatory adhesions, hypertrophy of the pyloric ring, or spasm of the musculature of the pylorus. In such cases the efforts of the stomach to empty itself become very forcible, and the increased peristalsis may, in thin subjects, become visible on the surface of the abdominal wall. Should the stomach, in spite of its more powerful contractions, be unable to force its contents onward within 'the usual time, its muscle gradually weakens and dilatation supervenes upon the motor inadequacy.

Motor insufficiency, or atony of the stomach, is a not infrequent condition, and almost invariably becomes associated with **dilatation.** It may be acute or chronic. The chronic form is usually the result of some form of obstruction to the outflow of the gastric contents through the pylorus, or to habitual overeating or overdrinking. The causes at work are either operative over a prolonged period of time and are gradual in their effects, or are frequently repeated.

The acute form may supervene upon the chronic, but is more often spontaneous. Here pyloric obstruction is rare, the fault in most cases being in the duodenum. Compression of the duodenum by the root of the mesentery, or by the traction of adhesions, or kinks leading to obliteration of its lumen, are the usual lesions found. Not a few cases, how many we cannot very well say, appear to be the result of a primary paralysis of the gastric muscle, either due to some toxic effect upon the nerve terminals, or to disease of the vagi, or, again, to inhibition of the cerebral centres. Conditions predisposing to acute gastric dilatation are anesthesia, prolonged and wasting disease, indiscretions in diet, deformity of the spine, injuries to the head, back, and abdomen.[1]

The results of motor insufficiency depend largely on the cause of the condition and its extent. In the milder grades, beyond some slight delay in the discharge of the gastric contents, the consequences are but slight. Should, however, food particles remain continuously in the stomach, decomposition sets in, with the production of abnormal acids and gases, and leads to serious disturbance of the secretory power of the mucosa,[2] and to dilatation of the organ. Gastritis is, also, a not infrequent result. The presence of an excessive amount of food, the retention of fluid, which is normally secreted by the stomach in considerable quantity, the degeneration of the muscle fibers, all contribute to the production of dilatation. In cases of functional obstruction, such as may be due to spasm, the dilatation is not necessarily associated with inability of the stomach to discharge its contents. Examples of this are found in connection with chronic gastritis, peptic ulcer, and carcinoma, and in hyperacidity and hypersecretion.[3] Possibly, here, the condition is an intermittent one, giving the gastric musculature time to recover. It should not be forgotten, either, in this connection, that, like other organs, the stomach has a certain amount of reserve force, so that for a time a slightly dilated stomach may be able to empty itself within a reasonable period, and, so, continuous retention of food does not occur.

Where obstruction to the onward flow of the stomach contents is complete or nearly so, death will eventually take place from inanition, unless the condition be relieved by operation. In the less extreme instances, in which there is stagnation of food and the products of secretion and digestion, conditions are favorable for the growth of microorganisms, so that we have abnormal fermentations going on with all this implies. Not only is the normal process of secretion impaired by the retention of products that should be removed, but the abnormal production of fatty acids, gases, and other chemical substances, leads to irritation of the mucosa, dilatation, pain, eructations, and vomiting. When the decomposed materials, with the enormous accumulation of bacteria that accompanies them, is in course of time passed on into the intestine, further irritation and further decomposition are initiated.

In the acute cases a lethal termination comes on more or less rapidly in cases that are not recognized and treated judiciously, apparently from the combined effects of inanition, shock, and collapse.

[1] Nicholls, Acute Dilatation of the Stomach, International Clinics, 4: 1908: 80.
[2] Kausch, Mittheil. aus d. Grenzgeb., 4: 347.　　　　　　[3] Kausch, Ibid., 7.

Some curious nervous effects are produced by gastric dilatation, such as tetany, epileptiform convulsions, tetanoid muscular contractions, general depression, and collapse. Whether these are the result of systemic intoxication owing to the absorption of poisonous substances from the alimentary tract, or to more mechanical causes, such as the distension of the gastric muscle, or the loss of fluids from the body, is by no means definitely established. The striking observations of Verstraeten, Vander-linden, Halstead, Loeb, and the MacCallums,[1] however, suggest an explanation for a hitherto obscure condition, for they have proved conclusively that the important factor in the etiology of tetany and various convulsive phenomena is a deficiency of calcium salts in the system, in some cases, at least, dependent on parathyroid insufficiency. Possibly we may have to do with, in the gastric cases, insufficient absorption of the calcium in the ingested foodstuffs.

Vomiting is a common feature in dilatation of the stomach. In the slowly progressive chronic cases it occurs at comparatively rare intervals, an enormous quantity of offensive material, consisting of undigested food, fluid, fermenting and decomposing matter, being brought up, the accumulation of several days. The vomiting in the acute forms is essentially different, being more of the nature of a regurgitation, the material coming up with little effort and at brief intervals. Food has no time to accumulate, as it is immediately rejected, and the vomitus consists chiefly of watery secretion from the stomach, with greenish or blackish, curdy flakes, bile, and often a diastatic ferment. The amount brought up is quite enormous, as the vomiting is persistent and uncontrollable.

The act of vomiting is a somewhat complicated one, and is governed by a special "vomiting centre" in the medulla, situated not far from the respiratory centre. This centre may be stimulated directly by toxic substances circulating in the blood, and by a variety of intracranial conditions. It may, also, be affected reflexly by stimuli reaching it from other organs, such as the nose, stomach, peritoneum, and uterus. Vomiting begins with a deep inspiration. The glottis is closed, the diaphragm is depressed and fixed, and the abdominal respiratory muscles are contracted. The stomach, in some cases at least, undergoes antiperistaltic movements, and a small amount of its contents is aspirated into the oesophagus. Finally, the abdominal muscles contract vigorously and the contents of the stomach and oesophagus are forcibly expelled through the mouth. The act of vomiting, however, includes more than this, for it has a profound systemic effect. Salivation and sweating are common occurrences at its inception, the blood pressure falls, and the pulse is slowed, owing to vagus stimulation. Later, the blood pressure and the rate of the pulse are markedly increased.

Vomiting is always an indication of disordered function, whether of the stomach itself or of some remote organ with which it is connected by nerve paths. It is essentially a nervous phenomenon, the stimulus of

---

[1] W. G. MacCallum, Johns Hopkins Hosp. Bull., 9:1908:91.

which is either peripheral or central. Organic disease is not necessarily present, and many cases are purely functional. The power of unpleasant sights or smells, for example, is well known. The influence of the mind is, therefore, apparent.

Akin to vomiting is **belching**, by which is meant the expulsion of gas through the mouth. This gas is either air that has been swallowed or the product of fermentative processes going on in the stomach. Very often the gas brings with it small quantities of liquid, containing fatty acids or hydrochloric acid, which gives rise to unpleasant burning sensations in the mouth and gullet. This is known as *pyrosis* or "heart-burn." Apparently, there is a preliminary relaxation of the cardiac sphincter of the stomach, which permits gas to be forced through in consequence of compressive action of the diaphragm, abdominal muscles, or, possibly, of the stomach wall itself. The eructation of gas in certain hysterical persons may attain extraordinary proportions, the belching being almost explosive in character and recurring at frequent intervals. The condition appears to be due in these cases to the habit of "air-swallowing." Reflexes from the stomach and peritoneum play an important role in the causation.

Hiccoughing is somewhat similar, but is due to a clonic spasm of the muscles in question. As in the case of belching, it may be initiated by reflexes from the stomach or abdominal cavity. The remarkable barking hiccough, sometimes met with in hysterical conditions, is perhaps due to central causes.

4. **Intestinal Peristalsis.**—During periods of complete fast the entire gastro-intestinal tract is at rest. With the initiation of the digestive function, however, movements are instituted having for their object the thorough mixing of the food and its subjection to the action of the various digestive ferments in turn. The peristaltic movements of the bowels are normally unobtrusive, although the individual is often conscious of their presence. In thin persons they may be seen and felt in consequence of transmitted undulations of the anterior abdominal wall. Usually no sound is produced.

Under abnormal conditions these **peristaltic movements** may be greatly **increased**, both in force and frequency. This is especially well seen in those cases where there is some obstruction in the lumen of the bowel to be overcome. As illustrations of this, may be cited kinks in the bowel, volvulus, cicatricial contracture of the lumen, new-growths in the bowel, hernias and other causes of external pressure. When the obstruction comes on suddenly, violent cramp-like movements of the bowel above the seat of the trouble are induced. Should the condition be not relieved, however, these cease in time, giving place to an atonic and dilated condition of the bowel, which leads quickly to toxemia, collapse, and death. In cases where the obstruction comes on more gradually, the increased work of the bowel, in attempting to force its contents past the point of narrowing, results in hypertrophy of its muscular wall, though in the later stages a certain amount of dilatation is present as well.

More common, and, fortunately, less serious, are those cases of increased peristaltic action that come on in the absence of obstruction. To understand these we must bear in mind that the motor activities of the bowel, like the secretory functions, are initiated by and are largely under the control of the nervous system. Peristalsis is commonly reflex, the stimulus being the presence of solid and liquid matter within the lumen. In some instances, however, the stimulus appears to be central, as in those cases due to emotion, excitement, fear, worry, and the like. The influence of the mind over the activities of the stomach and bowels is a well-recognized fact. Excessive peristalsis, then, may, conceivably, be due to an increase in the normal stimulus within the bowel, to an increased irritability of the bowel wall, whether nervous or muscular, or to impulses proceeding from the cerebrum.

Usually the condition is accompanied by **diarrhœa**, though not invariably so. In elderly persons and hysterical subjects it is not uncommon to have gurgling sounds (*borborygmi*) produced within the intestines, which may be audible at a considerable distance, without diarrhœa. This is more apt to occur when the bowels contain gas but a relatively small amount of solid matter. The normal stimulus to the contraction of the bowels comes from the coarser, indigestible constituents of the food. Should these be in excess, increased peristalsis and diarrhœa will result. More often chemical irritants are at work, either introduced with the food or the result of faulty digestion and of abnormal fermentation. The organic acids and the various gases resulting from decomposition are the chief offenders. An interference with the absorption of water by the bowel, in some instances, will cause diarrhœa.

Any condition that leads to increased irritability of the intestine, either of its mucosa, muscle, or nerves, favors the production of diarrhœa, for here normal stimuli may produce excessive response. In many forms of acute enteritis such an increased irritability is present, though we have to reckon with the stimulating effects of the products of abnormal fermentation as well. It is singular, however, that a considerable degree of inflammation of the bowel may be present in some cases without diarrhœa, when we might reasonably have expected it. Typhoid fever, for example, is, in this country at least, more often associated with constipation than with diarrhœa. The same thing is true also of many chronic inflammations of the bowel, even when associated with ulceration. Such conditions are often remarkably sluggish.

We have seen that, normally, the movements of the gastro-intestinal tract are more or less influenced by the central nervous system. This operates probably through the agency of the vagus and splanchnic nerves. In hysterical and neurasthenic subjects comparatively slight stimuli are sufficient to bring on overaction of the bowels. Even the fear of a diarrhœa may be enough in certain susceptible individuals. In persons of a nervous type, worry, anxiety, fear, or surprise, in fact, any sudden emotion, will bring on a watery evacuation of the bowels. Under such circumstances the slightest indiscretion in diet, also, may be enough to precipitate an attack, though at other times it might be insufficient to produce this result. Organic disease of the central nervous system may, occasionally, produce diarrhœa, as, for example, locomotor ataxia during an intestinal crisis.

The act of defecation is to a considerable extent dependent on peristalsis of the bowels. The descending colon acts as a storehouse for the unused residue from the ingesta, the rectum being ordinarily a closed tube, owing to the action of the so-called third sphincter situated at its upper end. With the entry of feces into the rectum the stimulus comes, and leads to a desire for evacuation. As has been stated previously, the act of defecation is more or less under the control of the will, but not entirely so. The act may be delayed for a time, but eventually the call becomes imperative. In cases of diarrhœa the contraction of the external sphincter cannot for long be voluntarily maintained, and evacuation takes place, either as a gentle oozing, or with explosive force, according to the strength of the expulsive movements and the retaining power of the external sphincter. In some inflammatory affections of the bowel, such as dysentery, the acts of defecation are greatly increased in number and are accompanied by painful sensations or *tenesmus*. Hemorrhoids, fissures of the anus, and fistulæ also render the act exceedingly painful.

Involuntary evacuation of the bowels, or **incontinence of feces**, is, also, not infrequently met with. It may result, for example, from organic disease of the brain or cord, during delirium and coma, in sleep and intoxication, and from strong mental impressions, as fright or fear. It is presumed in these cases that the cerebral control is inhibited.

Deficient action of the bowels is a common complaint, being, indeed, with many an almost habitual condition. The term **constipation** implies somewhat more than a mere infrequency of evacuation, connoting, as it does, an alteration in the character of the feces. Owing to the fact that the food remains too long within the intestine, the fluid parts are, to a large extent, absorbed, or, it may be, the fluids in the food may have been deficient from the beginning. Consequently, the feces become firmer in consistency, and, in some cases, even dry, hard, and stony. The latter result is in great part an effect of pressure, and the fecal masses often are moulded to the shape of the intestinal cavity. What constitutes the condition of constipation is somewhat hard to define. Some persons have an evacuation of the bowels regularly once or twice daily, often at a stated time. Others may go without a movement for two or three days. Still others, women especially, may go a week or ten days, or even longer. Many persons affected in this way with sluggishness of the bowels preserve the manners and appearance of perfect health. They may not perhaps suffer from the abdominal fulness, the sallow, earthy complexion, the furred tongue, the loss of appetite, and the headache that are so often the accompaniments of this condition, but in the more marked cases it would be unsafe to assume that no harm was being done. A certain amount of slow poisoning may be going on, which will make itself manifest in the end, or may so sap the vital energy that the individual will fall a prey to disease of other kinds.

Infrequent evacuation of the bowels may result from obstruction to the passage of feces through the lumen, or from causes unassociated with such obstruction.

Gross causes of obstruction are found either in the intestinal tube itself or in structures external but adjacent to it. Thus, in the first class of cases, the passage may be blocked by fecal masses, gallstones, bones, or other foreign substances that have been swallowed, or may be completely obliterated at a given point by volvulus. The lumen may be narrowed as a result of chronic inflammation, cicatricial contraction, intussusception, tumors, or hemorrhoids.

In the second class, the obstruction is caused either by pressure or traction exerted from without. The lumen may, for example, be encroached upon or obliterated by hernial sacs, fibrous adhesions, a retroverted uterus, or other misplaced organs, or tumors. The traction of adhesions, the dilatation and descent of the stomach, and the prolapse of certain portions of the bowel owing to the weight of tumors in the wall, may result in kinking and obstruction.

Much more common are those cases of constipation that are unassociated with mechanical obstruction. As we have seen, the function of peristalsis is commonly reflex, the stimulus being the presence of food in the bowel of sufficient bulk, and especially the presence of an indigestible residue. An insufficient stimulus, affections of the muscular wall of the bowel interfering with its contractility, and derangements of the nervous apparatus, have all to be reckoned with in a discussion of the etiology of constipation.

Unsuitable diet plays an important role in many cases. Food that is too concentrated and easily assimilable, such as milk, eggs, and meat, will often produce constipation. A deficiency in the watery constituents or of the organic acids will have the same effect.

Deficient muscular power is a potent cause of constipation. We see this in elderly persons and those of a sedentary disposition, and, also, during the convalescence from acute disease. The muscle in these cases seems to undergo a certain amount of degeneration or atrophy, which considerably lessens its effectiveness. It should be pointed out in this connection that muscular contraction of the intestines often exhibits a definite periodicity, the call for evacuation and the resulting peristalsis occurring at about the same hour each day. Neglect of these calls is one of the most potent causes of constipation. The stimulus becomes increasingly ineffective, and, owing to the accumulation of feces, the lower portion of the large bowel becomes dilated, its muscle thinned, and its power of contraction correspondingly diminished. Ultimately, the power to evacuate by natural means is entirely lost, and can only be excited by the use of cathartics. It has been found by experiment that a certain amount of material within the bowel is necessary to induce its contraction, but if the bowel be greatly distended the contractility is lessened and finally abolished. The power to contract will, however, return if the dilatation be relieved. The constipation that accompanies peritonitis appears to be due to a combination of causes, cloudiness and degeneration of the muscle fibers, inflammatory œdema, and inhibition of the nervous impulses. A somewhat similar association of morbid conditions is met with in enteritis and colitis.

Reference should be made here, also, to a form of constipation thought by many authorities to be due to a condition of hypertonus of the intestinal muscle. Thus, persons enjoying robust health may be the subjects of constipation. This may, in part, be due to the fact that the assimilative functions of the bowel are particularly active, but, perhaps, also, to an increased tone of the whole intestinal tract. Relaxation of the bowel is rendered more difficult, and the wave-like, propulsive movements characteristic of peristalsis are not so easily set up. Sometimes this hypertonus is so excessive as to lead to actual spasm of certain portions of the tract. The condition is often associated with colic, and the propulsion of the feces for the time being is rendered impossible. This form is met with also in chronic lead poisoning.

The disorders of the nervous mechanism of the bowel and their relation to peristalsis are as yet very imperfectly understood. The ganglia and plexuses of nerves in the intestinal wall govern peristalsis, and changes in these structures have been described in connection with lead poisoning and constipation,[1] but similar appearances have been observed in other affections.

Constipation is occasionally met with in both functional and organic diseases of the central nervous system, as, for example, in hysteria, neurasthenia, melancholia, and meningitis. Why this should be we do not know. Perhaps some centrifugal impulse is interfered with which is required to bring about normal peristalsis. Or, again, an inhibitory mechanism is possibly set in action.

Constipation may, in some cases, be unattended by obvious signs of disorder, but the condition undoubtedly interferes with the proper conduct of digestion. Abnormal fermentation of the intestinal contents takes place, leading to flatulency. Poisonous substances are produced which may enter the circulation and produce far-reaching results. Inflammation and even ulceration of the bowel may occur, or, again, the weight of the retained material may lead to prolapse of the bowel and traction on important structures.

DISORDERS OF SECRETION.

Foodstuffs, when reduced to their simplest constituents, consist of proteins, carbohydrates, fats, water, and certain mineral salts. The digestive fluids concerned in the transformation of food are the saliva gastric juice, bile, pancreatic secretion, and the succus entericus. The food materials and the different ferments act and react upon one another variously in different parts of the alimentary tract, so that it is convenient to discuss the process of digestion as it takes place in the mouth, stomach, and intestines.

---

[1] Jürgens, Berl. klin. Woch., 23: 1882: 357; Maier, Virch. Archiv, 90:1882:455.

The Saliva.—In the mouth the digestive fluid is the saliva. This consists of the secretions of the various salivary glands discharging into the buccal cavity, and contains mucin and a digestive ferment—ptyalin. The chief function of the saliva is, apparently, to facilitate deglutition, for the ptyalin, the only chemically active substance, is absent in certain of the lower groups of animals, notably the carnivora. In the course of mastication the food is ground into small particles, thus assisting the action of the saliva. The watery constituents of the secretion render the food of softer consistence, and the mucin provides it with a slippery coating, so that swallowing of the bolus is greatly facilitated. The saliva, further, dissolves certain mineral substances that are soluble in weak alkaline solutions, feebly emulsifies fats, but exerts no action upon proteins, except that of maceration. The active constituent of the saliva is the ptyalin, which is a diastatic enzyme acting on the starches. In the chemical transformation that ensues, the ptyalin initiates hydrolysis of the complex starch molecule, so that it is reduced to simpler constituents. The first action of the ptyalin is to render the viscid starch more fluid, and then to convert it into a variable mixture of dextrin, maltose, and isomaltose. The conversion of the starch into a thin, watery fluid takes place very rapidly, only a few seconds being required to bring about the result. Thorough mastication of the food and its admixture with the saliva are very important, for the amount of salivary digestion is quite considerable, and renders the food to that extent more suitable for the action of the gastric juice. In fact, the conversion of the starches into dextrin and sugars continues for some time after the food enters the stomach, even when there is considerable acidity of the gastric contents.

A diminution of the amount of saliva, then, materially interferes with the rapidity of the digestive process, and, moreover, interferes with mastication, deglutition, and speaking. It occurs in many febrile conditions, notably in typhoid fever and pneumonia, as Mosler has pointed out, and in all conditions in which there is an increased elimination of water from the system, as, for example, diabetes, cholera, and chronic interstitial nephritis. Some few cases are definitely nervous in origin, *e. g.*, those due to certain paralyses of the facial nerve involving the chorda tympani. As is well known, in many emotional states, such as fear and "nervousness," the mouth becomes for the time being quite dry (**xerostomia**). Dryness of the mouth frequently leads to the retention within the buccal cavity of small particles of food which decompose and lead to a great multiplication of bacteria. In this way irritation and eventually inflammation are not infrequently produced. Not only do the bacteria produce their local effects in the mouth, but they may be introduced into the stomach in such numbers that this organ is unable to cope with them, and serious disturbance may be set up. The tongue, lips, and gums are dry, coated with decomposing secretion, desquamated cells, and decaying food (*sordes*), and may then become fissured and inflamed.

An increased flow of saliva (**ptyalism**) may be produced experimentally by irritation of the chorda tympani nerve or by cutting the salivary nerves. The nervous element is of considerable importance, for we find a notable increase in the saliva in cases of bulbar paralysis, in which there is a degeneration of the ganglion cells of the medulla. This has been considered by some authorities as being analogous to the paralytic secretion that results when the salivary nerves are cut. Krehl[1] is inclined to think, however, that this is not the correct explanation, but that the phenomenon is an irritative one due to the degeneration of the cells in the medulla. Very susceptible people will also manifest salivation at the sight or thought of food, or even when they think they have taken calomel. Other cases are undoubtedly reflex, as, for example, those associated with ulcer of the stomach, pregnancy, and trifacial neuralgia.

Ptyalism is also met with in all forms of stomatitis and in mercurial poisoning. In these cases not only does there seem to be a reflex stimulation of the salivary and mucous glands, but there are local changes in the mucous membrane, in the form of degeneration of cells, hyperemia, and inflammatory exudation.

Ptyalism must be carefully distinguished from the apparent increase in the salivary secretion which is present in some forms of paralysis of the muscles of the mouth, in which the patient is unable to swallow and the saliva simply dribbles out.

In cases of ptyalism the character of the secretion may be altered. Thus, in the reflex varieties, the secretion, while it is increased in amount, is deficient in solids. In others, the amount of ptyalin may be reduced. Occasionally, as has been noted in diabetes, fevers, and certain dyspeptic conditions, the reaction is acid instead of alkaline. This is due to the activity of microörganisms, whereby lactic acid is produced. The alteration in the characters of the saliva occasionally leads to curious results, such as the formation of calculi in the ducts of the salivary glands. Probably, infection and inflammation are here the primary causes, and lead to abnormal chemical reactions.

The swallowing of large amounts of secretion may be injurious, especially when alkaline, by diluting the gastric juice and neutralizing its acidity. Where multitudes of septic microörganisms have been swallowed, serious changes in the stomach may occur, as Hunter has pointed out, in the form of catarrh and atrophy of the glands.

The Gastric Juice.—The primary function of the stomach appears to be to serve as a storehouse for the food ingested. This is proved by the fact that the stomach has been removed in dogs and digestion goes on perfectly, provided that food is supplied in small particles and frequently. After a time the bowel distends at the site formerly occupied by the stomach, to accommodate increased quantities of food. This view is corroborated by the results in the few cases where the stomach has been successfully removed in man. An important, though secondary, duty of the stomach is to thoroughly mix the food with the gastric juice and pass it on to the intestines in quantities which they can comfortably deal with. Thus, the delicate mucosa of the bowel is protected from contact with,

[1] Principles of Clinical Pathology, 1907: 248: Lippincott.

and possible injury from, coarse masses of food. Only a small proportion of the food ingested is absorbed in the stomach. With the single
exception of alcohol, little more than traces of substances in solution,
such as albumoses, dextrin, sugars, and salts, are taken up, and practically none of the water. Almost everything is passed on to the
duodenum.

The ferments of the gastric secretion are pepsin and rennin. Some
authorities believe, also, in the existence of a fat-splitting ferment, but
others dispute this. Pepsin acts only in an acid medium, and this is
supplied by the production of hydrochloric acid.

It is extremely difficult to study the phenomena of digestion in the
human subject, inasmuch as it is rarely possible to obtain pure gastric
juice unmixed with food. Pawlow's work on dogs[1] has, however,
thrown a flood of light on the problem, and many of his conclusions
have been substantiated by later observations on human beings, who were
the subjects of gastric and œsophageal fistulæ. The normal stimulus
to the secretion of gastric fluid in the dog is the appetite, but it is probable
that this element has a much slighter influence in man. Here, the chief
factor is the direct stimulation of the gastric mucous membrane by the
presence of food in the stomach. As the French proverb has it, "L'appetite vient en mangeant." Pawlow found that beef extracts and small
quantities of alcohol produced the same effect, but that alkalies inhibited
the secretion. The stimulation of the special nerves of taste and smell
also seems to play an important role in this connection. The mere
act of chewing probably produces no effect. Nevertheless, there is a
close correlation between the appetite and the gastric secretion. Under
ordinary circumstances, the majority of people can digest the food they
have a fancy for. The hungry man is rarely a dyspeptic. Shakespeare,
then, had an insight into a deep physiological truth when he made
Macbeth exclaim, "Now good digestion wait on appetite, and health,
on both." The influence of the central nervous system is here again
apparent. The benumbing of the sensorium in fevers lessens the
demand for food, in spite of the fact that the tissues are being rapidly
burned up and the cells have every need for increased nourishment.
The emotions also play an important role. Anger lessens the flow of
gastric juice. Worry, anxiety, hysterical and neurasthenic conditions
often cause a loss of appetite (*anorexia nervosa*).

When the food is swallowed, after the preliminary mastication and
insalivation, there is a perceptible interval before the gastric juice begins
to be secreted. During this period, which averages from twenty to
thirty minutes, depending upon the nature of the meal, the thoroughness
of the insalivation, and the vigor of the secretion of the hydrochoric acid,
the conversion of the starches into dextrins and sugars proceeds rapidly,
for ptyalin is even more effective in a neutral solution than in an alkaline
one. With the appearance of hydrochloric acid, however, the alkalinity
gradually gives way to acidity and ptyalin digestion stops.

---

[1] Pawlow, The Work of the Digestive Glands. Eng. edit., C. Griffin & Co., London,
1902.

The further steps in the process of digestion may be briefly stated to be as follows: The hydrochloric acid provides a suitable medium for the operation of the peptic ferment, which it thus assists in hydrolyzing the proteins. It also converts cane sugar into dextrose and levulose. It inhibits the growth of microörganisms and thus prevents or lessens the acetic and lactic fermentation of the carbohydrates.

Rennin exerts its special action on milk, coagulating it and thus promoting its digestion by causing it to be retained for a longer time in the stomach.

The pepsin acts on proteins, and, assisted by the hydrochloric acid, converts them into acid albumin and eventually into albumoses. According to Neumeister, there are two sets of albumoses, proto-albumose and hetero-albumose (primary albumoses), which are gradually converted into deutero-albumoses (secondary albumoses). Finally, some of the deutero-albumoses are transformed into peptones.

Hammersten has noted the presence in the gastric mucous membrane of an oxidizing ferment (oxidase) which converts milk sugar into lactic acid.

At the height of the digestive process the hydrochloric acid is present in various conditions. Some of it is free and uncombined; some has united with the inorganic bases or basic salts of the food, and has broken up salts of the weaker acids; some, again, has combined with organic basic compounds, of which the proteins are the most important. Toward the close of gastric digestion, the stomach contains a variable mixture of starches, dextrin, sugars, peptones, and unconverted albumoses.

The length of time that the food remains in the stomach varies considerably in different cases. The character of the food, the state of health, and the type of animal have much to do with it. Under ordinary circumstances, the stomach in the herbivora is never empty. In the carnivora the food may pass on within one or two hours. The interesting observations of Cannon with the x-rays after giving a dose of bismuthi show that from the point of view of motor function the human stomach is bicameral. The ingested materials are retained for a time in the fundal portion, and as they are passed along in small masses to the pyloric region this latter gradually dilates to accommodate them. In man, with his mixed diet, this process takes from four to six hours, fatty materials being retained longest in the stomach, and carbohydrates the shortest. Under pathological conditions, however, food may be retained very much longer than this. In chronic dilatation of the stomach from pyloric carcinoma, for example, the stomach may be found to contain food that was taken days before. In such cases the power of gastric digestion is much impaired, and the retained peptones and albumoses cause direct irritation of the mucous membrane.

The subject of disorder of the gastric secretion is an extremely difficult one to deal with. Our knowledge of the normal phenomena of digestion is still imperfect, for it is gathered from observations carried out on experimental animals and but rarely on human beings, in all cases under conditions which present wide deviations from the normal. Our ideas, therefore, are based on insufficient data and, not infrequently, on inference rather than fact. This being the case, it is not surprising that our discussion of the various disturbances of secretion will be quite inadequate.

Disorders of gastric digestion involve the quantity or the quality of the gastric juice, or both. Thus, the *total amount* of the secretion may be *less than normal* or it may even be *absent* altogether. Or, again, it may be *increased*. The qualitative changes have to do with the proportions of hydrochloric acid and the ferments. As a rule, the zymogens of pepsin and rennin continue to be produced, even if the secretion of the acid has partially or completely ceased. But in advanced organic disease of the stomach both acids and ferments may be lacking.

As we have seen, the secretion of the gastric fluid is chiefly reflex, the stimuli, which are rather complex in nature, being the presence of food in the stomach, the excitation of the nerves of taste and smell, and the appetite. Conceivably, then, a defect in the necessary stimuli would result in a diminished secretion. Thus, organic or functional disorders of the special nerves of taste and smell, a benumbing of the cerebral centres, certain emotions, like anger, insufficient or uncongenial food, would all play a part. In this category may be placed most of the acute infective diseases associated with high temperature, in which anorexia is a well-marked feature; delirium and coma; tumors at the base of the brain; hysteria, neurasthenia, and melancholia. Deficient secretion (hyposecretion) and absent secretion (achylia gastrica) are known to occur in neurotic individuals. The same thing has been observed in certain cases of tabes dorsalis. Here, possibly, the cause is to be referred to interruption of the reflex arc.

In a second set of cases, organic changes, involving more or less destruction of the secretory glands, may be demonstrated. Thus, extensive carcinoma of the stomach, amyloid disease, atrophy of the mucosa, whether senile or that form resulting from chronic inflammation, may be cited as examples in point.

In still another series of cases there is some serious systemic disease. Thus, profound anemias result in diminished gastric secretion. Or there may be an excessive output of fluid from the body, as in diabetes and chronic interstitial nephritis. Or, again, a deficiency of chlorides is the cause at work.

When the amount of hydrochloric acid in the gastric juice is diminished or absent, we speak of **subacidity** (hypochlorhydria) and **anacidity** (achlorhydria) respectively. The total quantity of acid produced appears to bear some relation to the quantity and character of the food ingested. How much acid should be found normally appears to be still under discussion, for different authorities give different statements in this regard. According to Krehl,[1] the secretion probably continues until the free and combined hydrochloric acid in the gastric contents amounts to about 0.2 to 0.3 per cent. Bickel[2] gives considerably higher figures. He found, in individuals the subjects of œsophageal and gastric fistulæ, that the pure gastric juice contained from 0.35 to 0.5 per cent.

---

[1] The Principles of Clinical Pathology, 1907: 254, Lippincott.
[2] Kongr. f. in. Medizin, 1906.

It is important to remember in this connection that our ordinary clinical analyses of the stomach contents are made on mixtures of food and gastric juice. Consequently we are apt to underestimate the extent of acid production. An estimation of the free hydrochloric acid is of little or no practical value. We can only obtain accurate information by determining the total quantity of acid, both free and combined. To do this, we have to find out the total quantity of chlorides in the gastric contents and subtract from this the quantity of chlorides contained in the food. When the hydrochloric acid in the gastric contents is found to be diminished, we have to exercise some care in the interpretation of our results, for the condition may be accounted for in two ways, either there is a diminished secretion of the acid, or else it is neutralized in some abnormal way after its secretion.

In cases where the gastric secretion is inhibited, either partially or completely, the amount of hydrochloric acid will, of course, be proportionately diminished. The ferments will naturally be diminished in quantity as wel . But instances are not infrequent where the secretion of the acid alone is defective.

Free hydrochloric acid may be absent in a variety of conditions. For example, certain acute functional and organic disturbances of the stomach, notably, the acute infectious diseases, may be mentioned. Perhaps more often, anacidity is found in chronic conditions affecting the integrity of the mucous membrane, such as atrophy, carcinoma, and amyloid disease. Curiously enough, diseases in parts external to the stomach may produce the same result. Pernicious anemia, abdominal carcinoma, advanced tuberculosis, and cachexia are cases in point. The exact condition of things has been more carefully studied in connection with gastric carcinoma than in other diseases. Where a large amount of the secreting surface is involved in the newgrowth, especially where there is marked ulceration, it would not be surprising to find a total defect or a diminution in the amount of acid secreted. In some instances, however, it is unquestionable that hydrochloric acid is secreted, though it is not found in the free state, for the total amount of the combined chlorides may equal or exceed the normal. Apparently, the carcinoma produces substances that have the power of neutralizing the acid produced. These are presumably of the nature of enzymes, inasmuch as they are destroyed by heat.[1] Moore has laid down that in all carcinomatous states there is a reduction of acid; this needs confirmation.

A deficiency in the amount of hydrochloric acid secreted will of necessity inhibit to a corresponding extent the activity of the pepsin, and so delay gastric digestion. Provided, however, that the motility of the stomach be not impaired, the nutrition of the individual thus affected need not be seriously disturbed. With a suitable dietary, the intestine may be able to compensate the inefficiency of the stomach. It is, further, worthy of note that carcinomas of the stomach are able to produce ferments competent to digest proteins more quickly even than the normal gastric fluid.

[1] Emerson, Arch. f. klin. Med., 72: 426.

One of the most important results of diminished gastric acidity is the multiplication of bacteria within the stomach. It is well established that the stomach, under normal conditions, contains numerous microorganisms derived from the ingested food and external air. Provided that gastric motility is unimpaired and the food is passed regularly along into the intestines, no great multiplication of these organisms can occur. Should, however, stagnation of the stomach contents be present, more or less growth takes place and fermentative processes are set up. Thus, for example, sugar is converted into alcohol and carbon dioxide; alcohol, into acetic acid; dextrose, into lactic acid, butyric acid, hydrogen, and carbon dioxide. Gases are set free, such as carbon dioxide, hydrogen, and methane, which, together with the air that has been swallowed, produce flatulency and distension of the stomach. These fermentative processes, however, are kept within bounds by the presence of the hydrochloric acid, which has decidedly antiseptic properties. A 0.2 per cent. degree of acidity in a culture medium will, in time, destroy many bacteria, though some, and especially spores, are not greatly affected. It should be remembered, however, that the conditions in the stomach are by no means so favorable for this inhibitory action. Some of the hydrochloric acid secreted is neutralized by alkalies, or enters into combination with the proteins, which combinations are much less effective than free acid. Moreover, many portions of the food do not come in contact with the gastric juice at all, for they may be passed rapidly along into the intestine or lie in the centre of large masses. Consequently, the antiseptic powers of the gastric juice are somewhat limited, and many active microörganisms gain entrance to the bowel.

In cases of subacidity and anacidity an opportunity is afforded for the enormous increase of bacteria, both in numbers and variety, with a concomitant increase in the amount of fermentation. Under these circumstances, processes, similar to those just referred to, are set in operation, but there is a special tendency to the formation of lactic, butyric, and other volatile organic acids. Lactic acid fermentation is a chief and characteristic feature of anacidity with stagnation of the stomach contents. In fact, the lactic acid may be so abundant as to restrain the development of other bacteria that ordinarily would produce their own peculiar form of fermentation. In such cases, the Oppler-Boas bacillus is usually present in the stomach in enormous numbers and is the cause of the lactic acid production. In marked cases of anacidity putrefaction of the proteins may occur as well. In some few instances fermentation occurs in the stomach in the absence of subacidity and impaired muscular power. Possibly, here we have to do with the ingestion of excessive amounts of fermentable material together with agents that are competent to produce fermentation.

It should be pointed out that, in the present state of our knowledge, there is no pathognomonic relationship between any one kind of bacterial decomposition and any particular clinical state. Our findings have to be interpreted in such cases in the most general way. The chief factors are, the character of the food, impaired gastric motility, the amount of hydrochloric acid secreted, and the multiplication of bacteria. On the correlation of these depend the result.

Abnormal fermentation in the stomach is injurious in a variety of ways. The mucous membrane may be irritated and inflamed, leading to anorexia, pain, regurgitation, and vomiting, and, possibly, spasm of the pylorus. Gases accumulate and produce distension, flatulency, and belching. Toxic substances are formed, which may be absorbed and lead to systemic disorder. The condition is not without its effect on the bowel as well, for diminished acidity in the stomach usually leads to increased putrefaction in the intestine.

Theoretically speaking, we are able to make a distinction between increased acidity of the gastric secretion (**hyperchlorhydria**) and **hypersecretion**. In the former there is a relative increase in the amount of acid produced; in the latter there is an absolute increase proportionate to the increase of the gastric secretion as a whole. In view of the gaps in our knowledge, however, as to the normal behavior of the stomach in digesting varying quantities and kinds of food, it is hardly possible to make this distinction in practice. As a result of his experiments, previously referred to, Bickel, indeed, concludes that what is usually designated by clinicians as "hyperacidity" is in reality hypersecretion. The effect of hypersecretion is to raise the percentage of hydrochloric acid in the mixture of gastric juice and food ordinarily submitted to examination, and the result may, therefore, be wrongly interpreted. The total amount of acid in the stomach contents in so-called "hyperacidity," as a matter of fact, does not exceed that present in normal gastric juice. Under the circumstances, we cannot, perhaps, do better than use the terms hyperacidity and hypersecretion in the ordinary sense in which they are employed by certain clinicians. Hyperacidity may, then, be taken to mean an increased secretion of the hydrochloric acid with the gastric juice, occurring during digestion. Hypersecretion is an excessive secretion of the gastric fluid, usually hyperacid, occurring not only during digestion but in the intervals also. Both conditions are to be regarded as symptoms rather that actual disease entities.

The diagnosis of hyperacidity depends on the detection in the stomach contents of an increased amount of hydrochloric acid. The chief causes of the condition are dietetic errors, overwork, worry, the various neuroses, and the abuse of tobacco. The condition is found also in cases of ulcer of the stomach. Disease elsewhere in the body, such as chlorosis, cholelithiasis, and renal calculus, may be at work in some cases.

Hypersecretion may be a transient condition, may recur periodically, or, again, may be continuous. Transient and periodical hypersecretion is met with in certain nervous affections, such as locomotor ataxia, hysteria, and neurasthenia, or it may occur more or less independently (*gastroxynsis* of Rossbach). It is apparently due to irritability of the gastric mucous membrane, of its secretory nerves, or, in some cases, to stimulation of the cerebral centres.

Continuous hypersecretion (*Reichmann's disease*) is found particularly in young neurotic individiuals. Dietetic errors, emotions, and motor insufficiency are the chief causes. The condition is met with also in association with certain forms of chronic gastritis. An important factor in the causation is dilatation of the stomach, with its concomitant muscular insufficiency, whether this be due to a primary paresis of the stomach wall or to the many forms of obstruction to the evacuation of the gastric contents. In the chronic forms the hypersecretion is probably to be attributed to the stimulation of the mucous membrane by the retained food. In the acute forms of gastric dilatation a relatively enormous amount of fluid may be secreted. As much as several quarts have been removed in some instances with the stomach tube. Here, as in the earlier stages vomiting is persistent and no food can be retained, it is impossible that the stimulus can be stagnated food. Unfortunately, very few complete studies of the gastric secretion have been made in these cases, so that we are somewhat in the dark. Hydrochloric acid has been found present in some cases, but not invariably. It would seem reasonable, however to think that the gastric fluid in acute dilatation is not a true secretion. Other factors may enter into the question. Owing to the stretching of the stomach wall, the vessels are elongated and thin-walled, and lack tone; furthermore, there is the depreciating effect of the toxins present within the stomach. Consequently, it would not be surprising if the bloodvessels should become more permeable and allow a considerable quantity of fluid to exude and enter the cavity. Organic obstruction, too, promotes the condition by preventing the normal discharge of the stomach secretions into the bowel. In some cases, also, in which obstruction of the duodenum below the bile papilla has been demonstrated, the gastric fluid has contained bile and a diastatic ferment. We pass on now to the consideration of the subject of intestinal digestion.

The Intestinal and Related Secretions.—The strongly acid chyme, when it leaves the stomach, passes into the duodenum, where it meets with an alkaline medium, composed of pancreatic secretion, bile, and succus entericus. The hydrochloric acid is neutralized and the chyme is thus prepared for the action of the pancreatic ferments, which can act only in the presence of alkalies.

The old view that an acid reaction of the chyme persists for a considerable distance down the intestine, and that the acid is only gradually neutralized, is almost certainly erroneous. Mere traces of hydrochloric acid are enough to destroy the activity of the pancreatic ferments, which are poured out only in the duodenum. Consequently, it is impossible to understand how pancreatic digestion could be carried on under such circumstances. As a matter of fact, only small amounts of food pass through the pylorus at any one time, and they come in contact with a much greater bulk of alkaline secretion in the duodenum, so that the acid is immediately neutralized. The chief digestive agents in the intestines are the pancreatic secretion and the succus entericus. Some authorities describe also, another, maltase, which converts maltose into dextrose.

The Succus Entericus.—Comparatively little is known about the intestinal juice. It has been determined, however, usually by the employment of the Thiry-Vella fistula, that, in addition to mucus, the cells of the intestinal wall elaborate and discharge into the lumen of the bowel a fairly copious alkaline fluid. This secretion can, apparently, to some extent, dissolve casein, but, more particularly, contains an amylolytic ferment (invertase) which can invert cane sugar and convert maltose into dextrose. This supplements the action of the pancreas, which cannot so operate upon maltose. Furthermore, the work of Cohnheim,[1] Glassner, Hamburger, Bayliss and Starling, and Hekma[2] has brought out the important fact that the succus contains an activating substance or hormone, called by Oppenheimer "enterokinase," which has the striking property of rendering trypsin active. Presumably, the proteolytic ferment of the pancreas is secreted as a zymogen which, under the influence of the specific hormone, is converted into trypsin. In some similar way, also, the fat-splitting action of the pancreatic ferment is intensified by the succus entericus.

The Pancreatic Secretion.—By far the most important part is played by the pancreatic secretion. This contains three ferments: amylopsin, which converts the carbohydrates; trypsin, which peptonizes proteins; and steapsin, which hydrolyzes fats. Amylopsin in every way resembles ptyalin in its action except that it is more powerful. Steapsin is the only ferment in the body that has a specific chemical action on fat. It is true that some observers have described a fat-splitting ferment in the gastric secretion, but their conclusions are by no means as yet generally accepted. Steapsin acts by breaking down neutral fats into fatty acids and glycerin. It has been usually held that only a small portion of the fat undergoes this decomposition, and that the fatty acids produced combine with the alkalies of the intestinal contents to form soaps, which soaps emulsify the unconverted fat. The chemically unaltered fat is then absorbed by the columnar cells of the intestinal villi. There is considerable evidence for thinking, however, in view of later experimental work, that this view is incorrect, and that practically all of the fat (84 per cent.) is hydrolyzed into fatty acids and glycerin and in this soluble form absorbed.

The action of trypsin is similar to that of pepsin, but is more rapid and more complete. The proteins are first converted into alkali-albumin, and this into deutero-albumoses. Whether primary albumoses are formed is questionable. If they are, they appear to be very unstable and undergo rapid conversion. The deutero-albumoses are transformed into peptone and the latter, for the most part, into amido-acids and organic nitrogenous bases. Only about half of the peptone present is converted, the more stable moiety remaining being known as anti-peptone. Those substances that are partially peptonized in the stomach will, of course, only require to undergo the later stages of tryptic digestion. The manner of production of the pancreatic secretion, as revealed by recent experimentation, is of the most interesting and even startling

[1] Zeitschr. f. Physiol. Chemie, 36: 13: 1902.
[2] Jour. d. Physiol. et d. Pathol. générale, 1: 1904.

character. The older view, as developed by Pawlow and his pupils, is to the effect that this secretion is due to a nervous reflex, the stimulus being the acid gastric juice, acting upon the sensory nerve terminals in the wall of the duodenum. The work of Bayliss and Starling, before referred to (vol. i, p. 364), has completely overturned this conception. According to these observers, and there appears to be nò reason to doubt their conclusions, the cells in the mucosa of the duodenum and upper part of the small bowel produce a substance which they call "secretin," that, injected into the veins, sets up the flow of pancreatic juice. Wertheimer, further, has proved that the stimulus to the production of secretin is to be found in the action of the acid contents of the chyme upon the duodenal mucosa. Curiously, too, the pancreatic secretion experimentally produced is devoid of proteolytic action. What appears to be the natural sequence of events is this: The action of the acid in the chyme stimulates the cells of the duodenal mucosa to produce secretin. This is absorbed into the circulation. When it reaches the pancreas the pancreatic cells produce their excretion, either through direct stimulation, or, possibly, indirectly through an effect upon the nerves. This secretion contains a pro-enzyme (trypsinogen), which under the influence of the enterokinase in the bowel contents is converted into trypsin. Here we have a striking exemplification of the close correlation existing between the various parts of the alimentary tract and of the potential influence of the body at large (through the blood). The importance of the nervous system, then, is not an initiative or all-controlling one, but rather, at most, is regulative.

The Bile.—The bile has no zymotic action on foodstuffs, but is valuable as an adjuvant to the pancreatic secretion, in that it renders more soluble substances which would otherwise be quite insoluble in water. It can, for example, dissolve to some extent lecithin and cholesterin, and thus aids in their elimination from the body. It also aids in the solution of the soaps and free fatty acids. Its antibacterial properties, referred to by some, are decided, though not powerful.

The purpose of the milk-coagulating ferment, said by certain authorities to be present, is not clear, any milk in the food being acted upon by the rennin in the stomach.

The effects of a deficient secretion of the pancreatic ferments cannot be stated precisely. One would expect, and it undoubtedly is a fact, that undigested proteid matter and unconverted fats are to be found in the stools in increased amounts in certain cases of pancreatic disease Yet clinical studies on patients having extensive degeneration of the pancreas, and the experimental extirpation of the pancreas in dogs, have given contradictory results in the experience of different observers. Some have found that the absorption of proteins and fats in the bowel is considerably diminished, while others did not. In the same way, some have noted a diminished cleavage of fats in the bowel, while others did not. It is probable that these discrepancies in the results of clinical studies are to be explained in this way. Unless the pancreas were extensively damaged and its secretion lessened almost to the vanishing point, not much alteration in the normal processes of digestion need result. For it is clear that the pancreatic secretion is normally secreted in an amount much greater than is absolutely necessary to digest any meal that is ordinarily taken. The contents of the small intestine at a point just above the ileocecal valve have been shown to be exceedingly rich in amylolytic and proteolytic ferments, and it is altogether probable that these are not absorbed but destroyed in the large bowel. An extreme amount of degeneration would be requisite, then, to produce notable changes in the constitution of the feces. In a similar way, the pancreas must be extensively diseased before diabetes will result. In any case, a compensatory mechanism is not unlikely to be at work in some cases, for the intestine is competent to some extent to absorb unaltered proteins and fats and would be still more likely able to absorb those partially converted. Hydrochloric acid, too, can invert sugars. Given sufficient time, a very fair amount of intestinal digestion may take place, even if the pancreatic secretion were reduced to a minimum. The experiments on dogs are, moreover, scarcely comparable to the conditions prevailing in man, for the extirpation of the pancreas is attended with much shock, and we have no information how the secretion of bile is influenced by this operation. The fact, however, that the administration of pig's pancreas to the animals deprived of their pancreas increased the absorption of food goes to prove that a deficient pancreatic secretion may inhibit absorption.

The conditions which might be expected to seriously interfere with the action of the secretion are those which extensively damage the structural integrity of the pancreas. Such are atrophy, fibrosis, chronic inflammation, and carcinoma. Obstruction to the duct, unless due to the presence of a new-growth in the head of the pancreas or a calculus, is not likely to be often a cause. Opie[1] has shown that in about two-thirds of all cases there is a patent duct of Santorini in man. It would be extremely unlikely for both the duct of Wirsung and that of Santorini to be obstructed at one time, though it is not impossible. The most likely site for obstruction is at the papilla of Vater, and here the common bile duct would be occluded as well.

In one other way the pancreas can suffer severe injury, and this is from the entry of bile into the duct of Wirsung. This occurs most often where there is a biliary calculus impacted at the bile papilla, of such a size and shape as to prevent the discharge of bile into the intestine, while permitting a regurgitation into the pancreatic duct. Acute hemorrhagic pancreatitis may result[2] or, in less extreme cases, chronic pancreatitis. The same result can be produced experimentally by injecting bile, hydrochloric acid, or certain other substances into the duct.

The modifications in the composition of the bile that occur as the result of disease are by no means well understood. Nor is their practical significance, if any, at all times evident. Only in the case of the forma-

---

[1] Diseases of the Pancreas, Lippincott & Co., 1903.

[2] Opie, Johns Hopkins Hospital Bulletin, 12:1901:182.

tion of gallstones have we anything like an adequate conception of the processes that take place and the important results that may eventuate from them.

The *modus operandi* in cholelithiasis has been sufficiently considered elsewhere in this work (vol. i, p. 946), so that we need not occupy space by discussing the subject again here. Suffice it to say, that the chief factors at work are: (1) An infectious catarrh of the biliary passages; (2) stagnation of the bile; (3) the secretion of cholesteryl oleate and calcium salts by the inflamed mucous membrane; (4) the splitting up of cholesteryl oleate, under the influence of alkalies, into cholesterin and oleic acid, with the precipitation of the former and the formation of more or less soluble soaps; (5) the combination of the calcium salts with bile pigment to form bilirubin calcium.

The stagnation of the bile and the injury to the walls of the bile passages, that so commonly result from the presence of calculi, lead often to secondary infection and other widespread results. These will be dealt with later, and we shall simply content ourselves here with considering the effects of a deficiency of the supply of bile in the intestine upon the processes of digestion.

Bile may be prevented from entering the bowel by obstruction of the common or hepatic ducts by calculi, the pressure of enlarged glands or inflammatory adhesions, by catarrhal inflammations of the passages, and by new-growths.

The results that follow depend upon the position of the obstruction. If at the bile papilla, the outflow of the pancreatic juice may be more or less interfered with as well as that of the bile. If higher up, the supply of bile alone is cut off. Complete absence of the bile from the intestine is evidenced clinically by jaundice, more or less malaise and constitutional disturbance, and a peculiar coloration of the stools. The discharges are pale gray or "clay-colored," owing to an excess of fat and an absence of the bile pigments. It has been found, as a result of experimentation on dogs,[1] and observations on man (Fr. Müller), that the process of intestinal digestion is considerably interfered with. The absorption of carbohydrates is practically normal, that of proteins only slightly, if at all, diminished, but about 60 to 80 per cent. of the fat ingested escapes absorption. This effect is, in part, explained by the fact that, to be absorbed the fats must be first hydrolyzed and rendered soluble, and the cholates are excellent solvents for fatty acids. Should the bile be deficient, the solution is rendered correspondingly difficult. Hewlett,[2] also, has shown that bile has the power of accelerating the fat-splitting action of the pancreatic secretion eightfold or more. Lack of bile, therefore, will greatly diminish the activity of the pancreatic juice in respect to fats.

While the bile has no great antiseptic properties, so that an absence of

---

[1] Voight, Beiträge z. Biologie, Stuttgart, 1882; Röhmann, Pflüger's Archiv 29: 509.

[2] Johns Hopkins Hospital Bulletin, January, 1905.

bile in the intestine is not attended by any notable increase in its bacterial flora, yet it is possible that in the condition of biliary obstruction the processes of fermentation may be more or less abnormal. On this point, however, we have little accurate information.

The practical application of these facts is that in cases of this kind, the diet should consist mainly of proteins and carbohydrates. By keeping out the fats, we not only avoid giving a food that cannot be digested and absorbed, but lessen the possibility of abnormal decompositions and consequent irritation.

DISORDERS OF ABSORPTION AND ASSIMILATION.

By the term absorption, as we shall use it in the present discussion, we mean the process by which the various nutritive substances contained within the alimentary tract are taken up into the circulation. The substances to be absorbed are the reduction products derived from the primitive constituents of the food, proteins, carbohydrates, and fats, as a result of the action of the various ferments. These are, in the main, peptones, albumoses, dextrin, various sugars, glycerin, and fatty acids. To a slight extent proteins and fats are absorbed as they are without preliminary hydrolization. Water and salts also have to be considered. In our discussion of this subject we are concerned with the process as it occurs in the stomach and bowel. Absorption practically does not take place in the mouth and œsophagus. These structures, for one thing, are covered with a dense, comparatively impermeable membrane of squamous epithelial cells, which is, further, during mastication and deglutition, protected by a coating of mucus. It is true that under certain circumstances toxic substances may gain an entrance through the buccal mucous membrane, but the mastication of food is not a parallel case, for the food remains much too short a time in the mouth for such a result to follow and the different elements of the food are scarcely in a soluble state. The chief function of the stomach, as we have seen, is to be a receptacle for the ingested food. Its powers of digestion are comparatively limited and its powers of absorption are also limited. The carbohydrates, dextrin, saccharose, dextrose, lactose, and maltose, are absorbed fairly well, the better the more concentrated the solution. Peptones are absorbed with difficulty, and water hardly at all. Alcoholic solutions are taken up with fair avidity and seem to increase the power of the stomach to absorb other substances. By far the most important agent in the absorption of foodstuffs is the intestine, for, unlike the stomach, it is provided with special organs for the purpose, namely, the villi and solitary follicles. Peptones, sugars, emulsified fats, glycerin, and fatty acids are absorbed chiefly in the small and, to a much less extent, in the large bowel.

To gain anything like an adequate apprehension of the complicated processes concerned in absorption, we must acquaint ourselves with the physical and chemical conditions present during digestion. Let us take the small intestine as an illustration.

Here the organs specially differentiated for the purpose of absorption are the villi. Each villus is a minute elevation, projecting about 1 mm. above the general level of the mucosa. It is composed of a core of delicate areolar and adenoid tissue, covered with a basement membrane and a single layer of columnar cells continuous with those lining the intestine elsewhere. In the centre is a lacteal, or possibly two lacteals, connected by lateral channels, and an afferent bloodvessel. The wall of the lacteals is composed of a single layer of endothelial plates. About the lacteals can be detected a few fibers of unstriped muscle, whose function is, by their contraction, to empty the lacteals of their contents. Surrounding the lacteals is a freely anastomosing meshwork of venous capillaries, lying between them and the superficial epithelium. The total number of the villi is very great and has been estimated at 4,000,000. They are so closely packed, as a matter of fact, that the mucosa presents a velvety appearance. During digestion the blood capillaries are congested and the villi assume an erectile condition.

In regard to the process of absorption, the position of affairs may be briefly summarized in this way. In the villi the bloodvessels are, of course, filled with blood, and the other structures are bathed in lymph. The lumen of the intestine contains foodstuffs largely in solution. Between the two sets of fluids there is only a basement membrane and a single layer of cells. The diffusion of the fluids must take place through this barrier. To reach the circulation, furthermore, the resulting mixture must pass another obstruction, namely, the cells forming the walls of the lacteals. The old view was that this interchange was of the nature of an osmosis, but no physiologist of repute would indorse this idea now. One of the fundamental properties of primitive cells, the amoeba for example, is the power of taking up from the surrounding medium foodstuffs and other materials, assimilating what are necessary and useful, and rejecting those that are not required or positively harmful. There is no reason for supposing that the cells of the animal body, even when differentiated for special purposes, lose necessarily these early peculiarities. In fact, all the evidence that we possess points unquestionably the other way. Applying this to the subject in hand, we believe that absorption cannot be explained on a mere physical basis of osmosis, but are forced to conclude that the process is inseparably bound up with the vital properties of the cells concerned. Absorption and, for that matter, secretion are selective processes.

The investigation of the subject of absorption is one attended by great difficulties, and the finer details of the process are still to a large extent matters for conjecture. We have stated our belief that the phenomena of absorption are not to be explained on mere physical principles. The vital properties of the cells have also to be taken into account. As a matter of fact, it has been shown that extracts of the walls of the intestine are rich in ferments, and, consequently, that the tissue cells are by no means a negligible factor in the question of digestion and assimilation. Thus, there has been found a group of sugar-splitting enzymes, such as maltase, which converts maltose into dextrose; invertase, which transforms cane sugar into dextrose and levulose; and, possibly, lactase, changing lactose into dextrose and galactose. Moreover, as Cohnheim has shown (*loc. cit.*), there is a powerful proteolytic ferment—erepsin— which has the property of splitting peptones and proteoses into simpler crystallizable constituents, leucin, tyrosin, arginin, etc. Lipase (steapsin), the fat-splitting ferment, has also been detected. Some of these, like invertase, have been found within the lumen of the bowel, but there is little doubt that whether they commonly are thus excreted or not, they may be present within the epithelial cells, and possibly in the other tissues, after the fashion of internal secretions, and thus play an important role in the matter of intracellular metabolism, and, consequently, in assimilation and nutrition. So far as can be gathered from recent work, what takes place is briefly this: The various substances resulting from protein decomposition are taken up by the columnar cells covering the villi, pass through the cells into the subepithelial reticulum, and find their way into the blood capillaries, whence they eventually reach the portal vein and the liver. The farther the process of decomposition has been carried, the easier and more rapid is the absorption. Before this can happen, however, at least the major portion of the proteins must, apparently, be hydrolized into more soluble substances, such as albumoses. When these are taken up by the epithelial cells, according to Folin, they are further resolved. Conceivably, at all events, this may be brought about by the erepsin, which converts the albumoses into amido-acids. The NH_2 groups are split off and the ammonia and nonnitrogenous substances pass into the blood by diffusion. Something like this will explain the facts as we at present know them. It is likely, moreover, that these products of protein metamorphosis undergo some further modification in the tissue spaces before they enter the blood. In a similar manner, the greater part of the sugars reach the blood-vascular system, though possibly some small portion may be taken up by the lymph. The fate of the fats has been a matter of great discussion. It is a fact that globules of fat can be demonstrated by appropriate methods within the columnar cells. On the older theory, the cells in question took up the fats, which are in a finely emulsified state, bodily, by a sort of amœboid action. We know now, however, that the most of the fats ingested are hydrolyzed in the intestine into fatty acids and glycerin. These, with the soaps, are soluble, and are probably taken up in this form by the columnar cells and there recombined to form neutral fats. For, it has been shown experimentally, that if we feed an animal with fatty acids, neutral fats can be demonstrated in the epithelium. Apparently, then, the columnar cells can synthesize the products of fat decomposition, and even supply the glycerin for the purpose. The recombined fats are then taken up by the lymph-radicles and pass into the central lacteals, and eventually into the thoracic duct and general circulation. As in the case of the proteins, the fats undergo transformation in their passage from the epithelium to the lacteals, for a large part of the fat in the chyle is in a state of fine division or molecular disintegration.

The carbohydrates, chiefly in the form of sugars, are taken up by the epithelium and passed into the portal blood. To some extent, also, dextrin can be dealt with by the columnar cells.

The water is taken up by the mucosa of the small intestine, but the amount lost in this way is replaced by water excreted by the cells, for the contents of the bowel at the ileocecal valve are just about as fluid as those at the duodenum. The chief absorption of water takes place in the large bowel, so that the feces, when they reach the rectum, are firm and comparatively dry. In cases of constipation almost the whole of the water may be taken up and the stools become hard, stony, and scybalous.

The fate of the unused ferments is somewhat doubtful. Probably, they are not resorbed, but are destroyed in the colon.

We must not leave this part of the subject of absorption without a brief reference to the role played by the leukocytes in the process. During digestion numerous leukocytes can be seen in the subepithelial connective tissue, between the columnar cells, and on the surface of the mucous membrane of the intestine, which are apparently attracted from the vessels and tissue spaces by positive chemiotaxis. This fact was long ago pointed out by Heidenhain, and has been amply demonstrated by numerous observers since. One part, at least, of their function is connected with absorption, for fat and the precursors of fat can be detected in their substance by appropriate methods. A. B. Macallum[1] has very prettily and conclusively shown that the leukocytes can take up foreign substances, notably iron. Experimenting with the lake lizard (necturus), he took an animal that had fasted for thirty months (to insure that the intestine would be empty) and fed it on albuminate and peptonate of iron. Killing the lizard eight hours later, he found leukocytes laden with iron within the lumen of the bowel between the columnar cells of the mucosa, and even in the capillaries of the liver and spleen, showing that, through the agency of leukocytes, iron could enter the portal system and general circulation. Presumably the same would hold good for other substances, bacteria and foodstuffs. We must, however, interpret this attraction of the leukocytes to the mucous surface of the bowel with some caution, for the same thing occurs as a result of the exhibition of a saline purge, such as magnesium sulphate, where the process at work is quite the reverse of absorption. Still, this probably only means that in this case, also, we have to deal with an irritation and stimulation of the secreting cells, which determines the attraction of the leukocytes. It is altogether likely that the leukocytes play an important part in the function of absorption, perhaps not so much in the case of the neutral fats, but more especially in regard to proteins and the soluble products of digestion. There is, however, another way in which the leukocytes may, possibly, be important. According to Delezenne, enterokinase can be obtained from leukocytes and the cells of lymphatic glands. Whether the former have absorbed the substance from the intestinal contents or its wall, or whether they

[1] Jour. of Phys., 16: 1894: 268.

are capable of manufacturing it independently, we do not yet know, but either or both may very well be true. We have indications, at any rate, that ferment action is a universal property of protein molecules wherever found. Henriot has described a fat-splitting ferment in the blood serum, and Cohnstein and Michaelis find evidences of the existence of a similar one in the red blood corpuscles. Blood also is known to contain oxydases. Consequently, the question of the assimilation of foodstuffs carries us very much beyond the mere consideration of the alimentary tract itself. This aspect of the subject is new and the field almost untrodden, but the possibilities are immense.

We shall be helped to a better understanding of the disorders that may attend absorption if we bear in mind the chief factors in the mechanism of this function. It is evident, from what has been said above, that the structures mainly concerned are the columnar cells lining the mucosa of the gastro-intestinal tract, the bloodvessels, and the lymphatic system. Disorders of absorption would naturally, then, be likely to attend disturbance of any portion of this mechanism. But there is another way in which these disorders might arise. The stomach and intestine may contain abnormal substances that are actually deleterious to the economy, or secretions that are quite normal may be resorbed instead of passing away.

We must admit that our knowledge of the pathology of absorption is far from being complete, but some points seem fairly clear. The intestinal mucosa constitutes, as it were, a first line of defence. So long as the layer of columnar cells is intact, it is possible for secretory and absorptive processes to go on normally, and a powerful barrier exists against microbic invasion. Should a solution of continuity occur, or should the vitality of the lining cells be damaged, then infection and intoxication are likely to be induced. Yet this is not absolutely necessary, for it has been shown conclusively that under certain circumstances bacteria may penetrate a normal mucosa. Notably is this the case with the bacillus of tuberculosis. Similarly, soluble toxins may pass in. Some of these may be ingested with the food, while others are produced *in situ* by abnormal decompositions and bacterial fermentations. Thus, ptomaines, like neurin, mydalein, mytilotoxin, and tyrotoxicon, may be present in putrefying food. Specific bacteria, such as the typhoid bacillus, the cholera vibrio, the bacillus of tuberculosis, and the actinomyces bovis, may lead to infections of alimentary origin. Or, again, chemical substances, like the metallic salts, aromatic compounds, and the fatty acids, may cause trouble. In the vast majority of cases, however, these substances are distinctly irritating and lead to injury of the intestinal mucosa.

Normally, the gastro-intestinal tract contains bacteria in considerable numbers and some variety.[1] The excessive growth of these is held in check by the acid in the stomach, and by the biliary acids, the fatty acids resulting from the decomposition of fats, and the digestive secretions, in the intestine. Perhaps, of even more importance, is the regular and

---

[1] Strasburger estimated (Zeitsch. f. klin. Med., 46: 1902: 413) that about one-third of the dry matter of normal human feces consisted of bacterial remains.

frequent elimination from the body of fecal matter, whereby stasis is prevented and little time is allowed for development to occur. In the large bowel, where the refuse products are retained longest, the greater part of the nutritive material has been absorbed and there is less for the bacteria to decompose. Probably, too, those microörganisms that may be called the natural inhabitants of the alimentary tract perform a useful function in antagonizing the effects of foreign invaders.

Disorders may be brought about by excessive multiplication of the normal bacterial inhabitants of the tract or an increase in their virulence. Indigestible food, disturbances of secretion, and motility are competent to cause the former condition, while strangulation of the bowel may cause the latter.[1] Local inflammation and irritation of the bowel often then result. Pathogenic bacteria of extraneous origin, when ingested, do not always produce serious results, for they may be rendered inert by the various agencies already referred to. But if they gain entrance to the body in large numbers, or in small doses frequently repeated, or if their virulence be high, infection usually occurs. Their pathogenic powers will be aided by any diminution of vigor in the ordinary bacterial flora, or by diminished resistance on the part of the mucosa.[2]

Disturbances affecting the vitality of the lining columnar cells of the gastro-intestinal mucous membrane, if widespread, seriously interfere with absorption. Thus, in enteritis of a moderate grade, the absorption of fats is diminished, and in the most severe forms the absorption of all kinds of foodstuffs is difficult or impossible. Where only small isolated patches of the mucosa are involved this result does not follow. Thus, in most cases of typhoid fever the power of absorption is not notably diminished.

Passive congestion of the intestines will delay absorption and especially interferes with the absorption of fats. Obstruction of the lymphatics, such as occurs in tuberculosis of the bowels and mesenteric glands, notably hampers the absorption of the fats.

Increased peristalsis, as in diarrhœa, if affecting the small bowel, will seriously diminish absorption by lessening the time that the chyme remains in contact with the mucosa. When due to disordered conditions of the large bowel, the absorption of water is lessened, but the effect on the general nutrition is not so great, for by the time the foodstuffs have reached the colon the greater part of the nutritive material has already been extracted.

A number of serious disturbances may arise from the resorption of the secretions normally found in the intestines. A certain amount of resorption is, indeed, physiological. For example, the solidity of the feces found in the large bowel indicates that a considerable amount of water is taken again into the circulation. The increase in the viscosity of the bile contained within the gall-bladder, as compared with that found in

---

[1] Macaigne, Arch. gén. de Méd., December, 1896.

[2] The reader will find the subject of intoxication and infection originating in the digestive tract dealt with in vol. i, pp. 300 and 323, and may also consult Herter, the Common Bacterial Infections of the Digestive Tract, New York, 1907.

the ducts, points in the same direction. It is probable, too, that a considerable proportion of the bile salts and pigments are resorbed from the intestine. We have, in fact, to recognize a reversibility of cellular action. According to the direction of the forces exerted upon a cell or series of cells, either secretion or resorption will take place. Under ordinary circumstances resorption is followed by no noticeable effects, but should a given secretion be resorbed in excess, or should it be taken up by cells other than those that produced it, far-reaching disorders are certain to follow. The most important disorders that we have to consider here are those connected with the bile and pancreatic secretion.

Bile will be resorbed into the circulation if from any cause there be obstruction to its free discharge into the intestine. This may be brought about by calculi in the common or hepatic ducts, a catarrh of the finer bile channels (cholangitis), tumors of the common bile duct or the head of the pancreas, enlarged glands or abscesses at the hilus of the liver, and tumors of the liver itself. The condition is evidenced clinically by **jaundice**, slowed pulse, mental hebetude, itchiness of the skin, and lessened coagulability of the blood. According to the degree of obstruction, the digestive processes within the bowel are interfered with, as described above, and the stools are more or less devoid of their normal brown pigment. Bile can be detected in the urine. The immediate mechanical effect is dilatation of the bile passages, particularly the capillaries, with compression and, possibly, atrophy of the parenchymatous cells of the liver. The retained bile passes into the lymph-channels and the venous system and eventually reaches the general circulation. The resorption of the bile is dependent not only on the degree of the mechanical obstruction, but on the character of the secretion also. A thick, viscid bile may be resorbed even when the obstruction is comparatively slight, as might result, for example, from a catarrh of the finer bile passages or swollen hepatic cells. The icterus found in phosphorus and toluylendiamin poisoning, snake-bite, and certain infections and intoxications is of this type. The toxic symptoms are referable to the presence of the bile salts in the blood, as has repeatedly been demonstrated experimentally. The cholates, even in small quantities, stimulate the vagi, and larger amounts act upon the heart itself and produce convulsions. The resorption of bile from the intestines in such amounts as to produce jaundice, in the absence of mechanical obstruction to its outpouring, is hardly likely, though Quincke has considered this probable in the case of icterus neonatorum. Jaundice can be brought about, of course, in other ways besides obstruction, but this phase of the subject does not concern us here. For fuller information on this part of the subject, the reader is referred elsewhere in this work (vol. i, p. 967 et seq.).

Obstruction to the free outpouring of the pancreatic secretion may at times be followed by serious results. Dilatation of the ducts and the fine ramifications of the ducts within the acini are the immediate sequel, but a chronic interstitial inflammation with fibrosis is eventually set up. Obstruction of a lateral branch leads to cystic dilatation, provided that the cells of the affected lobule are capable of secretion. Some of these retention cysts attain a relatively enormous size. Should large areas of the secreting structure be destroyed by catarrhal inflammation and pressure, the internal secretion of the pancreas may be interfered with and a form of glycosuria result. Obstruction to the outflow of secretion may be produced by new-growths and fibrosis in the head of the pancreas, or a calculus impacted in the ampulla of Vater. Should the calculus be of a certain shape and size, and so placed as to allow the entry of bile into the pancreatic duct, acute hemorrhagic pancreatitis is apt to be set up. This is associated with a curious condition, known as **fat necrosis**, in which whitish opaque areas are to be found in the fatty tissues surrounding the pancreas, the omentum, the appendices epiploicæ, the mesentery, and peritoneum. It has been shown to be due to the action of the fat-splitting ferment of the pancreatic juice upon the fat, whereby glycerin, fatty acids, and calcium soaps are formed in the tissues. The diffusion out of the secretion appears to be due to pressure within the ducts or to actual injury to the cells. The condition has been met with in other forms of inflammation of the pancreas, but is rare in cases of suppuration (see vol. i, p. 982).

THE RELATIONSHIP OF DISEASES OF THE ALIMENTARY TRACT TO DISORDERS OF THE GENERAL SYSTEM.

As we have had occasion to point out already, the alimentary tract is brought into close connection with the other great systems of the body through the blood and lymph-circulation and by means of the nervous mechanism. It is not surprising, therefore, that disorders of other systems, or of the body as a whole, will often have a profound effect upon the digestive organs, and *vice versa*. The cells of the alimentary system being both absorptive and eliminative in their functions, we are prepared to find that intoxication and infection will bulk very largely in any consideration of this part of our subject.

It is a well-recognized principle in pathology that when one organ or system is from any cause inhibited in its action, others will attempt to take up the work and carry it on as perfectly as they may. This is known as the *law of vicarious function*. It is particularly well exemplified in the case of glandular organs, and the attempt at compensation is often manifested by structural change as well as increase or perversion of function. Instances might be multiplied and are not wanting in connection with the alimentary system. As a corollary to this, it can be laid down that the excessive secretion of any gland, if it result in a great loss of the body fluids, will be accompanied by diminished activity of other secretory organs. A familiar example of the first class is the elimination of urea and other substances by the skin and mucous membranes in cases of chronic Bright's disease. Here it is not uncommon to get stomatitis and diarrhœa as a result. Ulceration of the lower bowel is a not infrequent accompaniment also. The exposure of the body to alternations of heat and cold is frequently followed by diarrhœa in some people. This is, in part, due to the interference with perspiration, to splanchnic congestion, but, possibly also, there may be a nervous element as well. Suppressed menstruation, the absorption of abscesses, the retrocession of eruptions in smallpox, measles, and scarlatina, are occasionally followed by diarrhœa. Gout in many cases is associated with a looseness of the bowels; in fact, diarrhœa may be the only notable manifestation of the uratic diathesis (**diarrhœa arthritica**). Cases are known where checking the intestinal evacuations has been followed by the arthritic manifestations. Again, an example of the second group, the constipation of diabetes, often associated with dryness of the skin and mouth, is the result of the polyuria.

The diarrhœa that at times accompanies the infectious diseases, notably the exanthemata and pneumonia, is probably for the most part due to attempts at elimination and perverted excretion.

Other ways in which the stomach and bowels are affected in systemic diseases are through the circulatory and nervous systems. The diarrhœas met with in exophthalmic goitre and Addison's disease are apparently vasomotor in origin. That found in amyloid disease of the bowels is possibly due to interference with excretion and absorption, whereby irritation is set up. The vomiting, which is so often an early symptom of the onset of acute infectious disease, is due to efferent nervous impulses which cause excessive irritability. Constipation and diarrhœa may result from abnormal mental and nervous states, as, for example, in the acute infections, notably meningitis, in chronic lead poisoning, neurasthenia, and hysteria. Involuntary evacuations and diarrhœa occur in cases of coma, mental degradation, and hysteria.

The increasing number of studies that have been made in regard to the normal and abnormal digestive processes, especially in connection with bacterial activity within the intestine, serve to indicate our realization of the growing importance of this subject. While our knowledge is still far from complete, for the problems involved are of very wide range, sufficient has been gathered to prove that the absorption of deleterious substances from the gastro-intestinal tract is a frequent and most potent factor in the causation of disease elsewhere in the body. The list of affections that have, from time to time, been attributed by various authors to gastro-intestinal intoxication or infection is a formidable one, and, in our judgment, the relationship is in some instances based on inconclusive evidence. Yet in not a few cases the etiological association can be determined with some certainty. For example, we might cite the following affections of the various systems:

1. *Skin.*—Erythema; urticaria; dermatitis.
2. *Muscles.*—Polymyositis.
3. *Central Nervous System.*—Headache; mental hebetude; giddiness; insomnia; delirium; convulsions; coma; neurasthenia; various psychoses.
4. *Urinary System.*—Albuminuria; Bright's disease; oxaluria; cystinuria.
5. *Blood and Circulatory System.*—Chlorosis; pernicious anemia; eosinophilia; arteriosclerosis.

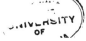

6. *Constitutional and Diathetic Conditions.*—Cachexia; glycosuria; uric acid diathesis.

In discussing this question it is not always possible to distinguish between the effects of intoxication and of infection. Bacteria are constantly present in the alimentary tract and their number and virulence are very rapidly increased under certain circumstances. Derangements of the digestive secretions and, above all, impaired motility are the most potent factors in this connection. In addition, then, to the toxic substances that may be introduced into the alimentary tract from without, or that may be produced by disordered function, we have to reckon with those resulting from bacterial metabolism and abnormal fermentation, and in many cases with the entry into the system of the microörganisms themselves. The majority of intoxications originating from the digestive system are of the exogenous type, though some few are of a mixed exogenous and endogenous nature (see also vol. i, pp. 300 and 302).

The toxic agents under discussion may, therefore, be divided into three main classes: (1) Those introduced from without; (2) those resulting from the action of the digestive ferments within the gastro-intestinal tube; (3) the products of bacterial activity.

1. In the first group we include (*a*) chemical and mineral substances, such as lead, copper, arsenic, acids, alkalies, numerous salts, alcohol, ptomaines, and other nitrogenous bases derived from the putrefaction of protein matter; (*b*) parasites, both vegetable and animal; and (*c*) saprophytes.

To take but a few of these by way of illustration. Lead, if absorbed in small quantities over a prolonged period of time, produces anemia, arteriosclerosis, interstitial nephritis, various paralyses, and mental degradation. Arsenic causes anemia and muscular paralyses. Alcohol has a special tendency to attack the nervous system and leads to the deposit of fat.

The products of bacterial fermentation, including the ptomaines, of which there are now a great number recognized, produce a variety of symptoms of an acute nature, but the chief features are gastro-intestinal irritation, colic, vomiting, and diarrhœa; later, headache, muscular weakness, collapse, coma, and death.

The second subclass includes moulds, yeasts, and bacteria of many kinds, trichinæ, and the eggs of various intestinal worms, which may contaminate the food.

Of alimentary infection with bacteria, typhoid fever and cholera may be taken as the types. It would seem, however, that a considerable quantity of the particular microörganism must be ingested, or repeated small doses during a prolonged period, before general infection can take place. An intact mucous membrane can apparently render inert a reasonable amount of bacteria, as experiments have shown, but infection at once takes place if there be a lowered vitality of the parts, such as may be produced by a gastro-intestinal catarrh. It is known, too, that on occasion bacteria may pass the barrier interposed by the mucosa without producing a local lesion, and set up disease elsewhere. Typhoid fever without intestinal ulceration can occur, and tuberculosis of the lungs may result from ingested bacilli without evidence of intestinal disturbance.

The various ways in which the larger intestinal parasites produce their effects have already been discussed (vol. i, p. 343).

Thirdly, saprophytes act by producing diffusible toxins which may be absorbed into the system. They are of little importance here. Perhaps the only ones deserving mention are the cholera vibrio and Oïdium albicans, and this latter is rarely so extensive in its distribution as to cause serious trouble.

2. Under the second category we have to deal with the effects of diminished or increased secretion of the digestive ferments, of resorption of the ferments and the products of ferment action.

Diminished secretion, by lengthening the time required for digestion, leads to the presence of undigested food in the stomach and bowel, causes irritation of the mucosa, and promotes the activity of bacteria. Thus, athrepsia may result in long-continued cases, and in the less severe ones, gastro-intestinal irritation, pain, tympanites, and diarrhœa.

Hypersecretion will produce pain, vomiting, and, in the end, malnutrition.

The resorption of the secretions, particularly the bile and the pancreatic juice, has already been dealt with in so far as the local effect on the liver and pancreas is concerned (P. 377). The resorption of bile produces systemic effects; the slow pulse, itching of the skin, mental dulness, coma, and hemolysis are to be attributed to the action of the contained biliary salts.

Whether the pancreatic secretion is ever resorbed into the circulation in sufficient amount to produce systemic effects has not yet been determined. Any result is probably indirect, the passage out of the pancreatic secretion into the substance of the organ leading to chronic irritation, fibrosis, and atrophy of the secreting structures, so that eventually glycosuria results.

The resorption of bile salts and pigments by way of the intestinal mucosa is believed to be a physiological process and is of no special importance. Jaundice and cholemia never seem to be produced in this way. The gastric and pancreatic ferments that are not utilized may also possibly undergo resorption, but observations made so far would seem to show that this rarely occurs to any extent.

Toxic substances are produced in the course of the ordinary physiological processes of digestion. Among these may be mentioned:

(a) Those derived from protein disintegration: Albumoses, peptone, indol, skatol, phenol, leucin, tyrosin, fatty acids, acetone, ammonia, cystin, carbon dioxide, hydrogen, sulphuretted and carburetted hydrogen, and methyl mercaptan.

(b) Those derived from carbohydrates: Formic, acetic, propionic, butyric, valerianic, lactic, and succinic acids, acetone, and various gases.

(c) Those derived from fats: Fatty acids and glycerin.

It is unlikely that, under normal circumstances, any of these substances are absorbed in sufficient quantity to cause disturbance, for the peristalsis of the intestine hurries them along, and they are either gradually neutralized as they reach the lower bowel or are quickly eliminated.

In cases of obstruction, however, they might be expected to play a part by causing irritation of the mucous membrane, and with the multiplication of the bacterial flora of the intestine which inevitably occurs in such cases, they join their forces with those of the similar substances resulting from putrefactive fermentation.

3. The activity of the microörganisms normally found within the gastro-intestinal tract is kept within bounds by the acidity of the gastric secretion, the presence of bile, and the regular evacuation of the intestinal contents. The bacteria that are present under these circumstances may be regarded as non-pathogenic, yet, on occasion, their numbers and virulence may be so increased as to produce pathological effects. This is particularly the case when there is constipation, strangulation, or some inflammatory affection of the bowel. The bacteria may actually pass through the wall of the intestine, if its vitality be lowered in this way, even at times without any solution of continuity, and may set up a general infection, or, in many instances, a peritonitis. In the same way, perforation or rupture of the bowel is followed by an infective inflammation of the peritoneum. The systemic effects of constipation, irritability, mental dulness, headache, malaise, and earthiness of the skin, are, no doubt, attributable to the slow absorption of toxins, in large part of bacterial origin, from the lumen of the bowel. Where actual organic obstruction exists, the symptoms are much more intense, namely, pain, headache, vomiting, intense prostration, lowered temperature, a weak circulation, coma, and perhaps death. The higher up in the bowel the obstruction is, the more severe are the manifestations, for the absorptive powers of the mucous membrane are much more active in the small bowel than in the large. In conditions of health, however, what might be termed the natural inhabitants of the gastro-intestinal tract probably exert a beneficent action in the economy, for they apparently have the power of inhibiting the activity of foreign intruders which may make their way into the bowel.[1] They may, however, be overborne in their resistance, should alien bacteria be introduced into the alimentary system in sufficiently large numbers, or if their vigor be diminished from any cause.

The bacteria in question produce their effects in two ways, by the excretion of the products of their own metabolism and by initiating abnormal processes of fermentation. In this manner are formed a variety of substances, such as the fatty acids, indol, skatol, phenol, compounds of the aromatic series, pyridin and chinolin bodies, diamins, toxalbumins, hydrogen, carbonic dioxide, and methane.

The effects produced may be local in the tract or its accessory organs. If acute, we may find degeneration, inflammation, or ulceration; if chronic, inflammation, atrophy, and fibrosis. At other times the resisting barriers are broken down, to the extent that toxins make their way into the circu-

---

[1] Bienstock, Arch. f. Hyg., 36: 1900: 335, and 39: 1900: 390. It is a matter of almost common knowledge now that bacteria of the lactic acid group, notably Bacillus Bulgaricus, have the power of inhibiting the action of harmful organisms in the bowel, which, according to Metchnikoff, are responsible for many degenerative processes throughout the body, and so tend to shorten life.

lation and set up general toxemia. Some of the substances absorbed, notably those resulting from protein decomposition, are rendered non-toxic by combination with sulphuric acid, glycocoll, and glycuronic acid, but, naturally, to this transformation there is a limit. We may gain a fair idea of the amount of putrefactive change going on in the bowel by estimating the amount of ethereal or aromatic sulphates in the urine, as they are both absolutely and relatively increased in amount in this condition. It should be remarked here, in passing, that it is possible that we have hitherto laid too great emphasis on the role played by the protein derivatives, for recent experiments would tend to indicate that the pernicious effects attributed to the products of protein decomposition are rather to be laid at the door of the potassium salts.

The interesting and very important attempts that have been made to elucidate the nature of hepatic cirrhosis, to take a familiar condition, will serve to illustrate the important part played by certain substances, products both of normal and abnormal fermentation. Hanot[1] was of the opinion that cirrhosis of the liver is due to the irritation produced by the absorption of certain substances resulting from disordered digestion. Hanot and Boix, in support of this theory, showed that atrophic cirrhosis of the liver could be produced in rabbits by the administration of lactic, butyric, and valerianic acids. The deleterious effects of potassium salts is well shown by some experiments of Lancereaux.[2] He noticed that in Paris cirrhosis of the liver was more common in those drinking wine than in those using other alcoholic beverages. This he attributed to the fact that many of the wines contained sulphate of potassium to render them "dry." Some of these "plastered" wines contained as much as four to six grams per liter of this substance. By feeding rabbits, guinea-pigs, and dogs with sulphate of potash for from six to eighteen months he could produce typical portal cirrhosis.

While the attention of these observers was concentrated on the determination of one particular point, it may be remarked, in criticism of their conclusions, that one cannot exclude the influence of bacteria in contributing to the result. That bacteria and their toxins play an important role in this connection cannot be doubted. Krawkow[3] has noted that cirrhosis could be induced by giving bacterial toxins by the mouth. Ramon,[4] also, tried a number of feeding experiments on different series of animals, giving (1) alcohol, (2) microbic toxins, (3) living cultures of bacteria, and (4) alternate doses of alcohol and bacterial toxins. The animals to whom the cultures were administered died of septicemia, with fatty degeneration of the liver. Those fed on alcohol alone developed fatty livers. In one case, in which alternating doses of alcohol and toxins were given, the animal, after surviving ten months, exhibited signs of hepatic cirrhosis. The influence of alcohol in the pathogenesis of cirrhosis has been the subject of much debate. Some have held that it sets up a gastro-intestinal catarrh, and that then the toxins elaborated are carried to the liver and set up the disturbance. Others think that

[1] Arch. gén. de Méd., i:1899:3.   [2] Bull. de l'Acad. de Méd., 38:1897:202.
[3] Arch. de Méd. expér. et d'Anat. path., 1896:106 and 244.
[4] Presse Médicale, April 21, 1897:178.

the alcohol, being quickly absorbed, is carried directly to the liver and leads to irritation and degeneration. Still others, like Ramon, take an intermediate position, holding that gastro-intestinal catarrh alone does not explain the condition, but that alcohol promotes the absorption of toxins from the bowel, and, moreover, lessens the power of the liver to resist them. Further, Bindo de Vecchi[1] was able to produce proliferation of the interstitial connective tissue of the liver by introducing certain germs into the intestine. His experiments point to the pathogenicity of the B. coli. Weaver[2] obtained similar results by the subcutaneous injection of a germ belonging to the colon group, which he isolated from guinea-pigs dying spontaneously, and Hektoen,[3] with a bacillus of the pseudodiphtheria type. Very recently, too, W. C. Mac-Callum has shown that chloroform is competent to produce degeneration of the liver parenchyma, but not cirrhosis. But where injections of B. coli are employed as well, cirrhosis could be produced. The preponderance of evidence, therefore, goes to show that certain products of fermentation in the bowel are competent to produce cirrhosis. Bacteria, also, while in general they are likely to produce acute lesions of a suppurative type, or even septicemia, can, if sufficiently attenuated, lead to a slow proliferative change. Apparently, however, before bacteria can act, there must be a lowering of the vitality of the liver parenchyma. This can be produced by alcohol, bacterial toxins, and certain organic fatty acids.

The hemolytic action of certain microörganisms and their toxins has now, for some years, been widely recognized. It is not at all improbable, and there is a certain amount of evidence in favor of it, that certain forms of severe anemia and the deposit of iron pigment in various parts of the body are due to gastro-intestinal intoxication and infection. Hunter,[4] for example, is a strong upholder of the view that pernicious anemia is infective in origin. His earlier observations tended to the conclusion that this disease is due to the hemolytic action of some special toxin elaborated in and absorbed from some part of the alimentary tract. This toxin is not simply the product of ordinary fermentative and putrefactive processes, but is of a special infective origin. Later, he showed that the region of the greatest absorption was the stomach, but to some extent the buccal and intestinal mucosæ. The important etiological factors in the disease are carious teeth, stomatitis, and glossitis, which lead to an infective gastritis. Certain local conditions in the stomach, such as malignant disease, gastritis, and atrophy of the mucous membrane, also predispose. The nature of the infecting agent is not clear, but it is possibly of a mixed kind.

One other phase of this subject, in conclusion, demands a few words. There is now abundant evidence to show that microörganisms are constantly gaining an entrance into the system by way of the alimentary tract. Ruffer,[5] on examining sections taken from the small intestine of healthy rabbits, found that leukocytes were present on the surface of the mucosa; others, again, between the epithelial cells, that had engulfed

[1] Lo Sperimentale, An. 53:3. [2] Trans. Chicago Path. Soc., 3:1900:228.
[3] Jour. Path. and Bact., 7:1901:214. [4] Lancet, London, i:1900:221, 296, 371.
[5] Brit. Med. Jour., 2:1890:491.

bacteria. ·The Peyer's patches contained immense numbers of micro-organisms, apparently within the lymphoid cells. Bizzozero[1] and Ruffer found an analogous state of things in the case of the rabbit's tonsil. Further, the leukocytes, travelling back from the surface to the lymphoid follicles, were taken up by certain large cells (macrophages) and eventually digested, together with any bacteria or foodstuffs they might contain. One of us (A. G. N.[2]), also, has demonstrated that microörganisms can be found in various stages of disintegration within the capillary vessels of the mesentery in rabbits, cats, dogs, and in the human subject at postmortem. Others, again, may be detected in the meshes of the tissues, grouped about the nuclei of what are presumably wandering cells, and within the lining endothelia of the vessels. Carrying the thought one step farther, Bizzozero and Ribbert[3] showed the presence of bacteria within the normal mesenteric gland. Finally, Nicholls[4] and Ford[5] have proved that bacteria can be recovered from healthy organs by cultivation. Recently, Wrosczek has brought forward a pretty confirmation of these studies. Feeding healthy animals on food contaminated with non-pathogenic pigmented microörganisms, he regained these by cultures from the internal organs without there being the slightest evidence of any lesion of the alimentary tract. These observations, taken together, prove beyond question that micro-organisms are constantly passing into the recesses of the organism from the gastro-intestinal mucous membrane. These do not, as a rule, lead to infection, for they are quickly rendered inert by the action of the leukocytes, the various endothelia, and, probably, the body juices. Still, a certain number of them may retain a limited degree of vitality, a potentiality for harm that on occasion may be called into activity. This latency of germs, termed by one of us (J. G. A.[6]) "subinfection," and noted also by others, particularly Schnitzler,[7] probably explains those puzzling cases of terminal and "cryptogenic" infection occasionally met with. Less intense than this action, we must recognize, we think, a "condition in which, as a consequence of chronic inflammatory disturbances in connection with the gastro-intestinal tract, there may, for long periods, pass in through the walls of the stomach or of the intestine a greater number of bacteria; and while the bacteria undergo the normal and inevitable destruction by the cells of the lymph-glands, the liver, the kidneys, and other organs, nevertheless the excessive action of the cells and the effect on them of the bacterial toxins liberated in the process of destruction may eventually lead to grave changes in the cells and in the organs of which they are part—changes of a chronic nature." Probably, in this way we should explain many of the forms of chronic fibrosis which occur so insidiously in the various organs.

[1] Centralbl. f. d. med. Wiss., 23:491.   [2] Jour. Med. Research, 11:1904:2.
[3] Deutsche med. Woch., 11:1885:197.
[4] Canadian Jour. of Med. and Surg., 6:1899:405.
[5] Trans. Assoc. Amer. Phys., 15:1900:389.
[6] Jour. Amer. Med. Assoc., 33:1899:1506 and 1572.
[7] Arch. f. klin. Chir., 59:1899:866.

CHAPTER XVII

THE MOUTH.

CONGENITAL ANOMALIES.

ABNORMALITIES in the structure of the oral cavity and its associated parts are not infrequent. Certain of them are of great practical importance, inasmuch as they interfere with speech or the proper manipulation of the food.

Astomia, or complete absence of the mouth, is very rare. It is usually associated with other defects of development, and is, of course, incompatible with life. The mouth may be excessively large (**macrostomia**), or exceptionally small (**microstomia**). The buccal cavity may be present but the external orifice wanting (**atresia oris**).

Abnormal shortness of the frenum of the tongue (**tongue-tie**) is by no means uncommon. All newborn infants should be examined for this condition, as it may seriously interfere with nursing. The tongue may be **double**, or cleft at the tip (**snake-tongue**).

Among the commonest and most important anomalies are **harelip** and **cleft palate**. Harelip is unilateral or bilateral, the fissure or fissures being situated to one side of the median line at the lines of junction between the intermaxillary and the supramaxillary bones. Various grades of the condition are met with, from a slight notching of the edge of the lip to a deep cleft sometimes reaching into the nasal cavity (**Cheilognatho-palatoschisis**). The defect may also extend into the hard palate or even into the soft palate. In the latter case the fissure assumes a median position.

Anomalies in the development of the jaws, such as **agnathia, brachygnathia, hemignathia, ateloprosopia**, are occasionally met with.

Defects in the teeth are common but relatively unimportant. Hutchinson has described certain peculiarities associated with congenital syphilis. The upper central incisors are the teeth affected. They are peg-shaped, short, and thin, the top being smaller than the crown. There is a small concave notch in the cutting edge. The affected teeth are often yellow in color. The condition is not absolutely pathognomonic, being found in other conditions, notably rickets.

CIRCULATORY DISTURBANCES.

The structures forming the buccal cavity are among the most vascular in the body. Consequently, alterations in the quantity or the quality of the blood are easily recognized and afford valuable clinical evidence of disease.

Hyperemia.—Active Hyperemia.—Active hyperemia occurs physiologically with the act of mastication, but as a pathological condition is an evidence of local irritation or a manifestation of certain of the infective fevers.

Koplik's sign in measles is an eruption of irregular hyperemic spots of bright red color, often having a small, bluish-white centre, which appears on the buccal or labial mucosa some hours or even days before the appearance of the skin exanthem. Occurring as it does so early, sometimes even before the catarrhal symptoms have developed, it is a valuable aid in diagnosis.

Passive Hyperemia.—Passive hyperemia is met with especially in obstructive cardiac and pulmonary affections. The lips and buccal mucosa assume a dull reddish-purple color.

Anemia.—Anemia may be one manifestation of severe general anemia. The mucous membrane appears pallid or even quite bloodless in such cases. Anemia of the soft palate is frequently associated with pulmonary and laryngeal tuberculosis.

INFLAMMATIONS.

Inflammation of the lips is termed **cheilitis**; of the mouth, **stomatitis**; of the tongue, **glossitis**; of the gums, **gingivitis**.

Stomatitis.—Catarrhal Stomatitis, Cheilitis, and Glossitis.—These affections are usually brought about by the action of mechanical, thermic, or chemical irritants. Excessive indulgence in alcohol or tobacco are of importance in this connection. Catarrhal glossitis is a constant accompaniment of all febrile conditions, and catarrhal inflammation of the whole buccal mucosa is often observed in infectious fevers. The mucous membrane of the lips, cheeks, tongue, and alveolar processes is reddened, swollen, and covered with secretion. The papillæ of the tongue may swell, giving it a granular appearance. The secretion contains leukocytes and desquamated epithelial cells. If it be allowed to remain, the exudate collects upon the tongue and about the roots of the teeth in the form of a dry, dirty, grayish-white, or brown coating (*sordes*). The lips and tongue often become dry, fissured, and ulcerated.

Aphthous Stomatitis.—This presents all the features of the catarrhal form, but is further characterized by the formation of small grayish or yellowish-white spots, either single or in clusters, usually upon the lips and tongue. The spots in question have a dull, opaque appearance, and are bounded by a bright red hyperemic zone. They may coalesce and form large patches. According to E. Fraenkel, the process is essentially a fibrinous inflammation.

The affection is usually found in children who are badly nourished and whose mouths are not kept properly clean. It has been met with in women at the menstrual periods, during pregnancy, and in the puerperium.   It is not uncommon also in those who have been on protracted sprees.

Ulcerative Stomatitis.—Ulcerative stomatitis is an acute affection, rarely chronic, which begins in the gums near the roots of the teeth. The tissues are at first red, swollen, and œdematous, and may form warty projections.   The gums tend to loosen from the teeth.   Later, the parts become pale, spongy, and friable, bleeding at the slightest touch, and eventually necrosis sets in.   The ulceration may extend to the lips and cheeks, and may penetrate deeply, leading to sequestration of the bone of the jaw.   The teeth not infrequently fall out.   Salivation is a marked feature, and the breath possesses a peculiarly offensive, penetrating odor.

The disease attacks by preference those who are badly nourished or who are weakened by long-standing disease.   It is found in diabetics, in persons suffering from scurvy, and in those who have been poisoned by mercury, phosphorus, lead, or copper.

Somewhat similar to this is the affection known as **pyorrhœa alveolaris**. This disease is, however, more chronic in its course, and is apt to progress insidiously with occasional acute exacerbations.   The gums are swollen, reddened, and spongy, bleeding readily, and show a tendency to retraction.   Gentle pressure will cause thin pus to exude from about the roots of the teeth.   In time the teeth loosen and fall out.

Single ulcers under the tongue are not uncommon in whooping-cough. A local ulcer, with irregular borders, situated near the frenum of the tongue, occurs epidemically and endemically in certain parts of Italy (Riga's disease).

Suppurative Stomatitis and Glossitis.—Suppurative processes, like erysipelas, may extend to the buccal cavity from without.   **Suppurative gingivitis and glossitis** may also result from direct trauma and infection. They may be met with as complications in certain infective fevers and in Bright's disease.   Suppurative glossitis is a rare complication of typhoid fever.   One of us (A. G. N.[1]) has recorded a case of hemiglossitis in this disease, and Thomas McCrae has published a similar instance and collected five others from the literature.[2]   The whole tongue or any portion of it may be affected.   The condition may be diffuse or phlegmonous, or multiple small abscesses may be found.

Gangrenous Stomatitis.—Gangrenous stomatitis (*noma; cancrum oris; cancer aquaticus; Wasserkrebs*) is a peculiarly rapid and fatal form of gangrene affecting the face, almost certainly of infective nature.   With few exceptions the disease is met with in badly fed and uncared-for children, especially when debilitated from disease.   It not infrequently complicates one of the acute infective fevers.   Rarely, it originates independently, or supervenes upon acute ulcerative stomatitis.   Children between the ages of two and twelve are those usually attacked.

The affection begins with the formation of a livid, swollen patch in

---

[1] Nicholls, Montreal Med. Jour., 25:1896:104.
[2] McCrae, Johns Hopkins Hosp. Bull., 9: 1898: 118.

the buccal mucous membrane, usually near the angle of the mouth, but sometimes in the gums. Small blisters form and the tissues present a grayish-yellow inflammatory infiltration that quickly becomes gangrenous. The structures in the neighborhood are infiltrated and œdematous. The gangrenous process quickly spreads until the whole thickness of the cheek is converted into a reddish-black necrotic material. The condition is usually unilateral, but may extend to the opposite side, and may even penetrate so deeply as to involve the bones of the nose and jaw. Septic infection of the whole system usually sets in and death soon results. In the rare event of healing taking place, the necrotic tissue separates and cicatricial contraction gradually ensues, often leading to considerable deformity.

No particular germ has as yet been proved to be the specific cause. Bishop and Ryan and Schimmelbusch have demonstrated the presence of a bacillus resembling that of diphtheria in some cases. It is not always to be found, however. The Klebs-Loeffler bacillus appears to be at fault in some cases.

Chronic Stomatitis.—Here the mucous membrane is infiltrated, the lymph-follicles enlarged, and the epithelium thickened and keratinized. Grayish or bluish-white flattened plaques (plaques opalines) are to be seen on the tongue and inner sides of the lips and cheeks. The cause is chronic irritation and the affection seems to have a particular relationship to syphilis and smoking. The condition is important, as it may afford a starting point for the development of carcinoma.

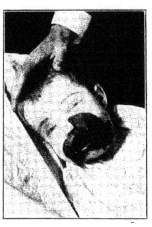

FIG. 79

Noma of the face or cancrum oris. (Case of Dr. A. T. Bazin.)

Specific Stomatitis.—**Thrush.**—Thrush is a mycotic stomatitis due to the action of a special fungus, Oïdium albicans. It is found usually in infants during the first year of life, but occasionally also in debilitated adults. The use of milk and starchy foods, with imperfect cleansing of the mouth, favors the process. The affection begins with diffuse reddening of the mucosa and the formation of a glistening, slimy, somewhat adhesive exudate of grayish appearance. Small, whitish dots next appear, which stand out prominently against the hyperemic background. These patches gradually increase and may coalesce to form a membrane. When this is removed, the underlying mucosa is greatly reddened and often eroded. The membrane quickly reappears upon the denuded surface. The disease usually begins on the tongue and the inner sides of the cheeks, but in bad cases may spread to the palate, lips, pharynx, œsophagus, or even to the stomach and intestines. The growth of the fungus begins in the epithelial layers and extends to the deeper structures. Exceptionally, mycotic emboli may find their way to the internal viscera.

Gonorrhœal stomatitis has occasionally been observed.

Diphtheria.—Diphtheria of the mouth is usually secondary to the ordinary pharyngeal diphtheria.

Tuberculosis.—Tuberculosis of the buccal cavity may be primary, but much more often is secondary to tuberculosis of the lungs or larynx, or to lupus of the face. In the secondary form the condition is set up by the passage of infective sputum over the mucous membrane. One or more small isolated nodules of grayish-yellow color are found on the dorsum of the tongue, usually near the tip, which eventually break down. A typical tuberculous ulcer of the tongue is round, oval, or irregular, and painful. The edges are slightly indurated and raised above the general level, inverted or undermined. The base is uneven and nodular, and covered with reddish-gray granulations, or a grayish or yellow shreddy slough. Smaller tubercles may form about the periphery of the main ulcer, which break down and coalesce with it. Primary tuberculosis occurs most frequently on the tongue, palate, and tonsils.

Syphilis.—The primary chancre is occasionally found upon the tongue, lip, or tonsil, but secondary and tertiary manifestations are far more common. The mildest form of the affection in the secondary stage is a simple erythema or *angina*, but the more characteristic appearance is the presence of small, flattened patches of grayish-yellow color situated on the gums or near the angles of the mouth (*mucous patches*). Not infrequently, the superficial epithelium assumes a peculiar bluish-white, pearly appearance, somewhat resembling the corrosion produced by nitrate of silver (*plaques opalines*). These are found ordinarily on the lips, cheeks, and tongue, but at times also on the gums, tonsils, and pharyngeal wall. Such lesions may go on to superficial ulceration and small fissures be produced. In young children radiating scars at the angles of the mouth (*rhagades*) are characteristic of syphilis. *Gummas* are situated most frequently in the posterior wall of the pharynx, the palate, gums, and tongue.

Gummas of the tongue generally occur about the centre of the dorsum, and give rise to deep, irregular excavations, having thickened, slightly concaved, or undermined edges, and a base covered with yellowish slough. They are generally bounded by a reddish areola.

The ulcerative lesions of tuberculosis, syphilis, and epithelioma, affecting the tongue, are not unlike one another, and an error of diagnosis may easily be made, a mistake which will, of course, have serious consequences to the patient. Tuberculous ulcers are usually situated on the dorsum of the tongue near the tip or toward the root; syphilitic gummas, on the dorsum near the middle; epitheliomatous ulcers, usually on the edge of the tongue, opposite the molar or bicuspid teeth. Epithelioma is more common in men than in women, and rarely occurs under the age of forty. The epitheliomatous ulcer has irregular, raised, hard, and everted edges, and the tissues about it are much indurated. It spreads rapidly, and is attended with neuralgic pain and much salivation. Tuberculous and tertiary syphilitic ulcers are not indurated and the edges are not everted. Glandular involvement is not found, while it is common in the case of epithelioma. The history often affords a clue to the nature of the lesion. In the case of tuberculosis of the tongue there is usually evidence of tuberculosis in the lungs or elsewhere; in

FIG. 80

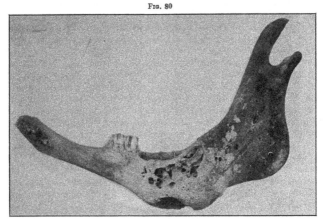

Actinomycosis ("lumpy jaw") of the lower jaw of a cow. Note the overgrowth of bone and the inflammatory osteoporosis. (From the Pathological Museum, McGill University.)

FIG. 81

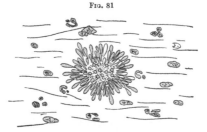

Actinomycosis fungus in pus. Fresh, unstained preparation. Magnified about 500 diameters. (Abbott.)

gummas of the tongue, we may have a history of specific infection and of gummas in other situations; in epithelioma, we have the irritating influence of a pipe or tooth, or again, the new-growth may originate from an old scar, from a primary luetic sore, or from leukoplakia.

Actinomycosis.—This disease is not uncommon in cattle, giving rise to the condition known as **"lumpy jaw."** The jaw becomes hard and wooden, or, in the more acute forms, may be riddled with sinuses. Rarefaction and hyperplasia of the bone may take place. The disease is occasionally seen in man, and is perhaps more common than has been suspected.

The disease is due to infection of the tissues with a ray fungus, the *actinomyces bovis*. The usual point of entrance is the mucous membrane of the mouth and pharynx, especially in the neighborhood of a carious tooth. Israel and Partsch have demonstrated the presence of the fungus in the cavities of decayed teeth. The actinomyces is believed to be present on the stalks of certain kinds of grass. Infection has followed the practice of picking the teeth with a stalk of hay, or with a needle. A few instances are on record in which granulomatous tumors have been formed upon the tongue (Claisse[1]). When the jaw is attacked, the appearances produced are not unlike those of periosteal sarcoma, but when the looser tissues of the neck are reached growth is very rapid, following the line of the fascia. From the face and neck the process may invade the meninges and the brain and cord, or the thoracic organs. If an incision be made into the mass, before suppuration has occurred, minute yellowish dots are to be seen, which are the actinomyces. If there be a discharge, careful search should be made for the fungi, which appear as yellowish masses (sulphur grains) the size of a pin-head or smaller. These may be picked out and examined with a low-power lens, or a film may be made and stained by Gram's method. In human actinomycosis the filaments are apt to lack the characteristic clubbed appearance.

PROGRESSIVE METAMORPHOSES.

Occasionally, the squamous epithelium covering the tongue becomes thickened and gives rise to plaques of a firm, somewhat glistening appearance (**leukoplakia** or **psoriasis linguæ**). Some attribute this condition to chronic inflammation, notably syphilis. The affection occasionally goes on to the formation of epithelioma.

The lingual papillæ may be hypertrophied so that the tongue has a warty appearance, being lined by intersecting furrows. Exceptionally, the filiform papillæ become so elongated as to resemble hair, and may give the upper surface of the tongue a greenish or blackish furry appearance (so-called **hairy tongue**).

Tumors.—**Hemangioma** and **lymphangioma** are met with in early life. The former is usually found on the lips, where it forms bluish-red, somewhat elevated blotches. The so-called **macroglossia** and **macrocheilia** are examples of cavernous hemangioma or diffuse lymphangiectasis affecting the tongue and lips respectively. In some cases both conditions are combined. A neurofibromatous macroglossia has also been described.[2] The structures are greatly enlarged, owing to increase in all the com-

---

[1] Presse Med., Paris, 1897: 789.
[2] Abbott and Shattock, Trans. Path. Soc. Lond., 54: 1904.

ponent elements, fibrosis, or, again, actual new-growth of lymph-vessels. In macroglossia the tongue may be so much enlarged that it projects beyond the lips. It often becomes dry, fissured, and ulcerated, owing to exposure to the air and the pressure of the teeth. From its size it may interfere with feeding and respiration. Microscopically, the organ shows increase in fibrous tissue and contains numerous small cavities lined with endothelium— the dilated lymph-channels and bloodvessels. Actual cysts may be formed. Among the benign new-growths appearing at birth or soon after may be mentioned the **fibroma, lipoma, myxoma, chondroma,** and **teratoma.**

Teratomas usually develop from the palate or vault of the pharynx. They arise either from embryonic "cell inclusions" or are possibly examples of polar hypergenesis (vol. i, p. 238). Tumors having the structure of thyroid substance occasionally have been met with in the base of the tongue, originating from "rests" of thyroid cells situated along the course of the fœtal thyroglossal duct.

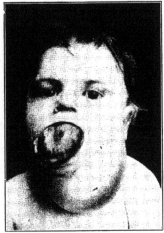

Fig. 82

Macroglossia. (Dr. Shepherd's case, Montreal General Hospital.)

Adenomas, often showing colloidal degeneration, may be found arising from the mucous glands of the lips and tongue.

The malignant tumors, **sarcoma** and **carcinoma,** are more common in adult life. The term **epulis** is a clinical one applied to a tumor situated on the jaw, which springs usually from the gums. Some of these have the structure of a fibroma (*fibrous epulis*); others are sarcomatous (*myeloid epulis*); still others are epitheliomatous (*epitheliomatous epulis*). *Myeloid* or *giant-celled sarcomas* originate in the periosteum or bone marrow, and form rounded, nodular growths of rather firm consistence. On section, they often have a brick-red color, owing to hemorrhage. Other forms of sarcomas—*round spindle-celled, hemangiosarcoma,* and *lymphangiosarcoma* of the tongue have been met with.

Epithelioma is found upon the lip, tongue, or gums. It begins as a small, elevated papule, or as a firm, circumscribed, whitish-gray infiltration of the tissues. The surface ulcerates and the ulcer quickly enlarges, invading the neighboring structures and the regional lymph-nodes. Epithelioma of the upper jaw has a special tendency to involve the antrum. Histologically, epitheliomas are of the squamous-celled variety. Finger-like down-growths of the superficial epithelium are to be seen, which are united by lateral processes in such a way as to form a sort of meshwork. Here and there, epithelial "pearls" or cell-nests may be seen. Round-celled infiltration is common.

FIG. 83

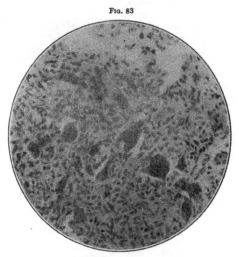

Giant-celled sarcoma, from the periosteum of the jaw. Winckel No. 6, without ocular.

FIG. 84

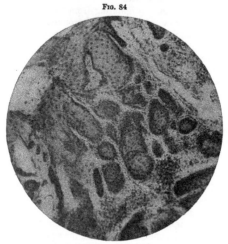

Epithelioma, starting from the lip. Winckel obj. No. 3, without ocular
(From the collection of Dr. A. G. Nicholls.)

Cysts.—Cysts are not uncommon in the mouth. They are usually of the nature of *"retention"* cysts (*ranula*) and are caused by the blocking of the duct of one or other of the glands discharging into the buccal cavity. Cystic degeneration of the fungiform papillæ of the tongue is recorded, but is rare. **Dermoid cysts** are also met wth.

Fig. 85

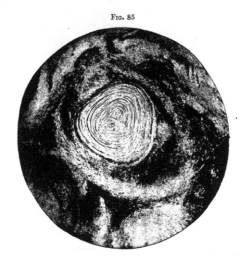

Epithelial pearl or "cell-nest" from an epithelioma of the lip. Winckel No. 6, without ocular. (From Dr. A. G. Nicholls' collection.)

THE TEETH.

Caries.—Caries is the most important affection. This begins with the formation of an opaque, white, or, more often, greenish or greenish-black speck upon the enamel, the result of disintegration and destruction of the enamel prisms. The process, if not interfered with, steadily advances until the centre of the tooth is excavated, and the whole tooth eventually undergoes decalcification. It thus becomes soft and is apt to break. Very commonly caries is accompanied by inflammation of the pulp (**pulpitis**), or of the alveolar periosteum.

Hypertrophy.—Excessive growth of the teeth occurs as a result of insufficient attrition. Loss of the opposing teeth or mal-apposition, as from fracture of the jaw, are the usual conditions at work. The tusks of the wild boar are a familiar example.

Tumors.—Among tumors may be mentioned the **odontoma, odontinoid, fibroma, myxoma,** and **sarcoma.**

The odontoma is formed during the period of growth and arises from the pulp or forms excrescences about the crown or root. Odontinoids develop later in life from the dentin. Sarcoma and the other connective-tissue tumors usually arise from the periosteum of the jaw or about the teeth. Rarely, they start from the pulp, during the period of develop-

FIG. 86

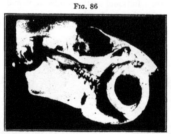

Head of a woodchuck: showing hypertrophy of the incisor teeth from lessened wear; the cause, fracture of the lower jaw. (Pathological Museum, McGill University.)

ment. Falkson has called attention to a multilocular cyst or **cystade-noma**, lined with cylindrical epithelium and containing teeth, which develops from embryonal tooth follicles.

INFLAMMATION.

Inflammation may occur in the pulp (**pulpitis**) or around the root of the tooth. The condition is due to infection. According to Miller, acid fermentation of the particles of food clinging about the teeth assist the pathogenic action of the bacteria. Pepsin and various vegetable acids are said to be responsible for the destruction of the dentin

FIG. 87

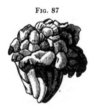

Odontoma. (Garretson.)

(Schlenker). The inflammation may be *acute* or *chronic, suppurative,* or *non-suppurative.* Acute suppuration may occur in the pulp of the tooth or deep down in the periosteum surrounding it. It leads to inflammation of the alveolar process and the formation of a local abscess (**parulis.**) If not relieved, fistulæ, necrosis of the bone, phlegmon of the neck and floor of the mouth, or even general septicemia may result. In certain cases infection of the antrum of Highmore occurs. In chronic, non-suppurative inflammation of the pulp and periosteum, granulation tissue, new bone, and dentin may be produced.

PALATE, PHARYNX, AND TONSILS.

The mucous membrane of the palate, pharynx, and tonsils is not unlike that of the other portions of the buccal cavity, but has these peculiarities, namely, that its character as a mucous membrane is still more pronounced and that it is particularly rich in lymphoid elements, both in the shape of follicles and the larger aggregations known as the tonsils. Consequently, exudative processes are of more importance than are desquamative ones.

The tonsils appear to have an important function. While the lymphoid cells are themselves, to a limited degree, phagocytic, polymorphonuclear leukocytes in considerable numbers make their way from the bloodvessels to the surface through the epithelial covering. These leukocytes are strongly phagocytic and their activity suggests that the tonsils form one of the barriers against the invasion of the system by pathogenic microörganisms.

INFLAMMATIONS.

Pharyngitis.—The term **angina** or **pharyngitis** is a general one used to designate inflammation of the posterior part of the buccal cavity, pharynx, tonsils, and palate. The condition is comparatively common, and is usually the result of irritation from mechanical, thermic, or chemical agents. It is found also in association with certain of the infectious diseases, such as scarlatina, measles, acute rheumatism, diphtheria, and variola. When the tonsils are chiefly or alone involved the affection is called **tonsillitis, or amygdalitis.**

The inflammations of this region may, according to their severity and duration, be divided into *acute* and *chronic;* or, according to their morbid peculiarities, into *catarrhal, herpetic, phlegmonous,* and *membranous.*

Acute Catarrhal Pharyngitis.—Acute catarrhal pharyngitis is characterized by redness and swelling of the mucous membrane, which becomes glazed, owing to the inhibition of the secretion. Later, there is an abundant discharge of a mucoid or mucopurulent exudate, sometimes tinged with blood. Microscopically, the secretion contains mucus, pus corpuscles, blood cells, and desquamated and degenerated epithelium. In the more severe cases, small abrasions may be noted on the back of the pharynx. The lymph-follicles are often also hyperplastic and appear as small, rounded or oval, elevated, and reddish nodules, projecting through the membrane.

Phlegmonous Pharyngitis.—In this form the inflammatory process is less marked upon the surface than in the deeper parts. The cases are due to infection with pyogenic microörganisms, in some instances assisted by traumatism. Not infrequently, they arise as secondary complications of certain of the infective diseases, such as scarlatina, diphtheria, erysipelas, and syphilis. The mucosa is of a deep, purplish-red color, swollen, tense, and shiny, presenting occasionally superficial vesicles. In the erysipelatous form the infiltration is diffuse and the exudate seropurulent rather than purulent. In other cases the process is localized and quite large abscesses may form. **Retropharyngeal abscess** sometimes results from tuberculous caries of the cervical vertebræ. **Peritonsillar abscess is** a common complication of acute tonsillitis and may occur on one or both sides. Such collections of pus may burst into the pharynx, or may erode the internal carotid artery or one of its branches, and cause fatal hemorrhage, or, again, if deep down may be absorbed with the formation of a scar. If the discharge of the abscess occur during the night, suffocation may result. General septicemia may also occur. Gangrene is a rare terminal event.

Membranous Pharyngitis.—Membranous or "croupous" pharyngitis may arise directly from traumatism, as, for example, the inhalation of irritating gases (steam, ammonia), but much more commonly it is due to infection with pathogenic microörganisms, such as Streptococcus pyogenes, Bacillus diphtheriæ, Pneumococcus, and Bacillus coli. Apart from diphtheria, membranous pharyngitis is, as a rule, met with as a complication of certain infective fevers, such as scarlatina, measles, typhoid, and variola.

Diphtheria.—True diphtheria may be taken as the type of this form of pharyngitis. Here, the inflammation is due to the action of the Klebs-Loeffler bacillus. The affection begins with marked congestion and swelling of the mucosa, which quickly assumes the character of a membranous inflammation. In the earlier stages small, grayish or grayish-white opalescent spots appear on the tonsils, uvula, or other parts of the pharyngeal wall. These gradually become distinctly membranous and of a dirty yellow or yellowish-brown color. They are bounded by a hyperemic zone, and may be slightly separated and elevated at the edges from the underlying tissues. If the membrane be removed a superficial erosion is left, which bleeds readily. On this area the membrane may reform with great rapidity. In the severer cases the patches become confluent, and thick, laminated sheets of membrane are formed on the posterior portion of the pharynx, which may extend into the trachea, larynx, and bronchi, into the nasal passages, or even to the skin. In the most virulent cases extensive necrosis takes place, and large gangrenous excavations may be found about the pillars of the fauces. The tonsils and lymph-nodes of the neck are usually enlarged.

By examining a series of sections taken at different periods, it has been made out that the mucous membrane is at first congested and more or less infiltrated with inflammatory products; the superficial epithelium degenerates and is cast off either wholly or in part; the cellular exudate coagulates, forming a fibrinous deposit both in the superficial layers and on the exposed surface of the part affected. This material, composed of leukocytes, fibrin, and degenerating tissue, gradually undergoes a form of coagulation necrosis and fuses into a more or less homogeneous mass, the diphtheritic membrane. In the deeper parts the bloodvessels and lymphatics are distended, there are numerous areas of cellular and fibrinous infiltration, and the glands are blocked with exudate and desquamated cells. In cases that recover, the membrane is exfoliated in large shreds or *en masse*, especially when antitoxin has been used, or, again, may be gradually absorbed. The lost epithelium is regenerated, and healing takes place without scarring.

The specific bacilli are usually superficial and, as a rule, do not enter the circulation, at least to any great extent. Severe symptoms are, however, not infrequently present, resulting from absorption of the toxin. Death may occur during the active stages of the disease or during convalescence, from vagus paralysis. A commoner form of paralysis is that affecting the muscles of the throat, especially those of the palate. Paralysis of accommodation, monoplegia, hemiplegia, and paraplegia may occur. In the more intense cases of intoxication practically all the muscles of the body may be involved with the exception of the diaphragm. Another complication of diphtheria is abscess formation, the result of secondary infection by pyogenic microörganisms.

The membranous pharyngitis due to streptococci is likely to be more acute than diphtheria in regard to its immediate symptoms. It is not followed by paralyses, but the cocci penetrate deeply and are apt to be carried to distant parts, setting up a generalized septicemia or multiple abscess formation.

Vincent's Angina.—This term is applied to a feebly contagious form of pharyngitis, characterized by superficial ulceration and the formation of a membrane. The affection usually begins on one or both tonsils and spreads to other parts of the pharynx, or may start at the edge of the gums, involving the lips and cheeks. It is associated with the presence of the Bacillus fusiformis and Spirochæta dentium in large numbers, and most authorities attribute the disease to the symbiotic action of these two organisms.

Chronic Pharyngitis.—Chronic pharyngitis may arise insidiously or may result from a succession of acute attacks. The abuse of tobacco and alcohol are common causes. Many cases, too, represent the extension of a chronic rhinitis. The mucous membrane is more or less congested and presents numerous distended venules. Often, it has a granular, warty appearance, due to hyperplasia of the lymphoid follicles (**chronic granular pharyngitis**). The secretion is mucoid, mucopurulent, or purulent, and often adheres in the form of dry scales or crusts, which decompose and emit an offensive odor. In other cases, secretion is scanty, and the mucous membrane is of a reddish-brown color, thin, smooth, and shiny. This is known as **chronic atrophic pharyngitis** (pharyngitis sicca).

Acute Tonsillitis.—In acute tonsillitis the inflammation may be a superficial one or, again, may involve the parenchyma of the glands, causing considerable swelling of the parts. The tonsils are swollen, red, and hot, and covered with an abundant secretion of creamy mucopus. When the tonsillar crypts are distended with secretion, yellowish-white, rounded spots can be seen on the surface of the tonsils, and the condition is then commonly known as **follicular** or **lacunar tonsillitis**. In severe cases, the inflammatory process may go on to suppuration, either in the tonsil or in the cellular tissue about it (**quinsy, peritonsillar abscess**).

Histologically, in acute tonsillitis, we find marked congestion of the glands, hyperplasia of the lymphoid elements, exudation on the surface, and desquamation of the epithelium.

Occasionally, in addition to the ordinary manifestations of catarrhal inflammation, minute vesicles are formed upon the mucous membrane, which rupture, leaving painful ulcers—**herpetic tonsillitis or pharyngitis**.

Chronic Tonsillitis.—In chronic tonsillitis the organs are permanently enlarged and, except for their size, often appear to be normal. Sometimes there is a dusky redness of the palate and fauces. The crypts are small and the surface smooth. The enlargement may be so great as to interfere with swallowing, respiration, and speaking, and is important also in that it tends to perpetuate the inflammation, owing to the increased susceptibility of such tonsils to irritation. Children with a rheumatic taint seem to be specially liable to this disorder. Chronic tonsillitis and pharyngitis predispose to bronchitis and other lung affections.

In another form of chronic tonsillitis the tonsils are not enlarged, but the crypts are more roomy than normal and are filled with secretion, desquamated cells, food particles, and microörganisms of various kinds. This material becomes inspissated and may be extruded spontaneously or by pressure in the form of cheesy, whitish-yellow plugs, which have a peculiar, characteristic, offensive odor. Sometimes the masses are retained and become infiltrated with lime salts, forming concretions.

Hyperplasia of the tonsils and of the pharyngeal or Luschka's tonsil is often met with in children, and seems to be in many cases the result of a chronic inflammatory process. **Adenoid vegetations** are papillomatous or polypoid growths occurring in the vault of the pharynx and posterior nares. When of any extent, breathing may be interfered with, and children so affected complain of headache and earache, breathe through the mouth, and are apathetic and backward at school. The condition is often associated with enlargement of the pharyngeal tonsil and sore throat. Deafness and inflammation of the middle ear may result from interference with the Eustachian tubes through pressure or catarrh. In long-standing cases the chest shows a characteristic deformity.

Histologically, the condition is due to hyperplasia either of the lymphoid elements or of the connective tissue. In the former case the adenoids are soft and friable; in the latter, firm and tough.

Tuberculosis.—Tuberculosis of the tonsils and pharynx can occur as a primary infection, but is almost always secondary to pulmonary or laryngeal tuberculosis. Owing to their exposed position the tonsils are liable to infection of all kinds, especially from the food, and it has been possible to produce experimentally tuberculosis in these glands by feeding animals on infected material. In tuberculosis of the pharynx the mucosa is injected·and contains numerous small tubercles, that ultimately break down and form shallow ulcers. These may in time coalesce and lead to extensive loss of substance.

Syphilis.—Syphilitic sore throat usually takes the form of a *catarrhal inflammation* that is difficult to distinguish from the simple variety, or of *mucous* or *opaline plaques*. *Gummas* are not uncommon. The *primary chancre* has been found upon the tonsil.

Typhoid.—Superficial ulceration of the posterior pharyngeal wall is not very uncommon in typhoid fever.

Actinomycosis.—Cervical and prevertebral actinomycosis may originate in the tonsils and the pharyngeal mucous membrane.

PROGRESSIVE METAMORPHOSES.

Tumors.—Connective-tissue tumors, carcinoma, sarcoma, and **teratoma** occur in this region. Sarcoma of the tonsil is occasionally met with.

THE SALIVARY GLANDS.

These are glands of acinous structure, and in the human subject are of serous or mixed serous and mucous type. Their ducts discharge into the buccal cavity.

Parotitis.—**Acute Parotitis.**—Acute parotitis and analogous inflammations of the other salivary glands are usually due to infection with microörganisms from the mouth. They may also complicate many of the infective fevers, such as typhoid, diphtheria, pyemia, cholera, and syphilis. Parotitis has been observed as a complication of certain abdominal conditions and after operations on the abdominal viscera. When pyogenic organisms are at work suppuration of the glands may follow, or even gangrene. In such cases *salivary fistulæ* sometimes result. Milder inflammations may lead to increased secretion and later to fibrous induration of the gland with, possibly, stenosis of the duct. In such cases concretions composed of phosphate or carbonate of lime are not uncommonly found within the duct (*sialoliths*), sometimes causing or associated with cystic dilatation of the ducts and acini.

Epidemic Parotitis.—Epidemic parotitis (*mumps*) is an infectious disease, characterized by great swelling of the parotid gland and to some extent of the submaxillary and sublingual glands, associated with slight febrile disturbance. The infecting agent, which has not as yet been absolutely determined, presumably enters through the excretory duct. In the course of two or three days the inflammation subsides and the gland gradually resumes its normal state. The inflammatory exudate is mainly serous. Suppuration rarely occurs. The affection is occasionally complicated by orchitis or oöphoritis.

Angina Ludovici.—Angina Ludovici is a somewhat rare and peculiar form of phlegmon or septic cellulitis, occurring in the floor of the mouth and sides of the neck. It may eventually spread down the neck to the mediastinum and pericardium. The affected parts are swollen, dusky red in color, and present a brawny induration. Abscess formation and gangrene may supervene. Cases are not infrequently fatal from general septicemia. Angina of this type may originate in inflammation of the submaxillary gland, but is more common as a result of trauma or infection from carious teeth. Cases occasionally are met with in scarlatina.

Parasites.—Parasites are rare. *Echinococcus* has been recorded.

Tumors.—Among tumors of the parotid may be mentioned **fibroma, myxoma, chondroma, adenoma, rhabdomyoma, sarcoma, endothelioma,** and **carcinoma.** The most common tumor of the parotid gland is *mixed* in character, consisting of chondroma together with fibrous and myxomatous elements, and is probably to be attributed to the overgrowth of misplaced embryonic tissue. It has a distinct tendency to undergo sarcomatous transformation. Carcinoma is rare.

CHAPTER XVIII.

THE ŒSOPHAGUS.

AFFECTIONS of the œsophagus are relatively uncommon. Some of them are of great clinical importance, however, inasmuch as they may interfere with the passage of food into the stomach and thus lead to malnutrition. Owing to the special function of the œsophagus it is peculiarly liable to suffer from the effects of mechanical, chemical, and thermal irritation. It may also be affected by disease of neighboring structures—larynx, trachea, mediastinal and peribronchial glands, and vertebræ.

CONGENITAL ANOMALIES.

Malformations may occur alone or associated with other defects. The most common event is for the upper third of the tube to end in a blind **cul-de-sac,** often dilated, while the lower portion forms a **fistulous communication** with the trachea or a bronchus. Any part of the tube may be **absent** either completely or the defective portion may be represented by a fibrous cord. Local areas of **stenosis** have been met with. Rarely, the lumen is partially **occluded** by a diaphragm-like fold of mucous membrane.

A localized **dilatation** of the œsophagus, the so-called "fore-stomach" or "antrum cardiacum" has been observed. It is decidedly rare. In acardiac monsters the œsophagus may be completely **wanting.** Partial or complete **reduplication** is found in double monsters.

ALTERATIONS OF THE LUMEN AND SOLUTIONS OF CONTINUITY.

Simple contracture of the lumen of the œsophagus from spasm is occasionally observed in hysterical persons and hypochondriacs, and also in chorea, epilepsy, and hydrophobia. **Stenosis** of the œsophagus may be developmental or acquired. In the latter form the lumen may be narrowed from extrinsic or intrinsic causes. Thus, pressure from enlarged mediastinal glands, aneurisms, tumors of the lung and pleura may bring it about. Local inflammatory swellings, phlegmon, growths of the thrush fungus, tumors, cicatricial contraction of the wall from trauma, corrosive poisoning, syphilis, and diphtheria are among the intrinsic causes. **Foreign bodies** may also lodge in the tube and obstruct its lumen.

Dilatation.—Dilatation may be developmental or acquired. The first-mentioned variety is rare. The condition is general throughout the tube.

Acquired dilatation is usually secondary to stenosis and may be general or local. Generalized dilatation is either *cylindrical* or *fusiform* and results from stricture or chronic œsophagitis. The œsophagus may be enormously dilated, the lumen measuring 30 cm. or more in circumference. The muscular coats usually hypertrophy in these cases. Rarely, "idiopathic" dilatation, without stenosis, is observed.[1] It has been attributed to spasm of the muscle at the cardiac end, or to paralysis of the muscular fibers of the wall. A similar condition can be produced experimentally in the dog by cutting both vagi in the neck. Kraus[2] has described a case of this kind in the human subject, where, at autopsy, the vagi were found to be diseased.

Local dilatations or diverticula[3] are of two kinds, *pressure diverticula* and *traction diverticula*. The first form is due to pressure from within the lumen; the second, to external force pulling out the wall.

Pressure diverticula are rare. They generally are situated on the posterior wall at the junction of the pharynx and œsophagus, at the point where the muscular wall is normally weakest, most often slightly to the left. The swallowing of large boluses of food leads to a local bulging which gradually increases until a sac is formed extending downward between the œsophagus and the vertebræ sometimes extending into the thorax. Microscopic examination shows that, as a rule, the muscular fibres are lacking in the wall of the sac, so that the condition might be regarded as a hernial protrusion of the mucosa and submucosa through the muscularis. In some few cases the muscular fibres have been found to be continuous in the wall. In the latter case the condition is usually regarded as an ectasia due to a disturbance of the closure of the fetal cleft at this point. Food and fluid tend to enter the sac and become lodged there, undergoing decomposition, thus giving rise to maceration of the epithelium, ulceration, inflammation of the œsophagus and neighboring structures. Pressure symptoms on the rest of the œsophagus are common.

Traction diverticula are not uncommon. They are usually to be found on the anterior wall about the level of the bifurcation of the trachea. They result from inflammation, usually tuberculous in nature, of the neighboring lymph-nodes, which become adherent to the œsophageal wall and, from subsequent cicatricial contraction, exert traction upon it. The sac is comparatively small and funnel-shaped. The remains of the diseased gland can be detected at the apex. Such diverticula may be single or multiple. Perforation of the sac may take place, leading to suppurative pericœsophagitis and extension to the pleuræ, pericardium, and lungs. The wall of the sac may consist of all the elements of the œsophageal wall, or the muscularis may be partly or completely defective.

[1] V. Bergmann, Ges. de Charité-Aerzte, 7, November, 1907.
[2] Leyden Festschrift.
[3] Riebold, Virch. Archiv, 192: 1908: 126.

Rupture.—Rupture of the œsophagus occurs, but is rare. It may result from trauma or increased internal pressure. It is said to have occurred from severe vomiting after a full meal and in the state of intoxication. Probably, in such cases some pathological condition in the œsophagus has existed previously to render this accident possible.

Perforation.—Perforation of the œsophageal wall may result from traumatism, the rupture of peptic, syphilitic, and cancerous ulcers, the pressure of foreign bodies within the lumen, from suppuration, or tuberculous caseation in the neighboring parts, or, again, from aneurism.

CIRCULATORY DISTURBANCES.

Hyperemia.—Owing to the comparative scarcity of bloodvessels in the œsophagus, hyperemia is seldom a striking condition.

Active Hyperemia.—Active hyperemia may be due to the irritating properties of certain articles of food, alcohol, and so on. It occurs also in newborn children, in the early stages of inflammation, and in various infective diseases.

Passive Hyperemia.—Passive hyperemia occurs in all cases of general congestion, in obstructive disturbances of the circulation in the heart, lungs, and liver. In portal cirrhosis of the liver, the veins of the lower portion of the œsophagus often become enormously distended (*œsophageal varices*), and may form nodular or papillary masses projecting into the lumen. The appearance produced is very similar to that in rectal hemorrhoids. The veins are dilated and tortuous, sometimes reaching the size of a lead pencil. Rupture of these varices may lead to serious and even fatal hemorrhage.

Hemorrhages.—Œsophageal hemorrhages may be caused also by traumatism, ulceration, or malignant new-growths. The effused blood may be vomited up or, again, digested and passed on into the intestine. An aortic aneurism may erode into the œsophagus and rupture there.

INFLAMMATIONS.

Œsophagitis.—**Catarrhal Œsophagitis.**—Catarrhal œsophagitis is the commonest form of inflammation. It is due to the action of thermal or chemical irritants in the ingesta, to extension of inflammation from the pharynx or stomach, or arises as a complication of certain of the infective fevers, measles, scarlatina, typhoid, and variola. It is characterized by congestion of the mucosa and exfoliation of the superficial epithelium, together with increase in secretion, which, however, is usually scanty on account of the paucity of mucous glands. Shallow erosions commonly result, situated for the most part on the top of the longitudinal folds, which, when healing, leave small scars.

If the cause persist or be frequently brought into play, *chronic catarrh* will result. This condition is found also in the œsophagus above a stenosis, and as a result of prolonged passive congestion. The mucosa is of a livid red color, the epithelium is thickened, resulting in the formation of papillomatous or polypoid outgrowths or plaque-like patches of leukoplakia. The surface is covered with tenacious mucus or mucopus. The muscular wall is thickened, both from hypertrophy and from productive fibrosis. The lumen is usually dilated, but may be narrowed. Superficial ulceration is common.

Follicular Œsophagitis.—In follicular œsophagitis the mucous glands are involved. The lumina are obstructed and there is an excessive production of mucus, which leads to the dilatation of the glands and ducts into small cysts. Round about the glands there is a small-celled infiltration. This may result in abscess formation and, from rupture of the abscess, ulceration.

Phlegmonous Œsophagitis.—Phlegmonous, or *diffuse suppurative œsophagitis*, may be primarily due to the action of foreign bodies or corrosive substances, but most commonly arises by extension of suppurative inflammation from neighboring structures, such as the pharynx, stomach, periœsophageal lymph-nodes, the vertebral column, and the cricoid cartilage. It occurs also in advanced pulmonary tuberculosis without any obvious cause, and occasionally supervenes upon the follicular form. The affection begins as a purulent infiltration of the submucosa, leading to the formation of localized or diffuse collections of pus. The mucosa is reddened and undermined, and fistulous openings may be formed in its substance, which give vent to the pent-up exudation (*œsophagitis dissecans profunda*). The tissues about the œsophagus are sometimes involved and the abscesses may discharge into the larynx or trachea, or, more rarely, into the mediastinum or pleura.

Pustular Œsophagitis.—Pustular œsophagitis is the name given to an eruption of papules in the mucosa of the œsophagus occurring in smallpox. As in the skin, the papules become pustules, and when they rupture form small ulcers.

Membranous Œsophagitis.—Membranous œsophagitis accompanied by superficial necrosis is not very uncommon in variola, measles, scarlatina, typhoid, typhus, pyemia, cholera, chronic Bright's disease, pneumonia, tuberculosis, and the gastro-intestinal catarrh of infants. The fibrinous deposit is rarely generalized, but usually confined to the tops of the folds. Ulceration may occur with stenosis of the lumen of the œsophagus from cicatricial contraction. True *diphtheria* of the œsophagus is rare.

Exfoliative Œsophagitis.—Exfoliative œsophagitis (*œsophagitis dissecans superficialis*) is characterized by the desquamation of the lining epithelium in large flakes or even as a complete cylinder. The etiology is not clear. Some cases may be due to the action of corrosives. The disease usually occurs in neurotic individuals.

Corrosive Œsophagitis.—Corrosive œsophagitis is that form due to the action of corrosive poisons, chiefly acids or alkalies. Concentrated lye, carbolic and sulphuric acids are the agents commonly at work. The lesion produced is a necrotising inflammation. The epithelium is swollen, shreddy, and desquamating in patches, or in the more severe cases is converted into a yellowish, grayish-white, or blackish eschar. The tissues are congested, extravasations of blood are to be found in the submucosa, and a line of demarcation is formed between the living and the dead tissue. The necrotic portion is eventually cast off, if the patient live. Suppuration occurs, and, as healing takes place, serious contracture of the lumen results. The inflammation may extend to the neighboring tissues.

Tuberculosis. — This is always secondary to advanced tuberculosis in other parts. Most commonly it is due to extension of the disease from the peritracheal lymph-nodes, from the larynx or pharynx. Less often, it results from swallowing infected sputum. Miliary tuberculosis of the œsophagus also occurs, but is rare. Tuberculous ulceration is usually superficial, but perforation may take place. The borders of the ulcers are thickened, and small tubercles can be made out in the substance. The bases are smooth or irregular.[1]

Syphilis.—Ulceration of the œsophagus may occur both in the secondary and tertiary stages. Gummatous infiltration is the most frequent lesion. It leads to ulceration, perforation, and cicatricial contraction of the lumen.[2]

Actinomycosis. — This affection is rare. Primary actinomycosis of the œsophagus has been described in a few cases. Extension to the thoracic viscera is the rule.[3]

Parasites.—Thrush.—This is most commonly met with in poorly nourished children and in those suffering from prolonged disease and cachexia.

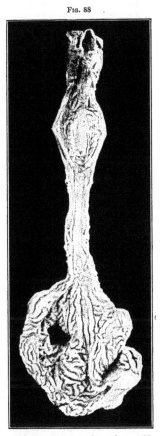

Fig. 88

Stricture of the œsophagus in a child, due to swallowing lye; above the stenosed portion the tube is dilated. The perforation in the stomach below marks the site of a palliative gastrostomy. (From the Pathological Museum of McGill University.)

[1] Claribel Cone, Johns Hopkins Hosp. Bull., 80: 1897: 229, Tileston, Amer. Jour. Med. Sci., 1906.

[2] See Kraus, Nothnagel's Handbook, article on the Œsophagus, xvi: 1902.

[3] A. Poncet, Province Médicale, Lyon, 9: 1895: 205; Bull. de l'Acad. de Méd., 15: 1896; see also v. Baracz, Arch. f. Chir., 68: 1902: 1050.

As a rule, the infection extends from the mouth or pharynx, but sometimes arises independently. It may may be associated with tuberculosis of the œsophagus.[1] **Trichinosis** has also been observed.

Foreign Bodies.—The chief foreign bodies that are at times found more or less completely obstructing the œsophagus are: bones, fish, needles, plum-stones, leeches, and false teeth. Phlegmonous œsophagitis commonly results. Hard, angular, or sharp substances of course do more damage to the wall than do others, and may lead to ulceration, abscess formation, or even gangrene, sometimes followed by perforation. Septic matter, at times mixed with food, may thus be discharged into the mediastinum, pleura, pericardium, or into a bronchus or a large vessel, such as the aorta.

RETROGRESSIVE METAMORPHOSES.

Atrophy.—Atrophy of the wall may occur in general marasmus and, locally, as a result of pressure. Various forms of degeneration are met with also. They are rare and have been but little studied. The most important are **necroses**. Pressure from foreign bodies impacted in the lumen, or from aneurisms or tumors from without, lead to ischemia, atrophy, and eventually loss of substance. What may be termed a "bedsore" of the œsophagus is occasionally met with in cachexia and prolonged fevers as a result of pressure of the larynx upon the organ.

A **round** or **peptic ulcer,** analogous in all respects to the peptic ulcer of the stomach, has been described. It is rare.

Œsophagomalacia.—Œsophagomalacia has been oberved as an agonal manifestation in cases of cerebral disease. It is, however, not uncommon as a postmortem phenomenon as a result of the digestion of the tissues by the gastric juice which has regurgitated through the cardia. The epithelium is macerated, desquàmated, and the muscular coat may be discolored, softened, or liquefied. Perforation of the wall sometimes occurs with escape of the stomach contents into the pleura.

Gangrene.—Gangrene of the œsophagus may be associated with noma of the cheek or pharynx, gangrenous tonsillitis, or gangrene of the lung. It may also result from the action of corrosive substances and severe inflammation.

PROGRESSIVE METAMORPHOSES.

Hypertrophy.—Hypertrophy of the muscular wall is produced by any cause that tends to obstruct the free passage of food into the stomach. Muscular spasm, carcinoma, and strictures are the most important conditions to be mentioned in this connection.

Leukoplakia.—Leukoplakia, similar to that occurring upon the tongue,' is common. Multiple, small, rounded, or oval, plaque-like

[1] Cf. Maresch, Zeitschr. f. Heilkunde, 28: 1907: 145.

elevations of a pearly white color are observed upon the mucosa. Microscopically, they consist in a simple local hyperplasia of the squamous lining epithelium. They are found in cases of passive congestion, and, as our late colleague Wyatt Johnston was wont to emphasize, in chronic alcoholism.

Tumors.—New-growths are, on the whole, not common. They originate in the œsophagus itself or in the neighboring parts, and are rarely, if ever, metastatic. The benign growths are usually small and of but little practical importance. The most common are the **polypoid** or **papillary fibromas**, and the **intramural fibromas. Lipomas, myxomas, myomas,** and **polypoid adenoma** (one case) are recorded.

Sarcoma.—Primary sarcoma of the œsophagus is quite rare. *Spindle-celled, round-celled,* and *alveolar* forms are described, and also *lympho-sarcoma.* One or two cases of *rhabdomyoma* are also recorded. As a rule, sarcoma invades the œsophagus by extension from some of the neighboring structures.

Carcinoma.—The most important growth is carcinoma, which may be primary, or secondary to carcinoma of the cardia of the stomach, pharynx, or thyroid gland.

Primary carcinoma of the œsophagus is usually of the *squamous-celled* type, *adenocarcinoma* being distinctly rare. The latter form may originate from the mucous glands, from developmental cysts lined with columnar cells, which are sometimes present in the wall, or again from the persistent islands of columnar epithelium, which, as Schridde and others have shown, are constantly to be encountered in the mid region of the tube. Glandular carcinoma may be simple, medullary, or scirrhous in type. We have met with one instance of a glandular cancer, approximating the scirrhous form, which formed a small, isolated growth and led to complete obstruction. The favorite sites for carcinomatous growths are at the narrowest parts of the lumen and where there is transitional epithelium. They, therefore, occur most often at the level of the cricoid cartilage, opposite the bifurcation of the trachea, and at the entrance into the stomach. The tumor tends to encircle the lumen and thus produces stenosis, a condition that is not entirely relieved even when ulceration takes place. In some parts there may be sufficient proliferation of connective tissue to form a scirrhous-like growth, but in others the mass is softer and more fungating. The mucous membrane in the neighborhood is usually inflamed and the œsophageal wall above the stricture is hypertrophied and the lumen dilated. The new-growth may extend through the wall of the œsophagus to the trachea, bronchi, lung, mediastinum, pleura, pericardium, or large bloodvessels. Metastases occur in the regional lymph-nodes, the liver, lungs, and bones.

Carcinoma occurs most often in males, between the ages of fifty and sixty years, particularly often, it is said, in smokers and drinkers.

Dermoid Cysts.—Dermoid cysts are very rare. They occur at a point near the junction of the œsophagus and pharynx. The congenital cysts lined with ciliated columnar epithelium sometimes found in the œsophageal wall are of *teratoid* nature. They represent the remains of the original communication between the œsophagus and trachea.

CHAPTER XIX.

THE STOMACH.

ANOMALIES.

Congenital Anomalies.—Complete absence of the stomach has been reported in connection with other grave anomalies, such as acephalus. It is rare. The organ may be abnormally **small,** even in otherwise well-developed individuals. The pyloric opening may be completely or, more often, partially **occluded,** and attached to the duodenum by

Fig. 89

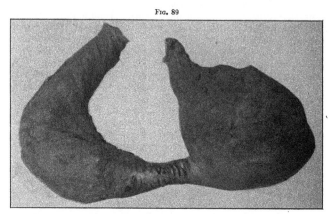

Hour-glass stomach. (From the Pathological Museum of McGill University.)

a fibrous cord. **Diverticula** are rare. The stomach may be divided into several chambers by intersecting septa. It may also be composed of two chambers, owing to a constriction about the middle (**hour-glass deformity**). In complete transposition of the viscera the stomach may be **reversed,** the pylorus being situated to the left. Occasionally, the stomach assumes a **vertical position,** possibly a persistence of the embryonic condition.

Another type of congenital displacement is that found in connection with defect of the diaphragm. There may be absolute defect, with free communication between the thoracic and abdominal cavities (**congenital false hernia**); the diaphragm may be congenitally weak at some point, so that violence or muscular strain subsequently applied may cause it to give way, with protrusion of the abdominal viscera into the thoracic cavity (**acquired false hernia**); or there may be thinning of the diaphragm so that the abdominal organs are dislocated into the thoracic cavity, but are contained in a sac of diaphragm or peritoneum (**true diaphragmatic hernia**). The second variety mentioned is the most common, 224 of Leichtenstern's 252 cases being of this type. True diaphragmatic hernia is a rare form, occurring in only 11 per cent. of all cases.[1]

FIG. 90

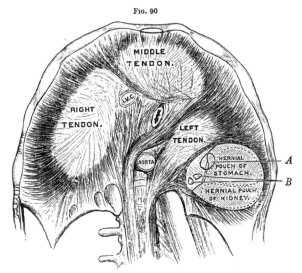

Congenital diaphragmatic hernia in man, aged fifty-seven years; partly false, there being at *A* and *B* direct communications between the peritoneal and pleural cavities, from the edges of which fatty omental folds of tissue passed into the thorax; partly true, the serous membrane forming a covering over the stomach and left kidney as they lay in the pleural cavity. The muscle of the diaphragm is shaded dark.

Congenital Hypertrophic Stenosis of the Pylorus.—Congenital hypertrophic stenosis of the pylorus is somewhat rare, although undoubtedly more frequent than has been thought. There may be a pre-existing congenital stenosis of the orifice with subsequent hypertrophy of the muscles. In some cases the condition is thought to be due to pyloric spasm. The microscopic examination of the pylorus shows merely hyperplasia of the muscle with some fibrosis. There may also be slight catarrh of the mucosa. The affection is important, as it occurs in infants usually under four months old, and may lead to death from starvation if unrelieved.[2]

---

[1] F. M. Fry, Diaphragmatic Hernia, Mont. Med. Jour., 24:1895–6:101.

[2] Rolleston and Crofton-Atkins, Congenital Hypertrophy with Stenosis, Brit. Med. Jour., 2:1900:1768. See, also, Scudder, Boston Med. and Surg. Journ., 1905:494.

ACQUIRED DISPLACEMENTS.

Displacement of the stomach may be upward (*vide supra*), downward (gastroptosis), or to the side. In all cases the cardia is a fixed point, the pylorus or some other portion moving upon this as on a hinge. A common form is that in which the middle portion of the organ sags downward, the pylorus and the cardia remaining in their normal position.

Dislocation is sometimes due to causes inherent in the stomach itself, such as dilatation or contraction, but is often, also, the result of extrinsic factors. A loaded colon, the weight of tumors, the traction of adhesions, will, on occasion, tend to drag the organ down. The pressure of corsets or an enlarged liver may force it downward.

Gastroptosis is nearly always part and parcel of a general prolapse of the abdominal viscera (splanchnoptosis). The term Glénard's disease originally referred to prolapse of the intestines alone (enteroptosis), but has been used more comprehensively to include cases of enteroptosis combined with prolapse of other organs as well. Besides the stomach and intestines, the liver and the right kidney may be displaced (hepatoptosis, nephroptosis).

In *Glénard's disease* there is a peculiar symptom complex, nervous dyspepsia, and atony of the stomach, constipation, or constipation alternating with diarrhea, dragging sensations in the back, anemia, and in the later stages, neurasthenia. Anatomically, there is relaxation of the hepatic and hepatopyloric ligaments. Glénard, who originally described the condition, thought he had discovered the anatomical basis of neurasthenia, but this view is not generally accepted. Bouveret and Charcot considered that the prolapse was rather the result than the cause of the neurasthenia, due to the loss of muscular and nervous tone. The causes of splanchnoptosis are, pressure upon the abdominal contents from above. as from corsets; the cramping effect of a long, narrow, or phthisical chest; an enlarged liver; relaxation of the supporting ligaments; weakening of the abdominal walls from pregnancy; the pressure of tumors or cysts; nervous depression; and conditions which tend to drag the viscera down.

ALTERATIONS IN THE SIZE AND SHAPE OF THE LUMEN.

Contraction of the stomach is found in certain forms of chronic gastritis and in diffuse scirrhous carcinoma. The cavity of the stomach in the latter case may not be large enough to contain more than a cupful of fluid.

Hour-glass.—Hour-glass contraction, when acquired, may be due to the cicatrization of an ulcer, torsion of the stomach, tumors, hernia, or adhesion to displaced viscera.

Dilatation.—Dilatation of the stomach is a not uncommon condition. The two main factors in its causation are a deficiency of muscular tone and difficulty in evacuation of the organ. The affection often comes on slowly and insidiously, and it may be long before clinical symptoms manifest themselves. Overeating and drinking are potent causes and act by bringing about a gradual distension of the organ, with sometimes descent. In not a few cases the stomach is considerably enlarged, but is able to digest and discharge its contents in the regular space of time. Such a condition is termed *megalogastria*, and probably should be differentiated from true dilatation, in which the muscle is overstretched and functionally weak. Among the causes that act by obstructing the onflow of the gastric contents may be mentioned carcinoma of the pylorus, stenosis and hypertrophic stenosis of the pylorus, pyloric spasm, external pressure of new-growths or enlarged glands, the traction of inflammatory adhesions, gastroptosis, and tight lacing.

A considerable number of cases of *acute dilatation* of the stomach are now on record, and the condition is probably much more common than has generally been realized. Acute dilatation comes on with great suddenness, and unless promptly relieved by appropriate measures usually runs a rapidly fatal course. The chief etiological factors of a predisposing nature are: (1) operations under general anesthesia; (2) severe and prolonged disease; (3) indiscretions in diet; (4) disease or deformity of the spine; and (5) traumatism. A few cases have come on without obvious cause. Now and then one will supervene upon chronic dilatation. The direct causes appear to be primary paresis of the gastric musculature, and obstruction to the onflow of the gastric contents. In about half the recorded cases definite mechanical obstruction has been found, occasionally at the pylorus, but much more frequently in the duodenum, just below the bile papilla. Kinks, the traction of adhesions, and the pressure of misplaced organs may bring this about. The most constant anatomical lesion, however, is compression of the duodenum by the root of the mesentery.[1]

Volvulus of the stomach has been observed.[2]

CIRCULATORY DISTURBANCES.

The amount of blood in the stomach varies widely within physiological limits, depending upon the degree of functional activity for the time being. Consequently, postmortem appearances must be interpreted with some degree of caution.

Œdema.—Œdema is rare, even in inflammatory processes.

Anemia.—Anemia occurs as a manifestation of general systemic anemia, and in association with atrophy of the mucosa. In the latter case it is difficult to determine whether the atrophy is the result of the anemia or *vice versa*.

[1] Nicholls, Acute Dilatation of the Stomach, Internat. Clinics, Lippincott, 4: 1908: 80.

[2] Pendl, Wien. klin. Woch., 1904: 476.

Hyperemia.—Active Hyperemia.—Active hyperemia occurs physiologically during digestion and imparts a delicate rose-pink color to the mucosa. It also results from the action of irritating or corrosive substances and from inflammation. In such cases the congestion is very intense and is present in irregular patches, localized especially to the tops of the rugæ.

Passive Hyperemia.—Passive hyperemia is found in connection with portal obstruction, particularly that occurring in cirrhosis of the liver, and, more remotely, with vascular obstruction in the heart and lungs. The pyloric portion is the part chiefly affected. The mucosa is of a dull, purple red color, and the veins are often distended. The stomach wall is often also œdematous. Extravasations of blood occur, so that patches and spots of a yellowish or brownish color are not infrequent. In long-standing cases the mucous membrane becomes markedly pigmented.

Hemorrhages.—Hemorrhages into the stomach wall are quite common. According to Birch-Hirschfeld, they are found in about 50 per cent. of cadavers. He regards them as due to severe and protracted vomiting just before death. In general, extravasations are due to increased vascular tension, blood dyscrasias, or disease of the vessel walls. They are found in cirrhosis of the liver, leukemia, pernicious anemia, the hemorrhagic diatheses, scurvy, acute yellow atrophy of the liver, thrombosis, embolism, and in some acute infections; also, in poisoning from phosphorus, strychnine, and morphine; and in severe vomiting.

Hemorrhage into the cavity of the stomach may be due to the erosion of a vessel from a simple or cancerous ulcer, traumatism, or, rarely, leukemia, hemophilia, or vicarious menstruation. When the bleeding is at all extensive the blood is usually vomited (*hematemesis*), or, again, may be passed by the bowel (*melena*). When recently effused the blood is acid, bright red, pure or mixed with food; when the hemorrhage is of some standing, however, the blood assumes a turbid brown appearance like coffee-grounds, owing to the action of the gastric juice. It is worth while pointing out that all blood vomited does not necessarily result from gastric hemorrhage. It may be due, for example, to bleeding from the nose, mouth, or œsophagus, the blood being subsequently swallowed, or to the oozing from an aneurism. In young infants pus and blood from a suppurating breast may be swallowed and later on regurgitated, an occurrence that sometimes gives rise to an erroneous diagnosis.

Hemorrhages into the mucosa lead to weakening of the local resisting power of the stomach, and areas so affected are not infrequently converted into shallow ulcers, owing to the eroding action of the gastric secretion (hemorrhagic erosion).

INFLAMMATIONS.

Gastritis.—Inflammation of the stomach in the vast majority of instances is due to the irritating action of substances that have been ingested; some few cases are attributable to the agency of the toxic substances circulating in the blood; a few, also, to the extension of inflammatory processes from neighboring parts.

Ingested substances act as irritants largely owing to their physical or chemical properties. Foodstuffs may on occasion act as the excitants of gastritis (**dyspeptic gastritis**). An excessive amount of food is a common cause, owing to the inability of the stomach to digest and pass it along quickly enough. This is particularly apt to occur when the function of the stomach is impaired, as from muscular atony, pyloric stenosis, carcinoma, or fibrous induration. Should food from any of these causes be retained, it undergoes abnormal fermentation. Putrid gases, irritating fatty acids, and bacterial toxins are produced in notable quantities and lead to severe disorders. The ingesta also may be too hot or too cold, or otherwise irritating. The abuse of alcohol is a potent cause of inflammation. Gastritis, too, is a common accompaniment of the acute infectious fevers. Pus, infected sputum, and foul material from the buccal cavity may also induce the affection.

The most severe cases of gastritis are brought about by **corrosive poisons**, the conditions resulting varying according to the character of the destructive substance and the length of time that has elapsed since its ingestion. Strong corrosives lead to extensive necrosis of the mucous membrane. The slough produced by sulphuric acid is hard, dry, brittle, and of a grayish color. Nitric and hydrochloric acids give a yellowish tint. Caustic alkalies produce a transparent, pulpy, digested appearance. The morbid appearances resulting depend considerably upon the amount of food in the stomach at the time, being, of course more intensely marked in the fasting organ. The effects of caustics are usually more pronounced at the fundus and posterior wall, and especially on the tops of the rugæ. The remainder of the mucosa may be free from necrosis, but may show signs of a more or less intense inflammation, often hemorrhagic in character.

Hematogenous Gastritis.—Hematogenous gastritis arises more especially in the course of infections and intoxications, as in septicemia, typhoid fever, pulmonary tuberculosis, and variola. Metastatic abscess formation is, however, rare.

Gastritis per Extensionem.—Gastritis of this type may result from any localized inflammatory condition in the neighborhood of the stomach. Simple adhesion to adjacent structures may occur or perforation of the stomach wall, with discharge of inflammatory products into the cavity. Fistulous communications with other viscera may thus arise. Cholelithiasis, empyema of the gall-bladder, suppurative pancreatitis, may be mentioned in this connection. A perinephritic abscess has been known to rupture into the stomach. One of us (A. G. N.[1]) has recorded an apparently unique case of this kind in which the patient vomited pus and blood for three days before death.

Acute Catarrhal Gastritis.—Acute catarrhal gastritis is characterized by swelling and hyperemia of the mucous membrane, together with the

[1] Nicholls, Mont. Med. Jour., 27:1898:110.

production of a viscid adhesive exudate, consisting of mucus, desquamated epithelium, and leukocytes. Here and there, small hemorrhages may be seen and also superficial erosions.

Histologically, the secretory cells of the glands are cloudy and are desquamating, while goblet cells are very numerous. The epithelium of the peptic glands is more granular than usual and is often detached from the basement membrane. On the surface can be seen a stringy deposit of mucus, entangled in which are clumps of gastric epithelium, red blood-cells, and leukocytes. There is a round-celled infiltration between the tubules and in the submucosa, and the interstitial bloodvessels are congested. The endothelium of the lymphatics also may show signs of proliferation. These changes are usually confined to the region of the pylorus, but may be generalized.

Membranous Gastritis.—A more intense, though somewhat rare, condition is membranous gastritis. In its typical form it occurs most frequently in children. The membrane lies in small patches on the tops of the rugæ, or, more rarely, covers the whole stomach, forming, as it were, a cast of the interior. The membrane is loosely attached to the mucosa and is of a grayish color, or, again, is brownish from hemorrhage.

Membranous gastritis occurs most commonly in newborn children, in cases of septic infection of the umbilical cord, and in those suffering from scarlatina, measles, diphtheria, and variola, rarely in other infective fevers. True *diphtheria* of the stomach occurs, and, curiously enough, the infection may pass from the throat to the stomach without attacking the œsophagus. Necrosis and suppuration may cause a more or less extensive loss of substance in the mucosa, and deeply eroding ulcers may be formed.

Phlegmonous Gastritis.—Phlegmonous gastritis is rare. It occurs idiopathically, particularly in drunkards, and occasionally in general pyemia. More or less localized pus collections are formed in the stomach wall which may reach a considerable size and rupture into the cavity of the organ.

Follicular Gastritis.—Follicular gastritis is also rare. It is due to inflammation of the lymph-follicles, which are present in small numbers in the stomach. Suppuration may occur, giving rise to small, rounded ulcers.

Chronic Catarrhal Gastritis.—Chronic catarrhal gastritis may result from repeated acute attacks, but not infrequently arises independently. It is most common in those addicted to excess in alcohol or tobacco, in cases of long-standing passive congestion of the stomach, and as an accompaniment of gastric ulcer, carcinoma, and dilatation. It may also complicate anemia, Bright's disease, tuberculosis, and gout.

Several different forms have been described, but they are all probably to be regarded as stages in one and the same process. The mucous membrane is of a brown or grayish-brown color, owing to the deposit of an iron-containing pigment derived from the blood in the secreting cells and interglandular tissues. Congestion is not necessarily present, and may, in the later stages at least, be completely lacking, except in those cases originally due to passive hyperemia of systemic origin. The mucosa is covered with a thick, adherent layer of mucus, mixed with leukocytes and altered desquamated epithelial cells. In not a few cases numerous flattened, elevated plaques are produced (*état mamelonné*), and the proliferation of the interglandular fibrous tissue may be so great that warty outgrowths result (*gastritis polyposa*). In still another class of cases the productive change is most marked in the glandular elements, so that outgrowths resembling adenomas are produced. The last two forms are often grouped together under the term **hypertrophic gastritis.**

Again, the overgrowth of the interstitial connective tissue may lead to sclerosis and contraction of the organ (**atrophic gastritis**). Here, the mucosa is thin, hard, and of a grayish color. The other coats may also show fibrous hyperplasia, so that the thickness of the stomach wall is greatly increased while, at the same time, its capacity is diminished.

FIG. 91

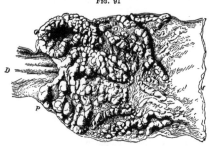

Multiple adenomatous polyps (adenitis polyposa) of stomach: *D*, duodenum; *P*, pyloric ring. (Orth.)

Occasionally, the contraction of the tissues is most marked in the neighborhood of the pyloric ring, and may lead to stenosis at this point and subsequent dilatation of the organ.

Microscopically, the most striking feature is a cellular infiltration in the interstitial areolar tissue, more especially in the outer layers of the mucosa. This leads to more or less separation of the gland-tubules. The ducts are catarrhal, often tortuous, dilated, or even cystic, the secreting cells being increased both in size and number. These changes lead to thickening of the mucous membrane giving it an irregular appearance.

Specific Forms of Gastritis.—**Thrush** is occasionally present in small, isolated, whitish patches on the mucosa, in cases where the fauces are extensively involved.

Tuberculosis.—Tuberculous infection of the stomach is, on the whole, rare, probably owing to the fact that the acid character of the gastric secretion is inimical to the growth of the tubercle bacillus, as of other germs. Tuberculosis of the stomach in human beings is almost invariably associated with advanced tuberculosis elsewhere, usually in the lungs.

Van Wart[1] has recorded one case, however, which is an exception to the rule. Orth, by feeding rabbits on tuberculous material, was able to produce typical lesions in the intestines in seven cases and in the stomach in one. Alice Hamilton[2] has recorded three cases of tuberculous ulceration of the stomach and has collected 16 more from the literature. Tuberculous ulcers are generally multiple and situated near the pylorus. Some are little more than superficial erosions of the mucosa, the discovery of the specific bacillus alone deciding the nature of the case, while others have a more typical appearance, with infiltrated edges and an irregular base containing caseous tubercles. It is remarkable that in many cases the intestines escape the infection. The stomach may, also, be involved along with other organs in a miliary dissemination of the disease.[3]

Syphilis.—This disease is also rare. Ecchymoses, hemorrhagic erosions, and chronic gastritis have been described among the lesions occurring. The most characteristic manifestation is the gumma, which may give rise to ulcers that may perforate. Cicatricial contractures of the affected part may also result.[4]

Typhoid.—Typhoid ulcers are reported, but are still rarer than tuberculosis.

Actinomycosis.—Actinomycosis is also excessively rare.

Inflammation of the stomach, more particularly the ulcerative and phlegmonous forms, may extend through all the coats and involve adjacent structures (**perigastritis**). If the infection be a mild one, simple fibrinous adhesion takes place between the contiguous surfaces, as, for example, those of the stomach and liver or anterior abdominal wall, with subsequent organization. Or, if the condition be more severe and of a septic nature, local abscesses may be formed about the stomach. Perforation of the stomach wall and adhesion to a hollow viscus, such as the colon, may lead to the formation of a fistulous track. Communication may thus be opened up between the stomach and the pleura.

Parasites and Abnormal Contents.—Any of the ordinary intestinal parasites may find a lodgement in the stomach. *Pentastomum denticulatum* and *Echinococcus* are met with in the stomach wall, but are rare.

It is not uncommon to find **foreign bodies** in the stomach which have got in with the food or have been swallowed by accident or design. Buttons, needles, spoons, scissors, hairpins, nails, false teeth, knives, forks, coins, stomach tubes, and many other articles are at times swallowed by insane and hysterical patients or by circus performers, and may give rise to serious trouble. *Hair-balls* (trichobezoar) are frequently

[1] Johns Hopkins Hosp. Bull., 14: 1903: 235.

[2] Ibid., 8: 1897: 75.

[3] See, also, Arloing, Des ulcer. tuberculeuses de l'estomac, Thèse de Lyon, Paris, 1903; and Poncet and Leriche, Rev. de Chir., 1: 1909.

[4] For literature, see Oberndorfer, Virch. Archiv, 159: 1900: 179. Brunner, Deutsche Chir., 46c: 1907.

found in cattle and, rarely, in human beings, Schopf[1] has collected 16 cases. The McGill Museum contains two examples.[2] The hair-ball is composed of the patient's own hair, or, as in one case reported, a mixture of that of the patient and that of a pet dog, felted into a compact mass by the muscular action of the stomach. The individual hairs composing it may be quite long and vary somewhat in color. As

FIG. 92

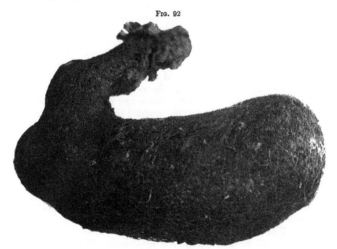

Hair ball in the stomach. The hair forms a complete cast of the stomach and duodenum.
(Case of Dr. James Bell, Royal Victoria Hospital, Montreal.)

a rule, they are somewhat darker than the patient's hair, probably owing to chemical action in the stomach cavity.   The hair may, in time, accumulate to such an extent as to form a complete cast of the interior of the stomach and duodenum.   Inflammation of these viscera not infrequently results, which may lead to perforation.   An analogous accumulation of vegetable fibre is known as *phytobezoar*.   Resinous concrements are recorded found in painters and others who have consumed spirit varnish.

RETROGRESSIVE METAMORPHOSES.

Atrophy.—Simple atrophy is met with in cachexia from any cause, marasmus, pernicious anemia, and as a senile change. The stomach is small, the wall thin, and the mucous membrane thin, pale, smooth, and shiny. The glands are granular and diminished in size. Diffuse or patchy fatty degeneration is a not uncommon associated condition.

[1] Wien. klin. Woch., November 16, 1899.
[2] See Montreal Med. Jour., 32:1903:94.

Degeneration.—Fatty Degeneration.—Fatty degeneration occurs in typhoid fever, septicemia, variola, pernicious anemia, leukemia, and in poisoning with phosphorus, arsenic, and lead, and occasionally in chronic gastritis.

Hyaline, Colloid, and Amyloid.—Hyaline, colloid, and amyloid transformation are not common.

Calcification.—Calcification of the mucosa has been observed in cases of rapid absorption of the lime salts from the bones in corrosive sublimate poisoning.

Postmortem Gastromalacia.—A brief reference should be made to the condition known as postmortem gastromalacia. The condition is not common in our experience in bodies sectioned within twenty-four hours of death. Local areas of softening, usually situated on the posterior wall of the fundus or at the cardia, may be found, which, from their appearance and special characters are to be attributed to the action of the gastric secretion, assisted probably by processes of decomposition. These areas are gelatinous, of a dirty, reddish-brown or green color, and often give rise to perforation and escape of the stomach contents. Much difference of opinion has been expressed over the question whether or not this softening is exclusively a postmortem appearance. The determining factors appear to be the condition of the secretory function of the stomach at the time of death and the length of time that has elapsed since death. It is quite possible, however, that in certain diseases where the resisting powers of the mucosa is diminished the phenomenon may be an agonal one.

Peptic Ulcer.—Of more practical importance is the so-called **peptic ulcer**, found both in the stomach and duodenum. When in the duodenum it is never situated below the bile papilla, being confined to that portion acted on by the gastric juice.

Peptic ulcers are single or multiple, and when in the stomach are usually situated at the pylorus, preferably on the lesser curvature. They may be mere superficial erosions, round or oval excavated ulcers, or may be so large as to girdle the stomach. The causes are many, but seem to depend mainly on defective circulation in the part, the result of thrombosis, embolism, spasm, or disease of the vessel walls. Small areas of hemorrhage or anemia predispose to their formation. The not infrequent association of gastric and duodenal ulcers with severe burns of the skin is well recognized. Here, the condition appears to be analogous to the necrotic changes that occur in the lymph-nodes from the action of toxic substances derived from the injured region. Once the protecting mucous membrane is damaged or destroyed, the digestive action of the gastric secretion comes into play and leads to further loss of substance.

The typical ulcer is round or oval, extending more or less deeply into the wall of the viscus. It has a characteristic funnel shape, the edges being terraced, more or less sharply cut, and gradually narrowing as the base is approached. In chronic cases, however, the edges may be rounded and the whole wall thickened. The ulcer is occasionally deeply pigmented, owing to the action of the gastric secretion upon the blood. Sometimes a number of superficial erosions tending to coalesce are found, a circumstance that throws some light on the etiology of the condition.

Microscopically, a recent ulcer shows but little. Except for the loss of substance and the terraced condition of the edges there may be no further change, or at most only a fine granulation of the cells. Only exceptionally is there a marked inflammatory reaction. Even in ulcers

Fig. 93

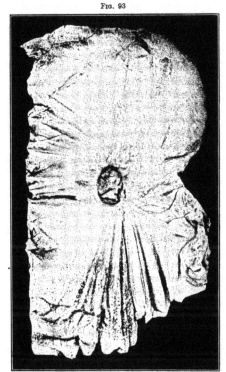

Peptic ulcer. (From the Pathological Museum of McGill University.)

of long standing the reactive phenomena are by no means pronounced. There is merely slight diapedesis of leukocytes, the muscularis shows fatty changes, and the vessels exhibit proliferating endarteritis.

Peptic ulcers are essentially chronic and give rise to a variety of symptoms. Repeated small hemorrhages will produce systemic anemia; larger ones may cause death. Pain after food and dyspeptic symptoms are quite common, but the condition not infrequently is entirely latent and unsuspected. A serious event is perforation of the ulcer resulting in general peritonitis. An ulcer on the posterior surface may rupture into the lesser peritoneal sac, a relatively favorable event. This may lead to fibrous perigastritis. Rarer sequels are perforation into the colon, spleen, gall-bladder, through the abdominal wall, into the left pleural cavity, into the left lung, and into the pericardium. In chronic ulceration, fibrous adhesion between the affected part and neighboring organs, such as the pancreas, liver, and adjacent lymph-nodes, is a common event. Finally, ulcers may heal, with the production of minute fibrous scars or larger stellate, contracted cicatrices. Stenosis of the pylorus and hour-glass constriction of the stomach are some of the results of this occurrence. Carcinoma may develop at the site of an old ulcer.

Simple Erosion.—There is one form of ulceration of the stomach, found not infrequently at autopsies, about which a word or two should be said, especially as the condition is one that has not as yet attracted much attention. The ulcers are very numerous and take the form of small, irregular, shallow pits, giving the mucosa a somewhat "moth-eaten" appearance. There is no infiltration and no surrounding congestion. The lesions resemble simple erosions. They may extend down to the muscle coat. Little is known about the etiology. The slighter cases may be of postmortem or agonal development. The more severe we have encountered in acute sepsis, and more especially in children.

PROGRESSIVE METAMORPHOSES.

. **Hypertrophy.**—Hypertrophy of the muscular wall of the stomach is met with in association with stenosis of the pylorus, chronic gastritis, and tumors. The whole wall may be affected or merely the portion near the pylorus. The congenital hypertrophy of the pylorus has already been referred to. Most cases are probably to be classed as hypertrophies from overwork. In chronic gastritis, there may be an overgrowth of the mucosa in the form of flattened sessile nodules (*état mamelonné*) or polypoid or papillary excrescences (*gastritis polyposa*). A somewhat similar condition is found occasionally in the neighborhood of chronic ulcers. The proliferation in these cases may begin in the interstitial fibrous tissue or in the glands.

Tumors.—Connective-tissue new-growths are rare and comparatively unimportant. **Fibromas, neurofibromas, lipomas,** and **myomas** have been met with. We have seen one case of a pedunculated *fibromyoma* springing from the serous surface at the fundus.[1] **Lymphangioma** beneath the serous covering of the stomach has been recorded.

Sarcoma is rare. Corner and Fairbank[2] have collected 58 cases. Gastric sarcomas may be subserous and pedunculated. Some of them

---

[1] Nicholls, Mont. Med. Jour., 32:1903:326.

[2] Practitioner, 72:1904:810. For the most recent study, see Donath, Virch. Archiv, 195:1909:2.

contain unstriped muscle fibers and are called by some observers **malignant myomas.**[1] In one such case Korinski found fibres of unstriped muscle in the metastatic growths in the liver.

Secondary sarcomas are occasionally met with.

Of the epithelial new-growths, **adenoma** (true polyps) has already been noted; **carcinoma** is by far the most frequent and important.

FIG. 94

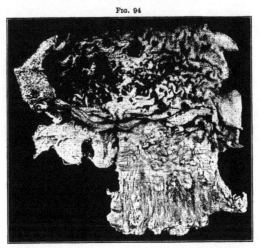

Secondary melanotic sarcoma of the stomach. (From the Pathological Museum of McGill University.)

Carcinoma.—Carcinoma of the stomach usually arises after middle life, and is somewhat more common in men than in women, the relative proportion being 52 to 48 per cent. According to Reiche, of 4759 cases of carcinoma, 50.2 per cent. occurred in the stomach.[2] The growth may originate from an apparently healthy mucosa or (some hold, often), in an old peptic ulcer. With regard to position, more than one-half the cases are situated at or near the pylorus. Next in frequency is the lesser curvature, and next, the cardia. Gastric carcinomas vary considerably in external appearance, some being soft and fungating, some papillomatous, some ulcerating, and others scirrhous or gelatinous.

Gastric carcinomas fall into five main classes—*medullary, adenocarcinoma, scirrhous, colloid,* and *squamous.* In 1348 cases of gastric carcinomas collected by Fenwick and Fenwick, 863 were medullary, 447 scirrhous, and 38 colloid.[3]

[1] Ghon and Hintz, Ziegler's Beiträge, 45: 1909.
[2] Deutsche med. Woch., 1900: 135
[3] Cancers and Tumors of the Stomach, 1903.

.The **medullary form** is characterized macroscopically by the formation **of** a soft, spongy mass, with smooth surface, but divided into flattened

Fig. 95

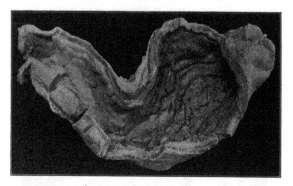

Diffuse scirrhous carcinoma of the stomach. Note the great thickening of the wall. (From the Pathological Museum of McGill University.)

Fig. 96

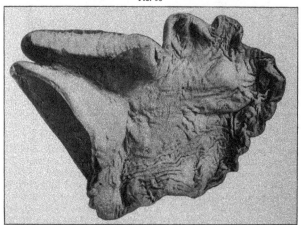

Scirrhous carcinoma of the pyloric portion of the stomach. (From the Pathological Museum of McGill University.)

nodes. Occasionally, the tendency is to infiltrate rather than to form projecting outgrowths. It is usually situated near the pylorus. When of any size, it may ulcerate, owing to lack of nutrition. **Histologically,** the new-growth consists chiefly of masses of cylindrical or isodiametric cells, with relatively little connective tissue. Fibrous induration of the stomach wall is a frequent accompaniment.

The **adenocarcinoma** forms large, soft, fungous masses, having a shreddy almost papillomatous appearance. Microscopically, the epithelial cells are arranged in atypical glandular masses, preserving a more or less complete resemblance to the gland-tubules from which they spring. There is a small amount of stroma, often infiltrated in places with round cells.

Fig. 97

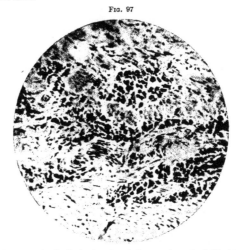

Carcinoma of the stomach. Section is taken through the muscular coat. Reichert obj. 7a, without ocular. (From the collection of the Pathological Department of McGill University.)

Scirrhous carcinoma involves the whole wall of the stomach or merely the pyloric region. The affected portion is much thickened and fibrous. The mucous membrane may be intact over the growth, but is not infrequently absent. In the diffuse form the stomach may be so contracted that its cavity can contain only about a cupful. Scirrhus at the pylorus often leads to cicatricial stenosis, with dilatation of the organ.[1] Histologically, the main portion of the growth is formed of dense connective tissue, the epithelial elements being scanty. Fibrous induration of the muscular coat is a marked feature.

Colloid carcinoma is found in nodular masses or as a diffuse infiltration of the stomach wall. When incised, the tumor is composed almost

[1] We have encountered two cases, confined to the pyloric ring, in which the cancer cells proper had undergone almost complete degeneration and absorption, the remaining dense stroma causing a doubtful diagnosis of congenital or acquired hypertrophy and stenosis.

entirely of gelatinous material, sometimes collected into cysts. Microscopically, it is a cylindrical-celled carcinoma, as a rule, but the marked feature is the tendency to colloid change exhibited by the cells, not only the epithelial cells, but those of the stroma as well.

Squamous epithelioma is rather rare. It occurs at the cardia, and probably originates in the mucosa of the lower end of the œsophagus, whence it invades the stomach.

A very uncommon form of cancer is the **Carcinoma sarcomatodes,**[1] in which the stroma shows sarcomatous transformation.

Carcinoma of the stomach may infiltrate all the coats of the organ and even bring about adhesion to neighboring structures, pancreas, colon, liver, omentum, which may, in turn, be invaded. It is not uncommon to find dilated lymphatics on the serous surface of the stomach filled with carcinoma cells. The lymph-nodes about the lesser curvature, the retroperitoneal, inguinal, thoracic, and supraclavicular nodes are in time involved. In a large proportion of cases metastasis takes place through the blood-vascular system, somewhat in contravention of the general rule. Secondary growths are common in the liver, invasion taking place through the radicles of the portal vein.

Medullary and especially colloid cancers tend to invade the peritoneum and give rise to numerous and widely distributed secondary growths resembling in type the parent growth. The omentum is often infiltrated and distorted, and may sometimes be recognized as a transverse band crossing the upper part of the abdomen. One of us (A. G. N.[2]) has reported a somewhat unusual case of diffuse scirrhous carcinoma of the peritoneum and omentum, with contraction of the mesentery and chronic peritonitis, originating in a scirrhous carcinoma of the stomach.

When situated near the pylorus, gastrectasis, with all that that implies —retention of food, fermentation, gastritis, excessive vomiting—supervenes. Ulceration may lead to erosion of a vessel and fatal hemorrhage, or to perforation and peritonitis.

---

[1] Lindemann, Zeitschrift f. Krebsforschung, 6: 1908.
[2] Nicholls, Jour. Amer. Med. Assoc., 40: 1903: 696.

CHAPTER XX.

THE INTESTINES.

CONGENITAL ANOMALIES.

TOTAL absence of the intestines and similar gross defects are found only in connection with other serious malformations. Partial or complete defect of the appendix has been observed. Sometimes portions of the bowel are defective. Thus, the anus with more or less of the rectum may be absent; or the anus may open into a sac which does not communicate with the colon above. Membranous septa, transverse or longitudinal, may be present. Defects of the lower bowel and urogenital sinus are rather common. Thus, there may be a large cloaca into which the bladder and rectum discharge. The bladder may be divided and the large intestine absent, so that the ileum empties into the bladder. In less extreme cases there may be merely incomplete closure of the septum that exists between the rectum and urogenital sinus. The rectum, when defective, may end blindly or discharge into the bladder, urethra, vagina, or perineum. Congenital narrowing (stenosis) or imperforate areas (atresia) occur. Inverted positions of the various portions are recorded, both with and without inversion of the other abdominal or thoracic viscera. An abnormal course of the colon is common. It may pass diagonally across the abdomen, without forming an hepatic flexure, or there may be accessory loops. Perhaps the most frequent form is a downward loop of V-shape, which is found in 9.5 per cent. of autopsies. Hernial protrusions may take place through a fissure of the abdominal wall, a patent inguinal canal, or a defect in the diaphragm.

A common anomaly is the Meckel's diverticulum, occurring in our experience in about 2.7 per cent. of autopsies. It is found usually in the ileum, ordinarily, in adults within a meter of the ileocecal valve. The diverticulum is cylindrical, funnel-shaped, or larger at the distal end. The apex is sometimes rounded, bifid, or lobulated. The average length is about 7 cm. The pouch is situated on the opposite side from the mesenteric attachment, and represents the remains of the omphalomesenteric duct. All degrees of patency of this duct may exist. Thus, it may remain open for its whole length, giving rise to what is known as an omphalomesenteric fistula; it may be open at the umbilical end—omphalic fistula; it may be closed at both ends, forming a cyst, when situated in front of the peritoneum called a preperitoneal cyst, when attached to the intestine called an enterocystoma. Not infrequently, the Meckel's pouch is attached to the umbilicus by a fibrous cord, the remains of the involuted duct.

Structurally, the diverticulum consists of all the layers of the intestine, although the muscular coat may be somewhat thinned at the apex. It may have free communication with the bowel, or may be partially shut off by a valve.

The importance of the condition lies in the fact that the diverticulum may become strangulated and inflamed, or, again, may perforate. Where the fibrous attachment persists, coils of intestine may be caught and strangulated. Exceptionally, even adenoma and carcinoma may develop at the umbilicus from inclusions of the mucous membrane.

Congenital Hypertrophy and Dilatation.—Congenital hypertrophy and dilatation of the colon (*megacolon;* Hirschsprung's disease[1]) is a peculiar condition affecting mainly the ascending colon, but sometimes also to a lesser degree the transverse. The cause is unknown, though many cases are undoubtedly developmental peculiarities. In one reported by Formad, the colon contained 22 kilos. of feces. The irritation of the retained feces leads to inflammation and ulceration of the bowel, and sooner or later to a fatal termination. The condition has been found at birth, but frequently develops during early childhood.

ACQUIRED ANOMALIES OF THE LUMEN.

Acute Dilatation.—Acute dilatation of the intestines (*enteroplegia*), is strictly comparable in regard to causes and results with acute dilatation of the stomach. Many cases arise from acute obstruction, as from foreign bodies, adhesions, volvulus, or hernias. An important etiological factor is infection, either local or systemic. The influence of local infection is seen in the cases that occur in connection with peritonitis, appendicitis, cholecystitis, or other inflammatory conditions of the abdominal viscera. The gastro-intestinal paralysis accompanying pneumonia, typhoid, scarlatina, and meningitis is probably to be attributed to the influence of toxins circulating in the blood. Blows on the abdomen and falls have been followed by the condition. Some cases, again, have followed upon anesthesia. Some few have come on apparently without cause, and have been attributed to nervous influences. A not inconsiderable number follow surgical operations on the abdominal viscera, no doubt, as experimental work has shown, the result of prolonged handling and the exposure of the intestinal coils to the air.

Chronic Dilatation.—Chronic dilatation begins insidiously and may take months to develop. Perhaps the most common cause is partial obstruction of the lumen of the intestine. The intestinal wall is usually hypertrophied as well as the cavity dilated.

Acquired Diverticula.—Acquired diverticula of the intestine are not uncommon. They differ from the true diverticula, of which the Meckel's is the type, in that they are often multiple, situated between the layers of the mesentery or near to the mesenteric attachment, and are usually

---

[1] Hirschsprung, Jahrbuch f. Kinderheilkunde, 27: 1888; for discussion and literature see Petrivalsky, Arch. f. Chir., 86: 1908: 318.

composed of one or two coats of the bowel, the muscular layer being often wanting. In many cases the condition is really a hernia of the mucosa into the serosa, or, again, the serosa may be the only constituent. Most cases are associated with chronic pulmonary affections in old people. The strain of coughing is apparently the exciting cause, the bowel wall giving way at its weakest point, namely, where the mesenteric veins leave it at the mesenteric attachment. After middle life there seems to be a physiological tendency to weakening at these points. Other cases are associated with ulceration of the mucosa, or are due to the traction of adhesions or tumors attached to the bowel. Hansemann[1] has recorded one in which there were about 400 diverticula, varying in size from that of a hemp-seed to that of a pigeon's egg.

Stenosis.—Stenosis of the lumen may be brought about by cicatrizing processes in the wall of the intestine, as in tuberculosis, syphilis, dysentery, or uremic ulceration; new-growths; compression of or traction on the bowel from without, as from tumors, healing peritonitis, or a coil of intestine loaded with feces. These are common causes of chronic obstruction.

Volvulus.—Volvulus occurs generally between the ages of thirty and forty years. In this condition the bowel is more or less completely obstructed owing to a twist and kink about its long axis. In other cases, a loop of intestine is twisted upon itself much as in the case of a handkerchief used as a tourniquet, or, again, one coil of bowel may be twisted about another. Half the cases occur in the sigmoid flexure. The next most common site is in the small intestine. McFarland notes having met with one case involving a Meckel's diverticulum. Volvulus occurs in the movable portion of the intestines, and is thought to be brought about by excessive peristalsis caused by unequal filling of the coils or by contusions. An abnormally long mesentery would no doubt predispose.

Intussusception or Invagination.—This is the condition in which one portion of the bowel slips into another, much as one might invert the finger of a glove. It is comparatively frequent, and is usually met with in the young, 34 per cent. of cases occurring in children under the age of one year. Irregular peristalsis and muscular spasm are believed to be the direct causes. Active purgation, diarrhœa, intestinal irritation, intestinal ulcers, and polypi are believed to predispose. Intussusception may be acute or chronic, single or multiple. Multiple intussusceptions are quite common at autopsies, and are probably an agonal manifestation. They are readily distinguishable from the pathological form from the fact that they are readily reduced and there is no sign of severe constriction of the bowel or of inflammation. They are frequently ascending, while the true intussusceptions are almost invariably descending, that is to say, the upper portion of the bowel is invaginated into the lower. Various grades of invagination occur, and if unrelieved the condition tends to become aggravated.

---

[1] Virch. Archiv, 144: 1896: 400. See also Fischer, Jour. Exp. Med., 5: 1901: 333.

The following varieties are recognized: The *ileocecal*, in which a part of the ileum and the ileocecal valve enters the colon; the *ileocolic*, in which a portion of the ileum passes through the valve; the *ileal*, in which the ileum is alone involved; the *colic*, involving the colon alone; and the *colicorectal*, involving the colon and rectum. The portion of the intestine involved forms a sausage-like tumor with a curved outline. On further examination of the mass three layers of bowel are recognizable, an outermost or receiving layer—the *intussuscipiens;* an innermost or entering layer, and a middle or returning layer, both together constituting the *intussusceptum*. At the point where the intussusceptum enters the intussuscipiens there is generally a constriction, termed the neck. The part of the intussusceptum farthest away from the neck is the apex. Intussusception may also be double, the originally invaginated portion being carried bodily into the intestine below. As the condition progresses the inner and the middle layers increase at the expense of the outer. As a result of the constriction the circulation is interfered with and often entirely arrested. In the early stages there is slight reddening of the affected region, with possibly the exudation of a little plastic lymph. Later, the part is greatly swollen and congested, and the various layers are glued together with inflammatory exudate. Finally, necrosis and gangrene result, and the patient often dies from obstruction, peritonitis, or shock. If operative measures be undertaken, the invagination can usually be reduced in the large majority of cases (94 per cent.) during the first twenty-four hours, but the longer operation is delayed the more difficult does this procedure become. By the fourth day only about one-third can be relieved. The amount of intestine invaginated is often of great extent. The ileum has been known to pass through the ileocecal valve and appear at the anus. An uncommon event is separation of the necrotic portion and spontaneous healing. One instance is on record (Hermes) in which 60 cm. of the bowel came away and the patient recovered. In the Pathological Museum of McGill University are seventeen inches of small intestine passed *per anum* by a boy who had all the symptoms of strangulation of the bowel and recovered. In such cases inflammatory lymph forms a union at the point of constriction, which subsequently becomes organized.

ACQUIRED ANOMALIES OF POSITION.

The term **hernia** or **rupture** is used generally to denote the dislocation of one or more viscera with partial or complete passage through the limiting body wall. In a more restricted sense it is applied to the intestines and associated structures.

Hernias of the intestines may be *external* or *internal*. In the former, the intestines enter the inguinal or femoral canals, the umbilicus, the abdominal wall, or the obturator foramen, and eventually present externally beneath the skin and subcutaneous tissues. In the latter, which are rarer, the intestine passes through openings in the omentum, mesentery, the foramen of Winslow, or into pockets of the peritoneal sac.

The chief causes operating to bring them about are weakness of the peritoneal sac at some particular point, either acquired or congenital, as in patency of certain canals that are normally closed; and internal pressure, brought about by strain or the weight of the contained viscera. In some few cases a tumor or local adhesion may exercise traction upon the peritoneum and lead to the production of a sac.

The structures entering into a hernia are various. As a rule, they are the small intestine, mesentery, and omentum; less often, the cecum, large intestine, or other viscera, such as the stomach, spleen, liver, gall-bladder, ovary, uterus, ureter, and urinary bladder. As the intestine or other organ prolapses or descends, it carries before it a prolongation of the peritoneal membrane. This covering is absent only in cases in which the membrane is torn, or when portions of the intestine that, like the cecum, are extraperitoneally situated are prolapsed through an opening in the fascia and muscles of the abdomen. In the early stages the sac is represented merely by a shallow concavity, but later, owing to pressure, is converted into a globular or pear-shaped receptacle communicating with the abdominal cavity by a narrow neck. Occasionally, only in a small portion of the intestinal wall is caught in the sac, the main portion of the loop being free (*Littré's hernia*). In such cases there may be the same evidences of obstruction as in the ordinary type.

External Hernias.—*Inguinal hernia* is the most common form of hernia, and is more frequent in men than in women. The etiological factors are, congenital weakness or patency of the inguinal canal, or descent of the intestines or other viscera with the peritoneal membrane through the canal. If the organs in question pass through the internal ring and enter the canal, but without escaping from the external ring, the condition is termed an **incomplete inguinal hernia**. If it passes outside of the external ring it is called a **complete inguinal hernia**. If the descending organs enter the scrotum it is a **scrotal** or **inguinoscrotal hernia**. In women the hernial protrusion may occur into the labium majus, forming an **inguinolabial hernia**.

Several subvarieties are recognized. Thus, if the organs present at the external abdominal ring without having traversed the canal, it is called a **direct inguinal hernia**. If they pass in the ordinary way through the canal, the hernia is termed an **indirect** or **oblique inguinal hernia**. Hernias are further divided into **external** and **internal inguinal hernias**, according as the prolapsed organs pass to the outer or inner side of the deep epigastric artery.

Femoral hernia is also comparatively frequent, and is more common in women than in men. In this form the intestines are prolapsed along the course of the femoral vessels and make their appearance on the inner side of the thigh just below Poupart's ligament.

Obturator hernia is not common. It occurs at the obturator foramen, along the course of the obturator artery and nerve.

Umbilical hernia may be congenital, but perhaps is more frequent in women who have borne children. Prolapse takes place through the umbilical ring or into the cord. The hernia is often large and usually contains intestine with omentum. Rarely, the liver may be extruded as well. At times the condition amounts to an actual evisceration.

Abdominal hernia is a term applied to prolapse of the viscera through the abdominal wall in regions other than at the usual foramina. The hernia often takes place between the recti muscles in an abdomen rendered lax by childbearing, or into the scar of an operation wound.

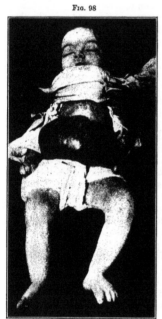

Fig. 98

Ischiadic hernia occurs at the great sacrosciatic foramen.

Perineal hernia is rare. It takes place between the bundles of the levator ani muscle.

Lumbar hernia consists in a protrusion of the intestine into the space bounded by the crest of the ilium, the external oblique, and the latissimus dorsi muscles.

Vaginal hernia is very rare, and consists in a descent of the bowel between the rectum and uterus.

Internal Hernias.—The most frequent form is said to be that in which the intestine passes through a hole in the mesentery. Hernias may also occur through the foramen of Winslow, through openings in the omentum, into the fossa duodeno-jejunalis, the subcecal fossa, and the fossa intersigmoidea. **Diaphragmatic hernia** may occur as a result of congenital defects in the diaphragm or as a result of traumatism (see p. 410).

Hernia through the umbilical region of the liver, appendix, and part of the colon; child, aged eight months. (Dr. A. E. Vipond's case.)

According to the structures entering into the hernia, various types are recognized. An **enterocele** contains some part of the intestine; an **epiplocele**, a portion of the omentum; a **cystocele**, a portion of the bladder; a **cecocele**, a part of the cecum; a **rectocele**, a portion of the rectum; a **hysterocele**, the uterus.

Hernias probably never are cured spontaneously. When the prolapsed organs can be replaced in their normal relations the hernia is spoken of as **reducible**; when the hernial contents cannot be returned, the hernia is **irreducible**. Hernias may be temporarily irreducible, owing to the presence of gas, fluid, or feces, or permanently irreducible from the formation of inflammatory adhesions. If a hernia has lasted any length of time secondary changes set in, chiefly of a mechanical or inflammatory nature. The hernial sac becomes thickened and its constituent elements fuse together so that it may no longer be possible to distinguish the original layers. The inner surface is smooth and pearly, often traversed by elevated ridges. The coils of intestine and omentum in acute conditions may be adherent to each other or to the wall of the sac with fibrinous lymph or, in old cases, by firm fibrous bands. The mesentery is often shortened and deformed from old inflammatory thickening. Acute infection with inflammatory exudation may occur in an incarcerated or strangulated hernia, or in any long-standing case. The mobility of the intestines gradually becomes so much impaired that the intestinal contents cannot·be passed on and severe derangement of the circulation sets in (*incarceration*). Pressure may be exerted through the elasticity of the tissues forming the neck of the sac or from the weight of feces within the coils. If the pressure be so great as to hinder the venous return, the intestine becomes greatly congested. The coils assume a purplish-red color, and are swollen and œdematous, though they may for a time preserve their lustre. If the condition be not relieved the hernial contents become greatly inflamed and finally gangrenous. The bowel then presents an intense blackish or bluish-red appearance, with possibly suppurative foci here and there which lead to perforation. At the point of constriction, which is usually the neck, the tissues are of a pale grayish-white color (*strangulation*).

INTESTINAL OBSTRUCTION.

Intestinal obstruction results from any condition which impedes or prevents the passage of the bowel contents. The chief etiological factors are hernia, strangulation, intussusception, volvulus, paralysis of the bowels, stenosis and atresia, tumors, and abnormal contents. Hernia and strangulation are the most frequent causes. In an analysis of 1000 operative cases, Gibson[1] found 35 per cent. were due to hernia, 19 per cent. to constricting bands, 19 per cent. to intussusception, and 12 per cent. to volvulus. The fibrous adhesions resulting from peritonitis may cut off pockets from the general abdominal cavity or form bands and loops through which coils of the intestine may become prolapsed. Slits in the mesentery or great omentum, and an attached Meckel's diverticulum, sometimes act in the same way. Owing to peristaltic action or to distension, the prolapsed bowel may become kinked at some point and obstruction ensue. The intestine may also be obstructed by the pressure of tumors, cysts, wandering organs, or the traction of cicatricial bands. Polypi, cysts, tumors, gallstones, and healing ulcers may obstruct the bowel from within.

The lumen of the bowel may be occluded by the accumulation of feces which have become inspissated. Intestinal worms seldom cause trouble, but tangled clusters of ascarides have sometimes led to obstruction. Foreign bodies occasionally are introduced through the rectum, but usually enter through the mouth, either by accident or design. A great

[1] Annals of Surgery, 32: 1900: 486 and 676.

variety of substances have been found, fruit stones and seeds, hair, false teeth, needles, pins, hairpins, and tacks.

Below the point of obstruction the bowel is empty or nearly so, while above it is distended enormously by gas and fecal accumulation. At the occluded part the mucosa is often eroded and the bowel wall anemic as a result of pressure, while the proximal portion of the intestine is congested, inflamed, eroded, or necrotic. Not infrequently a considerable amount of transudate is found free in the abdominal cavity. In chronic cases the intestinal wall is considerably thickened as well as dilated, owing partly to functional hypertrophy and partly to inflammatory infiltration. In obstruction of the bowel, the virulence of the contained microbes is greatly increased, while at the same time the resisting power of the tissues is low, so that not uncommonly peritonitis results, even in the absence of any solution of continuity of the bowel wall.

CIRCULATORY DISTURBANCES.

Hyperemia.—**Active Hyperemia.**—Active hyperemia occurs physiologically during digestion, and, pathologically, as a result of irritation, infection, or dilatation of the vessels under the influence of nervous stimuli. The intestines are also congested in cases of peritonitis. The mucosa becomes markedly reddened, but the condition quickly passes off after death, so that the appearances at autopsy may not be very striking.

Passive Hyperemia.—Passive hyperemia arises in the course of obstruction in the general systemic circulation, as well as from hepatic cirrhosis or similar interference with the portal circulation. Local passive congestion is also met with as a result of the compression of the mesenteric veins in the conditions of hernia and strangulation. The affected bowel in these cases is swollen, œdematous, purplish-red, or blue in color, and the serosa is possibly slightly roughened. In chronic congestion the mucosa may be somewhat pigmented.

Varices.—Varices occur occasionally. The commonest site is the rectum, the condition being induced by stasis in the inferior hemorrhoidal vein. The varices are to be found within the rectum or externally around the anus, in the form of small, globular or polypoid swellings of a dull, bluish color (*hemorrhoids*). The chief causes are sedentary habits, chronic constipation, the pressure of tumors in the pelvis or of the pregnant uterus, and obstruction within the portal circulation. The hemorrhoids often become inflamed and ulcerated, and may lead to hemorrhage. Repeated loss of blood in this way sometimes gives rise to severe anemia, the cause of which may sometimes be overlooked.

Œdema.—Œdema results from active or passive hyperemia, acute and chronic inflammations, peritonitis, or is a manifestation of general anasarca. The walls of the intestine are firm and thickened, giving a sensation to the fingers resembling that of wash-leather. The muscle is pale and gelatinous, and the mucosa is anemic and swollen, with a sodden, watery appearance. The natural folds are accentuated.

Hemorrhage.—Hemorrhage into the mucosa is a not uncommon event in cases of active and passive congestion, in embolism or thrombosis of the mesenteric vessels, in pernicious anemia, hemophilia, and the hemorrhagic diatheses.

Hemorrhage into the lumen results from inflammation, ulceration, necrosis, injuries, foreign bodies, and new-growths. Dysentery, typhoid fever, peptic ulcer, ulcerating carcinomas, hemorrhoids, are the most important causes. When the blood is effused high up it becomes black and tarry as a result of the action of the digestive juices and the sulphuretted hydrogen in the feces; when escaping lower down it is usually red. Severe bleeding into the lumen of the intestine may occur, and may even prove fatal without the blood escaping externally. This is termed *occult* or *concealed* hemorrhage.

Embolism and Thrombosis.—Embolism and thrombosis of the mesenteric arteries or veins lead to infarction of the whole area of the bowel supplied by the obstructed vessels.[1] Hemorrhage, often extensive, takes place into the intestinal wall, which undergoes necrosis and even gangrene. Peritonitis often supervenes, owing to infection from the intestinal contents. The symptoms are mainly those of intestinal obstruction. Melena may occur. Some of the ordinary causes of embolism are present, endocarditis or arteriosclerosis. Thrombosis is usually the result of an infective thrombophlebitis of the mesenteric veins.

Several observers recently, notably Ortner, have drawn attention to the clinical importance of **mesenteric arteriosclerosis.** The condition gives rise to colic with alternating attacks of diarrhœa and constipation.

INFLAMMATIONS.

The inflammatory disturbances of the intestines are, on the whole, strikingly like those of the stomach, both etiologically and anatomically. Any differences are to be explained by variations in function and mechanical conditions. Most cases of inflammation of the intestines are due to the irritative action of the intestinal contents, which may be unsuitable, may have undergone abnormal fermentation, or, again, may contain toxic substances of an animal, vegetable, or mineral nature. Some cases, also, are due to infectious or toxic agents carried to the intestine by the blood-stream or body juices. These probably act by depressing the vitality of the specific tissue cells, by modifying secretion, and by increasing the virulence of microörganisms contained in the feces, which, under ordinary circumstances are devoid of pathogenic properties.

The portions of the intestinal tract most apt to suffer from inflammatory disturbances are (1) the duodenum, owing to its close association with the stomach, and the diverse influences to which it is subjected during the acid and alkaline 'tides' respectively; (2) the large bowel, where feces and other irritating substances are liable to accumulate, and (3) the lower end of the ileum, where the development of fecal bacteria attains its maximum.

[1] Matthes, Mediz. Klinik, 16: 1906.

Enteritis.—Inflammation of the small intestine is termed **enteritis;** of the large, **colitis;** of both, **enterocolitis.** If the stomach be involved as well, we speak of **gastro-enteritis.** Any portion of the bowel may be inflamed, but it is rare for it to be affected throughout its whole extent. Therefore, we speak of **duodenitis, jejunitis, ileitis, typhlitis** or **cecitis, colitis, appendicitis, sigmoiditis,** and **proctitis.**

Acute Catarrhal Enteritis.—This is due to indiscretions in diet, or food containing bacteria of certain kinds or bacterial toxins. Climatic conditions and change of diet also seem to have a considerable effect in inducing the disease. Acute catarrhal enteritis and gastro-enteritis is especially common in young children, in whom it is produced by overfeeding and the use of milk laden with microörganisms. B. dysenteriæ, B. enteritidis, B. coli, B. proteus, and the streptococcus are the germs usually present in these cases. Catarrhal enteritis also accompanies or complicates certain of the acute infective fevers, such as typhoid and pneumonia. The cholera vibrio produces an acute serous enteritis.

The postmortem appearances in acute catarrhal enteritis are not constant, for a notable amount of catarrh may exist without producing any gross lesions that are recognizable after death. In some cases there is a patchy congestion of the mucosa in the neighborhood of the lymph-vessels, on the top of the rugæ, and, in severe cases, of the serosa. Punctate hemorrhages are occasionally to be seen. The mucosa is often swollen and presents a dull, cloudy, grayish appearance, so that the folds are more in evidence than usual. Generally, though not invariably, the surface is covered with a mucous or serous exudate (*serous enteritis*) containing relatively few leukocytes. In other cases the white cells are more abundant and the exudate assumes a mucopurulent or purulent character. The exudate may contain, also, desquamated epithelial cells in varying stages of degeneration. This may, possibly, be to some extent due to postmortem maceration of the tissues.

Microscopically, there can be made out marked hyperemia of the mucosa and submucosa, with some œdema. The secreting cells of the tubular glands show evidences of increased functional activity in the presence of great numbers of goblet cells. Slight erosions of the mucosa may occur and the surface is covered with more or less exudate. In the severer forms collections of leukocytes are to be seen in the mucosa about the gland-tubules and in the submucosa around the bloodvessels. The condition of simple catarrh may pass almost imperceptibly into *suppuration,* and considerable portions of the mucosa may slough away, leaving sharply defined *ulcers* with infiltrated walls. The submucosa contains leukocytes in great numbers. Suppurative enteritis may lead to a diffuse *phlegmonous* condition or to the formation of localized *abscesses* in the submucosa, which burst into the lumen, leaving small ulcers. A purulent peritonitis is an occasional sequel.

Desquamative Enteritis.—In the so-called desquamative enteritis the mucosa is cast off *en masse* in the form of a tubular cast. This occurrence has been described in the large bowel in connection with the summer diarrhœas of children. It is found also in cases of dysentery, cholera, and in poisoning by arsenic.

Follicular Enteritis.—The part played in enteritis by the solitary and agminated glands is a varying one. In many instances these structures show no marked changes, but in others they are so greatly affected that the disorder may properly be termed **follicular enteritis.** In this type of intestinal inflammation, the follicles are swollen and project above the general surface of the mucosa, where they are recognizable as dots of a grayish or grayish-white color on a more or less hyperemic background. When the Peyer's patches are affected, owing to the unequal swelling of the lymphoid and connective-tissue elements, the surface becomes somewhat reticulated or traversed by shallow grooves. Follicular enteritis is not infrequently found as a result of cholera, typhoidal or tuberculous infection, and is particularly common in diphtheria.

Histologically, the swelling of the follicles is due to hyperemia and proliferation of the lymphoid cells. There is, in addition, a perifollicular cellular infiltration and the neighboring lymph-vessels are filled with cells. The follicles usually present no further change, but now and then undergo necrosis. In this way small, rounded abscesses are formed which discharge their contents and give rise to one form of ulcerative enteritis.

Membranous Enteritis.—Under the term membranous enteritis are classed those severer forms of inflammation of the intestines which lead to coagulation-necrosis and ulceration. There may be produced a "croupous" or fibrinous exudation upon the surface of the mucous membrane, which becomes fused, as it were, by coagulative changes into a more or less homogeneous mass—membranous inflammation, or the exudate may be both on and within the substance of the mucosa—diphtheroid inflammation. It is impossible always to separate these forms one from the other, since they are produced by the same causes, and the croupous may pass imperceptibly into the diphtheroid.

The chief causes are dysentery, various infections, such as pyemia, cholera, typhoid, and tuberculosis, rarely diphtheria, coprostasis, uremia, and poisoning by ptomaines, arsenic, quicksilver, and bismuth.

Membranous enteritis is usually met with in the large intestine (*membranous colitis*), but occasionally also in the ileum. It probably begins as an ordinary catarrh, with congestion and swelling of the mucosa, which rapidly progresses into a more severe inflammation. The mucosa becomes deeply reddened and a brawny sort of film of a whitish-gray color appears upon the surface, especially upon the top of the rugæ. At first this membrane can be scraped off with the knife, but later this becomes impossible, owing to the fact that the mucosa undergoes a form of coagulation necrosis and the exudate and mucous membrane become welded into an indistinguishable mass. As the disease progresses, the redness and swelling increase, the patches of membrane tend to coalesce, and the coagulated substance assumes a dirty, yellowish-green, or brown color through contact with the feces.

In course of time portions of the membrane and necrotic mucosa may be exfoliated, giving rise to ulcers which may coalesce and reach a considerable size. They may extend superficially, or, again, penetrate deeply. The denuded tissues in such cases may become infected by septic microörganisms and a local suppurative condition or a diffused phlegmon may be the result. If the condition heal, the ulcers cicatrize, the mucosa is in large part regenerated, and more or less fibrous thickening of the intestine remains.

Special Forms of Enteritis.—Dysentery.—Under the term dysentery are included a number of intestinal inflammations, which, while they differ considerably, have this in common, that they are characterized clinically by colic, severe and persistent diarrhœa with tenesmus. Pathologically speaking, they are all forms of colitis. Dysentery occurs epidemically, endemically, and sporadically, more especially in tropical and subtropical climes, but also occasionally in temperate regions. The disease may be acute or chronic. The difficulties in the way of making an adequate classification of the forms of dysentery are great, owing to the fact that the etiological factors are not entirely understood, nor is it as yet possible to satisfactorily correlate our knowledge of the subject. While it is certain that the majority, if not all, the dysenteries are to be attributed to the activity of microörganisms, it is equally certain that a variety of differing infectious processes have been grouped under the one head. It is probable also that the dysenteries occurring in different countries are characterized by specific differences.

The multitudinous investigations which have been made into the subject of dysentery during the past few years seem to have determined that there are three main types: (1) A form due to irritation from unsuitable food, preformed poisons, and similar causes; (2) a form due to bacterial activity; and (3) a form due to protozoan parasites. We know little as yet in regard to the irritative or chemical dysentery, and it seems to have little to differentiate it from other forms of colitis.

Acute dysentery of the second order for the most part is due to infection with some member of the group of dysentery bacilli. Some few cases have been found to be associated with the B. pyocyaneus (Calmette,[1] Lartigau[2]) and with a spirillum (Le Dantec[3]).

Epidemic Dysentery Due to Shiga's Bacillus.—This disease affects the large intestine and the lower portion of the ileum, though in some cases the lesions are confined to the rectum, sigmoid flexure, and lower portion of the colon. In mild cases the mucous membrane is intensely congested and swollen and the rugæ are unusually prominent. Numerous small hemorrhages may be noted in the mucosa and the surface of the bowel is covered with viscid, blood-stained mucus. The lymph-follicles are swollen and there are often superficial erosions. The process may eventually assume an ulcerative or membranous character. The colon may be of a grayish or greenish color, and presents brownish-black sloughs or eschars. When present, the membrane may be confined to the tops of the rugæ or may affect larger areas of mucosa. In the

---

[1] Quoted by *Lartigau*.   [2] Jour. of Exper. Med., 3: 1898: 595.
[3] Comptes rendus de la Soc. de biol., 1903: 16.

very severe cases, the wall of the intestine is softened and thickened, while the submucosa is densely infiltrated with pus cells. Peritonitis may supervene.

The specific cause is the B. dysenteriæ of Shiga,[1] a non-motile bacillus somewhat closely resembling that of typhoid. It is present in a large proportion of cases of epidemic dysentery, is pathogenic for experimental animals, and is agglutinated by the serum of immunized animals or those suffering from the disease.

Epidemic Dysentery Due to Flexner's Bacillus (Institutional Dysentery or Pseudodysentery).—This form is due to a bacillus first isolated by Flexner[2] from cases of epidemic dysentery occurring in the Philippine Islands in 1900, and later by Kruse[3] and others in cases occurring in Germany. In America, epidemic dysentery appears to be more often caused by Flexner's bacillus than by that of Shiga. Flexner's organism is evidently closely allied to that of Shiga, but is differentiated from it by minor cultural peculiarities and by the fact that the two types react differently toward immune sera prepared from the two strains.

Park, Collins, and Goodwin[4] drew attention to a form intermediate between the Shiga and Flexner types, and, indeed, the more recent exact bacteriological studies in different parts of the world have drawn attention to the existence of a score and more forms or strains, differing from each other in their actions upon the various sugars and glucosides and in their agglutinative properties. Many cases of summer diarrhœa in children have been shown to be due to Flexner's organism. Some also are due to infection with the B. pyocyaneus.[5]

Endemic or Amœbic Dysentery.—Amœbic dysentery is a form endemic in Egypt and other tropical and subtropical regions, due to the Amœba coli or Amœba dysenteriæ (Kartulis; Losch;[6] Kruse and Pasquale;[7] Councilman and Lafleur[8]). It has been found in southern Asia, the Philippines, in Italy, Russia, and North America. Small epidemics have been noted in New York and Baltimore, and one case has recently been observed in Montreal in a patient who had never been outside of Canada.[9] The lesions are found usually in the large intestine, particularly in the neighborhood of the cecum and appendix, and, occasionally, in the lower part of the ileum. In the earlier stages the mucous membrane is œdematous, swollen, and hyperemic, and there are local infiltrations that manifest themselves as hemispherical elevations above the general surface. Later, the mucous membrane covering these becomes necrotic and sloughs away, leaving an ulcer with thickened undermined edges,

[1] Centralbl. f. Bakt., 23:1897:599; ibid., 24:1898:817, 870, 913.

[2] Ibid., 28:1900; and Philadelphia Medical Journal, 6:1900:414.

[3] Deutsche med. Woch., 26:1900:637; ibid., 27:1901:370.

[4] Jour. Med. Research. (6 N.S.):1904:553.

[5] K. Cameron, Montreal Med. Jour., 24:1895–6:673.

[6] Virch. Archiv, 65:1875:196.

[7] Zeitschr. f. Hyg. u. Infect., 16:1894:1.

[8] Johns Hopkins Hosp. Rep., 2:1891.

[9] Finley and Wolbach, Montreal Med. Jour., 6:1910:389.

the base of which is formed of infiltrated submucosa of a grayish-yellow, gelatinous appearance. It is this infiltrated, yellowish mucosa and submucosa that is the most distinctive gross feature of this form of colitis. The amount of softening in the submucosa is often far in excess of the superficial necrosis, so that a kind of abscess communicating with the lumen of the bowel by a small sinus is produced. In severe cases the ulcers may coalesce, forming sinuous tracks bridged by strands of comparatively healthy mucosa, or large portions of the mucosa may disappear leaving only small islets of intact membrane. The ulceration extends more or less deeply and may eventually reach the serous coat. Perforation of the bowel is rare. As a rule, in the advanced cases the wall of the bowel is greatly thickened. Occasionally, the condition may be complicated by a membranous inflammation.

Histologically, there is a more or less extensive necrosis of the cells, beginning in the submucosa, and an infiltration of the deeper layers with leukocytes. There is also proliferation of the connective tissue. The walls of the vessels in the affected area are infiltrated, while the vessels themselves are filled with leukocytes or are thrombosed. The amœbæ are found in the tissues in the base and edges of the ulcers, also in the lymphatics and bloodvessels, but rarely in parts in advance of the active lesions.

Plasma cells and fibrin may be abundant.

The stools in amœbic dysentery are frequent, bloody, and mucoid, later of a greenish-gray color, fluid, and containing mucin. Amœbæ are to be found in the dejecta.

Among the complications are focal necroses in the liver and liver abscess. The frequency with which liver abscess occurs in dysentery is somewhat uncertain. Manson,[1] in 3680 cases of tropical dysentery, found liver abscess in 21 per cent.; Hirsch,[2] in 2377 autopsies on tropical dysentery, noted the condition in 19.2 per cent. Probably in these statistics dysenteries of bacterial origin are included with the amœbic form. Dysenteric abscesses of the liver may rupture into the pleural cavity and into the lung. The necrotic substance is of a peculiar anchovy sauce-like appearance and contains the amœbæ.

Cholera Asiatica.—Cholera is an acute infectious disease characterized by cramps, diarrhœa, vomiting, fever, and collapse. The specific cause is the cholera spirillum or "comma bacillus" discovered by Koch.[3] The lesions are chiefly confined to the lower portion of the ileum. In general they are those characteristic of a serous enteritis. In the early stages the mucosa of the small intestine is more or less congested and covered with a slight amount of fibrin. The contents of the bowel are thin and watery, cloudy, alkaline, and of a grayish color. On standing, this material deposits a quantity of small, whitish flakes (rice-water discharge), in which the specific microörganism may be detected. The

[1] Quoted by Robinson, Jour. Amer. Med. Assoc., 36:1901:1319.
[2] Handb. Gen. and Hist. Path., London, 3:1886:412.
[3] Vierteljahrschrift f. öffentl. Gesundheitspflege, 16:1884.

mucous membrane is usually pale and anemic, except perhaps in the neighborhood of the lymphoid follicles, where it is hyperemic. The Peyer's patches and the solitary follicles are swollen and rather pale. Later, they shrink somewhat and assume a reticulated appearance. In the more advanced stages, the hyperemia becomes less marked and the wall of the intestine is more or less swollen. The bowel may also be nearly empty. The lymphoid elements sometimes present a slaty pigmentation. Membranous enteritis may supervene as a secondary manifestation.

Histologically, one sees little more than desquamation of the superficial epithelium, with some coagulation-necrosis of the villi. Leukocytic infiltration in the mucosa is but slight and is generally absent in the deeper layers. The epithelium of the glands shows mucoid change.

Mucous Colitis.—Mucous colitis is a curious affection of the large bowel in which tubular and membranous casts are discharged in the evacuations. The condition appears to be due to hypersecretion with inspissation of the mucus and proteins produced. It is found most often in hysterical women and is probably a secretory neurosis. Only rarely is it due to inflammation of the bowel.

Typhoid Fever.—Typhoid fever is an acute infectious disease due to Bacillus typhosus (Eberth-Gaffky). Properly speaking, it is a disease of the body as a whole, but the most constant and characteristic lesions are to be found in the intestines. The portal of infection is usually some part of the bowel, but exceptional cases have been recorded where infection has taken place through the lungs (Roux, Sicard, Dufaud).

As a rule, the lesions are to be found in the last three feet of the ileum and in the first part of the colon. In a few cases the colon alone is affected (Hodenpyl[1]). In rare instances typhoid assumes the character of a generalized bacteriemia, the characteristic lesions in the intestine being wholly wanting. Cases of this kind have been recorded in America by Flexner and Harris,[2] Nicholls and Keenan,[3] Lartigau,[4] McPhedran,[5] Opie and Bassett,[6] and others.

In typical cases of typhoid, the mucous membrane of the intestine is swollen and congested, presenting all the signs of an acute catarrhal inflammation. The characteristic lesions, however, are to be found in the Peyer's patches and solitary follicles. The lymphoid structures are invaded by the specific microörganism, become inflamed, and proliferate actively. The Peyer's glands, therefore, are enlarged, soft, and intensely reddened, and project above the general surface as flattened plaques. The solitary follicles also may be so much swollen that they

[1] Brit. Med. Jour., 2:1897·1850.
[2] Johns Hopkins Hosp. Bull., 8:1897:259.
[3] Mont. Med. Jour., 27:1898:9.
[4] Johns Hopkins Hosp. Bull., 10:1899:55.
[5] Phila. Monthly. Med. Jour., October, 1899.
[6] Phila. Med. Jour., 7:1901:99.

appear like little polyps on a slender pedicle. At the height of the first stage the surface of the affected plaques presents a curious grooved appearance (plaques à surface reticulée). This appearance is due to the unequal swelling of the connective-tissue stroma and the lymphoid elements.

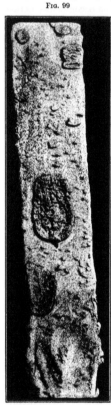

FIG. 99

Small intestine. Peyer's plaques showing tumefaction and superficial ulceration. Typhoid fever. (From the Pathological Museum of McGill University.)

Histologically, at this period, the mucous membrane is in a catarrhal condition and there is intense congestion of the vessels both of the mucosa and the submucosa. The lymphoid elements show hyperplasia, and there is a perifollicular infiltration with lymphocytes and leukocytes. Lenkocytes may be discovered in all the coats of the bowel, even in the serosa.

At the beginning of the second week, portions of the affected follicles undergo a form of coagulation necrosis. The central parts slough away, leaving superficial erosions, which often assume a brownish color from bile staining. In the course of the next few days the sloughing process gradually extends until well-defined ulcers are produced, having a fairly smooth base and swollen and infiltrated edges. The ulceration tends to penetrate into the depths, and usually extends as far as the muscularis mucosæ, which may be recognized by its clean, ribbed appearance. The well-defined, typical, typhoid ulcer is somewhat oval, the long axis running the long way of the bowel, the base is smooth, the edges comparatively thin and undermined. Small ulcers may be irregular, especially when they do not involve the whole extent of the Peyer's patch, or, again, may be small and round, when involving a solitary follicle. As a rule, the most advanced ulcers are to be found in the region of the ileocecal valve and become less marked as one passes up the ileum. In very severe cases the last foot or so of the small bowel, together with the head of the cecum, may be converted into a large, gangrenous eschar, in which may be recognized here and there small islets of the original mucosa, the ulcerating process having extended far beyond the limits of the Peyer's glands.

The process of healing varies naturally with the intensity of the process. The plaques that are merely hyperplastic become soft again and hyperemic through gradual absorption of the inflammatory products.

Not uncommonly there is an extravasation of red corpuscles from the vessels, so that hemorrhagic infiltration occurs. Where ulceration has occurred, the border of the necrotic areas becomes less swollen and again suffused with blood. Not infrequently there is hemorrhagic infiltration of the tissues, a fact that probably accounts for those cases of intestinal hemorrhage which occur later on in the stage of beginning convalescence. The glandular elements of the still intact mucosa poliferate and gradually spread over the denuded area, thus restoring the original continuity of epithelium. When the ulceration has been very extensive, the glandular regeneration may be incomplete or absent, so that the floor of the ulcer is covered by a layer of connective tissue containing no or relatively

FIG. 100

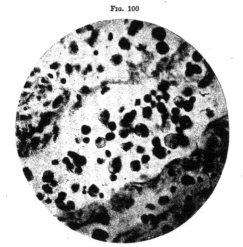

Intestine in typhoid fever. Section shows a sinus in a Peyer's patch with the great proliferation of the epithelial cells. Zeiss obj. $\frac{1}{12}$, oil immersion, ocular No. 1. (From the Pathological Laboratory of McGill University.)

few imperfectly formed glandular elements. Healed ulcers may often be recognized as oval patches, which are smooth, pigmented, and somewhat depressed below the general surface of the bowel. During the first eight or ten days the specific bacilli can be recognized in the Peyer's patches in well-marked clumps. Coincidently with the intestinal involvement, the mesenteric glands and spleen are swollen, hyperplastic, and inflamed. They may, as a consequence, be greatly softened. Spontaneous rupture of the spleen has occurred, but is rare. The mesenteric glands may undergo necrosis or suppurate.

Owing to the tendency of the typhoidal ulceration to penetrate deeply, perforation of the bowel is not uncommon, leading usually, unless recognized and dealt with early, to a fatal peritonitis. Because of the peculiar asthenic type of the typhoidal infection and the fact that leukocytes are scanty, the exudate is poor in fibrin and adhesions do not readily form. Only twice have we seen a typhoidal perforation closed by adhesion of the great omentum. Perforation occurred 54 times in 2036 cases of typhoid treated at the Royal Victoria Hospital, Montreal; that is, in 2.66 per cent.

Another dangerous complication is hemorrhage due to the erosion of some vessel in the ulcerated area. This accident occurred, including fatal and non-fatal cases, in 6.04 per cent. Other complications are pneumonia, pleurisy, nephritis, septicemia, periostitis, thrombophlebitis, thrombo-arteritis, cholecystitis, cholelithiasis, endocarditis, and meningitis. A general tendency to hemorrhage may occur.[1]

The pathogenesis of typhoid fever has been the subject of considerable discussion. Virchow thought that the swelling of the plaques was due to œdema and inflammatory exudation, a view subsequently modified by the researches of Rokitansky and Hoffmann. The more recent studies of Mallory[2] have thrown a flood of light upon the subject and have placed it on a more satisfactory footing. According to Mallory, the essential feature of typhoid is a proliferation of the endothelial cells throughout the body, a change which he thinks is due to the action of a diffusible toxin derived from the bacilli. The lesion in question is found in the Peyer's patches, mesenteric glands, liver, and bone-marrow, as well as in the lymphatics and blood-capillaries, but is proportionately more intense the nearer to the point at which the infecting agent gained entrance. The endothelial plates attached to the fibrous meshwork of the lymphoid follicles and mesenteric glands, as well as those lining the capillaries, proliferate, become fused into plasmodial masses or giant cells, and act as phagocytes. They ingest the bacteria and slowly eat up the lymphoid cells, which thus gradually disappear. A few leukocytes are to be seen in the follicles and within the crypts of Lieberkühn, but are not an important feature. Owing to the massing of these endothelial cells within the capillaries and the consequent obstruction to the blood supply, the parts deprived of their nutrition undergo necrosis. The focal necroses in the liver and spleen are to be explained in the same way.

Paratyphoid Fever.—Paratyphoid fever is an affection that can be differentiated with difficulty from typhoid, both as regards its clinical course and the anatomical lesions produced. The intestinal manifestations vary. As a rule, they resemble the lesions of dysentery rather than typhoid. In some cases they are absent. The specific micro-organism is a form (or forms) intermediate in properties between B. typhi and B. coli. The only conclusive point in the differential diagnosis between typhoid and paratyphoid fever is the agglutination test.

Tuberculosis.—This is one of the most frequent conditions found in the intestines. Three anatomical forms may be differentiated, the

---

[1] Nicholls and Learmonth, Lancet, London, 1: 1901: 305; also Meyer and Neumann, Zeitschr. f. klin. Med., 59: 1906: 133.

[2] Jour. Exper. Med., 3: 1898: 611.

ulcerative, miliary, and the *hyperplastic.* In the vast majority of cases the condition is a secondary one, being due to the infection of the bowel by bacilli derived from a more or less distant focus. The most common event of this nature is the ulceration of the intestines that accompanies pulmonary tuberculosis, the result of swallowing infective sputum. Occasionally, caseous glands rupture into the œsophagus or intestines and bring about infection. A hematogenous origin is certainly rarer.

With regard to primary tuberculosis of the intestines, statistics are conflicting, and it is difficult to get reliable information as to its frequency. The preponderance of the evidence at present available goes to show that the milk of tuberculous cattle often contains virulent bacilli which are competent to produce intestinal disease in animals fed upon the infective material. It is, therefore, fairly generally held that tuberculous cattle are a grave menace to the health of the community, and more especially to children in whose dietary milk forms such an important part. At present it seems impossible to decide with certainty to what extent primary infection of the intestine takes place, though we must undoubtedly agree with Koch that it is comparatively rare. In 1230 autopsies at the Royal Victoria Hospital, Montreal, potentially infective tuberculous lesions were found in 285 cases, but only two were undoubted instances of primary intestinal infection,[1] although seven others were probably of this nature. During five years at the Charité Hospital at Berlin, Koch only met with ten examples. Kossel,[2] in 286 consecutive autopsies on children, of whom 22 had died of tuberculosis, in only one found the affection confined to the intestinal tract. Hunter[3] in 5142 autopsies in China found only five instances. On the other hand, Spengler[4] refers to 92 cases of tuberculosis, in 4 of which the intestinal tract was alone affected. Still,[5] in 269 autopsies on cases of tuberculosis in children under twelve, found that where the course of infection could be determined with some certainty the lungs were attacked primarily in 105 cases, the intestines in 53, the ear in 9, the bones and joints in 5. Shennon[6] in 355 cases of tuberculosis in children found the primary seat of infection to be intestinal in 28.1 per cent. Apparently primary intestinal infection is more common in England and France than it is in America and Germany.[7] The relative frequency of human and bovine infection is further indicated by the statistics of isolation of bacilli of the human and bovine type respectively.

Park and his associates on the staff of the New York City Board of Health have studied cultures of the bacilli from a number of cases of tuberculosis, not greatly inferior to that studied by observers in all the other laboratories throughout the world combined, in order to determine the relative frequency of human and bovine infection by the isolation of the human and bovine types. From the remarkable report

[1] Nicholls, Mont. Med. Jour., 31:1902:327.   [2] Zeit. f. Hyg., 12: 59.
[3] Brit. Med. Jour., 1:1904:1126.   [4] Zeit. f. Hyg., 13:1893:346.
[5] Brit. Med. Jour., 2:1899:455.   [6] Edin. Hosp. Rep., 1900.
[7] A useful resumé of recent work on this controverted subject will be found in the British Medical Journal, 1:1909:epitome, 7.

by Park and Krumweide[1] giving their results, we have compiled the
following table:

	Adults over 16 Years.		Children, 5–16.		Children under 5 Years.		Total.
	Human.	Bovine.	Human.	Bovine.	Human.	Bovine.	
Park and Krumweide . .	296	1[2]	45	9[3]	66	22[4]	436
Other responsible workers . .	381	8	54	24	99	37	606

In typical cases of tuberculosis of the intestines resulting from infection
of the alimentary type, the process begins in the Peyer's plaques and
solitary follicles in the form of small nodular elevations beneath the
mucous membrane.   These are tubercles or specific granulomata.   In
a short time the central portion changes to a yellowish-white color,
an evidence of central necrosis and caseation.   Later, this softens and
is discharged, so that a small ulcer with infiltrated borders is produced,
in the neighborhood of which other minute caseous foci appear.   These
ultimately coalesce, forming a larger ulcer.   A typical tuberculous ulcer
of the intestine has the following peculiarities: the edges are irregular,
infiltrated, but not usually undermined; the base is uneven, ragged,
and necrotic, and in it can often be seen small, yellowish, rounded masses,
which are caseous tubercles; the ulcers tend to encircle the bowel, owing
to the fact that extension of the infection takes place along the course
of the lymphatics; the ulcers do not tend to perforate; small isolated
tubercles can often be seen upon the serous surface of the bowel; the
mesenteric lymph nodes are often caseous.   The tissues about the
ulcer usually show little disturbance, but there may be, in addition, a
catarrhal enteritis.   Certain catarrhal and ulcerative processes in the
bowel and even membranous and gangrenous enteritis have also been
attributed to the action of the tubercle bacillus, but it is uncertain in
how far these may be due to associated microörganisms.   We have
met with one case of follicular enteritis in which the puriform material
from the inflamed follicles contained tubercle bacilli.
The tuberculous process usually extends into the muscular coats and
even into the serous membrane, infection taking place along the course
of the lymphatics.   Thus, we may find a small crop of tubercles on

[1] Jour of Med. Research, 23: 1910: 205–368.
[2] Of these 297 cases, 278 cases of pulmonary tuberculosis without exception
afforded bacilli of the human type.
[3] Here, again, all the pulmonary tuberculosis cases afforded the human type.
Of 27 cases of cervical adenitis, 19 gave the human type, 8 the bovine.
[4] 5 cases of pulmonary tuberculosis all afforded the human type. Of 18 cases
of cervical adenitis bacilli of the human type were isolated from 6, of the bovine
type from 12.

the serous surface, surrounded by congested and newly formed capillaries. Not infrequently there can be seen also about these a little knot of dilated lymph-channels filled with clear fluid or cellular and caseous material, vessels which have become blocked from the tuberculous infiltration. In the neighborhood of these subserous tubercles there is often a local peritonitis, evidenced by a slight dulling of the peritoneal membrane and possibly a deposit of delicate fibrin. As the ulcers coalesce and enlarge, they tend to extend transversely around the bowel, forming a girdle-shaped area of erosion. In cases where the Peyer's patches are involved, especially where the process has not had time to progress very far, the ulcers may resemble the typhoidal form, in that they are oval or rounded, their long axes running the long way of the bowel.

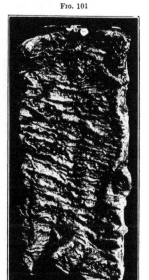

FIG. 101

Histologically, the structures at the edges and base of the ulcers present the ordinary features of granulation tissue. In this can be made out a varying number of tubercles, composed of the usual leukocytes, epithelioid and giant cells, with a certain amount of central caseation. In the more advanced cases similar tubercles can be found between the muscle bundles and along the course of the lymphatics in the serous coat. Great numbers of "Mast-zellen" are also to be seen in the submucosa and muscularis. The muscular coat shows a certain amount of fatty degeneration. By appropriate methods tubercle bacilli can be demonstrated in the granulomatous areas.

Tuberculous ulceration of the bowel. (From the Pathological Museum of McGill University.)

An interesting and important form, that has of late been attracting some little attention, is the so-called *chronic productive* or *hyperplastic* tuberculosis of the intestines. In this type tissue destruction is trifling, while cell proliferation is in excess. The condition may involve the peritoneal membrane as well, either wholly or in part, or, again, may be one manifestation of a widespread tuberculosis of all the serous sacs.[1] When localized, the lesions are generally found in the cecum and appendix or in that neighborhood. Occasionally, certain coils of the large or small intestine are matted together, thickened, and rolled up into a ball, owing

[1] Nicholls, Some Rare Forms of Peritonitis Associated with Productive Fibrosis and Hyaline Degeneration, Jour. Amer. Med. Assoc., 40:1903:696.

to sclerotic induration and retraction of the mesentery, and the omentum may be converted into a thick cord. The wall of the affected bowel is enormously thickened, sometimes measuring as much as 1 cm. The infiltration may in fact be so great that a tumor-like mass is formed which can be felt through the abdominal wall. This has been mistaken for carcinoma. The infiltrated bowel may be surrounded by [dense fibroid adhesions, which may anchor it to the parietes. If caseation be at all active in such cases, fistulous communications may be formed with the exterior of the body and between the loops of the gut. The lumen of the intestine is sometimes narrowed to such an extent as to cause obstruction, but there is rarely ulceration of the mucosa. Histologically, the main

FIG. 102

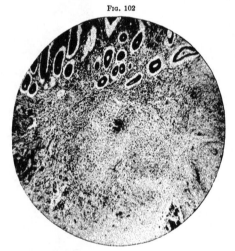

Intestine showing two small caseous foci of tubercle in the submucosa. Zeiss obj. DD, ocular No. 1. (From the Pathological Laboratory, McGill University.)

feature is extensive hyperplasia of the connective tissue in which typical tubercles are scanty or even absent. Caseation is rarely extensive, and the specific bacilli may be hard to demonstrate. A striking feature in some cases is a hyaline degeneration of the exudate and of the newly-formed connective-tissue fibrils.[1]

Syphilis.[2]—Syphilis of the intestines may be hereditary or acquired.

[1] The following papers may be consulted on this subject: Lartigau: Jour. of Exper. Med., 6: 1901-5: 23; Koerte: Deut. Zeit. f. Chir., 1894 to 1895: 60: 562; Coquet: Thèse de Paris, De la variété chir. de Tumeurs cecales tuber., 1894: 28; Itié: Thèse de Montpellier, De la tuber. intest. à forme hyper., 1898: 12; Shiota, Arch. f. Chir., 87: 1908.

[2] For literature, see Oberndorfer, Virch. Archiv, 159: 1900: 179.

In the hereditary form, the small intestine is perhaps the part most frequently involved, and, moreover, unlike what occurs in other infectious diseases, it is the upper portion, usually the jejunum, that is affected. Cellular infiltrations and gummata have been observed, which lead to ulceration, peritonitis, and rarely to perforation.

The lesions of acquired syphilis are most frequently localized in the rectum, rarely in the colon and small intestine. The chancre has under certain circumstances been found in the rectum, as well as specific condylomas and papules. The common lesion is, however, the gumma. Here the inflammatory process begins in the submucosa and leads to extensive ulceration. In severe cases the mucosa for a distance of 10 to 12 cm. above the anus may be almost completely destroyed, only a few shreds being left. In recent cases the ulcerated surface exudes pus. Later, extensive fibrous proliferation takes place, which eventually leads to marked stricture of the rectum, with all its attendant disorders of obstruction, dilatation, hypertrophy, and ulceration. Gummas may also develop in the perirectal cellular tissue and lead to the formation of external or internal fistule. About half the cases of stricture of the rectum are said to be of syphilitic origin. The condition is twice as common in women as in men.

Actinomycosis.[1]—Actinomycosis of the intestines in about 60 per cent. of cases is to be found in the neighborhood of the appendix and cecum. In many cases of abdominal actinomycosis with external sinuses and peritoneal adhesions it is impossible to determine the exact starting point of the process. Hinglais[2] has collected 120 instances of actinomycosis of the appendix and cecal region. In such cases the affection begins with symptoms of appendicitis, but subsequently large retrocecal abscesses or external fistulæ have developed. Actinomycosis of the intestines begins by the formation of whitish patches in the mucosa with proliferation of the submucosa. As the disease progresses, ulceration takes place, with not infrequently the formation of sinuses, in the discharge from which the characteristic "sulphur grains" or actinomyces can usually be demonstrated.[3] In other cases, instead of suppuration or ulceration, hard, tumor-like masses, sometimes pedunculated, may be produced.

The infection is supposed to be due to the use of contaminated water or vegetables.

Inflammation of Special Regions.

Duodenitis.—Inflammation of the duodenum—**duodenitis**—is nearly always associated with gastritis. In this affection, infective agents may travel up the common bile duct and the pancreatic duct. In this way a catarrhal or suppurative cholangitis or sialodochitis may be produced. Duodenitis not infrequently leads to acute interstitial hepatitis

[1] Leith, Edin. Hosp. Rep., 2: 1894: 128.   [2] Thèse de Lyon, 1897.
[3] Krasnobajew, Arch. f. Kinderheilk., 23: 1 to 3.

and occasionally to acute suppurative pancreatitis (q. v.). Catarrh of the ducts in question predisposes to the formation of calculi also. Catarrhal jaundice is due to a plug of mucus in the ampulla of Vater and probably is attributable always to a preëxisting gastroduodenitis.

Ileitis.—Ileitis is practically the same thing as the enteritis already described, the inflammation being commonly localized to this portion of the intestinal tract.

Colitis.—Colitis, or inflammation of the colon, is a comparatively frequent condition, being a notable feature in cases of dysentery. The colon may be alone involved or in association with other portions of the bowel. Ileocolitis is the ordinary lesion of the so-called cholera infantum. Many cases of colitis are associated with the infections and various forms of intoxication, and the affection is not uncommon in advanced Bright's disease. The reason why colitis is so frequent is perhaps not far to seek, when we consider the opportunities afforded for traumatism and infection. The feces tend to accumulate in the large bowel, they are harder there than elsewhere, and their progress is slower, and the antibacterial action of the digestive ferments is much lessened. A frequent cause, therefore, of the condition is the presence of dense, scybalous masses, the accumulation of which leads to dilatation of the intestine, with possibly the formation of diverticula. Hard, fecal masses are retained in the little pockets thus formed, and lead to ulceration through pressure necrosis.

Anatomically, we may recognize *catarrhal, follicular, membranous, hemorrhagic, mucous, ulcerative,* and *gangrenous* forms.

Typhlitis.—Typhlitis is inflammation of the cecum. When the cellular tissue about the cecum is involved as well, the condition is termed **perityphlitis.** When the inflammation is extraperitoneal and behind the cecum, it is spoken of as **paratyphlitis.** Typhlitis may occasionally be due to the presence of hardened feces in the cecum, but apart from this, the three conditions are nearly always the resultants of inflammation of the appendix vermiformis. We have met with a membranous typhlitis in the case of a cerebral lesion, however, where the patient had been unconscious for some days before death. It is also met with in mercurial poisoning and uremia.

Appendicitis.—Not many years ago the terms typhlitis, perityphlitis, paratyphlitis, and the still vaguer appellation, "inflammation of the bowels," were employed to designate almost all affections of an inflammatory character occurring in the right iliac fossa. We owe to Fitz's classical monograph the recognition of the fact that the vast majority of these cases have their origin in a diseased appendix vermiformis, from which naturally followed the adoption of more rational measures of treatment.

Inflammation of the appendix—**appendicitis**—is much more common in males than in females. Most cases come to operation between the ages of twenty and thirty. Where previous attacks have been recorded in the histories they have occurred in the second decade of life.

We shall perhaps be better prepared to understand the etiology of inflammation of the appendix if we consider the anatomical structure and the situation of the organ concerned.

The appendix is situated at the head of the cecum; its cavity is continuous with that of the large bowel, being divided from it by a more or less inconstant fold of mucous membrane, the valve of Gerlach. It is long and narrow and apt to be somewhat curved upon itself. The structure appears to be the relic of a large cecal pouch, such as is still to be found in the ruminants and others of the lower animals, and considerable evidence has been adduced to show that it is gradually involuting. Ribbert, in a study of 400 appendices removed at post mortems, found retrograde and atrophic changes in about 25 per cent. in the absence of any indications of previous inflammatory change. A. O. J. Kelly[1] has found more or less obliteration of the lumen in about one-quarter of the cases. Being an organ, therefore, that is disappearing one need not be surprised that the appendix is a common seat of disease. In view of its situation, moreover, it is apt to be a depository for foreign bodies or inflammatory exudates, which, owing to its dependent position and narrow lumen, are almost certain to be retained within it. A slight inflammation or kinking at the neck will also favor the retention of its contents. Thus, the appendix becomes at times practically a culture tube for various microörganisms, and a ready subject for traumatic and chemical irritation.

Considerable stress used to be laid upon vascular disturbances as a cause of appendicitis, but the importance of these has undoubtedly been overestimated. Thrombosis and embolism might conceivably bring about anemic necrosis of the organ, which would thereupon become an easy prey to pathogenic microörganisms, but this appears to be a very rare occurrence. Breuer has shown that the artery of the appendix is not an endartery, and that, contrary to the usual opinion, there is a fairly effective anastomosis in the various coats of the organ. Again, the endarteritis and periarteritis held by some to be a chief cause in bringing about necrosis have not been found constantly or even frequently present. In any case, to bring about the condition in question, obstruction of the vessels would have to be somewhat widespread. The vascular changes are more reasonably to be interpreted as the result rather than the cause of the inflammation. Possibly, however, kinks or other constrictions of the appendix at its orifice, by interfering with the free outflow of blood, may in some few cases play a leading role.

At one time it was almost universally held that foreign bodies or fecal concretions within the appendix were the important factor. Apart from fecal concretions, foreign bodies are quite rare in the appendix and when present are to be classed as accidental occurrences rather than causative agents. James Bell,[2] in between 900 and 1000 cases of appendicitis operated upon, found foreign bodies within the appendix in only 7, and thinks that this is probably more than the usual pro-

---

[1] Phila. Med. Jour., 4: 1899: 928, 983: 1032.
[2] Mont. Med. Jour., 31: 1902: 765.

portion. Foreign bodies have also been met with in appendices that presented no obvious appearances of disease. Among the substances found may be mentioned apple-pips, grape-seeds, hair, bits of bone, pins, bits of glass, gallstones, wood-fibre, segments of tænia, thread worms, and round worms. In the Pathological Museum of McGill University is an appendix containing a large number of shot, the owner of which never suffered from appendicitis. Sharp substances, such as pins or glass, might, however, be expected to give trouble. Concretions consist of fecal material, desquamated cells, and leukocytes, inspissated in a mucoid matrix, and sometimes infiltrated with calcium salts. They are found in normal appendices, and in themselves appear to be comparatively unimportant. It is quite likely, however, in appendices that are inflamed and swollen, concretions may bring about necrosis through pressure and, as a matter or fact they are more numerous in appendicitis of the ulcerative and gangrenous type. E. W. Archibald,[1] in his analysis of 89 cases, found concretions in only 3 out of 38 non-perforative cases, while in 41 perforative cases they were found in 22. It should be pointed out that concretions are an expression of a previous or co-existent inflammatory process rather than the exciting cause of inflammation. As in the case of biliary or urinary calculi, there must have been a preëxisting catarrh of the mucosa producing an excess of mucus with exudation and desquamation of cells to provide a nidus in which the salts may be deposited. Once formed, of course, the concretion might be expected to perpetuate or aggravate the condition. As a rule, however, it is only the larger masses which, by pressure upon the mucosa and obstructing the free discharge of retained secretions, lead to trouble.[2]

Another point of etiological moment is that the lymphoid elements of the appendix undergo involution along with the other structures. The appendix, at first, is much more rich in lymphoid elements than the rest of the intestine, the cells in question being diffused throughout the mucosa or aggregated into follicles. These elements are probably concerned in the manufacture of substances that immunize the body against bacterial infection from the lumen of the bowels. Ribbert and Kelynack have pointed out that this lymphoid tissue is most marked in childhood and atrophies after the thirtieth year or in exceptional cases as early as the twentieth. The fact, therefore, that the defensive powers of the appendix against infection under these circumstances are beginning to wane will explain the greater prevalence of appendicitis after early adult life.[3]

The most important single cause of appendicitis is infection, the activity of the microörganisms being aided by the anatomical peculiarities just detailed. Aschoff,[4] the most recent investigator of the subject, holds

[1] Mont. Med. Jour., 29:1900:81.
[2] This question is discussed by Aschoff, Mediz. Klinik, 24: 1905.
[3] See v. Hansemann, Festschrift f. Mayer, Berlin, 1905.
[4] Die Wurmfortsatzentzündung, Jena, Fischer, 1908.

that the disease begins as an enterogenous infection, beginning at the bottom of the crypts. To produce this result only the slightest abrasion of the epithelium is necessary. Of the bacteria at fault, the most important are B. $_{coli}$ communior (in Montreal), Staphylococcus pyogenes albus and aureus, Streptococcus pyogenes, Diplococcus pneumoniæ, and B. pyocyaneus. In Kelly's 400 cases the B. coli was present in 92 per cent.

Tavel and Lanz, Barnacci, and Welch have pointed out the frequency of mixed infection. Probably the vast majority of appendicitis cases are due to mixed infection, and the reason that this is not generally realized is to be looked for in faulty bacteriological technique. The B. coli readily overgrows and destroys less vigorous germs. Therefore, plate cultures should be made at the time of operation in order that the various forms may be properly isolated. Cultures should also be made under anaërobic conditions. It is likely, also, that during life the same destruction of the weaker organisms by B. coli takes place, so that the culture methods may reveal only a single germ when the disease has really been brought about by several. It may be shown that microscopic sections of the appendix, appropriately stained to show bacteria, often reveal the presence of microörganisms within the lumen which have failed to develop in the cultures taken. Where mixed infection can be recognized, B. coli and Staphylococcus are usually found together. In a few cases, Staphylococcus, Pneumococcus, or B. pyocyaneus have been found alone.

In regard to the extent of the inflammatory process itself, the whole appendix may be involved or only a portion of it, usually the distal part. It is difficult to give an accurate classification of the forms, inasmuch as the types met with pass imperceptibly one into the other. The following may be suggested as a convenient grouping:

Acute	*Catarrhal.* *Diffuse, suppurative, or phlegmonous.* *Ulcerating* { *Perforated.* / *Non-perforated.* *Gangrenous.* *Specific (e. g., typhoid).*
Chronic	*Catarrhal.* *Diffuse or sclerosing.* *Specific* . { *Tuberculous.* / *Actinomycotic.*

Acute Catarrhal Appendicitis.—Catarrhal appendicitis may be acute or chronic. In the acute form the appendix is swollen, the external venules are congested, and the organ is often kinked or twisted. The mucous membrane is swollen, succulent, congested, with possibly minute hemorrhages, and there may be even slight roughening of its surface. The cavity contains thin mucus with a few leukocytes, and there may be concretions. Occasionally, there are a few old adhesions about the organ. On histological examination, the mucosa is congested, œdematous, and the epithelium is in a state of catarrh. The lymphoid follicles are proliferating and the submucosa is also œdematous.

Acute Diffuse Appendicitis.—This form is more severe. The appendix is swollen in all its thickness and may be covered with fibrinous lymph externally. All the features of the acute catarrhal form are present, but in addition there is a diffuse infiltration of leukocytes in all the coats, which, therefore, are greatly thickened and œdematous. The lymphoid elements are also actively proliferating. Here and there there may be small superficial erosions of the mucosa. The cavity may contain mucopus. The meso-appendix is often involved as well.

FIG. 103

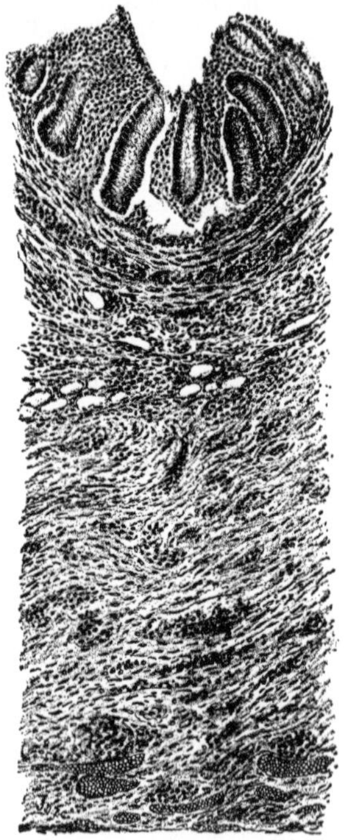

Acute appendicitis, with extensive round-celled infiltration of all of the coats of the appendix. (Stengel.)

Acute Ulcerating Appendicitis.—In the acute ulcerative type there is at some point or other an area of necrosis, usually corresponding to the situation of a fecal concretion. This ulceration may be of varying depth, and not infrequently perforates. The appendix is often discolored at the point of necrosis, and is bathed externally in pus.

Gangrenous Appendicitis. — Gangrenous appendicitis is an extreme and fulminating variety, in which the whole appendix or some part of it rapidly necroses and is converted into a blackish, sloughy mass. This form may be primary or may be engrafted upon other types of appendicitis. It is due to a particularly virulent form of infection or to vascular obstruction.

Typhoidal ulceration of the appendix resembles typhoidal ulceration elsewhere. It may lead to perforation and peritonitis.

Chronic Appendicitis.—Chronic appendicitis may be insidious in its development or result from an acute or subacute attack. In not a few of the cases we find a succession of attacks of more or less acute inflammation, in any of which ulcerative and gangrenous processes may supervene, placing the patient's life in jeopardy. Both the chronic and the relapsing cases lead to proliferation of connective tissue, whereby the appendix becomes indurated and the lumen in some cases entirely obliterated, so that the whole organ is converted into a fibrous cord (*sclerosing appendicitis*). Here and there collections of round cells may be seen in the various coats, relics of a more active stage of inflammation. Obliteration of the proximal portion may lead to the retention of secretion and inflammatory products, so that the remainder of the appendix becomes dilated into the form of a cyst of cylindrical or globular shape. The contents of the cyst are either serous, mucous, or purulent, and may become inspissated. In all chronic and relapsing cases fibrous adhesions form in the neighborhood of the appendix. By obliteration of the lumen spontaneous cure may result. This, however, is not to be expected.

Fig. 104

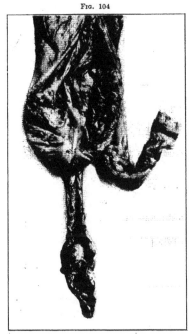

Gangrene of the appendix vermiformis in acute appendicitis; concretion. (Pathological Museum, McGill University.)

The danger from appendicitis is largely dependent on perforation, which occurs sooner or later in a large proportion of acute cases. If the inflammation be a fulminating one and adhesions have not formed, a septic peritonitis supervenes, which, in the vast majority of cases is fatal. A general peritonitis due to B. coli, or in which the cultures are sterile, appears to be less virulent and some few cases get well after appropriate surgical treatment. Where fibrinous adhesions have formed, perforation of the appendix leads to the formation of a localized abscess in which concretions or portions of the appendix may be found. The patient will frequently recover in such cases if the abscess be promptly evacuated and drained. More favorable still are those cases in which dense, fibrous adhesions wall off the diseased appendix from the general abdominal cavity. The appendix may lie behind the cecum, pointing upward, and lead to the formation of an abscess in the region of the liver. In other cases the organ lies in a little pocket of peritoneum or even entirely behind the peritoneum. Such cases are relatively favorable. Periappendicular abscesses may burst into the bowel, giving rise to fecal fistulæ, or may evacuate themselves externally. Septic thrombosis of the mesenteric and omental veins is a common accompaniment, as are also septic portal pylephlebitis and abscesses in the liver. Empyema of the right pleural cavity is occasionally met with.

Tuberculosis.—Tuberculosis of the appendix is found in association with tuberculosis of other parts of the intestinal tract, and does not differ in any way from it. Here also the hyperplastic form has been observed.

Proctitis.—Proctitis, or inflammation of the rectum, is commonly brought about by traumatism, such as may be caused by impacted feces, fruit-stones, fish-bones, or foreign bodies introduced through the anus. Dilated hemorrhoidal veins may also become thrombosed and infected, thus leading to inflammation. Proctitis is also caused by gonorrhœa, syphilis, tuberculosis, and certain mineral substances such as arsenic and mercury. Ulceration is a common feature, but is of chronic type and leads to thickening of the wall, polypoid outgrowths, and more or less atresia. The ulcers may penetrate deeply and give rise to abscesses about the rectum (*periproctal abscesses*), which may burst into the peritoneal cavity, bladder, or vagina (*rectovesical* and *rectovaginal fistulæ*), or make their way to the external surface (*complete* or *external fistulæ*). Where the abscess communicates only with the lumen of the bowel and has no external opening, the condition is termed by surgeons *blind* or *internal fistula*.

RETROGRESSIVE METAMORPHOSES.

Atrophy.—Atrophy of the intestines is not uncommon. It may affect the mucosa only or the whole thickness of the bowel.

Degeneration.—Fatty degeneration and hyaline degeneration are occasionally met with in the muscular coat.

Amyloid Infiltration.—Amyloid infiltration is not uncommon in advanced cases of amyloid disease. It affects the walls of the smaller bloodvessels, principally of the mucosa and submucosa.

Necrosis, ulceration, and **gangrene** are not uncommon in the intestine, and result from inflammation, pressure, and circulatory disturbances.

Enterolithiasis.—The curious condition known as enterolithiasis includes the formation of large concretions within the cavity of the bowel, and of fine granular particles, or intestinal sand.

Intestinal sand is composed of a large proportion of organic matter with about 33 per cent. of calcium salts. Myer and Cook[1] have shown that, in some cases at least, certain articles of diet, notably bananas, may be responsible for the condition. A vegetable resin together with tannic acid is found in this fruit and under the influence of digestion an insoluble tannate is produced which appears in the feces.

Concretions or **enteroliths** are usually found in the appendix or diverticula of the intestine and consist of inspissated feces and desquamated cells, which have formed a nidus for the deposition of calcareous salts.

PROGRESSIVE METAMORPHOSES.

Hypertrophy.—Hypertrophy of the intestinal wall occurs as the result of chronic obstruction.

Tumors.—Benign tumors are comparatively rare and of no great importance. The forms met with are the **adenoma, fibroma, lipoma, myoma, myoadenoma, osteoma, hemangioma, lymphangioma,** and **chylangioma.** The connective-tissue tumors usually spring from the submucosa and project outward into the peritoneal cavity. Polypoid or pedunculated masses are not infrequently produced, which may break loose, forming free bodies in the abdomen, or may be passed *per anum.* Occasionally, they induce intussusception and intestinal obstruction.

The **enterocystoma** is a curious cystic growth resulting from a developmental anomaly in the form of partial persistence of the omphalomesenteric duct.

A rare condition is the presence of an **accessory pancreas** lying concealed in the substance of the intestinal wall, or forming a small nodular mass projecting on the serous aspect. Such tumors are the result of developmental errors, and are usually found in the upper alimentary tract, duodenum or jejunum. When in the jejunum they may be situated at the tip of a diverticulum.[2]

Polypoid outgrowths, often pedunculated and having the general structure of adenoma, are not uncommon in the intestine, especially in the duodenum and in the large bowel near the ileocecal valve or the rectum. They are found especially at the margins of chronic ulcers and in connection with long-standing enteritis. It is questionable whether they are ever true tumors, and they should, in our opinion, be classed with the inflammatory hyperplasias.[3]

The malignant growths are **sarcoma, lymphosarcoma, endothelioma,** and **carcinoma. Sarcomas** are *round, spindle-celled, alveolar,* and *melanotic.* The round-celled form is the commonest of the primary sarcomas, but is still rare. It usually occurs between the ages of forty and fifty. E. A. Robertson[4] has recorded a case in a child of four. The growth

---

[1] Amer. Jour. Med. Sci., 137:1909:383.

[2] Nicholls, A Case of Accessory Pancreas, Mont. Med. Jour., 29:1900:903.

[3] Munk, Beiträge f. klin. Chir., 60: 1908.　　　- [4] Mont. Med. Jour., 27:1898:31.

was situated in the neighborhood of the ileocecal valve. Melanotic sarcomas are single or multiple, and are found studding the serous surface. They are usually secondary to melanotic sarcomas of the skin or choroid of the eye, but may be primary.[1]

Lymphosarcoma[2] may be primary or secondary. It usually starts in the lymph-follicles, but may begin independently of them. Sooner or later the new-growth extends beyond the limits of the follicles and invades the mucosa and other coats of the intestine.

The bowel may also be invaded secondarily from sarcomatous mesenteric glands.

Carcinoma.—By far the commonest new-growth of the intestine is the carcinoma. In the large majority of cases it is found in the large intestine, and usually in the rectum. It is occasionally met with about the ileocecal valve, the iliac, splenic, and hepatic flexures, and the cecum. Of late years a considerable number of cases of primary carcinoma of the appendix have been recorded.[3] They are curious in that they do not tend to form distant metastases. Primary, round-celled sarcoma of this structure has also been described.[4] When in the small intestine, a rare occurrence comparatively, the site of election is in the neighborhood of the bile papilla. A noteworthy fact is the relative frequency with which intestinal carcinomas are met with in young people. This perhaps is to be explained by the not infrequent occurrence of mucous polyps of the intestines in children.

FIG. 105

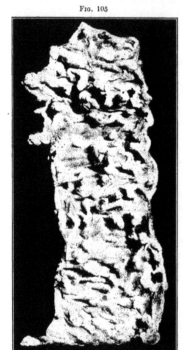

Chronic colitis with polypoid outgrowths. (From the Pathological Museum of McGill University.)

The carcinomas of the intestine are of the *medullary*, *scirrhous*, or *colloid* type. Histologically, with the exception of the squamous-celled form starting at the anus and that originating in the Brunner's glands, they are cylindrical-celled and of glandular appearance.

[1] Sanduer, Inaug. Diss., Erlangen, 1904.   [2] Glinski, Virch. Archiv, 167: 1902; 373.

[3] Elting, Annals of Surgery, 37: 1903: 549; also, Harte, Annals of Surgery, June, 1908, and Rolleston, Lancet, Lond., 2: 1900: 11

[4] Paterson, Practitioner, 70: 1903: 515.

PLATE V

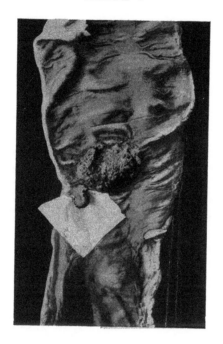

enoma (Papillomatous) of the Colon with Early
Carcinomatous Change. (Nicholls.)

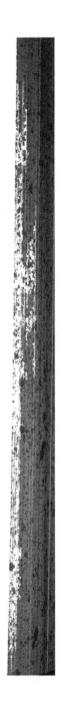

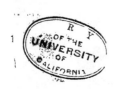

The new-growth forms a solitary, localized, sharply defined, fungating mass, or, again, may involve a considerable area of the bowel. The softer cancers have little tendency to obstruct the lumen. In some cases, the infiltration is more restricted, but forms a ring-like mass encircling the bowel. The muscular wall is infiltrated and hardened, so that the intestine is converted into a stiff, uncollapsible tube. The surface generally ulcerates, producing a shallow erosion, the edges and base of

FIG. 106

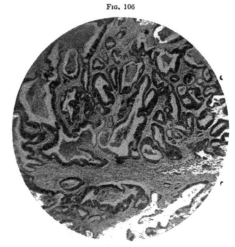

Carcinoma of the rectum. Zeiss obj. A, without ocular. New formation of tubules is seen well below the muscularis mucosæ. (From the collection of Dr. A. G. Nicholls.)

which are densely fibrous, leading to a cicatricial constriction of the bowel. The affected part may become adherent to neighboring structures, or the ulcer may perforate, leading to peritonitis. Metastases in the liver (through the portal system), lymph-nodes, and peritoneum are common. Secondary carcinomas are as rare as the primary are common. They are metastatic or arise by implantation from carcinomas of the pancreas, stomach, uterus, and vagina.

CHAPTER XXI.

ANOMALIES.

Congenital Anomalies.—The liver may be completely **absent**, or may deviate considerably from the normal in form and size. The organ is occasionally thin and flat, or the shape of a short truncated pyramid. A somewhat common anomaly is for the left lobe to be prolonged backward and downward in the form of a **lingula**. The lobes may be increased in number and **aberrant lobes** attached by a narrow pedicle have been found in hernial sacs at the umbilicus, where they have been mistaken for tumors. **Accessory livers** are occasionally met with, situated in the suspensory ligament. The liver may be **reversed** and situated on the left side of the abdomen in the condition of transposition of the viscera. It may also be **dislocated** in various forms of congenital hernias.

The gall-bladder may be absent or buried in the liver substance, or, again, directed backward. The biliary ducts may be absent, abnormally dilated, or occluded at some point. The ductus communis choledochus may be reduplicated and the single or double duct may discharge into the stomach or at some unusual situation in the bowel.

Acquired Abnormalities of Shape and Position.—Of acquired deformities the most common is the so-called "**lacing-lobe**." The pressure of a tight corset forces in the lower portion of the thoracic wall, so that a transverse fissure is produced, which divides the right lobe into an upper and a lower portion. The Glisson's capsule over the fissure is thickened and of a pearly white color, while the subjacent acini are atrophic. A portion of the liver may be almost if not quite separated from the main mass, being connected merely by a fibrous band. The lacing-lobe is generally seen in persons having a short thorax, tight lacing in those with long waists being more likely to produce a movable kidney.

The so-called **Liebermeister grooves** are common also, occurring in our experience in 7.26 per cent. of all autopsies. These consist in a variable number of parallel grooves on the outer convexity of the right lobe, which are directed forward. They do not correspond in direction with the ribs. Several explanations have been offered for their occurrence. Liebermeister thought they were due to pressure from difficult respiratory movements, while Zahn attributed them to the action of a hypertrophied diaphragm. In some cases the depressions can be shown to correspond with thickened bands of muscle. Possibly a few instances are congenital.

Owing to a laxness of the suspensory ligament the liver may be more or less remote from its natural position (**hepatoptosis; mobile** or **floating** liver). The organ may be anteverted, its anterior border passing downward and forward, the posterior border remaining practically unaffected. The displacement may also be oblique, the left lobe descending, or, again, the whole organ may be affected. The condition of dislocated liver is commonly associated with gastroptosis or enteroptosis.

The liver may be pushed downward by the pressure of pleural exudates or effusions, intrathoracic growths, or emphysema. It may be forced upward in cases of ascites, intra-abdominal cysts, or tumors. The traction of intra-abdominal adhesions also may pull the organ out of its natural position.

CIRCULATORY DISTURBANCES.

Anemia.—Anemia of the liver is either a manifestation of a generalized or systemic anemia, or is due to some local disturbance, such as pressure upon the organ or swelling of the parenchyma.

Hyperemia.—**Active Hyperemia.**—Active hyperemia is met with as a physiological condition after a meal, and, pathologically, in the early stages of acute inflammations of the liver, and in all cases of congestion of the gastro-intestinal vascular system.

Passive Hyperemia.—Passive hyperemia is brought about by any cause that raises the blood pressure within the hepatic vein and inferior vena cava. Among the important conditions that should be mentioned in this connection are stenosis or insufficiency of the mitral or tricuspid valves, cardiac weakness, emphysema of the lungs, indurative pneumonia, right-sided pleural effusions, aneurisms, tumors, or enlarged glands pressing upon the inferior vena cava.

In the early stages the liver is enlarged, often attaining a considerable size, soft, and full of blood, which drips out of it on section. In color it is dark, purplish-red. After the blood has been drained out the organ will be found to be somewhat shrunken (*red atrophy*). Later, the liver is more or less diminished in size, firm, with a finely granular surface. On section, the appearance is like that of a nutmeg, whence the term "*nutmeg-liver.*" This is due to the fact that the central portion of the lobule is congested and somewhat depressed below the general surface, while the periphery is pale yellow or yellowish-brown, and swollen, owing to the presence of fat within the secreting cells. Here and there redder patches are to be seen which are regenerated lobules. In the most advanced stage the liver is small and hard, owing to the production of fibrous tissue (*cyanotic induration*). In this way a form of cirrhosis may be produced—the "cirrhose cardiaque" of the French writers.[1] In our experience this condition is rare.

On histological examination, the main changes are at first to be found in the central portion of the lobules. The centrilobular veins with their capillaries are distended with blood, and the columns of liver cells between are compressed. The secreting cells, therefore, become atrophic,

---

[1] Cornil and Ranvier, Manuel d'histologie pathologique, Paris, 1901.

and contain yellowish-brown granules of pigment, together with minute globules of fat. The degeneration is, as one might expect, most marked in the central and intermediate zones of the lobules. Here and there groups of cells are seen, much larger than the ordinary parenchymatous cells, having also large nuclei, which take an intense stain. These indicate an attempt at regeneration. In the more advanced forms practically all the capillaries of the lobule are congested and the great bulk of the liver cells disappear, being represented only by fragmented nuclei and masses of pigment. In certain cases, where the congestion is gradual in its onset, concomitant with the degeneration there is proliferation of connective tissue, leading to induration (replacement fibrosis), a condition found usually about the radicles of the hepatic vein, but to some extent also in the periportal districts. The portal sheaths may present evidences of a round-celled infiltration.

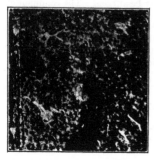

Nutmeg liver. (From the Pathological Department of the Royal Victoria Hospital.)

Leukemia.—In leukemia the capillaries everywhere are filled with leukocytes, and particularly large accumulations may be noted in the

Fig. 108

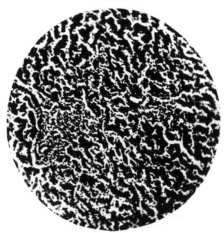

Leukemia of the liver. The capillaries are filled with leukocytes. Zeiss obj. A, without ocular. (From the collection of the Pathological Department, McGill University.)

portal districts. There has been a debate whether these represent a hyperplasia of lymphoid tissue normally present there or a multiplication of leukocytes that have migrated there.

Œdema.—Œdema of the liver is met with occasionally and leads to enlargement of the organ. The condition has not attracted much attention, but is more common than has usually been thought. The liver substance is more succulent than usual, and on section has a pale, dull, shiny appearance. Microscopically, one can see clear spaces between the capillaries and the parenchymatous cells of the liver. The condition can be reproduced experimentally by stimulation of the liver, and apparently may be readily brought about. Birch-Hirschfeld attributed icterus neonatorum to compression of the bile ducts by œdematous connective tissue.

Hemorrhage.—Hemorrhage into the substance of the liver may result from traumatism, the hemorrhagic diathesis, infarction, acute yellow atrophy, and various infections.

Embolism and Thrombosis.—Embolism or thrombosis of the hepatic artery or its branches, especially when associated with cardiac weakness, leads to the formation of a white or red infarct (Chiari). The infarction is rarely typical, for the reason that the liver is well supplied with blood also from the portal vein.

Thrombosis of the portal vein is a not uncommon condition. In the majority of instances it is really a thrombophlebitis. The main trunk of the vessel or any of its branches may be affected. Infective processes occurring in the organs or structures included in the portal system, as, for example, the spleen, intestines, stomach, or mesentery, particularly when septic in character, may lead to it. It is especially common in connection with appendicitis. Inflammations, too, about the bile ducts, or in the retroperitoneal tissues in that neighborhood, may extend to the portal vein and induce thrombosis. If septic, the thrombus may break down and lead to the formation of an abscess, and minute particles of infected material may be carried as emboli into the liver. Or, again, if non-infective, the thrombus may gradually soften and disappear, or may organize. In one case, with ascites, which we observed, following typhoid fever, the main trunk of the portal vein was completely occluded, and here and there in the smaller branches strands and tags of fibrous tissue could be detected, the remains of the previously existing thrombus.

Thrombosis is also occasionally observed in cases of portal cirrhosis, and where pressure is exerted upon the portal vein by tumors extending from the biliary passages, pancreas, stomach, or intestines. Where the obstruction to the circulation is complete, ascites comes on rapidly and may be intense. Important structural changes in the liver do not usually occur in the liver itself, since it is supplied with blood from the hepatic artery.

Infarcts.—Infarcts of the liver of the same type as those occurring in other organs are rare. They may be produced by embolism, thrombosis, or other causes leading to occlusion of the portal vein, hepatic artery, or hepatic vein.[1] The condition seems to be more common after

[1] See Hess, Amer. Jour. Med. Sci., 130; 1905: 986.

occlusion of the artery than of the vein, and in this case is of the anemic variety. Hemorrhagic infarction, so-called, is believed to be more frequently due to portal embolism, though it may also result from obstruction of the hepatic artery. The condition is not always a true infarction, however, inasmuch as the liver cells may still retain their staining properties. More properly it is an intense capillary congestion. When the obstruction involves the vessels in the intermediate portion of the lobules, formed by the union of the capillaries of the portal vein and hepatic artery, it leads to the production of one variety of focal necrosis. Schmorl[1] and Prutz have described this condition in connection with eclampsia. Such necrotic areas are usually demarcated by a zone of reactive inflammation. If the part be infected, abscess formation will follow, but if not, and the patient survive, the degenerated cells are absorbed and replaced by connective tissue.

INFLAMMATIONS.

Hepatitis.—The subject of hepatitis, or inflammation of the liver, is one of the most abstruse in the domain of special pathology. This, in part, arises from the fact that we are still to some extent ignorant of the etiology of many of the diseases coming under this category, and, in part, from the circumstance that the terminology has been and still is greatly confused. It is impossible, therefore, at present, to establish a classification that is entirely satisfactory, and any that may be proposed must be largely tentative.

From the standpoint of the morbid histologist, we may divide hepatitis into the acute parenchymatous, the acute interstitial, and the chronic interstitial, an arrangement that is, perhaps, as little open to cavil as any. It should be remarked, however, that these types are not always sharply defined one from the other, and that various combined or mixed forms occur.

Acute Parenchymatous Hepatitis.—Acute parenchymatous hepatitis, an affection with difficulty distinguishable from cloudy swelling, is a fairly frequent occurrence in the course of the infective fevers, particularly typhoid, tuberculosis, pneumonia, and septicemia. The liver is slightly enlarged, and on section is pale, grayish, and friable. Microscopically, the parenchymatous cells are swollen and granular, while the nuclei are slightly obscured. Not infrequently, one can see in the portal sheaths small collections of leukocytes, which may even extend for some little distance between the columns of liver cells. At the height of the process the parenchymatous cells become fatty, hyaline, and often vacuolated. While certain of them necrose and disappear, others seem to proliferate, as there is an increase in the number of the nuclei and also in their size. The condition approximates to the type of the inflammatory necroses accompanied by a reactive and reparative inflammation.

[1] Path. *Gesell.*, 5: 1902.

Allied to this affection is the rarer condition in which necrosis and atrophy are the prominent features, the regenerative processes being for a time at least in the background. Wasting is marked and the shrinkage of the liver can be watched clinically day by day. Of this the type is the so-called *acute yellow atrophy* of the liver. This disease begins with all the signs of a severe systemic intoxication—high fever, delirium a quickly-developing jaundice, multiple hemorrhages, and finally, convulsions and coma. A fatal termination generally takes place. In the early stages the liver is usually enlarged, but quickly diminishes in size. The liver may be reduced to one-half its natural size, its consistency is increased, and the capsule is thrown into folds, owing to the shrinkage

FIG. 109

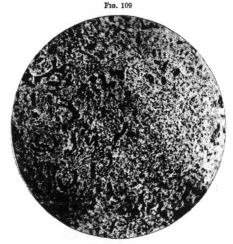

Acute yellow atrophy of the liver. Section shows atrophy of parenchymatous cells, fragmentation of nuclei, and pseudobile ducts. Zeiss obj. A, without ocular. (From the collection of the Royal Victoria Hospital.)

of the parenchyma. On section, the surface is of a bright, lemon-yellow color, with numerous patches of a darker brownish red. The reddish color usually predominates in the left lobe. The yellow areas are soft and somewhat swollen, while the red are firmer and rather of a leathery consistency. Small hemorrhages are common throughout the substance. The vessels contain thin blood and the bile capillaries thin bile.

Histologically, the parenchymatous cells in the yellow patches show extensive fatty changes, together with an accumulation of bile pigment and crystals of bilirubin. The fatty droplets can be found not only within the cytoplasm, but also within the nucleus. The reddish areas are composed mainly of a network of capillaries, in the meshes of which can be seen isolated, degenerating liver cells, and a detritus of broken-down cells, fragmented nuclei, masses of pigment, chromatin, and blood. Where death has been more than usually delayed, some evidences of regeneration can be made out. Small nodes of newly-formed liver cells may be found here and there, recognizable by the fact that they are larger than normal, stain more intensely, and have large, deeply-staining nuclei, some of them exhibiting mitosis. A round-celled infiltration can be made out in the portal sheaths together with some proliferation of the connective tissue. Pseudobile capillaries may also be present in considerable numbers, giving the section somewhat the appearance of a cirrhosis.

Acute yellow atrophy, in most cases, is almost certainly an acute degeneration, the result of a circulating toxin. From the fact that cases sometimes occur in epidemic form, though rarely, this toxin is, probably, in some instances, bacterial in origin. The disease is most common between the ages of twenty and thirty, and is usually found in women during the puerperium. Secondarily, it may occur in connection with certain of the infectious fevers, such as variola, erysipelas, typhoid, septicemia, and osteomyelitis. Very similar forms of acute degeneration and necrosis of the liver parenchyma occur in connection with poisoning by phosphorus, arsenic, and chloroform. Several cases have been reported lately resulting from chloroform anesthesia. They usually are met with in children, the subjects of long-standing and debilitating disease.

Acute Interstitial Hepatitis.—Acute interstitial hepatitis may be simple, but is more often suppurative. It is due to infection of the liver by microörganisms that gain entrance to it through the general blood stream, the portal vein, or the bile passages. In newborn children infection through the umbilical cord is an occasional cause. In rare cases a retrograde metastasis of bacterial agents may take place from the superior vena cava.

Simple interstitial hepatitis is occasionally seen in the livers of persons dying from infectious disease, notably typhoid and tuberculosis. Besides cloudy swelling of the parenchyma, small collections of inflammatory round cells, of greater or less extent, are to be found in the portal sheaths. Some authorities are inclined to attribute some importance to this manifestation of infectious disease in the etiology of cirrhosis.

Acute *suppurative interstitial hepatitis* may be primary or secondary. The primary form is rather rare in temperate regions but is more common in the tropics, where it is known under the name of tropical abscess. The cases occurring in this country are almost invariably due to trauma, such as severe crushing injuries to the liver, or are examples of wound infection. The vast majority of cases, as we meet them here, are secondary to infection elsewhere, and are either metastatic in nature or arise by direct extension. In the metastatic forms the infective agents reach the liver by way of the hepatic artery and vein, the portal vein, or the bile ducts. In 1474 autopsies of which we have notes, performed at the Montreal General and Royal Victoria Hospitals, there were 46 cases of liver abscess; 22 were due to portal infection, 8 were biliary, 7 occurred from extension, 3 gave a history of dysentery, 3 cases were arterial, and 1 was apparently primary.

Suppurative Hepatitis of Arterial Origin.—This form is usually but one manifestation of a generalized septicemia, the infective agents reaching the liver by way of the hepatic artery. The etiology of this form is, therefore, that of septicemia in general. The disease may complicate all kinds of wound infection, ulcerative endocarditis and aortitis, osteitis, osteomyelitis, putrid bronchitis, gangrene of the lung, infection of the puerperal uterus, and suppurative lesions about the bladder, prostate, and urethra. It has been known to follow carbuncle and whitlow. The infective agents usually at work are Streptococcus pyogenes and Staphylococcus albus and aureus.

Suppurative Hepatitis of Venous Origin.—Infection of the liver may take place through the hepatic vein. Undoubted instances appear to be rare, and arise usually from retrograde embolism. Some cases are traceable to pylephlebitis or cholecystitis.

Suppurative Hepatitis of Portal Origin.—Here the infective agents come from any part of the district drained by the portal system. Septic processes in the appendix, cecum, small intestine, stomach, pancreas, and spleen are important in this connection. The most frequent single cause is appendicitis (perityphlitis). Combining the statistics of Armstrong,[1] Einhorn, Langheld, and Fitz, in 546 cases of appendicitis that were examined *post mortem*, pylephlebitis and abscess of the liver were found in 28, or rather more than 5 per cent. Exceptionally, in cases of cholecystitis and pericholecystitis, extension of the process to the portal vein may result in an embolic infection of the liver. The lesion is in many instances essentially an acute thrombophlebitis of the portal vein or a purulent infiltration of the vessel wall and adjacent parts—*suppurative portal pyelephlebitis*. In a typical case of septic portal infection the liver contains multiple abscesses of varying size. These are grouped about the branches of the portal vein, after the fashion of currants upon a stem. The larger abscesses are usually irregular or lobular in appearance, owing to the fact that they result from the confluence of smaller foci. Small, isolated abscesses are often to be found grouped about the larger ones, but separated from them by a small amount of comparatively unaltered liver tissue. The abscesses are filled with yellowish-green, viscid pus, often mixed with blood, having a foul odor, and sometimes containing sequestra of liver substance. Round about the abscesses is a narrow zone of a yellowish-white color, or, in cases of a gangrenous type, of a dirty green appearance. The portal vein and its branches within the liver usually contain more or less dirty-looking septic clot. The abscesses are chiefly to be found in the right lobe. Where the infection has taken place through the hepatic artery the foci of suppuration are usually smaller and more widely and evenly distributed.

Histologically, in the more recent lesions, the smaller branches of the portal vein are packed with microörganisms. Round about are extensive

[1] Brit. Med. Jour., 2:1897:945.

accumulations of inflammatory leukocytes, tending to stain badly toward the centre. In the larger abscesses the central portion has broken down and the cells composing it are in various stages of necrosis and disintegration. At the periphery the leukocytes gradually lose themselves between the liver cells. The parenchyma of the liver in the neighborhood presents the appearance of coagulation necrosis. The specific cells are swollen, hyaline, or compressed, containing nuclei that stain badly. When the abscesses are near the surface, the Glisson's capsule is often infiltrated, the endothelial cells are in process of desquamation, and there may be a deposit of fibrinopurulent exudate (*perihepatitis*). The liver, as a whole, is congested and more or less swollen and cloudy. The

FIG. 110

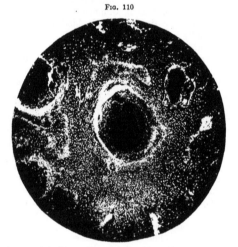

Multiple abscesses of the liver. Zeiss obj. DD, without ocular. (From the collection of Dr. A. G. Nicholls.)

cases are usually fatal, but instances are on record where the abscesses have ruptured into the lung or intestine with spontaneous cure. Healing may take place with the evacuation or absorption of the pus and the formation of fibrous scars.

Suppurative Hepatitis of Biliary Origin.—Here infection takes place through the bile passages. The most common cause is cholelithiasis with associated cholangitis; in other cases the infection results upon obstruction of the bile duct from tumors or cysts. The bile passages may occasionally be infected from the intestine, as in dysentery and typhoid. Lannois[1] has recorded a case of liver abscess occurring in typhoid. Rarely, ascarides may invade the ductus communis and,

[1] Revue de Médecine, 15:1895:909.

dying there, give rise to marked disturbance. Leick[1] has collected 19 instances of this kind.

The description of the various abscesses just given above holds fairly well for this variety. The pus, however, is usually mixed with bile, and may contain gritty matter or concretions.

Suppurative Hepatitis Arising per Extensionem.—This is a fairly common form of suppuration in the liver. The process is usually superficial, affecting the capsule and that portion of the liver immediately beneath it. Diaphragmatic and subdiaphragmatic abscesses, empyema, suppurative cholecystitis and choledochitis, perinephric abscess, abscess of the head of the pancreas, perforating ulcers of the stomach and duodenum invade the liver. Foreign bodies, such as fish-bones, needles, or other sharp-pointed articles, may pass through the stomach or intestines and become lodged in the liver, where they may set up suppurative inflammation.

Tropical Abscess.—This variety is characterized by the formation of one or more foci of necrosis and softening in the liver, either with or without a relation to dysentery. Unlike the forms of abscess we have been describing, the rule here is for one large or at most but a few abscesses to be developed.

The cases are met with usually in tropical and subtropical countries, whence the name. The etiological factors are as yet but imperfectly understood. Some few cases appear to be due to dietetic errors; free living, the excessive use of animal food, and particularly excess in alcohol, are thought by some to be particularly potent causes. We must, in these cases, assume that there is some previous deterioration of the resisting power of the liver that renders it a more easy prey to toxins and invading microörganisms. The great majority of cases are associated with tropical dysentery. In this connection Kartulis[2] states that in 500 cases of liver abscess coming under his notice, from 50 to 60 per cent. gave a history of dysentery. There must be something peculiar about the condition, for in the catarrhal and ulcerative dysenteries found in temperate climes liver abscess is excessively rare. The studies of Kartulis, Lösch,[3] Kruse and Pasquale,[4] Councilman and Lafleur,[5] have shown that a fairly large proportion of cases of dysenteric origin are due to the amœba coli. What this proportion is is uncertain. Flexner is of the opinion that the great majority are of amœbic origin. In a large experience he did not find a single case due to the Shiga bacillus. A few writers, however, refer to the discovery of a typhoid-like bacillus which possibly was this organism, and Pansini and Babes seem to have obtained it or a similar germ in several cases of liver abscess.

The amœbic abscess in about 75 per cent. of the cases is solitary, and in about the same proportion is situated in the right lobe, usually in

---

[1] Deutsche med. Woch., 1898; see also v. Saar. Path. Gesellsch., 1904.
[2] Centralb. f. Bakter., 2:1887: 745. Virch. Archiv, 118:1889.
[3] Virch. Archiv, 65:1875:. 196. [4] Zeitschr. f. Hyg. u. Infectionskrankh., 16:1.
[5] Johns Hopkins Hosp. Rep., 2:1891.

the dome or under surface near the hepatic flexure of the colon. In early cases the necrotic area may be scarcely liquefied, and is hyperemic, spongy, and infiltrated with a glairy tenacious material. Later, a regular abscess is formed, its walls formed of necrotic liver substance and shreddy connective tissue. The contents of the abscess vary much. In some few cases the fluid is serous, but in most there is a mixture of pus and necrotic material. The pus is somewhat glairy and translucent in some cases; in others, grayish or brownish-red, so that its appearance has been compared to anchovy sauce. The quantity varies from a few ounces to many pints. Practically the whole of the right lobe of the liver has been found in some cases to be occupied by a huge abscess enclosed in a thin shell of liver substance. In long-standing cases, the abscess becomes walled off by pyogenic membrane or a fibrous capsule. The liver substance in the neighborhood is generally congested, softened, cloudy, and friable, and shows other signs of degeneration, but in some cases has been found to be practically normal.

Histologically, the contents of the abscess are a finely granular detritus, broken-down liver cells, red and white blood-corpuscles, and hematoidin. There is usually a more or less widespread necrosis of the liver parenchyma. The amœbæ are found chiefly at the periphery of the abscess, in the capillaries, and about the portal sheaths. They are more numerous in the smaller foci. An important point is that leukocytes are scanty in the contents of the abscess and in the wall, except in cases where secondary infection has taken place, showing that the lesion is essentially a non-suppurative one. In many cases bacteria are found in the abscesses, notably staphylococci and streptococci. The earlier observers were of the opinion that the necrosis was due to the pyogenic cocci, while some others held that the amœbæ acted as carriers for the germs and by their growth and movement, which ruptured the capillaries, paved the way for bacterial infection. The preponderance of evidence at the present day, however, is in favor of the view that the amœbæ are the direct cause of the lesions.

Most untreated cases end fatally, but if death do not take place soon, or if the condition be not relieved by operative interference, the abscess may rupture and give rise to further serious consequences. The most frequent event is for the rupture to take place into the right pleura or lung, the fluid subsequently being discharged through a bronchus; next to that, into the peritoneal cavity. More rarely, the abscess may discharge into the pericardium, sudden death being the result. Again, the abscess may point externally or empty into the transverse colon, stomach, or duodenum; very rarely, into the bile passages, the hepatic vein, the vena cava, or the pelvis of the right kidney.

In exceptional cases the process remains latent or comes to an end. Small foci of suppuration may be absorbed with the formation of a scar. In the case of larger ones, the fluid part of the contents is absorbed, and we get a small cavity walled in by a connective-tissue capsule and filled with a cheesy substance in which lime salts may subsequently be deposited.

Cirrhosis.—Under the terms *cirrhosis, chronic interstitial hepatitis, productive hepatitis,* are included a variety of morbid conditions, which, while they differ in regard to their etiology and the minuter details of structural change, have this in common, that there is a hyperplasia of connective tissue, which, in time, becomes sufficient markedly to interfere with the functions of the organ. Much confusion of mind has existed with regard to these conditions, owing to the difficulty of bringing clinical symptoms into harmony with the anatomical appearances found *post mortem,* but perhaps even more from the lax use of terms. Particularly unfortunate are the terms "hypertrophic" and "atrophic" as applied to cirrhosis, for at best they are merely relative, and, moreover, have been used erroneously as synonymous with enlargement or diminution in size.

All the evidence at our disposal, whether clinical or experimental, clearly indicates that cirrhosis or fibrosis of the liver is in most cases the result of the irritation of some toxin, bacterial or otherwise, which may reach the liver in one or other of three ways, *i. e.,* through the hepatic artery, through the portal vein, or through the bile passages. The occurrence of cirrhosis as a result of infection or intoxication operating through the hepatic artery, while theoretically possible, is not established by positive evidence. The cirrhosis resulting from the action of coal dust—**cirrhosis anthracotica**—may perhaps be of this nature. It is beyond question, however, that irritants may reach the liver through the portal vein and the bile ducts, so that we can at once recognize two important classes of cases—**portal cirrhosis** and **biliary cirrhosis**. A fourth form, one that is included with doubtful propriety among the cirrhoses, is called **capsular cirrhosis** or **perihepatitis with cirrhosis**, in which the irritants affect primarily the capsule. A few cases also are met with of fibrosis of the liver that are more akin to degeneration than to inflammation, of which the cirrhosis following chronic passive congestion is the most important form. The following classification, based mainly upon anatomical and histological grounds, will be found useful, and has at least the merit that it fits in fairly well with clinical observations:

I. Portal cirrhosis
    (*a*) with enlargement.
    (*b*) with contraction (Laennec's cirrhosis; hobnailed liver, gin-drinker's liver).
II. True biliary cirrhosis (Hanot's form).
III. Obstructive biliary cirrhosis
    (*a*) with enlargement.
    (*b*) with contraction.
IV. Pericellular or diffuse cirrhosis.
V. Capsular cirrhosis (perihepatitis with cirrhosis).
VI. Senile atrophy and arteriosclerosis.
VII. Cirrhosis from passive congestion.

Portal Cirrhosis with Enlargement.—The first form mentioned is in many cases, in our opinion, simply an early stage of Laennec's cirrhosis. We have met with one or two instances in which the liver was at first greatly enlarged, and at death, many months later, the ordinary, small, hob-nailed liver was discovered. This preliminary enlargement is not likely to be due to hypertrophy, but rather to acute congestion and inflammatory infiltration. Hypertrophy and hyperplasia of the liver cells proper undoubtedly occur in the various forms of cirrhosis, but are particularly marked in the contracted or hob-nailed liver, called improperly the liver of "atrophic" cirrhosis. Such hyperplasia occurs somewhat late in the disease and always falls short of the amount necessary to restore the perfect function of the organ. Conversely, hyperplasia is not a marked feature in cases of cirrhosis with enlargement, sometimes called "hypertrophic" cirrhosis. As a matter of fact, hyperplasia of the liver parenchyma and, more particularly, of the connective tissue is present in a variable degree in all forms of cirrhosis, so that it would conduce to clearness if the terms "atrophic" and "hypertrophic" were discontinued in connection with this subject.

FIG. 111

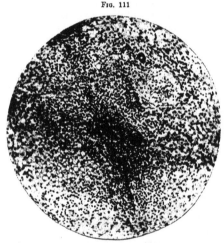

Slight cirrhosis of the liver with fatty infiltration. Zeiss obj. A, without ocular. (From the collection of Dr. A. G. Nicholls.)

A second and important form of portal cirrhosis with enlargement is the so-called *fatty cirrhosis*. Here, in addition to the ordinary anatomical changes characteristic of portal cirrhosis, there is more or less extreme fatty infiltration.

The organ, in a well-marked case, is much enlarged, with a smooth, or, possibly, a slightly granular surface. The edges are rounded and the color is yellow. The appearance is that of the fattily infiltrated liver, but with this difference, that the organ is very firm, is not friable, and cuts with difficulty, owing to the excess of fibrous tissue that is present.

Microscopically, there is usually a moderate amount of cirrhosis, of the type to be described under the next head, but the remaining liver parenchyma is more or less fatty, the cells being filled with large fatty globules. ᐧ In some instances there may be no normal liver cells left. The fatty cirrhotic liver may᾿ be latent, being found accidentally at autopsy but in some cases gives rise to a train of symptoms similar to those in Laennec's cirrhosis. This form of liver is met with usually in connection with pronounced alcoholism.

Portal Cirrhosis with Contraction.—This is the form variously designated as Laennec's cirrhosis, atrophic cirrhosis, hob-nailed liver, gin-drinker's liver, contracted liver. While alcohol has been credited with being the

Fig. 112

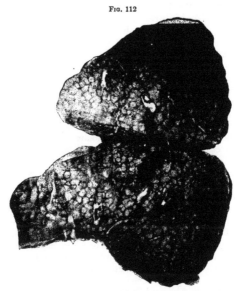

Laennec's cirrhosis, portal cirrhosis, hob-nailed liver, gin-drinker's liver. A transverse section is made through the organ and the upper portion is turned upward. (From the Pathological Museum of McGill University.)

etiological factor in about 60 per cent. of cases, experimental investigations do not bear this out. Probably alcohol acts not directly but indirectly, like a variety of other substances, in bringing about cirrhosis. Alcohol produces gastro-intestinal catarrh, this leads to abnormal fermentative processes and the elaboration of toxins, which toxins, in turn, act upon the liver. The finer details of the process have led to much discussion, but it is probable that the toxins lead primarily to degenerative changes in the parenchymatous cells, which necrose and are replaced by new connective tissue. It is not impossible, however, that a vicious circle is produced and that irritants in the blood act through the vessels upon the fibrous structure of the portal sheaths, stimulating it directly to hyper-plasia (cf. p. 383 et seq.).

To gross appearance the liver is more or less diminished in size, in advanced cases perhaps not weighing more than half the normal amount. The organ is deformed and the surface warty, being covered with granulations or nodules, ranging in size from that of a pin-head to that of a bean. The color is yellowish, orange, or yellowish green, whence the term "cirrhosis," according to the amount of bile-staining that has occurred. The granulation is often most marked in the left lobe and on the anterior border. The capsule is thickened, and there are often adhesions between the liver and the diaphragm. The gall-bladder is generally diminished in size. On section, the organ cuts firmly, with a resistant feel, and it can then be seen that the depressions on the surface are associated with bands of fibrous tissue which form a net-work throughout the liver, dividing the parenchyma into a great number of sharply defined islets. The fibrous bands are of a whitish or pinkish-gray color, slightly translucent in appearance, and project above the general level, thus giving the cut surface an irregular, granular appearance.

Histologically, the most striking feature is the enormous proliferation of the connective tissue which forms a series of connected bands enclosing the lobules. These bands may be distributed so as to enclose several lobules (polylobular cirrhosis) or to isolate each lobule separately (monolobular cirrhosis). Both conditions are usually to be made out in cases of Laennec's cirrhosis, and may be included under the terms "perilobular" or "interlobular" cirrhosis. In advanced cases, the fibrous tissue may insinuate itself between the individual columns of liver cells (intralobular cirrhosis); but this is never a marked feature, although it is not at all uncommon in the biliary forms. Where the inflammatory process is recent or active, the portal sheaths are more or less densely infiltrated with clusters of round cells, in part, fibroblasts, and, probably, in part leukocytes. In the older portions or where the disease has about run its course, the round cells are scanty, and we find dense bands of fibrous tissue having the characteristic fibrillation of the adult tissue, with relatively few elongated nuclei. In the bands of fibrous tissue are found groups of cells arranged in parallel rows closely resembling bile capillaries. Their origin is somewhat debatable. They are generally more abundant in the parts where cellular infiltration is conspicuous, for, as the fibrous tissue is formed it seems to crush them out of existence. These apparent bile capillaries may be fairly numerous, but in some cases, again, are scanty or even absent. Three modes of origin are possible: they may be new ducts derived by proliferation of the original bile capillaries; they may be bile capillaries that have persisted after destruc-tion of the lobules to which they belonged; or they may indicate rever-sionary degeneration of the liver cells. On careful examination, one will often see that these apparently newly-formed capillaries do not re-semble capillaries so much as they do columns of liver cells that have undergone atrophy, for the protoplasm of their component cells strikes a color with hematoxylin-eosin similar to that of the normal liver parenchyma. Further, certain of them will be found to be in direct connection with the cells of the periphery of the liver lobules. Such pseudocapillaries, therefore, probably represent columns of liver cells that have reverted to a more primitive condition.

In addition, bloodvessels can be made out in the fibrous septa, which are numerous, large, and thin-walled. These can be injected through the hepatic artery. The branches of the portal vein, on the other hand, either from external pressure or changes in the intima, are more or less occluded, thus accounting for the portal obstruction that sooner or later becomes so marked a feature in this form of cirrhosis. The liver cells themselves often present little alteration, but at the periphery of the lobules many of them show atrophic changes, being fattily degenerated or reduced to flattened plates, or, perhaps, little more than nuclei. The atrophy is to some extent due to the encroachment of the fibrous tissue, but also, no doubt, to the influence of circulating toxins and impaired nutrition. Occasionally, there is marked fatty infiltration, as in the fatty cirrhosis above described. Here and there attempts at compensation can be made out, for masses of liver cells, more or less perfectly reproducing the lobules, can be seen, composed of newly-formed cells, which are large, stain deeply, and show nuclei in various stages of mitosis. Pigment granules of a yellowish-brown or yellowish-green color are also to be seen within the specific cells, in the interstices of the connective tissue, and in the endothelial cells lining the vessels. Some of these may be biliary pigment, but not infrequently they can be shown to contain iron, probably, therefore, being hemosiderin derived from broken-down red blood corpuscles. Cases are on record where sufficient of this iron-containing pigment has been produced to stain most of the tissues of the body, including the skin, a bluish-gray or leaden color. This is the condition known as **hemochromatosis** (see p. 486).

In well-marked cases of Laennec's cirrhosis the portal vein and its branches are dilated. Dilated veins may often, also, be seen in the skin, especially on the sides of the abdomen and thorax and around the umbilicus (*caput Medusæ*). The œsophageal, gastric, and hemorrhoidal veins are usually dilated and may be varicosed. Rupture of the œsophageal vessels may give rise to fatal hemorrhage. The spleen is moderately enlarged, its capsule thickened, and it is sometimes embedded in adhesions. Not infrequently the pancreas is cirrhotic as well. The gastro-intestinal mucosa is in a state of passive congestion, and is apt to be thickened, presenting chronic œdema. Ascites is present in about half the cases. Jaundice occurs in about 27 per cent., and is usually slight. A not unusual complication is tuberculous peritonitis.

Hanot's Cirrhosis.[1]—Hanot's cirrhosis, sometimes called, though erroneously, hypertrophic cirrhosis, and sometimes "true" biliary cirrhosis, is a rare form in this country.[2] In fact, it seems to be uncommon outside of France. The disease is characterized by enlargement of the liver

---

[1] Hanot, Sur une forme de cirrhose hyper. du foie, Thèse de Paris, 1876.

[2] There is a tendency among clinicians to confuse the enlarged stage of portal cirrhosis with this type.

and jaundice, which persists for months or even years. The jaundice is often intense, as in the obstructive form, but the stools are usually colored. In some cases it comes on acutely and the disease runs a course like that of acute febrile icterus, or, again, of acute yellow atrophy.

The liver is greatly enlarged, weighing from 2 to 4 kg. The surface is smooth, or at most covered with flat prominences. On section, the organ is firm and grates under the knife. The cut surface is yellowish or yellowish-green, owing to bile staining, and has a finely granulated appearance resembling shagreen leather.

Histologically, there is an overgrowth of connective tissue, often rather poor in nuclei, which is diffuse in character, tending to invade the lobules (intralobular cirrhosis) or isolate small groups of liver cells. The islets of parenchyma remaining are small, and single cells or small groups of cells are seen separated one from the other by delicate strands of connective tissue. There is usually a considerable production of pseudobile capillaries. The cells contain bile pigment. The process seems to be essentially due to a catarrh of the finer bile capillaries and the portal system appears to be free. An infective origin is probable, but the etiology has not yet been thoroughly worked out.

Obstructive Biliary Cirrhosis.—This form is due to some gross obstruction to the free outflow of bile, either within the ducts, as from a calculus, carcinoma, or a fibrous stricture; or from without, as from a new-growth in the head of the pancreas or in the periportal lymph-nodes. Obstruction does not appear to be the sole cause, however, for complete occlusion of the ducts may occur without the production of cirrhosis. Another factor is usually operative as well, and this is inflammation, in the form of a cholangitis. This is easily set up, since bacteria are invariably to be found in the bile passages in such cases, a catarrhal inflammation, originally dependent on microbic infection, being the cause of the calculus formation in the first place. Exceptions to the rule may occur, nevertheless.

In the earlier stages of the disease the liver is much enlarged, closely resembling the liver in Hanot's cirrhosis. In one of our cases, in which a stone was found in the hepatic duct, the organ weighed 4850 grams. To gross appearance, the liver is enlarged, smooth, and bile-stained. It cuts firmly, the cut surface being finely granulated and of a yellowish-green color. The bile ducts can be seen to be dilated and their walls thickened.

Microscopically, the newly-formed connective tissue is both interlobular and intralobular in its distribution and is rather dense. It is characterized by the presence of central dilated bile ducts surrounded by chaplets of pseudobile ducts which are conspicuous by their numbers. Degenerative changes can be made out in the parenchymatous cells. Focal necroses may be found. Ascites is rare, and the spleen is not greatly enlarged. The portal circulation appears to be not notably interfered with. Pyogenic infection of the bile passages may occur with the production of a suppurative cholangitis and the formation of small abscesses along the course of the infected ducts.[1]

---

[1] For a useful consideration of this form of cirrhosis, see Ford, Amer. Jour. Med. Sci., 121:1901:60.

In another type of the affection, probably a later stage of that just described, the liver is contracted, bile-stained, and has a fairly diffuse granulation, the granulations being of medium size and rather even in character.

Pericellular Cirrhosis.—In this form of cirrhosis there is a singularly diffuse hyperplasia of connective tissue, which tends to surround and isolate very small groups of liver cells or even individual cells. The fibrous tissue is curiously transparent and almost hyaline looking, with but little fibrillation and relatively few nuclei. Degenerative changes in the parenchyma, save atrophy, are not pronounced.

FIG. 113

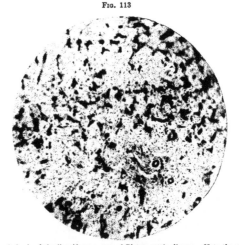

Pericellular cirrhosis of the liver from a case of Pictou cattle disease. Note the great relative isolation of the liver cells and the delicate connective tissue with scanty nuclei. Reichert obj. 7a, without ocular. (From the collection of Dr. J. G. Adami.)

Pericellular cirrhosis is met with occasionally in syphilis and tuberculosis of the liver (q. v.), and is also well exemplified in a curious affection of cattle, studied by Osler, Wyatt Johnston, and Adami,[1] known as "Pictou Cattle Disease." This disease, which at first was thought to be restricted to a particular district in Nova Scotia, now seems to be more widespread, having been recognized by Gilruth in New Zealand, and, according to Thomas, is similar to the Schweineberger Krankheit of Bavaria. Gilruth has found, and Pethick has confirmed this, that it can be brought about by feeding animals with Senecio jacobœa, one of the Compositæ. In some particulars it is not unlike Laennec's cirrhosis in human beings. There are a moderate ascites, a right-sided pleural effusion, without jaundice, and the abdominal and periportal lymph-

[1] Montreal Med. Journ., 31:1902:105.

nodes are enlarged and succulent.   There is a peculiar gelatinous œdema of the mesentery and the intestinal walls.   The liver is moderately enlarged, with a smooth, or occasionally a slightly granular surface. Recent and healing ulcers are found in the fourth stomach.

Capsular Cirrhosis (Perihepatitis; Pseudocirrhosis; "Zuckergussleber";[1] Glissonitis).—This is a somewhat rare affection of the liver, in which the surface is more or less completely covered with a thick, fibrous investment, of pearly white, cartilaginous appearance, and hyaline structure.   The liver is at first enlarged, but subsequently undergoes marked contraction.   In the majority of instances the affection is simply a peculiar form of perihepatitis, and is usually associated with a similar transformation of the capsule of the spleen, the peritoneum, and the other serous membranes.   In fact, the condition is often part and parcel

FIG. 114

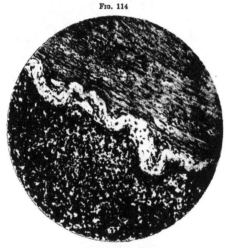

Chronic perihepatitis with hyaline transformation of the exudate (hyaloserositis). The Glisson's capsule is thrown into folds from atrophy of the liver parenchyma. Leitz obj. No. 7, without ocular. (From the collection of Dr. A. G. Nicholls.)

of a chronic progressive multiserositis, or, as one of us (A. G. N.) has called it, "hyaloserositis."   The relationship of cirrhosis of the liver to this form of capsulitis or perihepatitis is still somewhat obscure.   It is rare to find a true cirrhosis associated with the condition.   The liver, rather, shows brown atrophy and passive congestion.   At most, there may be a slight invasion of the liver substance by small fibrous bands passing down from and in connection with the capsule.   When cirrhosis is present in these cases, as it undoubtedly may be, it is more probably

[1] See K. Reimer, Inaug. Diss., Kiel, 1906.

due to passive congestion, or at all events is to be regarded as a condition quite distinct from the perihepatitis.[1]

Senile Atrophy of the Liver.—Here the liver is small and shrunken, the capsule thrown into folds, and the whole organ is firm. It is often also more deeply pigmented than normal. Microscopically, the connective tissue is increased. It is questionable whether this is not an apparent increase due to the paucity of liver cells, rather than a true hyperplasia. It is not to be denied, however, that the disappearance of the liver parenchyma may be accompanied by a compensatory new-growth of connective tissue, an example of what one of us (J. G. A.) has elsewhere termed "replacement fibrosis." If this be true, the condition might be termed an interstitial fibrosis or cirrhosis, though it should be remembered that it is primarily of a degenerative rather than an inflammatory origin. The atrophy in such cases may possibly be referred to lack of nutrition, due to thickening of the branches of the hepatic artery. It must be admitted, however, that we have practically no anatomical evidence in favor of an arteriosclerotic cirrhosis of the liver *per se*.

Cirrhosis from Passive Congestion (Cirrhose Cardiaque).—This is a form of cirrhosis described mainly by the French school of pathologists. The Germans in general are disposed to deny its existence. It is a fact, however, that in moderately advanced and long-continued cases of passive congestion of the liver, associated more especially with cardiac weakness, there may be a certain amount of fibrosis in the neighborhood of the centrilobular vein, following a preliminary atrophy of the liver parenchyma of these parts. This is, in our experience, a rare occurrence, but unquestionably does occur. It may well be doubted, however, whether such a fibrosis is ever sufficiently extensive to give rise to clinical symptoms.

Tuberculosis.—The occurrence of primary tuberculosis of the liver is doubtful. Cases of this disease can usually be traced to foci of infection in some other region of the body. The path of infection may be by way of the hepatic artery, the portal vein, the lymphatics, or by contiguity.

Anatomically, three forms can be recognized—*disseminated miliary tuberculosis, solitary tuberculomas,* and *chronic tuberculous sclerosing hepatitis*. If the liver be fatty, as it so often is in cases of advanced tuberculosis, miliary tubercles may readily be overlooked. When visible, they are present as minute, gray, or yellowish dots, often slightly bile-stained. The milia are situated for the most part in the periportal connective tissue and may encroach to some extent upon the lobules. Exceptionally, they are found within the lobules. The foci have the appearance of lymphoid nodules with epithelioid cells and possibly giant cells. Caseation is not uncommon. In the centre of the tubercle the liver cells are destroyed, while those at the periphery show fatty changes and atrophy. In some cases the tubercles are not fully formed, and we

---

[1] The relationship of perihepatitis to cirrhosis is discussed at some length by Nicholls, Studies from the Royal Victoria Hospital, Montreal, 1:3:1902:60.

find merely a round-celled infiltration in the periportal sheaths with some cirrhosis and the formation of pseudobile capillaries. The cirrhosis is often of the pericellular type.

Solitary tubercles, usually few in number, are occasionally observed, but are rare. They may be of considerable size, are caseous in the centre, and are enclosed in a more or less dense fibrous capsule. Occasionally, they soften or become secondarily infected, giving rise to abscesses.[1]

In the third form, the liver is the seat of a diffuse and extensive overgrowth of connective tissue, in which can be seen, here and there, gray or grayish-yellow tubercles.[2]

FIG. 115 [1]

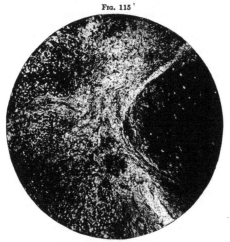

Gumma of the liver. Zeiss obj. A, without ocular. The gumma is the dark mass to the right. (From the collection of the Montreal General Hospital.)

Syphilis.—Both congenital and acquired syphilis may affect the liver.[3] The lesions of **congenital syphilis** in the main are comparable with those of tuberculosis. We can differentiate anatomically, *disseminated miliary gummas, large, well-formed gummas,* and *syphilitic cirrhosis.*

In the form with numerous miliary gummas the liver is often enlarged. The lesions affect either the whole organ or circumscribed areas of it. The milia, histologically, are identical with the milia of tuberculosis. The absence of the tubercle bacillus in the former is practically the only way to differentiate between them. There is usually marked

[1] For literature see Pertik, Tuberculose Referat, Lubarsch and Ostertag's Ergebnisse, 8: 1904: 279.

[2] Isaak, Frankfurter Zeitschrift f. Path., 2: 1908.

[3] For literature, see Herxheimer, Lubarsch and Ostertag's Ergebnisse, 11: 1907: 276, and 12: 1908: 549

fibrosis in the neighborhood of miliary gummas also. Large gummas are occasionally met with in congenital syphilis, but are more common in the acquired disease! They are of moderate size, as a rule, easily visible to the naked eye, and are scattered irregularly through the organ. They present a yellowish appearance, with broken-down centres, usually surrounded by dense, often radiating scars. In advanced cases the liver is greatly deformed and divided into numerous lobules of varying size by deep fissures, which represent contracting fibrous cicatrices, the sole remains of the previously existing gummas. This gives rise to the so-called *hepar lobatum*. The comparatively unaltered liver substance is often of a dark brown color.

Histologically, gummas closely resemble tuberculous granulomas, having a necrotic centre, a cellular periphery with giant cells, and being enclosed in a fibrous capsule. The capsule is somewhat irregular, sending out processes into the liver substance in the neighborhood, and contains collections of small, round cells, and, often, numerous pseudo-bile capillaries. The liver cells proper usually show brown atrophy, and there may be evidences of amyloid transformation. In advanced cases nothing but the scar is visible, the necrotic material having been completely absorbed.

In infants a diffuse cirrhosis is the common lesion of hepatic syphilis, and is of the pericellular and intra-acinous type. In the early stages, there is a cellular infiltration of the interlobular and intralobular connective tissue. This may be observed throughout the organ as a whole, or, again, may be restricted to scattered areas. The liver is somewhat enlarged, hard, and the capsule is smooth or, exceptionally, finely granular. On section, the color is yellow, yellowish or reddish-brown, somewhat recalling the appearance of flint. The lobules are not readily recognized. Histologically, there is a periportal proliferation of connective tissue, which tends to invade the lobules, destroying their substance, and containing numerous foci of round cells with pseudobile capillaries. The newly-formed connective tissue is delicate and translucent, containing relatively few nuclei, and is laid down diffusely, insinuating its way between the liver cells, so that they are found isolated one from the other, or in little groups of twos and threes. There is, apparently, not much tendency to contraction in this form. Hoffmann and others have demonstrated the presence of Spirochæta pallida in the livers of children dying of congenital syphilis.

The manifestations of **acquired syphilis** in the liver differ but little, on the whole, from those of the congenital form. Any differences are probably to be explained on the basis of time and the difference in the reactive powers of the liver at the different life periods.

The condition of the liver in the secondary stage is, of course, difficult to ascertain. The occurrence of jaundice and hepatic enlargement at this period suggests the presence of an acute interstitial hepatitis, perhaps associated with a cholangitis, or even a more severe affection, an acute parenchymatous hepatitis, closely resembling acute yellow atrophy.

The common type in the tertiary stage is the multiple gumma with cirrhosis. This is often associated with jaundice and gives rise to a nodular or fissured, contracted liver, which may be bile-stained. Occasionally, the gummas are so large as to be mistaken for malignant growths (*syphilomas*). In such cases there is a dense mass of fibrous tissue, with more or less gummy degeneration, surrounded by an outer layer of liver tissue, which is infiltrated with round cells. These seem to be derived from isolated gummas, presenting a reactive new-formation of liver substance at the periphery, which is dotted with numerous miliary gummas and eventually destroyed and replaced by fibrous tissue.

Actinomycosis.—Actinomycosis of the liver may be primary or secondary. There are but few undoubted cases of the primary disease on record.[1] The infection is generally thought to be from the intestine through the portal system. Less often it is from the peritoneum, kidney, or lung.

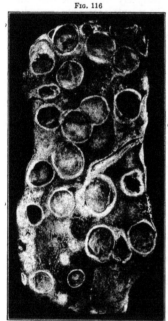

FIG. 116

The lesion takes the form of more or less numerous abscesses, which often assume a lobular arrangement, owing to the coalescence of smaller foci. With this there is a proliferation of connective tissue, giving the larger abscesses a curious and characteristic appearance. After the necrotic material is washed out, the larger cavities can be seen to be traversed in all directions by rather coarse communicating bands of connective tissue, so that an appearance rather like that of a loofah sponge is produced. The specific ray-fungus can be recognized in the tissues and in the necrotic and liquefied material. The liver becomes adherent to the diaphragm, abdominal wall, or a neighboring viscus, and fistulous communications may be opened with the exterior or some organ. Discharge of the abscesses into the lung is perhaps the most frequent occurrence. The infection in some cases becomes fairly generalized. In one case which we had the opportunity of sectioning, the liver was adherent to the diaphragm and the right lobe was occupied by a very large trabecular abscess of the type just described.

Echinococcus cysts in the liver of a hog. (From the Pathological Museum of McGill University.)

[1] See Moser, New York Med. Jour., 60: 1894: 176, and Auvray, Rev. de Chir., 28: 1903: 1.

Parasites.—The most important are *Echinococcus, Pentastomum denticulatum,* and *Distoma hepaticum.* The rarer parasites are *Cysticerci, Ascaris lumbricoides,* and *Psorosperms.* Echinococcus disease is not so frequently met with in America as in Europe. It is occasionally found, however, among the Mennonites of Manitoba and the Northwest. Echinococcus cysts are unilocular or multilocular, and are bounded by a laminated connective-tissue capsule. The liver cells in the immediate neighborhood of the cysts are flattened from pressure. Within the fibrous capsule is the gelatinous, transparent, echinococcus membrane, which, under the microscope is of hyaline appearance, with a characteristic concentric lamination. The contained fluid is clear, watery, or slightly tinted. It may contain numerous small bladders or daughter-cysts. Owing to absorption of the fluid and inspissation of the contents, the cysts may contain a caseous, gritty substance, resembling mortar.

RETROGRESSIVE METAMORPHOSES.

Simple Atrophy.—Simple atrophy of the liver, the result of malnutrition, is met with in marasmus, old age, and cachexia. The form due to pressure has already been referred to. Carcinoma of the œsophagus and stomach, by inducing starvation, has a special tendency to cause atrophy. In such cases the diminution in size may be very marked, the organ in some instances being only one-third of the normal weight. The atrophy affects the structure as a whole, but the anterior border suffers most. The liver is small, the edges are sharp, and the capsule wrinkled. The gall-bladder sometimes projects considerably beyond the liver margin. In advanced cases, little may be left at the borders but the connective-tissue capsule, recognizable as a thin, semitransparent membrane containing bloodvessels. The liver-substance remaining may be firmer than normal, owing to the relative increase of the connective tissue.

Histologically, the parenchymatous cells are shrunken, stain rather badly, and are somewhat pigmented (**brown atrophy**). The fibrous tissue appears to be increased, but this appearance is largely due to the disappearance of the liver cells proper. Frerichs has called attention to a form of atrophy—**melanemic atrophy**—believed to be due to blocking of the capillaries with black pigment. Atrophy of the liver is a marked feature in the disease known as acute yellow atrophy (q. v.).

Cloudy Swelling.—Cloudy swelling, a condition hardly distinguishable from acute parenchymatous hepatitis, is a common occurrence in the course of the infective fevers, particularly typhoid and scarlatina. It may also be due to the action of toxins, apart from elevation of temperature. A liver so affected is somewhat moist on section and the lobules are no longer distinguishable, the cut surface having a peculiar glassy appearance, as if smeared with thin glue. It is surprising, however, how little change can be recognized microscopically, the cells being at most a little swollen and rounded, while the nuclei tend to stain badly.

Fatty Liver.—Fatty degeneration of the liver is a common sequel of cloudy swelling and occurs in the course of severe anemias, such as pernicious anemia, in acute yellow atrophy of the liver, from congestion, and from the action of various toxic substances, notably phosphorus. In advanced cases the liver is diminished in size, feels doughy under the fingers, and the capsule is thrown into folds. The color is bright yellow or yellowish-brown. On section, the tissue is soft and friable, and fat droplets can be scraped off the surface with the knife.

Histologically, the liver cells, particularly those of the centre and middle zone of the lobules, contain a variable number of small clear vesicles, which represent the spaces occupied by the fat when the tissue was in the fresh state. Material hardened in formalin and cut on the freezing microtome may be stained by Sudan III, a selective stain for fat. The parenchymatous cells then appear filled with globules and granules of a carmine-red or brownish color. In the most advanced condition, it may be hard to recognize any normal liver substance except the portal sheaths. Slight grades of fatty degeneration can be seen in the centre of the lobules in cases of passive congestion of the liver, and in the neighborhood of inflammatory foci and new-growths.

Not unlike fatty degeneration in many ways is **fatty infiltration.** The liver is normally a storehouse for fat, especially that taken into the economy in the way of food, or elaborated from other nutritive substances. A certain amount of fat, therefore, can ordinarily be observed in every liver section, even under normal conditions, and, indeed, after a meal the amount may be quite noteworthy. An excessive amount of fat may, however, be deposited in the liver cells in cases where an excess of fat or of its precursors has been ingested, or where there is a lessened oxidation of the fat ordinarily supplied. The latter occurrence is seen in long-standing and wasting diseases, such as tuberculosis, anemias, and various cachexias. The use of alcohol is especially prone to induce this form of fatty liver

Macroscopically, the liver is enlarged and its weight increased. Its specific gravity, however, is diminished, and may be reduced to such an extent that the organ will float in water. The edges are rounded, the capsule smooth and tense, and the surface can readily be indented. The color is yellowish-brown or bright yellow according to the amount of fat present. On section, the organ is pale, yellow, bloodless, and distinctly unctuous.

Histologically, Klotz and McCrae[1] would draw a sharp distinction between globular fat and what they term "granular fat." With the older workers, they are inclined to regard the large globules as storage fat (infiltration). They find that the granules take on a lighter brownish stain with Sudan III, and when carefully examined are of irregular shape, with sharp angles. The cells are frequently packed with these irregular granules, which exhibit no tendency to coalesce, nor when these are present is the nucleus pushed to one side, as it is apt to be by the

[1] Jour. of Exp. Med., 12:1910:146.

large globules of fatty infiltration. They regard the fine granules as typical of fatty degeneration and found granular fat alone in forty cases, globular alone in eleven, while the two were combined in forty-seven cases. It may be noted, in addition, that in fatty degeneration the comparatively unaffected cells show cloudy and other degenerative changes, while in fatty infiltration, as with large globules, the cells devoid of fat present a practically normal appearance. In the former, too, the nucleus is apt to show degenerative changes.

Amyloid or Lardaceous Transformation.—This occurs under the same circumstances as amyloid disease elsewhere, that is to say, in connection with suppuration and prolonged wasting disease.

The organ is enlarged, its edges are rounded, and its consistence is increased, so that it has a somewhat elastic or rubbery feel. It does not lie flat on the table and looks as if forced into a capsule that was too small for it. On section, the cut surface, if the amyloid change be extensive, appears as if it were covered with a thin layer of gelatin, and the edges are translucent when held up to the light. The amyloid masses can be recognized by their semitranslucent glue-like appearance. The remaining liver substance varies in appearance according to the amount of fat present and the degree of congestion. The gall-bladder usually contains clear, thin bile.

Microscopically, in a moderately advanced case, the amyloid material is found to occupy by preference the intermediate zone of the lobules, the centre and periphery being free. The substance appears to be of the nature of a deposit and is laid down in glistening masses in the walls of the capillaries beneath the endothelium. In advanced cases the larger arterioles of the portal districts are affected, particularly in their middle coats. The parenchymatous cells, lying between the thickened capillaries, present various stages of fatty degeneration and atrophy.

Pigmentary Infiltration.—When we examine sections of liver under a high power, we find normally a certain amount of golden-yellow granular pigment within the secreting cells. This may be the natural coloring matter of the liver cells, bile pigment, or, as one of us (J. G. A.[1]) has suggested, bacteria in a dead or dying condition which have become bile-stained. Under pathological conditions, the pigment of the liver may be much increased and of very varying nature.

In *icterus* or *jaundice* the liver may be stained a bright yellow or green. The coloration is due to the retention of bile and its passage out of the bile capillaries, owing to some obstruction to the free discharge of the secretion. Cholelithiasis, cholangitis, tumors, and aneurisms pressing upon the bile ducts are among the main conditions to be mentioned in this connection. Icterus of the liver also occurs in some forms of cirrhosis, in severe blood destruction, and in acute yellow atrophy. In a well-marked case, the finer bile ducts on section are found to be distended and bile flows from them readily, while the central portion of the lobule shows a diffuse bile staining. Microscopically, the liver

[1] *Lancet*, 2:1898:293, 396, 492; Montreal Med. Journ., 27:1898:898.

cells are of a diffuse bright yellow color or contain yellowish or yellowish-brown granules, more rarely a crystalline deposit. According to Nauwerck and Fütterer, dilatation of the minute intracellular passages is to be observed. The pigment in question is bilirubin, believed to be identical chemically with hematoidin.

Another important form of pigmentation found in the liver is due also to a disintegration of the red blood-corpuscles, but beyond the normal. In such cases an excessive amount of hemoglobin is set free and carried to the liver, where it is metamorphosed in different ways. The pigments so derived are *hematoidin* (*bilirubin*) and *hemosiderin*. The principal point of difference between the two is that the latter contains iron. Should the blood destruction be moderate in degree, the liver appears to be able to cope with the condition to some extent, so that the hematoidin is excreted in the bile, while the hemosiderin is retained. A pathological increase of pigmentation is met with also in all cases of advanced passive congestion of the liver. **Hemosiderosis** occurs in severe sepsis, pernicious anemia, malaria, hemoglobinemia, in certain cases of cirrhosis of the liver, severe burns, and in various intoxications. The iron-containing pigment is deposited in the liver cells, particularly at the periphery of the lobules, but also in the tissue spaces. · It is of a golden color and may be differentiated from bilirubin by the fact that when sections are treated with hydrochloric acid and potassium ferrocyanide the Prussian-blue reaction is obtained (Perls' test). In exceptional instances, hemosiderin is found in the skin, mucous membranes, the intestinal wall, the pancreas, spleen, and other organs as well as in the liver. This condition has been termed **hemochromatosis** (v. Recklinghausen), and has been studied on this continent especially by Opie[1] and Maude Abbott.[2] Many cases are associated with cirrhosis of the liver (cirrhose pigmentaire) or pancreas (diabète bronzé), or both.

In malaria, the pigment found in the liver and other organs is, in part, hemosiderin and, in part, melanin, the latter a pigment elaborated by the protozoön that causes the disease.

Other pigments found in the liver are of extraneous origin, as, for example, coal dust (**anthracosis**) and silver (**argyria**). In some cases the amount of anthracotic pigment taken into the system has been excessive and has reached the general circulation, some of it, therefore, being deposited in the liver, or, an anthracotic lymph-node may soften and rupture into a vein. Welch has reported a case of cirrhosis of the liver due to coal pigment. One of us (J. G. A.) has met with a case of silicosis of the liver.[3]

Necrosis.—Necrosis of the type commonly known as coagulation necrosis is not uncommon in the liver. Large areas of a pale yellowish color and opaque appearance are frequently to be observed in connection with septic processes within the district drained by the portal system,

[1] Journ. of Exper. Med., 4: 1899: 279.
[2] Journ. of Pathology, 6: 1900: 315.
[3] Adami, Sajous' Encyclopedia, article Cirrhosis.

notably in cases of appendicitis. They are found also in eclampsia and acute yellow atrophy. Less extensive necrosis is seen in the various infective fevers, typhoid, diphtheria, variola, cholera, glanders and septicemia, and as a result of various intoxications. Sometimes multiple small areas of necrosis—**focal necroses**—are met with, which are visible to the naked eye as grayish or opaque yellow dots the size of a pin-head or less. These are small areas of necrosis of the liver cells, or perivascular collections of small round cells resembling lymph-follicles. The death of the cells appears to be due partly to the direct action of the toxin and partly to obstructive conditions within the capillaries (see vol. i, p. 980).

Fig. 117

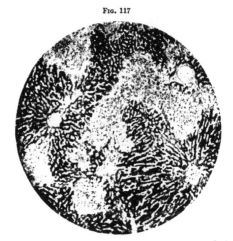

Multiple focal necroses in the liver of a rabbit subjected to experimental glanders. (Duval.)

PROGRESSIVE METAMORPHOSES.

Hypertrophy.—The liver may be enlarged in a variety of conditions, such as passive congestion, inflammatory infiltration, cysts, and tumors. Every increase in size, therefore, is not to be regarded as hypertrophy. The term hypertrophy, strictly speaking, applies to the enlargement of individual cells, and this is seen to a limited extent in many reparative processes going on in the liver, but the condition is practically always combined with an increase in the number of the cells—numerical hypertrophy or hyperplasia.

Hypertrophy of the liver in this sense is essentially a compensatory process, and, moreover, local. The existence of a generalized hypertrophy is doubtful. The liver is an organ that exhibits under certain circumstances a striking degree the power of repair. According to

Ponfick and von Meister, one-half to three-quarters of it can be removed, and, while the original shape is not restored, the remaining substance undergoes compensatory hyperplasia. The preëxisting lobules become greatly enlarged, there being, however, but little new formation of parts. Regeneration of this order is well seen in cases where portions of the liver are destroyed, as by traumatism, pressure, or various degenerative processes, for example, in advanced passive congestion, cirrhosis, acute yellow atrophy, and in the necrosis resulting from certain infective fevers. The nodular projections found in what is often spoken of as the "hob-nail" liver are to be regarded as local attempts at regeneration, rather than as the effect of the contraction of the newly-formed connective tissue, an explanation that has often been advanced. The proliferating liver cells are recognized by the fact that they are larger than normal, the cytoplasm stains deeply, the nucleus is large, rich in chromatin, and often shows evidences of mitosis. The regular arrangement of the liver lobules is, however, not altogether reproduced, with the possible exception of acute yellow atrophy where the new cells grow into the stroma and replace those that have undergone necrosis.

Fig. 118

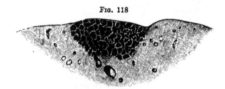

Cavernoma of liver.   Gross appearance.   (After Ribbert.)

Tumors.—The new-growths found in the liver may be primary or secondary, and are of connective-tissue or epithelial type. Primary tumors of all kinds are rare. The primary benign growths are the **angioma, cavernoma,**[1] **adenoma, fibroma, myxoma,** and **lipoma.**

The cavernoma (cavernous angioma) is of relatively frequent occurrence and usually is met with in the shrunken livers of elderly people. It is not strictly a newgrowth, as a rule, and is rarely of large size. It is recognized by its dark brown or purplish-red color and is sharply defined from the liver substance. It may be surrounded by a fibrous capsule. When cut into, blood can be squeezed out, leaving a spongy network of connective tissue, sometimes containing bands of muscle fibers. The tumor is formed by a relatively enormous dilatation of the capillaries which results in atrophy of the intervening liver cells. Proliferation of the vessel walls and the fibrous stroma can be made out in some few

---

[1] We would here, as elsewhere, note the distinction to be drawn between "angioma" and "cavernoma." The former is characterized by a new-formation of arterioles and is consequently a neoplastic tumor. The latter is merely a teleangiectasis, or relation of preëxisting vessels. Both are found in the liver.

cases, indicating the formation of a true **hemangioma**. The vascular spaces can be injected from the portal vein or the hepatic artery. Thrombosis is frequently observed in the enlarged vessels with consecutive organization of the clot. **Lymphangioma** has been described by Klebs.

Adenoma occurs in the form of single or multiple nodules of a grayish, yellowish-white, or reddish-brown color. These, microscopically, consist of branched and convoluted gland-tubules, or of bands and clumps of liver cells, which, however, are not arranged after the fashion of the normal lobules. Some of the tubules may possess a small lumen. Certain authors consider that adenomas are derived both from the epithelium of the bile ducts and from the liver cells proper, although Rindfleisch holds to the former view. Owing to dilatation of the tubules,

FIG. 119

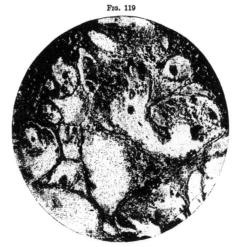

Cavernous angioma of the liver. Winckel No. 3, without ocular. Normal liver tissue is shown above and to the left. The fibrous trabeculæ of the blood tumor are well seen. (From Dr. A. G. Nicholls' collection.)

we may get an **adenocystoma** consisting of more or less numerous cysts or groups of cysts filled with clear fluid. Such tumors appear to be developed from outgrowths of the bile ducts in the periportal connective tissue.

We have recently met with a case of **lipoma**. The growth was the size of a green pea, situated on the dome of the liver, and was well encapsulated.

Primary **sarcoma**[1] is excessively rare in the liver. It occurs as a single large mass or as multiple circumscribed nodules. Round, spindle-celled, giant-celled angiosarcoma, and melanotic forms are described. They

[1] For literature see Carmichael and Wade, *Lancet*, Lond., 1:1907:1217.

seem to begin in the neighborhood of vessels. Ford[1] has recorded a case of primary sarcoma occurring in a cirrhotic liver.

In *lymphosarcoma* a large number of lymphoid cells are found in the portal sheaths and in the intralobular capillaries, while, in addition, lymphomatous nodules are scattered throughout the organ.

Secondary sarcomas are not uncommon in the liver, and are of all types. The pigmented forms are, however, the most important. With the exception of the lung, the liver is the most frequent seat of metastatic deposit in the case of the melanotic new-growths. We get then either circumscribed pigmented nodules, or a diffuse infiltration, in the form of yellow, gray, or blackish-brown streaks, which give the liver on section an appearance somewhat like granite.

FIG. 120

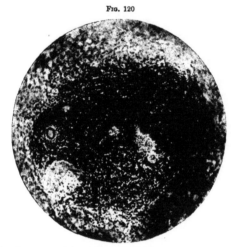

Liver. Lymphosarcoma nodule. Zeiss obj. A, without ocular. (From the collection of Dr. A. G. Nicholls.)

Mixed forms, *fibrosarcoma* and *myosarcoma*, are also described.

Block has described a **melanotic endothelioma.**

Hypernephromas are occasionally met with in the liver.[2]

Carcinoma.—By far the most important and frequent tumor of the liver is the carcinoma, which may be primary or secondary. The comparative frequency of the two forms may be gathered from Hale White's statistics. In 10,000 autopsies he found 10 cases of primary carcinoma and 240 of secondary. Primary carcinoma, therefore, is decidedly uncommon.

Three main types of primary cancer are described. In the first—

[1] Amer. Jour. Med. Sci., 120: 1900: 413.
[2] White and Mair, Jour. Path. and Bacter., 1907.

cancer massif—there is usually a single large mass of new-growth occupying the greater part of a lobe, usually the right. Not infrequently, in the neighborhood of this are to be seen a few isolated nodules representing local metastases. The tumor is of somewhat firm consistency and of a whitish or whitish-yellow color, occasionally somewhat reddened. Comparatively little cancer juice can be scraped away. As a rule, the mass is sharply differentiated from the liver substance, but at parts of the periphery some infiltration can be made out. The larger nodules of cancer often present degeneration and softening at the centre, and, if situated on the surface of the liver, may show umbilication. General metastasis is not common. The liver substance in the immediate neighborhood is compressed, atrophic, and the vessels are often occluded.

FIG. 121

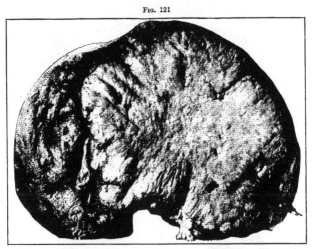

Primary carcinoma of the liver. (From the Pathological Department of the Royal Victoria Hospital. Case of Drs. C. F. Martin and W. F. Hamilton.)

The second form simulates cirrhosis. The liver is more or less enlarged, the capsule thickened, and the surface warty (*cancer nodulaire*). On section, numerous bands of connective tissue are to be seen, in which a few islets of liver substance still remain, but which contain nodules of cancer, the size of a pea or larger, of a whitish or pale red color, and of soft, juicy consistency. Where the nodules have originated in a preëxisting adenomatous new-growth they are of a grayish-brown color, firmer, and not so juicy. Invasion of the portal vein and liver capillaries is not uncommon; or, again, there may be a very diffuse infiltration with new-growth (*infiltrating carcinomatous cirrhosis*—Perls).

In the third, the rarest form, there is a carcinomatous infiltration of the Glisson's capsule originating from the larger bile ducts. The nodules

FIG. 122

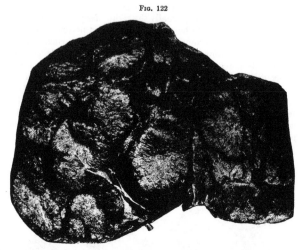

Secondary carcinoma of the liver: medullary form. The necrosis and softening of the cancer
masses is indicated by slight depression (umbilication) of their centres. (From the Pathological
Museum of McGill University.)

FIG. 123

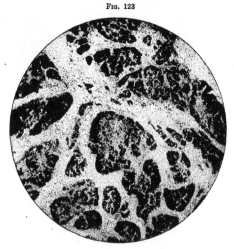

Secondary carcinoma of the liver. Winckel obj. No. 3, without ocular. (From the
collection of Dr. A. G. Nicholls.)

of new-growth in the portal districts are closely packed and often fused, gradually diminishing in size as one passes from the hilus to the peripheral portions of the liver. Icterus is common in this form, owing to compression and obstruction of the bile ducts.

As a curiosity may be mentioned a carcinoma with ciliated cells, described by Sokoloff.[1]

Carcinomas of the liver originate either from the specific parenchyma or from the epithelium of the bile ducts. According to their histological structure, we can divide them into the *cylindrical-celled adenocarcinoma, medullary*, and *scirrhous* forms. The carcinoma with cirrhosis, according to several observers (Hanot, Frohmann, Ziegler), is developed in a cirrhotic liver by atypical proliferation of the newly-formed liver cells.

Secondary carcinomas of the liver arise by direct extension or from metastasis. As the growth in the liver may attain to a considerable size and may dominate the clinical picture, it is sometimes difficult if not impossible to discover the primary focus. Carcinoma of the gall-bladder and of the bile ducts often spreads directly to the liver, but cancer of the pyloric end of the stomach only does so when there has been previous adhesion of the stomach to the liver. The occurrence of metastases in the liver is common in cancerous disease, particularly so when the primary growth is in the gastro-intestinal tract, pancreas, œsophagus, pelvic organs, or larynx They arise from small clusters of carcinoma cells, which have been broken off from the main mass, and have reached the liver as emboli through the portal vein, lymph channels, or the general circulation. Wherever they lodge they proceed to grow, infiltrating and destroying or compressing the liver tissue. At first they take the form of multiple miliary nodules scattered through the organ, but soon fuse into masses the size of the fist or larger. Where they reach the surface they project as whitish bosses covered with congested serosa. Not infrequently, softening and liquefaction take place in the larger nodules, which thereupon collapse somewhat, giving rise to the characteristic umbilication. The consistence of the nodes depends in general upon the character of the original growth. The liver, as a whole, may be enormously enlarged. Christian[2] reports one which weighed 15 kilos. On section the secondary masses are whitish in color, often somewhat broken down in the centre. The larger nodules are of an opaque yellowish color with, sometimes, radiating striæ, the result of degeneration. Mucinous, cystic, and calcareous degeneration are common, as well as hemorrhagic infiltration. Where the liver cells are pressed upon they are reduced to flattened scales of a brownish color (brown atrophy).

Cysts.—Apart from **parasitic cysts, blood cysts, retention** or **bile cysts, lymph cysts,** and **congenital** cysts should be mentioned. Congenital cystic disease of the liver is often associated with congenital cysts of the kidneys, a condition which it closely resembles.

[1] Virch. Arch., 162: 1900: 1.   [2] Amer. Med., 5: 1903: 131.

CHAPTER XXII.

THE BILIARY PASSAGES.

ALTERATIONS IN THE LUMINA.

Dilatation.—Dilatation of the bile ducts is due to obstruction to the free outflow of bile. The causes of this are very varied. The chief are: swelling of the mucous membrane; gallstones, parasites, and tumors within the ducts; external pressure from enlarged lymph-nodes or tumors involving the neighboring glands, duodenum, liver, or pancreas; inflammatory adhesions about the ducts; the pressure of aneurisms, a displaced kidney or liver. Obstruction is one of the predisposing causes of infection and inflammation.

The cystic duct may become occluded, leading to dilatation of the gall-bladder. Most of the biliary substances, including the pigment, are in time absorbed, so that the organ is found to be greatly distended with a clear, colorless, viscid fluid something like mucin (*hydrops vesicæ felleæ*). Occasionally, it is thin and limpid, like water. The wall of the bladder is usually thin and semitransparent, unless thickened by previous inflammation.

INFLAMMATIONS.

Inflammation of the bile passages (**cholangitis**), and of the gall-bladder (**cholecystitis**), is brought about by toxic or infective agents which may reach the liver in several ways. One very frequent mode is for bacteria to invade the passages from the intestine (*ascending infection*). In many cases the organisms are excreted by the liver through the bile (*descending infection*), as, for example, in typhoidal cholangitis and cholecystitis. Infection may also occur through the blood stream (*hematogenic infection*), or by the extension of inflammation from neighboring parts. The presence of calculi or carcinoma in the region, or of parasites in the biliary passages, will naturally predispose to inflammation and infection, and will aggravate any such conditions that previously exist. The microörganisms usually found are B. coli, pyogenic cocci, Diplococcus pneumoniæ, and B. typhi.

The type of inflammation is catarrhal, purulent, membranous, or gangrenous.

Cholangitis.—**Acute Catarrhal Cholangitis.**—Acute catarrhal cholangitis is a not uncommon affection. When secondary to gastroduodenitis, it is the usual anatomical basis of the disease known clinically as *catarrhal jaundice.* In some cases, cholelithiasis and hydatids in the liver or bile passages give rise to this form of cholangitis. In most, if not all, of them the infection is of the ascending type. Acute catarrhal jaundice is occasionally met with also in typhoid fever, pneumonia, secondary syphilis, and some other infectious diseases.

As patients rarely die while they are the subjects of this condition, it is rather difficult to say what are the anatomical appearances presented. The mucous membrane of the common bile duct is said to be a little swollen, but not particularly reddened, and the ampulla of Vater is filled with a grayish, slimy, mucinous plug, which is sufficient to obstruct the free outflow of bile and thus to produce jaundice. The liver is probably slightly enlarged, the bile capillaries dilated and full of bile. Should the process become *chronic* it is apt to spread to all the bile passages, including the gall-bladder. The cystic duct may in time become occluded. The wall of the biliary duct becomes thinned from dilatation and the mucosa presents polypoid outgrowths. Occasionally, the ramifications of the duct become thickened from fibrous hyperplasia and the process leads to interstitial hepatitis.

Suppurative Cholangitis.—Suppurative cholangitis, sometimes also called **phlegmonous cholangitis**, is due to pyogenic infection of the biliary passages. It is usually associated with or may supervene upon the catarrhal form. The causes are similar to those of simple cholangitis. Cholelithiasis and certain of the infective processes, such as pyemia, typhoid fever, pneumonia, and influenza, may be mentioned in particular. Probably in most cases the infective agents travel up from the intestine. One case that we have seen appeared to have originated from a phlegmonous duodenitis. In some instances, again, the infection is probably hematogenic, the pyogenic microörganisms finding in the damaged bile passages a favorable situation for their growth.

Cholecystitis.—Suppurative Cholecystitis.—The suppurative process is not uncommonly restricted to the gall-bladder (suppurative cholecystitis). The wall of the gall-bladder is œdematous, infiltrated with inflammatory products, and more or less distended with mucopus mixed with bile (*empyema of the gall-bladder*). The organ is not infrequently covered externally with a layer of fibrinous exudate, and may be adherent to the neighboring viscera. Such a condition may be the starting point of a septic peritonitis. Especially is this likely to occur if perforation of the gall-bladder have taken place. Fistulous communications with the hollow viscera or with the exterior sometimes result. Other complications are multiple abscesses in the liver and generalized septicemia.

The commonest cause is cholelithiasis, but the condition occasionally arises in the course of certain infectious diseases, such as typhoid, pyemia, dysentery, and cholera.

The occurrence of suppurative cholecystitis in the course of typhoid fever has received considerable attention. Chiari[1] noted that the typhoid bacillus sometimes persists in the bile passages for months after the

---

[1] Quénu, Rev. de Chirurgie, 6: 1906; also, Bader, Med. klinik, **47**: 1907.

apparent cure of the typhoidal attack, and recent observations have proved that it may remain even for years. This fact is of importance in connection with the etiology of cholangitis, cholecystitis, abscess of the liver, and gallstones. It may possibly also explain some cases of reinfection.

Membranous or fibrinous cholecystitis is exceedingly rare.[1]

Pericholecystitis and Pericholangitis.—Pericholecystitis and pericholangitis, or inflammation around the gall-bladder and bile passages, is usually to be traced to inflammation of the wall of these structures. It may be *simple, suppurative,* or *productive.*

Cholelithiasis.—The term cholelithiasis is applied to the condition in which calculi are found within the bile passages, together with the results that spring from them. Biliary calculi are found more than twice as frequently in females as in males, and usually after middle life. The most important single etiological factor is infection. In a large proportion of cases B. coli, pyogenic cocci, and not infrequently B. typhi can be demonstrated. Stagnation of the bile also assists by leading to the absorption of the alkaline substances and the production of an acid bile, which favors the growth of the microörganisms concerned. A slight catarrh is the result, leading to an outpouring of mucus in which the various pigments and salts are precipitated (see vol. i, p. 946).

The most common sites for calculi, in order of frequency, are the gall-bladder, cystic duct, cystic and common ducts, common duct, and hepatic duct. They are rare in the intrahepatic ducts.

Calculi in the gall-bladder may lead to catarrhal, fibrinous, or suppurative cholecystitis, with necrosis and even perforation. In this situation they are often single, and may be large enough to fill up the whole cavity. Sometimes they give rise to little or no disturbance, and at death the gall-bladder is found to be thickened and contracted about the calculus, with often adhesions about it. Fistulous communications at times occur. According to Courvoisier, communication with the exterior is the commonest event. Strümpell and Murchison, however, state that the cholecysticoduodenal fistula is the most frequent. An extremely rare form is the cholecysticogastric, an example of which one of us (A. G. N.) has had an opportunity of recording.[2]

Calculi in the common or hepatic ducts may lead to complete obstruction, the production of jaundice, dilatation of the ducts, inflammatory and productive changes in and about the ducts, with also inflammatory and cirrhotic changes in the liver and pancreas. Occasionally, large gallstones may ulcerate through and become impacted in the intestine. Carcinoma, usually of the cylindrical-celled variety, affecting the gall-bladder, may result from the irritation. It often spreads to the liver by contiguity.

---

[1] Rolleston, Trans. Path. Soc., London, 53:1902:405.
[2] Montreal Med. Jour., 27:1898:826.

PROGRESSIVE METAMORPHOSES.

Tumors.—Tumors of the bile passages are most common in the vicinity of the ampulla of Vater. **Papillomas** and **cystadenomas** are described.

Primary **carcinoma** occurs most frequently near the ampulla or at the junction of the common and cystic ducts. It is usually cylindrical-celled in type. Secondary carcinoma is due to direct extension of carcinoma of the duodenum, pancreas, stomach, liver, gall-bladder, or the neighboring lymph-nodes. Duval[1] has reported an apparently unique case of **melanoma** of Vater's diverticulum.

Primary connective-tissue tumors of the gall-bladder are rare. **Fibroma, lipoma, myxoma,** and **sarcoma** have been met with. Villous **papilloma** is occasionally found. The most frequent new-growth in this situation is **carcinoma.** It is of the *cylindrical* or *round-celled* variety, and usually associated with gallstones. Rarely, from metaplasia of the epithelium we get a *squamous-celled epithelioma.*[2]

[1] Jour. of Exper. Med., 10: 1908: 4.
[2] See Nicholson, Jour. Path. and Bact., 1908.

CHAPTER XXIII.

THE PANCREAS.

CONGENITAL ANOMALIES.

COMPLETE **absence** of the pancreas occurs, but only in fœtuses that present other serious defects. A portion of the head may be separate from the rest, constituting a **pancreas minus**, which lies upon the anterior surface of the duodenum. The organ may also be **divided** into two equal or unequal parts connected by the pancreatic duct. The tail may be attached to the head by a fibrous band containing the duct and vessels. Or, again, the pancreas may be **bifid** or **lobulated.** The duct of Wirsung may discharge into the stomach or into some unusual part of the intestine. Not infrequently it does not form a junction with the common bile duct at the bile papilla. An interesting, though rare, anomaly is the so-called **pancreas annulare**, forming a more or less complete ring about the duodenum, which may thereby be constricted. The most common anomaly is the presence of an **accessory** or **aberrant** pancreas. This is usually found in the duodenum or jejunum,[1] less often in other parts of the small intestine or in the stomach. Wright has recorded one case occurring in the abdominal wall in the region of the umbilicus.[2] Occasionally, the aberrant pancreas is found at the tip of an intestinal diverticulum.

A point worthy of note, inasmuch as it has an important bearing on the function of the gland, is the constant presence of the duct of Santorini (Opie[3]), which is patent in more than half ·the cases, and in a considerable proportion of these is effective as an outlet.

CIRCULATORY DISTURBANCES.

These are comparatively unimportant. **Active hyperemia** is met with during digestion and in the early stages of inflammation. **Passive hyperemia** occurs in conditions of general passive congestion. Hyperemia of the pancreas is said to be present also in cases of pernicious anemia.

Small **hemorrhages** may take place into the substance of the pancreas in passive congestion of the organ, in scorbutus and other hemorrhagic diatheses, and during the course of infective fevers. Massive hemorrhages also occur as a result of traumatism and in the affection known as hemorrhagic pancreatitis. This condition will be referred to later.

Anemia is present in conditions of systemic anemia.

[1] Nicholls, Montreal Medical Journal, 29:1900:903.
[2] James H. Wright, Jour. Boston Soc. Med. Sci., 5:1901:497.
[3] Diseases of the Pancreas, 1903:30: J. B. Lippincott Co., Phila.

INFLAMMATIONS.

Pancreatitis.—Inflammation of the pancreas—**pancreatitis**—is not very common. In 1750 autopsies of which we have notes acute inflammation was found in 9, in only 1 of which was it the cause of death.

Acute pancreatitis is usually due to infection with microörganisms, but may on occasion result from the action of toxic substances reaching the gland, the irritation of the pancreatic ferment or of hemorrhagic extravasation. The infective forms arise in three ways—through the blood stream, through the excretory duct, and by extension.

The hematogenic type is simply a manifestation of general septicemia, and is not common as compared with the frequency of general sepsis. By far the commonest cause of pancreatitis is the passage into the gland of bacteria, bile, or acid stomach secretions by way of the duct of Wirsung.

Ulcers of the stomach and duodenum, suppurative processes in and about the spleen and left kidney, occasionally extend to the pancreas.

Pancreatitis is *simple, suppurative,* or *specific,* and may affect the ducts, the lobules, or the interstitial tissue.

Fig. 124

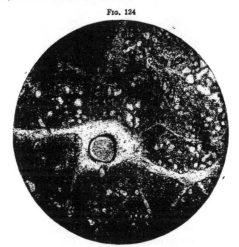

Acute sialodochitis with obstruction of the ducts leading to dilatation of the acini. Leitz] obj. No. 3, without ocular. (From the collection of Dr. A. G. Nicholls.)

Sialodochitis Pancreatica.—Catarrh of the ducts—sialodochitis pancreatica—which may be simple or purulent, is due to the action of infective microörganisms or toxic agents that have passed up the duct. Duodenitis seems to be the important predisposing cause. In one case that we have seen, the duct and its chief branches were packed with inflammatory leukocytes and the lining epithelium was in places desquamating. Owing to obstruction, the lumina were dilated and the acini converted into small cystic cavities, lined with flattened cells, which also in places were catarrhal. The condition suggested the dilatation of the tubules so often seen in the kidney of chronic nephritis. A slight amount of interstitial infiltration also had occurred. In such cases the main duct is not necessarily always occluded.

FIG. 125

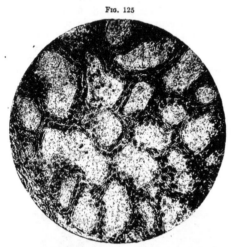

Sialodochitis pancreatica. Section shows the extraordinary dilatation of the acini with a certain amount of catarrh. The specimen is from the same case as the last, but under higher magnification. Leitz obj. No. 7, without ocular. (From the collection of Dr. A. G. Nicholls.)

Degenerative Parenchymatous Pancreatitis.—Orth describes a degenerative parenchymatous pancreatitis, which may possibly be the same condition spoken of by other writers as cloudy swelling. The pancreas is swollen and at first reddened, later assuming a whitish or grayish-yellow color. Histologically, the secreting cells of the acini present cloudy swelling, fatty degeneration, and necrosis. In a case reported by E. Fraenkel the organ was dotted throughout with a fatty granular material derived from the degenerating cells, while in the interstitial tissue there was a round-celled infiltration. This form of pancreatitis occurs in various infective processes, such as typhoid fever, pyemia, and variola.

Suppurative Pancreatitis.—Suppurative pancreatitis is by far the most important form of pancreatitis. It may be acute, even gangrenous, subacute, or chronic. Diffuse, purulent infiltration may occur, or definite abscesses may be formed. Abscesses are often multiple and of small size, but large single abscesses occur in some cases formed by the

confluence of smaller foci. The multiple pancreatic abscesses sometimes met with in generalized septicemia are hematogenic in origin,
due to the lodgement of infective emboli. Suppurative processes in
structures adjacent to the pancreas may extend into it. We have met
with one case in which an extensive perinephritic abscess had burst
into the peritoneal cavity, eventually discharging into the stomach.
Incidentally it caused gangrenous inflammation of the lower end of the
spleen and the tail of the pancreas. More frequent are those cases due
to the invasion of the pancreas by way of the duct of Wirsung. Since
the common bile duct and the pancreatic duct usually empty by a common
orifice into the intestine, it can readily be understood that inflammatory
processes in the duodenum and bile passages are apt to extend into the
pancreas. In such cases the symptoms are usually acute and are practically identical with those of the so-called hemorrhagic pancreatitis
(q. v.). The cases occur generally in young adult males and commonly
terminate fatally in from two to four days. There is usually an acute
duodenitis, which may also be associated with cholangitis, cholelithiasis,
and even acute interstitial hepatitis. Exceptionally, the affection
becomes chronic and life may be prolonged for some months or for a
year or more.

Pancreatic abscesses may rupture into the peritoneal cavity, giving
rise to a septic peritonitis, or may be discharged into the stomach or
intestine. In a case recorded by Chiari,[1] a sequestrum of the pancreas
was passed *per anum* with complete recovery. Small abscesses may
possibly become encapsulated or inspissated. Fibrosis is a constant
accompaniment of chronic suppurative pancreatitis.

Acute Hemorrhagic Pancreatitis.—Closely allied to the last-mentioned
form is the affection known as acute hemorrhagic pancreatitis, so-called
from the fact that the pancreas is more or less completely infiltrated with
blood. The pathogenesis of the condition is not entirely clear. Hemorrhage into the substance of the pancreas may result from trauma and
disease of the vessels, as, for example, arteriosclerosis, fatty degeneration of their walls, and embolism, quite apart from inflammation.
Of course, such extravasations of blood, if not quickly fatal and if not
so extensive as to destroy the pancreas, are followed by a certain amount
of reactive inflammation. The general consensus of opinion, however,
seems to be that in most cases the hemorrhage is secondary and not
primary. Quite often, fat-necrosis of the pancreas, peripancreatic fat,
the fat of the omentum and mesentery, is present also, and it may be
that the blood extravasation is to be explained on the ground of erosion
of the vessel walls by the liberated pancreatic ferment or the action of
suppurative inflammation.

Hemorrhagic pancreatitis is found most often in alcoholics and obese
persons, usually in those over thirty. The disease is ushered in suddenly
with intense pain in the epigastrium, nausea, and vomiting. The
abdomen becomes rigid and hypertympanitic. The temperature may

[1] Wiener med. Woch., 6: 1880

be moderately elevated. Constipation is the rule. The patient frequently dies collapsed in from two to four days. The disease may, however, become subacute or even chronic. Cases are often mistaken for gastric ulcer, biliary colic, or acute intestinal obstruction. Patients usually give a history of dyspepsia or of symptoms pointing to cholelithiasis. Fitz[1] has written an excellent monograph on the subject.

The pancreas is found to be enlarged, firm, and densely infiltrated with blood, often in large clots. The adjacent cellular tissue, the omentum, the root of the mesentery, and the lesser peritoneal cavity may contain blood. There may also be a small amount of blood-stained fluid in the general abdominal cavity. More or less extensive fat-necrosis is usually present. The inflammation, no doubt resulting from infection, may be intense, leading to suppuration or even gangrene of the organ. Death takes place probably from pressure upon the cœliac axis, as suggested by v. Zenker, from shock, or from sepsis. The nerve cells of the semilunar ganglia have been found to be degenerated with an interstitial leukocytic infiltration. Degenerative changes have also been observed in the peripancreatic Paccinian corpuscles. The common association of the condition with cholangitis and cholelithiasis,[2] suggests that bacterial infection is an important factor. The impaction of a gallstone in the ampulla of Vater may lead to the entrance of bile under pressure into the pancreatic duct. Fat-necrosis and hemorrhagic pancreatitis have been produced experimentally by the injection of bile, hydrochloric acid, and other irritating substances into the duct, or even by simple ligation of the duct. Alcohol and dietetic errors may act by setting up a duodenitis, which thereupon extends to the pancreas. Possibly, in some cases, the fatal attack is the last of the series of unobtrusive hemorrhages, for not infrequently microscopic examination shows pigment from old hemorrhages along with recent clots. Should the patient survive for any length of time, necrotic portions of the gland may become sequestrated and may lie in the centre of abscess cavities, which later may discharge into the abdominal cavity, the stomach, or intestine. .

Chronic Pancreatitis.—Chronic pancreatitis, like the acute form, may be *simple, suppurative,* and *specific.* There is always a more or less widespread production of fibrous tissue, which leads to induration of the organ (productive pancreatitis; sclerosis or fibrosis of the pancreas; indurative pancreatitis). Associated with this is usually a certain amount of atrophy of the secreting structure. The whole organ, therefore, becomes harder than normal. The most frequent causes are persistent inflammation of the ducts, obstruction to the free discharge of the excretion, and congenital syphilis. The association of cirrhosis of the pancreas with cirrhosis of the liver has already been referred to (p. 475).

In these cases the pancreas may be somewhat enlarged, but is usually considerably diminished in size. On section, it is hard and resists cutting, occasionally containing gritty material.

---

[1] Boston Med. and Surg. Jour., 120: 1889: 181.

[2] Opie, Jour. Exper. Med., 5: 1900: 397, 527.

Histologically, there is a notable increase in the amount of connective tissue, with more or less atrophy of the glandular elements. In the obstructive cases the newly-formed tissue is most marked about the ducts. Opie distinguishes two forms of fibrosis, a **chronic interlobular pancreatitis,** in which the connective tissue is most conspicuous between and around the lobules, the islands of Langerhans being involved only late or not at all, and a **chronic interacinar pancreatitis,** in which the fibrosis about the lobules is less pronounced, but connective-tissue proliferation is extreme round about the islands and even within them. Pearce has pointed out that in the lesions of congenital syphilis the islands of Langerhans escape.[1]

FIG. 126

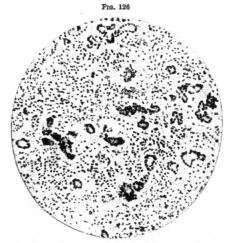

Syphilitic pancreatitis. Reichert obj. No. 7, without ocular. (Dr. H. D. Rolleston's case.)

Calculi.—The presence of calculi is one of the most potent causes of chronic interstitial pancreatitis and pancreatic abscess. Like biliary calculi, they are originally brought about by catarrh of the duct. When large they may lead to obstruction, with dilatation and even cyst formation. Pancreatic calculi are single or multiple, round, oval, or irregular in shape, and of a whitish or grayish-brown color. Chemically, they are composed of carbonate and phosphate of lime. They may be minute or quite large. One reported by Schupmann was 6 cm. long by 1 cm. broad. Owing to the proliferative inflammation resulting, a large portion of the secreting structure of the pancreas may be destroyed and glycosuria result.

Tuberculosis.—This disease is rare in the pancreas. One case of primary caseous tuberculosis is reported by Sendler, but this seems to be

[1] Amer. Jour. of Anat., 2: 1903: 445.

unique. Secondary tuberculosis is also rare. Disseminated miliary tuberculosis is recorded as affecting the pancreas, but the foci are small and few in number. Nearly all the cases are due to the extension of tuberculous disease from the lymph-nodes and other neighboring structures. It is the lymphoid structures within the pancreas which become involved. The organ seems to have special powers of self-defence, for it is surprising how often it escapes even when completely surrounded by tuberculous disease.

Syphilis.—This disease is also rare in the pancreas. Chronic indurative pancreatitis is observed in cases of the congenital affection (Fig. 126). Either the whole organ or the head only may be involved. Gummas are occasionally observed. When near the point of exit of the duct, jaundice may result from the pressure. Syphilitic endarteritis may also occur, leading to fibrosis of the organ. Reuter[1] has found Spirochæta pallida in the interstitial tissue in a case of chronic syphilitic pancreatitis.

RETROGRESSIVE METAMORPHOSES.

Simple Atrophy.—Simple atrophy occurs in old age and in the marasmus of infective or chronic disease. The pancreas is small,

FIG. 127

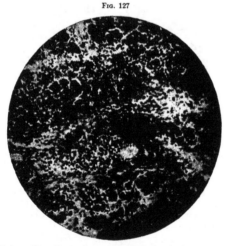

Pancreas. Diabetes mellitus. Section shows round-celled infiltration in the interacinar connective tissue. Zeiss obj. DD, without ocular. (From the collection of Dr. A. G. Nicholls.)

shrunken, and cylindrical on section. The surrounding fat is diminished. The organ cuts with somewhat increased resistance, the lobules are

[1] Zeit. f. Hyg. u. Infect., 54: 1906: 49.

small, and the interstitial connective tissue is relatively increased. When atrophy. is extreme, fatty globules and crystals make their appearance in the feces. According to Demme and Biedert, the fatty diarrhœas of children are associated with atrophy and fibrosis of the pancreas. Atrophy of the lobules may also be secondary to interstitial fibrosis. In many cases of diabetes the pancreas is found to be shrunken, but differs somewhat in appearance from the pancreas of simple atrophy. The organ is small, flabby, and relaxed. It is brownish in color and rather flat on transverse section. There may be a compensatory increase of the fat in the neighborhood. Histologically, the secreting cells are wasted while the interlobular connective tissue is distinctly increased. There is, in addition, an interstitial infiltration with round cells which extends from the periphery for some little distance into the lobule (Fig. 127). Opie[1] has shown that in a considerable proportion of cases the islands of Langerhans are in a state of **hyaline degeneration.** This he thinks is the cause of pancreatic diabetes, the degeneration interfering with the production of the internal secretion of the organ.

Fatty Degeneration.—Fatty degeneration of the secreting cells is common. It occurs in pancreatitis, passive congestion, in the course of infective fevers, and in poisoning from mineral salts.

Fatty Infiltration.—Fatty infiltration occurs in general obesity, and in cases where the intra-abdominal circulation is interfered with. It may also be compensatory to atrophy or fibrosis of the pancreas. On section, the organ is found to contain more or less numerous pads of fat, separating widely the lobules, which, as a result, are markedly atrophic. The condition predisposes to hemorrhage into the substance of the pancreas, possibly of the nature of an infarction.

Fat Necrosis.—This curious affection is characterized by the formation of areas of degeneration, varying in size from that of a pin-head to that of a pea, or larger, in the pancreas, omentum, or, in fact, in any of the fatty structures within the abdomen. The areas in question are of a dead white appearance, sometimes, but not invariably, surrounded by a hemorrhagic or inflammatory zone. They are soft, or have gritty centres. Occasionally the contents liquefy, forming small cysts. When in the pancreas the foci are situated in the interstitial stroma. Cases are on record, however, in which fat-necrosis affected the omentum, while the pancreas itself was free. The condition is usually associated with acute or chronic inflammation of the organ, tumors, or obstruction. The researches of Hildebrand,[2] Opie,[3] and Flexner[4] have proved that fat-necrosis is due to a liberation of the fat-splitting ferment of the pancreatic secretion, which acts upon the fatty substance of the pancreas and adjacent parts, converting the fats into fatty acids and subsequently into salts formed by the combination of the fatty acids with calcium. Severe cases are sometimes associated with extensive hemorrhage into the

[1] Opie, Jour. Exper. Med., 5: 1901: 397.   [2] Arch. f. klin. Chir., 57: 1898: 435.
[3] Amer. Jour. Med. Sci., 121: 1901: 27.
[4] Johns Hopkins Hosp. Bull., 11: 1900: 231.

pancreas, pancreatitis, or sequestration of large portions of the organ. Death, therefore, is not an uncommon result.

Calcification.—Calcification is observed in connection with fat necrosis, intrapancreatic extravasations of blood, pancreatitis, and fatty infiltration.

Self-digestion.—A condition to which more than a passing reference should be made is the so-called self-digestion. A pancreas thus affected has a peculiar dead white, sometimes slightly glazed, appearance. Under the microscope, in the milder grades of the affection, here and there through the pancreas can be seen lobules or portions of lobules in which the nuclei are undergoing fragmentation, appearing like small particles of pigment, while the outline of the cells is lost. In the most advanced condition, the whole substance of the pancreas presents a diffuse, opaque appearance, somewhat resembling ground glass, staining strongly with eosin. No nuclei are to be seen, and only the rough outlines of the lobules and ducts remain to indicate the character of the organ. The condition was first adequately described by Chiari, who attributed it to the action of the digestive ferment on the pancreas itself. It is frequently found, being present in 63 per cent. of autopsies. It is not unlikely, however, that in some cases it occurs as an agonal change, or even some little time before death. In general, the longer the time that has elapsed after death the more advanced the condition. But time is not the only factor. We have noticed that extensive self-digestion may be present as early as three hours after death, while in other cases the condition may be scarcely recognizable even at the end of from thirty to forty-eight hours. This suggests that the physiological condition of the gland at the time of death may be of importance. If the acini be loaded with ferment, we would expect to get rapid self-digestion. On the other hand, if the ferment has been discharged, the action would be lacking or retarded. We should remember in this connection that death does not at once arrest secretory action on the part of the glands, more particularly, that autolytic action may manifest itself specially in cells containing enzymes. Possibly, too, the relative acidity or alkalinity of the blood and tissue fluids, depending in some measure on the nature of the bacterial flora in the body, is a factor of no small importance. Bile and other fluids may also pass up the pancreatic duct and modify the conditions therein. Lastly, the amount of bodily heat and the degree of the external temperature would, no doubt, have some influence.

PROGRESSIVE METAMORPHOSES.[1]

Tumors.—Primary tumors of the pancreas are somewhat rare. Remo Segie,[1] in 11,500 autopsies at Milan, found 132 cases, divided as follows: carcinomas, 127; sarcomas, 2; cysts, 2; syphiloma, 1. In 1514 post mortems at the Montreal General and Royal Victoria Hospitals, primary carcinoma occurred 6 times and adenoma once. It appears

[1] Ann. univ. di med. e chir., 283: 1885: 5.

Fig. 128

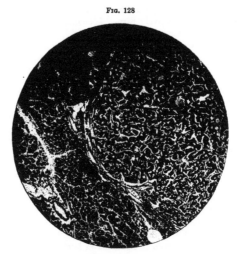

Adenoma of the pancreas arising from an island of Langerhans. Winckel No. 3, without ocular. The tumor lies to the right and is separated from the normal pancreatic tissue by a thin connective-tissue capsule. (From the collection of Dr. A. G. Nicholls.)

Fig. 129

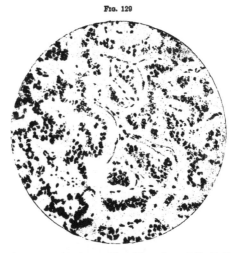

Adenoma of the pancreas arising from an island of Langerhans. Leitz obj. No. 7, without ocular. (From the collection of Dr. A. G. Nicholls.)

from this that carcinoma is by far the most common primary new-growth. Benign growths are excessively rare. **Adenoma** of a tubular character and **fibroadenoma** are described (Cesaris-Demel; Biondi). One of us (A. G. N.) has recorded for the first time a case of adenoma arising from an *island of Langerhans*.[1] A similar one has been reported recently by Helmholz.[2] Some of the so-called pancreatic cysts are to be classed as **cystadenomas**, of which there appear to be two varieties, multilocular cystomas and papillomatous cystomas.[3]

Lipoma, myxoma, and **chondroma** are recorded.

Sarcoma.—Primary **sarcoma** is but little less rare. It is usually situated in the head or tail of the pancreas.[4]

Lymphosarcoma.—Lymphosarcoma occurs.[5] In the only case we have seen that seemed to come under this category, the pancreas was much enlarged and nodules of new-growth, having a soft, white appearance, were found between the lobules. Microscopically, there was a diffuse infiltration of the organ with lymphoid cells, which, in parts, were aggregated together into definite clumps.

Carcinoma.[6]—Carcinoma is ordinarily met with in the head of the organ. It is usually of the *scirrhous* type, but *medullary* and *colloid* cancers are occasionally found. Carcinoma of the body or tail is, however, almost as common. We have observed two such cases lately at the Royal Victoria Hospital. Pressure upon the common bile duct from a growth of this kind results in icterus; pressure upon the duct of Wirsung, in dilatation and even cyst formation. In not a few cases, if the pancreas be extensively infiltrated, glycosuria makes its appearance.

Histologically, these growths are adenocarcinomatous or, occasionally, cylindrical-celled in type.

Secondary carcinomas usually arise by the extension of a primary growth in the stomach, duodenum, ampulla of Vater, or the biliary passages. Metastases by the blood or lymph-stream are not nearly so common.

Cysts.—Apart from the cystadenomas above mentioned, cysts of the pancreas may be due to obstruction of the ducts (*ranula pancreatica*) or of its intralobular radicles (*acne pancreatica*), to hemorrhage, to hydatid disease, or to congenital peculiarities.

Pseudopancreatic cysts are developed in structures in the neighborhood of the pancreas, with disease of which they are occasionally connected. They may be due to traumatism, colliquative necrosis, and effusions of fluid in the lesser peritoneal sac.

[1] Jour. of Med. Research (N. S., 3):1902:385.

[2] Johns Hopkins Hospital Bull., 18:1907:185.

[3] See Ransohoff, Amer. Med., 2:1901:138.

[4] For literature, see Geo. A. Boyd, Trans. Chicago Path. Soc., 4: 1899–1901: 191, and v. Halácz, Wiener klin. Woch, 52: 1908.

[5] Schirokogoroff, Virch. Archiv, 193: 1908: 395.

[6] Fuchs, Ueber carcin. Erkrankungen d. Bauchspeicheldruse, Inaug. Diss., Breslau, 1904; Herxheimer, Path. Ges., 7:1904; Grimani, Arch. per le Sci. Med., 6: 1905.

CHAPTER XXIV.

THE PERITONEUM.

THE peritoneum is a delicate, connective-tissue membrane, containing elastic fibrils, and covered with a layer of flattened endothelial cells. The deeper parts contain the bloodvessels and lymphatics, the latter of which are in functional communication with the abdominal cavity, which is thus to be regarded as a large lymph-space. The peritoneal membrane invests the diaphragm, abdominal wall, and the various organs contained within the abdominal cavity. Furthermore, the lymph-channels are in communication with those of the pleural sacs and anterior mediastinum. Consequently, the great majority of the disorders of the peritoneum are secondary to disease of the underlying viscera or contiguous serous sacs. In this connection, the most important factors are various infective conditions, notably of the digestive tract, less often of the liver and portal system, and of the female genital apparatus. The character and intensity of these infective processes are dependent largely on the nature of the invading microörganisms. The extension of the lesion is in many cases assisted by the movements of the intestines, and modified or localized through the agency of the great omentum and of adhesions.

CONGENITAL ANOMALIES.

Lawson Tait[1] has recorded a case in which the mesentery was completely **absent**, the peritoneal investment covering only a small portion of the circumference of the intestines and passing directly from one coil to another.

The mesentery may be abnormally **long** or **short**, or may present **defects** in its substance. The latter condition is of practical importance, since coils of the bowel may become prolapsed through the opening, resulting in obstruction or strangulation.

Pocket-like **diverticula, abnormal folds** and **duplications**, and **prolongation** of the membrane into persistent inguinal canals are not uncommon.

The great omentum varies much in size, being long or short, or, again, almost completely absent. **Bifurcations** and **partial defects** are more common.

CIRCULATORY DISTURBANCES.

Being in intimate relationship with so many of the viscera, and being itself vascular, local circulatory disturbances of the peritoneum are easily brought about. In this connection such conditions as inflam-

---

[1] Dublin Quart. Jour. of Med. Sci., 47: 1869: 85.

mation of the gastro-intestinal tract, hernias, obstruction, and tumors are of importance.

Hyperemia.—Active Hyperemia.—Active hyperemia is met with in the first stages of inflammation and as a result of the sudden diminution of intra-abdominal pressure, such as is caused by the removal of ascitic fluid or large tumors. Inflammatory hyperemia may be generalized throughout the peritoneal membrane or may be localized to special areas.

Passive Hyperemia.—Passive hyperemia results from obstruction to the portal circulation, either directly from disorders of the liver or indirectly from the heart or lungs. The vessels of the great omentum, stomach, and intestines become greatly distended, and in long-standing cases there is a transudation of clear, watery, slightly yellowish fluid into the abdominal cavity (*ascites; hydrops peritonei*), occasionally tinged with bile or blood-pigment. Not infrequently, soft gelatinous clots of fibrin or shreds of endothelium can be detected upon the surface of the intestines, indicating a slight grade of accompanying inflammation.

Interesting forms of intra-abdominal effusion are *chylous, chyliform,* and *pseudochylous ascites.* The distinctions between these have already been discussed (p. 111).

Ascitic fluid may be free in the abdominal cavity, when it tends to collect in the pelvis and flanks, if the patient be in a recumbent position, but when excessive may fill the greater portion of the abdomen. In children the fluid often collects between the layers of the great omentum (*hydrops omenti*). The presence of ascitic fluid leads to more or less distension of the abdomen, with pressure upon the contained viscera, and upward dislocation of the diaphragm. The thoracic organs may be interfered with and serious disturbance of circulation and respiration result. In long-standing cases the peritoneal membrane becomes thickened and presents a somewhat pearly appearance.

Hemorrhage.—Extravasations of blood occur into the abdominal cavity and into the substance of the peritoneum. The more extensive effusions occur, as a rule, from traumatic rupture of various organs, strangulation of the bowel, the bursting of an aneurism or of the sac in a tubal gestation, or, again, as the result of operations. Operations about the liver and bile passages, particularly where there is jaundice, are not infrequently followed by serious intra-abdominal hemorrhage. Large effusions often lead to death, while smaller ones may be absorbed, leaving blackish-brown stains on the peritoneal surface, the result of the chemical interaction of the sulphuretted hydrogen from the intestines and the iron contained in the blood-pigment.

Petechiæ or small ecchymoses occur in all forms of active and passive hyperemia, in sepsis and other infective processes, and in the hemorrhagic diatheses.

INFLAMMATIONS.

Peritonitis.—The inflammations of the peritoneum—**peritonitis**—are, generally speaking, not unlike those of the other serous membranes.

On the whole, however, they tend to be purulent or fibrinopurulent rather than fibrinous and serofibrinous.

We may, perhaps, with Grawitz, divide peritonitis into *primary* and *secondary* forms. Primary peritonitis is also called "idiopathic" or "rheumatic," owing to the difficulty of assigning the condition to a definite cause. Flexner[1] defines primary peritonitis to be "a condition in which the inflammation, usually diffuse, of the serous cavity takes place without the mediation of any of the contained organs, and independently of any surgical operation upon these parts." This form is due to microörganisms which reach the membrane through the blood stream or the lymph channels, or again, through the lumen of the Fallopian tubes. (See vol. i, p. 316.) It is conceivable that bacteria may pass through an intact intestinal wall and set up peritonitis, but whether this ever occurs is not easily proved. At all events, bacteria may on occasion pass through in the absence of any gross lesion of the intestine or any solution of its continuity, as, for example, in those forms which complicate ascites. It is theoretically possible that toxic agents of a chemical nature circulating in the blood might reach the peritoneum and set up inflammation in the absence of any other localization, but little or nothing is known in regard to this occurrence. The overwhelming number of peritonitides are secondary to disease elsewhere, usually of the abdominal viscera or of the adjacent serous sacs. Less often the inflammation is hematogenic in nature. It is, moreover, practically certain that all forms of peritoneal inflammation are due to the activity of pathogenic microörganisms. Trauma, by lessening the resisting power of the membrane, or by damaging the structure or continuity of the hollow viscera, is an important etiological factor.

Of 106 cases of acute peritonitis (not including tuberculous forms) studied by Flexner, 12 were primary. Microörganisms were found in 10 of these, in 9 of which there was but a single form of germ. In these cases, an inflammatory focus in almost any part of the body may provide the infecting agent.

Flexner also divides the secondary peritonitides into **exogenous** and **endogenous**. The former class are examples of wound-infection, the bacteria having been imported from without. In the endogenous form the infective microörganisms come from the intestinal tract. Of 34 cases of the former type, 25 were single and 9 were multiple infections. The organism most frequently found was Staphylococcus aureus, and next to that Streptococcus pyogenes. B. coli, when present, was generally associated with these other forms. In the latter type of peritonitis the infection is usually multiple. Here B. coli was most frequently found; next, Streptococcus pyogenes; and then both combined. As Flexner correctly points out, the few cases of primary peritonitis that do occur are examples of terminal infection.

The most common cause of peritonitis is some form of gastrointestinal disease, usually ulceration and perforation. In this connection

[1] Phila. Med. Jour., 2:1898:1019.

appendicitis, intestinal obstruction, strangulated hernia, gastric ulcer, typhoid fever, and dysentery are of importance.   Among other etiological factors may be mentioned cholecystitis, cholangitis, hepatitis, splenitis, mesenteric thrombophlebitis, infected mesenteric glands, suppuration of the pancreas and kidneys, and inflammation of the pelvic viscera. Occasionally, the infection spreads from the pleural cavities or pericardium, and the condition forms part of a multiserositis.   Some few cases are hematogenic, the primary focus of infection being in some other part of the body.

According to the character of the exudation, we can classify peritonitis as **fibrinous, serofibrinous, fibrinopurulent, suppurative**, and **hemorrhagic**. The character of the inflammation depends largely on the nature of the infecting microörganisms.[1]

The acute purulent exudates are commonly due to B. coli, Streptococcus, Staphylococcus, and Diplococcus pneumoniæ.   B. tuberculosis and Gonococcus are more apt to excite subchronic and chronic inflammation.

With regard to the distribution of the lesions in peritonitis, surgeons generally recognize *localized* and *diffuse* forms.   Whether an inflammation of the peritoneal membrane will spread and become generalized depends a good deal on the nature of the infecting microörganism and the resisting power of the individual.   Where B. coli, B. tuberculosis, and Gonococcus are at work, plastic or fibrous adhesions are apt to form about the primary focus of irritation, which more or less perfectly wall off the infective agents and prevent their extension.   In typhoid fever, on the other hand, peritonitis resulting from perforation is almost invariably fatal, owing to the lack of such reactive inflammation.   The omentum plays an important part, also, in peritoneal inflammations, as one of us (J. G. A.[2]), has pointed out.   Where there are inflamed areas in the abdominal cavity the omentum is apt to apply itself to them with relatively great rapidity, becoming adherent by plastic, and later by fibrous adhesions.   In this way, even where distant pelvic organs are concerned, undoubtedly the omentum often saves the situation and prevents a general peritonitis.   This apparently purposive action of the omentum is attributable to its constant motility as the result of a peristaltic action of the bowel, as also to its delicate nature and extreme vascularity, whereby any portion coming into a zone of toxin production and irritation rapidly becomes inflamed, and with a discharge of leukocytes gives origin to fibrin and plastic adhesions.   But also, as shown by Durham,[3] the irritated omental surface favors the adhesion of leukocytes that had been free in the peritoneal fluid, so that at the end of an hour after intraperitoneal injection of bacteria the free fluid contains relatively few free cells.   In animals that died within twenty-four to forty-eight hours after

[1] See *G*hon and Mucha and *G*hon and Sachs, Centralbl. f. Bakter., 1905 and 1906.
[2] The *G*reat Omentum, Phila. Med. Jour., 1: 1898: 373.
[3] On the Mechanism of Peritoneal Infections, Jour. of Path. and Bact., 4: 1897: 338.

inoculation with an efficient but not too great a number of bacteria, the peritoneal fluid was found to give no growth on culture media, though vigorous growths could be obtained from the omentum. This probably explains how it is that the fluid removed from the peritoneal cavity in operation cases so frequently is sterile. This protective power of the omentum is often well seen in cases of perforative appendicitis, and it is curious how it will search out and wrap itself about the diseased structure. In some cases, the protection is but temporary, however, the omental vessels becoming thrombosed and the organ itself gangrenous.

FIG. 130

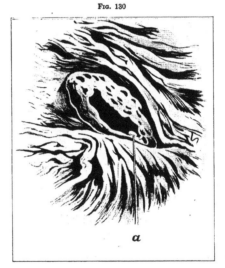

Exogenous perforation of the lower end of the ascending colon. The illustration, which is natural size, shows well the curious raised and perforated condition of the mucous membrane, and, at *a*, the opening through the muscle wall. (Adami.)

The morbid anatomy of acute peritonitis varies according to the nature and intensity of the infection. In cases of low virulence, such as are occasionally met with in ascites and passive congestion of the abdominal viscera, the serous surface of the intestines presents little more than a slight loss of lustre, with here and there a trifling deposit of delicate fibrin. In the ordinary form, during the first stage, there is marked congestion of the serous membrane, especially where the coils of intestine come into contact. A little later the serous surface becomes dull and lustreless and the contiguous surfaces become slightly adherent through the deposition of threads or yellowish-white flakes of fibrin. In some instances there is but little effusion of fluid, but not infrequently there is a moderate exudation of somewhat turbid fluid containing soft pultaceous masses and flakes of a yellowish color. This exudate tends to gravitate to the most dependent parts, namely, the pelvis and the flanks. In other cases the exudation is more turbid and definitely purulent. In cases which have lasted some little time, we may have relatively little fluid poured out, but we find small pockets of thick, yellowish-green pus between the coils of intestine, which are somewhat firmly adherent, or about the liver and spleen. It is not very uncommon for the pus to burrow through the intestinal wall and find vent in that way (Fig. 130). Or, the more fluid part of the exudation is absorbed, the pus deposits thus becoming inspissated or even calcified, while they become walled off by dense fibrous adhesions.

The peritonitis that supervenes upon perforation of the intestine is particularly virulent, and the exudation is feculent as well as purulent. The abdomen usually contains a considerable quantity of dirty, brown, turbid fluid having an offensive fecal odor. The intestines in peritonitis are usually much distended, owing to paralysis.

A peculiar form of peritonitis—the **acute hemorrhagic**—should be mentioned. Here there appears to be a subacute type of inflammation, in which a membranous deposit containing abundant, newly-formed capillaries is laid down. These capillaries readily rupture and there is usually a considerable outpouring of blood into the abdominal cavity. The condition is analogous to internal hemorrhagic pachymeningitis.[1]

Chronic Peritonitis.—Chronic peritonitis may result from the acute form, which has undergone a series of relapses or a gradual amelioration in its severity, or may develop insidiously from the first. Like acute peritonitis, it is usually at first local and is in almost every case secondary to disease of one of the abdominal viscera. Exceptionally, it may arise by extension from one of the other serous membranes.

We may conveniently divide chronic peritonitis, when well-developed, into (1) **chronic exudative peritonitis,** in which there is a considerable outpouring of serous, serofibrinous, or fibrinopurulent exudation, with loose, plastic adhesions, fibrous bands being few or absent; (2) **chronic exudative and adhesive,** presenting less fluid exudation, but with somewhat numerous and firm organizing adhesions, often leading to sacculation of the cavity; and (3) **chronic hyperplastic peritonitis,** where there is a serofibrinous or fibrinopurulent exudation of greater or less extent, the most striking feature, however, being the production of isolated plaques or continuous sheets of hyaline material, of whitish color and cartilaginous appearance (*hyaloserositis*), though ordinary dense fibrous adhesions are also numerous.[2]

The hyperplastic form is much rarer than the other two, but is of

---

[1] For a review of the literature on Peritonitis the reader may consult von Brunn, Centralbl. f. allg. path. Anat., 12:1901:1. For bibliography: Eichorst, Eulenberg's Real Encyclopedie.

[2] For literature, see Hale White, Guy's Hosp. Rep., 49 : 1895 : 1; A. O. J. Kelly, Trans. Coll. of Phys., Philadelphia, 1902; Nicholls, Some Rare Forms of Chronic Peritonitis, Jour. Amer. Med. Assoc., 40:1903:696.

considerable interest. The lesions may be confined to the abdominal cavity or may form part and parcel of a generalized multiserositis. The exudate, at first fibrinous or fibrinopurulent, gradually undergoes organization and hyaline degeneration, so that the viscera, but especially the liver (see Fig. 114) and spleen, are covered with a thick, pearly white, cartilaginous-looking membrane, which has been compared to porcelain or the icing on a cake (Zuckerguss). The serosa of the intestines and mesentery may also be involved, though usually to a less extent. The omentum is commonly found to be thickened and converted into a dense fibrous cord traversing the upper part of the abdomen. The mesentery is often also shortened, so that the intestines lie in a ball close to the vertebral column. Scattered adhesions may be found here and there. There may be a relatively large effusion of fluid, resembling that in ascites, but at times it is fibrinopurulent. Occasionally there is no fluid exudate, and the whole abdominal cavity is obliterated by the adhesion of the visceral and parietal layers of the peritoneal membrane. Where the capsule of the liver is chiefly involved (perihepatitis), the physical signs are very similar to although not identical with those of atrophic cirrhosis of the liver. Peritonitis of this type may be secondary to cholelithiasis and pericholecystitis (Nicholls; Hubler), trauma (Henoch), and passive congestion (v. Wunscheim). Occasionally, it is found as a result of tuberculosis or carcinoma of the peritoneum. Probably in all cases infection of a low grade of virulence is the direct cause.

Tuberculosis.—A common form of tuberculosis of the peritoneum is that in which small isolated tubercles are found scattered over the membrane, chiefly along the bloodvessels. This is usually a manifestation of a generalized miliary infection. The tubercles may be capped by a small amount of fibrin, and there may be slight congestion in their neighborhood. Local peritonitis is also met with in connection with tuberculous ulceration of the bowels. Fluid exudation may be scanty. In a few instances, the inflammation assumes the hyperplastic type, owing to the production of a serofibrinous exudate which undergoes organization and hyaline transformation (Strajesko;[1] Herrick;[2] Nicholls[3]). A few scattered areas of caseation here and there will often give the clue to the nature of the affection. A third variety is that which remains strictly localized, usually to the region of the appendix and cecum. There may be simply a diffuse thickening of the intestinal wall at this point without caseation, or there may be numerous fibrous adhesions about the affected part. Sometimes, also, the omentum and mesentery are thickened and contracted. The tissue hyperplasia about the cecum may be so great that cases have been mistaken for carcinoma. Lartigau[4] has studied this form.

In tuberculosis of the peritoneum the infection may be hematogenous or lymphogenous, or, again, may arise by extension from the intestines, Fallopian tubes, or pleural cavities.

---

[1] Allg. Wien. med. Zeit., 4: 1902. [2] Trans. Chicago Path. Soc., April, 1902.
[3] Jour. Amer. Med. Assoc., 40:1903:696. [4] Jour. Exper. Med., 6:1901–05:23.

Syphilis.—Little or nothing is definitely known with regard to syphilis of the peritoneum. Lancereaux[1] believed in the existence of a chronic adhesive and membranous peritonitis due to syphilis, occurring in children and occasionally in adults. Herringham[2] records two cases of chronic peritonitis with perihepatitis, which probably started from a gummatous liver. Probably all cases are secondary to syphilitic disease of the viscera. Primary gummas of the peritoneum are unknown.

ABNORMAL CONTENTS OF THE PERITONEAL CAVITY.

The abdominal cavity may contain **serous fluid, inflammatory exudates, blood, bile,** or **gas.**

Pneumoperitoneum, or gas in the peritoneal cavity, usually results from the rupture of some viscus in communication with the outer air, such as the stomach or intestine; less often from the action of gas-producing microörganisms, notably B. Welchii and B. coli.

Besides this, the contents of the stomach or bowels, gallstones, urine, feces, and parasites may escape into the peritoneal cavity. The so-called "**free bodies**" are derived from a variety of sources, appendices epiploicæ which have become detached, subserous fibroids of the uterus, ovaries, and mummified or calcified embryos. Swabs and gauze pads have occasionally been left in the abdominal cavity by mistake in the course of operations in this region. Some of these substances may produce "pseudo-tubercles" in the membrane.

PROGRESSIVE METAMORPHOSES.

Opaline Plaques.—Small, opaline plaques are occasionally found on the peritoneal surface as a result of chronic irritation or slight inflammation. They occur chiefly on the liver and spleen at points of pressure. The spleen may be covered with a thin, pearly sheet, or with numerous round, elevated spots, looking like drops of white wax or paraffin. Passive congestion of the spleen seems to be associated with the condition in many cases. Histologically, the patches are composed of hyperplastic connective tissue having a tendency to undergo hyaline transformation.

Tumors.—Apart from the new-growths originating in the various abdominal viscera that encroach upon the cavity, tumors of the peritoneum are most often situated in the great omentum, the retroperitoneal connective tissue, the radix mesenterii, less often in other parts. Among the benign growths may be mentioned **lipoma, fibroma, myxoma, chondroma, osteoma, hemangioma, adenoma, cystadenoma,** and **lymphangioma. Dermoids** and **teratomas** also occur.

One of the most important and interesting new-growths is the **retroperitoneal lipoma.** This is rarely pure, but is usually formed of an ad-

---

[1] Trans. New Syd. Soc., 1: 326.   [2] St. Barth. Hosp. Rep., 1893: 1.

mixture of fatty, fibrous, and mucinous constituents. The growth begins retroperitoneally, generally in the neighborhood of the left kidney, or in the root of the mesentery. It is difficult to diagnosticate and gradually increases in size, leading to more or less distension of the abdomen. It may become quite enormous. Waldeyer has recorded one sixty-three pounds in weight. When the tumor is of large size, the abdomen is swollen, soft, and fluctuating, giving the sensation of being filled with fluid. A dry tap, however, would exclude ascites and should always lead one to suspect retroperitoneal lipoma. A coil of intestine can often

FIG. 131

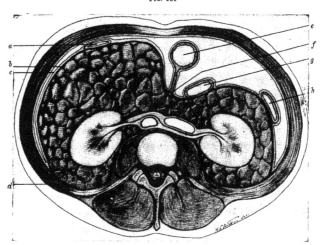

Semidiagrammatic cross-section through a perirenal lipoma at the level of the renal vessels, seen from above. The perirenal and retrorenal fascia unite to form the transversalis fascia. The whole intestinal tract lies in front of the perirenal fascia. *a*, descending colon; *b*, perirenal fascia; *c*, peritoneum; *d*, retrorenal fascia; *e*, small intestine; *f*, superior mesenteric artery; *g*, duodenum; *h*, ascending colon. (Reynolds and Wadsworth.)

be made out on percussion crossing obliquely over the front of the tumor. Cases are generally inoperable when discovered and invariably end fatally, partly owing to the enormous pressure and partly to a sarcomatous transformation to which this form of tumor seems particularly prone. One of us (J. G. A.[1]) has collected forty examples from the literature and has recorded two other cases, in one of which the tumor weighed forty-five pounds. These growths are probably to be referred to some congenital vitium.

Another important primary growth, although not at all common, is the **endothelioma.** This occurs in the form of multiple small plaques or

[1] Montreal Med. Jour., 25:1897:529 and 620.

warty excrescences, or, again, diffusely in more or less extensive sheets. It begins in a proliferation of the lining endothelium of the cavity or, possibly, from the perivascular lymphatics. The condition is sometimes associated with the effusion of fluid, occasionally bloody, together with the deposit of fibrin, so that it simulates a chronic productive inflammation. Metastases are not common. Histologically, the growth resembles an alveolar carcinoma.

Matas[1] has recorded a curious case of primary **myxosarcoma** of the great omentum, which produced extensive secondary growths throughout the peritoneum with a mucoid ascites.

Primary **colloid carcinoma**, originating in "rests" derived from the archenteron, has been observed (Birch-Hirschfeld).[2]

Secondary malignant growths are common, and here, again, the omentum is most likely to be involved. It may be converted into a short, thick, hard cord, running transversely across the upper part of the abdomen. In the case of carcinoma the primary growth is usually situated in the stomach, gall-bladder, pancreas, intestine, uterus, ovaries, and prostate. Colloid cancer, primary in the intestine, is peculiarly apt to bring about extreme involvement of the peritoneum and omentum, while even more extreme may be the development of secondary peritoneal growths in cases of malignant cystadenoma of the ovary, by implantation in cases of rupture of the primary cysts. Multiple **melanotic sarcomas** are also found, arising by metastasis from melanotic sarcomas of the choroid of the eye or of the skin.

Cysts.—The lymphangioma is said sometimes to assume the form of a **cystoma.** Other cysts are the **serous, chylous, hemorrhagic, dermoid,** and **parasitic.**

---

[1] Phila. Monthly Med. Jour., December, 1899.   [2] Text-book of Pathology.

SECTION IV.

THE NERVOUS SYSTEM.

CHAPTER XXV.

DISORDERS OF THE NERVOUS SYSTEM AND THEIR RELATIONSHIP TO FUNCTION.

It is a wellnigh hopeless task, in a work such as this, to deal at all adequately with the disturbances of nervous function. The subject is intrinsically so complex, its ramifications are so wide, and its manifestations are so elusive, that whole treatises, nay, a library, might be written without exhausting its problems or bridging the gaps in our knowledge. We must, perforce, content ourselves with the most general survey, and, far from emulating that great writer of whom it was said by perhaps a still greater "Nullum tetigit quod non ornavit," we shall aim merely to "point a moral" without attempting at the same time to "adorn a tale." For the sake of clearness, we shall change the order which we have usually adopted in these introductory chapters and shall deal first with the applied anatomy of the nervous system.

ANATOMICAL CONSIDERATIONS.

We shall take for granted a general acquaintance with the structure of the nervous system; its division into brain, cord, peripheral nerves, and sympathetic system; the investing membranes; the topography of the various lobes and convolutions of the brain; the ventricles and the various conduction paths, knowledge which, indeed, every third year student is presumed to possess. We shall, however, refer in some detail to the question of the nerve fibre, and especially "the neurone concept," as this is essential for a proper understanding of what is to come.

The nervous system in man is composed of nerve cells and fibres supported by a connective-tissue stroma of glia cells and fibres. These nerve cells, lying in the gray matter of the cerebrum and cerebellum, mid-brain, the medulla, and cord, form centres from which run fibres connecting the centres with each other and with the periphery of the body. The fibres are simply conductors, centripetal or centrifugal, of sensory or motor excitations. The centres are cells, or aggregations of many cells, in which force is stored up or transformed, so that a sensory stimulus is able to initiate a motor excitation. Thus, the entire nervous system is a reproduction on a large scale of its constituent elements, the neurones.

The Neurones.—The neurone is formed of a cell with its prolongations, the dendrites, and the axis-cylinder processes. Each neurone is anatomically independent. The cells are variously formed masses of protoplasm, with a large, round nucleus containing a large nucleolus. By means of special methods of staining (Nissl), the cell protoplasm of the majority of nerve cells (Nissl's somatochromes) may be seen to be studded with irregularly shaped granules (chromophilic or tigroid bodies; Nissl bodies), which are found also in the protoplasmic dendrites, but are not present in the cone of origin of the axis-cylinder, nor in the axis-cylinder itself. Other cells, as some in the olfactory system, contain none of these granules (Nissl's caryochromes). Certain facts, such as its diminution under overactivity and fatigue and its action under certain pathological conditions, make it probable that this chromophilic substance represents a nutritive element of the neurone derived, it may be, as a product of nuclear activity, its staining reactions being not dissimilar to those of the nuclear chromatin.

By means of other special stains (Apathy, Bethe, Beelchowski, Cajal) the spaces between these tigroid bodies may be seen to be occupied by fine fibrils, which form a network in the body of the cell surrounding the nucleus, and can be followed out into the dendrites on the one hand, and the axis-cylinder on the other.

The dendrites are protoplasmic processes, with, in many cases, very rich arborizations, large at their origin from the cell, gradually becoming thinner like the branches of a tree. They are simply an expansion of the cell-body, serving to increase and facilitate its connections with neighboring cells. The axis-cylinder process is usually single and of regular caliber from its origin to its termination, although some cells, *e. g.*, those of the posterior ganglia, have two axis-cylinders. It may give off collaterals at right angles which have the same characters as it has itself. On leaving the gray matter of the centre the axis-cylinder or axone becomes invested with a myelin sheath, and it is collections of these axis-cylinders with their sheaths which form the white matter of the brain and cord. Clothed in the sheath of Schwann, they form the peripheral nerves. Some nerves (sympathetic system) have the sheath of Schwann without the myelin covering.

The axone is made up of a bundle of fibrils, and on reaching its destination splits up into a terminal arborization about a second cell, terminating in small, button-like bodies (end feet), which lie in contact with the cell walls.

The neurone in this simple form, as an independent unit, is not without detractors, among whom may be numbered such authorities as Nissl, Apathy, Bethe, Durante, etc. Apathy, by means of his special method of staining, has studied the neurofibrils very closely, and asserts that they act in two ways. Certain ones penetrate into the ganglion cell and are then resolved into the elementary fibrils, anastomosing freely among themselves and thus forming an intracellular network, then reuniting to form the primitive fibrils of the axone. The second class, in entering the ganglion, do not penetrate into the cells of the ganglion, but resolve themselves directly into elementary fibrils and form an extracellular network. Later, they reunite into primitive fibres and enter the cells of the ganglion.

Apathy asserts that the motor fibres do not commence in the cells of the ganglion; they are nothing but the continuation of the sensory fibrils after the interposition of the nervous network, the ganglion cells being intercalated in the course of the conducting fibres like the battery in a network of telegraph wires. In other words, the fibrils do not commence nor terminate in any place, neither the sensory nor motor, neither at the periphery nor in the centres, but form a great system of continuous conduction paths, just as in the circulation the arteries through the capillary network are continuous with the veins. Bethe agrees with Apathy in these statements, but gives to the extra-cellular network a greater emphasis. He states that the greater number of fibrils go from one neurone to another; the sensory become motor without passing through the cells of the ganglion.

For a time it seemed as though the death blow had been given to the neurone theory by the discovery by Bethe, and later by Raiman, etc., of what is considered by them as autogenous regeneration in the peripheral part of a cut nerve. These observers maintain that, developmentally, the peripheral nerve fibres, including their axones, arise in the embryo by a fusion of long chains of cells placed end to end. This pericellular or catenary theory of the origin of peripheral nerves has been extended by some even to the dendrites and axones of the cells of the central nervous system.

Wilhelm His (1886) was the first to maintain from his embryological studies that the neurone is an independent unit, every nerve fibre being a process from an embryonic nerve cell (neuroblast). The researches of Golgi supported this view, and the recent work of R. G. Harrison[1] has most satisfactorily confirmed it. He found that cutting away a thin strip on the back of embryo tadpoles some survived and at the end of a week had no sensory ganglia nor sensory nerves, although they had motor nerves, but these, instead of showing cell chains along their course, as under normal conditions, appeared as naked, non-nucleated fibres, which could be traced as such all the way from the spinal cord to the extreme ventral part of the musculature, showing that the peripheral spinal nerves may develop in the absence of these sheath nerves.

As for the question of autogenous regeneration in the distal part of a sectioned nerve, this is by no means proved, and since Harrison's work, above quoted, we would not expect it.

Langley and Anderson[2] assert that if anastomosis with other nerves

[1] Reprint from Sitz, d. niederrhein. Gesell., Nat. u. Heilk., Bonn, 1904; Nerv. Versuche u. Beobachtungen über die Entwickelung der peripheren Nerven.

[2] Autogenic Regeneration in the Nerves of Limbs, Jour. of Phys., 31: 1904: 418.

in the limb and all possibility of outgrówth from the central stump be prevented no autoregeneration will occur. Lugaro[1] also has recently published the results of a most careful series of experiments, with the following conclusions:

1. In young dogs, in whom the lumbosacral cord and the corresponding posterior ganglia had been extirpated, no autogenous regeneration of the nerve fibres in the corresponding peripheral nerves could be made out.

2. Some non-myelinated fibres were found in the peripheral nerves which were proved to come from the sympathetic ganglia.

Finally, much doubt exists in the minds of many competent observers as to the existence of the extracellular neurofibrillary network that Bethe lays so much stress on, in spite of his brilliant experimental evidence to the contrary. This experimental evidence, it must be remembered, has not been confirmed. Cajal's stain and the new method of Donaggio, which show the neurofibrils very beautifully but do not stain the neuroglia, demonstrate the intracellular network perfectly, but give no evidence of an extracellular one. Certainly, the dependence of one neurone on another is not complete. Clinically, a lesion is often limited to one system, so that if there be a histological continuity between the neurones of the various orders, there is certainly a physiological and even a pathological-anatomical independence from the point of view of propagation of the lesions; and, as we have seen, there is an embryological independence.

FIG. 132

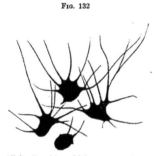

Glial cells with multiple processes, from a case of congenital multiple gliomatosis of the brain. (Stertz.)

These neurones, then, are gathered together into groups to form systems, which subserve different functions, each of these different systems being made up of several relays of groups or neurones. Barker has classified them as follows:

1. Neurones connecting the sense organs of the body with the central nervous system (peripheral centripetal neurones; sensory neurones of the first order; sensory protoneurones).

2. Neurones within the central nervous system, connecting the end-stations of the axones of the peripheral centripetal neurones with other portions of the central nervous system; and neurones which, in turn, connect the end-stations of the latter with still higher portions of the central system (sensory neurones of the second order and of higher orders).

3. Neurones connecting the central nervous system with the voluntary muscles of the body (lower motor neurones).

4. Neurones within the central nervous system which enter into

[1] Neurolog. Centralbl., September, 1906:786.

conduction relation with the lower motor neurones and throw the latter under the influence of other centres. Neurones connecting the pallium, cerebellum, etc., with the lower motor neurones.

5. Projection, commissural and association neurones of the telencephalon.

Neuroglia.—Neuroglia is the connective tissue of the central nervous system filling in the spaces between the nerve elements and forming a support for these and the vessels. It takes the place of the parenchymatous tissue, if this be destroyed, as does the fibrous tissue in other organs. In the adult, two main types of neuroglia cells are found, viz., spider cells, having a round nucleus and straight unbranching processes, and other cells with thicker processes profusely branching; the former are found chiefly in the white matter, the latter in the gray matter about the bloodvessels.

It has been asserted by Metchnikoff and others that in inflammatory and degenerative conditions, the neuroglial cells have a phagocytic action on the degenerated tissue. Marinesco maintained that whenever the achromatic substance of the nerve cell suffers injury there is a stimulation of the surrounding neuroglia cells to phagocytic activity. Certainly, where there has been a severe lesion of the nervous system, the neuroglia cells hypertrophy and proliferate secondarily and are frequently found increased in number about the degenerating nerve cells. But it is doubtful if this is evidence of a phagocytic action. Cerletti in his experiments could not satisfy himself of their phagocytic character. In a more recent communication Marinesco[1] limits the phagocytic action of the "satellite" (glial) cells to the removal of dead neurones and designates it *necrophagy* rather than *neuronophagy.*

Morbid Histology of the Neurone.—There is not a great variety of pathological changes seen in the neurone. Under the action of destructive agencies affecting the cell or its axis-cylinder, a series of changes in structure may occur, which may go on to absolute degeneration and necrosis. In the early stages of these retrogressive changes, which are confined to the finer histological elements of the cell and do not affect the nucleus, regeneration of these elements and return to normal appearance and function are quite possible. It is only when the disease has advanced far enough to affect the nucleus that the cell is doomed. Our knowledge of these degenerative changes is confined to what occurs in the large somatochrome cells of the motor nuclei, the spinal ganglia, etc. These changes may be summed up as follows:

1. A swelling of the cell-body with structural changes in the chromatin and fibrillary elements.

2. Ectopia nuclei; the nucleus no longer remains central, but wanders toward the periphery.

3. Vacuolization of the cell-body and granular degeneration of fibrils.

4. Total necrosis.

In the first stage there is a homogeneous swelling of the cell-body, the

[1] La Semaine Méd., 27: 1907: 145.

Nissl bodies become irregular in shape and size, and, later, are seen to be broken up into fine dust-like particles. This change commences in some cases in the perinuclear part of the cell; in others it begins about the periphery, or it may appear as a diffuse chromatolysis.

Simultaneously with these changes, or probably a little later, definite changes occur in the fibrillary network of the cell. It becomes less distinct and the fibrils themselves less regular. Up to this stage regeneration is possible, but if the process advance, the nucleus no longer holds its central position, but becomes eccentric; at the same time, the fibrils undergo a process of granular disintegration and fragmentation, vacuoles appear in the body of the cell, and the protoplasm has a granular appearance. The nucleus bulges out the periphery of the cell and is finally extruded, and the cell with its axone breaks up and is quickly absorbed.

Chromatolysis appears to be the primary stage of the retrogressive process. It occurs as an effect of overactivity and fatigue, in toxic blood conditions, febrile conditions, after section of the axone, etc., but, under favorable circumstances, the process may stop here and a more or less rapid return to the normal occur.

Specific changes in the cell dependent on the etiological factor have been described. Thus, Marinesco described (1) alterations due to indirect traumatism; (2) primary alterations in the cell due to direct action, mostly toxic, or of nutritive disturbances. The former, *e. g.*, after section of the axone, consists in central chromatolysis with displacement of the nucleus to the periphery. The latter, while they may involve the chromatic substance of the whole cell diffusely, are most marked in the more peripheral zone, and are, therefore, represented, at least temporarily, by a peripheral chromatolysis without displacement of the nucleus.

But these characteristics are by no means always distinct. Other observers have described specific alterations in the cells, dependent on the nature of the poison, maintaining that in the earlier stages, at least, of acute arsenical poisoning, the picture is quite different from that which is seen in acute phosphorus poisoning. In the later stages, and in chronic cases, these specific peculiarities are lost.

The structural changes in the nerve cell following solution of continuity in the nerve fibres are practically the same as those which follow the action of poisons, and may go on to total destruction of the cell. The intensity of the reaction depends on the severity of the lesion, being greater if the nerve is cut than when merely compressed, while a still more intense reaction follows if the nerve be evulsed.

After section, or, better still, evulsion, of a motor nerve, the cells first show an increase in volume; they may become almost double in size and rounder, and the fibrillary network shows certain indefinite structural changes. The tigroid bodies break up into fine, dust-like particles, first, perhaps, in the region of the nucleus, later about the margin; then the nucleus may wander toward the periphery.

Waller was the first to point out that the interruption in continuity of the nerve fibres, whatever be the cause, whether an incised wound or a vascular lesion, is followed by structural changes of a degenerative character in the fibre distal to the lesion; that is, in the part separated from its parent cell, or more exactly, as Cameron[1] maintains, from its parent nucleus, since the nucleus is the nutritive centre for the nerve cell. This is termed *secondary degeneration*. Thus, if we have a lesion of the motor fibres in the internal capsule of the brain, we get secondary degeneration in the direct and crossed pyramidal tracts, a descending degeneration. If the lesion be in the posterior roots between the ganglia and the cord, or in the course of these fibres in the posterior columns, we have an ascending degeneration in the posterior columns of the cord up to their terminal arborization about the cells of the second relay in the nuclei of Goll and Burdach.

These retrogressive changes begin immediately and apparently simultaneously in the whole extent of the peripheral fibre, progressing more rapidly the farther away from the nutritive centre the lesion is. First, the myelin sheath swells, then it breaks up into large and small globules, giving the fibres a varicose appearance. The globules are of a fatty nature and stain black with osmic acid (Marchi's method). These fat particles are carried away by leukocytes and probably other migrating cells which originate from the vascular connective-tissue elements.

Simultaneously with these changes in the myelin there is swelling of the axis-cylinders with a varicose appearance of the neurofibrils, which later become finely granular. They soon break up and are absorbed, their place being taken by proliferated glial tissue.

Secondary Atrophy of the Second Order.—Secondary atrophy of a nerve fibre may occur as a phase in secondary degeneration following separation from the parent cell. It may occur also in the central stump which still remains in connection with the cell, *i. e.*, a cellulopetal atrophy. Besides these forms, a definite reduction in volume of the greater number of the fibres in a tract may occur even when there is no interruption in their continuity, when they are in close anatomical and physiological connection with centres which have undergone secondary degeneration. This has been termed by v. Monakow, secondary atrophy of the second order. We would prefer to term it the atrophy of physiological inactivity (vol. i, p. 869), or disuse atrophy. Thus, we have changes of the neurone of the second order following destruction of the neurone of the first order, and *vice versa*.

Regeneration, in the sense of the formation of new nerve-elements, probably never occurs in the central nervous system. The regeneration of the chromatophilic granules has been mentioned. In the peripheral nerves, degeneration always occurs in the part distal to the section from the parent cell before regenerative processes begin. These consist in the growth of axis-cylinder processes out from the central end which push across the cicatrix and penetrate into the peripheral segment. Cajal describes the growing extremity of the young fibre as possessing a

[1] Brain, 1906: 332.

"terminal ball," which, if it becomes impacted in one of the tissue interstices, may become enormously swollen and enlarged. (See also vol. i, p. 628.)

Simple atrophy of the neurone may occur (1) in chronic conditions where a slowly acting toxin circulating in the system causes an impairment of nutrition in the cell, not sufficient, perhaps, to cause, in the first place very definite structural changes in it, but just sufficient to prevent it maintaining its long nerve-processes, which, therefore degenerate; this degeneration commences at the extreme periphery of the axis-cylinder; later on the cell itself atrophies. (2) The same thing occurs in conditions in which there is an inherent congenital lack of vitality in the neurone, in conditions of abiotrophy.

The morbid changes occurring in the **dendrites** have attracted comparatively little attention. They have been studied, however, by Coella, Creppin, Andriezen and others in dementia paralytica; by Hamilton Wright[1] in bromide poisoning; by Berkley in rabbits in serum poisoning; and, incidentally, in rabies, by Schaffer,[2] Babes,[3] Golgi,[4] Germano and Capobianco.[5] In all these affections the lesions described have been closely analogous; atrophy of the fibrils, varicose tumefaction of the same, and swelling of the nodes. Other changes are found, which are particularly well made out in the case of the pyramidal cells of the cortex and the Purkinje cells of the cerebellum, inasmuch as the lateral buds or gemmules are here specially well developed. The gemmules swell and are finally cast off, those situated over the nodes going first, until the whole twig may become denuded. These changes are of great importance inasmuch as when they exist, if even in a minor degree, the delicacy of the functional relations between the end-apparatus and the dendrone is marred, thereby more or less inhibiting the communication of impulses from neurone to neurone. With lesions of this character of a moderate degree in the cortex, mental hebetude and impaired motor activity inevitably result.

"Exhaustion" Conditions.—As we have already seen, fatigue and exhaustion of a neurone are characterized anatomically by a disappearance of the chromatolytic bodies in the nerve cell and degenerative changes in the myelinated fibres. According to the well-known hypothesis of Weigert and Roux, the tissues of an organ are normally in a state of equilibrium, and when one degenerates its place is taken by the surrounding tissue; if one becomes weakened, the energy of growth of its neighbors tends to crush it out.

This condition may be brought about either by increased consumption of the nutritive elements of the cell, or by a diminution of the reparative power of the cell, and is anatomically recognizable by the disappearance of cell and fibres and the secondary overgrowth of glial tissue filling in the space.

---

[1] Brain, Summer Number, 1898.	[2] Annales d. l'institut Pasteur, 3:1889:644.
[3] Virch. Archiv, 110:1887:562.	[4] Berl. klin. Woch, 1894:325.
[5] Annales d. l'institut Pasteur, 9:1895:625.

In such affections as occupation palsies, we have this state of an abnormal demand on the normal tracts or on the normal reparative power of the cells. In other cases, we may have a reparative power, relatively insufficient for the normal functioning of the cell. This is usually due to the action of toxins in the blood, alcohol, lead, syphilis, etc., and the result varies, depending upon whether the toxin has a selective action on any particular part of the nervous system and, again, on the relative activity of the various systems of neurones. Among diseases of this nature Edinger has classed peripheral neuritis, tabes dorsalis, lead palsy, subacute combined sclerosis, etc.

Gross Anatomical Considerations.—We come now to discuss certain gross anatomical relationships, a knowledge of which is essential to a clear apprehension of the pathogeny of many nervous affections. To begin with, the central nervous system is encased in and protected by a bony covering, the brain within the cranium and the cord within the vertebral canal. The head, being an exposed part of the body, is, of course, correspondingly liable to suffer from traumatic insults, but, inasmuch as the calvarium is a rigid covering, only the most violent forms of injury, such as penetrating wounds, fractures, and concussions are likely to affect the brain. Save only in the new-born, in whom the sutures are ununited, will slighter causes result in serious injury. Thus, the excessive overriding of the bones during the act of parturition sometimes results in laceration of the bloodvessels and damage to the brain, and is a potent cause of some of the infantile palsies, paraplegias, and diplegias, as well porencephaly, epilepsy, and even idiocy. The cord is somewhat better protected, being enclosed in a relatively large bony canal and covered with powerful muscles. Only gross forms of violence, such as fractures and dislocations of the vertebræ, are likely to be potent here.

The delicate tissues of the central nervous system are, however, doubly protected by the presence also of cerebrospinal fluid, in which they float. This fluid, inasmuch as it contains but little albumin, with a large amount of potassium salts, is clearly a secretion and not a transudate. It is produced by certain cells, probably those of the choroid plexus, and is absorbed by the Pacchionian bodies. While, no doubt, it is in large measure nutritive, a main function of this fluid is to act as a sort of buffer to prevent jar, and it does this very efficiently. The lymph in the perivascular lymph channels acts similarly in minimizing the effects of too sudden changes of blood pressure. On the other hand, it may be remarked that the influence of the cerebrospinal fluid is exercised not entirely for good, since, being continually on the move, it forms a ready means for the dissemination of bacteria and toxins throughout the whole length and extent of the cerebrospinal system.

The central nervous system is, further, brought into relationship with parts of the body external to it in several ways—by contiguity, through the blood stream, and by means of the peripheral nerve **trunks**.

Inflammatory lesions of the cranium and its cavities, as of the vertebral column, and also tumors, may extend to the nervous substance.

Infection, for example, may reach the meninges from the nose through the cribriform plate of the ethmoid; from the eye, by way of the orbit and optic nerve; from the middle ear, either directly or through the mediation of the lateral sinus. The last-mentioned event is particularly liable to happen where the squamosopetrosal suture remains open, as it does for a prolonged period in children in a considerable proportion of cases.

The circulatory apparatus also deserves a word. The arteries of the brain and cord are numerous and delicate and also somewhat poorly supported. Consequently, circulatory disturbances bulk largely in our consideration of the lesions of the nervous system. Sclerosis, thrombosis, embolism, and rupture are common and lead to important results. Arteriosclerosis leads to cerebral anemia, softening and necrosis, and is an important cause of thrombosis, aneurism formation, and hemorrhage. Rapid death, and, short of this, various paralyses, and mental degradation are liable to follow. The severity of the results depends upon the extent of the primary lesion, and particularly on its localization. In the event of the so-called "silent areas" of the brain being involved no symptomatic manifestations may be produced. In the case of the internal capsule, the pons, or medulla, the effects are most serious.

The vascularity of the tissues in question, moreover, is important in that it renders them particularly liable to be affected by circulating toxins, whether of mineral, bacterial, or metabolic character. And it is curious in this connection to see how certain regions are specially picked out. Thus, in poisoning by lead and other metallic substances, and in poliomyelitis, the ganglion cells of the anterior horns are apt to be involved. In chronic ergotism and locomotor ataxia, the spinal ganglia and posterior columns; in pernicious anemia, the posterior and lateral columns are attacked. Arsenic, lead, and alcohol, frequently involve the peripheral nerves. The explanation of this is not clear. Bacteria may be carried to the brain and meninges through the blood stream, as is notably the case in pulmonary inflammation.

Diseases of the peripheral nerves may extend to the central nervous system. Peripheral neuritis and atrophy may in time involve the posterior ganglia and the posterior columns. But the most notable example is found in tetanus in which the toxin, which has a notable affinity for nervous tissue, is undoubtedly conveyed to the brain and cord directly by means of the peripheral nerve trunks.

EMBRYOLOGY.

The central nervous system is formed by the invagination of the superior germinal layer of the embryo. Thus, there is produced a shallow furrow, the *medullary groove*, running axially along the dorsal aspect. The cells along the margin of this proliferate, so that two elongated ridges, the *medullary folds*, arise, which gradually meet and coalesce forming the *medullary canal*. This occurs very early, even before the twelfth day. Later, the medullary tube separates from the superficial ectoderm and becomes an independent structure. It is not, however, to be the final brain and cord but simply represents the axis about which these structures gradually form.

The primitive brain consists in a series of vesicles or dilatations of the anterior end of the medullary canal, while the rest becomes the cord. The lumen of the primitive medullary tube persists throughout life as the ventricles of the brain and the central canal of the cord. The hinder portion long preserves its communication with the primitive gut. It is lined by a membrane, the *ependyma*, composed of a single layer of ciliated epithelial cells, and a supporting structure of modified glia.

There are three chief vesicles from which the brain is derived, forming, respectively, the fore-brain, the mid-brain, and the hind-brain. The first is subdivided into two parts, the prosencephalon proper and the thalamencephalon. From the former arise the lateral ventricles, the cerebral hemispheres, the olfactory bulbs, and the corpus callosum. The second vesicle forms the third ventricle, the aqueduct of Sylvius, the nervous part of the eye, the epiphysis, the hypophysis, the optic thalami, the corpora quadrigemina, and the crura. The third primary vesicle is divided into two parts, the epencephalon, from which arise the pons and cerebellum, and the mesencephalon, forming the medulla oblongata. The fourth ventricle is derived from both portions.

In the production of anomalies of development it is a general rule that those structures which go to form the most highly differentiated portions of the brain are most likely to be involved. Therefore, we find anomalies most often and most extreme in the fore-brain, less often in the hind-brain, and very exceptionally in the mid-brain. In the case of the cord, it is the anterior portion of the primitive medullary tube which is completed first, so that anomalies are not so likely to occur here as in the other portions.

With regard to the bony structures, the bodies of the vertebræ appear first and the arches somewhat later. It is only at the end of the twelfth week that the lateral laminæ unite to close in the spinal cord, which takes place first in the dorsal region.

We do not intend to discuss here in detail the numerous and varied forms of errors in development, leaving that to another place (see p. 551), but shall merely draw attention to some general principles and point out the practical importance of the subject.

We would first remark upon the close relationship which exists between the various parts of the nervous system. Whether we believe or not in the perfect anatomical continuity of the neurone from the cell in the cerebral cortex to the peripheral nerve ending, there can be no doubt that excitations pass from one extreme of the system to the other, or, if we may so express it, that the functional continuity is complete. Consequently, it follows that defects in any one portion of the system are not merely local in their effects, but are followed by changes in the tracts physiologically related to them. More than this the nutrition and growth of skin, muscles, bones, and glands is largely dependent on nervous influences, so that the results are often far-reaching.

The congenital anomalies of development fall naturally into two classes. In the first, which we may term *primary*, there is a defect in the primitive "Anlage," so that certain parts are either not produced at all (agenesia) or remain stunted in their growth (hypoplasia). Or, on the contrary, the vegetative force is so excessive that it results in a form of giantism, an overgrowth (hyperplasia) met with, though rarely, in the brain, or in a numerical redundancy of tissues (notably in the cord). In the other, the *secondary*, somewhat analogous results may follow, but they are due to disease acting upon structures that are in the course of formation, leading to grave interference with growth and development. Thus, passive congestion, lymphatic obstruction, pressure of the amniotic sac, hemorrhage, and inflammation may bring about important results, not only through pressure and the actual destruction of tissue, but also through secondary sclerosis. As will be readily understood, it is sometimes difficult, if not impossible, to decide in a given case whether the defect of structures is due to imperfect growth or secondary atrophy. From the point of view of the clinician, however, this is of little moment, for the phenomena resulting are for the most part indistinguishable in either case. It is, further, worthy of remark that these congenital anomalies may involve the central nervous system alone, or the structures concerned in the closure of the primitive medullary groove, bones, muscles, and integument. The latter are associated with grievous deformities, and are usually incompatible with continued existence. Among them are such conditions as arhinencephaly, cyclencephaly, anencephaly, microcephaly, craniorachischsis, and spina bifida. The former include such conditions as partial and total hypoplasia (agyria; microgyria; atelomyelia, etc.), hydrocephalus, gliosis, and heterotopia.

Apart from these more obtrusive anatomical deficiencies, moreover, there are others of a more indefinite character, which are nevertheless the cause of well-marked disturbance. If we may put it so, these defects are of texture rather than material. Individual systems may be congenitally too delicate to carry out their normal function during the usual span of life. There is apparently an inherent lack of vitality in certain systems of cells, so that they die prematurely, their place being taken by glial tissue. To this condition Sir William Gowers[1] has given the name "abiotrophy." (Vide vol. i, p. 876.) It is seen in several members of a family being affected similarly without any apparent sufficient cause. The various types of Friedreich's ataxia, the family form of primary optic atrophy, peroneal type of muscular atrophy, amyotrophic lateral sclerosis, etc., are all to be included under this category.

APPLIED PHYSIOLOGY.

The disorders of nervous function naturally fall into two broad classes— those involving the mind and those involving the body. The distinction

[1] *Lancet*, London, 1:1902:1003.

is fundamental and yet the division between the two sets of phenomena is not always clear cut./ It is a matter of common remark and almost a truism to say that the mind has a great influence over the body and the body over the mind. To cite only a few examples by way of illustration, we have the bodily exhaustion that follows an acute maniacal attack, the muscular weakness associated with psychasthenia, and the imperfect mental concentration that results from excessive bodily exertion. The ancient maxim, "Mens sana in corpore sano," is a proof of the importance that has been attached to this correlation from time immemorial. To discuss the first group of disorders would be going too far afield, and our references to them will be entirely general and as it were incidental. They are more profitably relegated to special works on psychiatry. The latter group, inasmuch as they are closely correlated to disease of other systems, ought not to be overlooked in a work on systemic pathology.

Put briefly, the functions of the nervous system, in this restricted sense, are fourfold—to receive and transmit sensory stimulations, to initiate motion, to regulate secretion, and to promote nutrition. The symptoms resulting from disordered function are usually divided into two classes, *focal* and *general*. Focal symptoms are those due to lesions affecting particular portions of the nervous system. General symptoms result from causes which affect the system as a whole. Some of these causes definitely originate in some particular region, while the nature and localization of others cannot be made out. Not infrequently it happens, however, that general causes have a local manifestation owing to some particular idiosyncrasy or vulnerability of the affected structures.

General Symptoms.—These are in the main either *irritative*, as in delirium and convulsions, or *depressive*, as in syncope, collapse, and coma

Delirium.—Delirium is characterized by more or less dulling of the consciousness, with, in many cases, hallucinations of sense, and motor excitability. In mild cases the patient can be roused by speaking to him or by any procedure which causes pain. He lies comparatively still, continually babbling or muttering. There may be a slight tremor of the tongue and jaw, and of the skeletal muscles (*subsultus tendinum*). In more severe cases the patient is constantly picking at the bedclothes or attempting to grasp things in the air. The tremor is marked and almost constant, and insensibility is almost complete. Attempts may be made to get out of bed. The most intense forms resemble closely acute mania. Delirium is a common accompaniment of all the various infective fevers, if severe, notably, typhoid, typhus, variola, acute rheumatism, pneumonia, and meningitis. In some cases of typhoid and pneumonia it may be the first and most obtrusive symptom and may for a time mask the true nature of the case. Exceptionally, acute delirium is the earliest symptom of Bright's disease and acute endocarditis. While it is true that delirium is most apt to manifest itself when the temperature is high (104° or over), pyrexia is not the only cause. Toxemia seems to be equally potent, for delirium may occur with a low temperature. In fact, we have seen a severe attack of typhoid fever progress during the active stage without delirium, and when the temperature touched the red line delirium set in. Postfebrile insanity, fortunately, as a rule, of transient nature, is a well-recognized type. Delirium, it may be remarked, is particularly liable to occur in neurotic persons the subjects of febrile disease, even when not otherwise severely ill. *Delirium tremens* may be instanced as an example of the purely toxic form. Here irritative phenomena are in the ascendent. The patient is constantly on the move, talks incessantly, tremor is marked, there are hallucinations of sense, usually of a frightful character, there is often a slight fever, and insomnia may be intractable.

Convulsions.—Convulsions are due to the excessive action of the muscles. They may begin in a certain muscle or group of muscles, as in Jacksonian epilepsy, but frequently become generalized, or may be, so far as one can tell, generalized from the first. Two sets of phenomena are described—tonic spasms, in which the muscles for a time go into a tetanic contraction, and clonic, in which there are rapidly alternating periods of contraction and relaxation. The former type of contraction is seen in some cases of infantile convulsions, in tetanus, rabies and strychnine poisoning, in cerebrospinal meningitis, and occasionally in hysteria. Spasm of the diaphragm and the other muscles of respiration may occur and lead to difficulty in respiration, with engorgement of the heart and cyanosis. Consciousness is not necessarily lost. In general clonic convulsions complete insensibility usually occurs quickly, the face may be pale or more or less cyanosed, froth escapes from the mouth, and toward the end of the attack the muscles become gradually quiescent, the sphincters relax, and the patient passes into a state of coma of varying duration. In epilepsy, which may be taken as the type of general convulsions, the patient passes in turn from the stage of tonic spasm into general clonic movements, and finally into relaxation and coma. In such attacks there is great danger of the patient hurting himself, from falling in precarious places, from striking his limbs against hard substances, and from biting the tongue. Convulsions are due to a variety of causes, and are said to be more likely to occur in those of a neurotic type. We may, perhaps, classify them under the following heads: (1) *Of mechanical origin*, as those due to brain tumor, cerebral hemorrhage, and cerebral congestion. Of the latter type, probably, are the convulsions met with in cases of asphyxia and sunstroke. (2) *Of toxic origin*, such as those in chronic lead poisoning (saturnine epilepsy), uremia, acute yellow atrophy, alcoholism. Some of the cases, such as those due to meningitis and cerebral syphilis, for example, are probably attributable to both the above-mentioned causes, pressure from congestion, an increased amount of cerebrospinal fluid, and the destructive effect of the bacteria and their toxins. (3) *Reflex*, such as those from teething, otitis media, phimosis, gastro-intestinal irritation, and worms, causes so often operating in young children. Probably the convulsions due to gastro-enteritis are due as much to the absorption of toxins as to a reflex stimulus. (4) *From debility and malnutrition*, as in rickets, prolonged diarrhœa, the latter stages of whooping cough, and the like. (5) *Febrile*. This form is commonly seen in young children as the initial symptom in many of the infectious fevers, notably scarlatina, measles, and pneumonia. (6) *Functional*, as in hysteria major and hystero-epilepsy. Possibly, true epilepsy should be placed in this group, though the present tendency is to regard this disease as due to a toxic irritation of the cerebral cortex.

Syncope, Shock, and Collapse.—The first of these is a comparatively unimportant condition, inasmuch as it is transient and always recovered from (we are speaking now of the syncope or ordinary "faint" met with in healthy people). In its essence it is a vasomotor effect, the direct cause being anemia of the brain, but it is associated with such severe nervous manifestations that it may properly be discussed here. The person suffering from syncope falls to the ground without warning, save for a momentary feeling of giddiness, the face becomes pale, the muscles are relaxed, the pulse is small and rapid, and for a short interval may even be absent. Within a few moments the patient recovers. The causes are chiefly emotional, severe mental impressions, bad smells, disgusting or frightful sights, fear, and the like. We have once had a patient faint during the trivial operation of vaccination, and once again, while we were washing our hands and before the procedure was even begun. Severe pain will often cause a fainting attack. Also, in persons out of health, a sudden change of position, such as stooping and then rising, or, again, jumping out of bed quickly, will sometimes induce it. Naturally, the condition is more likely to supervene in those possessing an unstable nervous system.

Closely allied, but more severe, are collapse and shock. Here, the patient lies almost inert. While not unconscious he replies slowly and with difficulty to questions. The face is pale, haggard and drawn, the skin cold, clammy, and perspiring, the pulse rapid, small, or imperceptible, the pupils dilated, and the temperature is subnormal. There may be nausea and vomiting. If there be any difference between the two conditions, it is that collapse comes on gradually, while shock is usually immediate. Collapse is due to some cause which depletes the system, as persistent vomiting, diarrhea, and hemorrhage. Shock is seen, more especially, after severe and prolonged operations, particularly those on the nervous system and on the abdominal viscera, after severe concussion, pain, and emotion. Collapse is seen, therefore in such conditions as internal or external hemorrhage, the vomiting of pregnancy, cholera, acute dilatation of the stomach, acute pancreatitis, and acute peritonitis. We have also seen it recently in a case of typhoid fever in the fourth week, coming on without obvious cause, where with all the other cardinal features the temperature dropped within a few hours from 104° to 97°. The appearance resembled closely the collapse which we sometimes see in pneumonia after the crisis has set in. Shock is seen, in addition to the conditions above mentioned, in heat exhaustion, acute intestinal obstruction, and in perforation of the stomach or intestines. This condition may be rapidly fatal, and when recovered from convalescence is gradual. It is important to remember that one form of shock, that due to concussion, is a cause of certain functional disorders known as *traumatic neuroses*. (For further information see vol. i, p. 580.)[1]

Coma.—This is a condition of complete unconsciousness, it being impossible to arouse the patient. There is muscular relaxation, the breathing may be irregular and of the Cheyne-Stokes type, and accompanied by stertor. The pupils are dilated and insensitive to light. Occasionally the patient lies in a pseudo-wakeful state with the eyes open—*coma vigil.* Perhaps the chief cause is toxemia. Of this nature is the coma seen in Bright's disease, diabetes, alcoholic poisoning, cholemia, and in the terminal stages of the infective fevers. Other causes are perhaps mechanical, due to pressure upon the medulla. Such we find in cerebral hemorrhage, brain tumors, brain abscesses, and sinus thrombosis. The coma of cerebral concussion is probably due to the direct injury to the ganglion cells and the dissociation of the fibres and collaterals. Interference with the cerebral circulation, as from thrombi, may bring about coma. An instance of this is seen in the coma of pernicious malaria, in which the finer vessels have been found blocked with parasites. Some cases, again, are probably inflammatory, as in meningitis, sunstroke, cerebral syphilis, and general paresis. Where to class the coma of epilepsy is somewhat uncertain.[1]

Focal Symptoms.—These are manifested in particular nerve districts and are often due to a lesion localized to corresponding nerve centres or conducting paths. Examples of this we see in the paralysis of, say, a hand or foot, due to a tumor or inflammatory exudation over a portion of the cortical motor area, or in the wasting of certain muscles in cases of anterior poliomyelitis. Occasionally, too, general causes produce focal effects. Thus, in chronic lead poisoning, we may get a drop wrist; after diphtheria, a paralysis of the soft palate; or in alcoholic poisoning, an ataxic condition of the lower extremities. The precise result produced depends almost entirely on the particular nerve centres or nerve paths involved. We say "almost" for the statement is not true without some qualification. The nerve centre, the conducting fibre, the end-plate and the muscle form a functional whole. The centre may be perfectly healthy, but its influence destroyed by a break in the conduction path. The nervous mechanism may be perfect, but some local condition in the muscle may prevent its response. Examples of the latter condition are seen in the pain and disability of the muscles of the leg in intermittent claudication and myositis ossificans, the dystrophies, trichinosis, Zenker's degeneration and myotonia congenita. Indeed, both nerve centres, fibres, and muscle may be intact, but ankylosis of a joint may prevent proper functioning.

Focal symptoms, like the general, may be divided into *irritative* and *depressive.* The phenomena we have to deal with here do not differ so much in kind from those already discussed, as in distribution and

[1] For a clear, brief exposition of the various theories advanced to explain shock, the reader is referred to a paper by E. H. Falconer in the Montreal Medical Journal, 39:1910:678.

localization. We may conveniently deal with the subject under the following heads, representing the various functions of the nervous system: (1) Motion, (2) Sensation, (3) Secretion, and (4) Nutrition.

Disturbances of Motor Power.—The depressive manifestations that come under this category are all those which lessen the power of the muscles to carry on their wonted activities. Complete inability to contract is called *paralysis.* When weak contractions only can be produced we speak of *paresis.* When movements cannot be accurately carried out and, consequently, are more or less erratic, we have *incoördination.* All three sets of phenomena may involve both voluntary and involuntary muscle.

Motor impulses pass from the cerebral cortex to the muscles through two sets of fibres. The first, known as the upper motor neurones, begin in the cortical ganglia of the motor areas and pass by way of the pyramidal tracts to the ganglia in the anterior horns of the spinal cord, or to the corresponding nuclei in the pons and medulla. The second, the lower motor neurones, begin in the motor ganglia of the medulla and cord, pass down the pyramidal tracts to the peripheral nerves and thence to the muscles.

Lesions of the upper and lower motor segments have this in common, that they produce paresis or paralysis. We are able, however, to differentiate between affections of the two sets of elements by attention to special peculiarities. We have learned that the nutrition of a neurone depends, first, upon its continuity with its nutritive centre, the ganglion cell: and, secondly, on the condition of that ganglion cell. The upper and lower motor neurons are, furthermore, to be regarded as nutritional units. The secondary degeneration resulting from disease of the ganglion cell or the conducting fibre in large part gives us the clue to diagnosis.

Destructive lesions of the upper motor segment give rise to paralysis, but owing to the fact that the secondary degeneration in these cases stops at the beginning of the lower neurone, the paralyzed muscles do not manifest degenerative atrophy, nor is there any marked change in their electrical reactions. *The affected muscles become spastic, the reflexes are exaggerated, and the muscle tonus is increased.* Destructive lesions of the lower motor segment also lead to paralysis, but the muscles are flabby, their tonus diminished, and the reflexes are diminished or abolished. Inasmuch as the secondary degeneration involves the fibres running to the peripheral nerves and muscles, the muscles atrophy and exhibit the characteristic electrical reactions of degeneration.

We gain additional information on a consideration of the anatomical peculiarities of the two orders of elements. Lesions of the upper motor segment are apt to involve larger areas than are those of the lower. The reason for this lies in the fact that the component parts of the upper motor segment are much closer together than those of the lower. We see this very well, for example, in the internal capsule, which is a limited area through which the motor fibres pass. A relatively small lesion here, such as a hemorrhage, brings about destruction of a large number of fibres and we get a hemiplegia, or paralysis affecting one-half the body. Even in the motor cortex, while the separate centres are somewhat wide apart, they are still near enough to give somewhat extensive paralyses, more extensive in fact than those due to lower segment involvement. A small, well-localized lesion in the motor area may cause paralysis of a limb (cerebral monoplegia) or a portion of a limb. Similarly, lesions in the pyramidal tracts result in paralysis of all the muscles whose nuclei are situated below the point of injury. On the other hand, the nuclei in the lower motor segment are arranged in groups, extending from the peduncles of the brain to the termination of the spinal cord, and their axis-cylinder processes pass in the peripheral nerves to all the muscles of the body. Their component parts are, therefore, widely separated one from the other, and a local lesion produces at most paralysis of a single muscle or small group of muscles. From a consideration of. these points we are often enabled to say not only what segment is involved, but often also what particular part of it.

Before passing away from this part of our subject we should say a word in regard to the functions of the cerebellum. Without going into the question whether or not voluntary motor impulses pass through this organ, there can be no doubt that disease of the cerebellum may powerfully affect the muscles, quite apart from the matter of the sense of equilibrium. The function of the muscles is undoubtedly affected by centripetal impulses passing from them to the brain, which they do by way of the cerebellum. The fibres from the cerebellum to the cerebrum undergo decussation and cross the middle line again in their passage from the cerebrum to the cord, so that a unilateral lesion of the cerebellum will produce effects on the muscles of the same side of the body. We may, in fact, have a true cerebellar hemiplegia. We may also have a cerebellar ataxia without any disturbance of cutaneous sensibility.

Finally, we may have paralyses, due, so far as we are aware, not to gross organic lesions but to some interference with mental function. These are the so-called "physical paralyses" which are found in the hysterical and the insane. Such paralyses affect not single muscles but whole extremities, and, curiously, not all movements but only certain purposive acts.

The motor irritative symptoms comprise tremors, choreiform movements, associated movements, contractures, and convulsions.

Tremor is a series of regular oscillatory movements, of short amplitude, occurring about a fixed axis. The symptom is met with in a considerable number of diseases, and sometimes is of such a character as to be of diagnostic importance. We find it, for example, in chronic alcoholism, lead poisoning, exophthalmic goitre, in paralysis agitans, insular sclerosis, and hysteria. It is not uncommon in old age, and not unknown in childhood, in the latter case being an inherited peculiarity. It occasionally comes on without any obvious cause. The tremor varies, according to circumstances, in rapidity, in degree of amplitude, in distribution. It may be present only during voluntary movement, but may occur during rest also. It stops during sleep. Occasionally it is made worse during some purposive act. It is hard to say what is the cause of the phenomenon. The somewhat analogous fibrillary twitching seen in degenerating muscles is usually attributed to the irritative action of the products of degeneration either on the ganglia or on the nerve trunks. The twitching of the pectorals seen in cases of severe anemia and pulmonary tuberculosis when the chest is uncovered is possibly due to irregular response of the fibres to sensory stimuli. However, we know little about it.

Choreiform Movements.—The movements in chorea and similar affections are less regular than those of true tremor. They are not continuous, are more brusque and jerky, and are usually worse when the patient is excited. They, also, cease during sleep. Such movements are found in ordinary chorea, in Huntingdon's chorea, after a hemiplegia, and in hysteria and certain psychoses. Their origin is quite obscure. The posthemiplegic form is by some thought to be due to lesions in the superior peduncles of the cerebellum, interrupting the centripetal impulses that pass through the cerebellum to the cerebral motor cortex. Probably, irritation of the cerebral motor cortex has something to do with it, for in some instances, meningo-encephalitis has been discovered. In Huntingdon's chorea the irritation very possibly comes from the presence of dead and dying cells.

Associated Movements.—The nervous mechanism involved in the execution of a voluntary act is exceedingly complex. A great number of nervous stimuli pass out to a corresponding number of muscles. The muscular contractions resulting would often be erratic and to some extent superfluous were it not for the fact that their character is controlled by certain centripetal peripheral impulses. When, for example, in locomotor ataxia, the peripheral control is interfered with, we get sometimes associated with the performance of voluntary acts other unnecessary and purposeless movements, such as are ordinarily suppressed in the normal individual.

Contractures.—It not infrequently happens in the course of certain nervous affections that single muscles or groups of muscles become contracted. If such muscles happen to be concerned in the movement of a joint, there will be limitation of the excursion of that joint in a definite direction. Should such contractures occur during childhood, there is often serious defect in the growth or development of the bones and joints and there may even be notable deformity. Moreover, when a joint has remained in a fixed position for a long time the condition tends to become permanent owing to anatomical changes in the joint itself, the formation of adhesions, and alterations in the shortened muscles. The affections in which we get these contractures are numerous and of very varied origin. We may mention hemiplegia, transverse myelitis, anterior poliomyelitis, various paraplegias and diplegias, Friedreich's ataxia, hysteria, and certain joint lesions. Also, in fractures of the long bones, where splints have been applied for a long time, the muscles always become stiff, contracted, and painful on motion.

These contractures may be accounted for in more than one way. In one order of cases certain muscles become weak from disuse or from some disease of their intimate structure or from some disturbance of their innervation. The antagonistic muscles being then the stronger tend to move the joint into an abnormal position and hold it there, with the consequence that they tend to become permanently contracted. This form is known as *passive* contracture. In another class of cases the joints are maintained in an abnormal position by the tonic contraction of certain groups of muscles—*active* contracture. Here, the explanation is not quite clear and, indeed, the cause may not be the same in all cases. There is often, though not invariably, increase of the reflexes and we then speak of spastic contractures. It is possible in such an event that there is some reflex stimulation of certain muscles about the joint, or it may be that there is some common cause for the contractures and the exaggerated reflexes. In the case of posthemiplegic contractures it is usually the least paralyzed muscles that present this contraction. Mann would explain this peculiarity in this way. The nervous impulse that regulates a voluntary movement is of dual nature. It not only initiates contraction of certain groups of muscles but also inhibits the activity of the opposing sets of muscles. Consequently, a cerebral lesion will not only cause paralysis of the corresponding muscles but it interferes with the inhibitory impulses sent to their antagonists.

Convulsions.—We have already referred to generalized convulsions and then spoke of the two types, the clonic, in which there are alternate contractions and relaxations of the muscles with corresponding movements of the body, and tonic, in which the muscles maintain for a length of time their contracted condition and the parts involved become rigid. The exciting cause appears to be some irritative lesion of the cerebral motor cortex or of the descending motor fibres. While such convulsive attacks may involve the whole body they may be confined to certain parts of it and may not be associated with loss of consciousness. We then speak of Jacksonian epilepsy. Such attacks are usually associated with a lesion limited to a comparatively small area of the cortex. Thus, a tumor in the motor area, a hemorrhage, or, as in one case we sectioned, a small cluster of tubercles, may produce convulsive movements of only a small number of muscles. At other times, a whole limb, or one side of the body may be affected. When such seizures begin in some particular part we are able to get valuable diagnostic information. Not infrequently the process spreads from its original starting point and becomes more widespread or even general. Such movements seem to be explainable on the grounds of, in many cases, cortical irritation for they may be reproduced experimentally by stimulating parts of the motor area with an electrode.

Disturbances of Sensation.—The mechanism of our sensory perceptions is of the utmost importance. Our whole knowledge of the external world is due to centripetal nervous impulses. It is not too much to say that without these thought would be impossible and there could hardly be said to be any conscious existence. The influence of excitations of physical sense upon mental processes is among the most alluring problems of psychology and opens up a wide field which we regret being unable to enter here. But peripheral impressions exert a not inconsiderable effect upon the bodily processes. Light, sound, temperature, all influence circulation, respiration, muscular activity, and general metabolism. The external environment, particularly in matters of climate, physical resources and configuration of a country, have a powerful influence, as all students of ethnology are aware, upon the morale of a nation, their temperament, their endurance, their artistic sense, and even the color of their skin. Sensory impressions, moreover, set up reflexes of great importance to the general economy. Muscular effort is regulated, our sense of locality is developed, the various secretions and excretions are set in operation. The sight and smell of food stimulate the flow of saliva; chilling of the skin excites an increased discharge of urine, the presence of solid matter in the intestine bring about its contraction, to cite but two or three instances.

The sensory nerve apparatus consists of three parts: the terminal end-plate, the conducting fibres, and the receptive and perceptive centre in the brain. Disturbance in any one of these three structures results in disordered function. Damage to the end-plate, interruption in the conducting paths, destruction of the central receiving station or its connections, bring about either a perverted sensation or prevent it being perceived at all.

The resisting power of nervous tissue varies greatly. As a rule, sensory fibres are less susceptible to injury than are the motor. Thus, in a compression myelitis, while we may have a complete paralysis of the muscles innervated from the district affected, the sensory fibres are merely irritated and may at most convey the sense of pain (*paraplegia dolorosa*). While, again, the paralyses resulting from disease of the motor nerves gives us an accurate idea of the localization of the lesion, this is not always the case with the sensory nerves. Pain is not always referred to the point at which it is produced. Witness the pain at times experienced in the knee-joint from tuberculous disease of the hip, and the pains in the rectum, hips, and legs in chronic prostatitis. In general, where a lesion involves a sensory nerve trunk the pain is referred to its peripheral termination. There is, however, this analogy with the motor nerves that the disturbances are also paralytic and irritative.

We can best discuss this portion of our subject by taking up in turn the five primary sensations—sight, hearing, tasting, smelling, and cutaneous impressions.

Sight.—Anomalies of vision are due to disturbances in the refracting media, imperfect action of the various muscles, and lesions in the optic tract. The first-mentioned do not concern us especially here. Spasms or paralyses of the muscles controlling the movements of the eyeball are often of importance in the diagnosis of disease of the nervous system. They indicate often not only affections of the nerve trunks concerned in the innervation, but also abnormal conditions at the base of the brain or in the nervous centres. The superior oblique muscle is supplied by the fourth nerve; the external rectus, by the sixth nerve; the remaining muscles of the orbit, as also the iris and ciliary muscle, by the third. Gross lesions in the neighborhood of the pons, the floor of the fourth ventricle, and the aqueduct of Sylvius, are apt to involve one or more of these nerves. In this connection may be mentioned partieularly basal meningitis and tumors. Tabes dorsalis and general paresis not infrequently are accompanied by squint, inequality of the pupils, myosis, and the Argyll-Robertson phenomenon.

Lesions of the optic tract may involve its end-organ, the retina, the trunk of the optic nerve, the chiasm, and the cerebral centres. More or less diminution in the size and alteration in the shape of the field of vision may result from retinal lesions, particularly anemia, detachment, and the various forms of retinitis. Color vision may be affected in some cases more than light perception. The various lesions cencerned here are dealt with at length on page 666 *et sequitur.*

The changes in the optic papilla are also of great diagnostic importance. They are due to edema and inflammation, and we speak of optic neuritis, neuroretinitis, papillitis, or choked disk. Neuroretinitis occurs in Bright's disease and occasionally in diabetes. Papillitis and optic neuritis (see p. 676) are commonly the results of increased intracerebral pressure. They are seen, consequently, in meningitis, cerebral abscesses and tumors, in sinus thrombosis and in hydrocephalus When unilateral they may be due to orbital disease, various infections and intoxications, and in beginning tumor. Retrobulbar neuritis is met with in various infections (rheumatism) and intoxications (alcohol. tobacco, diabetes), in orbital conditions, insular sclerosis, and the extension of inflammation from the cranial cavity. In these conditions vision suffers considerably, and complete blindness from optic atrophy may result. Color vision is apt to be lost quicker than ordinary light perception.

We may, perhaps, at this point refer to certain terms which it is essential for us to be acquainted with. Complete blindness is spoken of as *anopsia* or *amaurosis*. It may affect one or both eyes. Defective light perception (due to nerve disturbances) is called *amblyopia* or *hypopsia;* increased acuity of vision (also of nervous origin) is *hyperopsia*. Small defects in the visual field, not reaching to the periphery, are known as *scotomata.* A central scotoma is one situated at or near the fixation point. A relative scotoma involves only the sensations of red and green and is due to a chronic retrobulbar neuritis limited to the papillo-macular bundle. It is most often due to poisoning with tobacco and alcohol. An absolute scotoma is one in which there is absolutely no perception of light over the defect. It is met with in diabetes, in insular sclerosis, and occasionally without any obvious cause. When one-half of each visual field is non-functioning we have *hemianopsia.* If the two right halves or the two left halves be involved we speak of *homonymous* hemianopsia. We see this in lesions of the visual sense area in the cortex, in occipito-thalamic radiation, or involvement of one optic tract. If the two nasal halves or the two temporal halves be affected we speak of *heteronymous* hemianopsia. In the latter case there is a lesion of the chiasm. Analogous defects affecting color vision rather than plain vision are called *hemichromatopsia.* .

Impairment of vision may, again, result from disturbance in the cerebral centres. This may be functional or organic. An example of the former is met with in some cases of hysteria in which the fields of vision may be notably contracted. This leads us to the consideration of some extraordinary phenomena which are classed under the term *sensory aphasia* or *apraxia*. *Mind-blindness* is the condition in which, while the patient is able to see perfectly, the visual image conveys no meaning to his mind or, in other words, fails to call up object memories. Such an individual may look at an object and have no idea of its name or use. Memory may be awakened, however, through another sense, as, for example, the sense of touch. In one particular form, *word-blindness*, the patient is unable to understand written or printed language. He can pronounce the words, may even write correctly, but is unable to read understandingly what he has written. In such cases the lesion is not in the nucleus of the optic nerve but in the so-called secondary or higher visual centre, situated in the posterior end of the inferior parietal convolution, particularly in the neighborhood of the the angular gyrus.

Hearing.—Total deafness is known as *anacusis;* partial, as *hypacusis;* increased delicacy of hearing, *hyperacusis.* Defective hearing is usually brought about by lesions in the internal ear, labyrinth and vestibule, or from occlusion of the Eustachian tube. Deafness may also be due to tumors or inflammatory deposits about the auditory nerve. The central auditory paths are bilateral in design, owing to the semidecussations at the corpus trapezoideum, the lemniscus lateralis on each side containing conduction paths from both ears. Lesions involving the lemniscus lateralis, or the colliculus inferior, or, again, higher up, affecting the medial geniculate bodies or the auditory radiations, cause partial deafness in both ears. Painful sensations, when sounds are heard, are observed in affections of the middle and internal ears, in otitic paralysis of the facial nerve, in trigeminal neuralgia, in migraine, and in some psychoneuroses. In *mind-deafness* the patient may hear sounds but is unable to recognize them. The most frequent form of this is word-deafness. The patient can hear spoken language but is unable to comprehend it. In such cases the lesion is in the first temporal convolution on the left side.

Taste.—Anomalies in the matter of taste have not been sufficiently studied for us to have much information. It is hardly possible for the nerve of taste to be involved without involvement of others in close association with it. While the question has been debated, it seems most probable that the nerves concerned in taste run along with the glossopharyngeal. Disturbances of taste have been observed in lesions of the middle ear, owing to involvement of the tympanic plexus. They also occur in some forms of hysteria and in association with gustatory hallucinations. Complete inability to taste is called *ageusia;* a deficient sense is *hypogeusia;* an overdelicacy is *hypergeusia.*

Smell.— Here we have analogous conditions, *anosmia, hyposmia,* and *hyperosmia.* Anosmia may be due to physical obstruction in the air passages, nostrils, fossæ and choanæ. Chronic inflammatory and atrophic conditions of the upper portion of the nasal mucosa may give rise to anosmia or hyposmia. Also, intracranial lesions involving the olfactory tracts and centres. The centre for smell is situated in the uncinate gyrus on the same side, and probably to a lesser degree on the opposite side. Lesions of this region have been observed in cases of epilepsy with olfactory auræ. The left-sided anosmia found occasionally in right-sided hemiplegia is said to be due to a lesion in the lateral root of the olfactory tract. Anosmia has also been met with in hysteria, cerebellar disease, and as a congenital anomaly.

Cutaneous Sensation.—The sensations derived from the skin are concerned with pressure, pain, and temperature. The fact that any one of these can be disturbed and the observation that certain portions of the skin are sensitive to pressure and certain others to pain, go far to prove that there exist special end-plates and nerve fibres for each kind of stimulation. Cutaneous sensations may be affected in three ways: by damage to the end-plates, to the nerve fibres, or to the cerebral centres. The character and the distribution of the sensory phenomena is often of the greatest assistance in diagnosis. Destruction of the peripheral sense-organs, or end-plates, occurs in a great many skin affections characterized by inflammation or fibrosis and must, naturally, interfere with the conduction of sensations from the parts, but comparatively little is known with certainty upon the matter. Lesions affecting the conduction paths may occur in the peripheral nerve trunks, the cord, or brain. In the case of first-mentioned, the different skin sensations may be affected in varying degrees and we consequently get partial anesthesias produced. But, apparently, the different orders of sensory fibres pass through different spinal tracts, and we find that a small, well-localized lesion may involve some of them and leave others alone. We do not know completely the course of the various fibres in question through the central nervous system. Some of them undoubtedly cross by way of the anterior commissure to the opposite side of the cord soon after they enter it. In this way we explain the Brown-Séquard phenomenon. If one-half of the cord be destroyed the muscles on the same side below the level of the lesion will be paralyzed, and there will also be a deficiency in the sense of position, and at the same time the cutaneous sensations on the opposite side of the body are interrupted. In the brain, the centripetal sensory fibres communicate with various reflex and automatic centres and some terminate in the cortex, apparently near the motor areas, for in lesions of the motor cortex we usually find a certain amount of diminution of sensibility in the paralyzed portions of the body, though this is far from being complete.

The delicacy of the central perceptions of peripheral stimulation varies, however, in different cases, being dependent apparently in large measure upon the number and distribution of the tactile corpuscles or end-bulbs. In regard to the skin the power of localization is quite accurate, though certain regions, such as the face, are much more sensitive than others, the back for example. In the case of the internal viscera, localization is somewhat defective and unreliable. Pain, for example, is not always felt in the region where it is produced. The sensation due to a lesion of a nerve trunk is often referred to the periphery (law of excentric localization). Instances of this might be multiplied. Thus, the pain produced by abscess of the liver is often felt in the right shoulder; that due to renal calculus may be felt down the leg; pain in the knee may be due to·disease of the hip joint; sensory stimuli may be referred to the opposite side of the body (*allocheiria*), as in tabes dorsalis.

Comparatively little attention has been given to the relationships existing between deep-seated visceral lesions and peripheral disturbances of sensation. While the subjective sensations of the patient in such cases are indefinite and often misleading, there can be little doubt that a careful examination of the cutaneous sensibility and the accurate delimitation of areas of referred pain will often give valuable information. Some years ago Head, in a most valuable and instructive series of papers,[1] pointed out that certain definite regions of the skin to which spontaneous pain was referred, which were also hypersensitive to pressure, were related to one another and also to visceral disease. Thus, particular areas in the scalp are correlated to definite somatic segments and both to affections of deeply seated organs. Lack of space prevents us entering into this subject farther, much as we would like to do so, but the reader is strongly advised to consult the original papers.

Complete lack of perception of sensory stimuli we speak of as *anesthesia;* diminished perception, as *hypesthesia;* increased perception, as *hyperesthesia;* perverted quality of the perception, as *paresthesia* or *dysesthesia.*

1. Anomalies of the sense of touch or pressure: It is questionable if true hyperesthesia of the sense of touch has been observed. The idea that overstimulation of the nerves of touch causes pain is erroneous. As above pointed out, the nerves concerned in pain production are different from those of touch. Anesthesia and hypesthesia to touch are observed in diseases like peripheral neuritis and tabes dorsalis, in which the peripheral sensory fibres or posterior nerve roots are involved, or where the posterior columns of the cord are diseased; in lesions in the posterior third of the posterior limb of the internal capsule; and in lesions of the motor cortex, for reasons adduced above; in hysteria, from central inhibition. The anesthesias of functional nature can often be differentiated by the fact that they present a distribution of so erratic or so extensive a nature that their presence connot be accounted for by any focal lesion. Thus, the whole body below the neck may be insensitive to touch or pain; or, again, both hands may be involved as far as the wrists ("glove anesthesia"). Under paresthesias may be classed pruritus or itching, which appears to be due to a toxic irritation of the nerve terminals; and formication, or creeping or tingling sensations.

2. Anomalies of the temperature sense: These sometimes accompany anomalies of the sense of touch but not necessarily so. Indeed,

---

[1] Brain, 16:1893:1; ibid., 17:1894:339; ibid., 19:1896:158.

this dissociation of sensations may extend to temperature, for a patient may have a diminished sensibility to heat and an increased one to cold (as sometimes in tabes dorsalis), or one temperature sense may be normal and the other abnormal. Subjective disturbances are common. We may cite the *chill* that is so often the initial symptom in infections, and the *hot flushes* that occur in some psychoneuroses, in exophthalmic goitre, in paralysis agitans, and at the commencement of the menopause.

3. Anomalies of the sensation of pain: These are common. Spontaneous pain is felt in many diseases, such as neuritis, tabes dorsalis, certain visceral affections, and psychoneuroses. Anesthesia to pain is called *analgesia;* hypesthesia is *hypalgesia;* hyperesthesia is *hyperalgesia.* When spontaneous pain is felt in an area insensitive to touch, we speak of analgesia dolorosa. In syringomyelia, in which disease tactile sensibility is well preserved, there may be complete analgesia, particularly of the extremities. Here the lesion is in the central region of the cord. A curious anomaly is delayed perception of painful impressions. In tabes dorsalis, for example, a pin prick may be felt as a simple tactile sensation some moments before the sense of pain is experienced.

Deep Sensation.—Under this heading we include all the various sensations derived from the muscles, bones, joints, and viscera. Most of these, as hunger, thirst, satiety, gastralgia, fatigue, and the libido sexualis, we can only mention here, reserving our remarks for the more important.

(*a*) The sense of position may be disturbed. If, for example, a limb be placed in a given position this can only imperfectly be reproduced by its fellow member. We see this in neuritis and tabes dorsalis.

(*b*) The sense of movement may be disturbed. Thus, either passive movements are not felt at all, or greater excursions than normal have to be brought about before the movement is recognized.

(*c*) The sense of resistance and weight may be disturbed. Weights, hardness, softness, and textures are misjudged. This often goes with alterations in the sense of movement.

(*d*) Stereognostic perception, the ability to recognize the nature of objects by feeling, may be disturbed. This sense may be lost even when the senses of touch, temperature, and pain are unaffected. Astereognosis is frequent in hemianesthesia due to cerebral disease, and is more likely to be present if the lesion be in the cortex, rather than in the internal capsule, pons, or medulla. It is found also in tabes and peripheral neuritis, provided that the sensory fibres from the upper extremities are involved, and may be a symptom of hysteria.

(*e*) The sense of perception of vibration may be disturbed. The test with the tuning-fork shows that insensibility of the bones in this particular exists in a considerable number of affections, such as tabes dorsalis, syringomyelia, hematomyelia, Brown-Séquard paralysis, myelitis, neuritis, cerebral hemianesthesias, and hysteria.

The Orientation of Our Bodies in Space.—We are now prepared to obtain a clear understanding of how we derive information as to the position of our bodies in space. This is done through the influence of coördinated peripheral sensory impressions. These impressions emanate from·the skin, muscles, tendons, bones, joints, the eyes, and the internal ear. We are not necessarily conscious of the operation of these various factors, but they all have more or less effect upon our powers of orientation. Perhaps the most important in this connection are the sensations derived from labyrinth of the ear and from the eye. The disorders at work may involve the peripheral sensory apparatus, the cerebral centres, or the cerebellum.

It is a well-known fact that when one sense is lost or diminished another will become more delicate through use and so compensate the disability. When this is the case the power of orientation in space may not be noticeably impaired. Thus, a blind man can move about with considerable precision provided he can use his sense of touch. A deafmute may, by education, become almost independent of his loss of hearing. Where education has not taken place notable results will follow disturbances of certain sets of impressions. Thus, a tabetic, who lacks some of his sensory impulses coming from the legs, depends greatly upon his sense of sight. If he shuts his eyes he immediately begins to sway (Romberg symptom) or may even fall down.

When one set of sensations conflicts with another we are apt to get a disturbance of equilibrium which we speak of as *vertigo*. This may result, for example, from the confusion of images produced by ocular paralyses of squints, or when the image in one eye is sharp while blurred in the other. Again, rotating the body about its axis, swinging, rolling, or pitching, as at sea, passing a galvanic current through the head from ear to ear, all will produce giddiness. owing to stimulation of the nerve of the labyrinth. In aural vertigo (Menière's disease) there is equally some disturbance of hearing as well, and the condition is due to some local irritation of the vestibular and cochlear nerves.

Vertigo may also be produced by cerebral irritation and pressure, cerebral anemia, and disturbances of cerebral circulation.

Associated with giddiness, not infrequently, are vomiting, muscular incoördination, and peculiar movements of the eyes.

We can pass on now with advantage to the consideration of reflex action, in which peripheral impressions play also a notable part.

On Reflex Action.—The pathologic disturbances of the reflexes often give us valuable information as to the nature of mental and nervous disease. In a pure reflex, sensory impulses produce an immediate excitation of the motor apparatus without the intervention of the will. The reflex arc consists of the sensory apparatus, the motor apparatus, and the connections between them. These connections are situated in the brain, the cord, or in the sympathetic system. Three classes of reflexes merit special consideration: the pupillary, the deep, and the superficial.

The eye reflexes are two, the light reflex and the reflex for accommodation and convergence. The light reflex may be abolished or absent in partial or complete blindness (amaurosis or amblyopia) and in paralysis of the sphincter muscle of the iris, that is to say, where there is a lesion of the optic tract or of the motor oculi. When the pupils do not react to light but react to accommodation and convergence we have what is known as the Argyll-Robertson pupil. The phenomenon is usually bilateral but may be unilateral. Its presence is of great diagnostic significance in tabes dorsalis and dementia paralytica. The pupils, again, may react neither to light nor accommodation (complete *ophthalmoplegia interna*). This is met with in brain tumor, tabes, and dementia paralytica, and not infrequently in cerebral syphilis.

Abnormal contraction of the pupils (*myosis*) occurs in opium poisoning, and in paralysis of the sympathetic nerve or irritation of the motor oculi. Abnormal dilatation (*mydriasis*) is seen in atropine and cocaine poisoning, in atrophy of the optic nerve, in irritation of the sympathetic nerve, and paralysis of the motor oculi.

Inequality of the pupils (*anisocoria*) may be due to unequal illumination or differing errors of refraction, but it may indicate a unilateral lesion of the optic, sympathetic, or motor oculi nerves. It is also often found in tabes dorsalis and dementia paralytica.

The reflexes that arise from the tendons, periosteum and bones are called the deep reflexes. The chief are, the knee-jerk, the Achilles reflex, and the periosteal radial reflex. Others are, the tibial, biceps and triceps reflexes, and the jaw-jerk. They tend to be increased during fatigue, and in marasmus and cachexia. Exaggeration may also be due to irritation of the sensory portion of the arc, as in neuritis and meningitis; to stimulation of the ganglion cells of the anterior horns, as in strychnine poisoning; or, possibly, to removal of inhibitory influences proceeding from the cerebrum or subcortical centres, as in neurasthenia and lateral sclerosis. The reflexes are abolished in all cases where the reflex arc is interrupted, whether in the sensory or motor portions or in the central connections. We find this, for example, in many forms of peripheral neuritis (*e. g.*, diphtherial and diabetic) in certain cerebellar lesions, in anterior poliomyelitis, and, notably, in tabes dorsalis. It should be remarked in this connection, however, that it is possible for the reflexes to be abolished without the reflex arc being completely interrupted. The path is only blocked sufficiently to prevent the elicitation of the reflexes under ordinary conditions. In such cases, a cerebral lesion which would ordinarily cause an exaggerated response may cause the lost reflex to return.

The superficial reflexes have quite a different significance from the deep ones. In fact, the former may be absent when the latter are exaggerated. On the whole, the responses are more powerful, slower, and more under the control of the will in the case of the superficial reflexes. The chief are: the plantar, the cremasteric, and the abdominal.

Normally when the sole of the foot is tickled the corresponding limb is drawn quickly up. More important is the fact that plantar stimulation is followed normally by plantar flexion of the toes. When the lateral tract is injured, however, we get dorsal flexion instead, and particularly dorsal flexion of the great toe (Babinski's phenomenon). In such cases, also, the great toe moves sluggishly, and there may be a spreading movement of the other toes.

Somewhat similar is Oppenheim's sign. This is elicited by rubbing the median aspect of the tibia downward toward the malleolus with the flat of the thumb or the handle of a percussion hammer.

The cremasteric reflex is obtained by stroking the inner side of the thigh in the adductor region. This is followed by elevation of the testis on the same side. The abdominal reflex is produced by stroking the skin of the abdomen on one side either above or below the level of the umbilicus.

The superficial reflexes, it is worthy of note, are particularly apt to be disturbed in unilateral cerebral lesions.

Before leaving this part of our subject we may perhaps refer briefly to nervous disturbances of the functions of defecation and urination. In the infant these functions are purely reflex, but through training the individual comes to manifest a considerable amount of cerebral control. The stimulus to contraction of the bladder or rectum comes in large part, though not altogether, from distension of these organs. The reflex centres are in the sympathetic system and not in the cord, as has usually been taught. If the impulses from the cerebrum are interrupted then voluntary control over urination and defecation is lost. We see this frequently in severe infectious diseases, such as typhoid, in which we often find incontinence. Or, again, the bladder may remain full and continually overflow (incontinence from retention). A lesion in the centripetal paths from the bladder may lead to slowness or difficulty in passing the stream, or may cause complete retention. A lesion in the motor path leading to paresis of the detrusor, will cause an identical train of symptoms, or if to a paresis of the sphincter, to a continuous dribbling. Irritation of the tracts connecting the reflex centre with the cerebrum may cause retention of urine from spasm of the sphincter.

Ataxia.—Closely connected with this subject of the reflexes and dependent upon it is that of incoördination or ataxia.

Every voluntary act is dependent for its perfect performance on the harmonious working of a most complex mechanism. Normally, to carry out any purposeful movement we require the simultaneous and successive action of certain groups of muscles which are accustomed to act together and are hence called synergists, contraction of some muscles (agonists) and relaxation of others (antagonists). The association of these contractions, their succession, and their force have all to be carefully regulated before we can attain the desired end. Disturbances of the regulating apparatus lead to those anomalies of movement that we call incoördination or ataxia. The movements that have to be executed differ considerably in character. There are some that can be performed at will, others can only be learned by practice. Repetition, however, tends to make even the most difficult movements easy. At first they are carried out under the conscious direction of all the senses, notably those of sight, touch, and position, and are executed clumsily, but by practice the various constituent movements of the act are carried out without conscious initiation or regulation; in other words, they become automatic. So, there is a gradation of movements from those that must be learned to those that are entirely volitional, and from these again, to those that are involuntary and reflex.

The movements under discussion may be initiated in three ways: by the will, by nervous impulses from the periphery, and by certain obscure internal chemical changes. In cases of ataxia the lesions at work operate upon some portion of the reflex arc or upon certain cortical centres, or, again, upon the sensory fibres passing through the cerebellum. As a rule, there is not much weakness in ataxic muscles, though they may be hypertonic, and both from clinical observation and from experiment it would seem certain that peripheral sensory impressions are of more importance in regulating muscular movements than are efferent motor impulses. Beevor and Horsley[1] have shown that electrical stimulation of the cortical motor area give rise to movements, not of individual muscles but of concerted groups, so that they conclude that in the cortex movements rather than individual muscles are represented. Other groupings of muscles occur in the cells of the anterior horns of the spinal cord and in the root fibres. The amount of coördinative power so derived is, however, not sufficient for the execution of the more complex acts. It is here that the importance of the afferent sensory impulses comes in. Not only the special senses, but both the superficial and deep sensations come into play. The most important of these for the purpose in hand are the sensations emanating from the eyes, the tendons, bones, and muscles. It is possible for ataxia to exist without demonstrable deficiency of the superficial sensations of pressure, pain, and temperature, but careful study, as Fränkel proved,[2] will show that in all cases some interference with the deeper sensory impressions exists, particularly those arising in the bones and joints. In tabes dorsalis, in which muscular incoördination is a striking feature, the loss of the tendon reflexes, the loss of the sense of position, and diminution in muscular tonus play a leading role. Contrariwise, it is possible for the most extreme anesthesias of the skin and deeper structures to be present without there being true ataxia. This has been noted in hysterical patients, but here the findings have to be interpreted with some caution. Probably in such cases there is an inhibition of the cerebral centres, so that the patients have been able, unconsciously, to make use of the sensory stimulations coming from the periphery.

It should be remarked that in cases of muscular incoördination an attempt is often made to compensate the loss of the centripetal impulses by directing the movements through the higher centres. Under such circumstances the act is usually performed with more difficulty than an automatically executed movement. Again, if the sensory impulses from the periphery be not all cut off the affected individual may learn to utilize those that are left to a greater degree than formerly and so a new automatic regulation may be developed.

Disturbances of the Nervous Mechanism of Secretion.—We have very little accurate information as to the true nature of the stimulation

[1] Philosoph. Trans., 181:129.
[2] Neurologisches Zentralbl., 15 and 16:1897.

resulting in glandular secretion. It has been shown beyond much question, in case of the salivary glands and the kidneys, at all events, that the nervous supply is in part vasomotor and in part secretory. It is a fact, moreover, that the function of secretion in a gland is accompanied by a condition of active hyperemia. Both hyperemia and secretion can be brought about, for example, in the submaxillary gland, by stimulation of the chorda tympani. Much seems to depend on questions of blood pressure and more even upon the rate of the blood flow, but experiment would seem to indicate that vasomotor influences are not everything. Probably they have to do with the production of the more watery constituents of the secretion, while the solid dissolved elements are the result of nervous stimulation of the specific secreting cells. We do not know altogether, however, how the latter form of stimulation is brought about, whether by reflex irritation or in some other way. Recent work would go to show that there are specific excitants or hormones which, circulating in the blood, are carried to the glands and bring about secretion. This, at least, is known to be the case in regard to the tryptic ferment of the pancreas. But as yet we cannot say whether this result is due to the action of the hormone directly upon the secreting cells or indirectly by stimulating the secretory nerve terminals. In some cases, as for example the salivary glands, the nerve fibres concerned are in part of cranial origin and in part derived from the sympathetic system. Wherever the centres governing the processes of secretion may be situated, it is a matter of common observation that they are to a large extent under the governance of the higher cerebral centres. Our mental states exert a great influence here. Many men can remember the horrors of their maiden speech, the mental inhibition, the dryness of the mouth, and the difficulty in articulation. "Nervousness" does not always, however, produce this inhibition of secretion, but sometimes the contrary. Witness the polyuria of the student waiting for his oral examination and the sweating of the witness under the searching cross-examination of the counsel. The flow and character of the gastric juice, also, is to some extent dependent on central conditions.

The Trophoneuroses.—A great variety of disorders are met with which are dependent on the loss of nutritive impulses emanating from the nerve centres. These involve particularly the muscles, bones, joints, and skin with its appendages. We have seen that when a nerve fibre is separated from its ganglion cell it immediately begins to degenerate. A similar thing occurs in other tissues wherever either the nutritive impulse is lacking or when it cannot be conveyed along the efferent fibres to the part in question. In anterior poliomyelitis, for instance, where the lesion is in the ganglion cells of the anterior horns of the spinal cord, we can get a pure neurotrophic atrophy of the corresponding muscular fibres. Not only this, if the disease occur in childhood, we find a notable interference with the processes of growth and development and sometimes a whole limb will remain stunted. In some cases, muscular atrophy may, to some extent, be attributable to disuse or to the extension of inflammation from the bones and joints, but these considerations cannot explain all cases. Furthermore, bones may become light and brittle, as in tabes and syringomyelia. Disintegration of the joints with effusions occur also in both the affections just mentioned. Atrophy of the skin takes place in certain affections of the peripheral nerves, in tabes and syringomyelia, and in some spinal affections. Blanching and falling of the hair, loss of the teeth, irregularities in the growth of the nails also result from atrophic disorders. The bed-sore, while in some cases due to pressure and infection, can undoubtedly occur as the result of trophic disturbances alone. Akin to this is the perforating ulcer of the foot in tabes and syringomyelia.

CHAPTER XXVI.

THE BRAIN.

CONGENITAL ANOMALIES.

Vices of development may be conveniently and naturally classified under the headings of (1) Agenesy, (2) Hypoplasia, (3) Hyperplasia, and (4) Heteroplasia.

Agenesy.—By the term agenesy we understand such conditions as are brought about by failure of the medullary canal to close, or the lack of formation of certain parts of the nervous system. It is not always possible to draw the line between hypoplasia, in which the parts are formed but lag behind in growth and development, and agenesy, for the two conditions are often associated. It is to be observed that we have

Fig. 133

Fig. 134

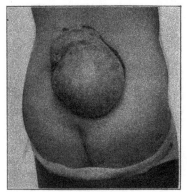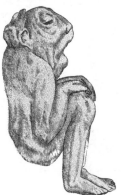

Spina bifida. (From the Surgical Clinic of the Montreal General Hospital.)

Anencephaly.

to do with two main types in agenesy, one in which the defect involves the bony structures as well as the nervous elements, and the other, in which the abnormality is confined to the nervous system.

Perhaps the most interesting and important condition here is that in which the medullary groove fails to close posteriorly. The vertebral arches, the muscles, and integument of the back are not formed, so that there is a broad furrow along the dorsal aspect of the head and trunk.

On the exposed surface there may be recognized rudimentary nerve substance, covered with cylindrical epithelium, which corresponds to that ordinarily lining the ventricles and neural canal, and the anterior portion of a highly vascularized pia-arachnoid and dura. The anterior portion of the brain is usually fairly well developed, but the base of the skull and the spinal column are abnormally curved. This condition is called **craniorhachischisis**. Frequently, the malformation is not so extensive, affecting only the head, **cranioschisis**, or the cord, **rhachischisis** (**spina bifida**, vide vol. i, p. 265).

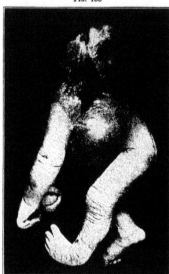

Iniencephaly.   (McGill Medical Museum.)

In cranioschisis (hemicephaly; acrania) the vault of the skull is completely or partially defective, giving to the head of the fœtus a characteristic cat-like or toad-like appearance. The brain substance may be absent (**anencephaly**), or present in rudimentary form. Several varieties of this malformation may occur.

In some cases the defect of the skull is not so extensive, but is limited to particular localities, while the integument is almost, if not entirely, closed in. In this way is formed a pouch or sac, which contains, according to circumstances, a diverticulum of the membranes together with fluid (**meningocele**), a portion of the brain (**encephalocele**), or both (**meningo-encephalocele; hernia cerebri**). The most common situation is in the median line, and usually in the occipital region (**meningo-encephalocele occipitalis**), or at the glabella (**meningo-encephalocele sincipitalis**, etc.). Occasionally, the defects are found at the vertex or the lateral and inferior portions of the cranium. Some of these cases probably differ etiologically from those just mentioned. They are believed to be due to traction of an adherent amnion on the skull.

In **encephalocele** the sac contains membranes and brain-substance, but no fluid. Sometimes an occipital encephalocele contains the greater part of the brain and forms a relatively enormous pouch hanging down the back (**notencephaly**).

Analogous to the malformations of the brain just referred to, we have a corresponding series confined to the cord and spinal column. These have already been discussed (vol. i, p. 265.)

Allied to the conditions we have just described is dilatation of the central neural canal. The ventricles of the brain may be dilated and filled with fluid (**hydrocephalus internus congenitus**), or there may be a diffuse dilatation of the central canal of the cord (**hydromyelocele; syringomyelocele; myelocystocele; hydrorrhachis interna**).

In congenital internal hydrocephalus, there is either a uniform or a cystic dilatation of the ventricles. The brain is distended, and its substance may be reduced to a thin sheet. The lining epithelium of the neural canal can usually be recognized here and there on the inner wall of the sac. The bones of the cranium are often separated one from the other, so that the head is enlarged, and defects of ossification may also be found. In rare cases, rupture of the sac takes place at birth or during intra-uterine life, thus producing a secondary cranioschisis. Virchow[1] has described local dilatations of the ventricles, analogous to the circumscribed dilatation of the cord known as myelocystocele. Of these may be mentioned, **hydrops of the fourth and fifth ventricles**, and **hydrops cysticus cornu posterioris.**

The local dilatations of the cord—**myelocystocele**—are associated with defects in the fusion of the arches or bodies of the vertebræ, and are due to accumulation of fluid within the central canal at such points. The wall of the sac is composed of spinal substance and the meninges. The cavity is lined with epithelium continuous with that of the central canal.

Anencephaly.—Complete absence of the brain, anencephaly, is usually associated with acrania, and occasionally with absence of the spinal cord (amyelia). At times there is an abortive attempt at the formation of a pons, medulla, and cord.

Cyclencephaly.—One of the most curious forms of agenesy is cyclencephaly, of which various degrees exist. In this, the anterior portion of the prosencephalon is the part involved. The normal division into two hemispheres does not take place and the cerebrum appears as a single cyst-wall enclosing a more or less enlarged ventricle. In some cases the eyes are fused into a single organ, situated in the middle of the forehead (*cyclopia*) and provided with a single optic nerve. The nose may be rudimentary or absent. The lower jaw and the bones of the face are absent, and the ears may be situated lower down than normal. In the less extensive deformity, the two eyes may be separate, although closely approximated and lying in a single orbit, or partially fused (**synophthalmia**). (Vide vol. i, p. 260.)

Arhinencephaly.—Defect of the olfactory bulbs—arhinencephaly—has been described. A great variety of malformations are frequently associated with this condition, such as rudimentary formation of the nose, harelip, cleft palate, and absence of the olfactory nerves, synotia, accessory auricles, anomalies of the heart and great vessels, umbilical hernia, defects of the diaphragm, and supernumerary digits.

Agyria.—Not uncommonly, defective development of the prosencephalon manifests itself in partial or complete absence of the convolutions (agyria), or of larger portions of the brain substance, or, again, of the commissures.

[1] Die krankhaften Geschwülste, 1:1863, Berlin; also Virch. Archiv, 27:1863:575.

Most frequently the corpus callosum, fornix, the soft commissure of the third ventricle, and the corpora candicantia are lacking. In absence of the corpus callosum, there is usually defect of the gyrus fornicatus and gyrus hippocampi, as well as other anomalies in the convolutions. Where considerable amounts of the external portion of the cerebrum fail to develop, we get fissures or deep excavations, usually in the central or lateral aspects of the brain, which are bridged over by the arachnoid, while the pia dips down and covers over the base. In such cases fluid accumulates in the cavity in the subarachnoid space, or sometimes in the meshes of the pia and in the subdural space. Defects of this kind, due to primary errors of development, constitute one form of what is known as **porencephaly.** Lesions not unlike them, however, are occasionally produced by trauma, vascular disturbances, or inflammation (*secondary porencephaly*).

Extensive defects of the brain, such as acrania and anencephaly lead to imperfect development of the cord (**atelomyelia**). In such cases it may be abnormally short. Again, when portions of the brain are lacking, the neurones of which are ordinarily continued into the cord, we get symmetrical or asymmetrical aplasia of the corresponding spinal tracts. The spinal cord may be entirely absent (**amyelia**). In this case it is said that the posterior ganglia and the sensory nerves may be perfectly developed (Lionowa).

Hypoplasia.—The weight of the adult human brain varies within wide limits. The average may be struck at 1400 grams in the male, and about 1300 in the female. As examples of extreme limits might be mentioned the brain of a Bushwoman (871 grams) and that of v. Turgenieff (2012 grams). Under pathological conditions, however, these figures may be widely exceeded. Thus, Ziegler[1] figures the brain of a microcephalic idiot, Helene Becker, which weighed only 219 grams, and Van Walsem[2] describes that of an epileptic idiot which reached the almost incredible weight of 2850 grams. In determining the proper weight of the brain in any given case, age, sex, race, and body weight should be considered. The brain takes on its most rapid growth during the first year of life, and reaches, practically, its maximum at the age of seven or eight. After about fifty it begins to decrease. The white races have larger brains than the black; the male than the female. In healthy human beings, according to Quain, the proportionate weight of the brain as compared with the body as a whole is 1 to 45.

Hypoplasia might be defined as a condition of the brain in which, while the parts present the normal configuration, the size and weight of the brain fall notably short of the normal average, laying, of course, due stress upon the considerations mentioned above. As a matter of fact, however, hypoplasia is usually associated with other peculiarities of development, such as local agenesy, imperfect or irregular formation of the convolutions, and structural changes in the nervous substance.

---

[1] Lehrbuch der speciellen pathologischen Anatomie, Jena, 1895:321.
[2] Neurol. Centralbl., 13 : 1899 : 578.

Microcephaly.—Hypoplasia of the brain, as a whole, occurs, and may be associated with a corresponding smallness of the cranium (microcephaly). The condition is often apparent at birth, but becomes more obtrusive as the general somatic development goes on. In some cases, the adult brain does not reach the size of that of the newborn child. As a rule, the skull presents premature synostosis of certain of the sutures with corresponding asymmetry, and other peculiarities of ossification, such as Wormian bones. The brain itself is not only small, but the scheme of the convolutions is much less complex than in the case of normal brains. The condition is often familial.

Micrencephaly.—In another class of cases the brain is disproportionately small, as compared with the size of the cranium (micrencephaly). This is generally associated with an abnormal accumulation of fluid in the subarachnoid space (*hydrocephalus meningeus* sive *externus; meningeal hydrops*), in the ventricles (*hydrops ventricularis* sive *internus*), or both. Some authorities have attributed the hypoplasia of the brain to the presence of this fluid, but while this may be true in some cases, it is more likely that the hydrops is secondary (*hydrops ex vacuo*) in most instances. Undoubtedly, hydrops is frequently associated with anomalies of development both of the brain and skull, such as arhinencephaly and cyclopia. When the brain is small we can speak of *hydrocephalic micrencephaly*. All the ventricles may be dilated or only certain portions of them.

Partial Hypoplasia.—Partial hypoplasia involves usually the hemispheres of the cerebrum and cerebellum, less commonly the corpus callosum and the structures at the base. In the case of the cerebrum, it leads to asymmetry and is generally associated with microgyria or even agenesy of certain convolutions.

Hypoplasia of the brain is most probably due to a primary vitium of development, but in some cases may be the result of pathological processes acting during intra-uterine life. Premature synostosis of the cranial sutures is at work in some instances.

Hypoplasia of the cerebellum may affect the organ as a whole, but is generally unilateral. The condition is associated with hypoplasia of the olivary bodies, pons, and medulla. The transverse fibres in the pyramidal tracts of the pons are absent. In one case, according to Hitzig, unique, the cerebellum was entirely wanting (Cruveilhier and Combetta)

As might be expected, microscopic study of the tissues involved in hypoplasia shows marked deviations from the normal. Certain of the ganglion cells of the cortex are lacking, and corresponding with this is an absence of neuraxones belonging to them. There may be a relative or compensatory increase (*macrencephaly*) in other parts.

Microgyria.—Occasionally, however, the convolutions are particularly numerous but diminutive (microgyria). Or, again, owing to defect of the nervous substance, the convolutions are represented only by membrane. While the hypoplasia is most marked in the cerebrum, the cerebellum and basal structures are to some extent involved. As a consequence we find lack of formation or defect in the medullation of certain fibres in the pons, medulla, and cord, particularly those that become medullated somewhat late, such as the pyramidal tracts and columns of Goll, less often of the anterior columns and cerebellar tracts (*micromyelia; atelomyelia*).

Hydrocephalus.—In not a few cases the accumulation of the cerebrospinal fluid, with dilatation of the ventricles, comes on after the brain is fairly well formed. The condition may arise during intra-uterine existence and the hydrocephalic head prove an obstruction during parturition. The enlargement of the head is not always marked at the first, but gradually increases and may become extreme. The cranium enlarges,

FIG. 136

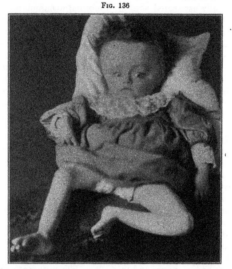

Hydrocephalus; child aged about four years.   Mental condition good.   Diplegia with talipes. Circumference of the head about 28 inches.   (Dr. A. E. Vipond's case.)

the skin is stretched, the subcutaneous veins are prominent, and the fontanelles are enlarged. Finally, the sutures give way, and the cranial bones become separated. The meninges are distended and tense. The dilatation of the ventricles may be so extreme that the substance of the hemispheres is transformed into a thin sac, little being left but the pia-arachnoid. The sulci are obliterated and the convolutions disappear. The basal ganglia are flattened, but the cerebellum usually is unaffected. The fourth ventricle is not, as a rule, dilated. The hydrops may be diffuse and symmetrical, or only one ventricle, or a portion of one ventricle may be involved. Dilatation of the fourth ventricle leads to pressure on the cerebellum, pons, and cord. The fluid in the ventricles is clear, colorless, or slightly yellowish.

The causes of hydrocephalus are not well understood. It has been attributed to inflammation of the ependyma and to interference with the return venous circulation, but the evidence for this is hardly convincing. The pia at the transverse fissure has been found to be indurated, and thus might conceivably press upon the veins of Galen. The normal channels of communication which exist at the transverse fissure between the ventricles and the subarachnoid space are occasionally obliterated. In unilateral hydrocephalus the foramen of Munroe may be found to be occluded. Probably obstruction of the lymphatics and transudation of lymph has a good deal to do with it.

Corresponding in some particulars to hydrops of the brain and its membranes, we have accumulations of fluid in and about the cord. A collection of fluid within the spinal meninges—**hydrorrhachis externa**—sometimes leads to atrophy or hypoplasia of the cord.

Hydromyelia.—Fluid within the central canal is called **hydrorrhachis interna** or **hydromyelia**. It leads to a diffuse or saccular dilatation of the central canal with more or less encroachment upon the substance of the cord. The condition may be merely microscopic or may involve the greater part of the thickness of the cord. The cavity is circular or irregular and situated in the centre of the cord, or it may extend into the posterior horns and columns.

The changes in the cord are referable to the effects of pressure, being chiefly atrophy, thickening of the vessels, and slight peri-ependymal gliosis. The cause is unknown. Some have suggested a secretory function on the part of the ependymal cells. Others think it due to vascular disturbances.

Hyperplasia.—Hyperplasia of the brain is usually associated with a corresponding developmental enlargement of the cranium (**macrocephaly**). Two forms may be differentiated.

In the first, there is a true hyperplasia of all the elements composing the brain, which differs, therefore, in no respect save that of size from the normal brain. The enlargement of the brain due to hydrocephalus should not be confounded with true macrencephaly. The weight of the brain in this condition may vary from 1500 to 2200 grams. Individuals possessing abnormally large brains have occasionally been noted for intellectual vigor, but this is by no means an invariable rule. Idiots and epileptics, on the other hand, occasionally have large brains. In moderate grades the membranes are put on the stretch, and the epidural space and the cavity of the ventricles are encroached upon.

In the second class, the enlargement is due to a relative increase in the amount of glia (gliosis). This may be generalized or confined to certain districts, convolutions, or parts of convolutions. The condition is referable to a primary peculiarity of development.

An interesting and somewhat obscure affection of the spinal cord associated with hyperplasia of the glia tissue is known as **syringomyelia**. This term simply means cavity formation in the cord ($\sigma\tilde{\upsilon}\rho\iota\gamma\xi$, a flute), and therefore might be taken to include such conditions as hydromyelia, hematomyelia, pyomyelia, and hemorrhagic, degenerative, and inflammatory softening. It is generally taken to mean, however, a condition, distinct from all these, which is attended by a somewhat variable, but still characteristic, train of symptoms. These are, in a typical case, muscular wasting of the Aran-Duchenne type, loss of thermic and painful sensations, with preservation of tactile sensibility. Irregular forms are also met with occasionally which recall amyotrophic lateral sclerosis, tabes dorsalis, and Friedreich's ataxia. The lesions are generally found in the cervical and upper dorsal portions of the cord, but may involve its whole length, and even extend into the medulla, pons, and internal capsule.[1]

To gross appearance the cord may present little change, although this is unusual. The dura is normal, the pia-arachnoid normal or but slightly thickened. The cord itself may present a natural configuration or may collapse on removal into a ribbon-like band, according to the extent of the pathological change. Sometimes there is slight enlargement, and

FIG. 137

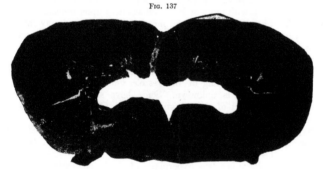

Syringomyelia   Dorsal cord, showing central cavitation.   (From collection of Dr. Colin K. Russel.)

there may be fluctuation on palpation. The cord not infrequently shows atrophy in certain tracts. On section, it is found to contain one or or more cavities, usually one, situated somewhat posteriorly to the central canal. The cavity has a predilection for the gray matter, usually of the posterior part and the dorsal horns, but not infrequently extends more or less widely into the white matter. It is round, oval, triangular, slit-like, or irregular in shape, and may be confined to one side of the cord. Its distinguishing features are asymmetry and irregularity. Occasionally, more than one cavity may be found occupying different sections of the cord without any attempt at communication. In a typical case, the cavity is distinct from the central canal, but in some instances is found to communicate with it at several points. The space is usually filled with the detritus from colliquative necrosis, cerebrospinal fluid, and, rarely, blood.

[1] Spiller, Brit. Med. Jour., 2: 1906: 1017.

Fig. 138

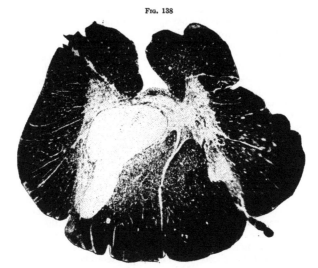

Syringomyelia, with extensive cavitation of the posterior horn. (From collection
of Dr. Colin K. Russel.)

Fig. 139

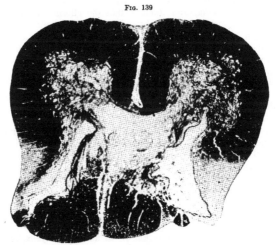

Syringomyelia. Lumbar cord, showing cavitation of both posterior cornua and descending
degeneration in the pyramidal tracts. (From collection of Dr. Colin K. Russel.)

Microscopically, the space is bounded by a zone of delicate neuroglia. Rarely, it has been lined by what appeared to be connective tissue, supposed to be derived from inclusion of the pia. Occasionally, it may be lined here and there with ependymal epithelium. The extent of the glial hyperplasia varies within wide limits. The central canal may be normal in size and appearance, or may be dilated (*hydromyelia*). The rest of the cord may show little or no change, but, as a rule, there is considerable ascending and descending degeneration. The nerve roots are often involved, and there is a descending degeneration of the peripheral part of the anterior motor neurones. The vessels commonly show hyaline degeneration and thickening of the intima. Diapedesis of cells, thrombosis, and rupture of the capillaries may take place.

These appearances have been variously interrupted. The generally accepted view at the present time is that syringomyelia is due to a primary hyperplasia of the neuroglia, followed by degenerative softening and cavity formation. The supporting structure of the central nervous system, or glia, is of ectodermal origin and is produced by the proliferation of the ependymal cells of the central neural canal. The original ependyma is represented in the human cord by the cuboidal cells forming the lining epithelium of the central canal, and small groups of cells in its immediate neighborhood. Syringomyelia is thus to be regarded as a central gliosis caused by the proliferation of the ependymal cells, the vascular changes which accompany it, such as thickening of the vessels, thrombosis, embolism, and hemorrhage, being responsible for the softening, which is largely of the nature of a necrosis from lack of nutrition. Virchow believed that syringomyelia was consecutive to congenital hydromyelia, and thought that the gliosis was due to the proliferation of inclusions of embryonic glia cells about the central canal. Such embryonic cells may take the form of diverticula from the neural canal, solid masses, or isolated cavities. The pressure of the fluid within the central canal is here supposed to play an important part in the production of the softening.

Another theory, held by certain French observers (Hallopeau; Joffroy), is that the process is essentially an inflammatory one, which directly and indirectly, owing to vascular changes, leads to softening and cavity formation (*myélite cavitaire*).

Still another view is that obstruction to the blood or lymph-circulation, due, for example, to the pressure of tumors in the posterior fossa of the skull or of the cord itself, and meningitis, lead to hydrops of the canal and secondary dilatation.

None of the theories propounded is entirely satisfactory, for cases have occasionally been met with which cannot be explained on any of the hypotheses. On the whole, the preponderance of evidence goes to show that errors of development are the most important factor.[1]

Diastematomyelia.—What might be called a numerical hyperplasia is seen in the cord, in the condition known as **diastematomyelia**, or redu-

---

[1] For one of the best monographs on Syringomyelia, with full bibliography, see Schlesinger, Die Syringomyelie, Wien, 1895.

plication of the cord. The reduplication occurs in the lumbar region. The two divisions are contained within the one vertebral canal, or are separated by a bony septum.

Diplomyelia.—Diplomyelia, or the formation of two cords, is met with in certain double monsters.

The cord may also be abnormally **long.** The spinal roots may be abnormally **numerous,** or, again, **defective.**

Heterotopia.—Heterotopia may be defined as the presence of normal constituents of the cord in abnormal situations. Thus, portions of the gray matter may be found in the white substance. Many of these appearances are due to artefacts produced in sectioning the cord, but there are undoubtedly cases in which the condition is due to an error of development. Of this nature are some forms of asymmetry of the cord. One pyramidal tract, for instance, may be small or even absent, while the other is correspondingly large. This is due to the failure of certain of the motor fibres to decussate.

THE CEREBRAL MENINGES.

The covering membranes of the brain are three in number: an outer, the dura; a middle, the arachnoid; and an inner, the pia. The last two are so intimately associated, anatomically and pathologically, that they practically form one structure. The membranes, owing to their relations, are liable to be involved in pathological processes originating in the brain and cranial bones; and, farther, being highly vascular and bounding spaces which are practically large lymph-channels, infective agents can readily reach them from distant or adjacent parts, and set up rapidly extending inflammation. It should be remarked that, while it is convenient for descriptive purposes to adopt the regional method of classification, it is almost impossible for one membrane to be diseased without to some extent involving the others and even the brain itself.

The Cerebral Dura Mater.

The dura mater is a tough, inelastic, connective-tissue membrane, lined on its inner surface by a layer of endothelium, of a grayish-white, glistening appearance, which serves the double purpose of a periosteum for the cranial bones and a protective covering for the brain. In adults it is only loosely adherent over the vault, while at the base of the skull it is much more closely attached. It sends three processes into the intracranial cavity for support and protection of the brain: first the falx cerebri, running longitudinally between the two cerebral hemispheres; second, the tentorium cerebelli, on which rest the occipital lobes separating them from the hemispheres of the cerebellum; and third, the falx cerebelli, running vertically between the two lobes of the cerebellum. It also sends prolon   ns enclosing the various cranial nerves and vessels as they make their exit from the skull. Around the margin of the foramen magnum it is closely adherent to the bone and is continous with the spinal dura mater. In certain situations the dura splits up into two layers to contain the various venous sinuses, which play an important part in connection with certain infective processes. Thus, in the superior border of the falx cerebri lies the superior longitudinal sinus, while the inferior longitudinal sinus is enclosed in its inferior border. The tentorium cerebelli encloses the two lateral sinuses in its posterior convex borders. In its anterior borders it encloses the superior petrosal sinus, and along the middle line of its upper surface runs the straight sinus. The occipital sinus runs in the attached margin of the falx cerebelli.

On the outer surface of the dura run the branches of the middle meningeal artery. The veins of the dura are connected with those of the scalp by numerous branches.

CIRCULATORY DISTURBANCES.

Congestion.—Congestion of the dura is commonly met with in association with inflammation of the various membranes, or where there is an increase in intracranial pressure from any cause, provided, of course, that that pressure be not excessive. In such cases, on removal of the calvarium, the dura weeps blood rather freely.

Anemia.—Anemia is met with in death by bleeding and in all forms of systemic anemia.

Hemorrhage.—Hemorrhage may take place upon the surface of the dura (*epidural*), into its substance (*intradural*), or beneath it (*subdural*). The commonest cause is traumatism, such as concussion and fracture, or, again, disease of the adjacent bony structures. The spontaneous rupture of sclerotic vessels is also a not infrequent finding. After falls, the bleeding is often due to rupture of the middle meningeal artery or some of its branches. The hemorrhage does not necessarily occur at the site of the blow, but may take place on the opposite side (by *contrecoup*) or at some other part. When the injury is severe, fatal consequences often follow, owing to compression of the brain. It is to be remembered that serious symptoms do not always come on immediately on receipt of the injury, but the patient may walk away after what is regarded as a trivial accident, and may die a few hours later, unless carefully watched and treated. The effused blood tends to gravitate to the floor of the cranial cavity, and may interfere with the vital centres there, although sometimes it remains curiously localized to the region of origin. Where the hemorrhage has been slow, or of the nature of an oozing, the blood is found clotted or even disintegrated. In such cases, especially if infection has taken place, a not uncommon event in the case of fractures, there may be more or less inflammation of the brain and meninges, and even abscess-formation. Extradural hemorrhage is occasionally met with in the newborn child as the result of a difficult or instrumental delivery. This is due to laceration of the vessels from the excessive over-riding of the cranial bones. If not immediately or quickly fatal it may give rise to a peculiar form of spastic paralysis, often associated with idiocy, known as *infantile cerebral palsy* or *cerebral diplegia*. The same condition occurring during intra-uterine life may cause *microgyria* or *porencephaly*. Hemorrhage into the substance of the dura is rare and usually of slight extent. It is sometimes associated with extradural hemorrhage in cases of traumatism.

Thrombosis.—Thrombosis of the venous sinuses of the dura is of not infrequent occurrence and is always of grave import. In one class of case the condition appears to depend upon general systemic weakness, where particularly there is deterioration in the quality of the blood. This leads to degeneration of the vessel walls, a condition which, with impaired vigor of the circulation, favors clotting (*marantic thrombosis*). Anatomical peculiarities are of some importance here also, particularly sudden enlargement of the vessels, which leads to slowing of the blood stream, and the unevenness of their walls due to the Pacchionian bodies. The condition is met with in marasmus, profound anemias, summer diarrhœa of children, and in the aged. The longitudinal sinus is the site of election for the process, but the transverse may be involved. Œdema, rupture of the meningeal or cerebral vessels and red softening are sometimes found as a result.

In another group the condition has an inflammatory basis (*thrombosinusitis*) and is analogous to thrombophlebitis. This is seen in meningitis and certain injuries to the cranial bones. Perhaps the most common cause is suppurative otitis media, complicated with necrosis of the petrous bone. Here the lateral sinus is apt to be involved. We have met recently with a case of thrombosis of both choroidal sinuses in puerperal septicemia.

There is at first inflammation of the wall of the sinus, followed by clotting of the blood. The vessel is filled with a dirty, necrotic-looking substance, of a grayish-red appearance, and its wall is often of a yellowish-green color. The process sometimes extends into the jugular vein. The dura is apt to be involved in the vicinity and there may be foci of suppuration between its layers. Supervening upon the affection we may get meningitis and abscess of the brain. As the condition is infective, metastatic abscesses may be formed in various parts and a general septicemia induced. When middle ear disease is the primary cause, the abscess is most likely to be found in the temporosphenoidal lobe or in the cerebellum. In marantic cases, or where the infection is mild, the thrombus may be absorbed or become organized, if the patient live long enough.

INFLAMMATIONS.

Pachymeningitis.—Inflammation of the dura is called pachymeningitis. It is divided into *external* and *internal* forms, according to the surface of the membrane chiefly involved.

Pachymeningitis Externa Acuta.—Pachymeningitis externa acuta is usually due to traumatism, such as fractures, gunshot injuries, and cutting wounds of the skull, or to the extension of disease from the neighboring bone, as in caries of the petrous bone and osteomyelitis. Occasionally, it is secondary to erysipelas of the scalp, owing to infection extending through the veins of the diploe. The dura is congested, swollen, and softened, and there is an exudate which may be serous, seropurulent, or purulent. The surface of the membrane is grayish white or grayish yellow, in some cases covered with extravasated blood. The process may spread to the pia-arachnoid or to the brain itself. When not fatal, the exudate may become absorbed or encysted. Not infrequently the membrane remains thickened and is adherent to the skull.

Pachymeningitis Externa Chronica.—Pachymeningitis externa chronica arises from trauma, local bone disease, and sunstroke, in cases where infection does not take place. The dura is thickened, owing to the proliferation of the connective tissue, and in some instances there is a formation of bone.

Pachymeningitis Interna Acuta.—Pachymeningitis interna acuta is usually dependent on external pachymeningitis. Certain affections of the brain, dural sinuses, and pia-arachnoid, also lead to it. The exudate may be simple or purulent.

Pachymeningitis Interna Hemorrhagica.—The most important form, however, is pachymeningitis interna hemorrhagica, which is not uncommonly met with. In the early stages, the disease is characterized by the formation on the inner surface of the dura of a delicate, homogeneous, granular or fibrillar deposit of fibrin, containing relatively few leukocytes. This, in time, becomes organized through the ingrowth of delicate capillaries, derived from the vessels of the dura, together with young fibroblasts. Thus, a delicate connective-tissue membrane is formed lining the dura, which contains an abundance of wide, thin-walled capillaries. Owing to the tenuity of the vessels, and probably also to the degeneration which their walls undergo, hemorrhage readily takes place, both by rhexis and diapedesis, into the substance of the newly-formed membrane and upon its surface. The extravasation is, in many instances, of the nature of a simple oozing, but not infrequently large effusions take place, which dissect the membrane away from the dura and collect in the circumscribed cavities thus formed (*hematoma duræ matris*). As the hemorrhages are apt to be repeated, we get an alternation of old clots, more or less disorganized, containing blood pigment, with a fresh deposit of fibrin, giving the whole a laminated appearance. The process is essentially sluggish and prone to relapse. The smaller extravasations may be absorbed, but the larger ones are only imperfectly removed, if at all, while from time to time a fresh exudation and another formation of membrane takes place. As the affection progresses, the new membrane becomes firmer and more densely organized and contains the remains of blood, blood pigment, fibrin, and even deposits of lime salts. The presence of so much foreign and irritating material excites inflammation, which tends to reproduce and perpetuate the condition. If the larger collections of blood are finally absorbed, we occasionally find traces of them in collections of fluid between the dura and the new membrane (*hygroma duræ matris; hydrocephalus pachymeningiticus partialis*). In the older and denser portions of the organizing membrane the vessels gradually become more or less occluded, but as new ones are being formed in other places the process hardly ever comes to a stop. As a rule, the affection is confined to the dura, but in some cases the pia-arachnoid is involved, and vascularized adhesions form between it and the dura.

Hemorrhagic pachymeningitis is most commonly seen in drunkards and the insane. It has been observed in general paralysis of the insane, senile dementia, Huntingdon's chorea, chronic heart and kidney affec-

Fig. 140

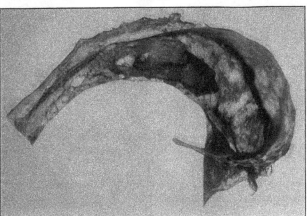

Osseous metaplasia in the falx cerebri. The bone is the dark irregular mass in the central portion. (Pathological Museum of McGill University.)

tions, and scurvy. It may be due to traumatism. Occasionally, it has been found associated with atrophy of the brain, apparently without any cause.

The etiology is not entirely clear. The majority of pathologists agree with Virchow that the process is an inflammatory one. It is possible that in some cases, owing to fatty and other degenerative changes in the walls of the dural capillaries, these give way and we get hemorrhage upon the surface of the dura followed by inflammation, exudation, organization, and membrane formation. Another view is that spasm and contraction of the vessels of the brain lead to diminution of the intracranial pressure and consequently hemorrhage.

Tuberculosis.—Tuberculosis of the dura is rather an uncommon condition. It is usually found in association with miliary tuberculosis of the pia, but occasionally is due to the extension of bone tuberculosis. It takes various forms, either a discrete miliary eruption of tubercles, a membranous deposit containing tubercles on the inner side of the dura, or large caseous masses or tuberculomas.

Syphilis.—In syphilis, multiple, small, cellular foci or granulomas, occasionally coalescing, may be formed, in some cases enclosing necrotic or gummy material. Adhesions may take place between the dura and the pia-arachnoid. The condition is most apt to occur at the base of the brain, and may involve the cranial nerves.

Fig. 141

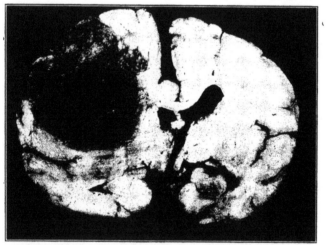

Endothelioma of the brain. The case is referred to in the text. The depression in the tumor resulting from the exostosis of the calvarium can be recognized. (From the Pathological Laboratory of the Royal Victoria Hospital.)

Histologically, the lesions consist in cellular and highly vascular granulation tissue which tends to go on to necrosis. The process usually begins in the adventitia of the vessels or in the epineurium. The nerve-fibres may eventually undergo atrophy.

PROGRESSIVE METAMORPHOSES.

Tumors.—Of the benign tumors, the most important are the **fibroma, lipoma, chondroma,** and **osteoma.**

Fibromas are rare. They are found on any part of the dura in the form of hard, nodular, spherical growths. **Lipomas** are still rarer. Small, gelatinous tumors, **ecchondromas,** are found occasionally near the clivus. So-called **osteomas** are met with in the tentorium and flax. They are more properly examples of metaplasia. The primary malignant tumors are the **sarcoma** and the **endothelioma**.

The sarcomas are generally spindle-celled, more rarely round-celled, mixed-celled, or alveolar. *Myxosarcomas* and very vascular sarcomas, or *angiosarcomas*, have been described. In certain cases, small spicules or nodular concretions of mineral matter are found in these growths. Hence, they are called *psammosarcomas*. Sarcomas of the dura may erode the bone and appear externally. They are sometimes of large size, and may produce serious pressure upon the brain.

Endotheliomas. — Endotheliomas are firm, flattened, or nodular tumors, originating from the endothelial cells covering the dura, or, possibly from the lining

Fig. 142

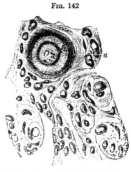

Portion of an endothelioma of the dura mater, showing the characteristic whorled arrangement of the tumor cells and at *a*, a concentrically arranged calcareous deposit or psammoma body. (P. Ernst.)

Fig. 143

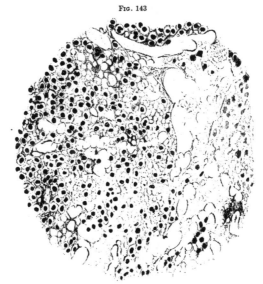

Section of a chordoma. To the right the cells are of the benign type, not unlike in arrangement those of cartilage; to the left, through active multiplication, the cells are taking on a more sarcomatous type and the growth is becoming malignant. (Fischer.)

membrane of the vessels of the subdural space. The growth readily implicates the pia-arachnoid, and may finally extend to the brain, which it compresses or invades. Irritation of some kind seems to be a potent factor in the causation. We have twice seen, post mortem, cases in which a spur of bone projecting from the inner surface of the parietal bone formed the centre about which an endothelioma developed. Occasionally, these tumors spring from the outer surface of the dura and erode the calvarium, finally appearing externally. Microscopically, they present the appearance of richly branching and anastomosing bands of flattened cells, tending to be spindle-shaped, with a characteristic concentric arrangement.

It is not infrequent to meet with tumors showing histological transitions from the endotheliomatous to the sarcomatous type (vide vol. i, p. 824). The commonest form of **psammoma** is a slow-growing, relatively benign endothelioma, with necrosis of the "cell-nests" and deposit of calcareous salts in the clusters of necrosed cells.

The secondary new-growths are **carcinoma** and **sarcoma**.

Chordoma is a curious tumor originating at the base of the skull in the upper termination of the notochord. It is situated near the clivus and invades the dura secondarily (see vol. i, p. 761).

The Pia-arachnoid.

The arachnoid is a delicate, connective-tissue membrane, devoid of bloodvessels, covering the brain, and lying in close relationship with the dura. The space between the two is known as the subdural space. The pia is also a delicate connective-tissue membrane, but vascular. It closely follows the contour of the cerebrum, dipping down into the sulci and sending prolongations, which carry bloodvessels and lymphatics, into the cortical substance. The arachnoid, on the contrary, passes from top to top of the convolutions. The space between the arachnoid and pia contains the cerebrospinal fluid, and is called the subarachnoid space. Passing from one membrane to the other are innumerable bands and strands of connective tissue, covered with a continuation of the endothelium lining the sac.

At the base, the pia and arachnoid are widely separated from one another, in certain situations. Thus, in the interpeduncular space and posteriorly between the posterior surface of the medulla and the inferior surface of the cerebellum quite large reservoirs are formed for the cerebrospinal fluid. The chief bloodvessels run in the subarachnoid space; the veins lie superficially, the arteries at the bottom of the sulci.

The pia mater is continued into the lateral ventricles through the transverse fissure in the form of the tela choroidea superior, and into the fourth ventricle in the form of the tela choroidea inferior, carrying with it the choroid plexus of vessels. The subarachnoid space is continuous with the ventricular cavities through the foramen of Magendie in the lower end of the fourth ventricle.

CIRCULATORY DISTURBANCES.

The circulatory disturbances affecting the pia-arachnoid will be more conveniently discussed when treating of the brain, inasmuch as there is such an intimate relationship between the brain and its membranes that the same causes often produce analogous and simultaneous results in both (see p. 577).

INFLAMMATIONS.

Leptomeningitis.—Inflammation of the pia-arachnoid, leptomeningitis, or, as it is usually more briefly termed, meningitis, may be acute or chronic.

Acute Leptomeningitis.—This is, in the vast majority of cases, produced by microörganisms, probably the only exceptions being those forms met with in sunstroke and the various intoxications. The germs usually at work are the pyogenic cocci, B. tuberculosis, Diplococcus pneumoniæ, Meningococcus intracellularis, and, occasionally, B. typhi, B. coli, B. Friedländeri, B. pyocyaneus, B. influenzæ, B. diphtheriæ, B. anthracis, Gonococcus, and Actinomyces bovis.

The infecting agents reach the meninges either through the blood (hematogenic infection), by extension from neighboring parts, or from the external air. The hematogenic form is well illustrated in those cases which complicate croupous pneumonia, endocarditis, acute rheumatism, pulmonary tuberculosis, typhoid fever, scarlatina, pleurisy, and bedsores. The second variety is due to the extension of an inflammatory process from the brain, dura, or bones of the skull. Of especial importance in this connection are affections of the middle ear, the mastoid cells, the soft tissues of the head and neck, and the accessory cavities of the nose. Those arising from external infection are the result of traumatism, such as fractures and penetrating wounds of the skull.

While in many cases the meningitis is due to the particular microorganism producing the primary disease, examples of secondary and mixed infection are not uncommon.

It is hardly possible for the pia-arachnoid to be inflamed without corresponding changes in the brain substance, at least, in the superficial layers of the cortex. This is, in part, due to the close apposition between the structures in question, so that lesions are readily produced by direct extension, but also in some measure to the dissemination of infective agents through the bloodvessels and lymphatics of the pia which send minute branches into the connective-tissue septa of the cortex. The cells of the gray matter, therefore, commonly suffer, showing fatty degeneration, vacuolation, and changes in the chromophilic bodies. Multiple, small ecchymoses are often to be seen in the cortex. In well-marked cases the condition would properly be termed **acute meningo-encephalitis.**

Acute Serous Meningitis.—Acute serous meningitis (Quincke[1]) is an important affection of the pia-arachnoid, often of the cortex, characterized by congestive hyperemia, œdema, and the production of a serous and cellular exudate. It is met with most frequently in children at the onset or during the course of certain of the infective fevers, such as scarlatina and measles. It is found, however, in adults also, as a result of traumatism, and in those suffering from obstructive cardiac disease, typhoid, otitis media, alcoholism, uremia and other intoxications. The causative factors are not always entirely clear.

The anatomical picture is not constant. In certain cases the inflammatory products are so scanty that the condition is only detected on microscopic examination. In the severer forms, the pia-arachnoid is congested, œdematous, friable, and the subarachnoid space contains a considerable quantity of watery exudation, sometimes clear, sometimes turbid and containing flakes. Along the vessels the fluid is apt to be of a yellowish color and gelatinous consistency. The dura is usually tense and injected, somewhat moist and shiny on the inner surface. If the exudate be at all considerable, the membranes are distended and the convolutions flattened. The extent of the disease varies and the lesions are, as a rule, irregularly distributed, being most marked along the course of the main vessels. At one time the involvement is most marked at the base, at another, over the sides and convexities. The arachnoid usually peels off readily, leaving a moist, congested, and œdematous pia. Minute hemorrhages may also be seen in the pia and the superficial layers of the cortex. Occasionally, the disease is localized to one part of the cortex owing to the delimitation of the exudation by adhesions. In addition to the meningeal involvement the disease may extend to the lining of the ventricles and produce a considerable accumulation of fluid there (*hydrops ventriculorum*).

Purulent Meningitis.—We may, further, recognize a *seropurulent*, *fibrinopurulent*, and *purulent* meningitis, according to the nature of the exudate produced. These include the majority of meningitis cases. The exudate is more cellular, consisting of a turbid serous fluid containing numerous leukocytes and, sometimes, flakes of fibrin, or it may be entirely purulent. The exudate tends to collect about the vessels and in the sulci, but in severe cases the brain may be bathed in exudate.

The distribution of the lesions is dependent largely upon the cause and the nature of the infecting agents. Hematogenic causes may affect the base, the convexity, and practically any part of the membranes. Traumatism, caries of the petrous bone, and infection of the accessory cavities lead to a local lesion, which may, however, become general. Again, the cranial cavity alone may be involved, or the whole central nervous system, as in the case of epidemic cerebrospinal meningitis.

The cerebral cortex, of course, suffers. It is œdematous, the vessels are congested, and there are frequently multiple minute hemorrhages.

---

[1] Sammlung klin. Vorträge (Volkmann), 67:1893.

The vessel walls and the connective-tissue septa are infiltrated with inflammatory products. The ganglion cells are swollen, vacuolated, and fatty, the axis-cylinders disintegrated. In cases where the process has extended to the ventricles, the choroid plexus is congested, swollen, bathed in pus, and infiltrated with inflammatory products. The ependyma and the underlying brain substance are œdematous and softened. Should the exudate be excessive, the ventricles are distended and the brain compressed. The gyri are flattened, the cerebrospinal fluid is squeezed out, and, as a result, the meninges, which were previously œdematous, now become drier.

As a rule, purulent meningitis is fatal, but the milder and more localized forms are sometimes recovered from. In such cases the only traces left of the trouble are a thickening of the pia-arachnoid, with possibly adhesions between it and the dura. This is due to absorption and the organization of the exudate into fibrous tissue. Purulent meningitis is, in most cases, a complication of disease elsewhere, and may usually be traced to pneumonia, acute endocarditis, infection of the nasal or aural cavities, traumatism, or to terminal infection in some chronic disease. Here the pyogenic cocci, Pneumococcus, and B. coli play the leading role, less commonly B. influenzæ, B. typhi,[1] B. diphtheriæ, B. Welchii, and Gonococcus.

Occasionally, cases crop up, either sporadically or in epidemics, which run a somewhat characteristic course, and cannot be attributed to any of the causes just mentioned. This variety is called *acute* or *epidemic cerebrospinal meningitis,* " *spotted fever,*" and *cerebrospinal fever.* Here the Meningococcus or the Pneumococcus, is found, either alone or associated with other pyogenic germs. At one time it was debated which of the two microörganisms above mentioned was the specific cause of the disease. Weichselbaum[2] was the first to recognize and describe a diplococcus in these cases, tending to be intracellular, which he regarded as specific and named Diplococcus intracellularis meningitidis. His observations were afterward confirmed by Heubner[3] in Germany, and Councilman, Mallory, and Wright[4] in America. Netter,[5] however, strongly maintained that the pneumococcus was the important agent, and held, though it now seems on inconclusive evidence, that the Weichselbaum organism is merely a degenerate form of this germ. At the present time the majority of authorities concede the specificity of Diplococcus intracellularis for most cases. The agglutination test and the favorable results following the therapeutic use of a specific serum (Flexner) place the distinction between the bacteria mentioned beyond question. The relative frequency of the two microörganisms in the

[1] T. Henry and Rosenberger, Proc. Path. Soc. of Phila., February, 1908: 52.

[2] Ueber d. Etiologie der acuten Meningitis Cerebrospinalis, Fortschr. d. Med., 5: 1887:Nos. 18 and 19.

[3] Deut. med. Woch., 1897.

[4] Jour. Boston Soc. Med. Sci., 2: 1897-98: 53.

[5] Bull. et Mém. Soc. Méd. d. Hôp. de Paris, 15: 1898: 407.

disease is not positively settled.	Combined infection seems to be a common event, and it has been thought that where Pneumococcus has been found alone Diplococcus intracellularis may have been present but have died out, as its tenacity of life is known not to be great.

In the form of cerebrospinal meningitis under discussion, the exudate is abundant and found throughout the whole extent of the central nervous system.	At one time the membranes of the cerebrum are chiefly involved, at another, those of the cord.	As a rule, the exudate tends to collect at the base of the brain and along the posterior aspect of the cord. It is largely serous, but turbid from the admixture of leukocytes and a small amount of fibrin.	On removing the skull-cap, the veins of the diploe, and the vessels and sinuses of the dura are congested.	The arachnoid is somewhat turbid and the pial vessels are injected.	The exudate is found chiefly along the course of the vessels, and fills up the cisterns at the base of the brain, and may even extend to the ventricles, which are often found to be distended.	The pus produced by Diplococcus pneumoniæ is somewhat different, being of a creamy yellowish-green color, more viscid and, rarely, mixed with blood.

Microscopically, the vessels of the cortex are congested and surrounded by aggregations of leukocytes.	There are multiple small hemorrhages and large areas of necrosis.

It is not uncommon to find lesions in other parts of the body as well as in the meninges.	Arthritis is comparatively frequent, being found more often in this disease than in other forms of meningitis.	Diplococcus intracellularis has been isolated from the joints in these cases.	Multiple abscesses, petechial spots, herpes and other rashes have been observed.	A rare complication is purulent pericarditis.[1]	These facts seem to indicate that cerebrospinal meningitis is really a systemic infection, the meningeal features of which dominate the clinical picture.[2] The distinction between the form just described and that due to a frank Diplococcus pneumoniæ infection is marked, pathologically speaking, for in the latter affection the exudate is thick, purulent, and of a greenish hue.

Meningo-encephalitis is sometimes met with in epidemics of influenza, and is one cause of hemiplegia and aphasia in young persons.

W. T. Howard, Jr., has reported a case of acute fibrinopurulent cerebrospinal meningitis with abscess of the brain due to the B. Welchii.[3]

Chronic Leptomeningitis.—Chronic leptomeningitis, etiologically speaking, is a somewhat obscure affection.	Some cases result from a previous acute attack, and are mostly of an infective nature.	They are met with as sequelæ of cerebrospinal meningitis, typhoid fever, acute rheumatism, erysipelas, and syphilis.	Others, again, are insidious in their development and are possibly in many cases to be regarded as degenerative

[1] Stewart and Martin, Montreal Med. Jour., 27: 1898: 159.

[2] For a very full consideration of this disease, see Osler, on the Etiology and Diagnosis of Cerebrospinal Fever, Cavendish Lecture, 1899.

[3] Johns Hopkins Hospital Bulletin, 10: 1899: 66.

manifestations, inasmuch as they seem to depend on vascular disturbances or circulating toxins rather than microbic influences. Such are the latent meningitides sometimes met with in chronic alcoholism and Bright's disease. They are apt to be combined with encephalitis (*chronic meningo-encephalitis*). Some few cases may possibly be attributed to excessive mental strain or nervous shock. Chronic leptomeningitis is at times associated with pachymeningitis interna proliferans.

The anatomical picture varies greatly in different cases. Local or diffuse thickenings of a whitish color, in the form of streaks or patches, may be found on the pia-arachnoid. They are composed of hyperplastic connective tissue and are often the sole relics of a previous acute inflammation. Some, however, are more probably the result of circulatory or nutritional disturbances. Proliferation of the lining endothelium is also to be seen in some instances. In the more severe forms cellular infiltration plays a more striking part. This is met with in the neighborhood of chronic suppurating foci, syphilitic and tuberculous bone disease, tumors, and areas of degeneration.

Tuberculosis.—Tuberculosis of the pia-arachnoid is a common occurrence, particularly in children and young adults. It is probably never primary, but in all cases is attributable to tuberculous disease elsewhere. The affection is brought about by metastasis, usually from some focus in the lungs or lymphatic glands, bones, genito-urinary organs, or by direct extension from the dura mater or bones of the skull.

Anatomically, two forms may be recognized, the disseminated miliary and the solitary tubercle. The first variety is due to the dissemination of considerable numbers of the specific bacilli through the arterial system. It is frequently, but by no means invariably, part and parcel of a systemic miliary tuberculosis. Diffuse tuberculous meningitis, or miliary tuberculosis of the pia-arachnoid, is characterized by the formation of whitish or grayish-white granules, the size of a pin-head or smaller, in the pia, which tend to be scattered along the course of the vessels. They are usually most numerous at the base of the brain, about the chiasm, at the anterior and posterior perforated spaces, the circle of Willis, and along the Sylvian fissures. The process frequently spreads by the Sylvian arteries and its branches to the convexity of the brain. The condition is usually bilateral, but it is not uncommon to find one side more affected than the other. Exceptionally, one side only is involved. It may, however, be still more restricted in extent. We remember seeing one case in which there were attacks of Jacksonian epilepsy due to the presence of a cluster of a dozen or more milia over a portion of the motor area. Associated with the efflorescence of tubercles is a more or less abundant exudate of a serous, seropurulent, or fibrinopurulent appearance, which accumulates not only in the meshes of the pia-arachnoid, but also in the various lymph-cisterns, the ventricles, and even in the brain substance. On removing the skull cap, the dura is congested and weeps blood. The pia-arachnoid is congested and œdematous, and along the course of the vessels can be seen minute tubercles, with sometimes petechial hemorrhages. The basal convolutions are often somewhat compressed. The cortex is swollen and œdematous. The ventricles contain a variable amount of fluid, similar to the exudation elsewhere, the choroid plexus is thickened, and the ependyma has a turbid granular appearance. Internal hydrocephalus is not an uncommon result. It may be due to involvement of the ependyma of the ventricles, or to obstruction of the communicating passage between the ventricles and the subarachnoid space. In some few cases the amount of exudate may be considerable, without obvious tubercles, but these can usually be recognized by the use of a hand-lens or on microscopic investigation. Occasionally, the granulations are the most marked feature, while the exudation is scanty (*dry tuberculous meningitis*).

The process begins by a specific inflammation of the walls of the smaller arterioles and capillaries. Small collections of leukocytes and epithelioid cells are formed in the vessel walls, which increase, gradually extending into the lumina and into the perivascular lymph-spaces. In the first stage there is a proliferation of the endothelial lining of the bloodvessels, leading to more or less obliteration of the lumina, but this is quickly masked by the exudative process. These changes at first are confined to the pial vessels but quickly extend to the superficial vessels of the cortex lying in the fibrous trabeculæ, and eventually invade the nerve substance (*tuberculous meningo-encephalitis*). This leads to swelling and degeneration of the cortical ganglia and nerve fibres. The main nerve-trunks passing out from the base of the brain may be similarly involved. The milia quickly undergo central caseation, thus becoming more opaque. Only in extremely chronic cases do the granules attain any considerable size. Tubercle bacilli can be demonstrated within the lymph-spaces and in the granulation tissue.

The disease is almost invariably fatal in a few weeks, although one or two authentic cases of recovery are on record, in one at least of which the tubercle bacilli were obtained by spinal puncture.

Should only a few bacilli reach the meninges through a single arterial twig, we get a small cluster of tubercles, which, in time, coalesce to form large nodular masses, varying in size from that of a walnut to that of a hen's egg. These are situated in the pia-arachnoid, but frequently encroach upon the substance of the brain or extend to the dura. Unless situated at or near the motor area, or in the parts connected with the special senses, they may remain latent and unsuspected for a long time. Such masses are nodular, firmer or softer, containing in their centres yellowish-white caseous detritus. Occasionally, owing to the infiltration of fluid, the degenerated material is partially liquefied, so that the tuberculoma resembles an abscess. In long-standing cases, the nodule may become calcified. As a rule, the necrotic mass is surrounded by a zone of grayish or grayish-white, semitranslucent granulation tissue, or, in the older cases, dense fibrous tissue. Where the affection is progressive, secondary tubercles may often be noted in this peripheral zone. Such tuberculomas are practically tumors and produce their effects by pressure and by interference with the circulation of the blood and lymph. They may also lead to the production of fresh tubercles in the adjacent parts of the brain or to a disseminated cerebral miliary infection. This result is due to local metastasis through the lymph-stream or to the discharge of infective material into the transverse sinus. Microscopically, this form does not differ from the small miliary focus, save in point of size and the relatively much greater amount of caseation, and in the peripheral fibrosis.

Syphilis.—The meninges are a rather common site for syphilitic processes. The parts most liable to be involved are the basal and, next, the frontal and parietal portions of the membranes. While the pia-arachnoid is chiefly involved, the process commonly extends to the cortex of the brain. It is rare for the central regions of the brain and cord to be invaded. Meningitis and meningocephalitis are met with usually in inveterate cases of syphilis, but also, although rarely, in the secondary stage.

The affection is characterized by two main features, the formation of gummas and involvement of the bloodvessels. The gummas resemble other infectious granulomas in that they are circumscribed foci of inflammation which pass through the stages of exudation and infiltration into that of degeneration. At first they appear as small, grayish, grayish-red, semitranslucent or gelatinous masses composed of a cellular granulation tissue, together with newly-formed vessels. Should the process advance, there is a gradual formation of cellular fibrous tissue accompanied by central necrosis. The gummas are produced first in the substance of the pia-arachnoid but later in its cortical prolongations, and even in the nerve-substance proper (*meningo-encephalitis syphilitica gummosa*). The bloodvessels are somewhat peculiarly involved. All the coats of the vessels are infiltrated with inflammatory products, which eventually give place to fibrous transformation. The striking feature, however, is the proliferation of the endothelium, brought about by division of its cells, followed by cellular infiltration, which frequently results in marked narrowing or even obliteration of the lumen. Such a state of things naturally predisposes to thrombosis, and this is an important factor in producing occlusion of the vessels. The gummas may be single or multiple, and are not infrequently localized to a comparatively small district. It is, moreover, not uncommon to find definite large masses or diffuse gummatous infiltration. Owing to growth by direct extension or by the coalescence of small, separate foci, nodular masses as large as a walnut may be produced, which are firm in texture and on section present yellowish streaks and patches due to degeneration. This form is commonly associated with proliferation of fibrous tissue forming dense bands about the gumma, and often leading to adhesion with the overlying dura. In progressive cases this fibrous tissue in its turn undergoes necrosis. The cerebral substance, as one would expect, manifests marked change. Advancing gummas lead to compression and destruction of the nervous tissue, while, owing to the vascular changes, ischemic necrosis and hemorrhages are not uncommon.

Actinomycosis.—So far as is known, actinomycosis is always secondary, arising by extension from the face and nasopharynx, or by metastasis. The meningitis produced is either localized or diffuse, and is accompanied by a serous or fibrinous exudate, in which the "sulphur grains" of the actinomyces may be discovered, and adhesion of the membranes. There seems to be in these cases a tendency to invade the walls of the veins and sinuses.

PROGRESSIVE METAMORPHOSES.

Tumors.—These are chiefly of the connective-tissue type, and are found not only in the external pia-arachnoid, but also in the telæ choroideæ and the lining membrane of the ventricles.

The benign forms, **angioma, fibroma, lipoma, myxoma, chondroma,** and **osteoma,** are rare. They form small, nodular or lobulated masses which compress the adjacent brain substance. A cystic **lymphangioma** has also been described.

A peculiar growth, the exact nature of which is somewhat obscure, is the **cholesteatoma** (Perlgeschwulst[1]). This is found especially in the meninges at the base of the brain, about the anterior or posterior transverse fissures, and, occasionally, in the substance of the brain. It forms a solitary tumor enclosed in a fibrous capsule, or else multiple free nodules in the pia or brain. On section, it is soft, of shining white appearance, with a silky sheen. Microscopically, it is composed largely of keratinized cells, resembling the horny epithelium of the skin. Most authorities seem to think that it is endothelial in origin, but Ziegler holds that it more probably arises from the external germinal layer or misplaced epithelium. This view is supported by the fact that hairs and sebaceous glands are sometimes found within the growth.

Dermoid Cysts.[2]—Dermoid cysts are found in the meninges, but are rare.

Not uncommonly multiple **cysts** containing watery or colloid material are met with in the choroid plexus.

Endothelioma.—The most important of the malignant growths found in the pia-arachnoid is the endothelioma, a tumor of somewhat variable structure, originating in the endothelial cells lining the bloodvessels and lymphatics or those covering the arachnoid and lining the subarachnoid space. Certain of these growths develop around vessels, presumably from the endothelium of the perivascular lymphatics, the so-called **peri-theliomas,** though it should be remarked that it is not always easy or possible to decide whether growths presenting this particular appearance originate in the adventitia (perithelium) of the bloodvessels or in the lining endothelium of the perivascular lymphatics.[3] No doubt, the majority of tumors arising in the pia arachnoid are endotheliomas.

---

[1] Chiari, Prager med. Woch., 1883.

[2] See Bostroem, Centralbl. f. allg. Path. u. path. Anat., 8:1897:1.

[3] A word or two of explanation and criticism may not be out of place here. The term perithelioma, meaning a tumor derived from perithelium, came into vogue some fifteen years ago. It was applied to a growth of a special histological type, the main feature being the grouping of the newly-formed tumor cells about the

Endotheliomas form circumscribed or diffuse, superficial, flattened masses, of firm consistence, and of grayish or grayish-red color. Rarely, they are melanotic. In general, they resemble the sarcomas, although in places they may present a somewhat carcinomatous appearance. Where the connection with the lymphatics or bloodvessels can be traced, the older cells composing the tumor are flattened or spindle-shaped, resembling endothelial cells, but in the newer, more rapidly growing parts, the cells lose this character and come to resemble closely the polymorphous cells of certain carcinomas. Solid strands or masses of such

FIG. 144

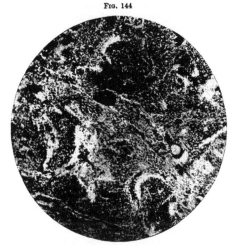

Endothelioma (psammoma). Winckel obj. No. 3, without ocular. (From the collection of A. G. Nicholls.)

cells in a connective-tissue stroma often give the tumor an alveolar appearance. Not infrequently the cells are laid down more or less concentrically in layers, after the fashion of whorls. Besides the endothelioma, ordinary types of sarcoma are met with, **myxosarcoma,**

bloodvessels in a radial fashion, recalling, to make a somewhat crude comparison, the relationship of the spokes to the hub of a wheel. The word later came to be applied in many quarters to any tumor having this peculiar arrangement. Strictly speaking, before we should term a tumor a perithelioma, we should be able to demonstrate the continuity of the tumor cells with those of the perithelium or adventitia Such a growth is not a lining membrane tumor, but is really a form of sarcoma. Perhaps, to avoid confusion, the old term "angiosarcoma" would be preferable Many of the growths, however, presenting this radiate arrangement originate from the lining cells of the perivascular lymphatics and should be called "perivascular" or "periangial" endotheliomas.

angiosarcoma, angiomyxosarcoma, melanotic sarcoma.[1] It is not uncommon to find in the choroid plexus small granular concretions, the so-called "sand bodies." On occasion, they are found in considerable numbers in tumors, notably endotheliomas and sarcomas, giving them a hard, gritty character (**psammoma, psammosarcoma**). They vary in size and shape, being laminated, rounded, irregular, or spinous.

Carcinomas.—Carcinomas have been described as occurring in the ventricles and generally arise from the epithelial layer of the choroid plexus, or more rarely from the ependyma.[2] They form soft growths composed of a fibrous stroma in which are nests of epithelial cells of cylindrical type. In some cases the stroma is vascular and proliferates, giving to the tumor a papillary appearance. The stroma often undergoes mucinous degeneration, so that the growth presents a peculiar appearance. Owing to the accumulation of the mucin, the papillæ are not infrequently converted into cysts. These are bounded by epithelial-cell masses, which in time may form a new fibrous stroma sometimes containing cell-nests, not unlike the "pearls" so commonly found in cutaneous epitheliomas. The neoplasm usually remains localized to the ventricle, producing its effects mainly by pressure, but occasionally secondary nodules are formed within the brain substance. They are, in our opinion, more correctly styled **"ependymal gliomas."**

Parasites.—Among the animal parasites may be mentioned *Echinococcus* and *Cysticercus*. Echinococcus leads to the formation of single or multiple cysts which press upon the brain substance and result in its degeneration. Cysticercus is met with usually in the form of a small cyst with a scolex, or as the so-called cysticercus racemosus. Here, there are large, lobulated, and generally sterile cysts, presenting internally and externally grape-like masses of secondary or daughter-cysts. In the neighborhood connective-tissue proliferation is to be observed. Such cysts may become calcified.

Blastomycotic infection has been met with, but very rarely.[3]

THE CEREBRUM AND CEREBELLUM.

CIRCULATORY DISTURBANCES.

The amount of blood present in the brain and its membranes varies widely even under normal conditions being dependent on increased or diminished function, emotion, and divers peripheral impressions.

Hyperemia.—Active Hyperemia.—Active hyperemia occurs pathologically in excessive action of the heart and whenever arterial tension is diminished. It may be general or local. Dilatation of the arterioles

[1] Thorel, Münchener med. Woch., 15:1907:725.
[2] See Kaufmann, Text-book of Special Pathological Anatomy, p. 1084:1909; Reimer, Berlin.
[3] Türck, Deut Arch. f. klin. Med., 90:1907:335.

with increased blood supply may be due to drugs, such as amyl nitrite, nitroglycerin, and alcohol, or to sunstroke.

Passive Hyperemia.—Passive hyperemia of the brain and its membranes, as of other organs, is commonly due to obstruction to the free outflow of blood from the part. This is met with in chronic cardiac and pulmonary diseases, and in the paresis of the cerebral vessels, which results from increased intracranial pressure. The condition is found in death by suffocation and in those dying in the status epilepticus. Local passive congestion is due to thrombosis or the pressure of tumors or exudates upon the efferent veins and sinuses, or, again, in some cases, to the recumbent position. Owing to the delicacy of the meninges and the comparatively unsupported condition of the vessels, hyperemia is more readily detected there post mortem than in the case of the brain. In the latter organ, one sees at most slight distension of the smaller vessels and capillaries with blood, which on section exudes in minute drops. Sometimes the substance of the brain presents a slight rosy flush. The appearances are, however, very inconstant; and congestion may disappear entirely after death.

Anemia.—Anemia of the brain is due to general systemic anemia, or any cause which interferes with the proper supply of blood to the part. Endarteritis, spasm of the vessels, cardiac weakness, aortic disease, increased intracranial pressure, as from exudate into the subarachnoid space, meningeal hemorrhage, hydrops ventriculorum, tumors, all play a part here. In other cases anemia may be collateral, due to an excessive accumulation of blood in some other part, the abdominal cavity, for instance. This is seen in the case of an ordinary "faint." Local anemia occurs also from partial or complete obstruction of the arteries, from emboli, thrombi, or pressure.

Œdema.—Circulatory disturbances, particularly changes in the vessel walls, lead to œdema of the brain in cases where the outpoured plasma is not promptly removed by the lymph-channels. On section, the brain is pale, moist, and shiny. The condition is brought about by heart weakness, obstruction to the general circulation, thrombosis of the sinuses of the dura. Local œdema is found in the neighborhood of hemorrhagic exudates, tumors, and thrombosed veins. Toxic causes, too, sometimes play a part, as in chronic nephritis. Œdema is a frequent accompaniment, also, of inflammation of the brain and meninges.

As a result of acute inflammation and passive congestion, it is not uncommon to find a transudation of fluid into the ventricles (*hydrops ventriculorum; hydrocephalus internus*), which leads to dilatation of the ventricles and compression of the brain.

Microscopically, the glia is looser and more reticular, and the lymphatic channels are distended with fluid.

Hemorrhage.—Cerebral hemorrhage is of comparatively frequent occurrence, as compared with hemorrhage into other organs. This is probably due to the facts that (1) the vessels of the brain possess scanty anastomoses; (2) they are given off from vessels of much larger caliber than themselves, and are therefore under higher pressure; (3) the muscular coat of the cerebral arterioles is very slight, so that they can offer only a weak resistance to a dilating force; and (4) the brain substance offers less support.

Two factors are chiefly concerned in its causation, degeneration of the walls of the bloodvessels, and increased blood pressure. It may take the form of hemorrhage *per rhexin* or *per diapedesin*. Rupture of vessels is most likely to occur in infancy, owing to inherited disease of the vessels, and after middle life, when the vessels are apt to be sclerosed. Another potent cause, traumatism, may, of course, occur at any age.

Small capillary hemorrhages are met with in congestive hyperemia and acute encephalitis, as well as in certain of the infective diseases, such as malaria, variola, anthrax, and the hemorrhagic diatheses. In some of the cases the extravasation of blood is brought about by fatty degeneration of the vessel walls or by the obstructive and necrotizing action of bacterial emboli, or even the blockage of vessels by simple emboli of broken-down tissue or blood cells. In such cases the hemorrhages are scattered along the vessels. They vary in size from that of a millet seed to a pea, and are present both in the brain substance and in the cortical prolongations of the pia. When in the latter situation, the hemorrhages have been regarded, but incorrectly so, as dissecting aneurisms. Obstruction of vessels by sclerosis may also lead to hemorrhages, usually of small extent. Hemorrhages are also due to congestion brought about by the pressure of tumors or exudates, and to trauma of various kinds.

Of more importance is *spontaneous hemorrhage* which is caused by rupture of an artery. In such cases there is almost invariably advanced degeneration of the vessel walls caused by sclerosis, calcification, or inflammation. In the common condition of arterial sclerosis the lesions may be fairly generalized, but in not a few cases some particular organ is specially picked out, such as the brain, heart, or kidney. Sclerosis, being primarily a degenerative process, leads in time to weakening of the vessel walls. The proliferative changes in the intima result in more or less obstruction of the lumen, which may indeed be complete, and this in its turn contributes to the dilatation of the other parts of the vessel. Miliary aneurisms are therefore rather common, being present, it is said, in one-third to one-half the cases. Rupture of the vessel is precipitated by increased arterial tension, such as may be caused by excitement, worry, mental or physical overwork—in fact, any condition which puts sudden strain on the vessel.

The most frequent site for this form of hemorrhage is in the basal ganglia. One of the penetrating branches of the Sylvian artery, usually the lenticulostriate, is the vessel at fault. Less commonly, the hemorrhage takes place into the pons, the peduncles, the cerebellum, the white matter, and, most rarely, into the convexity. This distribution is accounted for by the fact that the blood pressure is greater in the Sylvian artery and its branches, the latter coming directly off, and that arteriosclerosis is usually commoner and more extensive about the base of the brain. The effects produced depend on the extent of the extravasation.   Minute hemorrhages lead simply to pressure upon and dis-location of the adjacent brain substance without much further disturb-ance, and may be absorbed, leaving little or no trace, although the clinical symptoms may be striking, if temporary.   When large vessels give way, extravasations varying in size from that of a pea to that of a walnut, or larger, take place, leading to destruction of the brain tissue in the neighborhood and pressure on more distant parts.   In the most extreme cases, the whole of the corpus striatum on one side may be torn up and the blood may dissect its way through the white substance and destroy the greater part of the posterior lobe, or the blood may even find its way into the ventricle or into the meninges.   In such case the convolutions are compressed and the brain substance in other parts is anemic.

In the early stages one sees in the affected area a variable quantity of dark, soft, semifluid, or granulated blood, mixed with detritus from the destroyed tissue.   In the neighboring brain substance are numerous petechial hemorrhages, the result of the sudden disturbance of the vascu-lar equilibrium.   Later, the fibrin separates more completely and the serum is to some extent removed by the lymphatics, so that the pressure upon the brain is to that extent at least relieved.   The clot gradually contracts, becomes more granular, and changes from a red to a brownish color, owing to the transformation of the hemoglobin into hematoidin. The pigment is gradually diffused into the neighboring tissues, imparting to them a yellowish tinge.   In time, the greater part of the fibrin, cor-puscles, pigment, and detritus is transformed and absorbed, so that a cavity remains, containing a clear or slightly tinged fluid (*degenerative* or *apoplectic cyst*).   Sometimes, however, the tissues collapse to fill up the deficiency, and in such cases there is compensatory enlargement of the ventricles and the subdural space.   When the extravasation is not too extensive the damage is made good by the formation of a fibrous scar, either quite firm, or enclosing the remains of the destroyed tissue, together with pigment and cholesterin crystals. ˙ Old cysts eventually become walled in by fibrous tissue derived, it is believed, from the pro-liferation of the adventitia of the vessels.   We thus get a closed, smooth, fibrous sac, more or less pigmented, containing either clear fluid or fluid with granules of hemosiderin, crystals and amorphous masses of hematoidin.   As a secondary result, we find degeneration and atrophy of the neuraxones belonging to the affected area.

Encephalomalacia.—The arteries of the brain come largely under the category of "end" arteries.   Consequently, obstruction of their lumina, if at all marked, is followed by most serious results.   These consist in a peculiar form of infarct—necrosis and softening (encephalo-malacia)—in certain vascular districts, accompanied by more or less inter-ference of function, and followed often by death.   The occlusion of the vessels is commonly brought about by thrombosis or embolism.   Arterio-sclerosis, in the form of proliferating endarteritis, may also cause it, and in any event would predispose to the conditions just mentioned.   The causes of embolism and thrombosis are the same here as elsewhere.

Emboli are usually vegetations from diseased valves of the heart, dislodged portions of intracardiac, venous, or arterial thrombi, disintegrating tissue, or microörganisms. Thrombi are found in certain infectious diseases, marasmus, or form in diseased vessels or upon emboli.

Emboli generally reach the brain by the most direct path. Usually, it is the Sylvian artery or one of its branches that is involved, less commonly, the anterior cerebral, and less commonly still, the posterior cerebral. The left side of the brain is affected slightly more often than the right.

Arteriosclerosis, when present, is most marked in the circle of Willis and the Sylvian arteries. In advanced cases, all the arterioles of the cortex may be involved and look like small, white threads upon the pia. The sclerosis is commonly of the nodose variety. When the blood supply of the brain is gradually cut off, as in a slowly progressive arteriosclerosis, we get simple atrophy of the brain tissue, with, in time, a tendency to fibrosis.   This is well seen in aged people.   Under the designation "foyers lacunaires de désintégration," Marie[1] has described in cerebral arteriosclerosis small areas of colliquative necrosis about the vessels, particularly in the internal capsule lenticular and caudate nuclei, which are well defined and vary in size from that of a pin-head to that of a pea. The more frequent event of sudden anemia, brought about by embolism or thrombosis, or the circulatory disturbances in the neighborhood of inflammatory foci, produces local softening with rapid disintegration of the brain substance.

The older anatomists used to speak of three kinds of cerebral softening—white, red, and yellow. It should be remarked that these terms refer properly not to distinct pathological processes, but rather to special peculiarities or different stages of the one affection. In white softening there is a pure anemic necrosis, the tissues being absolutely cut off from the circulation. In red softening, hemorrhage takes place into the necrosed area, either by regurgitation or by rupture of neighboring vessels. Later, when fatty degeneration of the cells occurs, with transformation of the blood and liberated blood pigment, we have the so-called yellow softening.

In the early stages, extensive softening of the cerebral substance may be present with but few visible signs. The affected district is sometimes a little œdematous or turbid, but not infrequently it does not differ materially from the healthy tissue. On palpation, however, the part is found to be softer than normal and pulpy. The other regions of the brain often show slight hyperemia. In more advanced cases, the softened area may be of a reddish or yellowish color, and is of a pulpy, semiliquid consistence. In some cases there may be multiple small foci of softening in close juxtaposition, giving the part a cribriform appearance (état criblé). In other cases the destruction of tissue is complete, leading to the formation of cystic cavities containing fluid, fatty granules, and detritus (one form of porencephaly). Not infrequently, however,

[1] Révue de Médecine, 21:1901:281.

the cavity resembles a sponge, being traversed by small bloodvessels and fine strands of glial tissue.

Microscopically, in the degenerated area we see what has been termed "varicose" atrophy of the protoplasmic processes of the specific nerve cells, and chromatophilic changes in the ganglia, while the neuroglia is disintegrated, presenting numerous pigmented cells, droplets of fat and myelin, leukocytes, and corpora amylacea.

In course of time, the detritus is, to some extent, absorbed, the fluid thereby becoming thinner and clearer, and there is an attempt at cicatrization. In young persons and those with healthy vessels, provided that the lesion is small, there is a slight amount of proliferation of the glia about the softened area, leading to induration. In many cases, however, even this is wanting, and the cavity is surrounded by a more or less necrotic zone. When the cyst lies near the surface of the brain, the superficial boundary collapses, leaving a depression in communication with the subarachnoid space, which is filled with fluid (another form of porencephaly). The collapsed tissue is more opaque than normal, whitish, or pigmented.

The clinical symptoms produced by encephalomalacia depend upon the localization and extent of the lesion. In slowly developing cases of wide extent, there is apt to be gradual degradation of the intellect, amounting even to dementia. In the sudden local lesions we get various motor or sensory phenomena. A lesion in the internal capsule will lead to hemiplegia on the opposite side; one in the cortical motor area causes motor paralysis of the corresponding muscles. When the third left frontal convolution is involved motor aphasia results. Lesions in the posterior cerebral lobe and posterior part of the vertex cause interference with vision. It should be remembered that encephalomalacia accounts for a certain number of the cerebral birth palsies.

INFLAMMATIONS.

Encephalitis.—Inflammation of the brain is termed encephalitis Before entering on the discussion of this subject it should be observed that in many cases it is difficult, if not impossible, to be sure that certain lesions are of an inflammatory nature or not. The nervous tissue is the most delicate and highly specialized in the body, consequently, it is comparatively easily put out of gear, and, farther, its reparative powers are slight. Extensive lesions may be produced by trifling causes, are often quickly induced, and are followed by far-reaching results. Many conditions, such as embolic infection, abscess, traumatism, and tuberculosis, are frankly inflammatory and present no special difficulty. There are others, however, which are somewhat similar in appearance, due to intoxication with alcohol, bacterial or mineral poisons, to sunstroke and concussion of the brain, that are not quite so clear. The most obscure of all are those chronic conditions, of which disseminated sclerosis, system degenerations, Huntingdon's chorea, and general paralysis of the insane may be cited as examples. Some of these appear to be dependent on circulating toxins, and are, therefore, possibly inflammatory or degenerative, while others are more probably manifestations of developmental defects. The difficulty arises from the fact that degeneration and disintegration of the specific nerve elements are common to all these affections and are followed by insidious regeneration of glial elements. It is obviously, therefore, impossible, in the present state of our knowledge, to make a satisfactory classification. Any that we adopt must be based mainly on clinical grounds and on convenience.

Several forms of encephalitis can be differentiated according to their localization. In the majority of cases the cortex and peripheral portions of the cerebrum and cerebellum are involved, less frequently the basal ganglia. In many instances cortical encephalitis is associated with meningitis (**meningo-encephalitis**). When the gray matter is chiefly involved we speak of **poliencephalitis**. The medulla may be affected (**bulbomyelitis**), or both brain and cord (**encephalomyelitis**).

Encephalitis may be hematogenic, traumatic, or the result of the extension of inflammation from contiguous parts, as the meninges and cranial bones. According to the kind of exudation, it is simple or suppurative.

Acute Hematogenic Encephalitis.—This form occurs as a complication of certain infective processes, chief among which are acute endocarditis, septicemia, cerebrospinal meningitis. More rarely, it has been met with in typhoid fever, acute rheumatism, scarlatina, influenza, ulcerative pulmonary tuberculosis, and rabies. The condition may be due to the specific germ producing the primary disease, but is not infrequently brought about also by secondary infection. Some few cases are purely toxic, as in poisoning by carbon monoxide and illuminating gas.

The lesions are most commonly met with in the cerebral cortex, but any part of the brain may be involved. In the more strictly localized form, the gray matter in the floor of the third ventricle and about the aqueduct of Sylvius is often involved (*superior poliencephalitis*), or that in the neighborhood of the fourth ventricle (*inferior poliencephalitis*). The cerebellum is rarely involved. The foci of inflammation may be single, multiple, or evenly scattered throughout the brain.

The smaller areas of inflammation are often invisible to the naked eye and may only be discovered accidentally on making a microscopic examination. Larger ones appear as tumid patches of a diffuse reddish color and may present small hemorrhages.

Microscopically, the vessels are congested, surrounded by inflammatory leukocytes, and here and there may be small extravasations of blood. The nerve elements are softened and degenerated. The ganglion cells are also degenerated, and may disappear. The axis-cylinders swell up, become nodose, and disintegrate, while the myelin sheaths are converted into small droplets. The glia shows also retrogressive changes.

When there is a tendency to heal, the destroyed cells are to some extent absorbed, and at the periphery of the affected area there is proliferation of the glia. Small foci may heal completely, and even larger ones, if the patient survive, with the formation of a sclerosed area or a fibrous scar.

The most intense form—acute suppurative encephalitis—is usually due to the action of various pyogenic microörganisms, notably, the staphylococcus, streptococcus, and pneumococcus, and is met with, for example, in such conditions as gangrene of the lung, empyema, infected wounds, and ulcerating carcinomas. The condition is brought about by infective emboli derived from a primary focus, and is really a manifestation of a generalized septicemia. The lesions are usually multiple, and are found in the cerebrum and cerebellum, less commonly in the basal ganglia.

Fig. 145

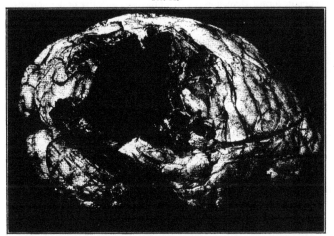

Extensive abscess of the brain. (From the Pathological Department of the Montreal General Hospital.)

The process begins with the formation in the brain of minute ischemic infarcts, with softening and hemorrhagic extravasation. To this is quickly added suppuration. Abscesses are thus produced, varying in size from that of a hemp seed or pea to that of a walnut or hen's egg, containing creamy, yellowish-white or yellowish-green pus. In exceptional cases a large part of one hemisphere is excavated. In the acute forms, after the pus is evacuated, the wall of the cavity is found to be covered with shaggy detritus, and the surrounding tissues are markedly œdematous and present multiple minute hemorrhages. The abscess may extend to the surface and induce meningitis, or may burst into a ventricle, so that severe and widespread inflammation is set up.

In the unlikely event of the patient surviving, it is possible that the smaller foci may heal with the production of scar tissue. Larger ones, after a lengthy period, become bounded by a zone of condensation, composed of a rather dense, fibrous capsule, lined with granulation tissue. So long as pus is being produced the adjacent brain substance is compressed and undergoes degeneration, although in time the process may cease to extend and the pus to some extent be absorbed. The encapsulation of the abscess does not entirely obviate the possibility of extension of the inflammation to neighboring parts. Diffuse meningitis or pressure on some important centre may induce a fatal termination. Abscesses in the cerebellum, by pressure on the veins of Galen and thrombophlebitis, lead to chronic hydrops of the ventricles.

Traumatic Encephalitis.—The description just given of the lesions found in acute hematogenic encephalitis will apply fairly well to the traumatic form. Here, however, the process is infective or non-infective. In the simple form, the pathological changes are local, corresponding, as a rule, to the point of injury, and the resulting inflammation is chiefly the attempt at removal of the destroyed tissue and its replacement. In the infective variety, germs have gained an entrance from outside, and the process may extend more or less widely into the substance of the brain (*abscess*) or along the meninges (*meningitis*).

Encephalitis per Extensionem.—Encephalitis per extensionem commonly originates in meningitis. As a matter of fact, leptomeningitis, so-called, is practically always a meningo-encephalitis. Many cases, 35 per cent., according to Collins, are the result of suppurative middle ear disease, which has led to necrosis of the petrous bone. In children, however, meningo-encephalitis may be due to an otitis without bone disease, owing to the fact that certain bony sutures remain unossified for some time, thus allowing direct communication between the middle ear and the cranial cavity. This channel of infection is still more effective since the dura frequently sends prolongations downward into the fissures. In such cases the temporal lobe and the cerebellum are most liable to be involved. In advanced and severe cases abscesses of considerable size may be produced.

Still other cases originate in infection from the nasopharynx, the frontal and ethmoidal sinuses, and the orbital cavity. Certain traumatic cases also come under the category of encephalitis by extension. In many instances extensive subdural collections of pus are found, together with sinus thrombosis.

Tuberculosis.—Tuberculosis of the brain occurs in the form of multiple scattered granulomas of small size (milia), and as the large solitary tubercle. The infection may be hematogenic, due to bacilli that have entered the circulation from some distant focus, usually the peribronchial, mesenteric, or retroperitoneal lymph-nodes. In many cases, but not all, the condition is part and parcel of a generalized miliary tuberculosis. As a rule, the meninges are involved as well—*tuberculous meningo-encephalitis* (see p. 574). In another class the infection is lymphogenic, originating in the petrous bone or the nasopharynx.

In the hematogenic type, the tubercles are distributed along the smaller arterioles and arterial capillaries, usually in the cortex, but to some extent in the central ganglia also. The process begins with the formation of minute foci of cellular infiltration, often with hemorrhage. These enlarge, undergo necrosis, and then appear as small grayish or yellowish-white nodules with caseous centres, frequently surrounded by a hemorrhagic zone.

When but a small area of the brain is implicated and the patient lives for some time, larger solitary tubercles are produced, varying in size from that of a pea to that of a walnut or larger. They form well-defined globular or nodular masses, of firm consistency, resembling tumors, and are in most cases due to the agglomeration and fusion of several separate foci. This is, perhaps, the commonest form of cerebral tumor found in young persons. On section, it is composed of a large central necrotic area, bounded by a zone of granulation tissue, in which can frequently be recognized small subsidiary tubercles. Occasionally, the caseous matter softens or liquefies, so that an abscess-like lesion is produced. Tuberculomas are found most commonly in the cerebellum, next in the cerebrum, more rarely in the basal ganglia, pons, and medulla.

Syphilis.—The syphilitic manifestations in the brain assume three types, **meningo-encephalitis** (see p. 575), **endarteritis**, and the **gumma**. Syphilitic endarteritis leads often to obstruction of the vessels and encephalomalacia, and possibly, also, to local atrophies, focal and system scleroses.

Gummas take the form of grayish or grayish-red, somewhat translucent nodules, of irregular shape. The central portion commonly shows degeneration and necrosis. When healing tends to take place, dense fibrous bands delimit and gradually substitute the mass. Gummas commonly begin in the meninges and extend to the brain. They may, however, develop in any part of the brain, but have a preference for the gray matter. The membranes overlying a gumma usually become adherent.

Uhle and Mackinney[1] report finding Spirochæta pallida in a gumma of the brain.

Actinomycosis.—Primary actinomycosis of the brain is excessively rare. One case has been recorded by Bollinger in a woman, in whom there was a granuloma the size of a hazelnut in the third ventricle, without evidence of actinomycosis elsewhere. More commonly, the condition arises by metastasis, or the extension of actinomycosis of the face, neck, or throat. In the metastatic form, which is usually only one phase of a general infection, multiple gelatinous-looking or necrotic foci are produced. In the cases due to extension, the actinomyces reach the cranial cavity through the various foramina and fissures.

As a rule, the meninges are involved in a more or less diffused suppurative inflammation, with the formation of numerous small necrotic foci that tend to invade the brain substance and the various sinuses. In the more chronic cases adhesion may take place between the membranes.

[1] Proc. Path. Soc. of Phila. (N. S), 9: 1906: 195.

RETROGRESSIVE METAMORPHOSES.

. **Atrophy.**—Atrophy of the brain is seen particularly well in old age. The brain, as a whole, is diminished in size, but the wasting is relatively most marked in the frontal and vertical regions. The convolutions are small and the sulci wide. In cases of moderate extent, when the brain is sectioned, little alteration may be noticed save that the gray matter of the cortex is somewhat thinned. In the more advanced cases, however, besides this, the perivascular spaces are enlarged, so that the vessels lie in wide channels, and small foci of degeneration are to be seen (état criblé).[1] It is not uncommon as a concomitant of the loss of substance to find enlargement of the subarachnoid space and of the ventricles, which are filled with fluid (*hydrops meningeus ex vacuo; h. ventriculorum ex vacuo*). The cerebellum, as a rule, is not involved to any extent, but occasionally has been found to be wasted.

Microscopically, the changes are referable to atrophy of the specific nerve cells, ganglia, and medullated nerve-fibres alike, with compensatory hyperplasia of the glia. There is granular disintegration with chromatolysis, and often pigmentation of the cells.

. Senile atrophy may, with considerable certainty, be attributed to several causes, chief among which are the normal tendency to retrogression of all tissues as advanced life is approached; impoverished nutrition of the body as a whole; and the local effects of imperfect blood supply, owing to sclerosis of the vessels. In accordance with the general rule that the more highly differentiated structures are the most liable to disease and degeneration, it is that portion of the brain containing the intellectual centres which chiefly suffers.

Other causes of atrophy are prolonged wasting diseases, alcoholism, and chronic lead-poisoning.

Fatty degeneration of the specific nerve-cells, **fragmentation** of the myelin sheaths, **disintegration** of the fibres, **necrosis,** and **liquefaction** are frequently met with in connection with injuries, inflammation, and circulatory disturbances. They need not be. more specially dealt with here.

We come now to discuss certain affections of the brain, which are introduced here largely as a matter of convenience, since their etiology is obscure. In these cases the most striking feature is atrophy of the brain substance. The difficulty lies in determining whether this atrophy is a primary degeneration or results from preëxisting inflammation. The fact that some of the cases occur in young persons, and in several members of the same family, suggests that inherited peculiarities or anomalies of development of the specific nerve elements may play a contributory, if not a leading, role. This need not imply that there is failure to reach anatomical perfection, but merely that there is a deficiency

---

[1] It should be noted that a somewhat similar porosity of the brain may be a postmortem manifestation due to gas-producing bacilli. See Chiari, Zeitschr. f. Heilk., 24:1903.

of vegetative force, so that the structures are after a time unable to meet the demands made upon them, or become unduly susceptible to deleterious influences. Whether we are to regard this condition of things as a disease in itself or as merely predisposing to other morbid processes must at present be left open. The most important affections coming under this category are general paresis of the insane, Huntingdon's chorea, and disseminated sclerosis.

General Paralysis of the Insane (Progressive General Paralysis; Dementia Paralytica).—General paralysis of the insane is a chronic affection of the nervous system, both central and peripheral, characterized clinically by a well-defined train of symptoms, chief among which may be mentioned, mental degradation and other disturbances of the intellect, delusions of a peculiar kind (délire de grandeur), muscular tremors and weakness, sometimes paralyses, disturbance of speech, and Argyll-Robertson pupil, with often special features referable to changes in the spinal cord. The disease is usually met with in those who have led the strenuous life, or who have been subjected to great mental stress and worry, especially if they have been alcoholics or have had syphilis. It is often met with in tabes dorsalis, inveterate epilepsy, and after trauma. Men are most often affected, especially those who are intellectually active. The disease is most common between the ages of thirty and fifty years. According to Edinger, dementia paralytica is an exhaustive disease comparable to tabes dorsalis, in which, owing to mental strain, shock, or worry, the cerebrum is primarily and most severely affected. As bearing on the etiology of the condition it may be remarked that Wassermann's precipitation test is positive in a large percentage of cases of this disease as it is in syphilis.

The lesions found are somewhat striking. The dura is often adherent to the calvarium, and there may be an internal hemorrhagic pachymeningitis. The pia is turbid and thickened, especially in the frontal region, and is often firmly attached to the surface of the brain, so that on attempting to remove it portions of the substance are torn away. The spinal pia is sometimes also adherent posteriorly, and there may be sclerotic changes in the posterior or lateral columns, or both. The cerebral convolutions are less distinct than normal, the brain substance is sclerosed, and the cortical gray matter is diminished. The frontal and parietal lobes are most markedly affected. Owing to dilatation of the vessels and enlargement of the perivascular lymph-spaces, the brain often presents a spongy or cribriform appearance. The ventricles are usually dilated, and the choroid plexus and ependyma are granular.

Microscopically, the pial vessels are surrounded by collections of small round cells, plasma cells, and, occasionally, "mast" cells, and there is proliferation of the connective-tissue trabeculæ penetrating the brain. The specific nerve-cells are swollen, cloudy, or granular, often vacuolated, atrophic, and pigmented. The neuraxones are altered in size and shape and the dendrites are wasted. The myelin sheaths are absent wholly or in part. The nuclei stain badly. The glia is greatly increased and the vessel walls are thickened. To the lesions in the brain are often added those of tabes dorsalis or combined sclerosis. The granulation of the ependyma is due to the subepithelial proliferation of the glia.

It is not unusual to find changes in the spinal meninges and cord as well—degeneration of the pyramidal tracts and posterior columns and chronic inflammatory infiltration of the membranes.

Disseminated Sclerosis (Multiple or Insular Sclerosis; Sclerose en Plaques).—The lesions in this disease are found scattered irregularly throughout the central nervous system. At one time the cord is chiefly affected; at another, the cerebrum. Occasionally, single foci are found in the brain which are probably of the same nature. The lesions consist, as the name implies, in the formation of islets of sclerosis, varying in size from that of a pin-head to patches two or three inches across. The larger lesions are apt to be found in the neighborhood of the ventricles and in the pons and medulla. When the foci are situated in the cortex or have extended through to the surface of the brain, slightly elevated nodules are to be seen, to which the pia may or may not be adherent. On section, the patches are rounded or irregular in shape, of a grayish-white or reddish-gray color, distinctly firmer than the normal brain substance. They can often be localized better by the sense of touch than by their appearance. When marked degeneration is going on, the areas appear somewhat variegated. In the cord, the cervical and lumbar enlargements are most likely to be involved.

Microscopically, the sclerotic areas are found to consist in the main of proliferated glia cells and connective tissue, in which can be seen remnants of degenerated nerve-cells and fibres. The axones show loss of their medullary sheaths, or may be entirely disintegrated, often leaving only a space to show where they were formerly present. At the periphery, these changes are most marked, and there may be found drops of myelin and fat, granule cells, and amyloid bodies. The vascular changes are not constant, but there are usually thickening and hyaline degeneration of the vessel walls, with distension of the perivascular lymphatics. Ribbert has described a new formation of vessels.

The causes of the disease are quite obscure. Some cases seem to be dependent on previous infection or toxic influences, and are probably due to a primary degeneration of the specific nervous elements, together with an attempt at repair on the part of the glial cells.

In other cases where the disease begins in early life, or there is a distinctly familial taint, it is probably due to defective embryonal development. The symptoms vary according to the distribution of the lesions. There is usually some impairment of emotional control with attacks of giddiness. Later, we get spasticity of the lower extremities, nystagmus scanning speech, extension tremor, and partial optic atrophy.

Huntingdon's Chorea (Chronic Degenerative Chorea).—Huntingdon's chorea is a curious and rare affection, characterized by irregular movements, disturbance of speech, and dementia. It usually occurs late in life, and is notably a family and local disease. This feature, together with the fact that the convolutions of the brain frequently show morphological deviations from the normal, has led most authorities to refer the affection to defective development. As the disease does not usually còme on until youth is past it would seem as if the "exhaustion theory" would apply here.

The brain is found to be atrophied, especially over the frontal and central regions, the meninges show patchy thickening and the vessels are sclerosed. Rarely, internal hemorrhagic pachymeningitis has been observed also. On section, the cervical gray matter is diminished.

Microscopically, there is atrophy and degeneration of the ganglion cells, especially in the large and small pyramidal layers. The cell bodies are granular, the nuclei enlarged and prominent, or, again, may stain badly. The processes are wasted. The vessels show slight nodular sclerosis, the perivascular lymph-spaces are dilated, and in their neighborhood there is some 'round-celled infiltration.

Local atrophy of the brain occurs as a result of the pressure of tumors or exudates, from inflammation and vascular disturbances.

PROGRESSIVE METAMORPHOSES.

The reparative powers of the specific nerve elements are strictly limited. In children and young people, in whom vegetative functions are in excess, we sometimes see in the neighborhood of destructive lesions an attempt at regeneration of the nerve-fibres, but it is of the slightest description, and authorities are not agreed on the interpretation of the appearances. Proliferation of the neuroglia is much more common, and is met with chiefly about old, inflammatory lesions. The so-called hypertrophy of the brain, in which the organ is considerably enlarged in all directions, is due to what may be called a diffuse gliomatosis, principally of the white matter, and is more properly included under the developmental anomalies (see p. 556).

Tumors.—The most important of the primary new-growths of the brain are the **glioma** and the **sarcoma. Angioma, fibroma, lipoma, osteoma, cholesteatoma,** and **dermoid cysts** have been described, but are much more rare.

Glioma.—The most frequent and characteristic tumor is the glioma, which is found in all parts of the central nervous system and its derivatives, as the retina. It is most frequently met with in childhood and adolescence, but is not uncommon after adult life. The usual situation is in the hemispheres just beneath the pia, but also, occasionally, in the corpus callosum, pons, medulla, and cerebellum. On removal of the calvarium, its presence may be at first unsuspected, for it is rare for it to be visible externally. At most, there may be slight fulness with, possibly, discoloration of the affected part. On section, the growth is indefinitely circumscribed, merging imperceptibly into the normal brain substance or separated from it merely by a zone of softening and degeneration. In consistence it is slightly softer or firmer than healthy brain substance according to circumstances. In appearance it is grayish, grayish-white, or reddish, somewhat translucent, and often streaked with reddish-yellow or opaque, white bands and patches. The tumor is vascular, and it is not uncommon for hemorrhage to take place into its substance. This may be so extensive as to mask the true nature of the growth and give it the appearance of an apoplectic focus. Owing to hemorrhage or colliquative necrosis the tumor may be converted into a series of cysts containing turbid-whitish or brownish fluid. In some instances it is extremely difficult to distinguish the mass from the brain substance, save that it is a little redder or paler than the normal structures. It is probable that some, at least, of the cases of hypertrophy of the brain described by the older writers were more properly gliomas. This tumor does not involve the membranes or the bone.

FIG. 146

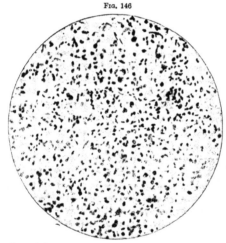

Medullary glioma of the cerebral vertex. Winckel obj. No. 6, without ocular. (From the collection of Dr. A. G. Nicholls.)

As its name implies, the glioma originates in the proliferation of the glial cells. Microscopically, we have a more or less cellular-looking growth, consisting of glial cells of the ordinary type which possess long branching and interlacing processes. The cell bodies vary considerably in size and contain large, deeply staining nuclei. The cells themselves are evenly distributed or aggregated into groups. The fibrils form a sort of meshwork, which at times is dense and at others rather loose, containing spaces which give the tumor somewhat the appearance of a myxoma (*myxoglioma*). The structure is in some cases not unlike a round-celled sarcoma, but its true nature can often be determined by teasing out a bit of the fresh tumor and discovering the branching cells. The use of a special stain for glia, such as Weigert's, gives much assistance. The bloodvessels and sinuses are often numerous and may be sò large and abundant as to warrant the designation of *glioma teleangiectaticum.* Hemorrhagès are frequent. The walls of the bloodvessels often present hyaline degeneration and the adventitia may proliferate, so that the vessels are surrounded by a zone of cellular or fibrocellular appearance.

In certain cases, a glioma of the structure just described contains cells, sometimes possessing more than one nucleus, which resemble closely the ganglion cells of the brain and cord. These are evenly scattered throughout the section or are massed into groups. Isolated medullated nerve fibres can also be made out. To this variety Ziegler gives the name of *neuroglioma ganglionare.* Many authorities, however, do not admit that in these cases there is a true new-formation of ganglion cells, or, more accurately, regard them as an overgrowth of congenital origin developing from a "cell-rest." (See vol. i, p. 753.)

At the periphery of a glioma the brain structure presents various grades of degeneration and necrosis, although it is remarkable how well it may be preserved in some cases. Not infrequently, the glioma sends out prolongations which gradually infiltrate and surround portions of the brain substance.

When a glioma is rapidly growing and so cellular that it resembles a sarcoma, it has been customary to speak of it as a **gliosarcoma.** As we have pointed out elsewhere (vol. i, p. 757), the term "sarcoma" must now be employed in a purely histological sense as indicating a hylic tumor of vegetative type, and thus we regard the term as perfectly correct, even while recognizing that gliomas are of epiblastic and not mesoblastic origin.

The etiology of glioma formation is somewhat obscure. The occurrence of the growth in early life, the peculiar localization, and the occasional presence of ganglion cells have suggested that errors of development, such as embryonic "cell-rests," may be at work. This view is supported by the observation of Stroebe,[1] who found in a glioma cystic cavities lined with cylindrical epithelium. The more delicate methods of staining devised by Weigert, and modified by Mallory and Beneke, have shown that in man the glia cells possess protoplasmic processes only during the embryonic stage, while the adult glia is composed mainly of fibres coursing between cells devoid of processes. Now the glia cells, or astrocytes, as they have been called, are derived ultimately from the ependyma, either directly or indirectly through less highly differentiated cells (astroblasts). Apparently gliomas exist which may be compared with glia cells in various stages, both embryonic and adult. Flexner[2] has described a glioma composed of ependyma-like cells. The gliosarcomas (medullary gliomas of Ziegler) possibly originate in the intermediate cells (astroblasts), which might readily persist in a latent form into adult life. The gliomas composed of branching and "spider"

[1] Enstehung d. Hirngliome, Centralbl. f. allg. Path., 5:1894:855.
[2] Glia and Gliomatosis, Jour. of Nervous and Mental Disease, May, 1898.

cells suggest a derivation from the primitive astrocytes, while the denser, more fibrous growths resemble the adult glia.

Sarcoma.—Sarcoma of the brain originates in the connective tissue forming the intracerebral prolongations of the pia or adventitia of the vessels. It takes the form of single or multiple growths of irregularly globular shape, which are fairly well defined from the brain substance or even encapsulated. In many cases, owing to the degeneration of the structures at the periphery of the tumor, it can be shelled out. The favorite site is in the cortex, where it forms a projecting nodular growth. On section the mass is of a grayish or yellowish appearance and presents numerous hemorrhages and foci of degeneration. Microscopically, the most common variety is the round or mixed-celled sarcoma, but spindle-celled forms are also found. In some cases the sarcoma is highly vascular, and seems to originate from the adventitia of the vessels. The tumor then consists of a series of whorls of spindle cells arranged radially and apparently continuous with the vessel walls (*angiosarcoma; perithelioma*). We have seen tumors of this type both in the cortex and in the corpus callosum.

Occasionally, there is a deposit of calcareous matter in the growth (**psammosarcoma**). The pia over the sarcoma is inflamed or infiltrated, while the adjacent brain substance is softened and degenerated. The ventricles may be dilated. Secondary nodules may be found in various parts of the central nervous system.

Angioma.—Of the primary benign tumors, the so-called angioma is not infrequent. This presents the appearance not of a tumor, but of a diffusely reddened patch, not unlike a congested area of inflammation. Microscopically, it consists mainly of dilated bloodvessels and sinuses, about which the brain substance is softened and degenerated. According to Virchow, angiomas are congenital, and are probably to be classed with the vascular nævi.

The **fibroma** is a rare tumor, taking the form of rounded nodules.

An **osteoma** of the corpus striatum has been recorded by Bidder.[1] **Lipomas** are rare.

The peculiar tumor, consisting of flattened epithelial cells arranged in laminæ, called **cholesteatoma,** has been met with in the brain, although more common in the meninges.

Dermoid cysts are decidedly rare. A few examples have been observed in the cerebellum.

The secondary tumors are, ordinarily, **sarcomas**. They arise by direct extension from the meninges, choroid plexus, cranial bones, tympanum, and orbit, and, along with¶**carcinomas,** may originate by metastasis. Metastatic **chorioepithelioma** has also been observed.

Parasites.—*Echinococcus* and *Cysticercus cellulosæ* have been met with. The resulting cysts are single and multiple. They are situated usually in the membranes, but may be found in the brain substance.

---

[1] Virch. Archiv, 88:1882:91.

TRAUMATIC DISTURBANCES.

Injuries to the brain are produced in a great variety of ways. Ordinarily, they are caused by great external violence, for the brain is particularly well protected, not only by the bony cranium, but by its several membranes, and, moreover, is supported by fluid. The most important injuries are concussion, compression, contusion, and laceration. The results are often serious, and depend upon the nature and extent of the trauma and its localization.

Concussion.—Concussion of the brain is brought about by falls or blows upon the head. Partial or complete loss of consciousness results, with muscular relaxation. The condition may be a transient one or end in death. The exact nature of the lesion is somewhat obscure. In some cases, although by no means invariably, multiple small hemorrhages have been noted in the brain substance. In some others, certain of the ganglion cells have been calcified. It is probable, therefore, that the injury leads to rupture of the finer capillaries, solution of the continuity of certain nerve paths, and degenerative changes in the fibres and ganglia.

Compression.—Compression of the brain is usually due to intracranial growths, hemorrhage, or excess of the cerebrospinal fluid. Up to a certain point the brain is able to accommodate itself to the abnormal condition of things, largely by the extrusion of a corresponding amount of the cerebrospinal fluid. It is often surprising what an amount of pressure the brain will bear without the production of structural changes or disordered function. Should, however, the compression exceed the limit, or be rapidly brought about, we get flattening of the gyri, interference with the free circulation of blood and lymph, resulting finally in anemia, softening and degeneration of the brain substance.

Contusions and Lacerations.—Contusions and lacerations of various kinds are produced by fractures, gunshot wounds, and cutting or stabbing injuries. Here the effects are mainly local. The slighter injuries lead to local softening; the more severe present, in addition to concussion, signs of disintegration of the brain substance. The remoter results depend, of course, upon the extent and localization of the injury. If none of the important centres are involved, provided that the site of the injury remain aseptic and the patient survive, the lesion, anatomically speaking, is not unlike those met with in anemia and hemorrhage. The tissue actually destroyed is gradually disintegrated and absorbed. the adjacent nerve fibrillæ and ganglia present various forms of degeneration, and about the periphery we find reactive inflammation with a slight proliferation of connective tissue, most noticeable along the course of the vessels. In time the granulation tissue may be converted into fibrous connective tissue. In the case of trivial injuries, healing may take place with the replacement of the dead material by a scar, composed mainly of fibrous tissue and bloodvessels, but also to a limited

extent of newly formed glia.   In the more extensive injuries, degene
tion is more widespread and persistent.

When infection of the wound has taken place, acute inflammat
is set up (*traumatic encephalitis*), with sometimes the formation of
abscess.   The meninges are apt to be involved in such cases.

CHAPTER XXVII.

THE SPINAL MENINGES.

INASMUCH as, anatomically and functionally, the spinal membranes do not differ materially from those of the brain, the discussion of the lesions affecting them will be somewhat sketchy, emphasis being laid only on such points as are of special interest.

The Spinal Dura Mater.

The dura mater spinalis is a tough connective-tissue membrane continuous with that covering the brain, completely enveloping the cord, and separated from the external vertebral column by what is known as the epidural space.

It forms a loose sheath about the cord, is adherent to the circumference of the foramen magnum and to the posterior common ligament in the extreme upper cervical region, and in the lower end of the spinal canal Below the level of the third piece of the sacrum it becomes impervious but continues down as a slender thread to the back of the coccyx, where it blends with the periosteum. The space between it and the bone is filled with loose, areolar tissue and a plexus of veins. On each side, opposite the intervertebral foramina, it has two openings, giving exit to the sensory and motor roots respectively of the corresponding spinal nerve. Prolongations of dura surround the roots until it is lost in their sheaths.

The pia-arachnoid of the cord is similar to that of the brain. The two membranes enclose between them the subarachnoid space, which contains cerebrospinal fluid. The outer layer, the arachnoid, is not normally adherent to the dura, except perhaps in the cervical region. The pia covers the entire surface of the cord, to which it is intimately adherent, and sends a septum down into its anterior median fissure. It also invests the spinal roots in their exit from the cord.

CIRCULATORY DISTURBANCES.

Hemorrhage.—Hemorrhage into the dura of the cord may arise from injury. It is met with sometimes in infants who have been delivered by instruments. It occurs also in asphyxia, strychnine poisoning, and tetanus. Minute petechial extravasations of blood are found in cases of meningitis.

INFLAMMATIONS.

Pachymeningitis.—Acute inflammation—pachymeningitis—is most frequently due to the extension of disease from the neighboring parts, the pia-arachnoid and vertebræ, or to trauma. The dura being rather dense, the resulting exudate, which may be cellular or fibrinous, is apt to collect on either the outer (**pachymeningitis externa**) or inner surface

Fig. 147

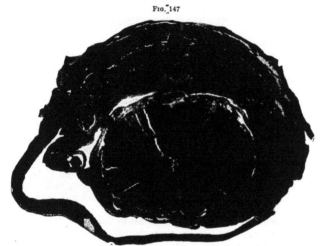

Pachymeningitis hypertrophica cervicalis of syphilitic origin. Secondary degeneration of the cord is well shown. (From the collection of Dr. Colin K. Russel.)

(**pachymeningitis interna**) of the membrane. In the severer forms, what are practically abscesses are produced, and may lead to compression and destruction of the cord at that spot. Where healing tends to take place, organization of the exudate is gradually brought about, with the formation of delicate vascular fibrous adhesions between the dura and adjacent structures.

A modified form of internal pachymeningitis is that known as **pachymeningitis interna hemorrhagica**, analogous to the disease of the same name occurring in the cerebral dura. Its etiology is rather obscure, save that it is apt to be found resulting from syphilitic or tuberculous disease of the vertebral bones or pia. In the severer forms adhesions are liable to take place between the dura and pia-arachnoid which result in degeneration in the cord.

Charcot and Joffroy[1] have described a **chronic hypertrophic cervical**

[1] De la pachymen. cerv. hyper., Thèse de Paris, 1873.

pachymeningitis, which leads to compression and degeneration of the nerve-roots and cord in the cervical region. The condition eventually involves the pia-arachnoid and the peripheral zone of the cord, with resulting fibrosis. Complete transverse softening of the cord, from occlusion of the vessels, may occur. Most cases seem to be due to syphilis.

Tuberculosis.—Tuberculosis of the dura is almost invariably secondary to Pott's disease of the spine, less commonly to tuberculosis of the pia-arachnoid and cord. In the earlier cases, scattered granular tubercles may form on the outer surface of the dura. These may coalesce, so that large caseating masses of granulation tissue are produced, which lead to compression and degeneration of the cord. Clinically, then, we get the features of a transverse myelitis. Delicate inflammatory membranes may in some cases be found on the inner surface of the dura. Or tubercles may make their appearance here, and eventually extensive tuberculous granulation.

Syphilis.—Syphilitic granulation may be primary, but is usually secondary to syphilis of the pia-arachnoid, less often of the bone. It leads to thickening and dense cicatricial adhesion.

Parasites.—*Echinococcus* and *Cysticercus cellulosæ* have been found both in the epidural and subdural spaces. These affections are usually secondary.

PROGRESSIVE METAMORPHOSES.

Tumors.—The primary tumors of the dura spinalis are the **sarcoma, psammoma, lipoma, fibroma, myxoma, chondroma,** and **teratoma.** They are all rare.

Carcinoma is met with in metastasis from carcinoma elsewhere, usually in the mamma.

The Spinal Pia-arachnoid.

CIRCULATORY DISTURBANCES.

Hemorrhages.—Hemorrhages into the meninges are due usually to trauma. *Petechial spots* are sometimes to be noted in infectious diseases and the hemorrhagic diatheses.

INFLAMMATIONS.

Leptomeningitis.—Inflammation of the pia-arachnoidea spinalis—leptomeningitis—is hematogenic, derived by extension from adjacent parts, or traumatic. According to the character of the exudate, we may recognize a purulent, a seropurulent, a fibrinopurulent, and a caseous form. The inflammation may be localized to a particular district may extend along the dorsal or ventral aspects of the cord, or may involve the whole length of the cord. In not a few cases it is combined with inflammation of the cerebral pia-arachnoid (*cerebrospinal meningitis*). It is common for the process to extend by the fissure and along the perivascular lymphatics to the cord, where small hemorrhages and infiltrations with round cells are not infrequent in the cortical portion (*meningomyelitis*). The nerve-roots may also be infiltrated (neuritis). As examples of hematogenic infection may be cited the so-called idiopathic or sporadic spinal meningitis, and the epidemic cerebrospinal meningitis (see p. 570).

Traumatic meningitis is due to infective agents, usually the pus-producing cocci, which are introduced into the spinal canal at the time of injury, or invade the wound subsequently.

Should the meningitis heal, it is not uncommon to find circumscribed areas of fibrous thickening, of a pearly white appearance, on the membranes, or the formation of more or less extensive adhesions between the neighboring structures. When the nerve-roots are involved in a cicatricial process we get secondary degenerations of the fibres. In meningomyelitis the peripheral portions of the cord may show atrophy and sclerosis.

Tuberculous Spinal Meningitis.—Tuberculous spinal meningitis is occasionally hematogenic, but in the great majority of cases arises by extension of tuberculous disease from the cerebral meninges, vertebral bones, or spinal cord. The most common is the cervical leptomeningitis that so often accompanies tuberculosis of the cerebral membranes; next, the form resulting from Pott's disease of the spine. In the latter case the infection probably extends inward from the dura. In the milder or less advanced conditions, one sees small, isolated, tuberculous nodules, arranged chiefly along the vessels. In more severe cases, however, there is a more widespread inflammation, with the production of a seropurulent or fibrinopurulent exudate, of yellowish-white color, sometimes mixed with blood.

The process may extend to the cord and nerve-roots, so that a tuberculous meningomyelitis or neuritis is produced. This leads to more or less widespread degeneration of the nerve elements.

Syphilitic Spinal Meni gitis.—Syphilitic spinal meningitis is rather rare. It takes the form of a circumscribed or flattened, diffuse, and superficial infiltration, which may extend to the cord, on the one hand (meningomyelitis), or to the dura, on the other. Occasionally, the process begins in the bone or dura and extends to the pia-arachnoid secondarily. The process in time leads to inflammatory induration and thickening of the pia-arachnoid, with the formation of adhesions between the various structures. In the central portions of the infiltrations, necrosis or gummatous degeneration is frequently observed. The sequelæ are in all respects similar to those in the tuberculous form.

PROGRESSIVE METAMORPHOSES.

Tumors.—Small, flattened plates of bone are not infrequently found in the arachnoid, which are supposed to be due to degenerative changes in the connective tissue. They are supplied with vessels from the dura. They must be regarded as metaplastic, or as embryonic inclusions, rather than as belonging to the category of true **osteoma**. **Cartilaginous plaques** are also found in the arachnoid.

Varicose dilatations of the veins of the pia, which occasionally assume the form of **cavernous angiomas**, are sometimes met with. They cause more or less extensive compression of the cord and nerve roots.

Of primary tumors proper, the **neurinoma, fibroma, myxoma, lipoma, angioma, psammoma, cholesteatoma, endothelioma**, and **sarcoma** should be mentioned. All tumors of the cord and its membranes tend to assume a flattened, elongated form, owing to the contracted and unyielding boundaries within which they lie. The **sarcomas** form circumscribed or flattened diffuse growths, which tend to invade the neighboring structures. The *alveolar endothelioma* is the most important variety. Owing to the abundant formation of bloodvessels in certain tumors, we may distinguish **angiomas** and **angiosarcomas**. Myxomatous degeneration is not uncommon in these cases, and hyaline changes may be so marked as to warrant us in calling the growth a **cylindroma**.

Neuromas or "multiple fibromas" are rounded or flattened, firmish growths, of pale color and smooth surface, which originate commonly from the perineurium of the nerve-roots. As we have seen in one case, they may lead to notable compression of the cord. (See vol. i, p. 758.)

Lipomas are found, commonly in association with spina bifida.

Secondary tumors of the spinal meninges are the **carcinoma, sarcoma,** and **myeloma**. As a rule, the vertebral column, nerve-roots, and the cord itself are involved as well, and the symptoms of compression myelitis are produced, root pains, spastic paralysis, increased knee-jerks, and bladder symptoms.

THE SPINAL CORD AND MEDULLA OBLONGATA.

CIRCULATORY DISTURBANCES.

Hyperemia.—**Active Hyperemia.**—Active hyperemia is commonly met with in the acute inflammations of the cord or meninges. In such cases the white matter presents a delicate, rosy flush, and the gray matter is somewhat brownish.

Passive Hyperemia.—Passive hyperemia is found in chronic cardiac and pulmonary affections, and in those who have been bedridden for prolonged periods.

Hemorrhages.—Hemorrhages into the substance of the cord are either punctate or massive. This condition is distinctly less frequent than cerebral hemorrhage. The causes are, however, much the same in both cases. Fatty, hyaline, or calcareous degeneration of the vessels, thrombosis, embolism, sudden alterations in blood pressure, and traumatism, play the leading role. With the exception of the traumatic forms, the lesions are more apt to be found in the medulla and upper part of the cord than elsewhere. Hemorrhage into the medulla is the main cause of the disease known as **acute bulbar paralysis.**

The minute, punctate, or capillary hemorrhages are commonly associated with the infections and intoxications, and are met with in such conditions as active and passive hyperemia, inflammations, tetanus, hydrophobia, strychnine poisoning, degenerative softening, and concussion of the spine. They are often met with, also, in the so-called **"caisson disease."**

The hemorrhages appear, on cross-section of the cord, as minute, reddish dots, scattered irregularly through the substance. In traumatic cases the lesions are generally found in the gray matter, and usually in the dorsal horns.

In the more extensive extravasations, the effused blood generally follows the line of least resistance. The whole thickness of the cord may be involved, local collections may be formed, or the blood may dissect its way along the fibers up and down the cord. Subsequently, degeneration of the nerve-substance takes place, with the formation of extensive cavities in the cord (*hematomyelopore*), Van Gieson). Occasionally the blood may escape into the central canal, which thereupon becomes dilated (*hematomyelia*), or into the membranes. Should the patient survive, the subsequent changes in the destroyed area are similar to those described in the case of cerebral hemorrhage. Van Gieson has, however, pointed out the fact that many of these cases are, in reality, artefacts.

Anemia.—Anemia, or, perhaps, more correctly, in the majority of instances, **ischemia,** is not infrequent, and is due to a variety of causes. The arteries of the cord are practically all end-arteries, so that their occlusion by endarteritis, thrombosis, or embolism is followed by local areas of anemia, softening, and necrosis. The pressure of inflammatory collections, effused blood, or tumors on the cord is followed by ischemia.

The cord is also ischemic in cases of pernicious and other systemic anemias.

INFLAMMATIONS.

Myelitis.—Myelitis in the stricter sense, or inflammation of the spinal cord, is due to hematogenic causes, to the extension of inflammatory processes from the meninges or vertebral column, less commonly from the central canal, and to traumatism. According as the process affects the gray or the white matter, writers have been accustomed to differentiate a *poliomyelitis* and a *leukomyelitis*. Several terms, also, are used to designate certain localizations of the inflammation, which sufficiently explain themselves. Such are *disseminated, diffuse, transverse, central,* and *annular myelitis.*

The earlier stages of the process are not precisely understood. It is probable, however, that many cases begin with degeneration or obstruction of the vessels, followed by the production of minute hemorrhages and the ordinary manifestations of inflammation. These changes may be brought about by bacterial or other toxins, such as ergot, lead, or arsenic, or by the actual localization of bacteria in the cord. The agents particularly concerned are the pyogenic cocci, Pneumococcus, the tubercle bacillus, and the toxic products of rabies, tetanus, leprosy, and syphilis.

Coincident with this, or following hard upon it, are well-marked degenerative changes in the nerve-fibers and cells, brought about, probably, by the combined action of the toxin, the interference with the circulation, and the pressure of the inflammatory products.

Acute Hematogenic Myelitis.—Acute hematogenic myelitis arises occasionally in the course of such affections as rabies, typhoid fever, dysentery, influenza, rheumatism, tonsillitis, pneumonia, and gonorrhœa. In some few cases, it appears to be due to infective emboli that have reached the cord from the cardiac valves, or from suppurative or other inflammatory foci in some distant part of the body. Occasionally, cases arise which are on analogy infective and hematogenic, yet a definite cause cannot be made out.

No particular rule is followed with regard to the distribution of the lesions. They are apt to be multiple, and may be confined to one small section of the cord, or may involve several segments. In some cases certain "systems" are picked out and the disease may extend rapidly along the cord.

According to the nature of the invading microörganism, we may distinguish *simple* and *suppurative* forms of myelitis.

When removed from the body, the spinal cord in these cases will present a variable picture according to the severity and extent of the process. The cerebrospinal fluid may be increased. The pia is commonly injected, especially over the affected areas. When palpated, the myelitic foci can readily be detected by their soft, pultaceous consistence, quite unlike the firm, resilient feel of the normal cord. On section, in advanced cases, these spots are semiliquid and the distinctive structure of the cord can no longer be made out. In color, the destroyed substance is reddish or reddish-brown (red softening). In the later stages it may be more yellowish (yellow softening). In milder forms, however, the cord may show only scattered patches of congestion, and the inflammatory nature of the lesions is first detected on making a microscopic examination.

We may now refer more in detail to the leading forms of acute hematogenic myelitis

Acute Anterior Poliomyelitis.—Acute anterior poliomyelitis, the *infantile palsy* of clinicians, is a disease of the cord in which the ganglion cells of the anterior horns, the axones proceeding from them, and the muscles supplied, are the parts chiefly affected. It is generally believed now that this affection is due to some hematogenic infection.

Recently, the work of Flexner and Lewis[1] in the United States and Landsteiner and Levaditi[2] in France has shown that the causative agent is a filtrable living virus, and that the disease is communicable by inoculation of this and of suspensions of the spinal cord of affected animals. It is found almost exclusively in young children, occasion-

FIG. 148

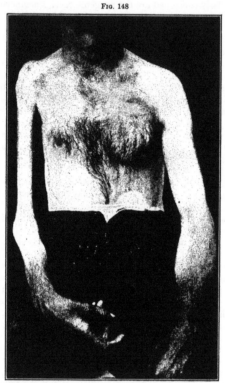

Old anterior poliomyelitis; hypoplasia of the right half of the shoulder-girdle, thorax, and right upper extremity. (From the Medical Clinic of the Montreal General Hospital.)

ally assuming an epidemic character. It follows exposure to cold, and is an occasional sequel of certain of the infectious fevers, such as measles and scarlatina. It seems probable that the causative agent acts first upon the bloodvessels and subsequently on the ganglia, contrary to what used to be thought. Clinically, the disease is characterized by

[1] Jour. Amer. Med. Assoc., 53:1909:639.
[2] Comptes-rendus Soc. de biol., 67:1909:592.

fever and a flaccid paralysis of one or more extremities, followed by atrophy of certain groups of muscles and eventually contractions and deformities. The reflexes are absent. Sensation is not impaired.

Post mortem, the cord presents congestion of the gray matter, particularly of the ventral horns, which are often the seat of red softening. The pia is injected, especially in its anterior portion, and the cerebrospinal fluid may be increased. With low magnification it can generally be made out that one horn is affected more than the other.

Microscopically, the most marked changes are to be found in the antero-exterior part of the ventral horn. Occasionally the anterior lateral tracts of the white substance are involved, rarely the posterior columns. The vessels of the affected region are congested with subadventitial infiltration with inflammatory cells, and there may be small hemorrhages, while the perivascular lymph-spaces are distended with inflammatory leukocytes. The glia is œdematous and infiltrated in places with round cells. The ganglion cells vary in appearance according to the age and intensity of the process. They may be swollen, turbid, and stain badly. The chromatin granules are arranged in irregular clumps, the nucleus stains diffusely, the nucleolus is vacuolated, and the protoplasmic processes are irregular. Later, the nuclei have disappeared, the cells are shrunken, deformed, and the protoplasmic processes have disappeared, leaving only a thickened axis-cylinder attached to the degenerated cell-body. Finally, many of the ganglia disappear. The fibres in the anterior roots present the usual features of nerve degeneration, the myelin sheath is breaking down into droplets of myelin and fat, the axis-cylinders are swollen and fragmented. The degeneration may extend down the peripheral nerves and lead to atrophy of the corresponding muscle groups. The glia is usually somewhat increased. Analogous changes may also be found in the medulla. There is usually an acute leptomeningitis as well.

As the disease subsides, or becomes chronic, the ventral horn is found to be considerably atrophied. The ganglion cells are diminished in number, and those that remain show evidences of degeneration. Certain fibers of the anterior roots have also disappeared. The perivascular infiltration with round cells is still noticeable, and compound granular cells may be found in fair numbers. Years after, when the disease has completely subsided, that portion of the cord corresponding to the site of the lesion is distinctly atrophied, and its contour is thereby altered. On section, one or both of the ventral horns is markedly atrophied. As a rule, one horn only is noticeably involved, while the other is normal or but slightly affected. Occasionally, the horn is about normal size, although the normal structure is lost, owing to what appears to be a colloid degeneration of the neuroglia. In certain parts the ganglia have entirely disappeared. Those that remain are usually normal. The bloodvessels are large and their walls thickened. The glia is considerably increased, and appears as a delicate meshwork containing abundant nuclei. Deiters' cells, or astrocytes, may be found in considerable numbers. The medullated fibres of the anterior roots have more or less degenerated, and the nerve-trunk looks thin and atrophic. Occasionally, a few fibres in the pyramidal tracts, in the immediate neighborhood of the primary lesion, may be degenerated, but this is only trifling.

The muscles innervated from the affected region of the cord rapidly atrophy, the fibres waste and disappear, the connective tissue is increased and may be infiltrated with fat. In children, not only the muscles, but the bones and vessels are markedly involved, and the limb may remain stunted or lag behind in its development.[1]

Acute Transverse Myelitis.—Acute transverse myelitis is occasionally met with in infectious diseases, but sometimes without very evident cause.

In the early stages, the whole thickness of the cord is swollen and softened for a short distance. On section, the affected part is reddened, œdematous, and may present hemorrhages. The cut surface assumes a convex form. Microscopically, the vessels are congested and are surrounded by clumps of leukocytes, chiefly of the polymorphonuclear variety. The interstitial substance is œdematous. The glia cells are swollen and increased in numbers. The axis-cylinders are swollen, fragmented, or atrophied, and the myelin sheaths are degenerating. The ganglion cells stain irregularly, their nuclei are dislocated, and the protoplasmic processes are varicosed or fragmented. Later, numbers of granular cells are found, which are probably connective-tissue corpuscles containing the debris of the broken-down tissue. "Amyloid" bodies may also be seen. This stage may be regarded as one of red softening. It soon gives place to yellow softening. The cord is somewhat swollen, and of a yellowish color. The gray matter is distinctly wasted. The microscopic appearances are similar to those just described, save that the neuroglia is more swollen and looser, consequently, in texture, the glia cells begin to show degeneration, granular cells are still more numerous, and the parenchymatous changes are more marked. The ganglion cells are swollen, irregular, and vacuolated, or, again, they may be shrunken, stain badly, and contain no nuclei. Some may be represented by a protoplasmic sac containing brownish pigment, and some have totally disappeared, as is proved by the fact that the number of ganglia is reduced. In very severe cases, the degeneration is so extreme that the affected portion of the cord is reduced to a pultaceous mass, composed of fat globules, granular cells, and detritus. In other cases, where the process has somewhat subsided in intensity, reparative changes make their appearance. The ganglia and nerve fibers have largely disappeared, the granular cells are less numerous and are found mainly about the bloodvessels, while the glia shows proliferation and is more abundant. Secondary degeneration may appear in certain tracts above and below the inflamed area.

Myelitic processes heal, when they do so, with the replacement of the destroyed nerve-elements by dense scar tissue, giving the cord at the

[1] A full study of this condition will be found in the following monograph: Pathologisch-anat. Untersuch. über akat. Poliomyelitis u. verwandten Krankheiten von d. Epidem. in Norwegen, 1903–06, Harbitz & Scheel, Christiana, 1907.

affected part a shrunken, grayish appearance and a somewhat hard consistence. This is, in part, due to hyperplasia of the glial cells, but in part, also, to proliferation of the connective tissue derived from the sheaths of the bloodvessels and the prolongations of the pia.

The clinical features depend on the position of the lesion. Transverse myelitis of the thoracic cord gives rise to spastic paraplegia of the lower extremities without atrophy, paralysis of the abdominal muscles, paralysis of the bladder and intestines, and anesthesia below the level of the lesion. A lesion of the lower cervical region causes flaccid paralysis of the arms with atrophy, spastic paralysis of the legs, loss of sensation in the arms and below the level of the second rib, pupillary changes, and respiratory embarrassment. When the lumbar region is involved we get flaccid paralysis of the legs with atrophy, paralysis of the bladder and bowels, and loss of the reflexes.

Acute Suppurative Myelitis.—Acute suppurative myelitis, when of hematogenic origin, is rare. It occasionally is found secondary to bronchiectasis, suppuration in the genito-urinary tract, and dysenteric abscess of the liver. The suppuration may be somewhat diffuse, following the line of the bloodvessels, or small abscesses may be produced. The pathological changes do not differ materially from those in other forms of acute myelitis, except that the process is more intense. When the abscesses are small and isolated, the degenerative changes are found only in the immediate neighborhood, while the intervening tissue is comparatively or entirely free.

Acute myelitis, arising by **extension,** can usually be traced to inflammation of the membranes and nerve-roots, or, rarely, to infection from the central canal. In the former case the disease is really a **meningomyelitis.** This may be suppurative, tuberculous, or syphilitic. Here, the infective agents probably travel by means of the bloodvessels and perivascular lymphatics. As would be expected, the lesions are most marked at the periphery of the cord.

Myelitis of central origin is generally due to abscesses or suppurative inflammation somewhere in the ventricles, the infective agents from which set up inflammation along the whole length of the cord. The changes produced are œdema, swelling, and disintegration of the cells in the gray commissure, extending into the ventral and dorsal horns, and occasionally even into the white substance.

Landry's Paralysis.—Apart from tuberculosis and syphilis of the cord, which will be described hereafter, perhaps the most important affection coming under this category is *acute ascending paralysis* (Landry's paralysis). This affection, as its name implies, is an acute one, characterized clinically by the occurrence of paralysis, usually extending from below upward, and ending quickly in death, owing to involvement of the bulbar nuclei. Sensory symptoms are in abeyance, and the affected muscles preserve their faradic irritability. The spleen is enlarged, sometimes also the various lymph-nodes, and the kidneys show degenerative changes. This would suggest a general systemic infection as the cause, although the nature of it is quite obscure. Probably a variety of agents may cause it. Judging from clinical features, the lesions may be primary in the cord and medulla, or may extend to them from the peripheral nerves.

The histological features of the disease have been much debated. Landry did not find changes in the central or peripheral nervous system. Others believe the cord to be extensively involved, while the majority regard the disease as primary in the peripheral motor neurones. The lesions apparently vary. In one case, they are practically those of an acute poliomyelitis. In another, there is an acute exudative inflammation in the connective tissue of the peripheral nerves, which may be simple, hemorrhagic, or suppurative, leading to extensive degeneration of the nerve-elements.

Traumatic Myelitis.—Traumatic myelitis includes all those forms which result from injuries, such as gunshots, cutting or stabbing, contusions, fractures, and dislocations of the vertebræ. These injuries lead to more or less laceration and compression of the cord, or even to solution of continuity or complete destruction of the cord at the affected region. The amount of inflammation, of course, depends on the nature and extent of the injury. The injury leads to the rupture and disintegration of certain of the nerve-fibres and ganglia, and this leads to secondary degeneration in the tracts functionally connected with the destroyed structures. The glia and connective tissue may also be involved. In severe cases the section of the cord affected may soften and become liquefied. Should there be but little blood, we get the well-known "white" softening. Where blood is effused, we have "red" and later "yellow" softening. Interference with the free flow of blood or lymph in the vessels may lead to foci of softening in districts remote from the injury. If infection with pyogenic microörganisms take place, we may have abscess of the cord with extension of purulent inflammation to the meninges. In the milder forms, healing may take place by sclerosis, or replacement of the destroyed tissue by proliferated glia cells. In the severer cases, especially where the membranes are involved, a dense connective-tissue scar may be produced.

Tuberculosis.—Tuberculosis of the cord is rarely primary. Collins[1] has met with one case of tuberculous myelitis in which no other tuberculous lesion was detected in the body. As a rule, however, there is tuberculosis elsewhere. The disease takes three forms—multiple *miliary granulomas*, larger single or multiple *nodules*, and *meningomyelitis*.

In the first mentioned form, numerous small tubercles, often of microscopic size, are found both in the gray and the white substance, usually about the vessels, indicating a hematogenic mode of infection. The obstruction to the circulation thus caused and the consequent lack of nutrition leads to areas of ischemic softening, and there may even be secondary degeneration of the fibres near by.

[1] American Text-book of Pathology, W. B. Saunders & Co., Phila. and London, 1901: 567.

In the second variety, granulomas sometimes as large as a hazelnut may be found, which present extensive central caseation or even lique-faction. The tubercles may extend to the meninges or break into the central canal, so that more widespread infection may take place. In some cases the continuity of the cord is practically entirely interrupted. Secondary degeneration of neighboring fibres occurs.

The most common form is the tuberculous meningomyelitis. Here the infection spreads from the meninges by means of the intraspinal prolonga-tions of the pia, through the perivascular lymphatics. Small tubercles are found about the vessels, which may in time reach a fair size, caseate, and lead to considerable destruction of the nerve-substance.

Syphilis.—Some writers are inclined to believe in the existence of a *simple acute myelitis* occurring in the earlier years of syphilis, which is not unlike the non-specific forms of diffuse myelitis before referred to. There is the same degeneration of the specific nerve-elements with cellular infiltration of the connective tissue. The bloodvessels appear to be specially implicated. They show endarteritis, may be thrombosed, and in their vicinity small hemorrhages may be seen. Less questionable, however, is *syphilitic meningomyelitis.* This is most common in the cervical and dorsal regions of the cord. The main characteristic is the thickening or degeneration of the vessels with, sometimes, the forma-tion of small gummas along their course. This leads to degeneration of the nerve-fibres and ganglia. Secondary degeneration is common. There is a small-celled infiltration about the vessels, and the glia is increased.

Leprosy.—In a few cases we find merely atrophy and degeneration of the nerve-elements, particularly the ganglia. As a rule, however, there are areas of softening and hemorrhagic extravasation. Micro-scopically, the nerve structures are degenerated, and the connective tissue shows inflammatory exudation and hemorrhage. The lepra bacilli have been found in the connective tissue, both of the gray and the white substance.

RETROGRESSIVE METAMORPHOSES.

We pass on now to discuss the various forms of atrophy and degenera-tion to which the spinal cord is liable. We have to premise, however, that the subject is beset with great difficulties. As has been before remarked, the nervous tissue is the most delicate and highly special-ized structure in the body. It is, consequently, particularly sus-ceptible to the action of all kinds of deteriorating agencies, while its recuperative powers are slight. This explains why it is that disintegra-tion and degeneration are the most constant and striking pathological changes which meet the investigator. These retrogressive phenomena are produced by the most diverse causes, and it is not always possible, in any given case, to determine the etiological factor chiefly or entirely to blame. Thus, the distinction between inflammatory and pure degenera-tions cannot always be made. Nevertheless, it is the custom among clinicians to apply the generic term *myelitis* (inflammation of the cord) to all forms of degeneration, irrespective of the cause, inasmuch as they are characterized by fairly definite and constant symptoms, depending on the localization of the lesion. The term "myelitis," in this wide sense, is a convenient one and thoroughly established by custom, but should be used with a certain mental reservation.

In order to get a clear understanding of degeneration of nerve-tissue and its results, it is important to bear certain facts in mind.

According to the "neurone" concept of the histological structure of the nervous system, commonly held at the present day, the brain and spinal cord, with their prolongations, the peripheral nerves, are to be regarded in the main as a peculiar aggregation of highly specialized cells, consisting of a large cell-body with dendritic processes (the ganglion cell) from which proceeds a single long and attenuated thread (axis-cylinder or neuraxone). The whole constitutes the neurone. Each neurone is, so to speak, self-contained, and has no communication with adjacent neurones, save by contiguity.

The various constituents of the neurone may act differently when subjected to abnormal conditions. In general, it may be said that a nerve-fibre or neuraxone when severed from any cause from its nutrient centre, the ganglion cell, will degenerate. The process begins at the distal extremity and extends gradually backward to the site of the lesion. In some cases the degeneration is *primary;* that is to say, it is due to some cause acting locally and directly on a fibre or bundle of fibres. The lesion may be chiefly or entirely confined to one physiological tract of the cord, and we then speak of a *primary "system" disease.* Or more than one tract may be involved and we have a *combined "system" disease.* In other cases, and probably the majority, the degeneration may be referred to some lesion at a distance, such as destruction of the ganglion cells nourishing the fibres, or anything which interferes with the conducting power of the fibres. This is called *secondary* degeneration.

In primary degeneration certain tracts appear to be specially picked out. These are the *sensory neurones of the cord,* which may be traced from the posterior nerve-roots into the column of Burdach, thence into the column of Goll, to end finally in the medulla in the nuclei of Goll and Burdach; the *central motor neurones,* starting in the pyramidal layer of the motor cortex, and passing through the internal capsule, the pyramids, into the pyramidal tracts; the *peripheral motor neurones,* beginning in the ganglia of the ventral horns, and extending through the anterior roots to the muscles.

Secondary degeneration is divided into *ascending* and *descending,* according to the direction it takes in the cord. Ascending degeneration is generally found in the *posterior columns,* the *direct cerebellar tract,* and the *anterolateral tract* of Gowers. It may be associated with lesions of the ganglia in Clarke's columns. The process terminates in the restiform bodies of the medulla. Descending degeneration mainly affects the *pyramidal tracts,* Thus, in the case of a unilateral lesion above the decussation, say, in ,the motor cortex, we find degeneration in the anterior pyramidal tract on the same side and in the lateral or crossed pyramidal tract on the opposite side. A few motor fibres appear not to decussate and pass down through the lateral columns. In long-standing cases, atrophy of the ganglion cells of the ventral horns has been observed.

Fig. 149

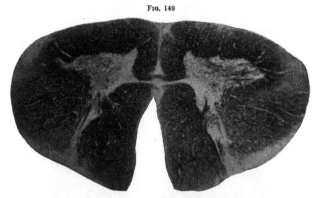

Compression myelitis. Cervical cord. Degeneration in the cerebellar and antero-lateral ascending tracts: to a slight degree in the postero-external columns also. Section taken above the site of injury. (From the collection of Dr. Colin K. Russel.)

Fig. 150

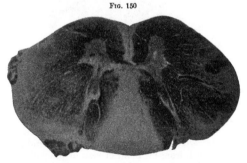

Compression myelitis. Dorsal cord. Degeneration in the postero-internal, lateral, and direct pyramidal tracts. Section taken from immediately above the point of compression. (From the collection of Dr. Colin K. Russel.)

Descending degeneration has at times been noted in the posterior columns. In the upper part of the cord it affects two small tracts passing outward and backward from a point slightly behind the gray commissure (comma-degeneration of Schultze). Lower down the fibres approach the posterior commissure, where they form the oval field of Flechsig.

Secondary degeneration is apt to be of considerable extent, since the nerve paths are so elongated and their correlation is close.

The causes of nerve degeneration are numerous. Chief among them may be mentioned mechanical trauma; circulatory disturbances, such as anemia, embolism, thrombosis, endarteritis, and hemorrhage; and toxins of bacterial, mineral, or vegetable origin. In some cases there may be a combination of factors at work.

Considerable difficulty is experienced when one attempts to decide upon a logical classification of the degenerative affections of the spinal cord. We have referred above to "primary" and "secondary" degenerations. Many authorities speak of "primary system disease," meaning by that a disease in which the lesions are confined to a definite "system"

FIG 151

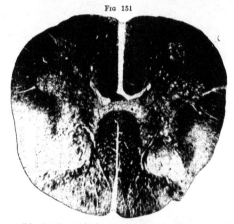

Compression myelitis. Lumbar cord. Degeneration in the lateral columns. Section taken below the site of compression. (From the collection of Dr. Colin K. Russel)

or nerve-tract, involving a greater or less extent of its course, which cannot be referred etiologically to any obvious or gross external anatomical change. This is certainly a convenient clinical generalization, but it may well be doubted, from the point of view of the pathological histologist, whether the lesions in question ever are restricted to one physiological nerve-tract. Again, in many cases, opinions are divided as to the propriety of the term "primary," inasmuch as our knowledge of the origin and course of the pathological changes is still imperfect, while primary and secondary manifestations are often so intimately associated.[1]

[1] We have adopted the distinctions between "primary" and "secondary" degeneration, as outlined above, out of deference to certain authorities. We feel bound to say, however, that in our judgment the points of difference are not well taken. We think that the terms "primary" and "secondary" should be used in the case of the nervous system in the same sense as they are used in other connections. Usage,

Of course, where it is possible, our classifications of disease should be based upon pathogeny and morbid anatomy, and it should be our aim to show the harmony between these and the clinical features. In many cases, however, as here, we must to a large extent be guided by expediency. It has been deemed wiser here, therefore, not to draw too fine distinctions, but to adopt a mainly "regional" classification.

Among the commonest forms of spinal cord degeneration is that due to pressure, the so-called **compression myelitis.** As a rule, the lesion is a *transverse* one, affecting all the elements of the cord in a comparatively restricted area. It may be caused by traumatism, such as fracture of the vertebral column with pressure of a lamina upon the cord, but is often also due to tuberculous caries of the spine, tuberculosis of the meninges, and primary or secondary tumors in the vertebral canal or in the cord itself. Central degeneration may be caused by the accumulation of blood or fluid in the central canal. Any of these conditions will cause marked destruction of the nerve-elements at the site of the lesion, with widespread ascending and descending degeneration in the associated tracts. The local effects produced may be referred in part to the direct influence of the pressure, but much more to the disturbance of the blood and lymph-circulation. The degeneration is first manifested in the white substance, the fibres of which swell up and disintegrate, much as has been described in the case of transverse section of the nerves. The axis-cylinders swell and become varicosed, and the myelin sheaths break down into fat. The ganglion cells are somewhat more resistant, but ultimately undergo vacuolation and chromatolysis. Granular cells appear early and in considerable numbers. In the course of a few days the degenerative changes may be traced to the extremities of the neurones. Later, both the fibres and their sheaths will have almost entirely disappeared, although degenerated and varicosed fibres may here and there be seen, the number of fibres remaining being, of course, dependent on the extent of the original lesion. The place of the degenerated fibres is taken up by newly-formed glial tissue, which eventually leads to contraction and sclerosis of the cord. The cord as a whole shrinks, becomes firmer, and assumes a grayish color.

It should, perhaps, be remarked that in cases such as tuberculosis of

in other words, should be uniform. A suppurating focus on the end of a finger is a primary lesion. It may lead to the production of, say, a liver abscess. The latter is a secondary lesion. Apply the same principle to the nervous system. A lesion of a neurone is "primary" if it occur independently of any extrinsic and remote pathological condition. Good examples of this are abiotrophic conditions and "exhaustion-atrophies," and toxic neuritides. If, on the other hand, a neurone degenerates because of the loss of its functional relationships with other neurones, because of the strangling action of a gliosis, or, again, from disuse, as in the case of ankylosis of a joint or the amputation of a limb, this would be a "secondary" degeneration. Inasmuch as all are united in regarding the neurone, central ganglion-cell, dendrites, and neuraxone as a unit, it seems illogical and artificial to draw fundamental distinctions between lesions which may affect these several components.

the meninges the resulting lesions in the cord may, in some instances, not be entirely due to pressure and circulatory disturbances, but to inflammation as well.

Multiple or Disseminated Sclerosis.—Multiple or disseminated sclerosis (see p. 588) is a disease which affects the nervous system as a whole. Not only may the spinal cord be involved, but the brain and peripheral nerves. The lesions are irregularly distributed, apparently without rhyme or reason, and may be chiefly localized in the brain, or, again, in the cord.

In the case of the cord, one finds multiple, grayish foci, generally in the white substance, but also to some extent in the gray matter, which may be the size of a pin-head or smaller, or may involve nearly the whole transverse thickness of the cord. These foci vary somewhat in appearance, being at one time rather soft and gelatinous-looking, of grayish-white color, rather badly defined from the normal tissues; at another, fairly firm, of a uniform gray color, and sharply differentiated. Occasionally, the lesions are to be found in relation with various bloodvessels.

Fig. 152

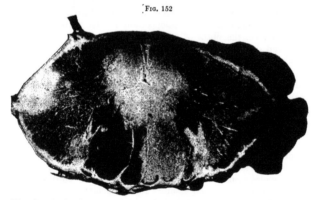

Disseminated sclerosis. The cord shows irregularly distributed patches of degeneration.
(From the collection of Dr. Colin K. Russel.)

The etiology of the disease is obscure. The affection of the vessels might suggest a vascular origin, such as a circulating toxin or infection, or, again, an ischemic necrosis. From the histological appearance of the lesions, Ziegler would recognize two varieties, *secondary multiple sclerosis*, which results from a previous focal degeneration or inflammation, and *primary multiple sclerosis*, due to a pathological hyperplasia of the glia, akin to what occurs in syringomyelia, and probably referable to some error in development. The latter type affects chiefly the posterior columns and the neighborhood of the ventricles, and is characterized by a peculiarly dense overgrowth of the glial substance, in which may be found scattered nerve fibres that present little or no degeneration.

Chronic Anterior Poliomyelitis.—In some instances the ganglion cells of the ventral cornua, together with the peripheral motor neurones, undergo degeneration. Chronic anterior poliomyelitis may be taken as the type.

This disease is similar in its clinical features to the acute anterior poliomyelitis described before (p. 603), save that it begins insidiously and runs a chronic or subchronic course. Some cases are believed to have an inflammatory basis, and the histological appearances are strictly comparable to those found in the acute form. In other cases the affection seems to be a pure degeneration, the lesions being atrophy of the cells of the ventral horns, with slight interstitial changes in the white substance, degeneration of the peripheral motor neurones, and wasting of the muscles supplied by them.

Progressive Bulbar Paralysis.—Analogous to this in all respects is the progressive bulbar paralysis, or glossolabiolaryngeal paralysis, in which the motor nuclei of the medulla, usually the nuclei of the hypoglossal, vagus, accessorius, facial, and glossopharyngeal nerves, are involved. There may or may not be degeneration of the pyramidal tracts. When degeneration in this situation is present we have really an amyotrophic lateral sclerosis. The nature of the disease is obscure. Sometimes it shows a familial distribution. It is most probably an abiotrophic condition.

Progressive Spinal Muscular Atrophy.—Closely resembling chronic anterior poliomyelitis, clinically as well as anatomically, is the disease known as progressive spinal muscular atrophy of the Aran-Duchenne type. Here, also, there is atrophy of the ganglion cells of the ventral horns, with degeneration of the peripheral motor nerve-fibres and the corresponding muscles. There are, however, in addition, more or less marked changes in the white substance of the cord, notably the pyramidal tracts and the anterolateral ground-bundle. The ganglia are found in various stages of atrophy, or may have disappeared. The anterior horns, as a whole, do not seem to shrink, as they do in chronic poliomyelitis, but are transformed into a fine reticulum, containing large numbers of spindle-shaped cells. The anterior roots are wasted, and many of the fibres forming the peripheral nerve-trunks are partially or completely degenerated. According to Gowers, the pyramidal tracts are invariably involved to some extent. In the most severe cases the degeneration can be traced upward as far as the motor cortex.

The affected muscles show simple atrophy, or fatty or vitreous degeneration. The muscle nuclei are often increased, and there may be increase of the interstitial connective tissue.

The process begins in the cervical region. The muscles affected are, first, those of the thenar and hypothenar eminences, the lumbricales and interossei, later, those of the forearm and shoulder. Besides this, the more usual Aran-Duchenne type, there are other forms, notably one in which the wasting begins in the lower extremities.

The cause of the disease is obscure. From the now well-recognized fact that certain mineral substances, such as lead, and bacterial toxins, like that of diphtheria, are occasionally productive of degenerative changes in the motor nuclei and peripheral nerves, it may be inferred that circulating poisons, either exogenous or, perhaps, of a metabolic nature, are at work.

Lateral Sclerosis.—Degeneration in the *lateral* or *pyramidal* tracts is commonly known as lateral sclerosis. It may be a descending degeneration, secondary to disease of the ganglion cells of the motor cortex of the brain or in any part of the upper motor neurone above the site of the lesion, or may be primary in the lateral tracts of the cord. The symptoms are entirely motor, consisting in paresis or paralysis of the muscles, hypertonus, and increased knee-jerks (*spastic spinal paralysis*). There is no muscular wasting. Somewhat similar phenomena are noted in the so-called "compression" myelitis, transverse myelitis, and certain cases of disseminated sclerosis, but here sensory symptoms are commonly observed, although less marked than the motor ones. Primary sclerosis of the lateral tracts is quite rare.

Posterior Sclerosis.—Posterior sclerosis (*locomotor ataxia; tabes dorsalis*) is, anatomically speaking, a degeneration of the sensory neurones of the posterior roots and posterior columns of the cord, with less constant changes in the spinal ganglia and peripheral nerves. The disease process is not confined to the spinal nervous mechanism, but involves the brain as well. The sensory nuclei and fibres in the medulla are not infrequently attacked, and degeneration of the nuclei of the oculomotor nerves and of the optic nerves may often be observed.

The symptoms in the first, or what is known as the preataxic stage, are chiefly lancinating pains in various parts, usually the lower extremities; loss of the knee-jerk; Argyll-Robertson pupil; occasionally, diplopia, myosis, and a "girdle" sensation. Later, we get, in addition, muscular incoördination (ataxic stage), diminution of sensibility to touch, pain, heat, and cold, sometimes atrophy of the optic nerve, and, finally, complete disability (paralytic stage).

To obtain a proper conception of the pathological changes that occur in tabes, it is necessary to bear in mind certain peculiarities in the embryological development of the cord.

The posterior columns are formed at a different period from the rest of the cord, and are developed from the posterior nerve-roots, and these from the spinal ganglia. The posterior columns must, therefore, be regarded as ingrowths into the cord of fibres of exogenous origin. There are, however, some few fibres of endogenous nature derived from cells situated in the gray matter of the cord.

It is now well known that the fibres composing certain tracts or nerve bundles, that are apparently homologous, become medullated at different stages of embryonic development. On this basis Flechsig and others would divide the posterior columns into the following components: (1) An anterior or ventral root-zone, next the posterior commissure and gray matter; (2) a middle root-zone, consisting of two sorts of fibres, known as the fibres of the first system and the fibres of the second system of the middle root-zone; (3) a middle zone, next the posterior fissure and distinct from the column of Goll; and (4) a posterior zone, being the dorsal portion of the posterior column, divided into a median part and a lateral part, the zone of Lissauer. The order in which these various zones are medullated is as follows: (1) The anterior root-zone, and soon after this the middle zone and the first system of the middle root-zone; (2) the column of Goll, the postero-internal root-zone, and the second system of the middle root-zone, all approximately about the same time.

Each fibre derived from the posterior root divides after entering the cord into two parts, a long, ascending branch and a short, descending branch. Each branch gives off collaterals which help to make up the posterior columns. The fibres entering the lower segments of the cord pass into the internal parts of the posterior columns to form eventually the columns of Goll. They terminate in the medulla in arborizations about the nucleus of Goll's column. The root fibres that enter the dorsal and cervical regions of the cord run in the other parts of the posterior columns and form their terminal arborizations about the nuclei in the posterior horns. The anterior root-zone contains fibres derived directly from the posterior roots, and commissural fibres which unite the gray substance at different levels. The first system of the middle root-zone is composed of fibres from the posterior roots, which run for a short distance in the posterior column and then enter Clarke's column. The second system of the middle root-zone consists of fibres from the posterior root-zone which form the column of Goll higher up. The formation of Flechsig's middle zone is not yet settled. The postero-external root zone of Flechsig (column of Lissauer) is composed of delicate, closely packed fibres, probably collaterals from the posterior roots, which, after running for some distance in the cord, enter the substantia gelatinosa.

The macroscopic changes in the cord in locomotor ataxia vary according to the extent of the disease. The earliest stage is, of course, rarely seen, except in those cases associated with general paresis. Here the cord presents little or no deviation from the normal save on microscopic examination. In a moderately advanced case the posterior portion of the cord is distinctly shrunken, firm, and of a grayish-white color. The posterior roots, as a rule, seem to be somewhat wasted, although not invariably so. The other parts of the cord are normal. The pia-arachnoid is somewhat thickened and opaque over the dorsal aspect of the cord. The dura is unaltered. The cerebrospinal fluid may be increased.

When stained by the Pal-Weigert or other method for myelin staining, marked abnormalities can readily be observed in the posterior columns. These vary somewhat in the different regions of the cord. In cervical tabes, practically the whole of the posterior columns may be involved. As a rule, however, the columns of Goll are affected, particularly in the posterior portion, or there may be two narrow bands just external to the columns of Goll and Lissauer. In the dorsal region there are usually two streaks of degeneration in Burdach's columns, and the process apparently tends to involve those fibres nearer the median line. In the lumbar cord, the degeneration commonly affects more or less completely the tracts of Lissauer. The fact that a portion of the Lissauer's tract lies ventrally to the posterior roots has given rise to the erroneous view that in tabes the lateral tracts are involved as well as the posterior ones, and that, therefore, the disease is a combined sclerosis. Embryologically and functionally, however, the ventral portion of Lissauer's tract belongs to the posterior column. Not infrequently the ventral portion of the posterior columns, or the anterior root-zones of Flechsig, escape. Owing to proliferation of the ependyma, the central canal is often obliterated.

FIG. 153

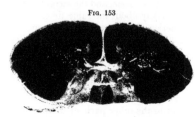

Cervical tabes dorsalis. Section through the cervical cord. (From the collection of Dr. Colin K. Russel.)

FIG. 154

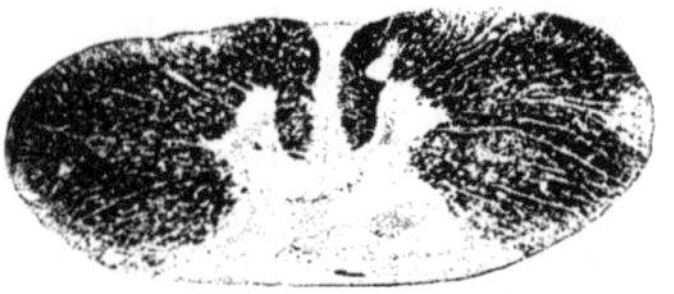

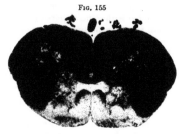

Tabes dorsalis. Dorsal cord. (From the collection of Dr. Colin K. Russel.)

FIG. 155

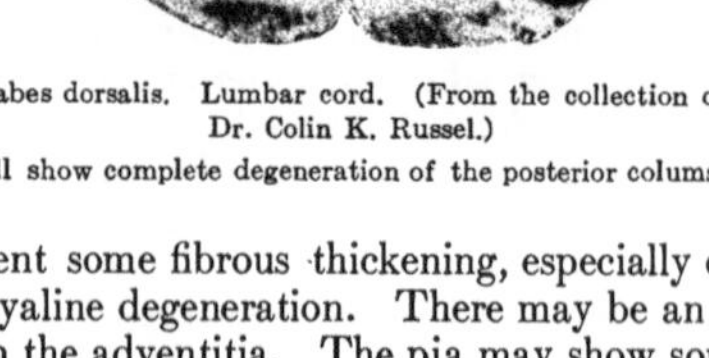

Tabes dorsalis. Lumbar cord. (From the collection of Dr. Colin K. Russel.)

All show complete degeneration of the posterior colums.

Besides the changes just described, there are others, less constant and important, in other parts, such as the gray substance of the dorsal and ventral horns, and the cell column of Clarke. The cells here show eccentricity of the nuclei and more or less chromatolysis.

The degenerative changes are much the same as in secondary degeneration elsewhere. The myelin sheaths break down, the axis-cylinders swell up, become fragmented, and disappear. To replace these the glia proliferates, and there is an increase of connective tissue, derived from the trabeculæ of the pia extending into the cord. The fibres which enter the gray matter from the posterior columns are occasionally degenerated. The vascular lesions are never extreme. The vessels in certain regions may present some fibrous thickening, especially of the adventitia, or may show hyaline degeneration. There may be an accumulation of granular cells in the adventitia. The pia may show some thickening and fibrosis.

The changes occurring in the spinal ganglia have not yet been established beyond cavil. It may be said, at all events, that they are rarely extreme and do not account for the extensive lesions found in the posterior columns. Stroebe found the cells of the ganglia to be shrunken, irregular in outline, many of them vacuolated and markedly pigmented. In advanced tabes, the ganglion cells had largely disappeared, the intercapsular space was distended, and the cells of the capsule were proliferating. The interstitial substance showed hyperplasia. The posterior roots external to the cord were markedly degenerated.

The changes in the peripheral nerves are inconstant and have been variously interpreted. The difficulty is to decide whether the degeneration that is sometimes present is primary or secondary. The small, cutaneous nerves are those usually picked out. The myelin sheaths are disintegrated, the axis-cylinders are swollen, and there is some increase of the interstitial connective tissue. The cranial nerves, particularly the optic, and the sympathetic fibres are similarly involved.

Atrophy of the cells in the motor cortex of the brain is sometimes met with.

The interpretation of the histological findings is, as one can readily understand, fraught with great difficulty, and much debate has taken place as to what constitutes the primary lesion. It may, first of all, be taken as certain that the degenerative process is essential to the nerve fibres and is not to be regarded as secondary to the increased formation of glia. Nor is there any evidence of a primary inflammatory disturbance. The main views are (1) that locomotor ataxia is a primary sclerosis of the posterior colums of the cord, and (2) that the changes in the cord are secondary to degeneration of the posterior roots. The latter is the one supported by the greatest amount of evidence, and is accepted by the majority of neuropathologists at the present time.

Déjerine would find the essential cause in endarteritis of the vessels supplying the intramedullary portions of the posterior roots, with consecutive fibrosis. In refutation of this opinion, it may be remarked that the vascular disturbances found in tabes are similar to those found in other degenerative diseases of the cord, and are never a striking feature in the histological picture. The vascular changes, moreover, are not uniformly distributed, and could hardly account for such a marked "system" sclerosis. The preponderance of evidence goes to show that the disease process begins in the extramedullary portion of the posterior roots. Some have described certain anatomical conditions that might account for this. Redlich and Obersteiner found a thickening of the pia and dense sclerosis of the peripheral zones of the neuroglia, which, in their opinion, lead to the degeneration in question by compression of the posterior roots at the point where they enter the cord. The medullary sheaths are much thinner here than at any other part of the fibre, which makes it probably the least resistant point. This meningitis, it need hardly be said, is not always present in tabes, and, conversely, we do not find the anatomical lesions of tabes in cases of meningitis and meningomyelitis.

It is not impossible, farther, that toxins circulating in the cerebrospinal fluid might affect deleteriously the nerve roots during their intrameningeal course.   Lesions in the cord, somewhat similar to those in tabes, have been described in connection with *chronic ergotism* and in *pellagra*. In ergot poisoning, the posterior roots are degenerated, and also the columns of Burdach in the cord.   The columns of Goll are not primarily affected, but may be secondarily involved in advanced cases.   The anterior root-zone, the median portion of the middle zone, and Lissauer's tract escape.   In pellagra, the posterior roots are not involved, and Marie, on this account, regards it as an endogenous disease of the cord. It is, in fact, a primary degeneration of toxic origin.

Oppenheim believes that the toxic agent at work in tabes dorsalis has a selective action on the posterior spinal ganglia and their homologues, the Gasserian and jugular ganglia, etc.   This toxin is just powerful enough to cause atrophy of the distal portion of the neurone in the posterior columns of the cord and in the peripheral nerves.

Marie considers that the disease is due to a syphilitic lesion involving the lymphatic channels of the posterior columns and of the corresponding pia-arachnoid, inasmuch as he has, in many cases, found a cloudiness and thickening of the pia-arachnoid on the dorsal aspect of the cord.

When such divergent views are expressed as to the exact meaning of the anatomical changes in tabes, it is not surprising that the etiology of the disease is not altogether clear.   It seems fairly certain that tabes is not a disease of the cord alone, but of the whole nervous system, involving the sensory neurones, and, probably, of exogenous origin.   We must bear this in mind, therefore, when searching for the cause.   Clinicians usually attribute the disease to syphilis, overwork, traumatism, exposure to cold, or sexual excess.   It is a fact, as Erb and many others have pointed out, that the majority of tabetic patients (from 50 to 90 per cent.) give a history or present signs of previous syphilis.   Recently, Wassermann has shown that his precipitation test, which is positive in active syphilis, is also positive in tabes dorsalis.   This is highly significant. It cannot be denied, however, that the affection occurs in those who have never had syphilis.   Tabes, moreover, rarely comes on during the active stages of syphilis, being usually found from five to ten or fifteen years, or even longer, after infection.   It is a matter of common observation, too, that antisyphilitic remedies have little or no effect on the course of the disease.   If, then, we admit the importance of syphilis, as we needs must, we have to regard tabes as a parasyphilitic affection, rather than as due directly to the infective agent of syphilis.   We must hold, therefore, with Obersteiner, who assumes a multiple causation for tabes, in which syphilis is the most frequent and important single cause.

Perhaps, the view that fits in most perfectly with the observed facts is that of Edinger,[1] the so-called "exhaustion theory."   This is based on the well-known idea of Weigert and Roux, that the constituent tissues of an organ are normally in a state of equilibrium, so correlated one to another that no cell can disappear without its place being taken by hyperplasia of the surrounding tissue, and when one constituent becomes

[1] Deut. med. Woch., 1904:1633, 1800, and 1921; 1905: 4 and 135.

weaker or less resistant, the energy of growth of its neighbors tends to repress it' still farther. According to this conception, cirrhosis of the liver is primarily a degeneration of the parenchymatous cells with a secondary overgrowth of the interstitial tissue. The gliosis that occurs in the spinal cord of an old hemiplegic case can be explained in the same way, and when a cell or fibre, or even a whole neurone, becomes so weak that it is unable to hold in check the proliferative capacity of the neighboring tissue, we must expect to find the same process going on.

Farther, function involves breaking down of the active tissue. Normally, the destructive process is compensated by a sufficient supply of nutrition, so that the production of living substance is constant. If this do not take place, the normal equilibrium of the parts is disturbed and a progressive degeneration is the result. Edinger applies this to the nervous system. He assumes that if the supply of nutrition be deficient, or if, though it be normal, excessive function be demanded of the cell, that is to say, if the normal relation between combustion and repair be disturbed, either by relative or by absolute superfunction, the energy of growth of the resting tissue will lead to a degeneration of the less resistant active parts, a result that will occur the more easily if both factors be at work. As examples of this, Edinger cites the hammer palsy of smiths and the atrophic paralysis of the forearm muscles in drummer boys, which, according to him, occur most frequently or only in badly-nourished subjects.

To apply this to tabes. The reparative processes in the specific cells are impaired, as a result of some toxin circulating in the system, this toxin in most cases being syphilitic in origin. The neurones which are normally most active, or are most constantly at work, are those which suffer. These are the sensory nerves from the muscles which play an important role in the regulation of muscular contraction, and are constantly submitting those stimuli by which we become aware of the condition of our muscular system and the position of our limbs. Clinically, this defect is manifested in the loss of muscular tone and the sense of position, and the consequent ataxia. Secondly, the purely sensory nerves which are constantly submitting sensations from the skin and mucous membranes would be likely to suffer and give rise to sensory disturbances. Thirdly, the eyes would suffer, and above all the constrictor of the iris, so constantly active in the reflex contraction of the iris to light, which must be almost constantly at work in comparison with the reflex for accommodation. In this way the Argyll-Robertson pupil can be explained. The paralysis of the external ocular muscles, the bladder disturbance, the occasional atrophic muscular palsies, may also all be explained in terms of this theory.

The peripheral motor neurones, which are normally capable of responding to two sets of stimuli, those from the upper motor neurone, which are relatively seldom at work, and those from the peripheral sensory neurone, keeping up the tone of the muscles, have the opportunity to repair when they are not at the service of voluntary impulses. They, therefore, would not be so likely to become exhausted as the sensory neurones. When, too, the sensory neurones have degenerated and they do not get stimuli from them, they have still more time to repair, though this is probably in part counterbalanced by the excessive energy that an ataxic patient puts into any voluntary movement.

In this way Edinger escapes the dilemma of believing that every person having tabes must be syphilitic. On this conception we can see how trauma, exposure to cold and wet, and excesses of various kinds may act as predisposing causes in bringing about depreciation of the nerve unit. The fact that tabes is more common in men than in women becomes explainable, also, men being more exposed to those deleterious influences which Edinger brings into the etiology of the disease.

Besides the degenerative diseases of the cord hitherto described, which affect the nerve elements of single tracts, there are others in which several neurone groups of differing function are involved. These are the so-called "combined system diseases," of which posterolateral sclerosis, Friedreich's ataxia, and amyotrophic lateral sclerosis are the most prominent members.

Posterolateral Sclerosis.—Posterolateral sclerosis, or *combined sclerosis,* the *ataxic paraplegia* of the clinicians, is characterized by sclerosis of the posterior and lateral tracts. In the posterior tracts, the postero-internal and the dorsal portion of the postero-external columns are the regions specially picked out. In the lateral tracts it is usually the crossed pyramidal tracts, but not infrequently the direct cerebellar tracts, the columns of Gowers, and the lateral limiting layers. Collins has recorded also degeneration of the cells of Clarke's column and of the fine, white fibres of the anterior horns.

The disease appears to be a primary one, but the exact pathogeny is not known. Many consider it a true combined "system" disease. Others think that the parts affected, owing to their comparatively poor blood supply, are less able than other parts to withstand the deleterious action of the morbific agent.

The disease occasionally follows exposure to cold. Syphilis plays an unimportant role in the etiology. The main clinical features are ataxia, muscular weakness, hypertonus, and gradually increasing rigidity. Sensory symptoms are rare and trifling. In advanced cases, owing to cerebral involvement, the disease may resemble general paresis.

Friedreich's Ataxia.—Friedreich's ataxia, or hereditary ataxia, is a curious disease first described by Friedreich.[1] It is distinctly a familial disease, but may or may not be hereditary. The great majority of the cases are met with in children before the age of puberty.

Clinically, the affection is characterized by ataxia of a swaying or staggering character involving all four extremities, nystagmus, scanning speech, and muscular contractions, giving rise to scoliosis and talipes equinus. The knee-jerks are usually absent.

The cord is found to be of less than normal thickness, a condition of

[1] Virch. Archiv, 70, 1877: 140. For literature see Oppenheim, Text-book, 5th edition, 1908.

things which is most marked in the cervical and upper dorsal region. Microscopically, the lesions are found chiefly in the posterior and lateral columns. The columns of Goll, the pyramidal tracts, and Clarke's columns are extensively involved, less so Burdach's and Gowers' tracts and the direct pyramidal tracts. There may, in some cases, be atrophy of the posterior roots and peripheral nerves. The lesions consist in degeneration and atrophy of the nerve fibers and their myelin sheaths, together with increase of the neuroglia. The pia is somewhat thickened, especially over the posterior aspect of the cord, which probably accounts for the peripheral or annular degeneration present in some cases. The bloodvessels are slightly thickened, but the vascular phenomena are not obtrusive. Dana has recently observed a peculiar porosis of the cord, both of the white and gray substance, which is due to dilatation of the perivascular spaces.

FIG. 156

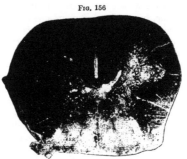

Friedreich's ataxia. Lumbar cord. Shows degeneration in the posterior columns, a relative amount in the pyramidal tracts, and a very little in the right direct cerebellar tract. (From the collection of Dr. Colin K. Russel.)

Many different opinions have been expressed as to the nature of the disease. The fact that the affection is most frequently met with in childhood, and is, moreover, apt to run in families, suggests that some anomaly of development is at fault. Some have held that this consists in hypoplasia of the third primary vesicle and neural canal, whereby the cerebellum, medulla, and cord lag behind in their development. Déjerine and Letulle have suggested as the cause a primary gliosis of developmental nature in the posterior columns. Others consider the degeneration of the nerve elements to be primary and the sclerosis secondary. Senator's idea that the essential lesion is atrophy or hypoplasia of the cerebellum has not been widely accepted.

Hereditary Cerebellar Ataxia.—Somewhat similar to the hereditary ataxia of spinal origin, just described, is what is known as hereditary cerebellar ataxia (cerebellar heredo-ataxia of Marie).

In this affection, which comes on somewhat later in life, the ataxia is less marked, and there is no scoliosis or club-foot. Atrophy of the optic nerves is frequent and the knee-jerks are increased. Spasm of the muscles comes on quite late. The most striking lesion found is hypoplasia of the cerebellum. The posterior and lateral tracts are not involved. At most there is atrophy of the anterior and posterior nerve-roots. The spinal cord, however, is somewhat smaller than normal. Transitional forms between hereditary cerebellar ataxia and hereditary spinal ataxia have been described.

The influence of toxic substances in bringing about degeneration is well illustrated by the spinal lesions which occasionally accompany such diseases as pernicious anemia, tuberculosis, diabetes, and carcinoma. The first-named condition may be taken as the type, the others being similar save that they are not so extreme.

Pernicious Anemia.—The lesions in pernicious anemia are most commonly found in the posterior and lateral columns of the cord, less frequently in the anterior. The posterior columns are more extensively and uniformly affected than are the others. In the early stages, the degeneration is systemic, but as the disease progresses the lesions become more irregular and extensive. Annular sclerosis may be found, or multiple scattered foci not unlike those in disseminated sclerosis. The lesions in the posterior columns are those of ascending degeneration in the cervical and upper dorsal regions. The postero-internal columns are much more markedly involved than are the postero-external. The ventral portion of the postero-external columns, the Lissauer's tracts, and the posterior nerve-roots escape, constituting a marked difference between this form of degeneration and tabes dorsalis. In the disseminated form, the lesions differ from those of disseminated sclerosis in that in the latter certain nerve-fibres within the sclerotic areas are to some extent at least preserved.

In the early stages the medullary sheaths are swollen and stain badly, but the axis-cylinders may be fairly well preserved. Later, the axis-cylinders are degenerated or have entirely disappeared, leaving small cavities in the myelin sheaths in which they formerly lay. The vessels are usually not much altered. In the most advanced cases the connective tissue is considerably increased, the walls of the smaller vessels are thickened, and there is proliferation of the cells of the adventitia.

The exact pathogenesis of the degeneration is unknown. It may be that the important element is the lack of nutrition due to the destruction of the blood corpuscles. Most observers seem to think that this is not the case, but that the degeneration of the nerve fibres and of the blood cells is referable to the same primary cause.[1]

Amyotrophic Lateral Sclerosis.—The last, and one of the most important, system diseases with which we shall deal is amyotrophic lateral sclerosis (Charcot). This disease is one of the entire motor

---

[1] Dr. Charlton, in our laboratory, by repeated sublethal inoculations of a strain of B. coli in the rabbit, induced disturbances of this type in the spinal cord—a result supporting Hunter's contention that pernicious anemia is an alimentary subinfection. Jour. Med. Res., N. S., 3:1902:344.

system, and, anatomically, presents the combined lesions of lateral sclerosis and progressive spinal muscular atrophy. The pathological

FIG. 157

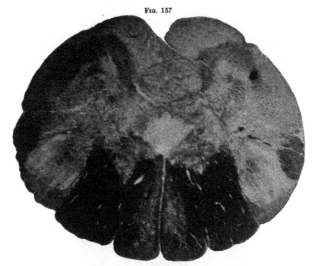

Amyotrophic lateral sclerosis. Cervical cord. Degeneration very marked in the cord except in the postero-external columns. (From the collection of Dr. Colin K. Russel.)

FIG. 158

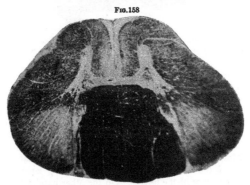

Amyotrophic lateral sclerosis. Degeneration is evident in all parts of the cord save the posterior columns. (From the collection of Dr. Colin K. Russel.)

changes are found especially in the cord and peripheral motor nerves, but extend frequently to the medulla, and in some instances to the internal capsule and motor cortex of the brain.

Clinically, the disease is characterized by muscular wasting, a variable amount of spasm, increased knee-jerks, with, in some cases, evidences of involvement of the motor nuclei of the medulla (glossolabiolaryngeal paralysis), and occasionally tremors.

The cord is firm and somewhat wasted looking, particularly in the cervical region. On section, the lateral pyramidal tracts are grayer than the rest of the white substance, and the gray matter is somewhat softened and reddened. Analogous changes, though less extensive, are sometimes to be observed in the medulla. The anterior nerve-roots, and often the hypoglossal and glossopharyngeal nerves, are atrophied. The corresponding muscles are atrophic, and there may be deformities and fixation of the joints.

FIG. 159

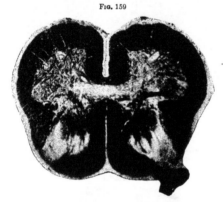

Amyotrophic lateral sclerosis. Lumbar cord. All parts are degenerated to some extent except the posterior columns. (From the collection of Dr. Colin K. Russel.)

Microscopically, as well as to gross appearance, it is in many cases evident that the most marked changes are in the lateral tracts. There is more or less marked degeneration of the direct and crossed pyramidal tracts. In some instances, the anterolateral column, the lateral limiting layer, and those tracts extending from the gray matter of the ventral horns to the surface of the cord are involved. Degeneration in the posterior columns, especially the columns of Goll, has been noted by Hektoen, Marie, and others. It must be remarked that, while the degeneration of the lateral columns is very striking when present, it is the most inconstant of the lesions. On the other hand, wasting of the motor ganglia of the ventral horns, or of their homologues, is invariably found. The substance of the ventral horns does not present much shrinkage, but the ganglia are greatly affected. They are not only diminished in number, but those that remain are wasted, stain irregularly or more diffusely than normal, and the nuclei may have disappeared. The protoplasmic processes are atrophied or absent. In some preparations the ganglion-cells may have dropped out, giving the horns a somewhat porous appearance. The bloodvessels are more or less thickened, the perivascular lymphatics are dilated, and there may be minute hemorrhages here and there. The changes in the fibres of the pyramidal tracts are those that have so often been described before. The glia is but slightly increased.

The involvement of the medulla is not so extreme as that of the cord. The nucleus of the hypoglossal nerve and the nucleus of Roller are degenerated, somewhat rarely the motor nucleus of the fifth nerve and the posterior nucleus of the vagus. The pyramidal tracts in this region are only slightly involved.

The degeneration of the pyramidal tracts has been in some cases followed into the brain. The large pyramidal cells of the motor cortex and the tangential fibres have been found to be degenerated. Some of the cells have disappeared. In the deeper layers of the cortex the cells may be atrophied, while the tangential fibres are unaffected.

The degeneration of the peripheral motor fibres is slight, not nearly so marked as that of the anterior roots.

The muscles corresponding to the affected ganglia are atrophied, while there is an interstitial lipomatosis.

Two main theories have been advanced to explain the process. The original view of Charcot, in which he has been followed by Erb, is that amyotrophic lateral sclerosis is a system disease, the main lesion being situated in the pyramidal tracts, the changes in the gray substance and peripheral nerves being secondary. Gowers, v. Leyden, Dana, and others regard the disease as a form of progressive muscular atrophy. The affection of the peripheral motor neurone is primary, that of the central motor neurone is secondary or associated. The question cannot be considered as settled. There is, however, reason to suppose, from the clinical course of some cases and the study of the cord in certain anomalous forms, that the degeneration of the pyramidal tracts may antedate the changes in the ganglion cells of the ventral horns and the peripheral motor neurones. Possibly, amyotrophic lateral sclerosis is one of the diseases to which Edinger's "exhaustion" theory would apply.

PROGRESSIVE METAMORPHOSES.

Tumors.—The most frequent and important new-growth found in the spinal cord is the **glioma.** This rarely forms a circumscribed tumor, but is usually met with as a diffuse proliferation of glial tissue (**gliomatosis**) in the neighborhood of the central canal, often extending for a considerable distance along the cord. At times it is composed of firm glia, and at others, of a more delicate, gelatinous, or mucoid glia (**myxoglioma**). Occasionally it is markedly vascular (**glioma teleangiectaticum**). The newly-formed glia seems particularly prone to softening and degener-

ation, and cavities are not infrequently produced which, if at all exten
sive, lead to the conditions known as *hydromyelia* and *syringomyelia*
Doubtless many cases of diffuse gliomatosis of this type are to be attrib
uted to errors of development; others are more akin to new-growths

Neurinomas, sarcomas, and angiosarcomas are rare. Multiple neurinoma
of the cord are sometimes associated with neurinomas of the periphera
nerves.

Secondary tumors are carcinomas, sarcomas, and myelomas.

CHAPTER XXVIII.

THE PERIPHERAL NERVES.

THE peripheral nerve-mechanism consists of three parts, the ganglia, the nerve trunks, and the end plates. The nerve trunks, which will concern us most, are composed of medullated fibres, continuous with the central nervous system, and of non-medullated fibres, derived from the sympathetic ganglia.

CIRCULATORY DISTURBANCES.

Anemia.—Anemia can be recognized with difficulty, but may be supposed to be present in cases of general systemic anemia, and, locally, in obstruction of the nutrient vessels, and from the pressure of exudates, tumors or dislocated bones.

Hyperemia.—Hyperemia is met with in cases of inflammation.

Œdema.—Œdema is rare. It may sometimes be observed where nerves pass through inflammatory foci.

Hemorrhages.—Hemorrhages, usually petechial in character, are found in inflammation and traumatism.

INFLAMMATIONS.

Neuritis.—Inflammation of the peripheral nerves, or neuritis, is due to circulating toxins or bacteria, to trauma, or to the extension of inflammation from adjacent parts. It has been customary with some writers to distinguish a **parenchymatous neuritis,** in which the primary lesion is degeneration of the nerve-fibres, and an **interstitial neuritis,** in which the changes begin in the connective-tissue portion of the nerve trunk. It should be again remarked here that degeneration and true inflammation of the nerve-substance cannot always be differentiated. For, atrophy and degenerative changes in the nerve-fibres may be followed by reactive inflammation in the interstitial substance of a secondary nature, while primary interstitial inflammation quickly leads to secondary wasting of the specific nerve-elements. In whatever way the condition may be initiated, degeneration of the nerve-trunks leads to well-defined results, and all such conditions are grouped indiscriminately by clinicians under the term neuritis. Primary parenchymatous neuritis is practically the same thing as atrophy of the nerve fibres, and is dealt with more precisely under the "Degenerations" later

(p. 632). In its causation, alcohol, lead, arsenic, and the toxins of the various infective diseases play a leading part. The disease, endemic in Japan and the Orient, known as Beri-beri or "Kakke" probably comes under this category.

Acute Interstitial Neuritis.—Acute interstitial neuritis, or **neuritis** in its restricted sense, is hematogenic or lymphogenic in origin, and may be produced by various infective agents or toxins. The affected nerve-trunk is swollen, œdematous, and hyperemic, with, sometimes, minute hemorrhages into the substance. Microscopically, we find in the endoneurium and epineurium all the ordinary signs of inflammation. The vessels are congested, the interstitial substance is infiltrated with serum and inflammatory leukocytes. If the process have gone on for some time, it is common to find the ordinary degenerative manifestations in the axis-cylinders and myelin sheaths. In suppurative cases small abscesses may be found here and there in the interstitial substance. Neuritis may also arise by direct involvement or lymphogenous extension, as in those cases where an abscess or infective granuloma has formed in the neighborhood of a nerve-trunk, or where meningitis involves secondarily the cranial nerves or the roots of the spinal nerves.

Traumatic neuritis arises from section of a nerve by accident or design, especially where the wound has become infected, from contusions or lacerations or from the pressure of tumors, fractured and dislocated bones.

Slight grades of neuritis heal without causing any permanent damage. More severe forms may lead to degeneration of the nerve elements, with consecutive atrophy of the associated muscles, or to actual necrosis or gangrene of the nerve trunk.

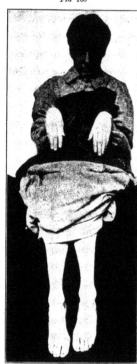

Fɪɢ 160

Multiple peripheral neuritis (wrist and foot-drop) in chronic lead poisoning. (From the Medical Clinic of the Montreal General Hospital.)

Chronic Interstitial Neuritis.—Chronic interstitial neuritis arises by hematogenic or lymphogenic infection or intoxication, and by the extension of chronic inflammation from neighboring parts. It may also occur without obvious cause. Microscopically, the connective-tissue cells have markedly proliferated, and the stroma may show collections of small round cells (*neuritis prolifera*). This overgrowth of the interstitial substance may be so great that the nerve trunk is considerably enlarged. Sooner or later, the nerve-fibres atrophy and disappear. Déjerine has drawn special attention to this form under the name *chronic hypertrophic neuritis*

Neuritis, especially those varieties due to hematogenic infection and intoxications, is apt to be symmetrical. It affects a number of nerve trunks (*multiple peripheral neuritis* or *polyneuritis*), and, moreover, the toxins are liable to single out particular regions. Where extensive degeneration has taken place we may, in some cases, find an ascending degeneration involving the posterior nerve roots, the posterior columns of the cord, or even the nutrient centres. The condition leads to paralysis and wasting of the muscles innervated.

Tuberculosis.—This is probably always secondary, and is found most commonly in the roots of the cranial or spinal nerves, as a result of the extension of a tuberculous meningitis. Occasionally, nerve-fibres are implicated in cases of "cold" abscess, tuberculous periostitis, and tenosynovitis. The process is an interstitial one, in which, in the perineurium and epineurium, there forms the characteristic granulation tissue, which eventually undergoes caseation. The infiltration may extend to the endoneurium and the fibres undergo secondary degeneration. In other cases there form areas of connective-tissue induration.

Syphilis.—Like tuberculosis, syphilis generally attacks the roots of the cranial and spinal nerves, inasmuch as the process commonly originates in meningitis. The interstitial substance is infiltrated with granulation tissue, which gradually is converted into dense, fibrous material. The nutrient vessels often show endarteritic changes, whereby the circulation is interfered with. This, together with the pressure of the newly-formed fibrous tissue, leads to marked degeneration of the fibres and serious interference with function, such as paralysis. Gumma of the nerves seems to be rare.

Leprosy.—Leprosy of the nerves constitutes one of the well-known clinical types of this disease. The disease appears to pick out more especially the cutaneous branches. Microscopically, we find cellular infiltration of the interstitial substance, with a marked tendency to proliferation, so that scattered spindle-shaped nodes are formed on the trunks. In the areas of granulation we find large, epithelioid cells, often vacuolated, in which the lepra bacilli may be readily detected, or the organisms may lie free. The process leads to degeneration of the nerve-fibres and thus produces the peculiar anesthetic and trophic changes in the skin characteristic of this form of leprosy. Where the ganglia are involved, the specific bacilli can be found also within them.

With regard to the ganglia of the sympathetic nervous system, it may be noted that they are apt to be involved in tuberculous processes. Thus, the solar plexus and semilunar ganglia may be attacked in tuberculosis of the suprarenals, kidney, or vertebræ.

RETROGRESSIVE METAMORPHOSES.

Atrophy.—Atrophy of nerves is of rather common occurrence. It may be due to any lesion which cuts off the nerve-fibres from their nutrient centres. Thus, destruction of the ganglion cells, either in the brain or in the cord, may lead to atrophy of the fibres proceeding from them. Pressure, also, exerted upon a nerve from any cause, if continued, will produce degeneration and atrophy. Severance of a nerve trunk and inflammation are frequent causes. Atrophy is also met with in old age.

Atrophy and degeneration of nerve-fibres usually begin at the point most remote from the nutritive centre and progress centripetally. As the type may be taken that form which results from the severance of a nerve-trunk by trauma (Wallerian degeneration), or follows continued pressure upon the trunk, as, for instance, from a tumor, enlarged lymph-glands, or constricting bands. (See Introduction, p. 524.)

Besides the degeneration caused by solution of continuity, just referred to, wasting of a similar kind may be brought about by the action of circulating toxins and bacteria, by certain circulatory disturbances, and by impoverished nutrition. Endarteritis and other obstructive lesions of the vessels and hemorrhages play a part here, largely by cutting off the nutrition, as do also systemic anemias and marasmus. Degeneration, affecting one or more nerve trunks, occurs sometimes in such conditions as diphtheria, influenza, typhoid, typhus, variola, tuberculosis, the puerperium, and intoxications with mineral substances, such as lead. Here we have, probably, in some cases at least, a combination of imperfect nutrition and the deleterious action of the poison. Occasionally, from some unknown infection or intoxication, the ganglion cells of the anterior horns are destroyed, followed by secondary degenerative changes in the fibres connected with them.

PROGRESSIVE METAMORPHOSES.

Regeneration of the nerve-elements after injury is possible under certain conditions. Provided that the nerve-centres or ganglia corresponding to the destroyed fibres are intact, restoration of structure and function is to be looked for. (For a full discussion of this subject the reader is referred to vol. i, p. 625.)

Tumors.—We have discussed the subject of the tumors of the peripheral nerves in our first volume (P. 758), and have there pointed out that the commonest of these tumors, the so-called fibroma or neurofibroma, is, according to the more recent studies, not developed from the connective tissue proper of the peripheral nerves, but from the cells which compose the sheaths of Schwann of the medullary nerves, cells which are of neuroblastic and not of mesoblastic origin. Following Verocay, these tumors should be spoken of as **neurinomas.** Here it may be noted that

Fɪɢ. 161

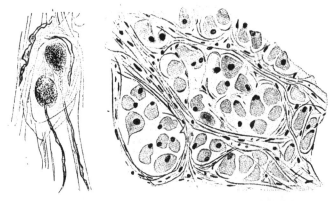

Cells from a benign and a malignant ganglioneuroma (a true neuroma) respectively; the former from the sacral region, the latter from the retroperitoneal region at the level of the pancreas. (R. Beneke.)

Fɪɢ. 162

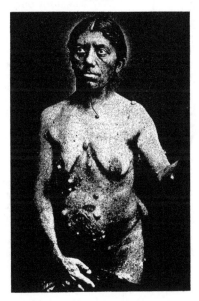

Multiple fibromatoid overgrowths along the course of the cutaneous nerves   (Herczel.)

FIG. 163

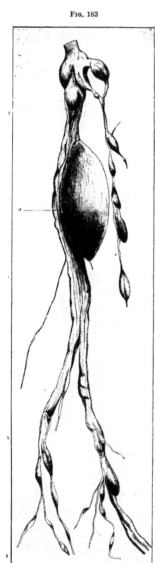

tumors of this nature are generally multiple, and are occasionally to be found in great numbers upon most of the peripheral nerves. We have, in fact, a condition of **neurinomatosis.** More particularly, this condition is liable to invade the cutaneous nerves, resulting in the appearance of multiple tumors of the skin (*fibroma molluscum*). Such tumors, on examination, are seen to contain nerve fibres proper, surrounding and compressed by the proliferating tissue. There may be a varying associated overgrowth of the connective tissue proper, so that, while in general soft, occasionally they assume a harder, more fiibromatous texture. They are liable, further, to exhibit various degenerations.

This neurinomatosis is evidently of developmental origin. The condition may show itself early in life. There is often a marked family predisposition. Rarely one or more of the tumors undergoes sarcomatosis transformation with the production of metastases.

Occasionally, also, a highly convoluted, tendril-like growth develops over a somewhat extended area. The nerve-trunks are diffusely thickened, and studded with nodules and spindle-like enlargements (*plexiform neuroma; Rankenneurom*). They are found particularly in the distribution of the spinal nerves and those of the head, and develop by preference in the skin and subcutaneous tissues. They sometimes form large, projecting, lobulated or folded growths, or may lead to a diffuse, rather indefinite thickening of the skin, which resembles closely elephantiasis or pachydermia (*elephantiasis neuromatosa*).

All forms of multiple fibromas of the peripheral nerves are probably to be referred to errors of development,[1]

Tumors of sciatic nerves and their branches. At *a*, large tumor connected with small intermuscular nerve. (Preble and Hektoen.)

[1] See Thompson, On Neuroma and Neurofibromatosis, Edin., 1900; and Adrian, Beitr. z. klin. Chir., 31:1901.

as they are commonly found in children, and there may also be a family predisposition. In rare cases, fibromas have been known to undergo sarcomatous transformation and produce metastases (Westphalen,[1] Recklinghausen, Larkin[2]).

FIG. 164

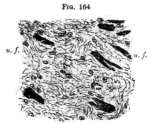

Section through a fibromatoid cutaneous nodule showing the nerve-fibres (*n. f.*) separated by fibroid overgrowth. (After Ribbert.)

Myxomas, lipomas, rhabdomyomas, and **sarcomas** are described. They are much rarer than the neurinomas, and form isolated, nodular, or spindle-shaped out-growths.

Striated muscle cells have been found in the interior of nerve-trunks. they have been attributed to misplaced embryonal cells, but little is known about them.[3]

[1] Virch. Archiv, 110: 1887: 29; ibid., 114: 1888: 29.
[2] Jour. Med. Research (N. S.), 4: 1903: 217
[3] Orlandi, Arch. p. le Scien. Med., 19: 1895.

CHAPTER XXIX.

THE SPECIAL SENSES.

THE EYE.

ANOMALIES OF DEVELOPMENT.

Defects and irregularities in development of the visual apparatus may involve the eyelids, the globe of the eye, or any of its component parts.

Complete absence of the bulb (anophthalmia) is rare. As a rule, microscopic examination will reveal traces of its substance. Anophthalmia is commonly bilateral, and frequently associated with other anomalies of development, coloboma, harelip, cleft palate, and imperfect closure of the cardiac septum. Ordinarily, while the bulb is extremely defective, the eyelids, conjunctival sac, muscles, and nerves are present, suggesting that at some period the growth of the bulb had been arrested, either as a result of a defect in development or of intra-uterine disease. A lesser grade of the affection is microphthalmia, in which the globe of the eye is fairly recognizable as such. All stages between anophthalmia and microphthalmia exist.

A curious and rare anomaly is cyclopia or synophthalmia, in which the entire visual apparatus is more or less perfectly fused into a single organ. This is one manifestation of the condition known as cyclencephaly, where the normal division of the prosencephalon fails to occur and the cerebrum remains· as a single cyst-wall enclosing a single, more or less dilated ventricle. In such a case, not only are the optic vesicles involved, but also the olfactory bulbs, the bones of the skull and face, and the soft parts. In the milder grades of the affection, two eyes may be formed, but they lie in a single orbit, or are partially fused. In the more marked form there is but one eye, situated in a single orbit, occupying the centre of the forehead, and provided with but one optic nerve. The various grades and the probable explanation of these states as due to polar hypogenesis have been discussed in Volume I (p. 260).

Hydrophthalmus.—Hydrophthalmus is a condition of early life, believed to be due to glaucoma occurring during intra-uterine existence. The globe of the eye is enlarged, and more or less fixed. The cornea is cloudy, the intra-ocular termination of the optic nerve is excavated, and the depth of the anterior chamber is increased.

Among partial defects should be mentioned congenital ptosis of the upper lid; epicanthus, a condition in which, together with flatness of the bridge of the nose, there is a fold of skin passing across the inner canthus from the upper to the lower lid (a moderate grade of this is normal in the Chinese race); lack of the iris (**irideremia**); **persistent pupillary membrane; persistent hyaloid artery.** Our colleague, Dr. Mathewson, has reported a case of **accessory eyelid.**[1]

Among the more striking anomalies is **coloboma.** This is a lack of substance, more or less complete, in one or more of the primary membranes of the eye, due to the failure of the primitive fœtal cleft to close. The retina and the pigment epithelium are derived from the secondary optic vesicle, about which are formed the choroid and scleral membranes. The primitive cleft in the secondary optic vesicle extends backward inferiorly into the optic stalk. Should it fail to close at its posterior part, coloboma of the optic nerve sheath results. If the middle portion does not close, the ordinary coloboma of the choroid results. Failure to close anteriorly results in defective formation of the lower part of the iris. According to this, several different forms and grades may be recognized. In complete failure to close, the choroid and sclera will be imperfectly formed, while the retina and pigment epithelium will be lacking. Should, however, the closure be merely delayed, both retina and pigment epithelium may be completed, but the choroid will be defective and the superimposed pigment epithelium will not become pigmented. In coloboma of the choroid, owing to thinness of the sclera, ectasia of this membrane is a not uncommon result. This ectasia, or staphyloma, of the sclera may be very marked, especially in cases of microphthalmus, and may indeed form a cyst as large as the eyeball itself.

In coloboma of the choroid, one finds, microscopically, in place of the proper retina and choroid, a thin connective-tissue membrane, in which are a few vessels and a scanty deposit of pigment. In other cases there may be present more or less perfect retinal elements.

Coloboma, when affecting the lower part of the vertical meridian of the eye is a purely developmental error. Coloboma in other directions, and the so-called coloboma of the macula, are due to inflammation occurring during intra-uterine life, the defect in formation being due to the mechanical effect of adhesions. Congenitally defective eyes are liable to other diseases, such as choroiditis and cataract.

The Conjunctiva.

The upper and lower eyelids are covered externally with skin, similar to that of the forehead and cheeks, but somewhat thinner and looser. Beneath this is a layer of loose, areolar tissue; next, the striated fibres of the orbicularis palpebrarum; then, the so-called tarsal cartilage, composed of dense, white connective tissue and containing the Meibomian glands, practically identical in structure with the sebaceous glands; a subconjunctival layer, containing more or less diffuse adenoid tissue; and finally

---

[1] Montr. Med. Jour., 37:1908:734.

the conjunctiva itself, composed of stratified epithelium. On the inner surface of the lids the epithelium is of the squamous variety and rather thin, but toward the fornix the membrane is looser, more vascular, and thrown into folds, while the epithelium is columnar. When the conjunctiva reaches the bulb, the superficial cells tend again to become flattened, and the membrane assumes more the appearance of that covering the cornea. The vascularity of the subconjunctival tissues and the looseness of their texture renders the membrane, and, indeed, the lid as a whole, particularly susceptible to circulatory and inflammatory disturbances, while the results of these conditions are usually striking.

CIRCULATORY DISTURBANCES.

Œdema.—Œdema of the lids and conjunctiva is a condition of clinical importance, as it is frequently an indication of serious disease. It is found, for instance, in chronic renal and cardiac affections, and in anemia. In such cases the conjunctiva is swollen, and has a glassy or watery look (*chemosis*). Œdema of the lids is, also, a common accompaniment of inflammation, not only of the eye itself, but of its associated structures.   Thus, it is met with in such conditions as conjunctivitis, panophthalmitis, dacryocystitis, retrobulbar abscess, and suppuration of the frontal sinuses.

Acute Hyperemia.—Simple acute hyperemia of the conjunctiva is a common symptom of irritation. A foreign body in the conjunctival sac, excessive crying, the exposure of the eyes to the wind or sun, "eyestrain," irritant gases, and the use of certain drugs, such as arsenic and potassium iodide, may all cause it. It is an early feature of many inflammations of the eyes, and is met with in acute rhinitis and facial neuralgia. Chronic congestion is most frequently due to errors ·of refraction and disorders of the ocular muscles, but may also be an indication of alcoholism, gout, nasal catarrh, and inflammation of the lacrimal ducts.

Hemorrhage.—Hemorrhage into the loose tissue beneath the conjunctival membrane may be the result of injury to the eye, fracture of the skull, or may come on without any particular cause. Severe attacks of sneezing, coughing, or vomiting have been known to cause it. Possibly, sclerosis or other degenerative change in the vessel walls predisposes to the condition.

INFLAMMATIONS.

Conjunctivitis.—Inflammation of the conjunctiva—**conjunctivitis** or **ophthalmia**—may affect the membrane as a whole, or any part of it. Acute and chronic forms are recognized. *Primary acute conjunctivitis* may result from exposure to wind and weather, heat, irritating gases, injury, or from the action of microörganisms. *Secondary acute conjunctivitis* may be due to the extension of inflammation from neighboring

Koch-Weeks Bacillus. (Weeks.)

FIG. 2

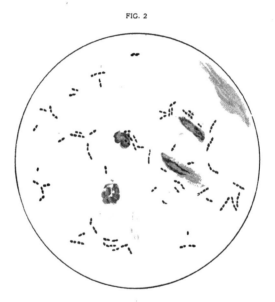

Morax-Axenfeld Diplobacillus. (Weeks.)

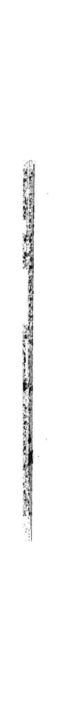

parts, face, eyelids, nose, or lacrimal ducts, or may accompany or complicate certain of the infectious fevers, such as measles, influenza, typhus and whooping-cough. .

Acute conjunctivitis may sometimes also be produced by the action of certain drugs. Simple catarrhal inflammation is a not infrequent occurrence in persons who are taking potassium iodide or arsenic. The external application of chrysophanic acid in psoriasis has been known to cause it. The local use of atropine, eserine, and hyoscyamine may also, if long continued, or in susceptible people, on occasion produce it.

A considerable number of microörganisms are now known to give rise to conjunctivitis. Chief among these are the Morax-Axenfeld diplobacillus, the Koch-Weeks bacillus, the pyogenic cocci, Gonococcus, and Pneumococcus. Exceptionally, Friedländer's bacillus, the Diphtheria bacillus, the Bacillus of Pfeiffer, and B. coli have been found. McKee,[1] in a study of 500 cases, gives the following proportions:

Morax-Axenfeld Diplobacillus in 200; Staphylococcus, 50; Streptococcus, 24; Pneumococcus, 13; Micrococcus catarrhalis, 12; Gonococcus, 10; McKee bacillus, 9; Koch-Weeks organism, 7; B. coli, 5; influenza bacillus, 3; Meningococcus, 1; Bacillus xerosis, B. Hoffmann; and saprophytes, 102; negative results in 64. Certain of these, the Koch-Weeks bacillus and Pneumococcus, are not infrequently to be found on the normal conjunctiva, and are usually innocuous. On occasions, owing to some increase of virulence or some injury to the membrane, they may assume pathogenic properties.

In all forms of conjunctivitis the process is essentially the same, though the intensity may vary. The conjunctival vessels are congested, the subconjunctival tissues are œdematous and infiltrated, the lymphadenoid follicles are enlarged, and the superficial epithelium is sodden, swollen, desquamating, or eroded. It is usual to classify the clinical varieties according to the character of the exudate, which may be serous or seromucoid, seropurulent, purulent, or membranous.

Acute Catarrhal Conjunctivitis.—In the milder grades of acute catarrhal conjunctivitis, the inflammation may be confined to the palpebral conjunctiva, which is swollen, reddened, and succulent. There is a slight mucoid discharge which tends to glue the eyelids together and accumulates about the inner canthus and the retrotarsal fold. In the more severe forms the bulbar conjunctiva is involved as well, and, owing to the congestion, assumes a reddish color. The conjunctiva is considerably thickened, particularly at the retrotarsal fold, where it may show papillary excrescences. The discharge is more abundant and is seropurulent or mucopurulent in character.

Acute Purulent Conjunctivitis.—Acute purulent conjunctivitis is a severe affection of the conjunctiva, due in the vast majority of cases to the Gonococcus of Neisser. The disease is most commonly met with in

---

[1] A Clinical Study of Five Hundred Cases of Conjunctivitis, Amer. Jour. Med. Sci., 134:1907:716.

newborn infants who have been inoculated from the maternal passages during birth (*ophthalmia neonatorum*), and next in adults the subjects of gonorrhœa of the urethra, vulva, or vagina. Occasionally, it is found in young, debilitated girls, who are suffering from non-specific purulent vulvitis and vaginitis. Sometimes, also, the acute catarrhal form, when passed rapidly from one individual to another, and occurring in weakly persons, may become intensified into the suppurative variety.

In purulent conjunctivitis the inflammatory process is extremely severe. There is intense congestion and chemosis of the conjunctiva, the lids are tense, swollen, and reddened. Small hemorrhages may occur into the conjunctiva, which bleeds at the slightest touch. The discharge, at first serous, soon becomes creamy and abundant, and is of a yellowish or yellowish-green color. In children, as a rule, both eyes are involved, as would be expected. In adults, one eye often escapes. There is great danger to sight in gonorrhœal ophthalmia, inasmuch as the cornea is apt to be involved in neglected, severe, or improperly treated cases. A diffuse opacity may spread over the cornea, or, in other cases, small ulcers may form, leading sometimes to perforation, with all this implies. More or less permanent thickening of the conjunctiva may result with scarring.

Membranous or **Croupous Conjunctivitis.**—Membranous or croupous conjunctivitis is characterized by the formation of a solid exudate in the form of a patchy or confluent membrane more or less firmly attached to the conjunctival tissues. Occasionally, owing to some peculiarity in the state of health of the affected person, a mucopurulent or purulent ophthalmia assumes this type. The too vigorous use of caustics may also cause it, as does also the solution of jequirity, commonly employed in the treatment of trachoma.

True *diphtheria* of the conjunctiva is rare. It occasionally arises by extension from the nasal passages, or by direct inoculation with infective material. Rarely, it may be primary. It has also been known to follow operative procedures. Both palpebral and bulbar conjunctiva are involved. The lids are greatly swollen and congested, while they are tense and brawny from infiltration. Owing to the interference with the circulation there is grave danger to the cornea in this form of conjunctivitis. The membrane is thick, firm, and adherent. The subconjunctival tissues are also considerably involved, and more or less deeply penetrating ulcerations are not uncommon. When healing takes place, this leads to the formation of scars, and not infrequently to incurvation of the lids. The discharge is at first scanty, thin, and ichorous, later purulent.

Variola.—Variola pustules are occasionally found upon the conjunctiva. They lead to purulent infiltration or ulcerations of the cornea. Staphyloma may thus result, or the condition may go on to suppurative choroiditis and panophthalmitis.

Parinaud's Conjunctivitis.—A curious, though rare, form of acute inflammation is Parinaud's conjunctivitis (**lymphoma conjunctivæ**). It is peculiar in that it is accompanied by local and systemic manifestations of infection.

The affection begins with slight symptoms of conjunctivitis, which, in a few days becomes worse, the lids become markedly swollen, and there is slight ptosis, with lacrimation and photophobia.   The conjunctiva of the lid is much swollen and reddened, and is studded with numerous papillary granulations, which are especially in evidence in the retrotarsal folds. The conjunctiva bulbi is not involved, save that it is somewhat injected. Soon the granulations enlarge, forming relatively enormous, papillary, and cock's-comb-like masses. The pre-auricular, inframaxillary, and cervical glands sooner or later become enlarged, and there is a slight evening rise of temperature. The secretion is scanty and mucopurulent in character. Ulceration does not take place, nor is a membrane produced. The enlarged glands may suppurate or may resolve. Stirling and McCrae,[1] in a case met with in Montreal, found a bacillus intermediate in properties between Bacillus diphtheriæ and Bacillus xerosis, which they regarded as probably specific.

Trachoma or Granular Conjunctivitis.—The most important of the chronic inflammations of the conjunctiva is the so-called trachoma or granular conjunctivitis. This affection is essentially chronic in its course, but manifests occasional acute exacerbations. Anatomically, it is characterized in the main by overgrowth of tissue, which in time, when absorption has taken place, is followed by cicatricial contraction. Although the disease is a common one in certain countries, and has been known for a long time, its etiology is still obscure. The disease is undoubtedly contagious, being transmitted from person to person by the secretion, usually by means of towels. Sattler has described a coccus which he regarded as the specific cause of the disease, but the evidence is as yet far from convincing.   Some hold that the disease is the chronic form of acute epidemic conjunctivitis, which is usually due to Gonococcus or the Koch-Weeks bacillus.

The process begins and is always most marked in the conjunctiva of the lids and retrotarsal folds, but may eventually extend to the tarsus and conjunctiva bulbi. At the onset and during the acute relapses, the lids are considerably swollen, the conjunctiva is much injected, and there is a moderate amount of mucoid or mucopurulent secretion. Photophobia and blepharospasm may be marked. Later, the conjunctiva is congested and considerably thickened, being studded with papillary out-growths (*papillary conjunctivitis*) and "granulations" (*follicular conjunctivitis*). The trachoma bodies or follicles are most numerous in the retrotarsal folds, and on eversion of the lids can be seen small, grayish, translucent nodules, resembling grains of boiled sago or frog's spawn.

Histologically, there is found a diffuse infiltration of the conjunctiva of the lids with lymphoid cells. The papillæ are much enlarged. The trachoma bodies are not typical granulation tissue, but due to a local hyperplasia of the lymphoid and connective-tissue elements, surrounded by a more or less perfect fibrous capsule. The subconjunctival tissue is also hyperplastic. Much interest has been excited of late by

---

[1] A Case of Parinaud's Conjunctivitis, Montreal Med. Jour., 33:1904:575.

the demonstration of peculiar minute intracellular corpuscles taking on a differential stain and lying in the neighborhood of the nucleus. They undoubtedly are to be met with in most early cases of the condition, but, unfortunately, they have been encountered also in cases of gonorrhœal conjunctivitis, and even (McKee[1]) in the conjunctival cells of a child a few days old. Thus they cannot be regarded as specific. In long-standing cases cicatricial contraction of the connective tissue takes place, with atrophy of the conjunctiva, so that the retrotarsal folds are gradually obliterated, the movements of the eyeball interfered with, and a condition of *xerophthalmia* is induced. The eyelids are often curved inward (*entropion*) so that the lashes are directed against the conjunctiva (*trichiasis; dystrichiasis*). From the combined results of friction and inflammation, the cornea sometimes becomes cloudy, the superficial epithelium somewhat roughened, and sluggish ulcers may become manifest. The corneal tissue may also soften and bulge outward. Not infrequently, the inflammatory process spreads under the subepithelial layer toward the centre of the cornea, the newly formed tissue gradually becoming vascularized (*pannus*).

Follicular Conjunctivitis.—Some authorities, notably Saemisch, describe a follicular conjunctivitis, which bears a strong resemblance to trachoma, at least in its early stages. The disease affects the conjunctiva of the lids only, and leads to the formation of nodes of hypertrophied lymphoid tissue. There are, however, no hypertrophied papillæ. The changes in by far the majority of cases are quite superficial and never lead to cicatricial contraction, ulceration, or pannus. The condition may heal without leaving any trace. The disease is said to be feebly, if at all, contagious. It must be said, however, that it is by no means proved that this affection differs essentially from trachoma, either etiologically, or in other particulars. In fact, transitional forms are by no means unknown. Some of the cases are attributable to atropine irritation.

Vernal Conjunctivitis (Spring Catarrh; Gelatinous Infiltration of the Limbus; Phlyctæna Pallida).—Vernal conjunctivitis is an apparently specific and extremely obstinate affection of the conjunctiva. The disease affects both eyes and is most common in children. As its name implies, it is most troublesome with the onset of warm weather, tending to disappear during the winter. It may last for years, and is believed by many to be feebly contagious. Both the ocular and palpebral conjunctivæ may be involved. The conjunctiva of the upper lid, which is the one usually involved, presents a peculiar bluish-white, milky appearance, characteristic of the disease, and is covered with flat, rounded elevations of almost cartilaginous hardness, giving it a curious tessellated appearance. When the bulb is affected, one sees flattened, elevated, gelatinous masses of a brownish-pink color, close to the limbus of the cornea. The growth may spread laterally, or occasionally may encircle the cornea, which may also be more or less encroached upon.

Microscopically, the patches are composed of connective tissue and

----

[1] Ophthalmic Record, June, 1910.

greatly thickened epithelium, which tends to send prolongations into the underlying structures. According to Fuchs, they consist of areolar connective tissue, which has undergone hyaline degeneration, covered with thickened epithelium. There is but little secretion in this form of conjunctivitis. There is no tendency to ulceration or the formation of pannus. Occasionally, the peripheral zone of the cornea undergoes fatty degeneration, producing an appearance similar to that in arcus senilis.

Eczema of the Conjunctiva.—Eczema of the conjunctiva (**conjunctivitis phlyctænulosa; conjunctivitis lymphatica sive scrofulosa**) is usually found in young children, especially those who are weakly or of the so-called "scrofulous" temperament. Unlike most other forms of conjunctivitis, it is invariably associated with some constitutional disturbance, furred tongue, loss of appetite, constipation. It is not infrequently seen in combination with eczema of the face, nose, ears, and hands. Ordinarily, one eye only is affected.

The disease is characterized by the formation of one or more papules or pustules, varying in size from that of a mustard seed to, in rare cases, that of a split pea. These are, histologically, composed of aggregations of inflammatory leukocytes, covered at first with the epithelial layer. Eventually, this may give way, so that an ulcer is the result. The papules, pustules, or ulcers are delimited by a zone of catarrhal inflammation, or the bulbar conjunctiva as a whole may be diffusely reddened and swollen. There is a mucopurulent exudation. Not infrequently, the cornea is involved in a similar manner. The conjunctiva of the lids almost always escapes. The affection may run an acute course, but often is chronic with occasional acute exacerbations.

Xerosis.—Xerosis of the conjunctiva (**pemphigus of the conjunctiva**) is a curious and somewhat rare disease, the exact nature of which is not entirely understood. It occurs under the guise of a chronic inflammation, in which the conjunctiva, chiefly that of the bulbus, slowly atrophies and contracts, owing to the formation in it of cicatricial tissue. The membrane itself is dry and lustreless, and is covered with fine, whitish, fatty scales. The process may resolve, but not infrequently progresses until the free edges of the lids are bound down to the globe and become continuous with the cornea, thus limiting greatly, if not entirely, the movements of the eyeball. The cornea, in turn, may become involved. The scales consist of stratified, keratinized, epithelial cells, often fattily degenerated, together with free fat-droplets. The desquamating material also contains a small bacillus, the so-called Bacillus xerosis, which bears some resemblance to the bacillus of diphtheria. Its specificity is, however, by no means beyond question.

Tuberculosis.—Tuberculosis is quite rare. So far as is known at present, it is always secondary to lupus of the face. In the connective tissue of the lids and bulb are formed more or less circumscribed, flattened outgrowths, recalling the fungoid masses seen in tuberculous synovitis. These are reddish, warty, and bear a close resemblance to granulations. In time they break down, giving rise to larger or smaller, irregular ulcers, in the floor of which grayish or yellowish, caseous tubercles may sometimes be seen. From the confluence of the tubercles, larger nodules may be formed. The irritation of the tuberculous process often, also, leads to enlargement of the follicles in the retrotarsal folds (*follicular conjunctivitis*).

Syphilis.—Primary and secondary lesions may occur, and also gummas. The condition is very uncommon.

Leprosy.—Leprosy is also rare.

PROGRESSIVE METAMORPHOSES.

Pinguecula.—Pinguecula, called so from the Latin "pinguis," fat, owing to an erroneous notion as to its nature, is a yellowish, elevated mass, situated in the conjunctiva bulbi and the subconjunctival tissue, usually to the nasal side, but occasionally, though rarely, to the temporal side. It is found in middle-aged people. Its position on the most exposed portion of the conjunctiva suggests that the condition may be the result of irritation, such as exposure to wind and rain. Microscopically, there is down-growth of the epithelium in places, with the formation of gland-like processes and even cysts. The connective tissue is increased and there is a marked development of new elastic fibres. Both fibrous and elastic tissue present hyaline degeneration.

Pterygium (πτέρυξ, a wing).—Pterygium is an overgrowth of the conjunctiva and subconjunctival tissues, usually occurring on the nasal aspect of the eyeball. It takes the form of a triangular elevation, more or less vascular, the apex being toward the centre and the base toward the periphery of the eye. The growth tends to encroach upon the cornea. The superficial epithelium is thrown into folds, and is composed of stratified cells, the deeper of which are cuboidal, while the others are more cylindrical or pointed.

The overgrowth of epithelium in places leads to the formation of gland-like structures and even cysts. Numerous goblet-cells are to be found in the shallower depressions. Beneath the epithelium there is an aggregation of lymphoid cells with numerous small vessels. The Bowman's membrane is substituted by a fibrillar layer of connective tissue, containing large blood- and lymph-vessels.

The cause or causes are not altogether clear. Most authorities attribute the tissue-overgrowth to irritation or hyperemia. Cases often follow exposure to heat, dust, or noxious vapors, and, also occasionally, traumatism. Eyestrain, by producing congestion of the vessels, may possibly be a cause. Pinguecula not infrequently precedes pterygium.

Cysts.—Cysts are due to dilatation of the lymphatics or to obstruction of the glands, with retention of the secretion. In lymphangiectasis, small, rounded vesicles, filled with clear fluid, are formed on the conjunctiva of the bulb, where they are arranged in little clusters or after the fashion of a string of beads.

Histologically, these formations consist of a number of intercommunicating cavities, containing a few lymphatic cells, and bounded by connective tissue, on which may sometimes be recognized the scanty remains of an endothelial lining.

Serous cysts may result from a lymphangiectasis in which the separating partitions between the spaces have given way, thus producing a single cavity. They are, however, occasionally found at birth, or result from injury, or, again, may be due to cystic degeneration of small, glandular lobules in the fornix. They form round, oval, or oblong swellings in the conjunctiva, of a somewhat yellowish color. Microscopically, they have a well-defined wall of connective tissue, usually lined with endothelial cells. *Teleangiectasis* of the tarsal and bulbar conjunctiva is occasionally me with, usually near the lachrymal caruncle.

Tumors.—Fibromas.—Fibromas spring from the palpebral conjunctiva or from the cul-de-sac, and are frequently pedicled. They may be flattened from pressure or may even assume a cup shape. Microscopically, they are composed of dense, fibrous tissue with relatively few vessels, although the smaller ones may be more cellular.

Papilloma.— Papilloma of the conjunctiva is extremely rare, and usually springs from the sclerocorneal junction. The tumor possesses a pedicle and is composed of a richly-branching core of connective tissue covered with a thick, stratified investment of epithelial cells, cuboidal, cylindrical, or spindle-shaped. Toward the periphery of the processes the core is more cellular and infiltrated with leukocytes.

Lipoma.—Lipoma is a rather rare tumor of the conjunctiva. It is congenital and appears in the form of an elevated, wedge-shaped mass, lobulated, and of a yellowish color, situated usually between the external and inferior rectus. Microscopically, it is composed of fatty and fibrous tissue, covered with thickened conjunctiva. It is supposed to originate in a hernia of the orbital fat.

Dermoid.—Another congenital tumor, occasionally met with, is the dermoid. As its name implies, it is composed of the elements of the skin. It is usually of small size, of a smooth, shiny appearance, and is situated at the corneoscleral junction, partly on the sclera and partly on the cornea. The corneal sector is commonly bounded by an opaque line similar in appearance to an arcus senilis. The superficial epithelium is somewhat similar to that of the skin, save that it does not become keratinized, but, on the contrary, is soft and swollen, apparently from maceration. Underneath there is a dense connective-tissue membrane, containing elastic fibres, bloodvessels, glands, and fat. Projecting from the surface are more or less numerous hairs. Alt[1] has described what he calls a **chondro-adenoma,** a congenital tumor, composed of gland-tubules suggesting those of the lacrimal gland, together with a mass of embryonic cartilage. The two elements were separated one from the other by, and enclosed in, connective tissue. The growth was the size of a split pea, situated on the bulbar conjunctiva. It was sessile, smooth, and of a whitish color. Probably this should be classed as a **teratoid growth.**

[1] Reference Handbook of the Medical Sciences, New York, Wm. Wood & Co., 4: 1902: 109.

Osteoma.—Osteoma has been met with in a few instances. It is found on the outer aspect of the eye, usually between the points of insertion of the superior and external rectus. It appears not to be congenital.

The malignant tumors of the conjunctiva are the epithelioma and the sarcoma. They may be primary, but are most frequently secondary to growths of the eyelids or orbit.

Epithelioma.—Epithelioma is the commonest tumor of the conjunctiva. It begins, usually, near the corneoscleral junction, with the formation of a small nodule covered with distended bloodvessels. The growth, if not removed, gradually spreads to the cornea, and finally invades the interior of the eye. Some of these new-growths may be pigmented (*melanocancroids*).

Microscopically, the tumor consists of a thickened epithelium, which sends out downgrowths of a finger-like, branching form into the deeper structures. The horny layer is often considerably thickened. About the periphery of the tumor the vessels are dilated and the tissues infiltrated with leukocytes.

Sarcoma.—Sarcomas are distinctly rare, and are usually pigmented Like the epithelioma, they commonly begin at the corneoscleral junction, or, rarely, in the fornix. They form rounded, sometimes lobulated, growths of a rusty brown or blackish color. They are very vascular and bleed readily. They do not tend to ulcerate, and appear smooth and shiny, owing to the fact that they are covered by epithelium.

Microscopically, the sarcomas are of the small, *round-celled* variety, more rarely *spindle-celled*. The vessels are numerous, and there are evidences of both old and recent hemorrhages.

TRAUMATISM.

The conjunctiva may be cut or torn, and such accidents usually give rise to considerable hemorrhage into the loose subconjunctival tissue, together with more or less œdema. The conjunctiva may also be injured by foreign bodies gaining a lodgement on it; or by the action of caustic substances, such as lye, lime, acid, or molten metal, which have sparked into the eye. More or less congestion results in all instances, and in the more severe injuries, inflammation. Occasionally, where the corresponding portions of the ocular and palpebral conjunctiva are involved, and there is loss of the epithelium, union of the eyelid with the eye may take place (*symblepharon*).

The Cornea.

The cornea of the eye is a stratified membrane, and is peculiar in that, under ordinary circumstances, it is perfectly transparent. It may be compared to a window placed in the frame of the sclera. It is elliptical in outline, being slightly broader than it is high. The outer and inner curvatures are, moreover, not parallel. The various layers of the cornea, beginning from without inward, are as follows. There is first a thin, stratified layer of epithelium, continuous with that of the conjunctiva, and similar to that of the skin, save that there is no stratum corneum. Next comes the anterior limiting, or Bowman's, membrane, a clear, anhistous sheet, which sends fibres of its substance into the deeper parts. The main portion of the cornea is composed of from sixty to sixty-five lamellæ of white fibrous tissue, the bundles of which are somewhat flattened and those of successive layers are arranged practically at right angles to each other. Between the bundles are numerous lymph-spaces or lacunæ, communicating with each other by means of delicate canaliculi, and continuous with similar spaces in the sclera. In the lacunæ are to be found the "corneal corpuscles," fixed cells which send delicate processes into the canaliculi, recalling in appearance the osteoblasts of bone. Besides these, wandering cells may be seen. Next comes the posterior limiting, or Descemet's, membrane, a clear, structureless sheet. At the edge of the cornea it is thicker, forming a ring-like zone (the annular ligament), and may be traced as far as the insertion of the iris as separate bundles of fibres (the pectinate ligament), bounded by minute clefts (the spaces of Fontana). The posterior component of the cornea is a single layer of flattened, endothelial cells, similar to those lining serous cavities, and continuous with those covering the anterior aspect of the iris.

The normal cornea is avascular, being nourished by the lymph system above referred to. Bloodvessels in the conjunctiva and subconjunctival tissues and in the sclera send out fine branches which pass in radially in the direction of the cornea. These branch dichotomously, and form an elaborate series of anastomosing loops in the limbus conjunctivæ, but do not encroach upon the cornea. The structure is so constituted as to be perfectly transparent, all its components possessing the same refractive index.

From its exposed position the cornea is particularly liable to injury and irritation, and, being avascular, is apt to suffer in all conditions of lowered vitality of the system. Under ordinary circumstances it is able to deal with moderate injuries and grades of inflammation without suffering much in the process, but all severe processes of this kind lead to extensive and permanent changes, often producing marked interference with the function of vision. Thus, opacity in the pupillary area interposes a physical impediment in the visual axis, and cicatrices of the cornea result in alterations in the angle of refraction.

CONGENITAL ANOMALIES.

Congenital abnormalities of the cornea are often associated with other defects of the eye. The cornea may be smaller than normal, as in microphthalmus. In this case it may also be somewhat flattened, or its curvature may be the same as that of the sclera, and its outline may depart more or less widely from the normal. The cornea is larger than normal in **megalophthalmus**, and, moreover, may be thinner than usual. The anterior portion of the sclerotic is also thinner than normal, giving it a bluish appearance. In such cases the anterior chamber is usually increased in depth (**hydrophthalmus anterior**). Partial or complete opacity of the cornea is also sometimes observed, and is a frequent accompaniment of microphthalmus, megalophthalmus, and hydrophthalmus. A condition resembling the arcus senilis is occasionally met with at birth—**embryotoxon.**

Congenital abnormalities in the curvature of the cornea are the cause of many cases of astigmatism.

INFLAMMATIONS.

Keratitis.—The various forms of inflammation of the cornea, known as keratitis, are of great practical importance, and, owing to the anatomical peculiarities of the part, present certain features which differ from those found in inflammations occurring in other parts of the body.

Being an avascular structure, the cornea is at some distance from its base of supplies, and is, therefore, comparatively poorly nourished. It is, consequently, but imperfectly able to resist acute disease, and is particularly liable to suffer from the deleterious influence of impoverished blood or circulating toxins. Ulceration of the cornea, therefore, may ordinarily be taken as an evidence of deficient vitality of the general system. Acute infectious keratitis, consequently, if not checked by treatment, is apt to proceed apace and bring about serious damage to the cornea, while the more chronic affections are liable to be sluggish.

Again, owing to its exposed position, the cornea is particularly exposed to traumatism and irritation of various kinds, and especially to infection.

Finally, any condition which interferes with the transparency of the structure, or its normal curvature, will seriously impair its function as a refractive medium.

Keratitis may be described as *partial* or *circumscribed, generalized* or *diffuse.* As a rule, the corneal substance proper is affected, but the epithelium on the outer and inner aspects may alone be involved. Keratitis, moreover, may be *primary* or *secondary* to disease of the conjunctiva or other parts of the eye, as, for instance, the iris—*iridokeratitis,* or sclera—*sclerokeratitis,* or, again, may be an expression of some constitutional deficiency or taint, such as syphilis.

The changes in the cornea produced by inflammation differ somewhat according to the nature, the localization, and the intensity of the process. Three main types are usually described, *infiltration, abscess,* and *ulceration.*

Inflammation of the cornea always results in diminution or loss of its transparency, the degree depending on the extent and the severity of the condition. Should the anterior layer of epithelium be involved, the cornea has a steamy, pitted appearance, somewhat resembling a mirror that has been breathed upon. Thickening of the epithelium, and, to a greater degree, infiltration, causes the cornea to assume a milky, somewhat opalescent appearance, passing on into a whitish, grayish, or yellowish opacity. This loss of transparency is due to an excessive accumulation of leukocytes within the lacunæ and canaliculi, the result of chemiotaxis. The infiltration may be superficial or deeply seated, localized or diffuse. Slight grades may resolve, leaving the cornea little or none the worse, but it is by no means uncommon to find some degree of opacity persisting. The condition may, however, be so intense as to give rise to ulceration or abscess with distinct loss of substance, which, on healing, results in the formation of a fibrous scar Prolonged keratitis of moderate severity frequently results in opacity, fibrosis, more or less and vascularization of the cornea.

Fig. 165

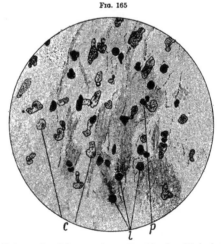

Mild grade of inflammation of the cornea in man (keratitis e lagophthalmo), characterized by enlargement and direct division of the nuclei of the corneal corpuscles *c*, with but slight invasion of polynuclear leukocytes *p*, and lymphocytes *l*. (Tooke.)

An abscess is a circumscribed infiltration in which the nutrition of the part has been so interfered with that local death has resulted. It may extend to the surface of the cornea and discharge externally, forming an ulcer; more rarely, it may evacuate itself into the anterior chamber.

Ulcers may be the result of infiltration or abscess, or may exist as such from the first. Perforation of the cornea may occur and the structure may be almost wholly destroyed. Adhesion and prolapse of the iris are not uncommon results. In not a few instances, the inflammation leads to the deposition of pus in the anterior chamber (**hypopyon**). Should the process heal, the loss of tissue is made good by the process of cicatrization. Milder grades are followed by slight opacity (**nebula**), more severe forms by the formation of a dense, fibrous, pearly scar (**leukoma**). The reparative material being softer than the normal corneal substance frequently gives way under the intraocular pressure and forms an anterior protrusion (**corneal staphyloma**). Sometimes, again, the loss of substance is not entirely repaired and the surface of the healed ulcer does not quite reach the general level of the cornea, while the regularity of the curve is disturbed (**corneal facet**).

Diffuse Keratitis.—Diffuse (interstitial or parenchymatous) keratitis is characterized by a more or less uniform inflammatory infiltration of the cornea throughout its whole thickness, which exhibits no tendency toward ulceration or abscess-formation. The epithelium presents a stippled appearance and the underlying cornea is opaque, somewhat resembling ground glass. The process generally begins with some ciliary congestion, followed by the formation of nebulous patches in the cornea, which gradually extend until the whole structure becomes involved. Delicate, closely-set vessels, derived from branches of the ciliary vessels, gradually make their way from the periphery into the cornea, which thus becomes both opaque and highly vascularized (*vascular keratitis*). These newly-formed vessels are in the substance of the cornea and, consequently, present a dull, reddish-pink color ("salmon patches" **of Hutchinson**). Salmon patches, when small, are often crescentic in shape, but when larger tend to assume the form of a sector. In other cases a narrow fringe of vessels is formed, continuous with the plexus at the corneal margin. This is one form of *marginal keratitis*. Mixed forms are, however, not infrequent. As a rule, the condition is bilateral, but days or weeks may elapse before the involvement of the second eye. The affection is a constitutional one, and, as a rule, due to syphilis. It is said to be met with also in strumous and gouty individuals. The disease runs a chronic course and relapses are common. Complete restoration of the transparency of the cornea rarely occurs. Cases of syphilitic nature are usually also complicated with iritis or iridochoroiditis.

Vascular keratitis may, however, at times be much more superficial and come on without obvious cause. It may also be secondary to trachomatous conjunctivitis or repeated attacks of phlyctenular keratitis.

The superficial epithelium becomes irregular from erosion and hypertrophic overgrowth, while new vessels are formed more or less abundantly between the epithelial layer and the Bowman's membrane and in the corneal substance itself (**pannus**). When the newly formed bloodvessels are few and scattered, the condition is spoken of as *pannus tenuis;* when so numerous as to give the cornea a reddish appearance, *pannus crassus.*

Neuroparalytic Keratitis.—Neuroparalytic keratitis is a form of diffuse keratitis of rather sluggish character, found in cases where the function of the fifth nerve is impaired or destroyed. Symptoms are largely in abeyance owing to the insensibility of the cornea. There may be merely infiltration of the tissue, but the process is very apt to go on to suppuration. The pericorneal congestion is comparatively slight.

Keratitis Bullosa.—Keratitis bullosa is a rare disease, characterized by the formation in rapid succession of transparent vesicles on the surface of the cornea, accompanied by marked paroxysms of pain. The vesicles are comparatively large, single or multiple. They may reach 4 to 5 mm. in diameter. When removed, the underlying cornea is found to be cloudy and the seat of parenchymatous keratitis. As a rule, the eye is diseased in other ways; for instance, from glaucoma or old iridochoroiditis. The condition is probably due to some disturbance of the lymph-channels of the cornea.

Not unlike this affection in some particulars is **herpes** of the cornea. Here, one or more small vesicles, containing clear transparent fluid, form on the surface of the cornea. When ruptured an excoriated surface is left. Severe neuralgic pains accompany the eruption of the blisters. There is often marked pericorneal injection. Herpes of the cornea may come on without obvious cause, or may be associated with catarrh of the respiratory passages. In *herpes zoster ophthalmicus*, which is probably due to some inflammatory disorder of the fifth nerve, ulceration and infiltration of the cornea are quite marked and the condition is slow in healing. The eruption of vesicles occurs in the district supplied by the fifth nerve and is accompanied by much pain and local anesthesia. The cornea is apt to be involved only in those cases in which the nasal branch of the first division of the fifth is affected. Complication with iritis and hypopyon is not uncommon in this form of herpes.

Ulcerative Keratitis.—Several varieties of corneal ulceration are recognized. The simplest form is the *small central ulcer*, met with in young badly-nourished children. It begins as a small, grayish-white elevation at or near the centre of the cornea. Sooner or later this breaks down in the centre, forming a minute excavation. The process appears to be somewhat sluggish, as the congestion is slight and the symptoms usually unobtrusive. The ulcer is most often single, but is apt to recur, or the other eye may become involved. Occasionally, we find, in anemic or strumous patients, somewhat similar ulcers, but even more sluggish, which run a chronic course with frequent relapses. There is little or no infiltration and the loss of substance is only imperfectly made good, so that a shallow depression or a flat facet is apt to be left, but without much damage to the transparency of the cornea.

Catarrhal ulcers are not infrequently met with as a result of catarrhal conjunctivitis in elderly people. The ulcer usually forms at or near the margin of the cornea as a shallow sulcus or there may be several minute delicate abrasions of the surface. There is a moderate amount of pericorneal congestion. The ulcer usually heals readily, unless it become infected, when serious suppurative inflammation may supervene.

Phlyctenular ulceration is closely related to phlyctenular conjunctivitis (q. v.), and is often associated with diffuse conjunctivitis. It begins with one or more superficial infiltrations about the size of a millet seed, either on the white of the eye near the cornea, or just within the corneal margin, or upon some other part of the cornea. The papule is circular, surrounded by a zone of congestion and opacity, and may assume the appearance of an acne pustule. The epithelium is soon destroyed, and a small abrasion or aphthous-looking ulcer is the result. Pericorneal congestion is always present and may be marked. Phlyctenular ulcers tend to advance in an almost radial direction toward the centre of the cornea, carrying with them a leash of vessels lying upon the track of opacity left by the ulcer (*phlyctenular pannus*). When the process ceases the vessels gradually disappear but more or less opacity remains. If this be present at or near the centre of the cornea, considerable disturbance of vision will result. Occasionally, the condition develops into a suppurative keratitis and may perforate. In extreme cases, the inflammation spreads to the vitreous and may destroy the eye.

Phlyctenular ulcers are met with usually in children, sometimes in apparently good health otherwise, but, as a rule, the subjects are strumous or suffer from grave errors in nutrition. Not infrequently, there is a history of measles or some other infectious disease.

Crescentic ulcers, close to, or actually upon, an arcus senilis, are sometimes met with in elderly debilitated subjects. They may form deep grooves around the cornea, which, if it be cut off from its nutrition, may thereupon exfoliate.

Suppurative Keratitis.—There are certain forms of suppurative keratitis which should be referred to. Abscess or infective ulcers may originate spontaneously or may result from some trifling injury. Probably the condition arises from the infection of the cornea rendered possible by the preëxisting injury, and assisted by debility and malnutrition of the patient. Such a condition tends to spread in one direction while healing in another, is unattended by the formation of new vessels so characteristic of healing inflammation, and is frequently complicated by hypopyon.

The Acute Serpiginous Ulcer.—Saemisch has described what he calls the acute serpiginous ulcer, a form which tends to penetrate deeply and extend widely, especially in one direction. It begins as a grayish spot, presenting slight ulceration, and having a sharply-cut border, one part of which is more opaque than the rest. The process is apt to extend rapidly, and may lead to perforation of the cornea. Iritis and hypopyon are common complications. Subacute and chronic serpiginous ulceration is also described.

Keratomalacia.—The so-called keratomalacia, met with in infants suffering from digestive disturbances, is a severe form of suppurative keratitis, due to infection with pyogenic cocci, notably Staphylococcus aureus. The affection begins apparently from the infection of some small fissure or abrasion of the cornea, which rapidly develops into an ulcer extending laterally and deeply into the substance of the cornea. This ulcer has a grayish base and yellowish edge and tends to perforate the cornea.

Abscesses.—Abscesses of the cornea are probably also in all cases the result of infection. They may occur as a primary infection, or may result from simple inflammatory infiltration, from traumatism, or ulceration. They usually form at the centre of the cornea as small, raised spots surrounded by a deeply congested area. The spots enlarge rapidly and break down, usually discharging forward, thus producing an ulcer covered with seropurulent exudation. When perforation of the cornea occurs posteriorly, *hypopyon* results.

In some cases of iritis the lower part of the cornea becomes secondarily involved, appearing somewhat hazy. Not infrequently, a number of minute dots, discrete, sharply defined, and of a whitish or grayish-white color, may be detected, especially by the use of a lens, on the posterior elastic lamina. These dots are arranged in the form of a sector with the apex toward the centre of the cornea, the smallest dots being near the centre (*keratitis punctata*). Keratitis punctata is nearly always the result of some affection of the cornea, iris, choroid, or vitreous.

The Results of Suppurative Keratitis.—Ulcers of the cornea, when they heal, not uncommonly leave behind them traces in the form of permanent *opacities* of the tissue or even *scars*. These, if situated over the pupil of the eye, may seriously interfere with vision, not only by introducing an opaque substance in the visual axis, but by altering the curvature of the refracting medium. In severe cases of ulceration, the whole or the greater part of the cornea may be *destroyed*, and the inflammation may spread to the iris, choroid, and the humors, leading to total destruction of the eye.

Smaller ulcers may *perforate* and lead to the escape of the aqueous humor through the opening. Occasionally a permanent *fistula* may result. This, according to De Wecker, is due to the eversion of Descemet's membrane, which forms a lining to the fistulous track. Occasionally, where perforation is not quite complete, Descemet's membrane may prolapse and present as a small, clear vesicle, resembling a glass bead, in the base of the ulcer.

Prolapse of the iris and *adhesion* of the iris to the region of the ulcer may occur.

Hypopyon.—Hypopyon, or pus in the anterior chamber, may occur with any ulcer, whether it has perforated or not, and with any suppurative condition of the cornea. The pus may be derived from an abscess or ulcer which has eroded through to the posterior surface of the cornea, or, occasionally, may be due to the extension of inflammation from the iris. In some severe cases of suppurative keratitis the pus sinks down between the lamellæ of the cornea (*onyx*). Onyx and hypopyon may co-exist.

Specific Keratitis.—Tuberculosis, syphilis, and leprosy only rarely give rise to circumscribed lesions in the cornea.

Keratomycosis aspergillina has been described, but is very rare.[1]

[1] *Leber*, v. *Graefe's* Arch., 25: Die Entstehung der Entzündung, Leipzig, 1891.

RETROGRESSIVE METAMORPHOSES.

Arcus Senilis.—Arcus senilis (**gerontoxon**) is a degenerative change in the cornea, found in elderly people. The condition begins with the formation of a light gray arc at the periphery of the cornea. It begins both above and below, the two arcs gradually extending until a complete circle is produced. The ring is sharply defined from the limbus and is separated from it by a narrow transparent band, while it gradually loses itself on the concave side in the clear cornea. The arcus is at first silvery gray in appearance, but later becomes denser and creamy. Both eyes are usually affected, although the condition may be unilateral. According to Fuchs, the condition is not, as has usually been taught, a fatty degeneration or infiltration of the cornea, but a *hyaline* degeneration of certain of the connective-tissue fibres. This is associated with the deposit of lime salts in minute particles in the superficial layers of the cornea near the limbus. The condition is to be attributed, no doubt, to the impoverished nutrition of the cornea due to senile changes in the vascular loops encircling the cornea.

Calcareous Degeneration.—Calcareous degeneration of the cornea is met with occasionally in the form of a transverse band of opacity, corresponding with the palpebral fissure. This is of a grayish or yellowish color, 2 to 3 mm. broad, and is found in elderly or prematurely aged people. It is also met with in eyes affected with deeply-seated disease, and in those with a tendency to glaucoma.

Pigmentation.—**Lead stains** not infrequently occur after the application of lotions containing salts of lead to an abraded or ulcerated cornea. The stains are dense, white, opaque, and sharply defined.

PROGRESSIVE METAMORPHOSES.

Tumors.—Primary tumors of the cornea appear to be unknown. Tumors of the conjunctiva, especially those which spring from the sclerocorneal junction, such as the **papilloma**, the **dermoid**, the **epithelioma**, and the **sarcoma**, may invade the cornea.

TRAUMATIC DISTURBANCES.

The cornea being firm and resistant, and supported by an elastic cushion, is never ruptured by a blow or by any sudden increase of intra-ocular tension. It may, however, be injured by the impact of foreign bodies, by abrasion, incised or punctured wounds, burns, scalds, or caustic substances.

Blows upon the cornea from small bodies may result in loss of the superficial epithelium, bruising, or even necrosis of the part. In the latter event, from the consecutive inflammation and infection which is so liable to occur, a corneal abscess often results. The various interstices and lymph-spaces become infiltrated with serum and pus cells. The conjunctiva is reddened, and there is ciliary congestion. In a few days the injured part becomes opaque and of a grayish color. The pus may form in the superficial layers or may extend more deeply. It may, therefore, discharge externally, internally, or in both directions. Pus may collect in the anterior chamber (*hypopyon*), and the condition may lead to *iritis* and *iridocyclitis*. If the abscess discharge externally, the lens or iris is apt to adhere to the damaged region and give rise to subsequent trouble in the form of irritation and inflammation, perhaps resulting eventually in *panophthalmitis* and *phthisis bulbi*. *Anterior staphyloma* is also a not uncommon result. Should the abscess heal, a dense, opaque, fibrous scar is formed, which, according to its position, will cause more or less interference with vision.

Slight wounds, where there is merely loss of the superficial epithelium or of a trifling portion of the deeper corneal substance, heal up without much trouble and without any serious after-consequences, except, possibly, in the case of weakly or debilitated persons and from lack of surgical cleanliness. Unless the injury extend to Descemet's membrane no scarring will result, but not infrequently the curvature of the cornea is altered and the refracting power of the structure correspondingly interfered with, a point of great practical importance when the injury is at or near the visual centre.

In the case of larger wounds, the vitreous may escape and the iris and lens become attached to or incarcerated in the wound, or may even be prolapsed through it. There is usually considerable loss of tissue, with the formation of a large cicatrix, to which the iris and lens may be permanently attached.

Burns, scalds, or caustic erosions are more serious than similar injuries to the conjunctiva, inasmuch as they lead to considerable reactionary inflammation, with opacity or scarring of the cornea, and even *symblepharon*.

The Sclera.

Scleritis.—The disorders of the sclerotic membrane are comparatively few. The most important is inflammation—**scleritis** (**episcleritis**). This is much rarer than keratitis and usually involves the anterior half of the membrane. It may exist alone or in association with inflammation of the cornea (**keratoscleritis**), iris, or choroid (**uveoscleritis**).

Simple scleritis occurs usually on the exposed portions of the ciliary region, generally to the outer side, but it may be found at any part of the circle, and may, exceptionally, extend widely and far back out of sight. The affection is subacute in character and relapses are the rule. The disease is generally met with in adults, especially in those exposed to cold, or who have a gouty or rheumatic tendency.

The process begins with one or more patches of congestion in the ciliary region, accompanied by swelling, and leading to elevation of the conjunctiva. The affected area appears reddish and rusty. The conjunctiva overlying the part is swollen, œdematous, and congested.

Microscopically, one finds infiltration of the tissue with leukocytes, especially in the neighborhood of the vessels, with some dilatation of the lymphatics. The inflammation may subside after a longer or shorter period, resolving entirely or leaving a grayish discoloration of the sclera. Occasionally, the inflammatory infiltration extends more or less widely into the cornea. Scleritis may also set up diffuse, interstitial keratitis or chronic iritis, or, again, choroiditis. Sclerochoroiditis leads to thinning of the tunics of the eyeball, with ectasia or dilatation of the anterior part (*staphyloma scleræ*).

Tuberculosis.—Tuberculosis of the sclera has only rarely been observed.

Syphilis.—Syphilis, especially the gumma, is somewhat more common.

The Iris.

The iris is composed of five layers. These are, from before backward: (1) The anterior epithelial layer, consisting of transparent, flattened, or polyhedral cells, having a spherical or slightly oval nucleus; (2) a delicate, hyaline basement membrane, continuous with the Descemet's membrane of the cornea; (3) the substantia propria, composed largely of bundles of fibrous connective tissue and bloodvessels; (4) a hyaline elastic membrane, extending over the ciliary processes and the choroid as the lamina vitrea; (5) the posterior layer of epithelium, composed of polyhedral cells.

The substantia propria contains in addition both circular (sphincter) bundles of unstriped muscle, and radiating fibres (dilator pupillæ). These are under the control of different sets of sympathetic nerve fibres, hence it is that the condition of the pupil in regard to contraction or dilatation is of great diagnostic value.

The color of the iris depends upon the amount of pigment which it contains. The epithelial layers are pigmented at birth, but the stroma does not become colored until later, so that the eyes of infants are always blue or gray. In the blue eye of the adult there is very little pigment in the stroma, while in the black eye all the layers are pigmented.

CONGENITAL ANOMALIES.

Albinism.—In albinism there is a marked lack of pigment in the iris as well as in the hair and other structures of the body. The iris is normal otherwise in structure, but appears of a lilac, rose, or yellowish-white color, according to the illumination. The pupil is always narrow. Owing to the lack of pigment to absorb the rays of light, photophobia is a marked symptom. The eyes are usually almost amblyopic, and nystagmus is common. The condition is undoubtedly due to a defect of development, and heredity plays an important role.

Heterochromia.—The irides in the two eyes may be of different color—heterochromia; for example, one may be blue and the other brown. Or, a blue iris may be dotted or streaked with brown.

Melanosis Oculi.—The iris, together with other parts of the eye, the conjunctiva, sclera, choroid, optic nerve, may contain areas of intense pigmentation, analogous to the pigmented moles of the skin—melanosis oculi. These may provide a starting point for malignant new-growths.

Persistent Pupillary Membrane.—One of the commonest anomalies of the eyes is persistent pupillary membrane. During fœtal life, the lens is surrounded by a vascular membrane, the tunica vasculosa, the bloodvessels of which are derived from branches of the arteria centralis, which pass around the edge of the lens and anastomose on its anterior aspect. As the iris is formed, its vessels unite with those of the tunica vasculosa. The portion of the tunica occupying what is eventually to be the pupil is called the pupillary membrane. As a rule, at birth, the membrane and its vessels have been absorbed, but occasionally portions of them persist as strands of tissue, often highly pigmented, which arise from the anterior surface of the iris and project into the pupil.

Corectopia.—The pupillary opening is situated normally a little to the nasal side of the central point. In corectopia the pupil is displaced outward and upward, and is small and irregular in outline as well. The iris may be otherwise normal and react perfectly to light, and in such cases the condition is usually unilateral. Often, however, there are other congenital defects in the eye, such as buphthalmos, microphthalmos, coloboma of the lid or iris, or albinism. Not infrequently, there is ectopia of the lens.

Dyscoria.—Dyscoria, or irregularity of the pupil, is a very common condition. It is due either to posterior synechia from fœtal iritis, or to a proliferation of the pigmented epithelium forming the posterior covering of the iris.

Polycoria.—Polycoria, or multiplicity of the pupil, does not occur in the sense of a number of pupils, each surrounded by a sphincter muscle. The term is commonly employed, however, to designate the condition in which an iris contains a number of openings in addition to the normal pupil. These openings usually appear as radial clefts, but may occur at the periphery of the iris. The appearance of polycoria may also be produced by a bridge-coloboma of the iris, or a persistent pupillary membrane.

Aniridia or Iridiremia.—Aniridia or iridiremia may, so far as clinical examination goes, be total or partial. In complete aniridia both eyes are involved, as a rule. The incomplete form is often difficult to distinguish from coloboma. Other congenital peculiarities, such as microphthalmos, ptosis, persistent hyaloid artery, may be present. The most frequent complication is cataract, but corneal and vitreous opacities, choroidal atrophy, and detachment of the retina may be met with. Luxation of the lens may occur. Glaucoma is another not uncommon complication.

Coloboma.—Coloboma of the iris is one of the most common developmental defects of the eye. The cause has already been mentioned (see p. 637). In this condition there is a cleft of the iris which extends into the pupil, forming with it a pear-shaped opening. The opening may be complete, the defect extending to the ciliary border, or incomplete, a bridge of iris remaining at the apex of the gap. The opening is situated downward, or downward and inward. The pupil is usually also displaced downward, less often upward.

CIRCULATORY DISTURBANCES.

Anemia.—Anemia of the iris occurs in all general systemic conditions associated with anemia or loss of blood.

Hyperemia.—Hyperemia is met with in the early stages of iritis and associated with tumors of the iris.

INFLAMMATIONS.

Iritis.—Inflammation of the iris—iritis—may occur as a primary affection or may be secondary to inflammation of other portions of the eye. The causes are local or constitutional.

Among the local causes may be mentioned, perforating wounds of the eyeball, especially if lacerated and complicated with injury to the lens; injury to the lens, without wound of the iris, and with only slight puncture of the cornea (*e. g.*, traumatic iritis occurring after cataract operation); superficial wounds and abrasions of the cornea; blows upon the eye; ulcers and other forms of keratitis, especially those complicated with hypopyon; and deep-seated disease of the eye.

The chief constitutional causes are syphilis, gout, and rheumatism. Iritis may also complicate the acute infections and other diseases which have generalized systemic manifestations. Gonorrhœal iritis, analogous to gonorrhœal arthritis, is occasionally met with.

Besides the causes mentioned there is another, viz., trophic disturbance, to which certain writers are disposed to attach considerable importance. Such disturbances may be reflex. In this category come those cases of iritis occurring in sympathetic ophthalmitis, in herpes zoster ophthalmicus, and as a result of dental or uterine irritation.

Acute iritis may be divided into three main varieties, according to the clinical features, **plastic iritis, serous iritis,** and **suppurative iritis.**

Plastic Iritis.—By far the largest number of cases of inflammation of the iris are to be included under the term plastic iritis. Most cases of rheumatic, gouty, traumatic, and sympathetic iritis belong to this category.

The condition is manifested by congestion of the whole eyeball, but particularly of the anterior ciliary vessels, and the conjunctival twigs which surround the cornea (ciliary and pericorneal injection). This results in the formation of a pinkish zone, from 3 to 6 mm. broad, just outside the peripheral margin of the cornea. The iris loses its clear, bright appearance and becomes somewhat muddy, turbid, and altered in color. An important feature is the formation of an inflammatory exudate both in the substance and on the surface of the iris which leads to the formation of adhesions between the iris and the lens-capsule (*posterior synechia*). The mobility of the pupil is, therefore, considerably interfered with, and under the influence of atropine the opening may be extremely irregular. In some cases the whole of the posterior surface of the iris becomes adherent (*total posterior synechia*). In the severer forms, the exudate may be very abundant, giving rise to occlusion of the pupil, turbidity of the vitreous, and even slight opacity of the cornea. The vigorous use of atropine may, in cases where the adhesions have not become fully organized, result in breaking them down, so that the pupil again becomes round. This procedure, however, generally results in some pigment being left upon the capsule of the lens. Pigment in this situation is pathognomonic of present or past iritis.

Serous Iritis.—Serous iritis is a not uncommon affection, the pathogeny of which is by no means clear. Some cases appear to be dependent on a rheumatic disposition, while others are reflex. In this form there is a special tendency for the whole uveal tract to be involved. The disease generally runs a subacute course and is not always very amenable to treatment. Pericorneal injection may be trifling and the iris is not greatly altered in color. The tendency to the formation of synechiæ is not so great as in the plastic form. The exudate is of a grayish or grayish-brown color and is found in the form of fine points on the lower half of Descemet's membrane. The vitreous may become somewhat cloudy and contain floating opacities. Not infrequently the ciliary body and the choroid are slightly inflamed (*cyclitis; iridochoroiditis*). It should be noted, however, that cases of iritis are occasionally met with which are intermediate in type between the plastic and the serous forms. Thus, iritis, which to gross appearance resembles the plastic variety, may be associated with considerable infiltration of the iris and the formation of adhesions, while the plastic type may lead to deposits of lymph on Descemet's membrane.

Suppurative Iritis.—Suppurative iritis is less common than the plastic variety. It may supervene upon plastic iritis, but is usually due to trauma, operations opening up the globe of the eye, and to ulcerative keratitis.

The inflammation is more intense, the congestion is greater, the exudate more abundant. The pus may collect in the anterior chamber (*hypopyon*).

Syphilis.—This resembles closely in anatomical features plastic or serous iritis, but mixed forms also occur. Sometimes minute gummas, from 2 to 6 mm. in diameter, are to be observed upon the iris, and by microscopic examination even those forms which appear to resemble simple inflammation can be seen to be of granulomatous type. Gummas of the iris do not differ appreciably from those elsewhere, and are made up of young, proliferating connective-tissue cells, newly forme and congested vessels, and the ordinary vascular changes characteristi of syphilis.

Tuberculosis.—Tuberculous iritis is rare, and, unlike syphilis, tend to affect only one eye. It may begin in the form of serous iritis, but smal grayish nodules can usually be seen on the iris near the ciliary proces and in Fontana's space. These nodules gradually enlarge and finally coalesce, so that we get a warty, grayish-red mass containing fine vessels, which encroaches more or less upon the anterior chamber. The cornea usually shows some fogginess and vascularization. The process at time may retrogress and finally come to an end, but very commonly the in filtration extends to the ciliary process and the adjacent sclera, resultin in caseation and total destruction of the eye.

RETROGRESSIVE METAMORPHOSES.

Atrophy.—Atrophy of the iris, characterized by thinning of its substance, loss of pigment, and fibrous transformation, occurs as a result of inflammation, especially if anterior synechia be present, and in chronic glaucoma. The bloodvessels are thickened and hyaline, so that their lumina are often obliterated.

Pigmentation.—The application of nitrate of silver and protargol to the conjunctiva has resulted in permanent staining (*argyria conjunctivæ*). The membrane becomes of an olive or slaty color. A similar result has been reported in the case of certain persons, who, from the nature of their occupation, have been exposed to the action of silver dust.

In cases of *icterus*, whether of the obstructive or toxic forms, the conjunctiva is invariably involved. In fact, so early and so characteristic is the staining that we always look there for the first evidence of jaundice. The "white" of the eye in such cases presents a more or less intense shade of yellow. A dull, earthy, or subicteroid coloration is also met with in obstructive cardiac disease, pernicious anemia, toxemias, and in the cachexia of chronic wasting disease.

PROGRESSIVE METAMORPHOSES.

Sarcoma.—Sarcoma, usually pigmented, is the only tumor originating in the iris and is the rarest form of intra-ocular sarcoma. Much more often sarcoma originates in the choroid.

The Ciliary Body.

Cyclitis.—Inflammation of the ciliary body—cyclitis—is commonly associated with inflammation of the iris or choroid. The process is evidenced by slight clouding of the aqueous humor and the anterior portion of the vitreous. With this there is a deposition of exudate upon the posterior surface of the cornea, with slight exudation into the pupillary area. The whole posterior aspect of the iris becomes adherent to the capsule of the lens with retraction of the ciliary portion of the iris, so that the anterior chamber becomes enlarged. The exudation which collects between the iris and the lens and between the periphery of the iris and the ciliary process gradually undergoes organization and leads by its contraction to dislocation of the iris backward. Similarly, the exudation before and behind the lens, as it is transformed into connective tissue, leads to traction upon the ciliary body away from the sclera and in the direction of the axis of the bulb. The involvement of the vitreous, which is a constant accompaniment of cyclitis, with the deposit in it of a cellular and fibrinous exudation, in the same way results in complete separation of the retina with cataractous transformation of the lens. Severe cyclitis may become suppurative and lead to the production of hypopyon, or even involvement of the whole uveal tract (**panophthalmitis**). Fibrinous cyclitis, inasmuch as it is not so severe an affection, leads gradually to **phthisis bulbi,** with more or less diminution of the intra-ocular tension.

Apart from inflammations which spread from the iris or choroid, the chief causes of cyclitis are injuries, especially such as are due to wounds or foreign bodies. Occasionally, wounds of the sclera near the margin of the cornea, when cicatrizing, cause tension upon the iris and ciliary body, and eventually inflammation.

One of the most important consequences of cyclitis and iridocyclitis, especially when the result of penetrating wounds of the tunics of the eye, as, for instance, stabs, incisions, or of rupture, ulcers, or foreign bodies, is the so-called **sympathetic ophthalmitis,** which affects the uninjured eye.

Sympathetic ophthalmitis usually sets in from six to twelve weeks after the primary injury to the fellow eye. It rarely occurs before three weeks after the injury, and exceptionally its appearance is delayed for many years. The process tends to relapse, and may continue with alternate exacerbations and ameliorations for months or even a year or two. Anatomically speaking, the affection takes the form of a plastic iridocyclitis or iridochoroiditis with exudation leading to total posterior synechia. In the early stages there is apt to be a dotted deposit on the posterior surface of the cornea, clouding of the vitreous, and often neuroretinitis. The vessels perforating the sclera near the ciliary region are congested. The intra-ocular tension is often increased. The mildest cases do not go farther than a chronic serous iritis, with keratitis punctata and disease of the vitreous, usually also with neuroretinitis. In more severe cases the eye remains glaucomatous, with total posterior synechia, corneal opacity, and a varying amount of ciliary staphyloma. In the worst cases the eye finally shrinks.

The Choroid.

CONGENITAL ANOMALIES.

Coloboma.—Coloboma affecting the lower part of the choroid may exist alone or in association with coloboma of the iris. Occasionally the coloboma is limited to a small area around the nerve, or it may be separate from it (see p. 637). **Albinism** has also already been sufficiently dealt with.

CIRCULATORY DISTURBANCES.

Hyperemia.—Hyperemia of the choroid is not infrequent. It occurs in cases of systemic passive congestion, congestion of the head, and in early inflammation of the choroid, retina, or associated parts.

Anemia.—Anemia is met with in general anemia, if severe.

Hemorrhages.—Hemorrhages into the choroid in the form of multiple minute extravasations are occasionally met with. They often lead to atrophy and pigmentation of the membrane. The cause is obscure. Larger hemorrhages may be due to traumatism, smaller ones to disease of the vessels.

INFLAMMATIONS.

Choroiditis.—The term choroiditis is often used in a loose way to include not only the frankly inflammatory affections, but also some forms of atrophy which are by no means closely, if it all, related to inflammation. We shall, however, in the course of the following remarks, employ it in the strict sense, namely, to designate *inflammation* of the choroid.

Owing to the close relationship that exists between the choroid and the retina, disease of one membrane is exceedingly apt to extend to the other. Thus, changes in the pigment epithelium which forms part of the retina may be due to deep-seated retinitis, or, again, to superficial choroiditis. It is, therefore, not always easy to determine in which membrane the inflammatory process has begun. Moreover, the retina, even if not directly implicated, often shows secondary atrophic changes as a result of choroiditis. On the other hand, in cases of equally severe choroidal inflammation, the retina, curiously enough, may escape.

The causes of choroiditis are not very varied. Some few cases are considered to be due to some systemic dyscrasia, such as gout; others are due to traumatism; others, again, and by far the larger number, are manifestations of infection, usually metastatic in type. In the last mentioned class syphilis is the most important single factor. Choroiditis may, however, be also found in other infections, such as tuberculosis, rheumatism, occasionally in typhoid and relapsing fevers, rarely, in leprosy and gonorrhœa.

According to the nature of the exudate produced, we can recognize purulent and non-purulent forms.

Suppurative Choroiditis.—Suppurative choroiditis is invariably due to infection with pyogenic microörganisms. This may be brought about by penetrating wounds of the eye, ulceration of the cornea or sclera, by embolism, or by extension from the meninges. The trouble begins acutely with chemosis of the conjunctiva of the bulb, moderate exudation into the pupillary area, and hypopyon. The exudation into the vitreous causes the appearance of a yellowish-gray reflex on optical examination. In the case of some of the milder forms of infection, such as that occurring in cerebrospinal meningitis, the disease may behave much as an ordinary cyclitis, but in many instances the process extends to the whole uveal tract, and finally results in **panophthalmitis.**

In this condition the inflammation is intense. The conjunctiva and the eyelids are usually enormously swollen, and the loose tissue of the orbit is infiltrated, so that the eyeball is pushed forward. The intraocular tension is usually much increased, leading to diminution in depth of the anterior chamber, but occasionally it is somewhat diminished. The cornea eventually is infiltrated and may even slough, allowing the exudation to appear externally in the form of discharge. After some days the severity of the process diminishes, and in three or four weeks the acute symptoms come to an end, with gradual shrinkage of the globe (*phthisis bulbi*).

Metastatic choroiditis is a manifestation of a generalized septicemia. The choroid of one or both eyes may be involved together with other parts of the body, or may be the sole area of metastatic deposit. Embolic or metastatic choroiditis is due, of course, to the dissemination of pyogenic organisms throughout the system and their deposit in the capillaries of the choroidal membrane. The primary source of the infection varies. It may be, for example, an infected wound, the puerperal uterus, acute endocarditis, smallpox, pneumonia, or erysipelas.

Serofibrinous Choroiditis.—Several forms of non-suppurative choroiditis are described, most of which are somewhat sluggish in their course. One of the most important is serofibrinous choroiditis. This affection begins somewhat suddenly and runs its course in from six weeks to six months. The choroid is injected and slightly œdematous, and the pericorneal vessels are occasionally engorged. There soon appears an exudation of serofibrinous material into the vitreous humor, obscuring the ophthalmoscopic picture of the fundus, which may eventually involve the anterior chamber and the posterior surface of the cornea. The condition may finally clear up with little or no impairment of vision, but not infrequently the choroid shows small patches of atrophy. Adhesion of the iris to the anterior surface of the lens-capsule may occur.

Chronic Choroiditis.—Chronic choroiditis may be *disseminated* or *diffuse.*

Choroiditis disseminata begins with the formation of rounded patches of exudation, rather poorly defined at the margins, in certain parts of the fundus, usually near the periphery. The patches multiply in number, and some of them may, in time, coalesce, involving a large part of the surface of the fundus. The retina overlying the spots in question is not elevated, but occasionally appears to be somewhat hazy, indicating some infiltration of its substance with inflammatory products (*chorioretinitis disseminata*). Usually the cornea and the humors are unaffected and remain clear, but occasionally, the condition may be complicated with parenchymatous keratitis. Gradually the exudation disappears, the patches become paler, and at the margins become irregularly pigmented, apparently owing to an increased deposit of pigment at certain points. Spots of pigment may often also be observed in the patches themselves. Occasionally pigmentation does not occur. Eventually the exudate disappears entirely or is partially organized,

FIG. 166

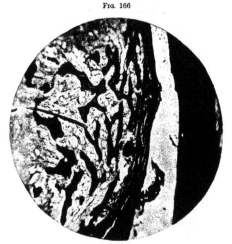

Formation of bone in the choroid, the result of chronic inflammation. Zeiss obj. DD, without ocular. (From the collection of the Royal Victoria Hospital.)

while the affected areas go on to complete atrophy with obliteration of the vessels and the formation of cicatricial tissue. The atrophic patches may, in time, increase in size, even when the inflammatory process appears to have come to an end, owing, apparently, to impairment of nutrition. The whole process may run its course in a few months or may be prolonged for years. Relapses are not infrequent. A curious feature, occasionally met with, is the formation of plates of bone as a result of the long-standing irritation.

Destruction of the choriocapillaris at the points of exudation probably always takes place. This, by interfering with the blood supply of the retina, leads to atrophy of that membrane, and, if extensive, may, in turn, lead to partial atrophy of the optic nerve. Degenerative changes, due to the lack of nutrition, may also take place in the vitreous and the lens.

Forster has described, under the term *choroiditis alveolaris*, an affection, usually found in children, which appears to be a form of choroiditis disseminata. This begins at or near the posterior pole of the eye with the formation of areas of pigmentation. These gradually become lighter in the centre and the plaques thin, until we get atrophic areas bounded by fairly dense rings of pigment. Such patches may coalesce. There may be only two or three patches of atrophy and pigmentation in this affection, or a large part of the fundus of the eye may be involved. The process may begin and remain more marked at the periphery of the fundus, or, again, may involve chiefly the central portion (*choroiditis posterior*).

Choroiditis diffusa begins gradually and progresses in a somewhat sluggish way. It begins with the formation in the choroid of large plaques of exudation, of a pale yellowish-pink or orange color. These are not pigmented. The overlying retina is slightly œdematous. The patches coalesce, forming large, irregular, map-like areas. The choriocapillaris and the pigment layer of the retina undergo atrophy and the vessels are thickened and become obliterated. The disk and optic nerve may occasionally show some evidences of atrophy. The deeper layers of the choroid practically always escape.

Syphilis.—Syphilis of the choroid may take the form of a serofibrinous choroiditis, or, again, a diffuse or disseminated choroiditis. Inasmuch as the retina is almost always involved, it would be more strictly correct to speak of these conditions as syphilitic chorioretinitis. In one form of syphilitic inflammation the vitreous chiefly appears to be involved and becomes cloudy, especially in the axial portion. In another variety the chorioretinitis is most marked in the neighborhood of the posterior pole. Atrophy and connective-tissue formation are marked features of syphilis.

Tuberculosis.—The usual form of choroidal tuberculosis is the miliary eruption, although massive tuberculosis is not unknown.

Miliary tuberculosis of the choroid is but one manifestation of a general miliary infection. The tubercles, which are similar in all respects to miliary tubercles elsewhere, may be few or very numerous and are situated under the choriocapillaris. The retina is not affected, save that it may be elevated somewhat where it overlies the milia. The vitreous is also free. The ciliary body and the iris are but rarely attacked by tuberculosis. The discovery of tubercles in the fundus of the eye by ophthalmoscopic examination is sometimes a valuable aid to the diagnosis of systemic tuberculosis.

In the massive form of tuberculosis, the choroid is the seat of larger nodules or tumor-like masses, which caseate in the centre. The process may lead to perforation of the sclera and the extension of the tuberculous process to structures outside the globe.

RETROGRESSIVE METAMORPHOSES.

Atrophy.—Atrophy may be the result of choroiditis or hemorrhages into the membrane, or, again, of imperfect blood supply, and occurs in small, scattered areas or in larger irregular patches. It is evidenced by pallor of the affected part of the choroid, with an increase in the amount of pigment. Atrophy also is met with in myopia.

There is, also, an affection called **"colloid disease" of the choroid** which may be discussed under this heading. Very small nodules, at first soft, later becoming hard like glass, are formed in the thin lamina elastica. The exact nature of these is not fully known. They are found in cases of partial atrophy after choroiditis and in eyes removed for old inflammatory disturbance.

TRAUMATISM AND ALLIED CONDITIONS.

Detachment.—Detachment of the choroid is rare, but may be met with as a result of hemorrhage or exudation of inflammatory products between the choroid and sclerotic. It may also be caused by a tumor and may accompany degeneration of the vitreous humor in the course of irido-cyclo-choroiditis.

Ruptures.—Ruptures of the choroid, either single or multiple, are occasionally met with as a result of blows upon the eye. They are accompanied by more or less hemorrhage and eventually exudation, which may find their way into the retina and the vitreous. When the extravasated materials are absorbed an atrophic patch is left. The rupture may be of almost any shape, but is usually arranged with the concavity toward the disk.

Wounds.—Wounds of the choroid may be of all kinds and usually involve other structures. If exudation take place into the vitreous, fibrous adhesions may be formed, sometimes leading to detachment of the retina. Infected wounds may bring about panophthalmitis.

The Retina.

The retina is the highly specialized terminal of the optic nerve. Owing to its preëminent importance in the visual apparatus, disorders which would elsewhere be of no consequence are here of the greatest practical moment. The retina is rarely diseased alone. Owing to its close proximity to the choroidal membrane and the nature of its blood supply, inflammation of the latter membrane and disorders of its vascular apparatus are particularly liable to involve the retina secondarily.

Again, retinal disease is very frequently an expression of some general systemic condition, and may be of great diagnostic value. Among such conditions may be mentioned general arteriosclerosis, pernicious anemia, leukemia, Bright's disease, diabetes, syphilis, and septicemia.

Finally, disorders of the optic nerve, particularly those which, like congestion, œdema, or inflammation, tend to hamper the blood supply of the part, often lead to serious disturbance of the retina.

CONGENITAL ANOMALIES.

The retina may be defective in the condition known as **coloboma oculi** (q. v.).

CIRCULATORY DISTURBANCES.

Anemia.—Anemia of the retina is of great practical importance. It may be due to extrinsic causes, such as general systemic anemia or loss of blood, or, again, to some local disturbance in the vessels, leading to a deficient supply of blood. General anemia must be of high grade before it will produce noticeable changes in the retina. The papilla is pale, the arteries are narrower than normal and imperfectly filled, while the veins are also somewhat diminished in size, although occasionally they may be overfilled.

The anemia of the retina resulting from extensive hemorrhage may lead to atrophy and fatty degeneration of the membrane. Blindness may result and be permanent.

Total anemia of the retina is due to obstruction of the central artery, whether by embolism, thrombosis, spasm of the muscular coat, hemorrhage into the optic sheath, injury to the artery within the nerve, or pressure upon it by a new-growth.

Embolism.—Embolism of the central artery of the retina is, according to recent investigations, considerably more uncommon than has usually been thought. The primary cause is to be looked for in endocarditis, aortic aneurism, or arteriosclerosis. The embolus usually obstructs the whole vessel before its bifurcation, although occasionally one of the terminal branches is alone affected. Instant blindness is the result.

On ophthalmoscopic examination a short time after the embolism has occurred, the retinal arteries are almost completely empty, the smaller branches being nearly invisible, while the larger ones present only a fine central thread of blood. The veins of the papilla and its neighborhood are also, though to a less extent, deficient in blood. The optic disk is pale, with sharp edges. In course of time a marked whitish turbidity of the retina becomes manifest, situated round about the optic nerve and fovea centralis. The contour of the papilla is thereby obscured and the whole of the macular region and its neighborhood becomes cloudy. In the centre of this area can be seen a reddish spot corresponding with, though somewhat larger than, the centre of the fovea. The affected portion of the retina gradually undergoes atrophy, so that the choroid shows through. Small hemorrhages may sometimes also be seen in the neighborhood of the papilla. Finally, the cloudiness disappears and the papilla and the retina atrophy and become functionless.

Thrombosis.—Thrombosis of the arteria retinæ centralis gives rise to a train of events similar to those in the case of embolism. The condition is rare and is probably in all cases to be attributed to arterial disease.

Spasm.—Spasm of the retinal artery and its branches has been observed in cases of migraine (Wagenmann), with the production of temporary blindness.

Hyperemia.—Hyperemia of the retina may be arterial or venous.

Arterial Hyperemia.—Arterial or active hyperemia results from inflammation of the retina, eyestrain, irritation of the eye, from keratitis, iritis, choroiditis, and is met with in cases of meningitis, Graves' disease, and neurasthenia. The arteries in this condition are overdistended, apparently lengthened, and varicose.

Venous Hyperemia.—Venous hyperemia, or passive congestion, is due to some interference with the return flow of blood from the eye. As a rule, the obstruction is referable to some diseased condition of the optic papilla, such as optic neuritis. Here, the swelling of the disk leads to compression of the central vein, and the same thing may be produced by glaucoma and by disease processes in the orbit, as, for example, tenonitis and orbital cellulitis. Occasionally, meningitis, intracranial tumors, or thrombosis of the cavernous sinus may be the causative factors. Congenital heart disease, when associated with general cyanosis, is associated with noteworthy congestion of the retina. Thrombosis of the central vein is one of the rarest causes of venous hyperemia. It is generally due to angiosclerosis, but occasionally has been obsevred in orbital cellulitis.

Venous hyperemia is characterized by distention and tortuosity of the veins, and the disks appear also to be hyperemic. In many cases the arteries look somewhat attenuated. In the severer forms, hemorrhages into the fundus may occur. Vision is not usually entirely impaired, and temporary improvement may take place. Relapses are, however, common, and the sight may ultimately be lost.

Hemorrhage.—Retinal hemorrhages are due to a great variety of causes. One of the most important is trauma. They are often also met with in certain constitutional diseases, especially those that damage the integrity of the vessel walls, and in some local affections of the eye itself.

A potent factor is passive congestion. We therefore are liable to get retinal hemorrhages in cases of suffocation, thrombosis of the central vein of the retina, in pressure upon the vein, such as may be produced by optic neuroretinitis and neuritis or glaucoma. Occasionally, hemorrhages are found in embolism of the central artery of the retina or infarction.

Vascular changes, sclerosis or endarteritis, predispose strongly to hemorrhage, and are met with in conditions such as general arteriosclerosis, Bright's disease, diabetes, gout, pernicious anemia, leukemia, scurvy, and in liver affections associated with jaundice. Among other general causes may be mentioned septicemia, malaria, relapsing fever, extensive burns of the skin, and poisoning with phosphorus and lead. Among rarer causes are mentioned disorders of menstruation and vicarious menstruation. Fatty, hyaline, and amyloid changes in the vessel walls may on occasion lead to extravasation of blood.

Retinal hemorrhages vary considerably in number, size, shape, and position. The patches are pale red, dark red, or black, according to the age, and frequently assume a radiate or "flame-shaped" appearance. This is owing to the fact that the extravasation often takes place into the nerve-fibre layer, where it follows the course of the fibers. The larger effusions of blood may force their way into the vitreous, which thereby becomes opaque, or between the choroid and the retina. Occasionally, the blood collects beneath the hyaloid membrane (subhyaloid hemorrhage).

The blood is often absorbed rapidly but leaves whitish patches in the retina, which are due to fatty degeneration and atrophy of the membrane, resulting from the interference with the nutrition. Not infrequently, such spots become pigmented, usually at the periphery, and may clear toward the centre. They may often, however, contain scattered blotches of pigment. In cases of hemorrhage into the vitreous the clots may remain attached to the retina and become organized, forming curious tags. This is believed to be the cause of the so-called *retinitis proliferans.*

The disturbances of vision which result depend, of course, on the extent and localization of the hemorrhages. Extravasations in the macula will lead to serious interference with the sight. Even moderate effusions of blood into the vitreous will produce cloudiness of vision. In other cases we may have metamorphopsia, less often, photopsia.

Hemorrhage into the sheath of the optic nerve may cause pressure upon the central artery and anemia. It has been known to follow trauma to the eye or hemorrhage at the base of the brain, the blood in the latter case forcing its way along the sheath of the nerve.

Aneurisms.—Aneurisms of the retinal arteries are very rare. They are usually miliary in size and multiple, though larger single ones may occur. Traumatic arteriovenous aneurism has been described.

Phlebectasia.—Phlebectasia is a rare condition in which the retinal veins present a markedly beaded appearance, due to alternate constrictions and dilatations. It has been noted in connection with suppressed menstruation.

INFLAMMATIONS.

Retinitis.—Under the term retinitis, which, strictly speaking, should be employed to designate inflammatory conditions of the retina only, are usually classed a number of affections, chiefly of a degenerative nature, that are only more or less doubtfully related to inflammation. Such are certain forms of fatty degeneration, atrophy, œdema, hemorrhage, and pigmentation.

Retinitis may exist *per se*, but is usually dependent on or associated with disease of the neighboring structures. When due to infection it may be brought about directly by trauma, or may be secondary to some disease process in a distant part. According to the type, we can recognize suppurative and non-suppurative forms.

Suppurative Retinitis.—Suppurative retinitis is, in a large proportion of cases, due to penetrating wounds of the bulb, whereby septic micro-organisms are imported into the eye. It may, for example, follow an operation for cataract extraction. Metallic substances, particularly copper, which have entered the eye and are disintegrating there, sometimes give rise to a mild form of suppurative inflammation. In other cases the infection is metastatic, the primary condition being puerperal septicemia or some acute infectious fever. In this variety the condition is apt to be a chorioretinitis. Where the inflammatory process has affected mainly the vitreous humor, the condition may give rise, in children, to the appearance known clinically as **pseudoglioma**. In the milder forms of septic retinitis, we find in the retina hemorrhages and white spots, not unlike those found in albuminuric retinitis without any marked evidences of inflammation, and apparently without the presence of microörganisms, while the severer cases go on to suppuration and exudation. In the latter class of cases staphylococci or strepto-cocci may be found.

In the earlier stages the retina appears to be swollen and cloudy with scattered hemorrhages. Later, the vitreous humor becomes turbid from exudation to such an extent as to interfere with further study of the case by ophthalmoscopic methods. Microscopically, the retina is swollen and œdematous, the nerve-fibre layer and later the ganglionic layer are infiltrated with leukocytes, and in the supporting stroma is a granular and fibrinous exudate, with, in severe cases, hemorrhagic extravasations. In course of time the radial fibres hypertrophy and elongate in the direction of the cornea. Ultimately the rods and cones atrophy and disappear. The process ends finally in panophthalmitis and phthisis bulbi.

Retinitis Simplex.—The mildest form of non-suppurative retinitis is that known as retinitis simplex (**serous retinitis; œdema retinæ**). The causes are not entirely clear. Some cases are attributed to the effect of eye-strain, others, again, follow blows upon the eye (commotio retinæ). The condition is also said to be one of the first manifestations of sympathetic ophthalmia. The retina is found to be congested and hazy, apparently from œdema, which may be either patchy or diffuse.

Albuminuric Retinitis.—Of much more practical importance, from the standpoint of the diagnostician, is albuminuric retinitis. In this form of retinitis the optic nerve papilla is usually involved as well (**neuroretinitis**). The changes, when well marked, are almost pathognomonic of nephritis, and it not infrequently happens that, in cases where the general symptoms are somewhat in abeyance, the diagnosis of Bright's disease is first made by the ophthalmologist. On examination, the optic disk is found to be reddened, swollen, and somewhat blurred at the margin, while in the neighborhood are numerous rounded or radially-disposed streaks of hemorrhage, together with larger or smaller;

irregular, white patches, which may coalesce and form extensive areas around the papilla. The retinal vessels, particularly the veins, are over-distended and tortuous. In the region of the macula can often be seen white streaks arranged in rows, having a characteristic, star-like form. Both eyes are usually involved, but one may be more affected than the other.

Microscopically, we find abundant lymph-corpuscles, especially along the vessels, and fibrinous exudate into the tissue spaces, together with hyperplasia of the supporting stroma. There is a widespread arteritis and capillaritis, resulting in thickening and sclerosis of the smaller vessels. The vascular changes, no doubt, account for the numerous small hemor-rhages that are found in this form of retinitis. The white patches above referred to are produced by dense accumulations of fatty granular cells, which are situated within and between the granular layers, and of hyaline and colloidal masses supposed to be derived from degenerating blood-extravasations and nerve-substance. The whitish streaks in the macular region are due to fatty degeneration of the inner ends of the radiating nerve-fibres. The optic papilla shows infiltration with lymph-cells, degeneration of its fibres, and hypertrophy of the interstitial sub-stance.

In albuminuric retinitis the power of vision is rarely lost completely, and this peculiarity is one of the most important means of distinguishing between this condition and the optic neuritis resulting from brain tumor in which the sight is always almost lost. The fact that the fovea cen-tralis is rarely affected in albuminuric retinitis accounts for the fact that central vision is almost constantly preserved.

Retinal changes somewhat similar to those occurring in Bright's disease are also met with in long-standing cases of diabetes, but are much rarer. In one form of the trouble, multiple small hemorrhages are to be seen in the retina and nothing more, the **hemorrhagic diabetic retinitis** of Hirschberg. This condition is probably not inflammatory in its nature. More characteristic is **central punctate retinitis.** Here, the retina presents numerous small, bright, shining spots, chiefly in the neighborhood of the optic disk and the macula, but not having the stellate arrangement of the spots in albuminuric retinitis. With these are to be seen multiple scattered hemorrhages. The retinal vessels seem to be normal and there is no œdema either of the papilla or of the retina. Not infrequently hemorrhage may take place into the vitreous, causing turbidity of that medium and considerable impairment of vision. Glauc-oma, secondary to the hemorrhage, may also occur. Vision is apt to be defective in diabetic retinitis, especially in the central portion of the field, and peripheral vision may also be impaired.

Chronic Diffuse Retinitis.—A chronic diffuse retinitis is described, resulting from inflammation of the uveal tract. It is marked chiefly by cellular infiltration, and, later, by the formation of new connective tissue in the deeper layers of the membrane. The radial fibres, together with the supporting stroma and the adventitia of the vessels, also show thickening. The increase in length of the radial fibres may attain such proportions that a layer of reticulated connective tissue is formed upon the inner surface of the retina. The nerve-fibres and ganglia ultimately atrophy and disappear, while the rods and cones are similarly affected, though to a less degree. In some few cases the rods and cones are, on the contrary, hypertrophied, becoming both longer and thicker than normal. This is particularly apt to be the case when detachment of the retina has taken place.

Disseminated Retinitis.—Somewhat akin to the last-mentioned form of retinitis is disseminated retinitis, which is analogous to disseminated chorioretinitis, above described. In many of the cases, in fact, it is not always easy or even possible to say whether the process has originated in the choroid and has subsequently spread to the retina, or whether it is primary in the latter membrane. Thin patches of exudation are found between the choroid and the retina, together with circumscribed destruction of the pigment-epithelium and of the layer of rods and cones. In some parts the retinal pigment tends to accumulate, so that it may be readily recognized on ophthalmoscopic examination. Ultimately the connective tissue of the outer layers of the retina and the supporting fibres proliferate and extend in the direction of the choroid. In this new material can be seen more or less altered fragments of the rods and cones, with masses of pigment and larger or smaller gland-like excrescences, derived from the lamina vitrea of the choroid. The connective-tissue formation and the pigmentation may eventually extend to the innermost layers of the retina, where the pigment is seen to be deposited along the course of the vessels.

Retinitis Pigmentosa.—In some respects comparable to the last-mentioned form is the so-called retinitis pigmentosa, an affection in which pigmentation is an early and characteristic feature. Inasmuch as the inflammatory manifestations are of the slightest description, and, in fact, are generally lacking, it is questionable whether the process is not more properly to be classed among the degenerations than among the inflammations. The ophthalmoscopic picture is characteristic. There is slight atrophy of the optic papilla, as shown by its yellowish-white appearance and sharp contour; the vessels, particularly the arteries, are shrunken, and there is a notable deposit of pigment in a zone intermediate between the posterior pole and the equator of the eye. The patches of pigment, which are more or less numerous, are small, irregularly indented, and arranged in large part along the course of the vessels. Where the pigmentation is more extreme the patches may coalesce to form large, deep black clumps, often containing rounded spots devoid of coloring. Hemorrhages do not occur, nor are the clear spots resulting from infiltration of the retina or atrophy of the choroid to be seen.

Histologically, one finds hyaline thickening of the vessels, with obliteration of their smaller branches, atrophy of the pigment epithelium, with the new formation of deeply-pigmented cells in the retina, where they become located in the vessel sheaths, and marked hypertrophy of the supporting stroma of the retina.

The disease affects both eyes, and can be inherited.

Among the rarer forms of retinitis may be mentioned **retinitis circinata** (Fuchs), **retinitis striata** (Nagel), **retinitis punctata albescens** (Mooren), and **retinitis solaris**.

Retinitis circinata is found only in elderly people and affects one or both eyes. On examination, a number of small, white spots can be seen arranged about the macula in a more or less perfect circle. The macula shows a grayish opacity. The white spots are deeper than the retinal vessels and may be slightly pigmented. There is diminution in central vision, contraction of the visual field, and a small central scotoma. In this affection one or both eyes may be involved.

Retinitis striata derives its name from the fact that there are a number of grayish stripes to be seen in the retina in front of the pigment layer but behind the vessels. These stripes may be three or four times as wide as the veins and may radiate from the disk like the spokes of a wheel, or, again, may have no particular arrangement. The retina may also show pigmentation. Vision is slightly reduced, but blindness does not usually result.

In **retinitis punctata albescens** the retina is studded with small, white dots, which are most numerous around the disk and in the macula. The fovea, however, is usually unaffected. Central vision is reduced, and there are sometimes nyctalopia and reduction of the peripheral field.

Solar retinitis is the result of exposure of the eyes to a bright light. There is found a central scotoma and, later, pigmentation of the macula.

Parasites.—*Cysticercus cellulosæ* has been met with in or beneath the retina. The condition is rare. Separation of the retina, clouding of the vitreous humor, and finally atrophy of the eye result.

RETROGRESSIVE METAMORPHOSES.

Atrophy and Degeneration.—Atrophy and degeneration of the retina occur not only as a senile change, but also as a sequel of various disease processes, among which may be mentioned, hemorrhage, sclerosis, of the retinal vessels, vascular obstruction from thrombosis or embolism, separation of the retina, chronic retinitis and neuroretinitis, chronic choroiditis. As a rule, the atrophy affects chiefly the nervous part of the structure, while the stroma and pigmented epithelium are not infrequently hyperplastic. The rods and cones at first show swelling and assume a club-shaped or pear-shaped appearance. They usually also elongate and tend to split at the ends, becoming converted into rounded or oval masses. The nerve cells of the external and internal granular layers, as well as the ganglion cells, may ultimately undergo fatty and colloid change and disappear. In this way the whole nervous mechanism may, at times, be destroyed and the retina replaced by a simple connective-tissue membrane.

In the eyes of old people the vessels of the retina are usually sclerosed, and there may be cystic degeneration in the anterior layers of the retina.

It is a common thing to find in choroidal and retinal disease marked changes in the pigment-epithelium. Certain of the cells lose their pigment, while others appear to take up more than the normal amount. Degeneration and alterations in the pigment layers are not infrequently found in the macular region after injuries of the eye and in old age.

Separation of the Retina (Amotio Retinæ).—Normally, the pigment layer of the retina is fairly firmly attached to the choroid, while the anterior portion appears to be merely superimposed upon the other and held in position by the pressure of the vitreous humor. In detachment of the retina, so-called, these two layers are separated, the pigmented layer being ordinarily left behind. Separation of the retina does not occur except in the most severe affections of the eye, such as advanced myopia, severe injuries, hemorrhages, choroiditis, iridocyclitis, cysticercus cysts, and intra-ocular tumors. Albuminuric retinitis, especially that associated with pregnancy, is one of the rarer causes of retinal separation. The condition may come on without obvious cause. When the separation is recent, the retina projects forward into the posterior chamber as a tremulous, translucent, grayish-colored membrane, thrown into folds, over which the vessels can be made out taking an irregular course. The separation tends to increase, and finally becomes complete, the retina remaining attached at the disk and ora serrata in the form of a plicated funnel. The separated retina is often œdematous and may undergo hyperplasia. Calcification, or, more rarely, ossification, may occur. The bloodvessels finally undergo sclerosis and become thrombosed. The nervous elements atrophy and eventually become macerated and disappear.

PROGRESSIVE METAMORPHOSES.

Tumors.—The only benign growths which have been found to originate in the retina are teleangiectatic and fibromatous tumors, which have been found in eyes after removal.

Glioma.—Glioma is the only malignant growth which is primary in the retina. Since it is found usually in early infancy and never later than the twelfth year, its development seems to be dependent on some congenital peculiarity. This view is supported by the fact that more than one of the same family may be attacked. In about 18 per cent. of cases both eyes are involved.

The new-growth begins at the back of the eye, pushing the retina before it into the anterior chamber. Comparatively early the sheath of the optic nerve is involved. It gradually spreads to the ciliary process and iris, and may eventually infiltrate the whole eye. Iritis and ulceration of the cornea occur, and, finally, the tumor penetrates the globe and appears externally, where it may attain relatively enormous proportions. It forms a soft, fungating mass, which is necrosed in parts and tends to bleed readily. In time the growth may involve the sclera, the eyelids, the soft parts and bones of the face, and may eventually reach the brain by way of the sheath of the optic nerve. Secondary growths may be found in the regional nodes, the parotid and submaxillary glands, in the liver, and other organs.

Histologically, the growth does not differ materially from the glioma occurring in the brain. It consists of numerous closely packed, mononuclear cells, embedded in a finely granular and fibrillated ground substance, which is abundantly provided with wide, thin-walled blood-vessels. The glioma cells are round and contain a single nucleus almost completely filling up the cell body, so that the tumor to some extent

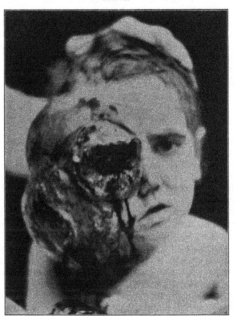

Glioma of the retina (from a patient of Dr. L. Webster Fox in the Medico-Chirurgical College, Philadelphia.) (McFarland.)

seems to be made up of granules, recalling the granular layer of the retina. By proper methods the peculiar spider-like cells of gliomatous tissue can be detected. In some specimens peculiar rosettes formed of rods and cones have been found and such tumors have been termed *neuro-epitheliomata.* The layer of rods and cones is homologous with the cells lining the central neural canal. Flexner would, therefore, term such tumors *ependymal gliomata.* Glioma usually starts from the outer portion of the retina, the granular layers, but, more rarely, may originate from the nerve-fibre layer.

The Optic Nerve.

CONGENITAL ANOMALIES.

Coloboma.—Coloboma of the sheath of the optic nerve has already been referred to (see p. 637).

CIRCULATORY DISTURBANCES.

Œdema and Congestion.—Œdema and congestion of the optic nerve either in the papilla or in the papilla and behind the bulb as well are found in the early stages of inflammation of the nerve, or as a result of the pressure of tumors. or inflammatory exudates upon the nerv trunk. These conditions will be more conveniently treated under the heading of inflammation.

INFLAMMATIONS.

Inflammation of the optic nerve may affect the retrobulbar portion of the trunk (**neuritis**) or the distal extremity (**papillitis**). Inflammation of the papilla—**papillitis**—may exist *per se*, but not infrequently is due to the extension of an inflammatory process from the retina (*neuro-retinitis*), from the nerve trunk, or from the brain, by way of the nerve trunk (*descending optic neuritis*).

Papillitis or Choked Disk (Stauungspapille).—Papillitis is commonly the result of meningitis, sinus thrombosis, intracranial tumors, and, occasionally, tumors and inflammatory exudates within the orbit. As to the essential nature of papillitis opinions differ. Some interpret it as the result of hydrops of the nerve sheath; others, as a true inflammation of the disk. It is a fact, however, that any condition which leads to increase in intracranial pressure, such as, for example, a new-growth or meningitis, results in forcing an increased amount of cerebrospinal fluid into the intervaginal space of the optic nerve. This induces pressure upon the central artery and vein of the retina which enter the nerve a few millimeters behind the globe. The papilla thus becomes swollen and œdematous.

The ophthalmoscopic examination in such cases shows the margin of the disk to be blurred and the retinal zone immediately about it to be dimmer than it should be. The papilla itself is cloudy, reddened, and swollen, particularly in the nasal portion. The veins of the retina are also somewhat congested. In the more intense cases of papillitis the infiltration of the tissues is still more marked. The papilla is greatly swollen and so cloudy that it is with difficulty recognizable. The retinal veins are also more indefinite, while numerous small extravasations of blood, arranged in radial fashion, are to be seen in the grayish-red nerve substance. In purely inflammatory cases the turbidity of the tissues is the most striking and characteristic feature. In the hydropic form the turbidity is not so great, but the disk is enormously swollen and the retinal veins are overfilled and distorted. While this is the rule, it must be admitted however, that it is not always possible to determine from the ophthalmoscopic examination alone the true nature and cause of the papillitis, whether due to pressure or to inflammation. The form met with in albuminuria is of the type of a neuroretinitis (see p. 670). Papillitis, when of mild grade, may pass away leaving the disk practically normal. The more severe or more prolonged cases usually result in loss of vision. This is due to atrophy of the nerve-fibres from the pressure of the inflammatory exudate or of newly-formed connective tissue.

Histologically, the choked disk from hydrops presents marked œdema, which is the sole cause of the great swelling, but sooner or later inflammatory infiltration is superadded and a picture results which cannot be differentiated from any of the forms of true papillitis. The tissues are infiltrated with small round cells, particularly along the course of the vessels, the nerve-fibres are swollen and nodular, and there are minute extravasations of blood and a deposit of finely granular detritus between the fibres. In the most advanced stages, there is a considerable increase of connective tissue and consecutive atrophy, more or less complete, of the nerve-fibres. In the latter case, the papilla is sharply defined, on ophthalmoscopic examination, of a dead white color, perhaps somewhat excavated, and the retinal vessels are shrunken looking.

Inflammation of the trunk of the optic nerve (*retrobulbar neuritis*) may affect the peripheral portion of the nerve and its sheath (*perineuritis*), the axial portion (*central* or *axial neuritis*), or various areas scattered through the nerve (*disseminated neuritis*). The parts involved are the intervaginal space and the interstitial fibrous stroma of the nerve. In the form above termed perineuritis, the intervaginal space is filled with an inflammatory exudate, consisting of serum, round cells, and often fibrin. Later, the endothelial cells, covering the connecting strands that traverse the space, proliferate. Accompanying this, the supporting stroma of the nerve may be found infiltrated with similar inflammatory products. Later, the inflammatory process may involve the nerve-fibres proper, so that, as the combined result of pressure and disintegration, they atrophy and finally disappear. The nerve-substance may thus be represented simply by masses of fragmenting myelin, fatty granules, and the so-called amyloid bodies. It is possible, too, that the inflammation and disintegration of the nerve-fibres may be primary—*neuritis medullaris* (Leber).

Retrobulbar neuritis may result in more or less complete loss of vision, according to the amount of nerve-substance that is destroyed. Where there is partial loss of vision, the condition is known as *scotoma*. We may have peripheral, axial, or disseminated scotomas. Perhaps in the majority of cases, the scotoma is situated in or near the centre. In chronic tobacco amblyopia there is a central scotoma with also some limitation of the peripheral field of vision.

Neuritis of the optic nerve trunk is often due to inflammation in the orbit, the extension of a basal meningitis, or an intracranial new-growth. Occasionally, it can be traced to a systemic infection or intoxication. In the toxic forms it is perhaps a question whether the inflammation is primary in the nerve trunk or whether the process begins in the retina, degeneration here leading to secondary ascending atrophy of the fibres.

Retrobulbar neuritis may disappear without serious damage being done, but not infrequently atrophy supervenes with more or less loss of visual power.

Tuberculosis.—Miliary tubercles have been found affecting the sheath of the nerve. Occasionally, also, the nerve has been destroyed by a diffuse infiltration of its substance with tuberculous granulation tissue.

Syphilis.—Syphilis may assume the form of a simple retrobulbar neuritis or a gummatous infiltration of the nerve. The whole trunk and even the chiasm may be involved. Syphilitic neuroretinitis (q. v.) is also a well-recognized condition.

RETROGRESSIVE METAMORPHOSES.

Atrophy.—Atrophy of the optic nerve occurs and is due to a variety of causes. In general, it may be said that any condition which interferes with the nutrition of the nerve-fibres or brings about destruction of the neurocytes, or nutritive nerve-centres, is competent to bring about atrophy. Pressure upon the nerve-trunk, as from inflammatory exudates, connective-tissue hyperplasia, congested vessels, or new-growths, is an important cause. Atrophy of the neurocytes in the retina, from inflammation, vascular disturbances, or other causes, leads secondarily to wasting of the nerve-fibres proceeding from them. Simple atrophy of the optic nerve occurs in tabes dorsalis and progressive paralysis of the insane. The cause is held by some to be a primary degeneration of the retinal cells. The various toxic amblyopias, notably that from quinine, are probably due to a similar condition, resulting from the induced ischemia of the retinal vessels.

PROGRESSIVE METAMORPHOSES.

Tumors.—Tumors of the optic nerve and its sheath are rare. They may be primary or secondary. The secondary new-growths, which are of course malignant, usually originate in other parts of the eyeball or in the orbit and involve the nerve by direct extension. Thus, glioma of the retina and sarcoma of the choroid may invade the disk, and carcinoma and sarcoma of the orbital cavity may attack the trunk of the nerve. Metastatic carcinoma has also been reported.

The primary tumors may, with Leber,[1] be classified into those affecting

---

[1] Die Krankheiten der Netzhaut und des Sehnerven. Handb. der gesammten Augenheilkunde, *Graefe* and *Saemisch*, 5:1877:910.

the intra-ocular, the intra-orbital, and intracranial portions of the optic nerve. They may further be divided into those that spring from the dural covering or the parts immediately adjacent to it—extradural new-growths; and those originating from structures within the dural sheath and for a time, at least, bounded externally by it—intradural new-growths.

The vast majority of primary intradural tumors have been reported as myxomas, fibromas, sarcomas, and various combinations of these elemental types, occasionally as gliomas. Many of these, however, were reported before microscopic technique was as perfect as it is today, so that Byers, who has written an exhaustive monograph on the subject,[1] holds that nearly all of these growths are of the nature of fibroma, of the type known as the false neuroma. They tend to involve the intra-cranial as well as the intra-orbital portions of the nerve, extending some-times into the chiasm. Owing to the wide distribution of the process, the association of the fibrosis with the lymph-channels, the œdematous appearance of the tissue that is so often present, Byers, further, compares the condition to elephantiasis and suggests the term *fibromatosis* of the optic nerve as the correct designation for the condition. Such tumors occasionally exhibit a limited tendency to malignancy, as do other fibrous growths. These new-growths occur in about 80 per cent. of the cases before the age of fifteen years. They are excessively rare after twenty-five. Females are slightly more often attacked than males, and the left eye is somewhat more often affected than the right.

Fibromas of the optic nerve start from the arachnoidal or pial covering, and are apt to extend anteroposteriorly rather than laterally. They tend to compress the nerve trunk, which early undergoes atrophy. Loss of vision and proptosis of the eyeball are characteristic symptoms.

A few cases of **endothelioma** have been recorded (Alt, Tailor, Kalt). These have been occasionally recorded, though incorrectly, as carcinoma, alveolar sarcoma, or fibrosarcoma. Cells of flattened appearance and of endothelial type are found aggregated into masses, separated one from the other by connective tissue. Occasionally, the characteristic cells are arranged concentrically or in whorls about a central, clear, refractile body. Such forms might, therefore, be included under the category of **psammoma.**

One case of **neuroma** has been reported, consisting both of medullated and non-medullated fibres.

The extradural tumors are the **fibroma, endothelioma,** and **sarcoma.** They originate from the connective tissue of the structure or its endothelial lining.

---

[1] The Primary Intradural Tumors of the Optic Nerve. Studies from the Royal Victoria Hospital, Montreal, 1: 1901: No. 1.

The Lens.

CONGENITAL ANOMALIES.

Several forms of partial congenital cataract are recognized. The opacity often assumes geometrical forms and usually involves both lenses. Remains of the hyaloid artery may be found in the form of fibrous strands or membranes of the posterior surface of the lens (**posterior polar cataract**), or on the anterior surface. Other anomalies are **congenital luxation** of the lens and coloboma.

RETROGRESSIVE METAMORPHOSES.

The anterior surface of the lens is covered by a single layer of epithelial cells which extend backward a short distance behind the equator of the lens and then gradually become converted into lens fibres. This epithelium is capable of overgrowth and may undergo a thickening known as **capsular cataract**. The transparent fibres of the lens proper, however, do not appear to be endowed with the same vitality, and are capable only of degeneration. Degeneration of the fibres gives rise to **lenticular cataract**.

Capsular Cataract.—Simple capsular cataract is usually due to the pressure of the lens upon the cornea in cases where the cornea has been perforated and the aqueous humor has drained away. We see it, therefore, in connection with ulceration of the cornea and in corneal staphyloma. Occasionally, a central capsular cataract is found in connection with ophthalmia neonatorum, even where there is no corneal perforation. Penetrating injuries of the lens may also bring about capsular cataract, but this is usually associated with lenticular cataract.

The histological appearances indicate that the epithelium of the capsule, usually about the centre of the anterior surface of the lens, undergoes proliferation, gradually becoming stratified. Eventually, the newly formed cells are converted into spindles and later into fibres, poor in nuclei and resembling connective-tissue fibres.

Lenticular Cataract.—This is often found in connection with affections of the retina and choroid, and in cyclitis. Other well-known forms are those resulting from traumatism, diabetes, and old age.

In injuries to the lens involving penetration of its capsule, we usually get a combined form of cataract. If the rupture be slight it may be covered by the iris or closed by the formation of a capsular cataract. Thus, a small localized opacity may result which may eventually be absorbed. In more extensive injuries, the capsule retracts and the aqueous humor soaks into the substance of the lens. The fibres of the lens begin to swell, become opaque and protrude through the opening. As the extruded tissue is absorbed or detached, other fibres in their turn prolapse, and this process goes on until, if the nucleus be not too hard, the whole substance of the lens is absorbed. Leukocytes may pass into the lens, also, and, later, vascular connective tissue, so that we get a fibrous cataract, in which calcareous salts are often deposited. A formation of bone may also take place.

In diabetes, the aqueous humor appears to undergo changes in its chemical composition which result in degeneration of the lens fibres. They become granular and disintegrate and the subcapsular epithelial cells degenerate and atrophy.

In **senile cataract** it is believed that the first step is the formation of a fissure near the equator of the lens owing to traction on the peripheral lamellæ and shrinkage of the nucleus. The clefts fill with liquid and the cortical fibres begin to swell up and become vesicular from imbibition. They next present small globules in their substance, and clear, homogeneous, myelin masses and fatty globules are found in the tissue spaces. Later, the superficial fibers become detached from the capsule and the cortex is converted into a soft, pulpy, or semifluid mass. This is the stage of tumefaction. Next, the liquid is absorbed and the lens returns to its normal size. The cataract is then said to be "ripe." The degeneration may go on farther, and the cataract is then said to be "over-ripe." The whole of the cortical portion may eventually be converted into a milky liquid in which the nucleus floats (**Morgagnian cataract**), or, again, the liquid may be entirely absorbed, leaving only the nucleus within the capsule (**membranous cataract**). In some cases of advanced senile cataract a capsular cataract develops also.

In the so-called **lamellar cataract** there is an opaque zone between the cortex and the nucleus. The condition is commonly met with in rickety children, and affects both eyes.

The Vitreous Humor.

The vitreous body is an avascular body, like the cornea, and like it may be the seat of an active infiltration with cells and inflammatory products, derived from the neighboring vascular structures. Primary **inflammation** of the vitreous is rare. The vitreous is also liable to undergo *fibrillation* and *liquefaction* as the result of the slightest lesion. Inflammations extending to the vitreous from other parts of the eye, the milder irritation produced by aseptic foreign bodies, or even the trifling changes present in myopia may bring this about. The vitreous in such cases becomes more coarsely fibrillated than normal, the fluid portion is to some extent forced out, and the whole body contracts and becomes detached from the adjacent structures. Detachment of the retina may be brought about in this way.

The vitreous, finally, acts as a passive receptacle for pus, blood, inflammatory exudations, and foreign bodies generally.

Parasites and Foreign Bodies.—The chief parasite is *Filaria sanguinis hominis*, which has been found both in the anterior chamber and in the vitreous. *Cysticercus* cysts have also been met with. All kinds of metallic and mineral substances may gain an entrance into the vitreous as a result of injury.

GLAUCOMA.

Glaucoma is an affection of the eye characterized by an increase in intra-ocular pressure. It may develop in a previously healthy eye (*primary glaucoma*), or in one that is already the site of gross disease (*secondary glaucoma*). The disease often begins slowly and insidiously, but may also set in acutely, in both cases with or without associated inflammatory disturbance. The cases in which the intra-ocular pressure increases slowly, though it may be intermittently, without reddening of the eye, are known as *simple glaucoma*. Those beginning acutely with all the signs of an ophthalmitis are called *inflammatory glaucoma*.

The pathogenesis of glaucoma is not altogether understood, for it is difficult to decide what are causes and what are effects. In general, it may be said that we have to recognize both atrophic and inflammatory changes. We have definite information which goes to show that if there be any impediment to the outflow of the aqueous humor the intra-ocular tension rises and the condition of glaucoma is initiated. In most cases this impediment is due to blockage at the filtration angle or to increased viscosity of the aqueous humor, which causes it to filter with difficulty. Thus, an inflammatory infiltration in the neighborhood of Schlemm's canal, which leads to the production of a cellular exudate in Fontana's space and on the anterior surface of the iris, is a potent cause. In fact, any condition which causes the periphery of the iris to press against the cornea may set up glaucoma, such as congestion or infiltration of the ciliary process, the traction upon the iris exerted by an anterior synechia, the pressure of the aqueous humor in cases of circular posterior synechia. Less often, the permeability of the filtration angle is interfered with by sclerotic changes in the pectinate ligament. Besides the factors just described as the causes of glaucoma, thrombosis of the choroidal veins (Klebs) and proliferation of the endothelium lining the venæ vorticosæ (Birnbacher; Czermak) have been regarded as of etiological importance. It is hard to say, however, whether the changes in question are not likely to be effects rather than causes. The etiology of simple glaucoma is quite obscure. The condition usually develops in hyperopic eyes and in individuals the subject of arterial sclerosis.

In a typical case of acute glaucoma, the conjunctiva is reddened and often œdematous; the cornea, cloudy, devoid of lustre, and with an uneven surface; the pupil is usually dilated. The faint, grayish-green appearance of the pupil of the eye suggested the term glaucoma for the condition. In the milder forms, the increased intra-ocular tension, though it may come on quickly, is accompanied by little more than hardness of the eyeball, opacity of the cornea, and slight pericorneal injection. The more severe cases assume the picture of an ophthalmitis. In some instances, in addition to the conditions described, we find hemorrhages into the retina, the vitreous humor, and the anterior chamber—*hemorrhagic glaucoma*.

As a result of the inflammation and the increased tension, widespread atrophic changes make their appearance. The sclera loses its elasticity, may be thinned, and may bulge at certain points. The lens may be cataractous. The iris is atrophic and its pigment may be gathered around the pupillary margin on the anterior surface. The ciliary body is flattened. The retina and choroid are atrophic and the vessels sclerosed or otherwise obstructed. The optic nerve presents the picture of an ascending degeneration and the bulging backward of the lamina cribrosa causes the so-called cupping of the disk.

The Orbit.

INFLAMMATIONS.

Inflammations of the orbit may be of the types of diffuse **cellulitis** or **abscess**. Cellulitis and abscess often result from injury, but may be

FIG. 168

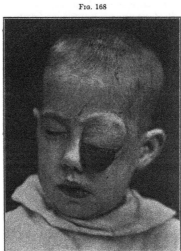

Exophthalmos from an intra-orbital growth. (From the Ophthalmological Clinic, Montreal General Hospital.)

spontaneous. Inflammation may extend to the orbit from the face in erysipelas, from the throat in tonsillitis, or from the socket of an inflamed tooth, or, again, from the lacrimal gland.

PROGRESSIVE METAMORPHOSES.

Tumors.—Tumors of the orbit may arise primarily from the connective tissue of the part, but much more frequently origina some of the contiguous structures. The benign tumors that have observed are the **angioma, lymphangioma, osteoma,** and various f of teratoid new formations, such as **dermoid cysts, rhabdomyoma, myoneuroma.**

Cysts of various kinds are also found, such as hygroma, meli(fatty and oil cysts, atheromatous, hematomatous, and steatom: cysts, many of which are congenital and perhaps related to the derm

The most common primary malignant growth of the orbit is **sarcoma,** usually the *round-* or *spindle-celled* form. *Osteosarcoma, m sarcoma, cylindroma,* and *myofibrosarcoma* are also described. **Chlo** occurs and apparently arises from the periosteum. Sarcomas endotheliomas originating in the antrum, brain, or pituitary gland involve the orbit secondarily.

Carcinoma is always secondary and originates from the eyelids, episcleral tissue, or the lacrimal gland.

New-growths originating in the orbit may lead to marked disloca of the eyeball (*proptosis; exophthalmos*).

Injuries.—Extravasations of blood may take place into the or tissue as a result of contusions, wounds, or fractures. Fracture of inner wall of the orbit opening up communication with the nose or n: duct often lead to emphysema of the orbital cellular tissue.

CHAPTER XXX.

THE EAR.

CONGENITAL ANOMALIES.

CONGENITAL defects of the ear may affect the whole auditory apparatus or a part of it. Malformations of the external and middle ear are generally unilateral, rarely bilateral, and are often associated with other developmental anomalies, such as harelip, cleft palate, club-foot, hernia, persistent branchial clefts, and facial hemiatrophy.

Complete **absence of the auricles** is exceedingly rare. It is said that in China there is a species of sheep, called the Yung-ti, in which this peculiarity is of normal occurrence. In the case of the auricle, the hélix antihelix, or tragus may be defective, or the whole structure is stunted (**microtia**). In other cases the auricle is exceedingly large (**macrotia**), either as a whole or in part; or there may be supernumerary auricles (**polyotia**). These additional auricles are usually unilateral, and are more or less perfect. As a rule, they are pre-auricular appendages, but may be found on the neck, cheek, or shoulder. Similar peculiarities seem to have been known from remote times, for there is in the British Museum the head of an Ægipan with an accessory auricle. The Satyrs are also represented with goat-like ears. Readers of Hawthorne's "Marble Faun" will remember the interesting way in which the story is made to centre around an inherited anomaly of this kind. Not infrequently, small, scar-like grooves, or *fistulæ*, discharging a creamy fluid, are found on the ear, remnants of the primitive gill-clefts (*fistula auris congenita*).

Complete **absence of the external auditory meatus** has been observed. It is generally unilateral, but may be bilateral. The condition is not necessarily associated with impairment of hearing. The site of the meatus is sometimes indicated by a shallow groove, but even this may be wanting. The atresia may be due to bone or membrane. Partial atresia, the presence of connective-tissue bands traversing the passage (Moos[1]), hour-glass constriction of the cavity, abnormal wideness or reduplication of the passage (Schwartze), have been observed. As a rule, these conditions are associated with other defects of the auricles, membrana tympani, or middle ear.

Congenital anomalies in development, configuration, and position of the membrana are fairly common.

Absence of the membrana is only found in connection with defect of the external auditory meatus and tympanic cavity. Small fissures of the

[1] Klinik der Ohrenkrankheiten, 85.

membrana, often bilateral, are occasionally met with as a result of non-closure and explain how certain persons are able to emit tobacco smoke from the ear.

The **middle ear** with its contained ossicles may be completely **absent** or **rudimentary**. Atresia may be present, partial or complete absence of the foramen, abnormal wideness or reduplication of the same. The incus and stapes have been found to be fused. In such cases the hearing may be practically normal.

The **Eustachian tube** may be **absent** in cases of defect of the external ears and rudimentary development of the tympanic cavity and labyrinth. **Kinking** of the tube or **abnormal position** of its pharyngeal opening are more frequent. **Stenosis** is rare.

Congenital malformations of the **internal ear** are occasionally met with. They are usually bilateral, and may be associated, though not invariably so, with other developmental anomalies of the auditory apparatus. The labyrinth may be wholly or partially defective, the cochlea may be undeveloped, or the modiolus or lamina spiralis. The aqueducts may be dilated or reduplicated. When the labyrinth is defective, the auditory nerve may also be absent or end in a bulbous swelling in the bone.

The External Ear.

ANOMALIES OF SECRETION.

Anomalies of secretion of the sebaceous and ceruminous glands are not infrequently met with. Secretion may be **scanty** with marked dryness of the surface of the canal. This is seen in association with certain affections of the middle ear (chronic sclerosing otitis media), and is apparently trophic in character. **Hypersecretion**, with its numerous unpleasant accompaniments, is of frequent occurrence especially in those suffering from chronic middle-ear disease. Under ordinary circumstances, the cerumen is gradually removed to the exterior by the movements of the jaw communicated to the meatus, and by the natural exfoliation of the epithelium. In certain cases, however, favored by excessive production of wax, collapse of the meatus, or change in the nature of the secretion, whereby it becomes tough and viscid, the cerumen accumulates and tends to become impacted. The hypersecretion is sometimes excited by persistent hyperemia of the meatus, but in other cases appears to be a trophic disturbance. Should foreign bodies be present, such as hair, epithelial plugs, cotton wool, etc., the secretion will tend to remain within the meatus and may be impacted by mis-directed efforts to remove it. The pressure of impacted wax rarely, if ever, causes any serious disorder of the auditory canal, although excoriation or inflammation of the canal and membrana tympani are of not infrequent occurrence. When enlargement of the meatus or destruction of the drum membrane is present, this is most probably to be attributed to antecedent suppurative processes

Keratosis Obturans.—Keratosis obturans (Wreden; Burnett) is a rather rare condition in which the meatus is obstructed by a material at first sight not unlike impacted cerumen. The substance is, however, tough and adherent, and of a lighter color than ordinary wax. After removal, which is difficult, the meatus is always found to be more or less eroded. The material in question is composed of an accumulation of the horny elements of the skin lining the cavity and the condition probably results from a chronic otitis externa. The condition is somewhat similar to, if not, indeed, identical with, the so-called cholesteatoma, which originates in the tympanic cavity.

CIRCULATORY DISTURBANCES.

Hyperemia.—Hyperemia of the parts may be due to inflammation or trauma, resulting from mechanical, thermic, or chemical insults. It is seen also in paretic or paralytic conditions of the sympathetic nerve and the vasomotor fibres of the cervical plexus.

Hemorrhage.—Hemorrhage, in the form of small **ecchymoses** or **blebs** in the skin, occasionally results from traumatism and occurs in severe inflammation of the auricle or middle ear.

Othematoma.—The most striking form is the extensive extravasation of blood known as othematoma, or **hæmatoma auris**, which gives rise to a bluish-red, fluctuating, tumor-like swelling. The effusion takes place between the cartilage and the perichondrium, or into the substance of the cartilage itself. Two forms are known—the *traumatic*, due to fracture of the cartilage, and the *spontaneous*. The latter is sometimes bilateral and symmetrical, and is found with most frequency in the insane, although it is also met with in severe blood dyscrasias, such as leukemia. Owing to the fact that section of the restiform bodies in experimental animals is sometimes followed by hematoma auris, Brown-Séquard[1] would refer the occurrence of spontaneous hematoma to lesions at the base of the brain. Degenerative changes in the cartilage and the formation of new bloodvessels is supposed to predispose to the condition. Cysts have been known to develop in the muscles of the auricle after a hematoma.

RETROGRESSIVE METAMORPHOSES.

The degenerative disturbances are not many, nor are they of great importance. In **gout**, small, nodular deposits of uratic salts (*tophi*) are not infrequently found in the auricle. **Fissuring, softening, necrosis,** and partial **calcification** are also met with.

[1] Bull. de l'Acad. de Méd., 34.

PROGRESSIVE METAMORPHOSES.

Exostoses and Hyperostoses.—The progressive metamorphoses are exostoses and hyperostoses, and various forms of tumors. Exostoses and hyperostoses may arise in any part of the external auditory meatus, but frequently grow from the upper or posterior part of the canal just in front of the drum-membrane. They form single or multiple growths, pedunculated or sessile, and of a spherical or conical shape. They are composed of cancellous or compact ivory-like bone. More or less occlusion of the meatus results. These growths are by some attributed to preëxisting subperiosteal abscesses which have made their way to the meatus. This is doubtful. Others, again, think that they are dependent on gout, excessive bathing, or hereditary peculiarities. It is possible also that they are due to anomalies of development.

Polypi.—Polypi, arising from exuberant granulations, are rather common in the meatus. They may be mucous, fibrous, myxomatous, and angiomatous. Some contain hairs; others, keratinous masses and giant cells.

Tumors.—Among tumors should be mentioned the **fibroma, lipoma, osteoma, angioma, chondroma, sarcoma,** and **carcinoma.** The sarcomas are usually *spindle-celled,* occasionally *round-celled, fibrosarcomas,* and *osteosarcomas.* The **chloroma,** a rare tumor of sarcomatous type and of pale green color, which sometimes originates from the temporal bone, may invade the meatus.

Sebaceous and Dermoid Cysts.—Sebaceous and dermoid cysts have also been described. Various forms of **warts** and **nevi** are found on the auricle but are rare.

INFLAMMATIONS.

Inflammation of the auricle may be primary or secondary to lesions in the neighborhood. Practically all the diseases in the skin may be found affecting this part. Most of these need only be mentioned here: Such are, the acute exanthemata, erysipelas, erythema, acne, ecthyma, eczema, herpes, impetigo contagiosa, psoriasis, pemphigus, seborrhœa, pityriasis alba, lupus, syphilis, actinomycosis, lepra, ichthyosis, elephantiasis, scleroderma, and gangrene.

Common affections of the auricle are **chilblain** and **frostbite (pernio).** Both conditions have this in common, that profound circulatory disturbances are induced as a result of extreme variations of temperature. In the milder form the auricle is swollen, bluish-red, and very itchy. When actual freezing has taken place, the organ is much reddened and swollen, intensely painful, and may be covered with blebs containing a yellowish or bloody fluid. In more severe cases ulceration or even gangrene may result, and more or less deformity remains.

Gangrene.—Gangrene is seen, rarely, in erysipelas and typhoid fever. **Noma** may occur in young, debilitated infants. Urbantschitsch has recorded a case of **Raynaud's disease** of the ear.

Perichondritis.—Perichondritis of the auricle and meatus is a rare affection. It gives rise to a fluctuating tumor on the concavity of the auricle, not unlike the othematoma. The process generally begins in the external auditory canal and thence extends to the concha and other portions of the auricle; the tragus alone escapes. The meatus is liable to be stenosed from inflammatory œdema. The fluid contained within the swelling is at first clear and serous, subsequently becoming purulent. The periosteum is stripped from the underlying cartilage, and necrosis of this structure may occur. Complete restitution to the normal may take place, but there is usually some shrinkage. Ossification occurs, but is rare. The left auricle is the one usually involved. Some cases, recorded by Haug, have been tuberculous.

Besides these frankly inflammatory disturbances, there is another affection that should be mentioned, characterized by a painless and afebrile collection of a clear, yellow fluid between the cartilages and perichondrium. After evacuation the condition readily clears up. These cysts are attributed by Hartmann[1] to previous degenerative softening of the part and formation of local collections of fluid.

Otitis Externa Circumscripta; Furunculosis; Follicular Inflammation.—Otitis externa circumscripta is a fairly common affection of the meatus in adults, though much rarer in children. It is usually caused by an infection of the sebaceous and ceruminous follicles with pyogenic cocci, but occasionally originates in the cartilage and perichondrium. The direct exciting factors are trauma of all kinds, chronic discharges from the ear, and chronic eczema. Anemia, gout, diabetes mellitus, and disorders of menstruation are said by some to be predisposing causes. Occasionally, pathological conditions of the nerves of the meatus cause a trophic or so-called "sympathetic" furunculosis of the opposite ear. This affection is characterized by the production of furuncles or boils, almost invariably in the cartilaginous portion of the canal. Several may appear together or may develop one after the other. In severe cases deep-seated abscesses may be formed, and the tissues around the ear are reddened and swollen. The neighboring lymph-glands are commonly swollen and tender, and even the parotid may be involved. Spontaneous resolution rarely occurs, and, as a rule, the abscess breaks externally. Polypoid granulations frequently form about the edges of the ulcer.

Otitis Externa Diffusa.—Otitis externa diffusa may be acute or chronic. It is rarely, if ever, idiopathic, but can usually be traced to various traumatic causes, chief among which is the instillation of irritating fluids. It occurs also in erysipelas, acute and chronic exanthemata, and suppurative otitis media. The affection is not uncommon, especially in weakly and badly nourished children. The condition should always arouse the suspicion of deeper-seated disease. The part affected is usually the osseous portion of the canal, but the process may extend to the membrana and the outer parts. The lining membrane of the meatus

[1] Zeitschr. f. Ohrenh., 15: 156; and 18: 42.

is reddened, swollen, and covered with discharge, at first serous but later purulent. Sometimes, from the presence of secretion, together with exfoliated cells, a kind of membrane is formed. In some cases the entire epidermis may be thrown off repeatedly, leaving each time a reddened, moist surface which quickly becomes covered with new epithelium (*otitis externa exfoliativa*).

Membranous Otitis Externa.—Membranous otitis externa is rare as a primary affection. It usually arises from an angina, such as that in scarlatina, which has extended to the middle ear. The osseous portion of the canal and the membrana tympani are first and chiefly involved, but the process may gradually extend outward. The parts are covered with a dirty white, firm, and adherent membrane, which, when removed, leaves a bleeding excoriated surface.

Diphtheria.—True diphtheria of the external auditory meatus is also rare as a primary affection. It has been observed in the course of epidemics of diphtheria of the throat, but in some cases there has been some previously existing inflammation or excoriation of the parts which predisposed to infection. Much more commonly the disease is secondary to diphtheria of the throat and middle ear.

Phlegmonous Inflammation.—Phlegmonous inflammation of the meatus arises from septic infection through a wound or abrasion of the surface.

Periostitis accompanies all forms of deep-seated or deeply penetrating inflammation, or may be due to an extension of inflammation from the middle ear.

Tuberculosis.—Tuberculosis takes the form of a nodular perichondritis or a miliary tuberculosis of the skin. The first form is found in the concha, the soft tissues of which are reddened and œdematous. Small nodules form resembling fibromas, which grow slowly and do not tend to soften. If, however, there be no operative intervention, after a considerable time tuberculous ulcers and fistulæ form upon the skin and portions of the cartilage may become sequestrated. The neighboring glands are swollen and tender. The infection is said by Haug to arise from the practice of piercing the ears, or from wearing the earrings of a tuberculous person.

Syphilis.—*Primary syphilis* of the auricle is rare, but has been described by Zucker. The auricle was greatly swollen and ulcers were present on the anterior surface of the tragus. The neighboring glands were enlarged. *Secondary syphilitic ulcers* are much more common. They form by preference at the point where the ear is pierced for an earring. Such ulcers are deep, crateriform, with sharp, indurated edges. In *tertiary syphilis* gummas form, or there is a perichondritis.

Parasites.—Otomycosis is a parasitic affection of the external auditory passage produced by various forms of moulds. As a rule, the aspergillus is the infecting agent. About 60 cases of **otomycosis aspergillina** have been recorded, mostly in Germany and the United States. It is a decidedly rare affection in Canada, only 4 cases having been recorded in Montreal in many years. The forms usually found are the

Aspergillus niger, the A. fumigatus, the A. flavus, and, exceedingly rarely, the A. glaucus. A case of the last-mentioned form of the affection has been recorded by Dr. H. S. Birkett and one of us (A. G. N.[1]).

The disease is most common in adults, and is liable to affect those who live in damp houses and under unfavorable hygienic conditions. Inasmuch as it has been found impossible to cultivate these organisms in the healthy ear, it is improbable that the disease is ever spontaneous, but more likely that some disease has preëxisted. Moisture and warmth appear to be the two essential factors. Maceration and loosening of the superficial epithelium, with the formation of a neutral or slightly acid medium, such as is produced by dermatitis, eczema,

FIG. 169

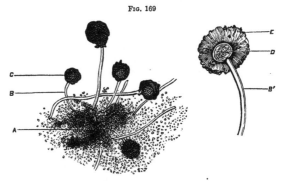

Aspergillus nigricans from the meatus. A, mycelium covered with numerous fallen spores; B, hypha; C, sporangium with ripe spores; B', hypha; D, receptaculum: E, sterigmata with spores. (Politzer.)

and psoriasis, so-called, provide the most favorable conditions. Infection probably takes place through the instillation of substances, such as oil, which contain the spores. The mycelium of the fungus grows in the rete Malpighii and gradually penetrates the deeper structures, while the hyphæ project into the cavity. Owing to the fungus extending to the sensitive parts, or possibly from the presence of some toxin, irritation and a certain amount of inflammation result.

On examination, upon the walls of the meatus, or even on the drummembrane (*myringomycosis aspergillina*, Wreden), can be seen membranous patches, or the meatus is filled with a dirty detritus of waxy consistence, like desquamating epithelium, covered with mould of a black-brown or dull grayish-green color, according to the nature of the fungus present. In several cases recorded, the disease has spread to the middle ear, and in two was apparently the cause of perforation

[1] Birkett and Nicholls, Otomycosis Due to the Aspergillus Glaucus, Montreal Med. Journ., 33: 1904: 338.

(Politzer, Bezold).   Among the rarer fungi that have been found in ear may be mentioned *Mucor mucedo, Mucor corymbifer, Trichothecer roseum, Ascöphora elegans, Otomyces purpureus, Pityriasis versicol* and *Oïdium albicans.*

Foreign Bodies.—A great variety of substances, provided o they be small enough, may be found in the auditory canal.   Such seeds, peas, nut-shells, beads, buttons, cotton, wool, sand, grav Matches or toothpicks, which have been inserted to relieve itchin have been broken off and portions left behind.   The *larvæ* of flies, even a living fly, have been found, as has also *Acarus folliculoru* Animal parasites are, however, much more common in the lower anim *Concretions* of carbonate or phosphate of lime are also met with somewh frequently in the lower animals but rarely in man.

Foreign bodies of all kinds are liable to excite congestion and infla mation, and may, by pressure upon the sensitive structures, give rise marked symptoms.   Some of these are of reflex character and aff the fibres of the trigeminus and vagus nerves.   Epileptiform convulsio vertigo, mental depression, neuralgic pains, and laryngeal cough ha all been found resulting from this condition.

The Drum-membrane.

The drum membrane forms the boundary between the exterr auditory meatus and the middle ear.   On the outer side it is cover by a thin layer of cutis continuous with the epidermis of the meatu and on the inner side, by the mucous membrane of the tympanic cavit As will be readily understood, from its position, it is especially liab to be involved in disease of either of the before-mentioned caviti(Primary lesions are rare.

CIRCULATORY DISTURBANCES.

Hyperemia.—Hyperemia may affect the external epidermal lay(the mucous surface, or both.   In milder grades the vessels are se(to be large and distended, while in the severer forms the membrana diffusely reddened.

Hemorrhage.—Hemorrhage into the membrana occurs on eith surface and takes the form of punctiform or linear ecchymoses.   Tho on the cuticular surface tend to spread upward and posteriorly towai the periphery.   They result frequently from traumatism.   In typhoi variola, endocarditis, and scurvy, bluish-red, sharply-defined elevatio may be found on the mucous covering.

INFLAMMATIONS.

Myringitis.—Inflammation of the tympanic membrane (myringiti is acute or chronic.   The membrane is rarely involved alone, but m;

be inflamed from injury, or by extension from the middle ear. Sea-bathing, foreign bodies, and careless instrumentation may produce it.

In the *acute form* the membrana is congested and swollen, and on examination the handle of the malleus and the short process can no longer be seen. Later, the superficial epithelium becomes macerated and is cast off. Microscopically, all the layers are swollen, œdematous, and infiltrated with round cells. The mucous membrane is especially congested and greatly thickened from the exudation of inflammatory products. In certain cases of intense inflammation, localized collections of pus are found in the cutis, giving rise to small, yellowish dots and streaks (*interlamellar abscesses*).

In *chronic myringitis* the membrana is swollen and infiltrated, the vessels much congested and varicose, while the surface is covered with small papillary or polypoid granulations (*myringitis villosa*).

Tuberculosis.—Myringitis may be due also to tuberculosis, in cases of tuberculosis of the middle ear. Small, miliary foci may be seen or a more rapidly caseating and destructive ulceration.

Syphilis.—*Condylomas* and *gummas* have been observed on the drum-membrane.[1]

RETROGRESSIVE METAMORPHOSES.

Atrophy.—Atrophy of the drum-membrane may result from severe and long-continued pressure upon it. This may be caused by foreign bodies or accumulations of detritus in the external auditory canal, or by the pressure of the external air in cases of obstruction of the Eustachian canal. The part chiefly affected is the lamina propria. The membrane becomes thin, more or less transparent, and sinks inward, or projects externally like a bladder.

PROGRESSIVE METAMORPHOSES.

Among the progressive disturbances may be mentioned the **polypoid outgrowths** that sometimes form on the cuticular or mucous surfaces. These are largely the result of chronic inflammation. Localized overgrowths of the epidermis of the outer surface are met with (**cornua cutanea**), or small, pearly nodules the size of a pin-head.

A rare and interesting growth is the **cholesteatoma,** which is found on the inner surface of the drum-membrane. It forms a tumor-like mass composed of more or less concentrically arranged scales and plates surrounded by a thin, vascular capsule. When of large size such growths may lead to atrophy of the bony parts, so that the auditory canal, tympanic cavity, and mastoid cells are thrown into one large cavity. The exact nature of this growth is still in dispute. Virchow considered

[1] Baratoux, Bull. et mém. de la Soc. d'Otol., 2:2.

it to be a true heterologous tumor; others refer it to a developmental defect—branchiogenic clefts.   Leutert believes that it is a retention-cyst, the squamous epithelium of the meatus or tympanic membrane having passed through a perforation and developed into an encapsulated mass. Rednew believes in a variable etiology, namely, that some of these growths are true tumors, while others are epithelial cysts, retained masses of tissue, or hyperplastic epidermis.

TRAUMATISM.

Rupture.—Rupture of the drum-membrane may arise from direct or indirect violence, as, for instance, from the introduction of pointed instruments, condensation of the air, concussion and fracture of the skull. In the cases due to the first-mentioned cause, the perforation is usually in the superior posterior quadrant.   In those due to condensation of the air, as from boxing the ears, concussions, explosions, working in caissons, pulling the auricle, fractures of the skull, sneezing or coughing, the rupture is in the anterior quadrant.   Some few cases are dependent on the weakening of the membrane from pressure atrophy.   Perhaps the most frequent cause is necrotic inflammation of the drum-membrane secondary to otitis media.   Only rarely does the form of inflammation restricted to the membrana (*interlamellar abscess*) lead to perforation. The membrana becomes eroded and infiltrated and, either by direct extension of the destructive process, or from the pressure of contained fluid, or both, finally gives way.   Any part of the structure may be involved.   There may be only one perforation or several, varying in size from one extremely minute to destruction of the whole structure. In the milder cases, the tear may heal without any obvious alteration in the part, but if extensive a scar is formed.   The lamina propria in such cases is not restored.   Large scars may sink inward and become attached to the wall of the labyrinth.   Occasionally, calcification of the membrana results, and rarely, ossification.

The Eustachian Tube.

Owing to the close relationship existing between the Eustachian tube, the nasopharynx, and the tympanic cavity, affections, especially the inflammatory ones, of these cavities are particularly liable to involve the tube by extension.   Primary involvement of the tube must be rare, if indeed it occurs. . The most important conditions met with are various alterations in the lumen, such as *kinking, stenosis,* and *dilatation.*

One of the common causes of obstruction is the nasopharyngeal or Luschka's tonsil.   The presence of this outgrowth in the young child may prevent the proper development of the tube, and in all individuals, owing to its close proximity to the nasopharyngeal orifice of the tube, may grow directly over it.   In many cases, from prolonged contact, or from the formation of inflammatory adhesions, union takes place, leading to traction upon the tubal lip and more or less kinking. In advanced cases, the obstruction may become even more extreme, inasmuch as the traction is greatly increased, owing to the fibroid involuton which the hypertrophied tonsil inevitably undergoes. Again, any obstruction in the nasal cavities which limits the supply of air to the nasopharynx, will tend to produce a partial vacuum in that cavity. Chronic congestion and more or less hyperplasia of the mucous membrane in the lower portion of the tube is thus induced and brings about stenosis.

Various inflammatory processes, both within and without the tube, or the presence of tumors, may lead to obstruction. Vegetations and polypi in the middle ear may press upon and occlude the upper end of the tube.

Where stoppage is complete, the air in the middle ear is gradually absorbed, the tympanic membrane is sucked in and thus rendered more tense, so that deafness results. In other cases, the tube is so large that its lumen is constantly patent, with the result that passage of air into the middle ear produces autophony, and sudden concussions of the air may lead to deafness and even rupture of the membrana tympani. Atrophy of the mucous membrane is a chief cause of this state of affairs.

Inflammation.—Catarrhal and purulent inflammation of the tube are not uncommon as a result of nasopharyngeal catarrh and otitis media and as complications of certain infectious fevers, prominent among which are scarlatina, measles, diphtheria, influenza, and typhoid. The lining membrane of the tube becomes hyperemic and swollen, so that the lumen is more or less completely obstructed and there may be abundant exudation.

Syphilis, variola, and **tuberculosis** may also produce lesions in the tube. Prolonged inflammation and congestion will, in time, lead to hyperplasia of the mucous membrane and the submucous connective tissue, and stenosis.

Foreign Bodies.—Foreign bodies in the tube may also cause obstruction. The condition is rare. A bougie may break off in the course of instrumentation. Pins, wire, and particles of food have also been known to enter the tube.

The Middle Ear.

The tympanic cavity is so closely connected by contiguity and the anastomosis of blood and lymph-vessels that it is particularly liable to be involved in any disease processes affecting the neighboring parts, such as the external auditory meatus, the nasopharynx, labyrinth, and cranial cavity.

CIRCULATORY DISTURBANCES.

Hyperemia.—Active **hyperemia** of the mucosa is met with in the early stage of inflammation.

Passive hyperemia may be found in general systemic congestion, such as may occur in the course of cardiac and pulmonary disease, or as a local effect of pressure, for example, in the case of tumors about the head and neck.

Hemorrhages.—Hemorrhages, either petechial in character or a free effusion of blood, may occur spontaneously, or as a result of concussion or fracture of the skull. They may also be caused by the severer forms of otitis media arising in the course of diphtheria, Bright's disease, or leukemia, and by embolism of the stylomastoid artery. Hemorrhages, so extreme that the blood escapes externally through the meatus or Eustachian tube, are met with in severe traumatism to the temporal bone, the spontaneous separation of polyps and in carious processes which cause erosion of important vessels, such as the carotid, the jugular vein, the transverse and superior petrosal sinuses.

INFLAMMATIONS.

Otitis Media.—Otitis media is of fairly frequent occurrence and arises from a great variety of causes. It may be divided into *simple catarrhal* (non-suppurative), *suppurative*, and *specific*, or, according to its course, into *acute* and *chronic*.

Among the primary causes may be mentioned, trauma, climatic changes, various forms of inflammation, and circulatory disturbances. Perhaps in the majority of cases microörganisms are at work as well. The chief traumatic causes are direct or indirect injuries to the drumhead, as from careless instrumentation, forcible syringing, concussion and condensation of the air, local irritants, contusions, and fractures of the skull. Exposure to wet and cold, sea-bathing, the aspiration of water, medicinal solutions, or infected secretions through the Eustachian tube should also be mentioned. External otitis of all forms, impacted wax, and foreign bodies may cause an inflammation that may extend to the middle ear. Infective secretions from the accessory cavities of the nose and nasopharynx may reach the cavity through the Eustachian tube. The pus from a retropharyngeal abscess has been known to burrow its way along the sheath of the tensor tympani and infect the cavity. In children perhaps the most frequent predisposing cause is the presence of adenoids. Many cases also are dependent on infective fevers, such as scarlatina, measles, variola, influenza, whooping-cough, and cerebrospinal meningitis. Gout, syphilis, and tuberculosis are also of importance. Some cases, finally, appear to be due to obscure circulatory disturbances, probably reflex in nature. In the vast majority of instances bacteria are present from the beginning, or make their appearance sooner or later. No particular germ can be regarded as the specific cause of otitis media, but nearly all the known pathogenic bacteria are capable of exciting it. The infection may be mixed or, again, one form may die out and be replaced by another.

With regard to the frequency of the various forms of microörganisms Orne Green's analysis of 101 cases may be cited. He found:

Staphylococcus (albus, 8; aureus, 9; not specified, 19) . . .	36
Streptococcus	19
Pneumococcus	10
Bacillus pyocyaneus	3
A capsulated bacillus	3
Bacillus diphtheriæ	2
Mixed infection	28

In many cases the infective agents reach the middle ear through the Eustachian tube, being introduced into it by the acts of coughing, sneezing, or gagging. When the drum-head is perforated the organisms may enter from the external auditory meatus. In the case of the infectious fevers, even in diphtheritic and scarlatinal angina, the invasion is most probably through the blood stream.

Acute Catarrhal Otitis Media.—In acute catarrhal otitis media the mucous membrane is reddened and swollen, while the submucous connective tissue is infiltrated with inflammatory products. The cavity is more or less filled with a serous or more viscid mucinous secretion, containing desquamated epithelial cells with a few mucous cells and leukocytes. Examination of the drum-membrane in the early stages will show congestion and beginning infiltration at the periphery, especially the upper part and near the manubrium mallei. Later on, small blebs containing serum or blood may be seen in the epidermis near Shrapnell's membrane. In other cases the drum-membrane, particularly the posterior portion, may bulge considerably, and even perforation may occur.

Chronic Catarrhal Otitis Media.—In the chronic form, the mucous membrane is thickened, firmer, of a grayish-white color, and presents here and there nodular and villous granulations. The thickening may affect the mucous membrane as a whole, or may be confined to certain localities, as the drum-membrane, the ossicles, the orifice of the Eustachian tube, or the labyrinth fenestrum.

Chronic catarrhal otitis media frequently supervenes upon an acute process, or may be chronic from the start. Most of the causes producing the acute form are competent to produce the chronic. Some cases of the chronic disease, however, originate independently in those of a gouty or rheumatic tendency or who have syphilis. The constant jarring from loud noises may also produce it. In such cases the lesion usually begins in the neighborhood of the tubal orifice. In other instances the affection begins about the base plate of the stapes and apparently depends on vasomotor conditions. In some it is said to be hereditary. Debilitating diseases play a part.

Acute Suppurative Otitis Media.—Acute suppurative otitis media occurs chiefly in the course of the acute infective fevers, as scarlatina, measles, variola, diphtheria and typhoid. It is not always easy to draw a hard and fast line between the catarrhal and the suppurative forms. Undoubtedly many cases of the latter originate in simple catarrhal inflammation.

The mucosa is greatly swollen and congested, while the cavity is filled with a purulent or mucopurulent exudation, sometimes mixed with blood. The drum-membrane becomes infiltrated, softened, and eroded, so that perforation is common. It is not usual for marked ulceration of the mucous membrane to occur except in disease of the most violent septic nature, but in such cases the ossicles and wall of the tympanic cavity may become necrosed and the infection extend to the cranial cavity, where it may lead to extradural abscess, meningitis, and thrombosinusitis. This is particularly liable to ocur in children in whom the petrososquamosal suture not infrequently remains patent for a long time, thus exposing the dura, which, furthermore, may dip down after the fashion of a hernia through the fissure. The inflammatory exudate tends to gravitate to the bottom of the tympanum, although cases are met with where, owing to œdema of the mucosa, the fluid remains pent up in the attic. Hence, it may dissect its way along the upper wall of the meatus and make its appearance externally behind the ear. In such cases the mastoid cells are almost invariably involved as well.

Chronic Suppurative Otitis Media.—Chronic suppurative otitis media is invariably the result of a previous attack or repeated attacks of the acute form. Here, the thickness of the lining membrane is greatly increased, owing to round-celled infiltration, congestion of the vessels, with hyperplasia of the tissue, chiefly of the subepithelial layer, and new-formation of bloodvessels. The secretion varies in amount and is usually foul-smelling, mixed with blood, and of a dirty brown color. When the secretion is retained, as it usually is, for this is one of the most frequent causes of an acute becoming a chronic process, it becomes inspissated, and, being admixed with cast-off epithelium, forms a tough, cheesy mass, possessing a peculiar laminated structure, known as cholesteatoma. The drumhead is perforated, more or less destroyed and deformed, and what remains of it may be greatly thickened and studded with granulations. In certain cases the epidermal layer of the drum-membrane penetrates through the perforation and tends to involve the cavity. Where the ciliated epithelium has been exfoliated, the exposed surface of the membrane is dark red and actively secretes pus, while here and there it is dotted with fungoid or villous-like granulations. These may proliferate to such an extent that opposite masses of granulations may fuse and give rise to cystic cavities or loculi lined with epithelium.

Sooner or later, the destructive inflammation, which has led to erosion and even ulceration of the mucosa, extends to the bony parts, which become carious and necrosed. The incus is usually first attacked, as it is somewhat imperfectly supplied with blood. Next, the malleus is involved, and later that portion of the tympanic ring on which the head of the malleus abuts, as well as the inner end of the Eustachian tube. When the wall of the tympanic cavity is affected the course is usually most marked at the tegmen. The wall of the labyrinth may be invaded so that the Fallopian canal and the cavity of the labyrinth are opened up, leading to paralysis of the facial nerve and sometimes infection of the cranial cavity. The lower part of the tympanic cavity and the anterior wall of the labyrinth are not so often involved.

In very severe forms of inflammation, such as those which in children complicate the infective fevers, extensive necrosis and sequestration of the bone may take place. The ossicles may, owing to necrosis and loosening of their attachments, be cast off and appear in the discharge from the meatus. The foot-plate of the stapes usually, however, resists the process. From the adjoining necrosing inflammation, together with the presence of retained secretions, the cavity of the middle ear becomes considerably enlarged. In course of time, owing to the stimulus of the inflammatory process on the periosteum and the bone-marrow, hyperostoses and exostoses are formed, usually on the promontory, the fenestrum rotundum, or the eminentia pyramidalis. Much more rarely, they form upon the ossicles and orifice of the Eustachian tube. In this way the cavity may in the end become notably diminished in size. In some cases the ossicles and other bony plates become sclerosed rather than necrosed. Invasion of the mastoid antrum is not infrequent in cases of chronic suppurative otitis media, and is always of serious import, as it may lead to extensive necrosis of the bone and infection of the cranial cavity, or to septic thrombosis of the lateral sinus. If unrelieved, or if operative measures be undertaken too late, the jugular vein may become thrombosed for a considerable distance and the patient die from general sepsis.

Besides the simple and suppurative forms of chronic otitis just described there are others of great practical importance, the etiology of which is not quite clear. These are the *adhesive* and *sclerosing* forms.

Chronic Adhesive Otitis Media.—In chronic adhesive otitis media there is a slowly progressive inflammation which leads to thickening and proliferation of the mucous membrane lining the tympanic cavity, and the formation of bands, membranes, and other adhesions binding the drum, the ossicles, and the tensor tendon together, or to the tympanic wall, or, again, traversing the cavity. The adhesions are composed of loose, avascular connective tissue, covered with epithelium.

Chronic Sclerosing Otitis Media.—Chronic sclerosing otitis media is perhaps of greater importance. In some instances there is a transformation of the infiltrated and hyperemic mucosa into dense, scar-like tissue. In other cases it is the deeper or periosteal portion of the mucosa that is sclerosed. In still others there may be a granular deposit of lime salts in the submucous tissue or in the drum-membrane. These changes may affect the whole lining membrane of the cavity, or certain structures may be more particularly affected, such as the drum-membrane, the ossicles, the promontory, and the window of the labyrinth. Naturally, when these lesions become pronounced, ankylosis, more or less complete, takes place between the ossicles. Most frequently the attachment of the stapes to the fenestrum ovale is involved, or, more rarely, the articulation between the malleus and incus. Ankylosis of the stapes, which in some cases is congenital, is due either to calcification of the annular ligament attaching it to the fenestrum ovale, or to cartilaginous or bony outgrowths. The ankylosis leads to pressure upon the endolymph of the labyrinth and serious interference with the circulation.

Diphtheritic Otitis Media.—Diphtheritic otitis media is usual secondary to diphtheria of the nasopharynx. It probably arises l way of the Eustachian tube, owing to the aspiration of infective materi.

Tuberculosis.—Tuberculosis of the middle ear is now a well-reco nized affection. It is probably never primary, but usually occurs la in the course of tuberculosis in some other part of the body. It is thoug by some that infection takes place through the Eustachian tube, althou it is not improbable that some cases are hematogenous. It is characte istic of the affection that it is insidious in its onset and of slow progressio so that the disease may exist for some time before symptoms arise draw attention to it. The first.sign is a discharge from the meatu and in a short space of time the membrane is completely destroye Then the cavity of the tympanum is found to be lined with an exuberai granulation tissue, secreting acrid pus, a condition which may persi for months. In other cases, when the patient lives long enough, or tl disease is more severe, the ossicles are loosened from their attachmen and cast off in the discharge, while large portions of the bony w. become carious, or even large sequestra may be formed. The micr scopic appearances of the diseased parts do not differ materially fro those in other forms of destructive inflammation, save that in the deep layers of the mucous membrane, giant cells and patches of caseati with bacilli can be seen. It is, however, a curious circumstance th tubercle bacilli frequently cannot be discovered in the discharge. Ho ever, the fact that there are advanced tuberculous lesions in other par of the body, the insidious nature of the otitis, and the rapid destructio of the tissues, is practically conclusive of the nature of the disease. I the severe forms where there is much destruction of bone, meningiti may develop, or, rarely, a local brain-abscess.

Syphilis.—Syphilis gives rise to forms of acute and chronic otit closely resembling those arising from non-specific causes. Neuralgi of the tympanic cavity is also, rarely, observed. Most authorities appea to be agreed that in syphilis there is a special tendency to implicatio of the auditory nerve.

PROGRESSIVE METAMORPHOSES.

Tumors.—Hyperplastic outgrowths and tumors are found mor frequently in the middle ear than in other parts of the auditor apparatus. They may arise from any part of the tympanic cavit' but generally spring from the wall of the labyrinth, the attic, or, occasior ally, from the membrana. The majority of these form polypoid masse either pedunculated or sessile, of a globular or nodular shape, and havin a smooth or papillary surface. They may attain such a size as to con pletely fill the tympanic cavity and even appear externally. They ai of importance, since they tend to perpetuate any suppurative proce that may be going on and to retain the secretion. Occasionally, a growt of this kind may be separated from its base and give rise to serious an even fatal hemorrhage.

These polyps are composed of a central core of varying nature, covered by ciliated epithelium, stratified columnar or squamous cells. Many of them are of the nature of inflammatory hyperplastic new-formations, while others are more truly tumors. Among the various forms may be mentioned **fibromas, angiofibromas, mucous** and **adenomatous polyps, angiomas,** and **myxomas,** which are rare.

Mucous polyps are soft, vascular growths, usually lobulated, resembling the mucous membrane in structure, but more cellular and containing gland-tubules.

Angiomas form red, slightly vascular growths, which may pulsate in accord with the radial pulse.

Myxomas are supposed to be derived from the remains of the mucoid substance which normally fills the cavity of the ear in the fœtal state.

Cholesteatoma has already been referred to (p. 693).

Sarcoma, osteosarcoma, and **carcinoma** have been described, but are rare. Most frequently they are secondary to malignant disease elsewhere. Malignant growths from the brain or dura may invade the ear. They may, however, be primary, and when this is the case, they can be traced to a chronic or neglected suppurative process in the tympanic cavity, or to necroses in the temporal bone. Large portions of the temporal bone may be destroyed. Meningeal and brain symptoms may result, or hemorrhage. In advanced cases there may be paralysis of the facial, abducens, and the first division of the fifth nerve.

The Internal Ear.

CIRCULATORY DISTURBANCES.

Anemia.—Anemia of the inner ear may be present in cases of general anemia, and in all conditions which lead to an imperfect supply of blood to the parts, such as endarteritis or embolism of the arteria auditiva interna, tumors pressing on it, or aneurisms of the basilar artery.

Hyperemia.—**Active hyperemia** is found in cases of early inflammation of the parts and inflammation of the associated cavities.

Passive hyperemia arises from generalized blood stasis in the head, as from heart and lung diseases, or struma. Local causes, such as tumor of the base of the brain or skull and sinus thrombosis, may also lead to the condition, owing to interference with the free outflow of blood.

Hemorrhages.—Hemorrhages, either punctiform or extensive, readily follow upon hyperemia and inflammation. Large doses of quinine and salicylic acid lead to hyperemia and hemorrhages in experimental animals (Grunert; Kirchner[1]).

These minute hemorrhages may be confined to certain parts of the cochlea or vestibule, or may be more extensive. They are seen particularly in severe otitis media and many of the infective fevers, such as typhoid,

---

[1] Berlin. klin. Woch., 1881: 49; 725; u. Monatssch. f. Ohrenheilk., 1883: 5.

variola, septicemia, acute tuberculosis, and mumps. They may also be caused by intracranial affections, such as meningitis and hemorrhagic pachymeningitis, and occur in severe blood dyscrasias, like pernicious anemia and leukemia. The more copious extravasations are due to trauma, as, for example, concussion and fractures of the skull. Such may become completely absorbed in time, or become organized or infiltrated with lime salts. The resulting structure is usually colored by altered blood pigments. Even moderate hemorrhages may lead to deafness, notwithstanding that in time they become more or less absorbed. This is due to the fact that inflammation frequently supervenes, leading to atrophy and degeneration of the connective tissue and nerve filaments. If infection occur, suppurative inflammation may set in and be communicated to the cranial cavity.

Inflammation.—Inflammation of the labyrinth is rarely primary, being much more commonly derived by extension from the middle ear or the cranial cavity. From the middle ear the infective agents invade the parts by means of the bloodvessels in the wall of the labyrinth, through fistulous openings, or through the fenestrum. In the earlier stages we see congestion and œdema of the labyrinth with round-celled infiltration. Later on, in the more severe infections, the cavity is filled with pus and the membranous structures are destroyed. In time the pus may become inspissated and the process be limited through the formation of adhesions in the porus acousticus internus; or the pus may burrow its way along the sheath of the acoustic nerve to the brain cavity.

In cases originating in the cranial cavity the inflammatory process extends along the sheath of the auditory nerve, or through the aqueduct of the cochlea, or both. Epidemic cerebrospinal meningitis plays an important role in this form.

Here, in the earlier stages there is hyperemia and hemorrhage into the labyrinth with more or less necrosis of the membranous structures. Later on, the softer parts are completely destroyed; the periosteum is stripped from the underlying bone, and the cavity is filled with pus and granulation tissue. Should the patient survive, this, in time, becomes organized into connective tissue or even, in parts, into bone. The intensity of the inflammatory process is most marked in the vestibule and semicircular canals and becomes less extreme toward the cochlea. As a result of the process we get in addition, atrophy and degeneration of the membranous structures and of the nerve-fibres, cells, and ganglia, while the cavity is filled with altered pus, detritus, cholesterin, and pigment. Thus, the whole auditory apparatus may become disorganized.

The productive or hyperplastic type of labyrinthitis is frequently associated with syphilis.

In **Ménière's disease,** an affection in which there is deafness, and severe vertigo, there is a hemorrhagic exudation into the semicircular canals and vestibule, but it is not quite clear whether here we have to do with simple blood extravasation or with inflammation.

Deaf-mutism is, by some, attributed to an internal otitis in early life, originating in meningitis which has extended along the aqueduct. Others, again, associate it with defects of the auricle, atresia of the meatus, immobility of the tympanic fenestra, and acquired lesions of the acoustic nerve.

The Acoustic Nerve.

Atrophy.—Atrophy of the nerve is frequently the result of pressure exerted upon it, as by internal hydrocephalus, tumors of the brain or base of the skull, fractures of the petrous bone, or hyperostosis about the porus acusticus internus. It may also be caused by hemorrhage and inflammation (neuritis). Cerebral causes, such as apoplexy and encephalitis, involving the nucleus of the nerve, may also be at work. According to Erb, atrophy occurs also in tabes dorsalis. Atrophy from inhibition of function (atrophy of inactivity) seems to be rather rare.

Tumors.—Primary tumors of the acoustic nerve are excessively rare, and our knowledge of them is strictly limited. According to Virchow, however, this nerve is more frequently the site of tumor growth than any other cranial nerve.

Fibroma, myxoma, psammoma, and **sarcoma** have been recorded.

As a rule, the malignant growths originate in some of the neighboring parts, usually the brain or dura. Politzer reports a case of **secondary carcinoma** originating in the mastoid region. Burkhardt-Merian[1] reports a **fibrosarcoma** originating in the inferior petrosal sinus, and Moos,[2] a **spindle-celled sarcoma** connected with the cerebellum which had invaded the acoustic nerve.

[1] Arch. f. Ohrenheilk., 12.   [2] Ibid., 4.

SECTION V.

THE DUCTLESS GLANDS.

CHAPTER XXXI.

THE FUNCTIONS OF THE DUCTLESS GLANDS AND THEIR DISTURBANCES.

In our first volume we have discussed, to some extent, the subject of the internal secretions, and the influence exerted by increase or diminution of the same upon the organism. It is not necessary, therefore, to bring forward at this point the evidence that has been accumulated demonstrating the existence of internal secretions. Such secretions, it may be recalled, are afforded both by typical glandular organs provided with ducts, such as the liver and pancreas (although in connection with the latter, there are those who hold that the specific internal secretion is derived from cell-masses unprovided with ducts—the islands of Langerhans), and again by atypical and ductless glandular organs—by organs which, having no ducts, must, if they be functionally active, abstract certain substances from the circulating blood and lymph, and, as the result of their metabolism, must discharge the products of their activity into the same. The organs usually classified under the heading of ductless glands may, from histological considerations, be classed under three headings: (1) those possessing alveoli or cell-masses of the accepted glandular type, namely, collections of cells of fair size and relatively abundant cytoplasm, of a cubical or polyhedral form, recalling those of the salivary glands, liver, etc.; (2) those possessing chromaffin cells and other elements which we now regard as derived from the nervous system; and (3) those composed in the main of lymphoid elements.

Such a classification is unsatisfactory because not a few of these ductless glands contain elements of more than one of these categories. The cortex of the adrenal belongs to the first type, the medulla to the second; the pituitary body likewise contains elements belonging to both of the two first categories; the thymus, while mainly formed of the third, contains in its Hassall's corpuscles, elements, rudimentary, it is true, of epithelial origin. It is, however, difficult to suggest any other classification, or perhaps it is more accurate to say that we here group together organs so widely different histologically that they defy classification, save as a group possessing the one common feature of being ductless At most, Gaskell, in his remarkable and strikingly suggestive work on the *Origin of the Vertebrates*,[1] traces the whole group of these ductless glands—pituitary, tonsils, thyroid, thymus, lymphatic glands, and adrenals —to a common origin, as one and all modified representatives of what were primarily duct-bearing, "coxal" glands, or excretory organs, situated at the bases of the segmental appendages of the protostracan forms, which, he holds, gave origin to the vertebrates as well as to the crustaceans and arachnids. While we gladly accept the results of his long-continued studies, as throwing light upon the peculiar structure and components of the pituitary body, adrenals, and thyroid, we confess to a difficulty in regarding the thymus and lymph-glands in general as metamorphosed "lepidic" structures, and that because lymphoid tissue is so widely and irregularly distributed throughout the organism that it seems impossible to regard it as the representative of an original chain of small, paired organs situated in each segment of the body. In fact, the tendency nowadays is to deny to the spleen and lymph-follicles the right to be termed glands. Their cells are neither of the accepted "glandular" form, nor do they show any trace of the characteristic glandular arrangement into clusters of the lepidic type. Conformably with this tendency, we have treated them apart and in connection with the vascular system. Yet another organ, this time of the true ductless gland type, namely, the corpus luteum, we discuss elsewhere; it is both more reasonable and more natural to deal with this in connection with the genital system.

Let us, then, as briefly as possible, sum up what we know regarding the structure and functions of the remaining "ductless glands," and of the effects upon the organism of disturbances of these functions.

THE THYROID AND PARATHYROIDS.

Anatomy.—The thyroid gland is composed of two lateral lobes, situated one on each side of the larynx, and connected by an isthmus. The average weight in the adult varies between twenty-five and sixty grams.

The organ is enveloped in a fibrous capsule sending prolongations inward to form the stroma, which contains numerous bloodvessels, lymphatics, and nerves. The vascular anastomoses are very abundant and the larger lymphatics have valves like the veins. Embedded in this stroma are numerous acini that vary somewhat in appearance. According to Wölfler, a cortical and a medullary zone are to be differentiated. The former contains solid bands and groups of cells; the latter is made up of closed vesicles lined by a single layer of cubical or cylindrical cells, and filled with a homogeneous gluey substance or colloid. The cells may contain minute drops of colloid or larger masses that force the nucleus to one side.

[1] London, Longmans, Green & Co., 1908: 418.

Between the follicles containing the colloid material may be observed groups and rows of epithelial cells that are considered by Wolfler[1] to be embryonic "cell-rests" which have not developed into the normal acini. They are especially common in the newborn. Embryonic cells may also be present in the capsule.

Embryology.—Embryologically, the thyroid is developed from three germinal centres, two lateral and one median. The median portion takes its origin in a diverticulum from the floor of the pharynx between the bases of the first and second branchial clefts. The lateral portions develop as evaginations from the posterior aspect of the fourth branchial arches. The fusion of the three parts usually occurs at about the seventh week. Originally, the organ resulting from this fusion connects with the pharynx by a duct called the thyroglossal duct. As a rule, this disappears after the eighth week, but it may persist either in the form of a fibrous cord or as one or more collections of cells, which, secreting fluid, are apt, eventually, to give rise to cysts either within the substance of the tongue or in the median line between tongue and upper end of the thyroid.[2]. Usually all that remains of the duct is a small depression on the surface of the tongue, known as the foramen cæcum. Not infrequently, however, judging from our postmortem experience, there is a pyramidal prolongation upward of the thyroid tissue of the middle, or more often of the left lobe, continued into a fibrous band which extends up to the middle of the hyoid bone, in the position, that is, of the thyroid duct.

Function.—The vesicles are lined by an epithelium of cubical glandular type, and are surrounded by an abundant network both of blood capillaries and lymph-vessels. The cells discharge their secretion into the lumina, and this tends there to become inspissated (colloid). But apparently there is also external discharge, for although its significance here is disputed, colloid matter has been detected in the surrounding capillaries and lymphatics. There is evidence that this colloid material contains the specific secretion of the gland. From the organ, Baumann and others have isolated a globulin having iodine in direct combination (iodothyrin). This body is by most held to be the active principle of the gland. It is, however, to be noted that the amount of iodine present in the organ shows wide variations and that the activity of the gland extract has not been clearly proved to be related to the amount of iodine present, although this view has been strongly supported by Oswald and Reid Hunt.[3] It is quite likely that this is not the only active principle; in treatment iodothyrin has been found less effective than the dried gland. The simplest hypothesis to account for this peculiar histological arrangement is that the thyroid cells are capable of a reversible action, and so normally regulate the amount of active principle present in the circulation; that when the active principle of the gland or its precursors are present

---

[1] Arch. f. klin. Chir., 29: 1885.

[2] See Erdheim, Ueber Cysten u. Fisteln des Ductus thyreoglossus, Arch. f. klin. Chir., 85:1908:212.

[3] Bulletin 47, Hygienic Laboratory, Washington, 1908.

in the blood in excess, these are taken up by the thyroid cells and stor
in the vesicles in a converted, less soluble state; when, on the contrai
these have become used up in the blood, and there is defect, now t
cells absorb the active principle from the vesicles, and discharge it in
the blood. On the one hand, we may find the contents of the vesicl
small in amount and distinctly fluid, with extensive congestion of t
organ, suggesting that the specific secretion is being discharged into t
blood rather than into the vesicles—as in ordinary exophthalmic goiti
or the regenerative hyperplasia that follows removal of part of the glan
on the other, as in colloid goitre, the vesicles may be found huge
distended, with dense, solid colloid, suggesting that the cells are d
charging into the vesicles with little reverse passage into the blood. It
interesting to note that in advanced stages of this condition we a
apt to get symptoms of myxœdema—of absence of thyroid secreti
(? through compression atrophy of the vascular epithelium); and contra
wise, when by operative handling of such an enlarged thyroid, a co
gestion of the gland is induced, symptoms of exophthalmic goitre a
apt to show themselves. It is eminently probable that, as indicated 1
Lucke, the activity of the secretion is controlled by the nervous syste1

Effects of Ablation and of Atrophy.—These are well known and ha
already been discussed. In the former case a condition of *cachex
strumipriva* may supervene (Reverdin, Kocher) identical in charact
with the *myxœdema* which Ord had noted as associated with atropl
of the gland and with Gull's *cretinoid cachexia*, Gull noting the rese1
blance between the symptoms of the atrophy of the thyroid in adult li
and those of *cretinism* in the young, associated with congenital lack
function of the gland. We shall revert to the effects of ablation wh
discussing the function of the parathyroids.

Thyroid Incompetence.—*Congenital atrophy* of the gland, or oth
disease associated with arrest of function, shows itself, as in creti1
more especially by delayed growth of the bones and tissues in gener
by non-development of the genitalia at puberty, sterility in adult life, a
by arrested mental development. Occurring in later life the inco1
petence is accompanied by depressed metabolism, heat production, a
gaseous interchange, slowed mentality, and listlessness. The hair ten
to drop out, the skin is thickened as though infiltrated by a firm œdem

Effects of Administration of Thyroid Extract.—Metabolism is marke
accelerated by giving raw thyroid of the domestic animals by the mou
or administering extract of the gland. The heart rate is increased, the
is a tendency to nervous excitement with muscular tremors. The f
of the organism become used up, and eventually there is evidence
increased breaking down of the proteins.[1] This is in striking contr
to the lowered metabolism and nervous depression of the myxœdemato
state. That this lowered metabolism is due to the lack of thyroid d
charge is demonstrated by the disappearance of the myxœdematous a
cretinoid conditions when thyroid extract is administered.

---

[1] Schorndorff, Pflüger's Arch., 67: 1897: 395.

The Parathyroids (Sandström[1]); (**Epithelkörperchen** of Kohn[2]).—The question of greatest present interest in this connection is the relationship of the parathyroids to the thyroid and to morbid states of the organism. And here there is wide diversity of opinion. There is, on the one hand, evidence that in a certain number of cases, both in man and in the animals of the laboratory, if the thyroid be removed and the parathyroids be left, few ill results ensue, whereas if both thyroid and parathyroids be removed, symptoms of **tetany** are liable to supervene, either rapidly or within a few days, with fatal result. This tetany may be induced if the parathyroids alone be removed. There is, thus, a tendency to regard the parathyroids as all important, the thyroid as of subsidiary importance, or, more exactly, to regard absence of the thyroid as leading to the relatively non-fatal myxœdema, removal of the parathyroids as inducing a rapidly fatal tetany. But, on the other hand, it is to be noted that not all of Reverdin and Kocher's cases, in which they extirpated the whole of the thyroids and the attached parathyroids, were followed by tetany and death within a short period. Our colleague, Dr. Shepherd, who has a large experience in the operative treatment of various forms of goitre, assures us that he has repeatedly removed the whole organ without leaving the parathyroids, and never once has he seen tetany supervene. It has been urged that in such cases accessory detached parathyroids have been present and have been left behind. Now, it is true, as we have observed from the studies of Dr. Freedman in our laboratory at the Royal Victoria Hospital, that there is a very wide variation both in the number of parathyroids in normal relationship to the larger gland, and in these accessory parathyroids. Swale Vincent,[3] who records a remarkable lack of after effects from removal of the thyroids and parathyroids in monkeys (contrary to Horsley, Murray and Edmunds, he never obtained myxœdema in these animals), states, however, that he made a most careful search for accessory parathyroids in his animals, and never encountered them. We have, in short, with the parathyroids, much the same problem that confronts us in connection with the Islands of Langerhans in the pancreas. Both have an embryonic, imperfectly developed, or latent appearance. With both there is evidence pointing to the assumption under certain conditions of an adult—developed state. The human parathyroids frequently, in place of the groups of cells (resembling those scattered through the adult thyroid between the vesicles) that are the common features of the bodies, exhibit well-formed vesicles filled with colloid; and in animals from which the thyroid has been removed, the parathyroids assume thyroid characteristics. This, however, is denied by the upholders

---

[1] Upsala Lakerforeningens Forhandlingar, 1880.

[2] Arch. f. mikrosk. Anat., 44:1895:366. For a full description of the site and histology of the parathyroids in man, see Welsh, D. A., Jour. of Anat. and Physiol., 32:1898.

[3] Vincent and Jolly, Journ. of Physiol., 34·1906:295, and Science Progress, 3:1909: January.

of the specificity of function of these bodies, who also regard the colloid vesicles encountered in certain apparently normal parathyroids as distinguished from those of the thyroid proper. Save for the small size of the former, we personally have been unable to recognize any histological difference between the two.[1]

Without denying specific function to the parathyroids, we are inclined to demand clearer and more certain evidence before accepting that they are absolutely distinctive organs. Amid the many contradictory observations, we are, however, impressed by the fact that these bodies arise from an *anlage* (the epithelium of the third and fourth branchial clefts) closely allied to, but nevertheless distinct from the lateral thyroid *anlagen*, as, again, that the symptoms of tetany, as shown by MacCallum, can be ameliorated by injecting emulsions of the parathyroids.

The most recent work, it may be remarked, strongly points to the importance of the parathyroids in regulating calcium metabolism;[2] upon their removal a rapid excretion, possibly associated with inadequate assimilation, deprives the tissues of calcium salts. The administration of soluble calcium salts to parathyroidectomized animals causes the disappearance of the symptoms of tetany.

THE ADRENALS.

Anatomical Features.—The adrenals, or suprarenals, are a pair of organs situated at the upper end of the kidneys, with which they lie in close apposition.

In shape the adrenal gland is generally compared to a cocked hat and consists of a cortex and medulla, enclosed in a fibrous capsule, which sends prolongations into the interior of the structure. The cortex is composed of three zones. The outer, or zona glomerulosa, consists of numerous spherical or oval masses of cells, of cylindrical or polyhedral shape, containing a spherical or oval nucleus. The middle zone, zona fasciculata, is composed of vertical columns of polygonal epithelial cells, having a spherical nucleus. The protoplasm is clear and pale, and the cell-bodies are usually loaded with fat. Between the columns are fibrous septa containing blood capillaries. The innermost layer, the zona reticularis, is formed of irregular masses of polyhedral cells, the various clusters of which anastomose one with the other. The cells are somewhat larger than those of the zona fasciculata, and are often distinctly pigmented. The medulla consists in cylindrical clusters of transparent cells, which are polyhedral, columnar, or branching. The cell-groups here also anastomose with each other. The medulla is particularly rich in bloodvessels, non-medullated nerve-fibres, chromaffin cells, and ganglia. In the centre is a large vein, surrounded by a comparatively large amount of unstriped muscle.

---

[1] An admirable presentation of the case for the distinction between the two organs is given by Dock in Osler's Modern Medicine, 5: 1909: 382.

[2] MacCallum and Voegtlin, Johns Hopkins Hosp. Bull., 19:1908:91.

The great vascularity of the organs and the close relationship of the capillaries to the groups of cells serve to indicate an important relationship between the secreting cells and the blood-vascular system. Further, the muscle bundles surrounding the central vein suggest a mechanism for controlling the amount of blood in the organ.

Embryological Considerations.—The embryogeny of the adrenals is not a little remarkable; the cortex and the medulla have wholly different origins; and, in fact, in certain lower vertebrates (elasmobranch fishes) constitute distinct organs. This suggests diversity of functions, even if the eventual fusion suggests also that the two are intimately dependent the one on the other. The cortex in different animals is, in fact, derived from the mesonephric or pronephric excretory organs; the medulla has a separate origin from the sympathetic nervous system. While the cortex is formed of columns of cells of glandular type in intimate association with a system of capillaries—so intimate that in places, according to some authorities, the cells actually abut upon the blood stream with no intervening endothelium—the medulla is characterized by an absence of gland-cells proper and presence of certain remarkable *chromaffin* cells. Such chromaffin cells are widely distributed throughout the body. They owe their name to their affinity for neutral salts of chromic acid, assuming with these a strong yellow or brownish color. They are derived from the nervous system, and from one portion of this, the sympathetic system. They are to be found in the sympathetic ganglia, in the pituitary, the carotid glands, and the organ of Zuckerkandl, situated on either side of the origin of the inferior mesenteric artery, and, according to some authorities, in the coccygeal gland, but are present in greatest abundance in the adrenal medulla.[1]

Function.—The Medulla.—The observations of recent years have demonstrated that, judged from the effects of their extract, these cells, wherever present, have the same properties. That extract has a powerful action upon the arteries and arterioles, leading to contraction of the same, and temporary pronounced rise of the blood pressure. These properties, as first noted by Oliver and Schäfer, are particularly marked in connection with extracts of the adrenal medulla. The active principle having these effects has been isolated in a crystalline form by Takamine and Aldrich independently, and by Abel. It is generally known as adrenalin, the name given to it by Takamine, but as his substance has become proprietary, Schäfer proposes *adrenin* as a more ethical name. It has an action upon skeletal and cardiac muscle as well as upon the plain muscles of arteries. Langley[2] has enunciated the view that in all cells a chief substance is present, to which is owing the chief function of the cell, and a more unstable intermediate or receptive body, which sets the chief substance in action when itself acted upon by nervous and

[1] For a study of the "Chromaffin System," see Gierke, Lubarsch-Ostertag's Ergeb. der allg. Pathol., Jahrg. 10: 1904 to 1905: 502; Wiesel, Internat. Clinics, 2: 1905: 288; and Kohn, Anat. Anz., 15: 1890: No. 21, and Arch. f. Mikr., 56: 1900: 81.

[2] Jour. of Physiol., 33: 1905 to 1906: 374.

other stimuli. The action of adrenin appears to be identical with that of the sympathetic nerves, and Langley suggests that adrenin, taken up by the cells, has the same effect on the receptive substance as have stimuli reaching it through the sympathetic nerve endings. Stoltz and others have prepared a synthetic adrenin having the same composition and effects as adrenin, but optically inactive, instead of being levorotatory, and, according to Cushing, not so powerful as the natural substance. Adrenin is soluble in water, and dialyzable, unaffected by boiling, but insoluble in alcohol, and non-acted upon by the gastric juice and by acids.

The Cortex.—As noted in our first volume little positive has been determined regarding the functions of the cortex.[1] There is a steadily accumulating body of evidence of an intimate association between it and the genital system, conditions of premature sexual maturity having frequently been found associated with the presence of cortical tumors. The abundance of lecithin and bodies of the nature of myelins is suggestive in connection with recent studies upon the importance of these bodies in relationship to the blood serum and the production of immunity.

The Relationship between Adrenal Function and Disease.— **Adrenal Incompetency.**—To repeat what was stated in our first volume, extensive disease of the adrenals (usually caseous tuberculosis), or atrophy of the same, is accompanied by the symptoms of **Addison's disease**—great muscular weakness, with low blood-pressure and soft pulse, anorexia, with gastric discomfort, and occasional vomiting, cerebral disturbances of a mild type, and cutaneous pigmentation. The vascular symptoms and lack of muscular tone are the very opposite of the result of injections of adrenin, and thus the generally accepted view is that normally the adrenal medulla affords the active principle to the blood whereby the vascular and muscular tone of the body is maintained. The French school, under Abelous and Langlois, uphold rather a theory of auto-intoxication, finding the blood of animals deprived of their capsules to possess curare-like properties, they regard the gland as removing or neutralizing this substance. These two theories are not, it may be noted, absolutely opposed; it is quite possible that adrenin may both neutralize the paretic action of such a substance, and itself act directly upon the muscle.

What has until now been a difficulty in understanding the relationship between the adrenals and Addison's disease, is the existence of a certain small number of cases in which either one or both adrenals and their medullas are apparently unaffected; and of another series of cases in which there might be complete replacement of the adrenals by newgrowth with no signs of Addison's disease. Many years ago it was suggested by Rolleston and others that in these cases not the glands, but

---

[1] See also Rolleston, Montreal Med. Jour., 36:1907:671; or Lancet, London, 2:1907:875; and Bulloch and Sequeira, Trans. Path. Soc. Lond., 56:1905:189. For the fullest collection of data bearing upon adrenal function, see Sajous, The Internal Secretions, 1:1902, and 2:1907.

the nearby semilunar ganglia and solar plexus, were involved. Very numerous nerves pass from these to the adrenals—and, indeed, besides chromaffin cells, the medulla contains ordinary sympathetic nerve cells. Thus some have held that nervous disturbances might lead to arrest of adrenal function. The recent studies upon the chromaffin cells have afforded a possible explanation. Here, Wiesel's observations are of distinct importance.[1] In seven cases of the disease he has examined, not merely the adrenals, but the whole chromaffin system—adrenals, the chains of sympathetic ganglia and plexuses, Zuckerkandl's organ, etc.—he has found a general absence of chromaffin cells, although now, as a compensatory process, the sympathetic ganglion cells may give the chromaffin reaction. If, as in the cases of cancer above mentioned, the adrenals alone are destroyed, the chromaffin cells elsewhere may be adequate to prevent disease, or there may be extensive destruction of the chromaffin cells in other areas, leading to symptoms of the disease, without extensive adrenal disease. As a matter of fact, Beitzke has reported a case of cancer involving the adrenals, without Addison's disease, in which he found the chromaffin cells intact elsewhere. Further confirmation is needed of these most suggestive observations.

But neither Wiesel's nor other studies upon ablation of the medulla have thrown light upon the specific pigmentation seen in Addison's disease. In the first volume (p. 971) one of us brought together the evidence that cell-pigment of the nature of melanin is a product of the disintegration of proteins, and is an oxidation product of bodies, like tyrosin, of the aromatic series, and Halle's observation that in the adrenal tyrosin is converted into adrenin through the action of an enzyme. Now, as extracts of all the tissues containing chromaffin cells have like effects upon the vessels, we may assume that adrenin is present in all, and is similarly produced. Thus, if Halle be correct, the absence of chromaffin tissue must tend to be accompanied by an accumulation in the tissues of members of the aromatic series, which, undergoing oxidation, become pigmented bodies of the nature of melanin, instead of undergoing conversion into adrenin. Along these lines of chromaffin inadequacy, with heaping up of members of the aromatic series, the pigmentation gains a plausible explanation.

There is still confessedly much to be accomplished before we have a thorough understanding of the bearing of adrenal changes upon the whole series of symptoms of Addison's disease. Yet the last few years appear to have carried us forward; the theory of adrenal or, more accurately, of chromaffin cell inadequacy would seem to be establishing itself.

Excessive Adrenal Function.—We said, in connection with the thyroid, that excessive production and discharge of the thyroid secretion led to a very definite syndrome. Is a like condition of excessive production of the adrenal secretion to be determined? We observed there that feeding or injecting thyroid extract brought about a series of symptoms

---

[1] Zeit. f. Heilk., 24: 1903, Pathol. Anat. Abt. No. 4; and Internat. Clinics, 2: 1905: loc. cit.

(hyperthyroidism) resembling in many respects, though not in all, the symptoms of Graves' disease (vol. i, p. 355). Is there any morbid state resembling in its symptoms the results of administering adrenalin or adrenin to man or the lower animals? As we have stated, the most striking feature of such administration is rise of blood pressure. As a matter of fact, hyperpiesis, or pronounced and continued rise of blood pressure, with accompanying disturbed health, is not uncommon. Is there any change to be observed in the adrenals in this condition? It may be objected that the administration of adrenin leads but to a transient rise of blood pressure; but, on the other hand, we must take into account that a difference is to be expected between the effects of experimental inoculation from time to time, and the steady outpouring of the active principle from an overactive gland; further, if experimentally we give repeated doses, each is followed by its rise; there is no accustomance. Now Roger and Gouget have noted hypertrophy of the adrenals in a case of experimental arteriosclerosis induced by lead intoxication, while Vacquez and Aubertin, Aschoff and Pearce,[1] Josué and Bernard, and others have called attention to the association between adrenal hypertrophy and arteriosclerosis, with distinct increase in the size of the medulla. Dr. Klotz, in our laboratory, has called our attention to the same noticeable hypertrophy. Whether this is primary or secondary must, for the present, be left an open question, as also it is not determined whether both states are to be encountered; a series in which the hypertrophy and increased secretion is the primary disturbance, another, in which, either through the agency of the nervous system, or through the absorption of foods, etc., acting by their disintegration products, increased production of adrenin is brought about. The rarity of high blood pressure and of hypertrophy of the medulla in early life is somewhat against the former. It has still to be determined whether this enlargement of the glands is purely associated with the arteriosclerotic or with all types of chronic interstitial nephritis, as also how far it is related to arteriosclerotic states in general. Further it must be recalled that authorities are far from being agreed as to the association here noted. Thus Mott[2] gives it as his experience that in advanced arteriosclerosis the adrenal medulla is more often atrophied than hypertrophied. It will be recalled that adrenin in itself leads to arteriosclerotic manifestations, and also that not all cases of this condition are associated with high blood pressure. It will thus be seen that much has still to be garnered before sure conclusions can be laid down. We have thought it worth while to mention these matters as an indication that the study of possible conditions of excessive adrenal activity is not being wholly neglected.

[1] Jour. of Exp. Med., 10:1908:735 (with bibliography).
[2] Allbutt and Rolleston's System, 6:1909:605.

THE PITUITARY BODY, OR HYPOPHYSIS CEREBRI.

Anatomical Features.—The pituitary body is a peculiar structure about the size of a pea, situated at the base of the brain, to which it is attached by a slender stalk. It weighs from 3 to 6 decigrams and fits snugly into an excavation of the floor of the skull, the sella turcica. It consists of three parts,[1] anterior, intermediate, and posterior. The anterior glandular lobe makes up the greater portion of the organ, surrounding most of the posterior, although separated from it by a cleft and the pars intermedia. It is a solid structure composed of columns of cells separated by large and abundant capillaries or sinusoids and a small amount of connective tissue. According to Berkeley, it is innervated by filaments from the carotid sympathetic plexus. The glandular cells are of three orders: (1) Small and polygonal with large nucleus; (2) a larger cell with nucleus of the same order as that of the preceding, with more abundant clear cytoplasm (*chromophobe* cells) which may show diffuse fine granules; and (3) cells which are full of material which stains deeply with eosin and hematoxylin (*chromophile* cells). Benda and Herring regard them as different stages in the growth and activity of one and the same cell. This portion probably furnishes a secretion directly into the blood. The narrow intermediate part has the same epiblastic origin as has the anterior. It is composed of small, clear, glandular cells, tending toward an alveolar or columnar arrangement, between which here and there lumina appear filled with colloid matter. It contains but few vessels. The colloid, it would seem, passes toward and into the posterior nervous portion, indeed, in the cat has been found accumulated in the infundibular canal. The posterior lobe appears at first sight to be composed of connective tissue, but more careful study by special stains confirms the view of Virchow (1857) that it is made up of neuroglia and ependymal cells and fibres, invaded in places by islets of epithelial cells from the intermediate body, with small masses of colloid and finer globules apparently of the same nature.

Embryological Considerations.—The explanation of this complicated structure is that the origin is twofold. The anterior and intermediate portions originate as a diverticulum from the primitive oral cavity. Traces of the original communication are frequently to be detected. Lanzert states that he has recognized the *canalis craniopharyngeus* in 10 per cent. of children examined. The Luschka's tonsil marks the site of the oral termination of the primitive duct. Occasionally cysts are found at this region, due to closure of the *pouch of Rathke*, which actually represents this oral termination, or to persistence of part of the channel. The cleft between anterior and intermediate lobes is ordinarily the sole remnant of the oral passage. The posterior lobe is formed by an evagination of the floor of the primitive mid-brain (third ventricle),

---

[1] We here follow the very full study of the histology of the pituitary by Herring, Quart. Jour. of Exp. Physiol., 1:1908:121.

the proximal portion of which constitutes the infundibulum, the dista
undergoing closure and forming the stalk and posterior lobe of the
pituitary body. If Gaskell[1] be right—and it is difficult to controver
the extraordinary volume of evidence he has brought forward in favor o
his contention—that the neural canal represents the original alimentary
channel of the invertebrate ancestors of the vertebrata. Like the thy
roid, embryological studies (Bela Haller) show that the glandular portior
is originally of a tubular type; Gaskell holds that these tubules represen
the coxal glands situated at the bases of the appendages (endognaths)
originally present around the original mouth. In the process of reduc
tion, the nervous elements of the old œsophageal tube and the surround
ing ring of gland-substance become intimately intermixed. In the cat

FIG. 170

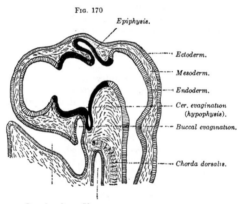

Epiphysis.

.... *Ectoderm.*

.... *Mesoderm.*

.... *Endoderm.*

.... *Cer. evagination*
     (hypophysis).

..... *Buccal evagination.*

.... *Chorda dorsalis.*

Buccal cavity.   Pharynx.

Origin of epiphysis (pineal gland) and hypophysis (pituitary gland). The blue part corresponds to the intermediate brain or thalamencephal. The red part is a portion of the bucca
ectoderm. The hypophysis is formed by the coalescence of two evaginations (after Mihalcovics
as modified by Charpy in Poirier's Traité d'anatomie Humaine).

the infundibular process within the posterior lobe retains its central
cavity and is lined by ependyma cells. The central canal has disappeared in other higher vertebrates.

Functions.—It is suggestive that like the adrenal the pituitary body
consists of a nervous and a glandular moiety. As with that organ,
physiological experiment has so far demonstrated no specific activity on
the part of the latter. But the former—the posterior lobe—affords
extracts having very definite properties (Howell), notably possessing a
direct action upon plain and cardiac muscle similar to that of adrenin,
but causing a more prolonged elevation of the blood pressure (Oliver
and 'Schäfer). There are indications, indeed, of the presence of more

[1] The Origin of Vertebrates, Longmans, Green & Co., London, 1908:321.

than one active principle. Thus, Schäfer and Herring[1] found that aqueous extracts had opposite effects upon the bloodvessels. In the first injections, the pressor or vasoconstrictor effects predominate; in subsequent injections, the depressor effects become manifest.[2] So, also, the same observers have discovered that from the posterior portion a substance can be obtained, soluble in water, and uninfluenced by boiling, having a specific effect upon the kidney, exercising, indeed, a diuretic effect more powerful than that of any known substance. As in the adrenal we observe some indications that the glandular cortex plays a part in the elaboration of the specific secretion, so here the colloid elaborated in the pars intermedia and discharged into the posterior lobe is regarded by many as having (like the colloid of the thyroid) active properties. Here it may be noted that Schnitzer and Ewald[3] and Wells find iodine in the pituitary, although in much smaller amounts than in the thyroid. Besides the depressor effects and the colloid, another suggestive relationship to the thyroid is seen in the compensatory hypertrophy of this organ noted by numerous observers[4] after thyroidectomy in the lower animals or atrophy of the thyroid in man; or to epitomize, the hypophysis cerebri possesses characters which in part associate it with the adrenals, in part with the thyroid. In acromegaly, to be immediately noted, changes have not infrequently been noted in the thyroid, while the disease may be complicated with symptoms of either exophthalmic goitre or myxœdema.

Relationship of Morbid Disturbance to Disease.—It is, however, difficult to associate these experimental results with the data of disease; in fact, we are but at the beginning of a knowledge of the function of the organ. One outstanding fact there is, that the remarkable conditions of **acromegaly** and **gigantism** are intimately associated with overgrowth, either simple or adenomatous, affecting more particularly the glandular portion of the organ.

Briefly, the morbid changes in the former of these rare diseases are that it shows itself in the second, or more often in the third, decade, less often in the fourth, as a progressive enlargement of the bony skeleton. All the bones are affected, but most strikingly those of the extremities and cranium, and more especially the lower jaw, which becomes enlarged in all directions, while the sella turcica, in which the enlarged pituitary is lodged, undergoes atrophy of its bony walls and great increase in its cavity. Along with this there is a thickening of the subcutaneous tissues, which, in a case of pituitary tumor described by one of us (J. G. A.), was the most marked feature, the condition approximating more to myxœdema than to acromegaly. The liver and spleen are often noticeably enlarged. The testes, ovaries, and uterus often exhibit atrophy or hypoplasia, although the external genitalia may be hypertrophied.

[1] Phil. Trans. Roy. Soc. Lond., 199:1906:29.

[2] The studies of Professor and Miss Meltzer point to the existence of similar depressor substances in thyroid extract.

[3] Wiener klin. Woch., 1896.

[4] Rogowicz, Boyce and Beadles, Hofmeister, Herring, and many others.

The pituitary in the majority of cases is greatly enlarged, either fro
a process of simple hypertrophy, or by neoplasia of the glandular portio
simple or malignant adenoma, or even, according to some authorities,
reversion to a sarcomatous type of growth. Benda, in four cases, recor
a marked increase in chromaffin cells. With these changes there m:
be nervous symptoms (blindness; paralysis of the oculomotor muscle
deafness, due, apparently, to pressure effects in the cranial cavity; ar
others that cannot so surely be ascribed to pressure, such as depressio
loss of memory, homicidal insanity, etc.). Glycosuria is not uncommo
(This has been observed in connection with other tumors of the base
the brain and cerebellum.) Polyuria, with or without glycosuria, m:
be a prominent symptom, a fact which is suggestive in connection wi
the existence above noted of an active principle promoting diuresis

FIG. 171

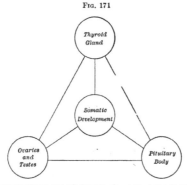

Diagram to illustrate the mutual relationship of certain of the ductless glands, and
their connection with bodily development.

the normal organ. We here would seem to see obscurely, as in conne
tion with both the thyroid and the adrenal, some relationship betwe
the activity of the epithelial elements of the organ and metabolism, a
more particularly the development of the proper organs of sex.
illustrating this latter point we may state that one of us (Nicholls) so
years ago performed an autopsy on a woman, about thirty years of ag
with a tumor of the pituitary, in whom there was a pronounced infant
condition of the sexual apparatus, and a similar state of things has be
noted in the male (Pechkranz[1]). Here, again, as in connection with th
adrenal, it cannot be said that the exhibition of the active extract of t
gland has brought about any uniform results. That occasionally, bo
in Addison's disease and acromegaly, it is followed by marked amelior
tion of symptoms, indicates, as suggested by Sajous, that we have not
yet conquered the right mode of dosage and administration.

[1] Zur Casuistik der Hypophysis-Tumoren, Neurol. Centralbl., No. 5: 1899: 203.

THE CAROTID BODIES, ZUCKERKANDL'S ORGAN, AND THE COCCYGEAL GLAND.

These may be dismissed briefly. All are organs of insignificant size. The first two are intimately associated with the vascular system on the one hand, with an abundant sympathetic network on the other, exhibiting columns or clusters of cells bordering upon the walls of an abundant capillary network.

The carotid gland is a small body, about 1 to 3 mm. in diameter, lying in the bifurcation of the common carotid artery, slightly to the posterior side of the internal carotid artery just as it leaves the main trunk. At first, it was thought to be of epithelial origin, derived, like the thyroid and thymus glands, from the branchial clefts. This is now known to be incorrect. It is formed from the primitive vascular *anlage*, from cells of epithelioid type, which become heaped up at this point and at first are continuous with those of the vessel-wall. The resulting nodule is enclosed in adventitia. Soon, capillary vessels, derived from the common carotid, enter the mass, and assume a form not unlike a glomerulus. When complete, the gland is enclosed in a fibrous capsule which sends in trabeculæ, dividing it into lobules. The unit of structure is the "cell-ball," composed of a tuft of capillaries that unite to form a vein. Several of these cell-balls are included in a lobule. The glomerule-like tufts are surrounded by epithelioid cells, arranged in cords or trabeculæ, which have an oval nucleus and nucleolus and a granular protoplasm. Besides this, the structure contains ganglion cells and sympathetic fibres derived from the cervical ganglion. There are also to be seen certain cells possessing the same affinity for chromic acid (chromaffin cells) that similar cells do which are found in the adrenals and Zuckerkandl's organ. The function of the carotid body is quite unknown, but it is undoubtedly connected with the sympathetic nervous system.

As regards the coccygeal gland, chromaffin cells are wanting (Störk[1]); according to Schuhmacher,[2] the specific cells of the organ are modified muscle cells of the wall of the median sacral artery. The gland, in short, cannot now be regarded as belonging to the same group. The carotid gland in man is situated in the posterior aspect of the bifurcation of the common carotid artery; Zuckerkandl's organ is closely attached to the adventitia of the origin of the inferior mesenteric artery; and the coccygeal gland lies close to the tip of the coccyx. Little is to be said in addition, save that these bodies may be the seat of tumors, growths of peritheliomatous type (see vol. i, Fig. 284, p. 824, and Fig. 289, p. 834).

[1] Arch. f. Mikr. Anat., 69:1907.
[2] Ibid., 71:1907.

THE THYMUS.

It is so usual to consider the thyroid and the thymus in associatic that, although personally we regard the latter organ as belonging to t lymphatic system, we have not ventured to depart from custom, ar therefore, must here note what is known regarding its function.

Anatomical Features.—The thymus lies in the upper part of t anterior mediastinum, extending from the pericardium almost to t thyroid, and is composed of two long, flat lobes, more or less intimat, united along their median aspects. The organ is enclosed in a connecti' tissue capsule that sends in trabeculæ dividing it into lobes and again ir lobules.

Microscopically, the lobules are composed of acini that bear a cl(resemblance to those of the lymphatic glands. In the peripheral zoɪ the connective tissue is richer and the lymphoid cells more numero' so that the lobules may be divided into a cortical and a medullary portic A striking feature of the picture is the so-called Hassall's corpuscles whi lie in the middle of the follicles and are composed of homogenec and, toward the periphery, concentrically arranged epithelial elemen These sometimes calcify.

The organ weighs about twenty-four grams at birth, and sligh increases in size until the end of the second year. It then remaɪ stationary until the age of puberty, and after that undergoes gradu involution. At the end of the twentieth year it is almost complet(substituted by fat. According to Waldeyer,[1] remains of the lymphc structure and of the Hassall's bodies are to be recognized throughout li Involution is, therefore, not always constant, and the gland in a m(or less complete form may persist into old age.

Embryological Considerations.—From their embryogeny there is ᴜ doubtedly ground for discussing the thyroid and thymus together. B(originate as segmental organs, as downgrowths of tubular type frc the mouth, or, more accurately, from the branchiæ, from the epitheliɪ lining the original gill-clefts. Originating thus, the thymus undergc a modification very similar to that seen in the faucial tonsils, whi(according to Gaskell, are of like origin, the epithelial cell-nests (Hassaɪ corpuscles) being the remains of the original epithelial downgrowtl The matter of the origin of the vertebrate leukocytes is still in dispu That Beard, extending certain observations of Kölliker, was too restrict in regarding them as derived primarily and essentially from the thyɪn epithelium, must, we think, be generally accepted. Gaskell[2] gathers ɪ gether much evidence showing that in lower forms the segmental tuɪ (nephridia) throughout the body may become modified into a lymphc and phagocytic tissue. On the other hand, the view is very widely h(that lymphoid tissue is essentially mesodermal and not hypoblastic epiblastic. The matter must be left open.

[1] Ruckbildung der Thymus, Centralbl. f. d. med. Wiss., 1890.
[2] Loc. cit., p. 425.

Certain it is that the thymus, when fully developed, prior to the end of the second year, is essentially a lymph-glandular organ, and that, so far, no specific active principle has been isolated from it, or recognized as existing. Later, the cells undergo a characteristic fatty change, and in addition come to contain hyaline droplets; and with this there is a slow progressive atrophy, until the gland is represented merely by fatty tissue with occasional small collections of lymph-cells.

It is interesting to note that there is an increasing tendency to ascribe the origin of the not uncommon **mediastinal sarcomas**, or **lymphosarcomas**, to overgrowth of this lymphoid tissue of the thymus. Weigert, in addition, has promulgated the hypothesis that the condition of **myasthenia gravis** is intimately related to neoplasia of the thymus. In an autopsy upon a case of this remarkable state of progressively increasing muscular weakness, he found present lymphosarcoma of the thymus, and, with this, scattered accumulations of lymphoid cells between and within the skeletal muscle fibres. These he regarded as metastases. Recent workers have confirmed the frequent presence of these "lymphorrhages" in the muscles and other organs in myasthenia, but only in 10 out of 180 cases of the disease have disturbances of the thymus been reported. Obviously, therefore, thymus neoplasia has no necessary connection with the condition, although it may be present along with other changes in the lymph-glandular system.[1]

Thymic Asthma.—The one severe condition in which we may regard the thymus as primarily at fault is thymic asthma, a condition of grave, rapidly progressive, and fatal dyspnœa in children, associated with hypertrophy and congestion of this organ. To this we have already referred (p. 245). But here if the gland be at fault—which some still strenuously deny—it is not by any internal secretion, but by the physical agency of its enlarged and congested state that symptoms are produced. Indeed, cases are on record in which cutting down upon and liberation of the enlarged thymus have alleviated the alarming symptoms of this disease. Wiesel points out that in two cases examined by him, in one of which (an adult) the thymus was the size of an apple, there was an accompanying hypoplasia of the chromaffin system in the adrenal medulla and elsewhere, and to this rather than to thymic enlargement he is inclined to ascribe the sudden death.

---

[1] For literature, consult Mandlebaum and Celler, Jour. Exp. Med., 10:1908:308.

CHAPTER XXXII.

THE THYROID AND THYMUS *GLANDS.*

THE THYROID GLAND.

CONGENITAL ANOMALIES.

COMPLETE or unilateral **defect** of the thyroid is rare. More frequent there is absence of the isthmus. Occasionally, **abnormal lobulati** is observed and the organ may be divided into several parts held togeth by bloodvessels and connective tissue. Very rarely, the isthmus pass between the œsophagus and the trachea. **Accessory thyroids are n** infrequently met with, and may be found at a considerable distan from the parent gland, viz., near the hyoid bone, behind the pharyr within the larynx or trachea, at the superior clavicular groove, and the aorta. Accessory thyroids in the base of the tongue, situated alor the course of the thyroglossal duct, have given rise to tumors.[1] Osl mentions having found accessory thyroids in the pleura.

Premature atrophy, or possibly **hypoplasia,** is the cardinal feature cretinism.

Congenital **enlargement**[2] is important, as it may lead to death fro pressure on the air passages. Not only may the normally-situated glar undergo this increase, but also the accessories. The causes are ve various, and include hyperemia, hypertrophy, teleangiectasis, cysts, fibro proliferation, and adenoma.

A strange anomaly is one mentioned by Wölfler, who found striat **muscle** in an otherwise normal gland.

CIRCULATORY DISTURBANCES.

Hyperemia.—Owing to the great vascularity of the thyroid, circulato disturbances are apt to be both frequent and profound. **Hyperemia m** lead to a surprising enlargement of the gland. Passive congestion met with in valvular and other heart affections, in suffocation, and obstruction of the veins of the neck from whatever cause.

Of much interest is the congestive hyperemia of neuropathic origi that is supposed by many to be the essential lesion of **Graves' diseas** The enlargement of the thyroid that occurs in females at puberty, durir

---

[1] J. C. Warren, Amer. Jour. Med. Sci., 104: 1892: 377.

[2] For the literature on congenital struma, see Demme, Gerhardt's Handbuch d Kinderk., 3:2.

menstruation, and in pregnancy is possibly to be placed in the same category (*struma hyperemica*).

Dilatation of the bloodvessels (struma vasculosa) is met with in two forms, an aneurismal and a varicose. In the former the arteries, not only within the gland but on its surface, are dilated and tortuous, resembling a cirsoid aneurism; in the latter the veins and capillaries are affected.

Hemorrhage.—Hemorrhage is frequent, especially in cysts and tumors, or when the vessels are dilated. It may also be due to trauma.

INFLAMMATIONS.

Inflammation may affect the otherwise normal thyroid (**thyroiditis**), or one that is chronically enlarged (**strumitis**). The latter event is the more common. The whole gland or any part of it may be involved. Both exudative and productive forms are recognized.

Acute Exudative Inflammation.—Acute exudative inflammation is rarely primary, but is due to disease elsewhere. It follows traumatism, or is a complication of affections like puerperal fever, typhoid fever, angina, septicemia, Bright's disease, pneumonia, ulcerative endocarditis, and acute rheumatism. The bacteria found include Streptococcus and Staphylococcus pyogenes, Diplococcus pneumoniæ, and B. typhosus.

The affected gland is swollen, hard, and painful. Resolution may rapidly take place or the condition may go on to abscess-formation. Large areas may undergo purulent softening, and if cysts be present they may fill with pus.

On account of the proximity of the large veins of the neck there is great danger of thrombophlebitis and general septicemia. The abscesses may rupture into the mediastinum, the most frequent event, or into the larynx, trachea, or œsophagus. When healing takes place fibrous scars may result, or the abscess may become encapsulated, and the contents inspissated and infiltrated with calcareous salts.

Chronic Productive Inflammation.—Chronic productive inflammation, or interstitial fibrous hyperplasia, is quite rare, except in the form that attacks a previously hyperplastic thyroid (*struma fibrosa*).

Tuberculosis.—Tuberculosis of the normal or enlarged thyroid is invariably secondary and due to hematogenous infection. The affection is more common than has been supposed. According to E. Fraenkel[1] it is usually present in general miliary tuberculosis. Both miliary and caseonodular forms are described.[2]

Syphilis.—Syphilis is rare.[3] Eleven undoubted cases are found in the literature (Davis).

Parasites.—*Echinococcus cysts* are rare. They may discharge into the trachea.

[1] Virchow's Archiv, 104: 1886: 58.

[2] Ruppanner, Ueber tuber. Strumen, Frankfurter Zeitschr. f. Path., 2:1909.

[3] See Mendel, Med. Klin., 32:1906; Davis, Arch. of Int. Med.; 5:1910:47 (with bibliography).

Actinomycosis of the thyroid, due to extension of the disease from th neck, has been observed. Occasionally, it is caused by metastasis.

RETROGRESSIVE METAMORPHOSES.

Atrophy.—Simple atrophy is a common condition in old age. Her the acini are wasted, the interstitial tissue is relatively increased, and th vessels are sclerosed. In some cases the atrophy is unilateral.

Two special forms of atrophy call for mention, namely, that due the continued exhibition of small doses of iodine and that found in my œdema. The explanation is by no means clear. In the former cas it would seem that iodine interferes in some way with the nutrition the cells, so that they become unable to assimilate foodstuffs and the undergo atrophy. With regard to myxœdema, as noted elsewhere, it difficult to regard the atrophy of the thyroid tissue as a primary cond tion; there must be some underlying cause, whether metabolic or (some have held) nervous. More recent workers, like Wilson, lay stre upon what may be termed "exhaustion atrophy;" they record cases i which atrophy and the myxœdematous state succeed glandular hype plasia and excessive activity of the gland with symptoms of Grave disease.

Degenerations.—The various forms of degeneration affect the thyroi but are most commonly found in association with other pathologic conditions of the gland. - Among them may be mentioned **fatty degener tion** of the glandular epithelium, **coagulation necrosis, hyaline degeneratio** and **calcification.**

Amyloid disease is met with under the usual conditions, but it interesting that it may affect "goitrous" nodules to a greater extent tha the rest of the gland.

Colloid degeneration is described as occurring in the thyroids of ol people. In some cases it appears to be a true colloid degeneration the cells which are small and tend to disappear, but in others it is simp an arrest in the development of a colloid struma.

PROGRESSIVE METAMORPHOSES.

In this category we place for convenience tumors and all those enlarg ments of the thyroid commonly known as "goitre," "struma," an "bronchocele," with the exception of those due to simple hyperemia.

Inasmuch as our knowledge of the growth and overgrowth of t gland is still somewhat defective, it is impossible to make a classific tion of the progressive metamorphoses that is entirely free from obje tion. That adopted here must, therefore, be regarded as mere tentative. It would be well in discussing "struma," when possible, draw a clear distinction between vascular disturbances, hyperplasia an hypertrophy, and true tumor-formation.

Goitre.—The most common and important condition that we have to deal with in case of the thyroid is the so-called **struma** or **goitre.** These terms, of course, strictly speaking, apply solely to increase in size, but have been so loosely employed that much confusion has resulted. The word "goitre" has been used indiscriminately for any enlargement of the gland, whether due to hyperemia, hypertrophy, cystic dilatation, fibroid induration, hyperplasia, or tumor-formation. Thus, anatomically speaking, the term is objectionable, for a great variety of etiologically differing conditions are arbitrarily grouped together, nor is it better from a clinical standpoint, since widely differing symptoms are associated

Fig. 172

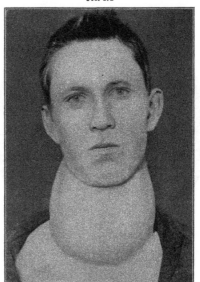

Parenchymatous goitre. (Dr. Shepherd's case, Montreal General Hospital.)

with enlarged thyroid. The size of the gland is the least important of its characteristics and is only of significance in those few cases where mechanical pressure is exerted on the air passages. It would, therefore, contribute to accuracy if the terms "goitre" and "struma" could be dropped from our nomenclature. For, it is certainly more scientific to discuss enlargements of the glands in the light of the etiological causes or anatomical peculiarities.

In attempting any classification of the goitrous enlargements of the thyroid, we are met at the outset with the old difficulty of deciding what enlargements are tumors (adenomata et al.) and what are merely hyperplastic overgrowths. Wölfler, in his classical studies on this subject, attempts, and rightly so, to make this distinction, but his classification is in several points open to criticism. He divides "goitre" into hypertrophic and adenomatous forms. In the first group, which would be more correctly styled "hyperplastic," he puts all those cases of enlargement due to increase of the specific glandular elements and vesicles or to increase in their contents; in the second, those forms where there are long, branching, cellular processes of embryonal type, which he regards as epithelial new-formations. His cardinal point is that the adenomas are derived from the activity of the interalveolar embryonic cells. It is certainly incorrect to call a simple collection of colloid within the

FIG. 173

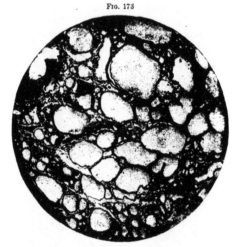

Colloid struma of the thyroid gland. The acini are greatly dilated and filled with colloid. Leitz obj. No. 7, without ocular. (From the collection of Dr. A. G. Nicholls.)

vesicles an hypertrophy, as Wölfler does (hypertrophia gelatinosa), and it is by no means certain that we are justified in making the wide generalization that adenomas are always derived from embryonic cells. More recent observers, notably Hitzig,[1] believe that new-formations resembling adult tissue are to be referred to the overgrowth of previously existing adult cells.

Hyperplasia.—Hyperplasia and regeneration of tissue are not infrequently found in the thyroid. When a portion of the gland is removed or is functionally useless, compensatory hyperplasia occurs. In such cases, as Halstead[2] has shown experimentally, there is metamorphosis

[1] Arch. f. klin. Chir., 47: 1894:464.
[2] Johns Hopkins Hosp. Rep., 1: 1896: 373.

of the lining epithelium of the acini into cylindrical cells that tend to assume a papillary arrangement, while the colloid material becomes more mucoid.

Hyperplasia may affect the glandular elements, the stroma, or both, and leads to considerable enlargement of the organ. How to class this form of goitre is difficult, for reasons already brought forward. Aschoff[1] points out that generalized diffuse overgrowth (hypertrophy proper) is to be sharply separated from the nodular overgrowths, all of which he regards as adenomatous. True goitres (here including Graves' disease) belong to the latter class alone. He holds, further, that the different forms of goitre or *struma nodosa*—parenchymatous, cystic, hemorrhagic, vascular, fibrous, and calcifying—are different stages in the life history of the one form of adenoma, the nodules developing by epithelial overgrowth of certain vesicles. With the peripheral or centrifugal growth of new tissue the central parts tend to undergo various forms of degeneration and necrosis.

Fig. 174

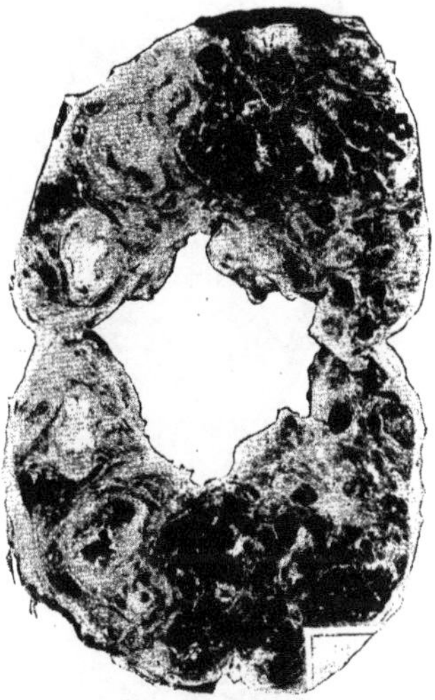

Colloid struma. The thyroid is divided vertically and the anterior portion turned upward. (From the Pathological Museum of McGill University.)

The first form to be noticed is that called by Virchow **struma hyperplastica parenchymatosa,** where the overgrowth is confined to the acini. The growth is often nodular, fairly well defined, and of a soft, yellowish-gray appearance.

Microscopically, it is composed of round, oval, and elongated, branching alveoli, often containing colloid. In other cases there is an increase of the fibrous stroma with atrophy and fatty degeneration of the secreting cells—**struma hyperplastica fibrosa.**

Colloid Goitre.—Another and one of the most frequent and important forms, is the **struma gelatinosa** or **colloid goitre.** Of these it is usual to distinguish two forms—(1) the *diffuse colloid goitre* and (2) the *nodular.* Careful study shows that at least a large proportion of the former, as a matter of fact, are of the nodular type, with nodules of great size.

Exophthalmic Goitre (Graves' Disease; Basedow's Disease).—This is an affection characterized by enlargement of the thyroid gland, protrusion of the eyeballs, rapid pulse, palpitation of the heart, nervousness, a tendency to flushing of the skin, and occasional attacks of diarrhea. In

[1] Deut. med Woch., 1910: No. 12.

the later stages we may get dilatation of the heart. The disease attacks usually youngish people and the female sex by preference. The etiology has been variously looked for in an intoxication or a vasomotor tropho-neurosis. Most of the manifestations of the disease can be reproduced by the injection of thyroid secretion, and can be alleviated by partial excision of the gland and by antitoxic medication, so that there can be little doubt that it is to be attributed to hyperthyroid-ism. What, however, is the cause at work behind this overactivity is still to seek.

Fig. 175

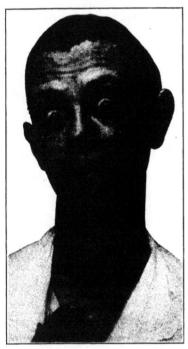

Exophthalmic goitre, or Graves' disease. (Case of Dr. Shepherd, Montreal General Hospital.)

The anatomical picture in these cases is not particu-larly characteristic. The gland is undoubtedly hy-peremic, as, indeed, is evi-denced by the presence of bruit over it during life. Next, it is goitrous. But beyond this the picture is somewhat inconstant. Per-haps, we may make one broad generalization and say that in some cases the lesions are local (adenomatous ?), in others, diffuse. In all there is more or less hyper-plasia of the alveolar par-enchyma. In the earlier stages, or the milder forms, the intra-alveolar prolifera-tion is slight, but the colloid secretion seems to be thin and scanty. Later on, the proliferation is more marked and the secretion more abundant though still thin. Later still, these features are even more marked and there is beginning degene-ration. Finally, the degeneration becomes very marked, the secretion again becomes thick, and there is exfoliation of the parenchymatous cells. Cases of Graves' disease have been known to supervene upon the ordi-nary colloid goitre after operative handling. Further details can be found in Wilson's paper, which is one of the recent studies of this subject.[1]

[1] Wilson, Trans. Assoc. Amer. Physicians, 23:1908:562. See also Haemig, Arch. f. klin. Chirurgie, 55:1897:1; Kocher, Mittheilungen aus den Grenzgebieten der Medizin und Chirurgie, 9:1903, and Brit. Med. Jour., 1:1906:1261; Ewing, Proc. New York Path. Soc., N. S. 6:1906.

Tumors.—Adenoma.—Here, microscopically, one sees vesicles of all sizes, from the small acinus of the normal gland to large cystic cavities lined with flattened epithelium. For the most part the connective tissue between the vesicles is scanty. Owing to the pressure of the accumulated colloid, the vesicular walls and the fibrous stroma are atrophic, and there is a tendency for the cavities to coalesce, so that a multilocular or even a unilocular cyst is the result. In the larger cysts, the colloid is converted into slippery, albuminous fluid. In another form of colloid struma there is a uniform enlargement of the thyroid, which on examination presents abundant colloid formation, cystic degeneration, and fibroid induration (*interacinous adenoma* of Wölfler). In still a third variety, both lobes of the gland are enlarged and on the surface soft, rounded elevations can be felt. On section, it is a colloid goitre, within the cavities of which there are large papillary outgrowths (*papillary cystadenoma*).

Fɪɢ. 176

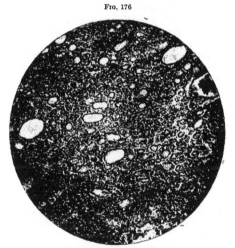

Fœtal adenoma of the thyroid. Winckel obj. No. 3, without ocular. (From the collection of Dr. A. G. Nicholls.)

There is one form, at all events, the so-called *fœtal adenoma*, in which Wölfler's view is probably correct. This growth is met with at any time from birth to the age of puberty, and its occurrence in young children argues for its origin in embryonic cell-inclusions. It forms multiple circumscribed nodules that are often extremely vascular.

A rare form of tumor that should also be mentioned is the *cylindrical-celled adenoma* which is found both in the normal and in the strumous thyroid.

It would be well to restrict the term adenoma to those cases where there is a more or less definite overgrowth of the glandular elements, which is nodular and sharply defined from the rest of the thyroid substance.

Among the benign tumors are the **fibroma,** an example of which has been recorded by Wölfler, **osteoid chondroma,** and **teratoma.** Whether **chrondroma** and **osteoma** occur is perhaps doubtful.

Sarcoma.—Sarcoma is the most common of the mesoblastic tumors, and is more liable to be found in cases where goitrous enlargement of the gland has preëxisted. It may be *round-celled, spindle-celled, giant-celled, alveolar,* or *angiomatous.* Rarely, in such tumors striated muscle fibres have been found (Wölfler). More uncommon are *fibro-, chondro-, osteoid-,* and *osteochondrosarcoma. Peri-* and *endotheliomas* are extremely rare. A *sarcomatous teratoma* has been met with. Sarcomas form nodular tumors that occupy more or less of the organ, but rarely the whole.

On section, the consistence varies and the surface is smooth and somewhat intersected by fibrous bands. The color is white or gray, or, again, admixed with red, according to the amount of blood present. The tumor grows rapidly and may penetrate the trachea or jugular vein, so that widespread metastases are quite common.

Carcinoma.— Primary carcinoma usually takes the form of *carcinoma simplex* or *c. medullare,* rarely, *c. scirrhosum,* and produces tumors varying in size from that of a hen's egg to that of a child's head. Billroth, however, has described cases where the thyroid was not enlarged. Carcinoma develops, as a rule, in glands previously enlarged and forms either grayish-white nodules surrounded by connective tissue, or a uniform, more or less diffuse, infiltration with only slightly altered parenchyma between the areas of new-growth. The nodular form is regarded by Wölfler as developing in a follicular-fibrous goitre, and the diffuse variety from the interacinar embryonal cells. *Cylindrical-celled carcinoma* is described as well as *papillary cystic carcinoma.* In certain cancers the stroma may undergo myxomatous degeneration (*carcinoma myxomatodes*).

Squamous-celled epitheliomas have been met with, due to the inclusion of epidermal cells during foetal life, but the vast majority are examples of secondary growths.

A few instances of *mixed* sarcomatous and carcinomatous growths have been described. They are more common in the thyroid than elsewhere.[1] An extremely rare and interesting tumor is a mixed form of *carcinoma* and *perithelial angiosarcoma,* of which an example has been reported by Woolley.[2] Only four cases are on record, one of them in a dog (Wells[3]).

Malignant tumors may also arise from the parathyroids.[4]

Inasmuch as many carcinomas contain colloid material, the secondary growths frequently produce the same substance. Any tumor containing

[1] Leo Loeb, Amer. Jour. Med. Sci., 125:1903:243.

[2] American Medicine, 4: No. 9: 1902: 331.

[3] Jour. of Path. and Bact., 7:1901:357.

[4] MacCallum, Johns Hopkins Hosp. Bull., 16:1905; Kocher, Deutsch. Zeit. f. Chir., 91:1908:197.

colloid, particularly if found in bone, should arouse the suspicion of a primary growth in the thyroid. Growths in the gland produce serious effects not only from extension, but also from pressure. The trachea or œsophagus may be compressed and the cartilages eroded, or paralysis may ensue from involvement of the recurrent laryngeal nerve. Invasion of the great vessels of the neck may lead to stasis, thrombosis, embolism, hemorrhage, and secondary growth.

A point of some importance in regard to tumors is that they are apt to be considerably altered in appearance by secondary changes. The connective tissue is frequently increased either diffusely, or about the nodules and cysts. It may also show hyaline or mucoid degeneration. Cystic metamorphosis is not uncommon, due to the overdistension and rupture of adjacent follicles or from colliquative necrosis.

Cysts.—A special form is the **hemorrhagic cyst**, formed by rupture of vessels and the discharge of blood into the cavities. Rokitansky[1] was probably the first to point out that hemorrhages occurred for the most part only in neoplastic growths of the thyroid. This observation has been confirmed here by Archibald.[2] There are two forms of hemorrhagic cysts: one in which hemorrhage takes place into an ordinary colloid retention-cyst, and another where extensive extravasation both into the vesicles and into the interstitial connective tissue occurs. The latter form has been more especially studied by Bradley.[3]

Calcification of the stroma and even of the vesicular contents has been observed. Amyloid and fatty changes, as well as inflammation, may also take place.

THE THYMUS.

CONGENITAL ANOMALIES.

Complete **absence** of the thymus has been observed in the case of monsters, and, rarely, in otherwise normal children. **Accessory glands** are not uncommon and are usually found just above the main thymus and near the thyroid. **Irregularity** in **shape** and **lobulation** are not rare. Enormous **enlargement** is sometimes met with.

CIRCULATORY DISTURBANCES.

Hemorrhages occur in death from asphyxia, in congenital syphilis, and in the hemorrhagic diathesis.

INFLAMMATIONS.

Primary **inflammation** is rare, if indeed it occur at all. Generally, the affection is due to extension from the neighboring organs.

[1] Zur Anat. des Kropfes, Wien, 1849.
[2] Montreal Med. Jour., 25:1897:780.
[3] Jour. Exp. Med., 1: 1896: 401.

Suppurative inflammation is found more particularly in septicemia. Care should be taken not to regard the yellowish cellular juice of the normal gland as pus, which it much resembles. *Multiple abscesses* are met with and, also, *diffuse purulent infiltration.*

Tuberculosis.—Tuberculosis is somewhat rare, and is found in miliary form and caseous masses.

Syphilis.—Syphilis takes the form of gummas or a diffuse fibroid induration.

RETROGRESSIVE METAMORPHOSES.

Focal necroses have been described by Jacobi[1] in connection with diphtheria.

Degeneration Cysts.—Degeneration cysts containing puriform matter, which has led to their being mistaken for abscesses (Dubois), have been described by Chiari.[2] They are due to postmortem softening or to the ingrowing of the thymus tissue into the Hassall's corpuscles, and were at one time thought, but erroneously so, to be characteristic of congenital syphilis.

PROGRESSIVE METAMORPHOSES.

Hyperplasia.—The thymus may participate in the general lymphatic enlargement that occurs in leukemia, pseudoleukemia, and the "status lymphaticus."

Hyperplasia may occur after birth and has been noted in connection with epilepsy (Ohlmacher[3]), exophthalmic goitre (Hektoen[4]) in acromegaly, myxœdema, and Addison's disease (Hart[5]). It is most commonly associated with a general lymphoid hyperplasia,[6] and is of interest on account of its relationship to cases of sudden death. The exact mechanism is not as yet determined. Some think that death is due to irritation of the inferior laryngeal nerves, or to pressure on the vagi and trachea. As before suggested it may be toxic. There have only been one or two cases in which compression of the trachea has been discovered post mortem, so that mechanical pressure does not appear to be an important factor. This much should be said, however, that it is not impossible, or even unlikely that the organ may be subject to sudden hyperemic enlargement, a condition that at times might pass off before the case came to autopsy.

Epithelial transformation of the thymus has been described by Lochte.[7]

[1] Trans. Assoc. of Amer. Phys., 3: 1888: 297.
[2] Ueber Cystenbildung in der Thymus, Zeit. f. Heilk., 4: 1894.
[3] Bull. Ohio Hosp. for Epileptics, 1898 and 1899.
[4] Internat. Med. Magaz., 1896.
[5] Wiener klin. Woch., 31:1908.
[6] Bartel and Stein, Arch. f. Anat. und Phys., 1906.
[7] Centralbl. f. allg. Path. u. path., Anat., 10: 1890: 1.

example has been described by Osler, and **dermoid cysts**. The latter
inate in persistent epithelial "rests" and contain yellowish-white,
y and granular material, together with hair.

he most frequent tumor is **sarcoma** in its various forms.[1] *Lympho-
:oma* may be recognized by its smooth homogeneous appearance,
forming to some extent to the normal outlines of the gland, in contra-
:inction to the more irregular and nodular arrangement of sarcoma
inating in the lymphatic glands. The presence of Hassall's cor-
cles in the former is said to be of importance in the differential
gnosis (Letulle).

arcinoma may be developed from the epithelial structures.

umors of the thymus are important, since they may grow rapidly
encroach upon vital structures like the heart, lungs, and great
sels.

[1] Schneider, Fibrosarcoma, Inaug. Diss., *Greifswald*, 1892

CHAPTER XXXIII.

THE ADRENAL *GLANDS*, PITUITARY, PINEA*L* AND CAROTID BODIES, AND COCCY*GEAL GL*AND.

THE ADRENALS.

CONGENITAL ANOMALIES.

COMPLETE defect and hypoplasia are rare. There seems to be some relationship between the development of the suprarenals and that of the brain and genitalia. In hydrocephalus, hemicephaly, and anencephaly, hypoplasia, partial aplasia, and fibrosis of the former organs have been found.[1] Hyperplasia and accessory glands have been noted in connection with hypoplasia of the ovary and hermaphroditism (Marchand).

Accessory adrenals form the most common anomaly. They may be found in widely distant parts, in the capsule of the adrenal, at the hilus of the kidney, on the renal and spermatic veins, in the liver, on the ovary and broad ligament. The accessories may be single or multiple, and are more common in children. Of special interest are those found in the capsule of the kidney, between the capsule and the cortex, or within the kidney substance, since, according to Grawitz and others, these misplaced "rests" may give rise to tumors (see vol. i, p. 810).

CIRCULATORY DISTURBANCES.

Hyperemia.—Passive congestion is common, and is met with under the same conditions as elsewhere.

Hemorrhages.—Hemorrhages into the substance of the gland, either minute or larger (hematomas), are met with from traumatism at birth, in passive congestion, fatty degeneration of the vessels, venous thrombosis, inflammation, leukemia, and the hemorrhagic diathesis. These constitute one of the causes of sudden, or relatively sudden, death. Chiari[2] has described a case in which the extravasation was as large as a man's head and weighed 2 kilos. In some cases *calcification* results and *phleboliths* have been observed. The blood may become encapsulated and a cyst form.

---

[1] Weigert, Virch. Archiv, 100: 1885: 176, u. 103: 1886: 204.
[2] Wien. med. Presse, 21: 1880.

Woolley[1] has recorded a case of hemorrhagic **infarction** of the right adrenal in the newborn, due to **thrombosis** of the central vein.

INFLAMMATIONS.

Hemorrhagic Inflammation.—Under the term hemorrhagic inflammation, Virchow has described a condition in which the adrenal is swollen, thickened, and infiltrated with blood. Microscopically, fatty degeneration is marked.

FIG. 177

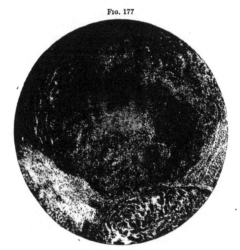

Early caseous tuberculosis of the adrenal gland. Leitz obj. No. 7, without ocular.
(From the collection of Dr. A. G. Nicholls.)

Small collections of inflammatory round cells are sometimes met with in the interstitial substance in cases of infection, pyemia and the like. They are probably due to embolic infection.

Suppurative Inflammation.—Suppurative inflammation, either localized or diffuse, is met with in general septicemia. Abscesses of considerable size may result, and sometimes burst into the colon or duodenum. The adrenal may be secondarily involved in inflammatory processes originating in the kidney, and (in the case of the right adrenal) in the liver.

Tuberculosis.—Tuberculosis of the adrenals is not uncommon in cases of advanced disease of the lungs and other organs. Small miliary granulomata may often be seen in the interstitial substance. Larger caseous

[1] Jour. of Med. Research, New Series, 2: No. 2; 1902: 231.

nodules may be found occupying the centre of the gland, which, spreading outward, may involve and destroy the greater part of the cortex. Tuberculosis of these organs is the usual lesion found in cases of Addison's disease.

Syphilis.[1]—Syphilis is rare. It usually takes the form of diffuse interstitial inflammation, less often gumma. Coagulation necroses resembling anemic infarcts have been met with in congenital lues.[2]

RETROGRADE METAMORPHOSES.

Atrophy.—Simple atrophy is met with in old age and general marasmus, and, occasionally, in Addison's disease. The chief feature is the narrowing of the cortex with great diminution in the amount of the lipoid matter which is normally present in all adult adrenals.

The gland is often found to be softened in the centre and cavitated. This is probably a postmortem change, although often induced by careless removal.[3]

Cloudy Swelling.—Cloudy swelling is met with here under the same conditions as elsewhere.

Fatty Degeneration.—A true fatty degeneration, associated with atrophy and disappearance of the nuclei, has been described in connection with marasmus, anemia, and affections of the heart, lungs, and vessels.

Amyloid Disease.—Amyloid disease is fairly common in all cases of widespread amyloid transformation. It affects, chiefly, the walls of the capillaries between the columns of the zona fasciculata.

Coagulation Necrosis.—Coagulation necrosis, either focal or diffuse, is a rather common condition, met with in puerperal eclampsia, chronic tuberculosis, and a great variety of infections and intoxications. The cells of the zona fasciculata are the ones usually picked out. They are opaque, turbid, have lost their clear vesicular appearance, and the nuclei stain badly or not at all.

PROGRESSIVE METAMORPHOSES.

Tumors.—These may be broadly divided into two orders, those of the cortex or of cortical elements, and those of the medulla. Of the first order Virchow[4] has described, under the term **struma lipomatosa suprarenalis**, a diffuse, or, more often, a nodular overgrowth of the cortical substance (**nodular hyperplasia; adenoma; benign hypernephroma; mesothelioma**). The nodules are single or multiple, sometimes bilateral, and may reach the size of a walnut. They are yellowish in color and

---

[1] Ribaudeau-Dumas and Pater, Arch. d. Med., 21:1909.

[2] Kokubo, Centralbl. f. allg. Path. und path. Anat., 14: Nos. 16 and 17: 1903.

[3] It deserves emphasis that, in our experience, most of the cavitation, so frequently described in autopsy protocols, is due to careless and rough removal of the organs. Removed with care and within eight hours after death the adrenals are not often found cavitated.

[4] Die krankhafte Geschwülste, 2.

are situated in the cortex, less frequently in the medulla. Microscopically, the growths are composed of long, sometimes branched, masses of cells, similar to those of the zona fasciculata, containing fat, and often pigment. In many cases the connective tissue is increased. Cystic degeneration and calcification sometimes occur.

Of the second order is the form also described by Virchow (as a **glioma**). It is, however, not a glioma proper, but a derivative of the cells of sympathetic ganglion cell origin, which form the specific constituent of the medulla—a form of **neuroma** or ganglionic neuroma (see vol. i, p. 809) which takes the form of a nodular mass in the medulla. The cells composing it are pale, irregular or stellate, faintly granular, with relatively large nuclei. The tumor may be as large as a raspberry. **Lipoma** is said to occur. **Angioma** and **cavernous lymphangioma**[1] are rare.

Among the malignant tumors that have been described are **sarcomas** of various types, *round-celled sarcoma, myxosarcoma, angiosarcoma, melanosarcoma, lymphosarcoma,* and *carcinoma,* so-called.

Those originating in the cortex are composed of cells varying more or less widely from those of the normal cortex, but, as a rule, it is possible to make out the transition. The cells are moderately large, polyhedral or flattened, containing a relatively large, oval, or irregular nucleus with a deeply staining chromatin-net. The interstitial stroma is not intercellular, but surrounds masses or columns of the cells. Multinucleated cells are numerous. Such tumors from their histological appearance might, therefore, be called carcinomas. In view of the recent careful studies of Minot,[2] Aichel,[3] and others, however, we have to believe that the adrenal cortex is derived from the Wolffian body and is, consequently, mesoblastic, or, more precisely, to use Minot's term, mesothelial. Unless it be kept in mind that the term can nowadays only be granted a histological significance, it is dangerous to speak of a tumor so derived as a carcinoma. As a matter of fact, these tumors, microscopically, present in some cases a carcinomatous appearance, and in others are more like the sarcomas. As illustrating this point, Woolley[4] has described a tumor of the adrenal, resembling a carcinoma, the metastases of which in the lung, brain, and lymph-glands were indistinguishable from sarcoma. The secondary growths in the lung were of transitional appearance, varying from a tumor composed of polyhedral cells in the younger portions to a spindle-celled form in the older. In the brain, the metastases were chiefly composed of round cells. Possibly it would be less confusing if, with Woolley, we speak of tumors arising from the parenchyma of the adrenals as *mesotheliomas,* irrespective of their histological appearance (see vol. i, p. 677).

The neuromas derived from the medulla may also assume malignant properties and the appearance of round-celled sarcoma.

---

[1] Oberndorfer, Beit. z. allg. Path. u. z. path. Anat., 29: 1901: 516.

[2] The Embryological Basis of Pathology, Science, New Series, 13: 1901: 481.

[3] Vergleichende Entwickl. u. s. w. der Neben. Arch. f. mikros. Anat., 65: 1900: 1.

[4] A Primary Carcinomatoid Tumor (Mesothelioma) of the Adrenals, with Sarcomatous Metastases, Trans. Assoc. Amer. Phys., 17: 1902: 627.

Secondary carcinoma, sarcoma, and *endothelioma* are met with in the adrenals.

The malignant tumors originating in the adrenals are particularly liable to invade the veins, and metastases are usually rapidly produced. It has been noted that they are liable to be associated at the same time with similar tumors of the thyroid or genitalia.

It should be remarked in concluding the discussion of tumors of these organs that the nomenclature is at present confusing. This is perhaps due to the fact that the exact nature of many of these new-growths is open to debate. It is the fashion nowadays, however, to speak simply of all tumors arising from the parenchyma of the adrenal or of adrenal "rests" as **hypernephromata** (Birch-Hirschfeld). Many of the growths called by the earlier writers "malignant tumor," "alveolar sarcoma," "carcinoma," would properly be classified under this head.

Parasites.—*Echinococcus* has been met with. It is rare.

THE PITUITARY BODY OR HYPOPHYSIS CEREBRI.

CONGENITAL ANOMALIES.

Partial or complete **persistence** of the ductus craniopharyngeus, and **cysts** in its course have already been referred to. **Absence** of the pituitary body is very rare.

CIRCULATORY DISTURBANCES.

Hyperemia.—Hyperemia is found in general cerebral congestion and in inflammatory and circulatory disorders at the base of the brain.

Hemorrhage.—Hemorrhage into the posterior lobe has been observed (Eppinger). It is often agonal.

INFLAMMATIONS.

Inflammation of the hypophysis is generally secondary to disease of the meninges or of the bones at the base of the skull. Stengel[1] mentions a case in which the anterior lobe was inflamed, apparently from infection which reached it from the parotid through the retropharyngeal lymphatics.

Tuberculosis.—Caseous tubercles have been described as occurring in the pituitary by Boyce and Beadles.[2]

Syphilis.—According to Lancereaux, the pituitary is enlarged and indurated in congenital syphilis. Gummas have also been met with.[3]

Parasites.—A few cases of *Echinococcus cysts* have been observed (Sommering, Lancereaux).

[1] Text-book of Pathology, 1900: 796, W. B. Saunders & Co., Philadelphia.
[2] Jour. of Path. and Bact., 1: 1893: 223 and 359.
[3] Hektoen, Trans. Chicago Path. Soc., 2: 1897: 129.

RETROGRESSIVE METAMORPHOSES.

Atrophy may occur. In cretinism and myxœdema, the sella turcica has been found to be enlarged, quite out of proportion to the gland resting in it. This has been explained as due to an involution of the hypophysis subsequent to a previous enlargement.

Large **colloid** deposits are sometimes found within dilated follicles and in the lymphatics. Whether this is to be interpreted as due to over-activity of the gland or as a degenerative manifestation is doubtful.

Fatty degeneration of the cells and **hyaline** changes in the vessels have been described in old people. **Amyloid** disease of the bloodvessels has been observed in advanced general amyloidosis. **Calcareous** deposits occasionally may be found.

PROGRESSIVE METAMORPHOSES.

Vicarious **hypertrophy,** often of considerable amount, has been noted in experimental thyroidectomy, fibroid goitre, cretinism, and myxœdema.

Tumors.—Struma[1] or **goitre** of the pituitary body is a condition not readily distinguishable from **adenoma.** In it the organ is considerably enlarged, owing to the cystic dilatation of the acini with an excess of colloid material, together with proliferative and vascular changes in the stroma. The enlarged pituitary may reach the size even of a hen's egg and produce marked pressure disturbances in the brain and floor of the skull.

Cysts, lined with ciliated epithelium and containing homogeneous or granular material, have been described by Weichselbaum.[2]

Considering the complicated development of the hypophysis, we should expect to find that **teratoid new-formations** were rather common, but this is not the case. *Dermoid cysts* have been described by Beck[3] and Weigert.[4] Hale White has reported a *neuromyoma* composed of striated muscle and medullated nerve-fibres.[5] Cystic tumors, presumably derived from the infundibular canal, have been noted by Rayer, Rokitansky, and Langer.

Of the simpler benign tumors may be mentioned **lipoma** (Weichselbaum), **angioma** and **chondroma** (Lancereaux).

The most important growths, however, are the **carcinoma** and **sarcoma.** These form diffuse or nodular masses, destroying the structure of the gland, and often leading to infiltration of the brain, optic tracts, and base of the skull. They may extend to the nasopharynx and orbit. The pituitary being mainly epiblastic, the new-growths originating

[1] *Löwenstein*, Virch. Archiv, 188:1907:44.
[2] Neubildungen der Hypophysis, Virch. Archiv, 75: 1879: 444.
[3] Teratom. Zeit. f. Heilk., 4: 1883.
[4] Teratom. Virch. Archiv, 75: 1875.
[5] Trans. Path. Soc. of London, 36:1885:37.

in the parenchyma are strict carcinomas in the usual acceptation of the term.   Sarcomas probably arise from the sheath of the vessels, the endothelial linings of the blood and lymph-channels, and from the pia.   We have met with one case of **endothelioma**[1] and another of **perithelial angiosarcoma.**

Secondary tumors may involve the hypophysis.   *Colloid carcinoma* and *melanosarcoma* have been met with.

In addition to the general symptoms of brain-tumor, growths in the pituitary rather early involve the optic tracts and other cranial nerves in the neighborhood, so that blindness and various local paralyses **are** met with.   Pronounced systemic anemia is a curious symptom occasionally found.   The explanation of this is not easy.   It should be noted

FIG. 178

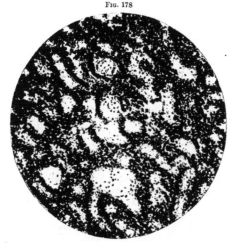

Perithelial angiosarcoma of the pituitary body.   Winckel obj. No. 5, without ocular.
(From the collection of Dr. A. G. Nicholls.)

that pituitary tumors may exist without the symptoms of acromegaly becoming manifest.   In such cases we must assume either that the growth has progressed so rapidly that death has occurred before this disease could appear, that compensation has taken place, or that the intact portion of the gland or perhaps the tumor itself has been adequate to supply the necessary secretion, or, finally, as is now more generally held, has not discharged an excess of internal secretion.   It is in association with adenomatous enlargement of the anterior lobe that acromegaly most often is found to develop.

[1] See James Stewart, The Symptomatology of Tumors Involving the Hypophysis Cerebri, Phila. Med. Jour., 3: 1899: 1169.

THE PINEAL GLAND.

The pineal gland, or epiphysis, is formed by a diverticulum from the roof of the posterior portion of the anterior cerebral vesicle. It is generally believed to have no function, or, at least, little or nothing is known about this,[1] and it is now regarded as the atrophied remnant of a central eye, which is somewhat better marked in certain of the lower animals. It may be remarked here, as bearing on the question of a possible internal secretion from the pineal gland, that Marburg[2] would connect certain types of adiposity (adipositas cerebralis) with tumors of this structure. The fact that adiposity (and genital hypoplasia) are associated directly or indirectly with disturbances of organs producing an internal secretion, such as the pituitary, thyroid, thymus, adrenal, genital glands, pancreas, and liver, is at least suggestive.[3]

Histologically, it consists of a connective-tissue stroma, in which are numerous alveoli, intersected by fine trabeculæ and filled with rounded cells, often possessing delicate processes. The follicles also contain considerable "brain sand." The organ is highly vascular and contains a plexus of sympathetic nerve-fibres.

The epiphysis is **congested** in inflammatory conditions.

Hemorrhage into its substance may occur with the formation of a hematoma.

Abscess has been met with in suppurative meningitis.

Hyaline degeneration of the vessels is described.

The calcareous matter may be notably increased (**psammoma**) and cysts may be present.

Hyperplasia and tumors occur.

Sarcoma[4] is the most important form. **Adenoma, chorioepithelioma**[5] and **dermoid cysts** also are described.

THE CAROTID GLAND.

Very little is written about the disorders of this curious little structure. Probably some of them escape observation on account of its small size and from the fact that it is but rarely examined. Some thirty cases of **tumors** have been described, all of them removed by operative procedure.

Histologically, they are **peritheliomas** and are highly vascular. They are composed of capillaries, about which are layers of epithelioid cells.

[1] Dixon and Halliburton, Quart. Jour. Exper. Physiol., 2:1909:283.
[2] Marburg, Arbeiten a. d. Neurolog. Inst. a. d. Wien. Univ., 17:1908:217.
[3] Lyon, Arch. of Inter. Med., 6:1910:28.
[4] Turner, Spindle-celled Sarcoma, Trans. Path. Soc. of London, 36:1885:27.
[5] Askanzy, Path. Gesell., 10:1906.

FIG. 179

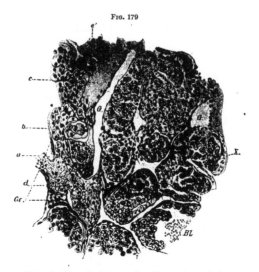

Tumor of the carotid gland; *Ge*, vessels; *Bl*, hemorrhage into a column of cells; at *d* the cells of the growth are taking on a more connective-tissue type; at *c*, hyaline degeneration.

FIG. 180

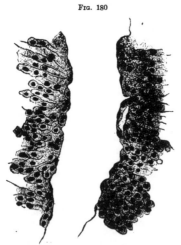

Portion of the same tumor more highly magnified to show peritheliomatous arrangement of the tumor cells in relationship to the vascular endothelium.   (Paltauf.)

The lobular arrangement of the gland is retained. So far, no case has been recorded in which there was recurrence or the formation of. metastases.[1]

THE COCCYGEAL GLAND.

The coccygeal gland, discovered by Luschka[2] in 1860, is a small body about the size of a pea, situated near the tip of the coccyx just above the coccygeal attachment of the sphincter ani, in the small tendinous interval formed by the union of the levator muscles of the anus. In structure, it somewhat resembles the carotid body, and is composed of numerous loops of bloodvessels, anastomosing freely with each other,

FIG. 181

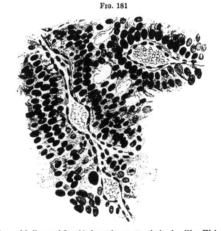

Section of a perithelioma of Luschka's or the coccygeal gland. (Von Hleb-Koszanka.)

derived from the middle sacral artery. These are enclosed in one or more layers of granular polyhedral cells, sharply differentiating it from the dense, fibrillar connective tissue round about. The whole structure is surrounded by a connective-tissue capsule, which sends in trabeculæ dividing the interior into a number of lobules. Sympathetic nerve and muscle fibres have also been demonstrated.

Its function is quite obscure. As already noted (p. 719), recent observations by demonstrating the absence of chromaffin cells and deficiency in sympathetic elements, as also by deriving its main cells from the plain muscle fibres of the arterial coat, place this gland in a cate-

---

[1] For literature see H. Gideon Wells, Ref. Handbk. Med. Sci., 8 : 1904 : 413. Another article is that of Paltauf, Ziegler's Beiträge, 11:1892.

[2] Die Steisdruse d. Menschen., Virch. Archiv, 18: 1860:106.

gory by itself.   But little, also, is known about its pathology.   Lus
thought that in it he had found the starting point of the various tu
of the sacral region.   Subsequent study has shown, however, tha
majority of these are to be classed as spinæ bifidæ, and new-gro
derived from misplaced "rests," or teratomas, and have no conne
whatever with the coccygeal gland.   Klebs has described a **cystosarc**
Fausto-Buzzi[1] an **angiosarcoma**, and Schmidt[2] a **teratoma**, appar
arising in this little body.

[1] Virch. Archiv, 109: 1887, 9.   [2] Ibid., 112: 1888: 372.

SECTION VI.

THE URINARY SYSTEM.

CHAPTER XXXIV.

THE URINARY FUNCTIONS AND THEIR DISORDERS.

THE kidneys are the chief excretory organs of the body. Their nature is glandular and their function is to secrete a fluid—the urine—and through it to eliminate the waste products of metabolism. Comparatively humble in size, they are nevertheless of importance second to none in the economy. As might be suspected from a consideration of the highly specialized character of their structure, disturbances of these glands are numerous, difficult to analyze, and far-reaching in their results. A knowledge of the development, of the anatomical peculiarities and relationships, of the normal functions of the renal organs, is an indispensable prerequisite, therefore, for the proper understanding of the various pathological processes to which they are subject. Of the development, because without it we cannot, for example, explain the incidence and character of many of the neoplasms found therein, or the striking association of the urinary and sexual organs in health and disease; of the anatomy, because it throws light on the origin and direction of disease processes; of the physiology, because disease is in a broad sense perverted function, and we can the better appreciate the relationships of the kidneys to other parts of the economy. Notwithstanding the immense amount of attention the subject has attracted for decades past, our knowledge has by no means attained finality. We are, unfortunately, still far from being assured about some of the most basal matters regarding the normal functions of the kidneys, and, as a consequence, there are many moot points in connection with the morbid disturbances of these organs and their significance.

EMBRYOLOGICAL CONSIDERATIONS.

The permanent kidney in man makes its first appearance about the fifth week of foetal life. At the cloacal end of the Wolffian duct there arises an evagination of cells, which project and finally invade a mass of mesoblastic tissue in the vicinity known as the blastema. As to the exact sequence of events, there has been considerable difference of opinion. The older view, to the effect that the primitive bud just referred to forms the ureter and the whole kidney tissue proper, including the glomeruli, has been displaced by that first advanced by Kupffer, Sedgwick, Gegenbaur and Wiedersheim, and more recently established by Herring, Schreiner, and Huber. The ureter, pelvis, calices and collecting tubules gain their origin from the Wolffian duct, the glomerular epithelium, the convoluted tubules, loops of Henle and junctional tubules from the blastema or nephrogenic tissue (see vol. i, p. 856, where also we discuss the bearing of these data upon the production of the congenital cystic kidney).

It is a striking fact that the great majority of the clinically important neoplasms of the kidney occur early in life, and are, moreover, of a very peculiar nature. They belong to the class of "mixed" tumors; that is to say, they are composed of a variety of tissues, glandular elements, muscle, connective tissue, fat, bone, and cartilage. They are, therefore, heterotopic and to be grouped with the terato-blastomas. The complicated evolution of the kidney. and its close proximity to the vertebral column and primitive myotomes provides at least a partial explanation of the frequency and distinctive character of these tumors (see vol. i, p. 661).

The close relationship existing between the Wolffian body and the genital gland, originating together, as they do, from the primitive genital ridge, explains why it is that developmental anomalies of the kidneys and reproductive organs are so apt to go together.

While the congenital vices of development of the kidneys and associated structures are numerous and for the most part of merely scientific interest, some few of them are of great practical importance, inasmuch as they may prove hazardous to life and may lead to errors in diagnosis and treatment. The various anomalies will be described later, but some few of them may be referred to now. For example, an ectopic or horseshoe kidney, if situated over the promontory of the sacrum, may be a cause of dystocia. Sudden congestion of a horseshoe kidney has led to pressure upon the underlying veins, with thrombosis and death. Again, a horseshoe kidney has been mistaken for an aneurism of the abdominal aorta. The puerperal uterus has compressed a displaced ureter and caused pyelonephritis. Worse than this, a patient's only kidney has been removed at operation, with, of course, disastrous results. A horseshoe kidney has been excised under the impression that it was a single misplaced organ. Cases of epispadias, hypospadias, extroversion of the bladder, and anomalous ureters often tax the resources of the surgeon.

ANATOMY AND ANATOMICAL RELATIONSHIPS OF THE KIDNEYS.

Some few points here call for brief consideration. The first is that the kidneys are relatively abundantly supplied with blood, and that at high pressure, for the renal arteries are short and directly connected with the aorta. The peculiar distribution of the vessels and its significance in regard to the secretory function will be referred to anon. The presently important fact is that the whole of the blood in the body passes sooner or later through the kidneys, and may, therefore, on occasion, bring about alteration in the local condition. Through the blood stream, too, the kidneys are brought into relationship with the heart, lungs, skin, muscles, and, indeed, with every part of the body Conversely, disease of the kidneys commonly produces a profound effect on other portions of the economy. Thus, it follows that toxins of all kinds and living microorganisms may readily be brought to the kidneys from primary foci elsewhere and set up serious pathological changes there. Such agents may act directly on the bloodvessels of the kidneys, thereby affecting the blood pressure and the rate of flow, factors which, as we shall see, are of primary importance in modifying the excretion of urine, or upon the stroma, or, more frequently, upon the parenchymatous cells. Again, circulatory obstructions in the heart or lungs lead to blood stasis in the renal organs, leading here, also, to changes both in the quantity and quality of the output. The lungs and skin, as important excretory organs, are complemental in function to the kidneys, and if extensively diseased would naturally throw more work on the latter. Affections of the kidneys which block the circulation or raise blood pressure are followed by hypertrophy and eventually dilatation of the heart, first and chiefly the left ventricle; those which cause substances ordinarily excreted to be retained bring about various degenerations elsewhere with vicarious action (and irritation sometimes amounting to inflammation) of the lungs, bowels, and skin.

A second point is that the kidneys are abundantly supplied with nerves, both vasomotor and secretory. Consequently, they are particularly susceptible to peripheral and central impressions. Mental states profoundly modify the amount of urine excreted (see pp. 546, 548), and various reflexes also, notably those from the bladder, genitalia, rectum, skin, and even the auditory and optic tracts.

A third point is that in the capsule of the kidney there is a plexus of unstriped muscle fibres, recalling those found in the spleen. This can hardly have any other significance than that, by contraction and relaxation, it promotes the circulation in these organs and thereby modifies excretion.

Fourthly, the kidneys are situated behind the peritoneum, usually surrounded by considerable fat, and comparatively remote from the other viscera. They are, therefore, well protected from injury and from those disease processes which spread by contiguity.

Finally, they are in communication with the external air, through the urinary passages, so that they may on occasion become infected from extraneous sources.

THE PHYSIOLOGY OF THE URINARY FUNCTIONS AND ITS APPLICATIONS.

We know, from a study of the liver, that some glands possessing excretory ducts may perform a double function—may discharge an internal as well as an external secretion, both being essential parts of their activity; they may so metabolize the material brought to them by the blood that some of the products are eliminated, others elaborated for the use of the economy. How far is this the case with the kidneys? It is difficult to say.

Upon general grounds it may be laid down that external excretion is the all-important function of these organs. Embryologically, the kidney of the higher animal is the homologue of the segmental ducts of the worms and other lowlier forms. And these segmental organs are tubes of direct communication between the body cavity and the exterior. There is no question regarding their function; they are primarily excretory, to discharge the excess body-fluid, nor are they of sufficient length to exercise extensive absorption from the fluid passing through them. Later, we find a stage in which the kidney possesses tubes having both a funnel-shaped orifice into the body cavity and glomeruli. Higher up again in the scale the funnels wholly disappear, the glomeruli taking their place. In other words, with the development of the blood-vascular system, the discharge of fluid is from the blood, and not from the body cavity. But simultaneously with the development of glomeruli, the relative length of the urinary tubules undergoes an extraordinary increase. What is the meaning of this? The cells lining these tubules assume further the character we have learned to associate with secretory cells; they do not form, at least so far as regards their cortical portions, a mere inert lining-epithelium. How do they act? Do they discharge material taken from the abundant surrounding capillaries into the lumen; or, on the contrary, do they resorb material useful for the economy which has been flushed out of the blood through the glomeruli; or, thirdly, do they accomplish both of those objects? Here, on general principles, we are forced to conclude that their *main* function is excretory, with discharge into the lumen of the tubules—and that because, when irritated or inflamed, we observe that it is the portion of the cell toward the lumen that undergoes well-marked breaking-down processes, with dissociation and discharge of its substance into the lumen, the discharge often taking the form of delicate fluid vesicles. So also it may, we think, be laid down as a broad principle that where a glandular surface has an absorptive function, there as large and not as small an area as possible is provided. The stomach, we know, has little absorptive, but active discharging powers, and in it we have abundant long tubules, but no villi; absorption of foodstuffs is at its height in the small intestine, and there we find abundant villous processes, affording the largest possible amount of surface. The structure of the renal tubules is the very reverse, the largest surface is exposed to the surrounding lymph, the smallest to the contained urine. The arrangement indicates that absorption from that lymph and discharge into the lumen is the main function.

It was considerations of this sort that led Bowman, in 1842, to propound his theory that the glomerulus "furnishes water to aid in the separation of the urinous products from the epithelium of the tube." Nor, must it be confessed, have we, in the last sixty years, advanced surely very much farther. Only two years later Ludwig enunciated the "mechanical theory," to the effect that under blood pressure a dilute fluid is filtered in abundance through the glomeruli, and that the function of the tubular epithelium is to concentrate this until it acquires the normal character of the urine. But, as pointed out by Heidenhain and his pupils, there are many objections to this theory. We shall not enter into the long-continued contest, or describe how, up to the present day, the battle has surged to and fro. For ourselves we cannot accept the Ludwig hypothesis, if only because, as Heidenhain pointed out, so small is the amount of urea in the blood that if this were removed by mere filtration, then no less than about 70 kilos of fluid would have daily to be filtered and resorbed by the tubules to explain the amount of urea present in the day's urine. This is asking altogether too much. Further, we have the fact, curiously neglected by the adherents of the filtration hypothesis, of the existence of hydronephrosis, and of its physiological cause, the fact that the pressure under which the urine is discharged into the pelvis is capable of being greater than the blood pressure; there is no escape from the conclusion that primarily this indicates an active excretory process. All the same, we have to admit that it is difficult to bring forward absolute evidence in favor of the secretory hypothesis. Heidenhain and others have attempted to prove the matter by demonstrating the passage into and through the cells of the convoluted tubules of indigo-carmine and other substances which are recognizable under the microscope, and in this and other ways, there has been accumulated a fair amount of evidence that the different regions of the renal tubules subserve different functions. But admittedly, it is difficult to obtain preparations by these means that are absolutely convincing and not capable of two interpretations; nay, with ordinary carmine, the bulk of evidence lies in the other direction.

Dreser's observations and the conclusions he has drawn from them present the same ambiguity. We know that the blood and lymph are alkaline in reaction, the normal urine in general acid. Dreser employed acid fuchsin as an indicator. This in acid solutions is of brilliant red color; almost colorless in weak alkaline solutions. Injecting the dye into the dorsal lymph-sac of a frog, the urine excreted in the course of an hour or two is of a brilliant red color. And now the glomerular regions of the kidneys on section were found to be almost colorless, *i. e.*, the discharge through the glomeruli was alkaline, the tubules below were filled with a bright red fluid. Here it will be seen there are two possibilities—either that the cells of the tubules excrete acid bodies, or that they absorb those bodies which give to the lymph its alkaline reaction. Were the latter the case, the cells of the tubules should be colorless. This they were, as a matter of fact, in the early stages of such experiments, but on repeating the injection, they assumed the red stain. On the whole, this staining must be regarded as favoring the secretion hypothesis. There is, however, indubitable evidence from Gurwitch's[1] experiments,

[1] Pflüger's Arch. f. d. Ges. Physiol., 91:1902:71.

that in the frog the convoluted tubules excrete pigment matter. In that animal there is a separate blood supply for the glomeruli and the **tubules** respectively. If the tubular blood supply (through the renal portal vein) be cut off, no pigment appears in the urine, although the pigment has free access to the glomeruli. The glomeruli and the cells of the convoluted tubules in the frog have the same general architecture as those in man, and this to a striking degree, and it would seem that if excretion occurs through the epithelium in the one animal, it must be the same in the other. Basler, by forcing pigment into the tubules from the ureter found no absorption, although under similar conditions sugar and ferro-cyanide solutions were absorbed and appeared in the urine of the other kidney. What is, however, most in favor of the secretion hypothesis is a consideration of the metabolic and constructive processes undergone in the kidney. One of these has been known for long. Hippuric acid is one of the normal constituents of the urine; it can be synthesized and excreted by the passage of glycine and benzoic acid through the vessels of the kidney. It is inconceivable that this conversion occurs in the glomeruli; we must conclude that it is brought about by the epithelium of the tubules. Uric acid, again, is a most insoluble substance; the abun-dance of the same in the urine of birds is such that we cannot believe that it passes out of the glomeruli in that form. In fact, we have indica-tions that it is not present in the blood as the acid, but as a more soluble sodium salt; while the researches of the late Sir William Roberts indicate that even in the renal tubules of the bird—and of man—it is first dis-charged as a compound salt, the "quadriurate," which undergoes disso-ciation with liberation and deposition of the uric acid. It is further note-worthy that uric acid introduced into the human economy appears largely in the urine as urea, while, contrariwise, urea fed to birds reappears as uric acid. When, further, as pointed out by Gowland Hopkins, we observe that the renal excretives are, as a class, more complex or less stable than their immediate precursors in the body, it is difficult not to conclude that the terminal steps of nitrogenous metabolism, whereby urea, uric acid, hippuric acid, creatinin and other bodies appear in the urine, are very largely controlled by the renal epithelium.

The Vascular Supply of the Kidney.—The distribution of the blood in the kidney is not a little remarkable, and possibly throws some light upon the mechanics of urinary excretion. In the first place the arterial supply of the cortex passes almost entirely to the glomeruli. A study of injected specimens shows that, with rare and inconsiderable exceptions, the interlobular branches of the cortical arteries pass to the glomeruli, constituting the afferent arterioles. The efferent vessels from the glomeruli break up into an intricate meshwork of capillaries around the convoluted tubules. On the other hand, in the medulla the blood supply of the collecting tubules is by a capillary network proceeding directly from the arteriæ rectæ. All are agreed that the main bulk of the water in the kidney passes out of the delicate walls of the glomeru-lar tuft. Cut off the glomerular blood supply, as in Nussbaum's well-known experiment upon the frog (which has a double blood supply through the renal arteries supplying the glomeruli, and the renal portal vein supplying the tubules), and the secretion of urine immediately falls to almost nil. It follows, therefore, that the blood circulating in the cortical capillaries, by having already passed through one capillary system (that of the glomeruli), is both more concentrated and under a lower pressure than that supplying the collecting tubules in the medulla. With a dilute urine, that is, in the convoluted tubules, and a low external blood pressure, we can imagine a resorption or reverse filtration of the urinary water from the tubules. These considerations would seem to favor Ludwig's theory, but the same line of thought would suggest that if this theory be accepted, when the urine reaches the collecting tubules its greater concentration, and the higher capillary blood pressure should favor additional discharge of water from the blood into the tubules.

That the discharge of urine is largely determined by circulatory conditions must be clearly accepted; reduce the general blood pressure by any means to 40 mm. Hg. or below, and the flow of urine ceases; increase the amount of blood circulating through the organ, as by ligaturing the arteries passing to important areas of the body, and the flow is greatly increased. Ludwig laid down that it is the blood pressure that mechanically determines the flow. Heidenhain, on the other hand, pointed out that if the renal vein be ligatured, the kidney becomes enormously congested, the blood pressure within it is greatly increased, and nevertheless there is a complete stoppage of urinary flow. It is, he postulated, the *rate of blood flow* through rather than the blood pressure in the glomeruli that determines the discharge. He concluded that with arrest of blood flow, the glomerular epithelium becomes asphyxiated, swollen and unable to function. Ludwig, on the other hand, explained the results as due to the intense capillary congestion causing compression and obstruction of the urinary tubules. The rapid resumption of urinary discharge in the inflamed and congested kidney which follows Edebohls' operation of decortication of the kidney, or excision of its capsule, favors Ludwig's explanation; but, on the other hand, it deserves note that the trend of modern work, as represented by the studies of F. Müller and Marchand and his school, is to ascribe the oliguria of acute nephritis more and more to glomerular lesions rather than to mechanical disturbances of the circulation.

From the above data it will be seen how difficult it is at the present time to reach any precise conclusion regarding the nature of the urinary discharge. On the whole, we conclude that while the water of the urine is in the main discharged through the glomeruli, along with sundry simple soluble salts and other substances (peptone, grape-sugar), that discharge is not a simple, but a selective filtration, and that while in the passage down the tubules there may be a resorption of certain constituents of the discharge, this resorption is of secondary importance compared with the active excretion of such substances as urea, uric acid, and other "extractives," bodies of the nature of toxins, coupled, it would seem, with active anabolic processes to form bodies like hippuric acid.

The Nerve Supply.—The nerves passing to the kidney form a fine plexus surrounding the renal artery. Various experiments have shown that these nerves are very largely vasomotor in function, although Berkeley, in his admirable studies of the terminal distribution of the nerve filaments within the organ, by means of Golgi's method, has demonstrated the existence of a wide network of filaments throughout the cortex and medulla with end knobs upon the Bowman's capsules and other terminations penetrating the membrana propria of the convoluted tubules, an arrangement which suggests strongly that these nerve-filaments are secretory in function. It is the vasomotor effects that have been most studied.

Section of the spinal cord in the cervical region, by removing the influence of the main medullary vasomotor centres, leads to a diffuse dilatation of the arteries of the trunk, and lowering of the blood pressure to 40 mm. Hg. or under, with which the urinary discharge is completely arrested. The renal vessels, along with the others, are relaxed, but at the same time the blood flow is so much diminished that the organ lessens in size. If, after such section the renal nerves be divided, and now the distal cut end of the cord be stimulated, there is pronounced general rise of blood pressure and resumption of the urinary flow. Such section of the renal nerves leads to vasomotor paralysis in the organ, and if practised alone, is also followed by increased flow of urine, in consequence of the augmented blood flow through the organ. Stimulation of the renal nerves, on the contrary, causes contraction of the organ and its vessels, and diminished urinary flow. The observations here are similar to what is observed with organs and vessels in general, namely, that disturbance of the tonic vasoconstrictor nerves may be demonstrated with fair ease. That vasodilators also exist has been shown by Bradford; appropriate stimulation of the anterior roots of the eleventh, twelfth and thirteenth dorsal nerves leads to definite expansion and congestion of the kidney without alteration in the general blood pressure. As Starling[1] points out, it is extremely probable that such vasodilator stimulation is the cause of the extreme hydruria encountered in hysteria and other nervous affections—and we may add, of the polyuria of emotional states. Similarly the anuria following catheterization is best ascribed to reflex extreme vasoconstrictor effects.

Recognizing, thus, the profound influence that the nervous system has upon the *amount* of the urinary discharge, it may be asked what is the mechanism whereby that discharge is controlled. The only satisfactory answer at the present time is that the amount of urine excreted is primarily dependent upon the glomerular blood supply, and this, in its turn, depends upon the tonus of the interlobular arteries. It is the relative contraction or dilatation of these arteries that determines the amount of blood entering the glomerular system. Histologically, a striking feature of the arteries in question is the good development of their muscular coat. Berkeley was unable to find any nerve-filaments

[1] Schäfer's Physiology, 1:1898:646.

passing into the glomerular loops; or otherwise, we have no evidence of independent contraction and expansion of the glomeruli; these are passive.

It is, to repeat, the afferent vessels that primarily determine the blood supply, and so the extent of excretion of the urinary fluid. Only secondarily the constituents of the blood as they act upon the capillary walls in the glomeruli may influence their filtration capacity. As with the arterioles in general (pp. 25 and 26), we have to recognize that contraction and expansion of these arterioles may be brought about either by central nervous influence, or directly by the action of substances diffusing out from the circulating blood.

The Relationship between Circulatory Disturbances and Chronic Interstitial Nephritis.—Where there has been a history of long-continued rise of general blood pressure, there we are apt to find the muscular coat of the cortical arteries hypertrophied—an indication of continued increased functional activity, and, whether from extreme contraction or from the later condition of "endarteritis obliterans," certain glomeruli undergo hyaline degeneration and become completely impervious. These now are represented as solid, shrunken, transparent bodies, and are a characteristic feature in the contracted areas of the granular contracted kidney of chronic interstitial nephritis. The simplest explanation of this hyaline degeneration is that it is a necrobiotic change induced by the progressive diminution of the blood supply, through arteriolar contraction and obliteration, preceded by a swollen state of the glomerular epithelium. It is to be noted that where certain glomeruli show this degeneration, others in their neighborhood exhibit the condition of (compensatory) hypertrophy, and may be of twice the normal diameter, with strikingly large capillary loops; and these it would seem are more pervious than normal, for in this condition of chronic interstitial nephritis, instead of there being a diminished excretion of urine, there is apt to be, on the contrary, an increased passing out of thin, watery urine of low specific gravity, containing a small amount of albumin, or, otherwise, these distended glomeruli permit an abundant discharge of fluid through their thinned walls, and with this, some escape of albumin from the blood plasma. Friedrich Müller is of opinion that this increased discharge is, in part, due to a modification in function of the epithelium of certain tubules. That epithelium becomes flattened and endothelial in type. This indicates, he holds, that now it permits the freer passage of fluid.[1]

We shall, in the ensuing chapter, describe the different forms of the contracted kidney—the postinflammatory, following upon an acute nephritis, the atrophic or senile, and the arteriosclerotic. It is this last, and the form allied to it, that we here refer to, pointing out that a similar sequence of changes occur in the cortex when there is intimal overgrowth with obliteration of the vascular lumen, and when, without such overgrowth, hypertrophy of the media and contraction of the

---

[1] Verhandl. d. Deutsch. pathol. Gesellsch., Meran, 9: 1905; 73.

arterioles lead to degeneration of certain of the glomeruli. In either case, if the glomerular supply be cut off, the capillary networks connected with the efferent veins of the affected glomeruli (1) receive no urine, and (2) have an impoverished surrounding blood supply. As a result, they undergo atrophy, and shrink until they are represented by columns of small cells with a scarcely visible lumen, and as they shrink there is some compensatory overgrowth of the surrounding interstitial connective tissue. Thus, as not all the interlobular arteries and their branches are similarly affected, we find areas of hyaline glomeruli and shrunken tubules with interstitial fibrosis alternating with other areas of distended glomeruli and large tubules with large lumina. This is the commonest type of so-called chronic interstitial nephritis, a contracted granular kidney, and, we would emphasize, in this the primary lesion would seem to be arterial.

Conclusions.—To sum up, it would seem that the quantity of urine discharged depends directly upon the quantity of blood flowing through the glomeruli. This blood flow depends in the first place upon the difference between the pressure in the renal artery, and that in the renal vein. If the arterial pressure be increased without increase in the venous, then the flow is greater, and the urinary excretion increases; if, on the contrary, through local obstruction or cardiac incompetence, the pressure in the renal vein be raised without corresponding rise in the arterial pressure, the urinary excretion is diminished. At the same time the size of the arterial channels in the kidney has to be taken into account; not only is there increased excretion when the general arterial pressure is raised, but without rise of this general pressure, if the interlobular and afferent arteries become dilated, there is increased blood flow and increased excretion, while, contrariwise, if without alteration of the general blood pressure the afferent arterioles undergo contraction, the glomerular circulation is diminished, and with this the urinary excretion falls.

As we need hardly remark, the primary duty of the kidneys is to separate out certain substances that are unnecessary or actually detrimental to the economy and to discharge them externally. These substances are in solution in the blood and are brought to the kidneys and dealt with there as we have just described. It is obvious, therefore, that the composition of the urine is dependent in large measure on the character of the blood. And here the important factors are the diet and the metabolic processes going on within the body. Variations in these will naturally produce marked effects. Yet we would emphasize that this is not the whole story. The secreting epithelium has to be taken into account. We have seen that even in health the epithelial cells exercise a selective function, permitting some substances to pass and retaining others, and, moreover, have the power to metabolize within themselves. These functions will undoubtedly be interfered with in the presence of kidney lesions, and so we have a third factor determining the character of the excretion, namely, the local condition within the kidney. The activities of the complemental organs, lungs, skin, and intestines, will also be of moment. It follows, therefore, that the composition of the urine is a valuable index to, and to some extent a measure of, the metabolic processes going on in the body and of the condition of the urinary apparatus. A thorough knowledge of urinary chemistry is, then, of the greatest value in diagnosis and treatment.

The disturbances of the urinary functions may conveniently be dealt with under the heads of excretion and conduction (or urination).

DISORDERS OF EXCRETION.

These may be classed into three groups: (1) The excretion of a urine normal as to composition but abnormal in quantity; (2) the excretion in abnormal amount of substances normally present in the urine; (3) the excretion of substances not normally found in the urine. With regard to the first possible group, it is conceivable, of course, that in any given sample of urine the percentage of the various constituents might vary considerably from the normal and yet the total output for the twenty-four hours might fall within natural limits; in other words, the urine might be increased or diminished, dilute or concentrated. It may well be doubted, however, whether the case is ever so simple as this. The quantity of the excretion, as we have seen, is to a large extent dependent on questions of blood pressure and the amount of blood circulating through the organs. In obstructive heart disease, for example, the total output of urine is often much diminished, but there are undoubtedly qualitative changes as well, to wit, among other things, the presence of albumin. From a consideration also of the various forms of polyuria, it is clear that in some cases at least the excretion of urinary salts does not occur necessarily in the same relative proportion as it does in normal states. Contrary to the general teaching, the degree of intracapillary blood pressure does not affect the rate of filtration, and we have to look for the explanation of the phenomenon in the different degrees of concentration of the urine in the matter of the individual salts or else in the selective properties of the kidney epithelium. Though our information is defective on this particular, it is quite possible that the excretion of urinary salts may exhibit specific difference in the cases, for example, of the polyurias of hysteria, cerebral disease, and diabetes insipidus. Nevertheless, the striking feature is the increase in the water, and it is, therefore, convenient to discuss here the quantitative variations of the urine, always, however, with a mental reservation.

Polyuria.—According to the general principles we have laid down, polyuria and increased excretion of urine may be brought about (1) by increase in the general arterial pressure without renal change, or (2) dilatation of the cortical arterioles without, of necessity, any rise in the general blood pressure. The condition of *diabetes insipidus* would seem to come under the second category. Here we encounter an excessive discharge of a thin, watery urine free from sugar. There is a tendency toward increased excretion of urea (in the twenty-four hours), although this is attributed to the increased consumption of food which, as in diabetes mellitus, is often present. A marked feature of this disturbance is the frequent presence of inosite in the urine.   Inosite, $C_6H_{12}O_6$, is a benzene derivative found in muscle, liver, and other organs, and, it may be added, seen also in the urine of other pathological conditions.[1] The condition has often been noted as affecting several members of the same family. In other cases brain lesions have been present, affecting the pons, cerebellum, or medulla.   This suggests that disturbance of the vasomotor centres in the medulla may play a role.   Experimentally, as shown by Claude Bernard, a similar polyuria may be brought about by injury to the medulla, and, as already noted, transient polyuria, evidently of the same order, is seen in hysterical and emotional states.

With this increased discharge there is, broadly speaking, a corresponding decrease in the total solids of the urine; the solids, that is to say, are reduced, although the reduction of the different constituents is not parallel, and individual cases show variation in its extent.   The total amount of sodium chloride, for example, is independent of the amount of urine, suggesting that ,the escape of the salt is governed, and is not a mere act of filtration.

These considerations lead to a reference to the action of diuretics, and the recognition of a very possible third factor in the production of polyuria. Of such diuretics there are two groups: those inducing heightened blood pressure plus improved circulation through the kidney, of which digitalis is an example; and those having little or no effect upon the general blood pressure, among which are to be included the soluble crystalloid substances—dextrose, urea, sodium chloride, and other saline diuretics. Regarding the former there is this to be noted, that drugs which cause heightened blood pressure accomplish this by contraction of the arterioles, and thus we must conclude either that the diuretic members of this group have a specific lack of action upon the renal vessels, or that the rise in blood pressure more than compensates the contraction of the renal vessels.   As a matter of fact, the drug that causes the most extreme arteriolar contraction—adrenalin—materially reduces the flow of urine, and digitalis is often without diuretic effect upon individuals in sound health. As regards the latter, it is still a matter of debate as to whether they act by local specific dilatation of the renal vessels (for the kidneys exhibit distinct enlargement), or directly stimulate the renal cells, their discharge through these being accompanied by an amount of water necessary to retain them in a state of solution.   It has been urged that all these salts abstract water from the tissues, render the blood more hydremic, and so favor increased filtration; the fact that these salts initiate excretion when added to the blood perfused through the extirpated kidney supports the other evidence we possess that these salts are largely discharged through the tubular epithelium, that they exercise a direct secretory influence. As shown by Schäfer and Herring, a direct diuretic action, independent of increased circulation, is exerted by pituitary extract.   ·

[1] See Meillère, Inosurie, Paris, 1906.

Oliguria and **Anuria.**—Along similar lines it is to be laid down that reduction or suppression of urinary flow can be brought about (1) by direct contraction of the afferent arterioles (as through the action of adrenalin), (2) by a lowering of the arterial pressure, or (3) a rise in the venous pressure. These last two may be combined and expressed by saying that a reduction in the difference between arterial and venous pressure leads to oliguria. Examples of lowered arterial pressure have already been given; of raised venous pressure, the oliguria accompanying obstructive heart disease is the commonest example. A fourth cause needs to be taken into consideration, namely, obstruction to the outflow, provided that this affects both kidneys. Such obstruction may occur within the renal tubules through blockage of the same with inspissated excretion, as in renal hematuria and hemoglobinuria, or along the course of the ureters and passages of discharge.

As we have stated, there is still debate as to how far the oliguria of acute nephritis is due to swelling of the tubular epithelium and obliteration of the lumen of the tubules as a result of congestion; how far it is due to glomerular disturbance. At the Meran meeting of the German Pathological Society, Friedrich Müller[1] laid down very precisely that the oliguria of acute nephritis is correlated to the extent of glomerulonephritis found present. The acute swelling of the glomerular epithelium, followed by proliferation of the same, arrests the function of these organs. Löhlein,[2] from Marchand's laboratory, has made an extended study of the glomerular changes in different forms of nephritis, and concludes that two types of acute nephritis are to be determined: (1) in which the tubular epithelium alone is involved (kidneys of cholera and diphtheria, of sublimate poisoning, and many kidneys of pregnancy; such kidneys, owing to the great regenerative power of the tubular epithelium, may undergo rapid and complete healing); and (2) what he would term acute nephritis proper, in which the glomeruli are characteristically involved. Of this the classical example is the scarlatinal kidney. Here the extent of the tubular change appears to depend upon the severity of the glomerular change. Of chronic forms of the disease, he lays down that chronic parenchymatous nephritis (chronic nephritis with dropsy) is a later stage of unhealed glomerulonephritis, or a septic glomerulonephritis of insidious origin. So also the "secondary contracted kidney"—the contracted kidney following upon acute nephritis—shows regularly changes in the glomeruli, exhibiting transition stages to those seen in the acute disease.

The substances excreted in the urine are of various orders and of very diverse origin. Some are the product of the ordinary processes of digestion and assimilation; some are the result of the normal metabolic processes of the body; some are the consequence of abnormal metabolic processes; some, again, are due to the action of extrinsic agents, bacteria,

---

[1] Verhandl. d. Deutsch. pathol. Gesellsch., 9: 1905: 64.
[2] Ueber die entzündlichen Veränderungen der Glomeruli der menschlichen Nieren, Leipzig, Hirgel, 1907.

for example, and various metallic and other poisons absorbed into the system; still others, possibly, though we have little information on this point, depend upon disturbances of the renal epithelium. The following is a list of the more important substances found normally in the urine, some of them, however, being present only in minute traces: Acetone, achroglycogen, allantoin, carbamic acid (rarely), chlorides, cholesterin, chondroitin, creatin (?), creatinin, diacetic acid, diastatic ferments, glucose, hematoporphyrin, indican, isomaltose, lactose, mucin, nucleinic acid, nucleoalbumin, orthocresol, oxalic acid, oxaluric acid, paracresol, paraoxyphenylacetic acid, paraoxyphenylpropionic acid, phosphates, pentose, pigments, proteolytic ferments, ptomaines, purin bases (?), pyrocatechin, sulphates, urea, uric acid, volatile fatty acids.

To take up the origin and the chemical relationships of these substances would demand more space than we can afford here, besides necessitating the consideration of questions of general nutrition and metabolism that have already been dealt with at some length in our first volume. We shall, therefore, confine ourselves almost entirely to the mention of some practical points in connection with a few of them.

Urea.—The excretion of this substance depends upon (1) the ingestion of nitrogenous foods, and (2) the breaking down of the organized albumin of the body. The amount eliminated in the urine of a healthy individual on a mixed diet varies from 20 to 45 grams daily. It is said that the quantity is increased in febrile diseases and diabetes mellitus; decreased in all conditions of malnutrition and in affections of the liver and kidney parenchyma. It should be noted, however, that the important question is not how much urea is eliminated through the kidneys, but the amount of nitrogen excreted by all channels. This phase of the subject will be referred to again.

Uric Acid.—A normal adult excretes from 0.2 to 1.25 grams of uric acid in the twenty-four hours. This is chiefly, if not entirely, derived from the katabolism of the nucleins contained either in the food or the body tissues. Pathologically, the uric acid of the urine is increased in febrile affections and wherever there is a loss of tissue albumin. The absolute increase found in leukemia is to be attributed probably to the katabolism of large numbers of leukocytes.

Creatinin.—This is present in the urine in amounts fluctuating between 0.6 and 1.3 grams for the daily output. The amount excreted depends largely upon the diet. A large intake of meat produces a relatively large output of creatinin. It also is produced by the disassimilation of the muscular tissue of the body. The amount of creatinin in the urine is increased by physical exercise, in diabetes and febrile disturbances; it is diminished in chronic nephritis, anemia, chlorosis, diabetes insipidus, tuberculosis, and in convalescence from acute disease. Its further exact significance is not well understood.

Oxaluric and Oxalic Acids.—These may be conveniently and properly dealt with together, for they are chemically and probably genetically related. Oxaluric acid by hydration splits up into oxalic acid and urea. The former occurs in the urine only in traces, usually as an ammonium salt. The latter is always to be found, most commonly as the calcium salt. Oxalic acid may be derived from sundry articles of food, such as rhubarb, asparagus, spinach, apples, and grapes. It is sometimes formed as an intermediate product in the breaking down of glucose. The normal amount of oxalic acid excreted in twenty-four hours is about 0.02 gram. This quantity may be increased in diabetes, and even without evident cause. Curiously, it sometimes happens in diabetes that as the amount of sugar in the urine decreases, the amount of oxalic acid increases.

Aromatic Bodies.—These are produced by the breaking down of albumins. They may be ingested as such in the food, may be absorbed from the intestine, where they are formed through bacterial decomposition, or they may be metabolized in the tissues with or without the intervention of bacteria. As a rule, they are met with in combination with sulphuric acid, glycuronic acid, or glycocoll, so we can recognize three main groups —(1) the conjugate sulphates, (2) the compound glycuronates, and (3) the compound glycocolls. To these we may add the aromatic oxyacids which occur free and uncombined. The chief substances in the first group are the *phenols*, including cresol, paracresol, pyrocatechin, and hydroquinon; *indican*, and *skatoxylsulphuric acid*. Paracresol is the most abundant in the urine, next to this, phenol, and the others are found only in small amounts. The average amount of phenol excreted is 0.03 gram *per diem*. It is increased in constipation, peritonitis, suppuration, pyemia, diabetes mellitus, and in phosphorus poisoning. Pyrocatechin and hydroquinone are found in the urine in cases of carbolic acid poisoning.

Indican, the ethereal sulphate of indoxyl, like the phenols, is a product of the putrefaction of albumin. Whenever, therefore, indican is present in the urine, we find phenol in somewhat parallel amounts. Conversely, however, the presence of phenol does not signify the presence of indican. On a mixed diet, from 2 to 50 mg. of indican can be recovered from normal urine. A meat diet increases the amount; a vegetable diet decreases it. Indicanuria, pathologically, is present in all conditions favoring intestinal putrefaction, as, for example, in ileus, peritonitis, appendicitis, cholera, typhoid, gastric ulcer, gastrectasis, and lead colic. Large amounts have been found also in empyema, putrid bronchitis, melanosis, and carcinoma of the liver, stomach, and uterus.

Glycuronic acid does not occur free in the urine, but only in combination with other substances, such as phenol, paracresol, indoxyl, and skatoxyl. It is presumably derived from glycogen (by way of glucose) and chondroitin-sulphuric acid. It is present in diabetic urine. In this connection it is important to remember that glycuronic acid can reduce metallic oxides, so that in certain cases a positive Fehling test may give rise to an erroneous conclusion. Unlike sugar, however, it is not fermentable.

Glycocoll (amido-acetic acid) combines with the aromatic products of albuminous decomposition to form *compound glycocolls,* of which the most important are hippuric acid and phenaceturic acid.

Hippuric acid may be derived from phenylpropionic acid and its oxidation product, benzoic acid, which substances are produced in intestinal putrefaction. Certain vegetables forming a part of our diet, notably those which contain cinnamic and quinic acids, and toluol, and thereby lead to the formation of benzoic acid, may cause an increased excretion of hippuric acid. Such are cranberries, plums, and prunes. The normal average excretion on a mixed diet (without any of the above-mentioned fruits) is 0.6 gram.

The chief aromatic oxyacids are paraoxyphenyl acetic acid and paraoxyphenyl propionic acid. They also are due to the katabolism of proteins, whether in the bowel or in the tissues. In acute poisoning by phosphorus or carbolic acid they may be present in greatly increased amount.

Hematoporphyrin.—The origin of this is quite obscure. It has been found in greatly increased amounts in the urine in cases of typhoid fever, Addison's disease, anemia, lead poisoning, cirrhosis of the liver, exophthalmic goitre, rheumatism, and gout.

For the significance of **diacetic acid, acetone,** and the various **sugars,** the reader is referred to vol. i, p. 380, of this work.

Among the substances not normally present in the urine we may mention albumoses, alkaptonic acids, β-oxybutyric acid, bile pigments, blood, cadaverin, chyle, cystin, fibrinogen, globulins, glycogen, hematin, hemoglobin, lactic acid, leucin, levulose, melanin, putrescin, serum albumin, tyrosin, and urobilin. With the exception of the important subject of albuminuria, our references to these must be very brief.

Albuminuria.—Various proteins may appear in the urine—unchanged from absorbed food, as egg-albumin after an excessive diet of raw eggs, mucins in inflammatory or degenerative states of the kidneys, nucleo-albumin and nucleinic acids from disintegration of the renal parenchyma (although these bodies may also be derived from the urinary passages and bladder). But these are inconsiderable in amount and frequency of appearance, as compared with serum albumin and the serum globulins. It is with these latter bodies that we are specially concerned when we speak of albuminuria. They are the dominant proteins of the blood plasma, hence their presence in the urine in the main indicates an abnormal escape of these colloidal constituents of the fluid of the blood.

This, in the first place, may be laid down with precision; unlike the ordinary capillaries, the glomerular loops do not normally permit the escape of the proteins of the plasma. Take, on the one hand, a perfectly healthy kidney immediately after death; cut off small pieces of the cortex, and plunge into boiling water or a solution of corrosive sublimate, and make sections; the capsule chambers of the Malpighian bodies are found perfectly free from any coagulum. Take, on the other hand, the kidney of an animal in which by one or other means albuminuria has been induced; repeat the process, and now in many of the capsule chambers larger or smaller menisci of coagulated albumin are to be seen. It is clear from this, in the first place, that albumin does not normally filter through the glomeruli to be subsequently resorbed in its passage down the tubes; and in the second, that, when albuminuria develops, the main discharge is through the delicate walls of the glomerular tuft. In the frog, and even in much higher animals, the presence of long cilia in the neck or first part of the renal tubule hinders regurgitation of urine from the tubule into the capsule chamber; this albumin, therefore, cannot have been excreted in the first place into the convoluted tubules.

Is this the only source of the albumin? Probably not. It is inherently probable, that is, that in acute nephritis, with the active disintegration of the tubular epithelium there occurring, the products of the broken-down cells swell the amount of albuminous bodies present in the urine. So, also, when the tubular epithelium becomes so disorganized that it is cast off and the naked basement membrane alone left, albumin-containing lymph may exude into the damaged tubules; and thus in acute nephritis with diminished urine, and that so full of albumin that in heating it clots into a solid mass, it may well be that the tubules as distinct from the glomeruli, have contributed a considerable proportion of the proteins. But in the milder and more chronic cases, we are safe to conclude that the bulk of the albumins have been discharged through the glomeruli. Here it is of interest to recall that cell-disintegration is not necessarily associated with the presence of albumin in the urine; casts, the coagulated products of cell-disintegration, may be present in urine that gives no reaction for albumin. Most often the albumin consists of serum albumin alone, but the proportion may vary within wide limits, and Maguire[1] and others have recorded cases in which the globulins alone were present, or with traces of serum albumin so small that they could not be estimated. And this notwithstanding that, according to Salvioli, the proportion of albumin to globulin in the blood plasma (roughly 3 : 2) is remarkably constant, and that from their constitution, the globulins should be the more diffusible. Here, we have some of the strongest evidence that the glomeruli are not simple filters, but exert a selective or controlling influence upon the fluid passing through their walls. What then are the conditions favoring albuminuria? This question is perhaps best answered by detailing the conditions under which albuminuria is encountered.

1. *Physiological Albuminuria.*—Albumin is apt to appear in the urine after cold baths, and violent exertion, the latter more particularly if partaken of in the morning, soon after change from the supine to the erect position. In these conditions it is supposed that glomerular congestion, with dilatation of the capillary loops, favors the exudation.

2. *Cyclical Albuminuria.*—This is noted more especially in boyhood and adolescence, although cases are on record in which it has continued into adult life. The subjects may appear to be in excellent health, but usually they complain of tiring easily. The characteristic feature is that albumin is absent from the urine passed on rising, but after this makes its appearance, rising rapidly in amount until the forenoon, dis-

[1] *Lancet*, London, 1: 1886: 1062 and 1100.

appearing in the afternoon. In some of these cases paraglobulin **alone** is present. Here, again, the change in the circulation accompanying the change from the resting to the erect, active state would appear to be a primary factor, although with it there must be assumed a peculiar sensitiveness or idiosyncrasy of the glomerular epithelium. The condition may follow scarlet fever, in which we know that the glomeruli are peculiarly liable to be affected, and has been noted after other fevers. There is no clear evidence that this form passes on to chronic nephritis, although Dukes, one of the first to call attention to its frequency among schoolboys, has placed on record cases in which, after disappearance, it has shown itself again years later under various stresses.

3. *Albuminuria from Circulatory Disturbances.*—Anything which materially slows the rate of blood flow through the kidneys favors the supervention of albuminuria, and this presumably by partial asphyxia, and, therefore, imperfect function of the glomeruli with or without dilatation of the capillary loops. Thus, on the one hand, contraction of the renal arteries, as in lead colic, or, more commonly, on the other, various obstructions (as from heart disease or local obstruction of the renal vein) is accompanied by a definite grade of albuminuria. In the former case there is lowered pressure in the glomeruli and renal capillaries, in the latter, heightened pressure. In both forms the amount of urine excreted is reduced. In both cases also it is possible that the malnutrition of the tubules leads to some disintegration of the parenchyma, and to a contributory albuminuria from this cause.

4. *Toxic Albuminuria.*—There are various drugs which appear to act more particularly on the tubules—to be excreted through those tubules and, indeed, to influence specifically particular regions of the same. Perhaps the most marked examples have been afforded from Ehrlich's laboratory, Levaditi[1] and Rehns[2] having shown that vinylamin and tetrahydroquinoleïne cause a necrosis strictly localized to the papillæ and collecting tubules. More often, as by sublimate and cantharidin, the convoluted tubules are involved. Some of these in their action induce a well-marked albuminuria. Here, we include chrome and various other metallic salts, cantharidin, various balsams, several bacterial toxins, and the so far unknown toxic substance of the eclamptic state. As already noted, Löhlein and others doubt whether the degenerative changes set up by these agents should be classed as true nephritis. With some of these there is evidence of accompanying glomerular disturbance, but in general the parenchymal disturbance is so severe that we may attribute the albuminuria mainly to this cause.

5. *Infectious Albuminuria.*—As laid down on page 757, the typical acute nephritis of infectious disease, notably of scarlatina and streptococcal conditions, is characterized by pronounced irritation and disturbance of the glomeruli, and here in general we find the most abundant discharge of albumin. The disturbance in some cases is so acute that

---

[1] Arch. internat. de Pharmacodynamie et Therap., 8: 1901: 45.
[2] Ibid., p. 199.

there is an escape of blood corpuscles through the glomeruli (acute hemorrhagic nephritis).[1] With these changes there develop also notable disturbances of the parenchyma, with cloudy swelling, fatty degeneration, necrosis and desquamation. More rarely, as in scarlatina, there may be associated an acute interstitial nephritis, with accumulations of plasma cells between the tubules.

Albumoses.—Most of the substances referred to by the older writers under the term "peptone" have been shown to be albumoses (hemialbumose; deutero-albumose; propeptone; histone). They appear in the urine in conditions in which the intracellular katabolism of proteins is perverted, as, for example, tuberculosis, suppuration, phosphorus poisoning, and osteomalacia. In the case of exudates it may sometimes be possible by testing for these substances to determine between purulent and simple effusions. A special form, that should be mentioned here, is *Bence-Jones' albumin*, which is an albumose, though differing in some respects from all other known albumoses. It is found in the urine in cases of multiple myelomata of bone. *Histone* and *nucleohistone*, derived from nuclei, are found where there has been much breaking down of leukocytes.

Hematuria.—Blood may appear in the urine from a variety of causes. These may be operative either in the kidney itself or in the urinary passages. When in large amounts it may be suspected by the dark or bright red color of the urine, or by the presence of coagula. Its presence may be determined with certainty by one of several tests, the spectroscope, the guaiacum or other chemical reaction, or the microscope. It occurs in certain forms of acute and chronic nephritis, in malignant tumors of the kidney, papillary angioma, polycystic disease, hemophilia, angioneuroses, nephrolithiasis, twist of the pedicle, trauma, and various inflammations of the ureters, bladder, and urethra.

Hemoglobinuria.—Besides the hematuria above mentioned, there may be escape of dissolved hemoglobin into the urine. Experimentally, this may be brought about in a variety of ways, by introducing substances into the circulation which cause hemolysis (large quantities of water, glycerin, pyrogallic acid, toluylenediamin, etc.). In disease, hemoglobinuria also follows acute hemolysis (after snake bite, potassium chlorate poisoning, and in paroxysmal hemoglobinuria). We have discussed these conditions in our first volume (p. 880), and only refer to them here to note that, as shown by one of us,[2] it is possible to demonstrate the discharge of hemoglobin through the glomeruli when the blood pressure is so low that anuria has set in, as also to obtain a urine containing three times the amount of hemoglobin present in the blood

---

[1] As Cornil well pointed out, the capsule chamber of the glomeruli may be compared with a serous sac like the pericardium or pleural cavity. It may be affected by the same series of acute inflammatory changes, and with continued subacute inflammation may show proliferative changes in its epithelium and the development of synechia and localized adhesions.

[2] Adami, Jour. of Physiol., 6: 1886: 382.

plasma. In other words, the presence of hemoglobin in the urine is due to active excretion, and not mere filtration.

Chyluria.—Rarely, we encounter cases in which the urine is diluted with lymph. Such chyluria may persist with exacerbations over long years. When due to renal disturbance, the cause is now generally regarded as a lymphangiectatic condition affecting the papillæ, with rupture of one or more of the dilated vessels.

Melanin.—This is occasionally found in the urine in persons the subjects of melanotic new-growth. The urine turns dark on standing. Before diagnosticating melanuria it is necessary to exclude the presence of indican and urobilinogen by appropriate tests.

Lactic Acid.—This is found in the urine in cases where the urea-forming power of the liver is impaired or in some perversion of glycolysis. We get it, therefore, in phosphorus poisoning, acute yellow atrophy of the liver, in asphyxia, carbon monoxide poisoning, trichinosis, excessive muscular strain, and epilepsy.

For the significance of **alkaptonic acids,** and **tyrosin** in the urine see vol. i, page 379.

DISTURBANCES OF THE FUNCTION OF URINATION.

Under this caption we have to consider the mechanism, muscular and nervous particularly, by which the evacuation of the excretion from the kidneys is rendered possible. The urinary passages, as distinct from those of the kidney, which are not dealt with here, are the pelves, ureters, bladder, and urethra. With the exception of the bladder, these structures act merely as conduits. The functions of the bladder are two—to act as a reservoir and to promote elimination. The kidney pelvis, while anatomically also a reservoir, has little to do with storage, but is to be regarded as functionally merely an amplification of the ureter necessary as a collecting surface. The disorders of the conducting apparatus are of importance mainly in proportion to the amount of obstruction they produce. The conditions to be thought of in this connection are: (1) Those obstructing the lumina, such as calculi, tumors, blood clot, necrotic tissue, kinks, twists, and parasites; (2) those producing thickening of the walls, such as tumors, inflammatory exudations, and hyperplasias; and (3) those operating from without, such as tumors, inflammatory exudates, misplaced organs, the pressure or traction of fibrous bands, ligatures, enlarged glands, and the like.

A rarer cause of disability is a solution of continuity somewhere in the conducting apparatus, whereby the urine is diverted from its natural course. This condition of things, known as **extravasation of urine,** is of great moment, inasmuch as it leads to inflammation, necrosis, and infection of the tissues involved.

The effects produced by obstruction depend mainly upon the degree and site of the lesion and upon whether one or both kidneys are concerned. Where the obstruction is partial (and urethral) urination may be conducted sufficiently well, but may be slowed or require straining. The passages above the point of blockage will at first be distended, but the walls quickly become hypertrophied under the strain of the increased work, and there may, for a considerable period, be very little further deviation from the normal. This hypertrophy is most marked in the case of the bladder. When the obstruction becomes excessive, hypertrophy gives way to dilatation, and the disability thereupon becomes aggravated. A common result of all this is that the resisting power of the tissues is lessened and infection is readily brought about. Where the urine stagnates it ferments, and we get a local irritation and inflammation of passages containing it, but more than this, an infection which is apt to travel upward and involve the kidney. We thus not uncommonly have the production of an "ascending" suppurative nephritis, the so-called "surgical kidney." The effects of dilatation are most strikingly seen in the case of the pelvis and kidney itself. Where some discharge of urine is possible, with intermittent increased pressure, the pelvis enlarges and there is a gradual compression and atrophy of the kidney substance, which continues until the organ is represented by a multiloculated cyst of great size, the walls of which, however, though but a millimeter or two thick, still present indications of glomeruli and tubules (**hydronephrosis**). If, on the other hand, the obstruction to the onflow of the urine be complete and permanent, the kidney rapidly atrophies and the amount of hydronephrosis is nothing like so great. The effect on the secretory activity of the kidney in such cases depends upon the amount of back pressure exerted. If the pressure above the point of obstruction amounts to 60 mm. of mercury, secretion comes to an end; if less, it is proportionately diminished. Apparently what happens is this. The retained urine at first causes merely distension of the various passages; then, with the increase of pressure, some of the fluid is resorbed by the kidney epithelium. The distended tubules and swollen cells then press upon the veins and capillaries, lessening the flow of blood through the kidney, and thereby diminishing the amount of secretion.

We now direct our special attention to the bladder, for this is the organ most concerned in regulating the function of urination. Were it not for the bladder, the urine would be continually dribbling away, a state of affairs that would be highly objectionable in more ways than one. It acts, first, as a reservoir, thereby greatly promoting our comfort; and secondly, as a mechanism for evacuation. Functionally, it consists of two elements, a detrusor muscle, which by its contraction drives the urine out, and a sphincter muscle, which enables this fluid to be retained. These actions are governed by the nervous system. In infants urination is entirely reflex, being set in operation by peripheral impulses, particularly the condition of distension of the bladder. Later, through education, the child is enabled to control and time the function. There are, therefore, a reflex centre and a cerebral centre. The former is situated in the sympathetic system and not in the lumbar cord, as used to be thought.[1] The sphincter is, to a large extent, a voluntary muscle. When the call comes for evacuation, the sphincter relaxes, a small amount of urine enters the membranous urethra (owing to the pressure the prostatic portion has previously become distended and funnel-shaped), the stimulus becomes imperative, and the detrusor contracts, expelling the contents. The factors governing the reflex irritability are the amount of distension of the viscus, the condition of the mucosa, and the character of the urine. An inflamed bladder will evacuate itself frequently even with a minimum of distension, and a similar result will be produced by highly concentrated acid urine. The intense desire to make water, associated with the ability to pass only a small quantity, and that with much straining, is known as *strangury*.

Retention of urine is due to one of several causes, apart, of course, from the cases due to actual physical obstruction of the urethra; lack of the necessary peripheral stimuli, paralysis of the detrusor, spasm of the sphincter, and loss of the mental control. Anesthesia of the bladder wall, lesions of the motor paths leading to the bladder, irritation of the tracts connecting the cerebral with the reflex centre, may be mentioned in this connection. The influence of mental inhibition is well seen not infrequently in certain neurotic individuals who are unable to urinate in the presence of others or on occasions when they are particularly anxious to do so. Cases are met with also quite often in acute febrile diseases, for example, typhoid fever and pneumonia. This is probably due to benumbing of the sensorium (in the earlier and more severe stages of the affections) or to general bodily weakness (in the later periods and during convalescence). The retention that occurs after childbirth and after operations upon the rectum or pelvic viscera is harder to analyze, and appears to depend on a combination of factors. In many cases, when the retention has led to overdistension of the bladder, the resulting pressure upon the sphincter may lead to a continual escape of urine, which may delude the patient and his friends into the belief that urination is sufficiently satisfactory (*incontinence of retention*). Gradually it may come about in such cases that the bladder empties itself reflexly, just as in infancy. The retention found at times in locomotor ataxia and amyotrophic lateral sclerosis is due probably either to diminution of the sensibility of the bladder or interference with the cerebral motor impulses. Milder grades of the various affections mentioned above, while not leading to complete retention, may produce delay in starting the act, straining, and weakness of propulsive power. Again, overdistension of the vesical

---

[1] L. R. Müller, Zeitschr. f. Nervenheilk., 21:86.

muscle may induce inability to contract. One variety of this should be mentioned, as it is not uncommon and of great practical importance. This is the local distension or sacculation involving the lower and posterior portion of the bladder wall met with in cases of enlarged prostate. Owing to the weight of the retained urine and the weakness of the muscle induced by the associated inflammation, the wall gives way at this point, and even if the expulsive power of the bladder be otherwise adequate, it becomes a physical impossibility to completely empty the organ. Thus, a certain amount of urine is always retained within (residual urine), which ferments, leading to irritation, inflammation, the formation of calculi, and even toxemia.

Incontinence of urine is the inability to retain it within the bladder. Two varieties of this are recognized—paralytic incontinence, in which there is weakness of the sphincter; and spasmodic incontinence, in which there is overaction of the detrusor. The former is met with in marantic states and convalescence from prolonged acute disease, from traumatism, the pressure of the fœtal head during parturition, the pressure of tumors on the base of the bladder and urethra, and as a consequence of an overfilled bladder. The latter is due to some form of irritation of the mucosa or muscular wall, such as may be found in cystitis, vesical calculus, and parasites.

Nocturnal enuresis is a form, found usually in young children, that is due to the excessive response of an unstable nervous system to some peripheral stimulus. Thus, the presence of intestinal worms, phimosis, a narrow meatus, anal fissures, adenoids, have all been regarded as producing the necessary irritation. It should not be forgotten, also, that nocturnal enuresis may be an indication of the occurrence of nocturnal epileptic attacks.

Relaxation of the sphincters, with resulting loss of urine, is met with also during states of insensibility and coma, epilepsy, and in high fevers.

THE INFLUENCE OF BODILY STATES ON THE PRODUCTION OF KIDNEY LESIONS.

From what has already been said in regard to the nature of the renal functions, it will readily be concluded that the chief factor in the production of kidney lesions is the blood. The amount supplied to the kidneys and its character largely determine the result. The circulatory disturbances of importance here are of two kinds: (1) Those leading to a diminished supply of blood to the kidneys, such as arteriosclerosis, arterial spasm, and a weak heart muscle; and (2) those producing an abnormal retention of blood within the organs, such as obstruction in the renal veins, conditions causing a general systemic blood stasis, and back pressure of urine upon the kidney tissues. As illustrating the first group of cases, we may cite the experiment of constricting the renal artery which leads to the production of albuminuria, and the arteriosclerotic kidney. The best example of the second is seen in the albuminuria found so often in obstructive heart disease. It is to be noted that in both sets of cases the blood, if not normal, is nearly so, there being at most a slight qualitative change, owing to the modified character of the flow and the alteration in blood pressure, whereby the metabolic interchange is somewhat interfered with. Both, however, have this in common, that there is a less than sufficient amount of nutriment supplied to the kidney cells and the toxic products of metabolism are not properly excreted and not rapidly enough carried off. The exact nature of the finer changes that conduce to the result is not thoroughly known, but it is almost certain that they are situated in the secreting epithelium and basement membranes. The glomerular structure in particular seems to be sensitive to deleterious influences of this kind. It is here, too, that the nervous system plays an important role. Disturbances of the reflex vasomotor mechanism, by modifying the amount of blood supplied, distinctly predisposes to the production of kidney lesions. A marked deviation from the normal in the quantity of blood present in the kidneys, especially if suddenly produced or frequently repeated, impairs their vitality and paves the way for infection and other forms of irritation.

But, further, the quality of the blood has to be taken into consideration. The blood may be vitiated by toxic agents of extraneous origin, such as bacteria and various drugs and chemical substances. Many cases of nephritis can be traced to infection, the bacteria in question gaining an entrance into the kidney tissue, as can be shown in many instances; or, again, acting from afar by means of their soluble toxins. Not a few, also, are due to substances ingested, such as lead, phosphorus, cantharides, chrome salts, balsams, and the products of abnormal putrefaction in the bowel.

In another class of cases the disturbance is traceable to disturbances in other structures exercising a complemental function. Thus, a retention of substances normally excreted by the skin, lungs, liver, and intestines of necessity throws more work upon the kidneys and often actually floods them with deleterious products.

Lastly, kidney lesions may result from the action of substances elaborated through faulty or perverted metabolism in the body at large. Here we would place those found in eclampsia, pancreatic diabetes, exophthalmic goitre, myxœdema, carcinosis, and various cachexias.

To repeat, then, we hold that an insufficiency of blood supplied to the kidneys, a deficiency in its nutritive value, and still more the presence of abnormal substances or of normal substances in abnormal amounts, are the chief factors of etiological importance in affections of these organs. The exact relationship of the lesions produced, however, has provoked much debate and difference of opinion. Fairly clear are the cases of so-called interstitial nephritis of the arteriosclerotic type, which have been before referred to (p. 753). Here we have to deal with, in the main, a simple atrophy of the parenchymatous cells from lack of nutrition, and later, perhaps, from diminished function, together with a gradual replacement of the destroyed structures by fibrous tissue. But the cases due to circulating toxins are more abstruse. From the pathologist's standpoint, we can, theoretically at all events, differentiate between two orders of phenomena, *degeneration* and *inflammation*. These two conditions are the keynotes to the clear understanding of the diverse affections grouped under the term ".nephritis." The former is manifested in the retrogressive changes, cloudy swelling, fatty degeneration, vacuolation, and necrosis met with in the secreting cells; the latter, in the congestion, exudation, and hyperplasia of tissue. We might, therefore, as Marchand did in reference to corrosive sublimate poisoning of the kidneys, employ the term "nephrosis" for the former class of cases in contradistinction to "nephritis." Klebs and Banti, long ago, drew attention to this distinction. It must be confessed, however, that the distinction between these two sets of disturbances cannot always be accurately drawn, either clinically or anatomically. The factors that are competent to bring about the one are quite as capable of producing the other. We have seen, for example, the most extreme coagulation necrosis of the cells of the contorted tubules in cases of carcinoma and certain of the infections without any evidence of exudation, as we have often noted the same degeneration in cases of undoubted nephritis. Possibly the explanation is to be found along these lines. Toxic agents in small amounts bring about the various retrogressive changes in the secreting cells we have just referred to, which changes may not progress farther, or the irritation may be sufficiently intense or sufficiently prolonged to excite reaction and an attempt at repair. Or, again, the kidneys may be so flooded with deleterious substances that a necrosis results severe enough to preclude the possibility of reaction, or the patient dies before inflammation has time to set in. In any case, the clinical effects are much the same, and it is practically immaterial whether we draw the distinction or not. Personally, we feel inclined to include both conditions under the term "nephritis," in one case the necrosis being primary, in the other secondary. We are the more led to this conclusion in that we consider, on the ground of our own and others' observations, that all cases of clinical acute nephritis, whether of the degenerative or exudative type, are partly of an infective nature; that is to say, while circulating toxins play an important role by lowering the vitality of the kidney parenchyma and producing irritation, the influence of bacteria reaching the organs as a result of systemic infection, or present there normally (as Ford has shown[1]), is not to be overlooked.

THE INFLUENCE OF KIDNEY LESIONS ON THE EXCRETION OF URINE.

We have just seen that circulatory disturbances and abnormalities in the composition of the blood profoundly affect the character of the secreting structure of the kidney. The lesions in point might be expected, in their turn, to modify the composition of the fluid excreted by these organs, and, moreover, the processes of systemic metabolism. As

[1] Trans. Assoc. Amer. Phys., 15:1900:389, and Jour. of Hygiene, 1:1901:276.

a matter of fact, this is the case, and we have to concern ourselves, consequently, with the consideration of what substances are excreted and what retained.

The examination of the urine is a routine procedure in the study of any case of disease, inasmuch as it gives us valuable information as to the condition of the kidneys and the nature of the metabolic processes going on in the body at large. The most striking features in the former case are a more or less marked deviation from the normal in point of quantity, specific gravity, and reaction of the urine; the appearance of substances not normally present, such as serum albumin, red blood cells, leukocytes, epithelium, casts, cell detritus, blood pigment, fat, shreds of tissue, urinary salts, and bacteria; and a variation in the amount of the chemical constituents discharged. We can refer here only to the most outstanding facts.

Acute Parenchymatous Nephritis.—In acute parenchymatous nephritis the amount of urine excreted in the twenty-four hours is greatly reduced, namely, to 300 c.cm. or even, in the earlier stages of the attack, to 100 c.cm. Complete suppression is occasionally met with. The urine is acid, of high specific gravity (1024 to 1030), turbid, and of high color. It may be smoky, or even bright red in appearance from the admixture of blood. It contains albumin, varying in amount from 0.3 to 1 per cent. (by weight, 5 to 10 grams daily). The sediment, which is usually abundant, consists of red blood-cells, leukocytes, renal and bladder epithelium, crystals of uric acid and oxalates, hyaline, granular, epithelial, leukocytic, and blood-casts. Hemoglobin may be present in the urine in cases in which severe blood destruction has taken place (hemoglobinemia). Blood and blood pigment may be present in considerable amounts in the forms known as acute hemorrhagic nephritis. It has been shown recently that the freezing point of the urine in cases of nephritis differs from that of normal urine. The process for the determination of this fact is called cryoscopy. The freezing point of normal urine has been demonstrated to be from 1.3° to 2.3° C. below that of distilled water, while that of the urine in nephritis is only 1° C. or less below that of distilled water. This is due to the molecular concentration of the urine, which is less in nephritis than in health.

The urine in acute embolic suppurative nephritis is practically that of acute hemorrhagic non-suppurative parenchymatous nephritis.

Chronic Diffuse Nephritis.—In the chronic diffuse nephritis (without induration), or large white kidney, the urine is also diminished in amount, varying between 300 and 700 c.cm., is acid, turbid, and of increased specific gravity (1018 to 1025). It is often highly colored, and may contain a notable amount of blood. There is always considerable albumin, from 15 to 30 grams in the twenty-four hours. The sediment may consist in any of the elements mentioned under the acute form.

Chronic Interstitial Nephritis.—In the chronic interstitial form (chronic diffuse nephritis with induration) the urine is increased in amount, from 1800 to 4000 c.cm. daily. It is acid, pale in color, and of low specific gravity (1002 to 1015). Albumin is trifling in amount and may even be absent for prolonged periods. Casts are few and usually hyaline in character. Occasionally a few erythrocytes may be found. The solids of the urine are generally diminished.

Pyelonephritis.—In the cases of pyelitis and pyelonephritis resulting from stone, granular and cellular debris, urinary salts, epithelium, and pus cells are often present in considerable amounts. Massive hemorrhage may also occur into the urine. Where ulceration takes place, shreds of tissue may be passed into the urine.

In many cases of nephritis, especially those complicating the various infectious fevers, bacteria, usually those specific for the primary disease, can by suitable methods be found in the urine. The bacteriology of chronic nephritis has not as yet been worked out. In tuberculosis of the kidney, the specific bacilli, often in considerable numbers, can be detected.

The question of the elimination of the various salts found in the urine is an extremely difficult one. Most of the statements in medical text-books are incorrect, or at least misleading, inasmuch as they are based on faulty analytical methods. Based on a long series of studies by himself and his pupils, Von Noorden gives the following as his conclusions: In acute nephritis and the acute exacerbations of chronic cases, urea, creatinin, pigments, hippuric acid, phosphates, inorganic sulphates are excreted with difficulty. Uric acid, xanthin bases, aromatic substances, ammonia, amido-acids, chlorides, and carbonates are excreted with ease. Water in the earlier stages is even more difficult to eliminate than urea, but later on the kidney may regain its power in this particular and may get rid of it with greater facility than normal.

The nitrogenous elements in the urine are derived from protein disintegration, and this follows the same rules in nephritis as in health. Observation has shown that the power of the kidneys to excrete nitrogen varies greatly both in acute parenchymatous inflammation and in chronic interstitial fibrosis. In some cases the amount found in the urine is practically normal; in others it may be less than the intake and the protein metabolism would warrant; here, unless eliminated by the lungs and skin, it will be retained in the system; in still other cases nitrogen appears in the urine in great excess, derived not only from the protein disassimilation going on at the time, but also from the retained products. As a rule, urea and other nitrogenous substances are retained in the earlier stages of acute parenchymatous nephritis, occurring in previously healthy persons, if the attack is at all severe. We do not know, however, to what extent this retention takes place or how long it persists. The cases studied have either improved or death has occurred within five to ten days. In the chronic interstitial forms the nitrogenous constituents may be retained, but sooner or later the period of retention is succeeded, gradually or suddenly, by one of free excretion. Considerable variations occur here in different cases. In a general way we may say that in parenchymatous inflammation the elimination of nitrogen proceeds *pari passu* with the excretion of water and in proportion to the immediate gravity of the case, and this relationship is more evident than it is in the chronic interstitial forms.

Since the publication of Hofmann's work it has generally been held that creatinin is excreted with great difficulty by the kidneys. This has not entirely been substantiated since. The studies of Tedeschi, Zanoni, Troitz, and L. Mohr go to show that this substance is excreted with more ease than most nitrogenous materials, and particularly urea. It seems probable, according to Zanoni, that the creatinin output is more disturbed in chronic interstitial nephritis than in the more acute forms.

We know little about the subject of the urinary pigments in relation to nephritis. Urobilin and hematoporphyrin are derived from the disintegration of hemoglobin, and a diet rich in this substance increases the amount of these pigments eliminated. As they are excreted with some difficulty, it might be wise to regulate the diet accordingly, and, as a practical point, to avoid giving substances which might cause hematoporphyrinuria, such as trional and sulphonal.

The synthesis of benzoic acid and glycocoll by the kidneys into hippuric acid has, on the basis of the work of Jaarsveld and Stocvis, Stocvis and Van der Velde,[1] and Kronecker,[2] been regarded as being carried out imperfectly by diseased kidneys. More accurate methods have somewhat shaken this conclusion. The subject, however, has lost much of its interest since it has been discovered that the synthesis in question can be carried out by other organs besides the kidneys.

The excretion of phosphoric acid rises and falls in nephritis as does that of other urinary constituents, though it is undoubted that in some cases there is considerable retention. This is not invariable, however.

With regard to uric acid, von Noorden concludes that the diseased kidney is relatively pervious to this substance. Yet it may be retained to some extent, but this retention is accompanied by a still greater retention of urea. A very small daily deficit in the amount excreted may result in a considerable accumulation in the blood. The matter is important inasmuch as uric acid and the purin bases are related chemically to caffeine, theobromine, and theocin, all of which act powerfully upon the heart and vessels, and it is possible that the circulatory disturbances so often found in nephritis are directly traceable to the accumulation of these substances in the system. As a rule, however, inflamed kidneys can react to a diet rich in purin almost as well as healthy organs.

Ammonia is easily excreted, though it may happen that the relative proportion of this substance may exceed the normal average (3 to 5 per cent. of the normal nitrogen). Where this is the case, however, it is due to a diminution in the total nitrogen, particularly urea, rather than an increased output of ammonia. In uremia both the absolute and relative amounts of ammonia is increased, yet it is, as a rule, less than 1 gram daily.

Generally the excretion of chlorides by nephritics is as free as in the case of healthy individuals; that is, it follows the intake to some extent. Numerous exceptions to this statement occur, however. It has been

[1] Experimental Archiv., 10:1879:268, and 17:1883:189.
[2] Ibid., 16:1883:344.

noticed that a particularly good excretion takes place when diuresis is **free and** there is a satisfactory elimination of the nitrogenous sub-stances, for example, in the later stages of acute nephritis, in the amelior-ations of parenchymatous nephritis, and in compensated interstitial nephritis. Yet the output responds less readily to the intake than in normal persons; in other words, there is a relative incapacity of nephritic organs to excrete. Their reserve power is slight. Retention of the chlorides is of special importance in that it is closely associated with the production of œdema in Bright's cases. A chloride-free diet will often clear up œdema in a wonderful way.

THE RELATIONSHIP OF KIDNEY AFFECTIONS TO GENERAL MET-ABOLISM AND THE STATE OF OTHER ORGANS.

Kidney affections, and particularly nephritis, may affect the bodily health in a variety of ways. While we find that local disturbances are produced in many other organs as a result of renal lesions, these are in large part to be explained in view of the disordered general metabolism thereby induced. It has long been known that hypertrophy (and later dilatation) of the heart, together with other vascular disturbances, are apt to accompany nephritis, together with high tension of the pulse. This increased blood pressure has at times been attributed to the diffi-culty that the heart finds in forcing the blood through the kidneys, the renal vessels being compressed by inflammatory exudation and the arterial vessels being to some extent sclerosed. This view is hardly an adequate one, inasmuch as the kidneys are small organs and one would expect that the relatively small amount of obstruction obtaining within them could readily be compensated in other ways. It is much more likely that the increased vascular tension and overwork of the heart is due to stimulation by toxic substances in the circulation (*vide supra*). The immediate effect of this is to produce contraction of the peripheral vessels, vascular degeneration, and sclerosis, and, later, myocardial changes. As a consequence, in advanced cases, we find not infrequently leakage of the cardiac valves, ruptured compensation, with all that implies, and hemorrhages into various organs, particularly the brain. In favor of this broader view is the fact that hypertrophy of the heart is not invariably present in chronic Bright's disease. The conditions just mentioned in their turn work detrimentally upon the structure and func-tion of the kidneys, so that bad is made worse.

A further result of the retention of substances that should be excreted by the kidneys is that they accumulate in the blood and seek another way of exit, through the lungs, skin, and the buccal, gastric, and intestinal mucous membranes.

For decades it has been part of the faith once delivered to the saints (of the medical persuasion!) that the inadequate elimination of the waste products of metabolism through diseased kidneys led to a vicarious excretion by other parts of the body. Consequently, purgation, sweat-ings, diuresis, and such like modes of derivation are commonly employed in the treatment of Bright's disease. Such a conception seems at first sight eminently reasonable. Unfortunately, study of the problem by more accurate modern methods has not tended to strengthen it. First, it may be well to be clear as to what we mean by "vicarious excretion." We can properly use this term only when we have evidence that, as a result of disease, those glands which ordinarily take up only traces of urinary excretives from the blood develop a capacity to attract these excretives similar to that possessed by the normal kidneys. Where, for example, a certain amount of urea is found in glandular secretions, owing to the fact that the blood contains a large quantity of it, this is not "vicarious excretion." Even in renal disease, when the retention of urea and other substances is considerable, the amount found in the sweat and saliva is too small to be regarded as an elective secretion. Ordinarily, there is practically no elimination of urea through the sudoriparous glands in nephritis, for, as is well known, nephritic patients scarcely perspire at all. According to von Noorden, when perspiration is artificially induced, it is rare to find much more than 1 gram of urea excreted by the skin in one day. The evidence is somewhat conflicting, but it would seem that while in some cases it has been possible to diminish the output of nitrogen in the urine by increasing the activity of the skin, yet this is by no means invariably the case. At all events, the amount of toxic matter retained within the system is so considerable that the small amount it is possible to eliminate through the skin is of little or no practical utility. In fact, free diaphoresis is not without its dangers, for the occurrence of sweating has so often coincided with a uremic attack that it is hard to avoid the conclusion that they are causally related. Von Leube and Walko[1] (and von Noorden corroborates this) have drawn attention to the fact that sweating promotes the excretion of water to a much greater degree than it does that of the solid substances, and that this may result in a rapid and dangerous concentration of toxic materials.

Both urea and uric acid have been found pathologically in the saliva. This occurs especially in chronic parenchymatous and interstitial forms of nephritis, and particularly when uremia has supervened. As much as 0.4 to 0.5 gram of nitrogen has been demonstrated by von Noorden to be excreted in this manner daily. Ptyalism and stomatitis occasionally are met with in uremia. This Barié attributes to the retention of some toxic agent, so far of unknown character, which irritates the salivary glands.

Perhaps the doctrine of vicarious excretion in nephritis derives more support from the condition of things in the intestine. Brauneck found in the feces of a nephritic patient ten times the normal amount of ammonia. A slight excess of ammonia is found in the saliva, gastric juice, and on the skin, but the main excretion takes place through the bowel. Apparently, what takes place is this: an excess of urea is excreted by the mucous membrane, which becomes gradually converted into ammonia. This phenomenon probably accounts in large part for the

[1] Zeitschr. f. Heilkunde, 22:1901:312.

diarrhœa that occurs in Bright's disease and for the intestinal ulceration found so often in uremia. The action is probably assisted by other agencies, for the increase of ethereal sulphates in the urine of nephritics (Biernacki, Von Noorden, Herter, and others) points to increased bacterial activity and abnormal intra-intestinal putrefaction.

The most striking and important manifestation of retained toxic matter is **uremia.**

The symptom complex, known as uremia, consists of increased blood pressure, cardiac hypertrophy, headache, and gastro-intestinal irritation (*petite urémie* of the French writers), with the addition, in the aggravated cases, of convulsions, coma, and death. There is no single substance in the urinary secretion to the retention of which these phenomena have not been attributed. Urea was the first. The injection of urea into the circulation will not, however, give rise to uremia. The well-known theory of Frerichs is to the effect that some ferment in the blood converts the urea into ammonia salts and that these are the cause of the trouble. This view has not been substantiated. And so with all the rest. Indeed, the toxic effect of all the known urinary substances combined does not completely account for uremia.

Most of the experimental work in this direction is vitiated from the fact that injection procedures bring about acute toxic states, while the production of uremia is a matter of months or years. As everyone knows, the manifestations of an acute toxemia are often quite different from those of a chronic one. Again, we know that certain tissues have an affinity for toxic substances; for example, some nerve cells for morphine, others for tetanotoxin. It is possible, then, that the condition of the tissues may be of moment in fixing the deleterious substances that are almost certainly at work in uremia, and determining the direction of the phenomena produced. On this point, however, we have no information. We must learn much more, also, in regard to the behavior of the various ductless glands, adrenals, thyroid, etc., in cases of nephritis; whether, for example, they produce an increased, a diminished, or a perverted secretion; whether, also, they produce substances that augment or neutralize the power of toxic agents of nephritis. Finally, the question of an internal secretion from the kidney substance itself will have to be considered, and the possible effects of nephrolysine, some interesting investigations on which are now being carried on.

In conclusion, we must refer to one thing more. The retention of toxic substances leads to irritation of various tissues, and in the end depresses the general vitality of the patient. Consequently, nephritics are particularly liable to complicating conditions of an inflammatory or infective nature. Among these we should note bronchitis, pneumonia, pleurisy, pericarditis, peritonitis, gastro-enteritis, colitis, and eczema. The tendency to many of these affections is increased by the blood stasis, the anasarca, the vomiting and diarrhœa, and the anorexia from which many of these patients suffer. Failing the onset of these complications, not a few cases of Bright's disease become "compensated," and the condition, with proper care, is not incompatible with a reasonably long life.

CHAPTER XXXV.

THE KIDNEYS AND URETERS.

THE KIDNEYS.

CONGENITAL AND ACQUIRED ANOMALIES.

THESE consist largely in defective development and abnormalities in size, shape, position, and anatomical structure.

Aplasia.—One or other of the organs may be absent (**aplasia**) in people otherwise perfectly formed. This occurred three times in one thousand autopsies of our series. According to Ballowitz,[1] in 57 per cent. of cases it is the left kidney which is lacking. The condition is usually of no great consequence, as the remaining kidney undergoes compensatory hyperplasia. The occurrence of the condition should be remembered in connection with surgical operations, however, for cases have been known where the only kidney was removed for disease, with, of course, disastrous results. As a rule, the corresponding ureter is absent, although occasionally a rudiment of it may be found connected with the bladder. Malformations of the genitalia are not infrequent concomitants. Where only one kidney is present it is often long and narrow, suggesting duplication (? compensatory), and may, moreover, be provided with a double pelvis and two ureters.

Both kidneys may be **absent**[2] in certain monsters, a condition which is, of course, inconsistent with life.

Hypoplasia.—Congenital hypoplasia of one kidney is rather common. The organ is small, surrounded by much perirenal fat, the secreting structure is scanty, and there may be considerable fibrosis. The vessels supplying it are also small. More rarely, both kidneys are thus affected.

Horseshoe Kidney.—An interesting anomaly, that is not infrequent, occurring, according to our statistics, in 0.4 per cent. of all autopsies, is the so-called "horseshoe" kidney. In this condition the kidneys are imperfectly separated one from the other. They lie close to the vertebral column, and are united most commonly at their lower end by kidney substance, or, more rarely, by a fibrous band. More rarely still, the union takes place at the upper or middle portion. The horseshoe kidney is usually situated somewhat lower than normal, and may be found upon the promontory of the sacrum. In the latter situation it may prove an impediment to labor. One of the component organs lies

---

[1] Virch. Archiv, 141:1895:309.
[2] Hauch, Soc. d'Obstetr., Paris, 19:1908.

somewhat higher than the other. The ureters generally pass out to the front and the vessels are abnormal in their origin. The condition is of no great moment and is usually discovered accidentally; but occasionally serious symptoms have resulted, such as thrombosis of the underlying veins and pressure upon the ureters giving rise to hydronephrosis or pyelonephritis. Such kidneys would seem to be more liable to disease than normal ones. We have met with one case in which one-half of the organ was tuberculous, and another in which it contained a large coral calculus.

FIG. 182   FIG. 183

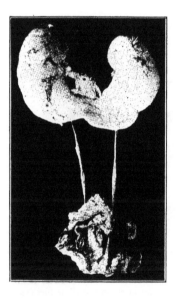

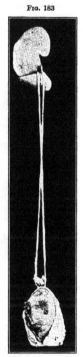

Horseshoe kidney. (From the Pathological Museum of McGill University.)

Complete double ureter. (From the Pathological Museum of McGill University.)

Kidneys are not uncommonly found which are **elongated, rounded, spleen-like,** or **hogbacked** in shape. The hogbacked kidney is probably not due to alcoholism, as used to be thought, but, rather, is congenital, for it is found often in children and in others who have never touched alcohol. In the spleen- or cake-like kidney the pelvis is frequently situated posteriorly.

Double Pelvis and Ureter.—Another fairly common anomaly is for one or both kidneys to be provided with a double pelvis and ureter. The ureters usually unite somewhere about their lower third and continue as a single channel, or may fuse at the point of junction with the bladder, or, again, more rarely, may empty by separate orifices into the bladder. When more or less separate, one ureter invariably crosses the other, the superior entering the bladder nearer to the urethral orifice. Such kidneys are often abnormally long, as if showing a tendency to reduplication in series.

The ureter of a normal kidney may, instead of emptying into the bladder, discharge into the colliculus seminalis, a seminal vesicle, the urethra, vagina, or uterus.

FIG. 184

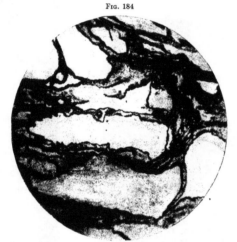

Congenital cystic kidney. Zeiss obj. DD, without ocular. (From the Royal Victoria Hospital collection.)

Fœtal Lobulation.—A very common anomaly is fœtal lobulation. Here, on the surface of the organ are numerous shallow furrows representing the original divisions of the various renculi. Rarely, the kidney is represented by a number of small separate organs.

Dislocation of the Kidney.[1]—Dislocation of a kidney is also fairly frequent. It may be congenital or acquired. In the congenital variety the vessels present an abnormal origin, while the ureter is usually shortened. In the acquired form, the vessels are normal in origin and distribution, though both the vessels and ureter are lengthened and tortuous. The adrenals usually occupy their normal position. The abnormally situated kidney may lie on the vertebral column, either on

[1] For literature see Sträter, Deut. Zeit. f. Chir., 83:1906:55.

its own or the opposite side, on the sacral promontory, in the pelvis, or beneath the anterior abdominal wall. The organ may be fixed in its abnormal situation by fibrous adhesions. Occasionally anomalies of the female organs of generation, more rarely of the bowel, are associated.[1]

Congenital dislocation, according to Kupfer, is due to a deficiency in the movement of the embryonic rudiments of the kidneys, which, up to a certain period, are formed just in front of the point of bifurcation of the aorta.

The acquired form (**nephroptosis; movable kidney**) seems to be due to deficiency in the amount of the perirenal fat, such as occurs in prolonged wasting disease; pressure, as from tight lacing; traumatism; heavy lifting; or to a relaxed abdominal wall, resulting in diminished intra-abdominal pressure. In most cases it is part of a general gastro-enteroptosis or splanchnoptosis. Occasionally, the dislocation is brought about by the weight of a renal tumor.

Dislocated kidneys may be mistaken for ovaries, Fallopian tubes, a retained testis, or tumors of the pelvic viscera, and in certain situations may be a cause of dystocia.

Cysts.—Congenital cysts of the kidney are not uncommon. The organs are greatly enlarged, warty, and on section are composed of numerous sacs containing thin fluid. The condition is supposed to be due to retention owing to imperfect fusion of the collecting tubules with the secretory portion[2] (see vol. i, p. 855).

CIRCULATORY DISTURBANCES.

Oligemia.—Generalized oligemia of the kidney is found in cases of general systemic oligemia, either essential or secondary. In the early stages, the organ on section is uniformly pale, of a grayish-yellow color and fairly translucent. In the advanced condition, as is well seen in pernicious anemia, the kidney is pale, yellow, and turbid-looking, owing to the resulting fatty degeneration.

Local anemia is met with in the white infarct.

Hyperemia.—**Active Hyperemia.**—Active hyperemia is met with in acute inflammations, a forcibly acting left heart, various intoxications, and in death from cerebral tumors, meningitis, and the like.

Passive Hyperemia.—Passive hyperemia is usually due to some obstruction in the general circulation, such as valvular heart disease, or some pulmonary disturbance. A unilateral lesion is rarer, and results from some obstruction in the inferior vena cava or renal vein, as from thrombosis or the pressure of enlarged glands, the pregnant uterus, or tumor-masses upon the vessel.

The kidney is enlarged, its consistency firmer than normal, and the capsule peels off with great ease. The stellate veins are injected and

---

[1] For literature see Pepere, Arch. di Obstet. e Ginecol., 6:1908.

[2] An excellent account of the various anomalies of the kidneys is that by Huntingdon, Harvey Lectures, 1906–07:222, Lippincott.

FIG. 185

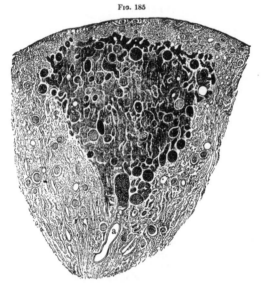

Anemic infarct of cortex of kidney to show coagulation necrosis, with surrounding zone
of congestion. a, artery. (Orth)

FIG. 186

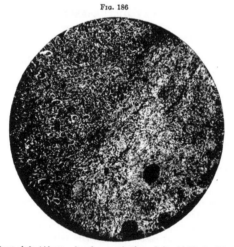

White infarct of the kidney undergoing organization.   Leitz obj. No. 3, without ocular.
The necrotic area is to the right. (From the collection of Dr. A. G. Nicholls.)

the surface has a dark purple red, or cyanotic appearance. On section, the organ is very firm, drips blood, and has a uniformly dark red appearance. In the milder grades, the straight vessels can be made out as red, converging lines and the glomeruli as minute reddish points in the cortical portion.

Microscopically, the vessels are all enlarged and congested, the Bowman's capsules contain albumin, with possibly a few red blood-cells, and the tubules contain a few hyaline casts. Certain of the epithelial cells, notably those of the descending loops, contain pigment granules derived from altered blood. In long-standing cases the capillary and venous walls appear thickened, there is increase in the interstitial connective tissue, and occasionally a round-celled interstitial infiltration—a condition known as "*cyanotic induration.*" In some instances the secreting epithelium is found to be fatty. Finally, atrophy may result.

Hemorrhage.—(See pp. 788 and 791.)

Infarction.—Infarction of the kidney is due to a sudden stoppage of the circulation in a portion of the organ, through embolism of one of the branches of the renal artery. It is usually anemic in nature. In the course of a few hours the part which is deprived of its blood-supply, becomes pale, grayish-white, and more or less opaque and granular. The area is usually roughly wedge-shaped, with the apex toward the boundary zone. The margin is well-defined by a zone of hyperemia or hemorrhage.

Microscopically, the affected area presents all the appearances of coagulation necrosis. The cells are swollen, granular, opaque, and take a diffuse muddy stain. The nuclei are pale or invisible. Round the margin the vessels are congested, there may be hemorrhage, and an accumulation of leukocytes due to a reactive inflammation. The infarcted areas vary in size from that of a bean to a third or even the whole of the organ. The necrosed portion may reach quite to the capsule: most often there is a small zone of healthy or relatively healthy kidney tissue between, depending on the amount of anastomosis with the vessels of the capsule. In course of time the affected cells undergo fatty and hydropic degeneration and are eventually absorbed and destroyed, their places being taken by proliferating connective tissue from margin. Ultimately, only a scar is left. The scar-tissue is grayish-white or reddish in color, sometimes pigmented. Where there have been numerous infarcts, the kidney is contracted, scarred, with a markedly irregular surface (*embolic granular kidney*).

The Arteriosclerotic Contracted Kidney.[1]—The arteriosclerotic contracted kidney is a form of granular kidney originating in a narrowing and eventual obstruction of the afferent vessels of the organ. The condition may be restricted to the renal artery and its branches, or may be part of a general arteriosclerotic process. The changes are of the nature of a chronic proliferation of the intima or media. This leads to collapse of the glomerular capillaries and atrophy of the tufts. The

---

[1] See Jores, Virch. Archiv, 178:1904.

glomeruli, through hyaline changes in the capillaries, become converted into rounded masses, at first relatively poor in nuclei but ultimately structureless or fibroid. The Bowman's capsules may be thickened, though usually not to any great extent. As a result of the degeneration of the glomeruli the efferent tubules become collapsed and atrophied. The process, as a whole, tends to affect certain vascular districts corresponding to the interlobular arteries. As the various structures atrophy, their place is taken by connective tissue, which gradually shrinks, leading to the formation of a scar. Thus, the surface of the kidney becomes more or less warty or granular, and the capsule is somewhat adherent. The atrophic process is more marked in some regions than in others, with

Fig. 187

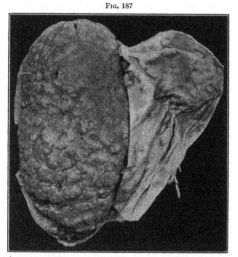

An arteriosclerotic kidney. The preparation shows well the irregular coarse granulations on the exterior of the organ. (From the Pathological Museum of McGill University.)

the result that localized rather sharply-defined depressed areas are to be seen on the surface. The interlobular vessels become also tortuous through sinking in of the cortex.

The arteriosclerotic kidney is usually bright red or grayish-red in color, or, owing to fatty degeneration, may be streaked with yellow. It is diminished in size, the capsule is adherent, and the cortex is narrowed and distorted. The organ cuts more firmly than usual and the glomeruli stand out as whitish dots. The smaller arterioles, through thickening of their walls, are easily recognized. The renal artery itself often shows marked sclerotic changes. A striking feature is the marked narrowing of cortex and medulla. The pelvis is relatively large and filled with fatty tissue.

The condition, though etiologically different, is not easily differentiated from the inflammatory contracted kidney. In the latter type, however, the process is more apt to be diffused and even in its character, and the signs of arterial sclerosis throughout the body are not so marked.

INFLAMMATIONS.

The subject of the classification of certain affections of the kidneys is one fraught with much difficulty. This is, in large part, due to the difficulty in determining the correlation between the etiology, the morbid anatomy, and the clinical manifestations in many cases of nephritis. On the one hand, the same etiological factor may bring about a diversity of anatomical changes, and, on the other, one and the same clinical picture may result from a variety of morbid causes. Again, the severity of the outward manifestations of the disease does not always bear a direct relationship to the apparent extent of the lesions. Time and again, we find at autopsy advanced renal disease in cases where from the clinical features we would not have expected it, and, conversely, we may have well-marked clinical evidence of disease with kidneys that are practically normal to gross examination. As a consequence, we do not find perfect unanimity among writers as to what constitutes nephritis and what does not.

There are three ways of classifying kidney affections: (1) according to etiology; (2) according to the location of the lesions; and (3) according to the nature of the inflammatory process.

The etiological method would be eminently scientific, but presents the practical difficulties that have just been mentioned. On this basis we might differentiate *congestive, toxic,* and *infective* disturbances.

The second, or topographical method, is theoretically possible and is not devoid of merit. We may, recognizing that the epithelium, the glomeruli, the interstitial stroma, and the bloodvessels may be affected, divide nephritis into parenchymatous, glomerular, interstitial, and arteriosclerotic forms. The first three of these forms may again be divided into acute and chronic; the last is, of course, always chronic. The chief objection to this classification lies in the fact that it is impossible to draw a hard and fast line between parenchymatous and interstitial inflammations. To indicate all the possible permutations and combinations would necessitate a cumbrous terminology.

According to the third method, we may recognize with Delafield, in the first instance, three types of kidney affections—*congestion, degeneration,* and *inflammation.* Inflammation may, again, be divided into *acute exudative nephritis; acute productive nephritis; chronic nephritis with exudation; chronic nephritis without exudation;* and *suppurative nephritis.* The considerations just detailed are sufficient to indicate the difficult nature of the problem before us.

That dropsy and albuminuria are, in certain cases, related to affections of the kidneys has been recognized for centuries. Aëtius (367 A.D.),

Avicenna (980 to 1036), and van Helmont (1577 to 1644) all held that certain cases of dropsy were due to disease of the kidneys. Cotunnius, in 1770, discovered that the urine of dropsical patients could be coagulated by boiling.

We owe our modern conceptions of kidney inflammations, however, to Richard Bright, of Guy's Hospital, who published, in 1827, the first thorough and scientific studies of this type of disease. Bright demonstrated the dependence of albuminuria and dropsy on disease of the kidneys. He accurately described the morbid changes in the kidneys, and showed the relationship of the clinical symptoms to the anatomical lesions. He, further, described many of the associated conditions and sequelæ, such as uremia and the cardiovascular phenomena, blindness, apoplexy, and inflammation of the serous membranes. So accurate and thorough was his work that most of it has stood the test of subsequent inquiry. As a result, the term Bright's disease has been adopted the world over as the designation among clinicians for the non-suppurative inflammations of the kidney usually associated with albuminuria and dropsy.

Further advances were made by Rokitansky, who described in 1842 the amyloid kidney. Johnson (1852) drew attention to the vascular changes in the kidney, work which was taken up and amplified in 1872 by Gull and Sutton in their study of what they called "arteriocapillary fibrosis," in which they emphasized the relationship of certain changes in the bloodvessels to cirrhosis and atrophy of the kidney.

A matter of some importance is to decide how much we should include under the term Bright's disease. Some authorities, such as Leyden, regard Bright's disease as embracing all forms of kidney disease associated with albuminuria and hydrops, and would, therefore, include in this category cases of degeneration of the kidney epithelium, pyelonephritis, and the amyloid kidney. Others, again, with Klebs, would separate the non-inflammatory degenerative manifestations from true Bright's disease. At the present time, it seems to be fairly generally agreed to differentiate the circulatory and degenerative disorders of the kidneys from the primarily inflammatory affections, or true Bright's disease. With regard to the forms of nephritis proper, Sir Thomas Grainger Stewart, in 1871, recognized three types—the inflammatory, the amyloid, and the contracting forms. Under the first he described three stages, that of inflammatory exudation, that of fatty degeneration, and that of induration, a classification practically coinciding with that of Bartels, who classified these affections into acute parenchymatous chronic parenchymatous, and interstitial nephritis.

In the classification that we have suggested here we have sided with those who would differentiate between congestive, degenerative, and inflammatory affections of the kidney. The further division of nephritis proper into *non-suppurative*, *suppurative*, and *specific* forms of inflammation is so convenient and accurate that it is hardly likely to arouse serious antagonism. More difference of opinion may, perhaps, arise over the various subvarieties of non-suppurative nephritis, but the forms mentioned here are all types well known to the pathological histologist, and, at any rate, do not conflict with clinical experience. They are, however, to be regarded merely as types, without it being understood that they are separated oné from the other by hard and fast.lines.

Under the affections of the kidney, ordinarily associated with either albuminuria or anasarca, or both, we recognize, therefore, the following:

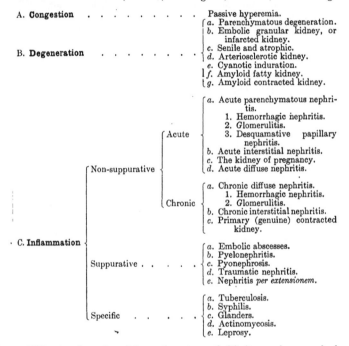

A. **Congestion** . . . . Passive hyperemia.

B. **Degeneration** . . . .
- *a.* Parenchymatous degeneration.
- *b.* Embolic granular kidney, or infarcted kidney.
- *c.* Senile and atrophic.
- *d.* Arteriosclerotic kidney.
- *e.* Cyanotic induration.
- *f.* Amyloid fatty kidney.
- *g.* Amyloid contracted kidney.

C. **Inflammation**

Non-suppurative

Acute
- *a.* Acute parenchymatous nephritis.
  - 1. Hemorrhagic nephritis.
  - 2. Glomerulitis.
  - 3. Desquamative papillary nephritis.
- *b.* Acute interstitial nephritis.
- *c.* The kidney of pregnancy.
- *d.* Acute diffuse nephritis.

Chronic
- *a.* Chronic diffuse nephritis.
  - 1. Hemorrhagic nephritis.
  - 2. Glomerulitis.
- *b.* Chronic interstitial nephritis.
- *c.* Primary (genuine) contracted kidney.

Suppurative . . . . . .
- *a.* Embolic abscesses.
- *b.* Pyelonephritis.
- *c.* Pyonephrosis.
- *d.* Traumatic nephritis.
- *e.* Nephritis *per extensionem.*

Specific . . . . . .
- *a.* Tuberculosis.
- *b.* Syphilis.
- *c.* Glanders.
- *d.* Actinomycosis.
- *e.* Leprosy.

With regard to the etiology of acute nephritis it may be remarked here that the most important single causal element is infection. We may recognize four main classes of this affection:

1. Those due to various intoxications, such as from alcohol, lead cantharides, phosphorus, chlorate of potash, and salicylic acid.

2. Those complicating the acute infections, such as scarlatina, small-pox, pneumonia, acute endocarditis, erysipelas, diphtheria, typhoid fever, septicemia, acute rheumatism, cholera, acute tonsillitis, vaccinia, septic wounds, epidemic cerebrospinal meningitis, and certain gastro-intestinal disorders.

3. Those associated with chronic diseases and cachexias, as diabetes, carcinoma, pulmonary tuberculosis, and syphilis.

4. The so-called "idiopathic" cases.

It has been abundantly demonstrated by experimental studies that a great variety of toxins, both mineral and bacterial, are competent to set up degenerative changes, of the nature of cloudy swelling, fatty degeneration, and even necrosis, in the secreting epithelium of the kidney. For example, as Wandervelde[1] has shown, toxins like those of cholera, cholera nostras, tuberculosis, diphtheria, pneumonia, influenza, and certain chemical substances, such as chromic acid, lead, phosphorus, mercuric chloride, when injected into laboratory animals, exert a harmful influence upon the glandular structure of the kidney, bringing about changes identical in appearance with those met with in the human subject. How far these are inflammatory is open to debate. Parenchymatous degeneration is doubtless an early stage of inflammation in many cases of nephritis, but, from the pathologist's point of view at least, can occur independently of inflammation, and, moreover, need not necessarily give rise to it. When inflammation does supervene in such cases it is quite fair to assume, in the absence of positive information, that it is as likely due to secondary infection as to the influence of the circulating toxin. Consequently, for the sake of clearness, while it is well to preserve in our minds the distinction between "degeneration" and "inflammation," practically, as we have before remarked, it is not always possible to distinguish between them.

We are, however, on more certain ground when we come to discuss the forms of nephritis occurring in the course of infective processes. Here a microbic origin can be traced in nearly every case. The bacteria found in the urine of such cases are usually those specific of the primary disease. Thus, streptococci and staphylococci have been found in the urine in cases of acute endocarditis (Weichselbaum, Mannaberg); the Typhoid bacillus, in cases of nephritis arising during the course of typhoid fever (Blumer); and Pneumococcus, in cases of pneumonia (Massalong, Klebs, Michelle). In a study of this subject made by one of us (A. G. N.[2]) some years ago, in 32 cases of acute nephritis of various forms, bacteria, usually the specific germs of the primary disease, were present in 28.

It is difficult, therefore, to avoid the conclusion that most cases of acute nephritis in man are due in large part to infection with microörganisms. The specific changes are produced, it may be presumed, in the course of an attempt on the part of the kidneys to eliminate the offending agents.

The acute forms of nephritis arising in the course of chronic diseases are largely of the nature of terminal infections.

The relationship of infection to chronic nephritis is, unfortunately, much more obscure. No doubt certain cases of acute nephritis pass imperceptibly over into the chronic type, and it is possible, and indeed likely, that in these instances the infective agents are still at work. As

---

[1] Act. d. pois. sur les cell. epithél. d. canalicules contournées, Brux., 1894.

[2] Nicholls, A Contribution to the Study of Bright's Disease, Montreal Med. Jour., 28: 1899: 161.

a proof of this, it may be pointed out that cirrhosis of the kidneys has been known to result from infective diseases, such as pneumonia and influenza. It is true that one important class of chronic kidney disease is due to arteriosclerosis, and another (primary contracted kidney) to the influence of alcohol, lead, and gout. (This latter form, however, may be at bottom but a variety of the arteriosclerotic type.) Yet, cirrhosis of the kidneys has been met with in children, in whom the influence of arteriosclerosis and chronic mineral intoxication could with certainty be excluded. The possibility of infection being the cause of many cases of chronic nephritis was pointed out in the paper just referred

Fig. 188

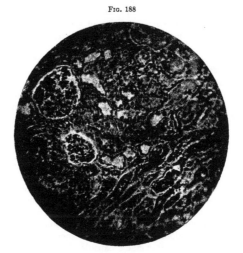

Acute parenchymatous nephritis. The section shows well the necrosis of the secreting tubules. Reichert obj. No. 7, without ocular. (From the Pathological Laboratory of McGill University.)

to. In eight cases of chronic parenchymatous nephritis minute diplococci were found in four; in one case of chronic glomerulitis the same diplococcus was present; in the chronic diffuse form (11 in number), bacteria were met with in all; in 10 cases of chronic interstitial nephritis, minute diplococci were found in every instance. Altogether, in 45 cases of chronic nephritis of all forms, minute diplococci were seen in 29 and bacilli in 4 more. The germs in question were usually found in the areas of interstitial round-celled infiltration, suggesting a causal relationship. The source of these bacteria is difficult to say, but it may be remarked that in nearly 41 per cent. of the cases there was a definite history of preceding gastro-enteric disturbance.

Simple or Non-suppurative Nephritis.—Acute Parenchymatous Nephritis.—(Synonyms: acute degenerative parenchymatous nephritis, acute tubular nephritis, desquamative nephritis, catarrhal or croupous nephritis, acute Bright's disease.)

This form of nephritis is of frequent occurrence and is characterized in the main by marked degenerative changes in the secreting tubules, such as cloudy and fatty degeneration. With this there is, however, congestion, exudation of serum, and desquamation of the secreting cells. In the earlier stages, the condition is, no doubt, identical with the simple parenchymatous degeneration that is so commonly found as a result of intoxications and infections of various kinds. In fact, it is sometimes impossible to draw the line between cloudy swelling and actual nephritis. The vascular changes, the desquamation of the cells, and certain characteristic changes in the urine, are usually sufficient, however, to make the diagnosis.

The kidneys are usually more or less enlarged and œdematous. The capsule peels off with more than normal ease, owing to the swelling of the kidney substance, which tends to bulge through the cut. The surface is pale, the stellate veins injected, and the lobules well indicated. The cortex is swollen, pale, and cloudy, presenting a marked contrast to the dark red or bluish-red medulla. In some cases the cortex is somewhat congested. Minute petechial hemorrhages can frequently be seen scattered over the cortical surface and throughout its substance.

Microscopically, the structures chiefly affected are the contorted tubules. The secreting cells are swollen, cloudy or granular, often vacuolated, while the nuclei stain badly or not at all. Within the lumina of the tubules, especially in the collecting portion, are to be seen hyaline or granular casts, and droplets of albumin. It is not uncommon to find the lining cells of the tubules lying free within the basement membrane in all stages of fatty and hyaline degeneration. In some cases the tubules contain blood. The glomeruli also show evidences of degeneration, the epithelium lining the Bowman's capsules being swollen and often desquamated, while structureless masses of albumin can be seen within the spaces. Hemorrhage into the capsules is noted in some cases. The amount of effused blood may be so great that free blood and blood casts appear in the urine, warranting the term *acute hemorrhagic nephritis.* The interstitial substance is swollen and œdematous, and there is sometimes, though not invariably, a small amount of round-celled infiltration and a deposit of fibrin in the interstitial stroma. The extent of the lesions varies in different cases. As a rule, the contorted tubules are the structures first and chiefly involved, but the loops of Henle and the collecting tubules do not always escape.

In certain cases, glomerular changes so dominate the picture that we can properly speak of *acute glomerulitis* or *glomerulonephritis.* This form is most commonly met with in scarlatina and diphtheria. To the naked eye the kidney, as a rule, shows very little change, at most being somewhat cloudy and hyperemic. The glomeruli are swollen and appear as reddish or pale grayish dots.

PLATE VII

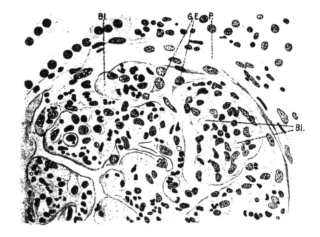

Acute Glomerulonephritis, Scarlatinal, of about the
Twenty-first Day.

tion of an affected glomerulus. The glomerular loops are plump, with
an increased number of nuclei.

blood within the capillaries, which exhibit also endothelial proliferation and contain some
:es. *G. E.*, swollen and proliferated glomerular epithelium, showing some desquamation. *P.*, capsular
tion with adhesion in part of glomerular epithelium to the capsule in regions devoid of capsular
ım. (After Lòhlein.)

Microscopically, both degenerative and productive changes in the glomeruli are found, so that, according as one or the other predominates, we may differentiate a degenerative and a productive glomerulonephritis. In the former variety, the capillaries of the glomeruli are congested or show hyaline degeneration, while the epithelial cells lining the Bowman's capsules are degenerated and desquamating. The Bowman's space is filled with degenerated epithelial cells, red and white corpuscles, albumin, and granular detritus. In the latter form, the lining cells and the various endothelia show proliferative changes.

Desquamative Papillary Nephritis.—A less important variety is the so-called desquamative papillary nephritis in which the lesions are chiefly confined to the tubules in the papillary portion, the cells of which are swollen and desquamating.

Acute Interstitial Nephritis.—(Synonyms: acute productive nephritis, "lymphomatous" nephritis of Wagner.)

This affection is found more especially in scarlatina and diphtheria. It also occurs in measles, pneumonia, whooping-cough, acute endocarditis, and epidemic cerebrospinal meningitis. The condition is probably due to the action of bacteria. The pyogenic cocci, B. coli, Klebs-Loeffler bacillus, and Pneumococcus are the microörganisms that have been found in association with it. Councilman,[1] in a study of such cases, would lay no stress upon the presence of these germs, as he found them in the kidney in the same proportions in cases other than interstitial nephritis. It may be remarked, however, that the production of nephritis probably depends on other factors than the mere presence of bacteria, namely, on the number and virulence of the germs and the vulnerability of the tissues, so that we need not refer any form of nephritis to the selective action of particular microbes. The infective origin is supported by the observations of Letzerich,[2] who has described an epidemic of acute interstitial nephritis due to a bacillus, which morphologically resembled B. tuberculosis and on injection into animals produced nephritis.

In this form the kidney is somewhat enlarged, the capsule strips easily, and its consistence is diminished. The cortical surface is mottled and of a gray, grayish-white, or grayish-red color. The stellate veins are injected. On section, the cortex is greatly swollen, paler than the medulla and of a streaky, opaque, grayish-white appearance. The striated appearance characteristic of the normal pyramids is lost. The kidney substance is soft, moist, and friable. The changes are most marked in the intermediate zone.

Microscopically, the degenerative changes in the secreting cells and the Malpighian tufts are reduced to a minimum and the characteristic feature is a more or less irregularly distributed accumulation of small

---

[1] Jour. Exper. Med., 3: 1898: 393.

[2] Untersuch. u. Beobacht. ueber Nephritis bacillosa interstitialis primaria, Zeit. f. klin. Med., 13: 1887: 33.

round cells in the interstitial substance. This infiltration is in small patches and is particularly marked at the bases of the pyramids, beneath the capsule, and around the glomeruli. The cells found are of the type of lymphocytes, with some plasma cells.

The Kidney of Pregnancy.—What may, for the present, be conveniently called the "kidney of pregnancy" is a peculiar condition met with in pregnant women. It has not yet been settled whether the condition is purely degenerative or whether it is in part degenerative and in part inflammatory, but the lesions on the whole correspond fairly closely with those found in what we have below called acute diffuse nephritis. It is important to note that the pregnant woman may be the subject of an acute nephritis exactly in the same way as other individuals may on occasion be attacked, and, again, that pregnancy may occur in one already suffering from Bright's disease. But, apart from these fortuitous associations, the kidney may become affected during the course of pregnancy, and apparently in some way as the result of it, without the ordinary etiological factors being discoverable. This is the condition of things which is so often associated with eclampsia. The affection in question usually arises during the latter half of pregnancy, and, preferably, in young primiparæ and in twin pregnancies.

The kidney varies somewhat in different cases, but is usually enlarged, the capsule peels off readily, the cortex is smooth, pale, and of a yellowish color. On section, the cortex is swollen. Microscopically, the lesions are those referable to an acute parenchymatous degeneration, while the interstitial substance is but little affected. Cases have occurred in which complete necrosis of the parenchyma occurred (Klotz,[1] Rose Bradford, Jardine).

The condition has been referred to auto-intoxication, the kidneys being inadequate to eliminate waste products for both mother and child; to infection and toxemia; to increased intra-abdominal and intra-pelvic pressure exerted upon the renal veins, the ureters, or the cœliac ganglia; to the absorption of toxic products derived from the placenta.

While for purposes of description it is convenient to refer to inflammation of the kidney as "parenchymatous," "glomerular," or "interstitial," according as the lesions are chiefly manifested in the secreting cells, the capillary tufts, or the supporting stroma, it would be far from correct to think that the pathological process in any case is confined to the structures named to the exclusion of the rest. Every acute and subacute nephritis is, in a sense, "diffuse," in that all parts of the kidney are involved, though it may be unequally. We name, therefore, the various forms according to the predominating features of the morbid changes. When we speak of *acute diffuse nephritis* in a specific sense we mean that type in which the inflammatory phenomena are more or less uniformly manifested throughout the secreting and the supporting structures of the organ. To cloudy swelling, fatty degeneration, and necrosis of the secreting tubules, are added œdema and leukocytic infiltration of the

[1] Jour. of Obstet., 58:1908:619.

interstitial tissue. As might be expected, however, the lesions are most marked in the cortical portion, that being the region of the greatest functional activity, and consequently, the most vulnerable. The congestion, which is a striking feature of all inflammations in their earlier stages, is chiefly manifested in the pyramids, the vessels of the cortex being rendered anemic owing to the swelling of the cells of the tubules and the pressure of the effused inflammatory products. The diffuse form is, perhaps, the most common type of acute and subacute nephritis.

Chronic Diffuse Nephritis.—The affection known as chronic diffuse nephritis (chronic parenchymatous nephritis, inflammatory fatty kidney; large white kidney; variegated kidney; chronic desquamative nephritis; second stage of Bright's disease) may occur as the sequel of the acute diffuse form, degenerative changes in the epithelium and interstitial infiltration becoming still more marked and the condition passing imperceptibly from the acute to the subacute and finally to the chronic state, or, more often, arising insidiously. The anatomical changes are strictly comparable to those found in the acute and subacute stages, but are more extreme. Thus, we may have *chronic parenchymatous nephritis, chronic hemorrhagic nephritis,* and *chronic glomerulitis.*

To gross appearance the most striking features are the inflammatory swelling and the peculiar color. The kidney is enlarged, somewhat soft and doughy in consistence, the capsule peels off readily, and the surface is smooth and of a grayish-yellow or grayish-white color, occasionally presenting dilated stellate veins or minute hemorrhagic spots. The pale color of the exterior may be uniform in intensity, but not infrequently is irregular, patches of congestion alternating with areas of pallor, giving the organ a somewhat variegated appearance. On section, the cortex is swollen, of a uniform or patchy pallor, similar to that of the surface, with occasional areas of congestion or hemorrhagic extravasation. The peculiarity in color is due, in part, to necrosis and fatty changes of the secreting cells of the tubules and in part to the anemia produced by the pressure of the effused inflammatory material. Until recently it was held that fatty degeneration of the tubular epithelium was a cardinal feature in this form. We know now, however, that in some cases, at all events, the fat is present, not as free fat, but combined in the form of soaps. The medullary portion is more or less congested, and of a dull red color, contrasting markedly with the pallid cortex. In the most extreme forms of this type the kidney may be of normal size, the surface slightly pitted, and the capsule somewhat adherent, indicating the onset of atrophy and fibrosis. When the amount of hemorrhage into the kidney substance is considerable it may justify the term *chronic hemorrhagic nephritis.*

Now and then cases are met with in which the organ is not specially enlarged and presents no marked deviation from the normal, at least so far as macroscopic appearance is concerned. These are the cases in which the inflammatory changes are chiefly confined to the glomeruli, while the rest of the tissues practically escape (*chronic glomerulitis*).

Microscopically, the morbid changes vary considerably. In the characteristic "large white kidney" the most notable feature is the presence of fat or soaps which are somewhat widespread in the epithelium of the glomeruli and the secreting tubules, and even in the lining cells of the bloodvessels. Myelin bodies of doubly-refractile appearance are found also both in the secreting cells and in their phagocytes. With this, there is to be observed a more or less extensive inflammatory infiltration, œdema, and leukocytic exudation into the interstices of the interstitial stroma. In the more advanced cases there may be indications of atrophy of the glomeruli and secreting cells, with, possibly, a slight amount of secondary fibrosis.

The glomeruli in many cases may show fatty degeneration of the epithelium of the tufts and the Bowman's capsules; in other cases, swelling, proliferation, and desquamation of the epithelial cells are more prominent, though not infrequently degenerative and reparative processes may be combined. In the Bowman's spaces there is an effusion of albuminous fluid which, owing to the method of hardening, has been coagulated into droplets, granular or fibrinoid masses. Leukocytes and, in the hemorrhagic cases, red blood-cells may also be found. The glomeruli themselves are often compressed from the accumulation of fluid and inflammatory cells, the epithelium is fattily degenerated, the capillary vessels are thickened, and may contain leukocytes and hyaline thrombi. The capillaries, being thus filled with inflammatory and degenerative products, become blocked and may in time be converted by organization into solid strands. Eventually, a certain number of the glomeruli shrink, are transformed into minute hyaline masses, poor in or devoid of nuclei, and surrounded by a contracted and thickened capsule.

The secreting cells, particularly those of the contorted tubules, show advanced necrosis and a deposit of fats and soaps in their substance, with consequent exfoliation, either in multiple isolated areas or uniformly throughout the cortex, though the collecting tubules do not entirely escape. The lumina of the tubules not infrequently are filled with degenerated cells, leukocytes, pigment and fatty particles, together with granular detritus. The lining cells are flattened, causing the lumina to appear relatively enlarged. They may, however, be dilated from obstruction. In hemorrhagic cases the tubules contain numerous red blood-cells. Casts of various kinds may be also detected. These changes in the tubules are usually conspicuous and are only of trifling extent in the form known as chronic glomerulitis.

The interstitial connective tissue is œdematous and presents here and there small areas of cellular infiltration. In the hemorrhagic forms the stroma also contains pigment granules. In the most advanced cases the supporting stroma is increased in amount and gives definite evidence of proliferation, while the Bowman's capsules are also thickened. Such changes are found in those kidneys which are beginning to show evidences of atrophy and contraction in their smaller size and slightly scarred cortex.

Chronic Interstitial Nephritis.—This form of chronic nephritis passes imperceptibly into the next, chronic interstitial nephritis (chronic productive nephritis; chronic indurative nephritis; granular kidney; chronic diffuse nephritis with induration; contracted kidney; secondary contracted kidney; fibroid kidney; cirrhotic or sclerotic kidney; third stage of Bright's disease).

It is generally held at the present time that the contracted kidney is of four types; the first arising as a sequel to the large white kidney (*secondary contracted kidney*); the second, originating in an acute nephritis and apparently not passing through the large white kidney stage (*primary contracted kidney*); the third, due to sclerosis of the renal vessels, and, therefore, of a degenerative rather than an inflammatory nature (*arteriosclerotic kidney;* see p. 781); and the fourth, the *senile.*

From the nature of the case it is extremely difficult, and in some instances impossible, to make out the exact sequence of events in these various forms. The doubtful points are hardly likely to be cleared up until we have the results of more extended experimentation at our command. Time, therefore, may modify our present conceptions of renal inflammation.

In a well-marked case of chronic interstitial nephritis of the secondary contracted type, the kidney is usually diminished in size. In consistence it is firm and hard, somewhat elastic, and cuts with more or less resistance, resembling in this other fibroid structures. The capsule is somewhat thickened and is, in places, adherent to the cortex. On removing it small portions of the cortex are torn away. The surface of the kidney is irregular, warty, or granular, being studded with prominences of somewhat uneven distribution, and of greater or smaller size. Occasional cysts, containing a clear colorless or straw-colored fluid, are usually to be seen. The color of such a kidney varies, and it may be mentioned in passing that the terms "small white kidney" and "small red kidney," which have been so often employed, do not indicate any important difference in type, the color of the organ being dependent largely on the amount of blood which it contains, though also to some extent upon the degree of atrophy and fatty changes that it has undergone. Generally, the kidney is somewhat translucent and of a dull red color, but it may be grayish or grayish-white, mottled, or even quite white and opaque. The superficial furrows are usually of a brighter red color than are the granulations. On section, the medullary portion is usually somewhat brighter colored than the cortex, but may, again, resemble it in hue. As a rule, the cortex is diminished in thickness and this is more especially the case in those parts immediately in association with the depressions of the surface. It may, however, happen that in other regions the cortex is of normal size, or even increased, owing to œdema. The larger vessels usually show some thickening.

The histological features may be epitomized as atrophy and degeneration of the secreting structures and relatively diffuse new-formation of connective tissue. The relative extent of these factors depends on the nature of the case and how closely the condition approximates to the chronic parenchymatous form. The glomerular epithelium is, in the less advanced cases, swollen and desquamating, but this is never so

FIG. 189

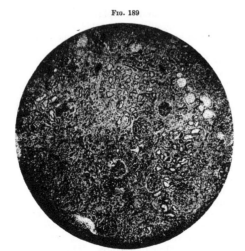

Chronic interstitial nephritis, showing atrophy of tubules and certain of the glomeruli; periglomerular fibrosis; dilatation of tubules. Leitz obj. No. 3, without ocular. (From the collection of Dr. A. G. Nicholls.)

FIG. 190

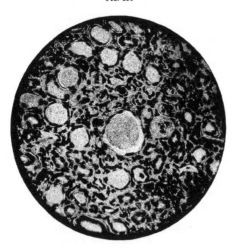

Chronic interstitial nephritis; dilatation of the tubules; hyaline casts. Leitz obj. No. 7, without ocular. (From the collection of Dr. A. G. Nicholls.)

marked as it is in the chronic parenchymatous form. Later, the glomerular tufts lose their epithelium and the vessels become thickened and impervious. Eventually, many of the glomeruli are converted into a structureless, hyaline mass, devoid or almost devoid of nuclei, and more or less lobulated, so that they come to resemble a trefoil or rosette. Not a few, however, can be seen which have evidently retained their functions and, in fact, have undergone a compensatory hypertrophy. The capsule at the same time shows evidences of proliferation and thickening. The changes in the epithelium of the convoluted tubules are strictly comparable with those occurring in chronic parenchymatous nephritis, but are rarely so pronounced. In many parts, where the interstitial tissue is increased, both secreting and collecting tubules may be compressed or collapsed, and are, therefore, smaller than normal, being lined with cubical cells. Not infrequently it will be found that certain tubules have entirely disappeared, or, again, their places are indicated by a ring or double row of simple nuclei. Such epithelial cells as remain are small, atrophic, granular, vacuolated, or fatty. In those parts of the kidney where the fibroid induration is less marked a different picture is to be seen. Here, the tubules are often dilated, some, indeed, being cystic. The lumina of such tubules are dilated and contain granular debris and, perhaps, an occasional cast, while the lining cells are flattened centrifugally from vertical pressure and are extended laterally to cover the increased surface of the basement membrane. The epithelium is also fatty and shows other evidences of degeneration. The dilatation of the tubules is to be attributed to obstruction of the lumina in some portion of their course, owing, either to the encroachment of the newly formed connective tissue, or, again, to blocking by casts, cellular debris, and precipitated salts.

In all cases, there is an increase of the interstitial connective tissue, the amount varying according to the nature of the case and the chronicity of the disease. The depressions of the surface are continuous with bands of connective tissue which extend deeply into the cortical substance and even into the labyrinth. These bands unite freely in the deeper portion, thus dividing the kidney into a series of lobules. In such areas of hyperplasia there may be seen accumulations of round cells, while here and there can be made out developing fibroblasts. In some few cases, the fibrous tissue is very dense and fibrillar. The glomeruli and tubules in these districts are in all stages of atrophy and degeneration and in large part have disappeared altogether. Between the fibrous patches the secreting structures that remain may be comparatively normal, but not infrequently show a certain amount of fatty change. Occasionally, evidences of regenerative hyperplasia can be detected. It is by no means uncommon, moreover, to find the lesions of an acute parenchymatous nephritis superimposed on those of the chronic interstitial form. The vessels in the fibroid areas show some thickening of the adventitia and usually of the intima also, leading to more or less obstruction of the lumina. Some of the vessels may indeed have disappeared.

An important form of chronic Bright's disease is that known as *primary chronic interstitial nephritis*. It has been called also the "gouty kidney," the "genuine contracted kidney," and the "red granular kidney." Anatomically, it resembles closely the other types of chronic interstitial kidney, and, indeed, it is difficult to separate it from them. The reasons for recognizing this variety as a separate entity are largely clinical. The disease begins insidiously, there being no history of any acute renal inflammation. When symptoms manifest themselves, the kidney is already contracted. The affection is, therefore, believed not to pass through the "large white kidney" stage. The process is primarily a chronic one. The etiology is often obscure. In most cases there is a history of alcoholism, gout, or lead poisoning. Sometimes the patient has suffered from some acute infective illness years before. Syphilis, diabetes, and mental strain, are also mentioned as causative factors. Heredity seems to play a part in some instances.

In this form the kidney is usually very small, smaller than that of secondary interstitial nephritis, hard, and granular. The granulations are unusually fine. The capsule is firmly adherent and the organ is generally of a dull red color. Cysts are present on the surface, containing modified urine or yellowish-green colloid material. The cortex is extremely thin, in places practically absent. The pyramids are also reduced in size, though relatively increased in proportion to the cortex. In the gouty cases calcareous and uratic deposits may be found in the substance of the organ. The branches of the renal artery are usually greatly sclerosed. The pelvis of the kidney contains, as a rule, an increased amount of fat, and the atrophied organ is also embedded in a large fatty mass.

Histologically, the pathological changes do not differ materially from those described in the secondary form, except that they are even more intense, and widespread. The newly-formed fibrous tissue is particularly dense. Compensatory regeneration is also met with here in the cells of the tubules.

Suppurative Nephritis.—In this form of nephritis, the inflammation is definitely due to the action of infective agents, usually the staphylococcus and streptococcus, which are brought to the kidney from some distant point. The pyogenic microörganisms in question reach the organ in one or other of four ways: (1) through the blood—hematogenic form; (2) through the urinary tubules; (3) by direct introduction from without—wound infection; (4) and by extension of inflammatory processes from adjacent parts—suppurative nephritis *per extensionem*. The most common methods of infection are through the blood stream (*descending inflammation*) and through the urinary passages (*ascending inflammation*).

Acute Hematogenic Suppurative Nephritis.—Acute hematogenic suppurative nephritis is usually the result or accompaniment of suppurative processes elsewhere in the body. It is, therefore, part and parcel of a generalized septicemia. The most important predisposing conditions to which this form of nephritis is secondary, are ulcerative endocarditis, osteomyelitis, puerperal sepsis, decubitus, pulmonary tuberculosis; less often, typhoid fever, dysentery, lobar pneumonia, scarlatina, variola, and actinomycosis. The offending microörganisms reach the kidney either in the form of definite emboli (*embolic metastatic* form of Orth), or singly or in small numbers, when they become entangled within the vessels and proliferate there (*simple metastatic* form of Orth).

In typical and well-marked cases of this affection, we have all the features of an acute parenchymatous inflammation plus the characteristic manifestations of a suppurative process, namely, abscess-formation. Both kidneys are usually involved, as might be expected. They are swollen and œdematous, and the capsule peels off with ease. The surface, which is paler than normal, is studded with a variable number of small abscesses that present as minute elevations of an opaque, yellowish-white color, surrounded by a congested or hemorrhagic zone. In many instances the abscesses are not larger than a pin-head in size or even less, and are equidistant one from the other throughout the cortex. This arrangement, when present, should always suggest the embolic nature of the case, inasmuch as the abscesses resulting from ascending infection from the lower urinary passages are massed in little groups, separated by areas of comparatively healthy tissue, corresponding to the clusters of papillary tubules.

On section, both the kidneys are found to be riddled with small abscesses chiefly in the cortical portion, but also, to some extent, in the medulla. The cortex is pale, cloudy, and swollen and presents in the neighborhood of the abscesses all the features of an acute parenchymatous inflammation. The abscesses in the cortex are rounded, while those in the medulla tend to be elongated, following the course of the tubules. Exceptionally, certain of them may reach the size of a hazelnut. In the simple metastatic form of Orth, the necrotic foci are usually found in the pyramids (*mycotic papillary nephritis*).

The histological appearances vary in different parts according to the age and intensity of the infective process. Thus, in the earliest stage of abscess-formation we can detect by suitable methods of staining clumps of bacteria within the glomerular and peritubular capillaries. In the immediate vicinity the epithelial cells present degenerative and even necrotic changes. When the lesion is more matured, numbers of leukocytes are found to be massed within the capillaries, within the Bowman's spaces, and in the interstitial stroma in the neighborhood of the tufts. When the abscess is fully formed, we get clumps of bacteria, surrounded by a zone of necrotic tissue, and bounded externally by a mass of leukocytes. In the immediate vicinity of the foci the kidney substance is markedly congested and œdematous, and the secreting cells are swollen, cloudy, and degenerating. In the mycotic papillary form the appearances are similar, but the bacteria are usually found in the secreting tubules of the papillæ and the median zone of the pyramids, indicating an attempt at excretion and elimination of the offending microörganisms.

Suppurative Pyelonephritis and Pyonephrosis.—The type of the ascending infection of the kidney is the disease known as suppurative pyelonephritis or "surgical kidney." In this form the infective agents reach the kidney by way of the urine. Inflammation of the urethra (urethritis), bladder (cystitis), ureters (ureteritis), or the pelvis of the kidney (pyelitis) may all, therefore, be the immediate precursors of suppurative nephritis. The liability to infection is, moreover, greatly increased by fermentative changes in the urine, obstruction to the outflow, the presence of animal parasites, or by mechanical irritation, as from the presence of calculi. In some few instances, the process is in the first instance a descending one, the offending microörganisms being excreted by the kidney into the urine, and exerting merely a passing influence on that organ, until they are resorbed from the lower urinary passages. Here we have the combined effects of soluble toxins upon the kidney substance and, later, of the actual growth of the germs within the kidney substance.

The bacteria chiefly concerned in bringing about this form of nephritis are B. coli, the various pyogenic cocci, and Gonococcus. The descending or excretory type of the affection is met with in such diseases as typhoid fever, scarlatina, variola, septicemia, cholera. The process may attack a previously intact kidney or, again, one the site of hydronephrosis. The cases in which the pelvis of the kidney is filled with pus are termed **suppurative pyelitis**. Sooner or later the kidney substance becomes involved, a condition that is spoken of as **suppurative pyelonephritis**.

In a case that is not too far advanced, one, and usually both kidneys, are swollen and œdematous, soft, and congested. On section, opaque, yellowish streaks can often be made out in the pyramids extending into the cortex, their long axes running in the direction of the collecting tubules, and bounded by a hyperemic zone. In the cortex, too, are similar areas of globular shape, aggregated into the little clusters, and separated from each other by comparatively healthy kidney substance. The streaks in question are due to the inflammatory products which have accumulated in the tubules and the neighboring lymphatics. The opaque areas in the cortex are minute abscesses in the connective-tissue stroma of those parts corresponding to the various lymphatic districts.

In more advanced cases, however, the abscesses are larger, more numerous, and the regional distribution is not nearly so evident. When the abscesses become confluent, they may attain a considerable size and may extend through the greater part of the thickness of the kidney. They may from the first communicate with the pelvis, and if the destructive process be extensive, the organ may be converted into a fluctuating sac containing pus and necrotic tissue, the walls of which are composed of the kidney capsule and shreds of disintegrating kidney substance (**pyonephrosis**). When the patient lives long enough the smaller abscesses may be encapsulated by the formation of fibrous tissue, but where the process is extensive the inflammation may extend to the capsule of the kidney (**perinephritis**) or even to the fat and connective tissue about the organ (**paranephritis**). Thus, the whole of the secreting substance may be destroyed, and the place of the kidney is indicated by a mass of connective tissue containing often inspissated pus and calcareous salts. In cases due to calculus we may find merely a fibrous contracted sac filled with stones.

Histologically, it can be made out that the inflammatory process begins through infection of the collecting tubules, beginning in the pyramids and extending up into the cortex. The kidney, as a whole, is congested, and especially so in the neighborhood of the infected areas. The lymphatics are often distended and filled with leukocytes, among which, by suitable methods of staining, bacteria can be detected. The secreting cells of the tubules near by are swollen, cloudy, and often degenerated. As the process goes on, leukocytes are massed at the part, central necrosis of the infiltrated area takes place and an abscess is formed, pushing aside the adjacent tubules. Later, in some prolonged cases, a certain amount of connective tissue hyperplasia can be made out at the periphery of the necrotic areas.

Traumatic Suppurative Nephritis.—Traumatic suppurative nephritis may result from stabbing or gunshot wounds, or, again, arise in consequence or as a sequel of surgical operations. In such cases the infecting agents are introduced directly from without (*wound infection*). The condition may also arise from contusion. This, by lowering the resisting power of the kidney, renders it an easy prey for microörganisms which may reach it from the lower urinary passages or by way of the blood stream.

Paranephritis.—Suppurative nephritis arising *per extensionem* is invariably associated with paranephritis, of which affection it forms one phase. The infection arises often from some quite remote part and attacks the kidney by way of the connective and fatty tissue surrounding it. The chief etiological factors are traumatism, lumbar and psoas abscesses, suppuration of the retroperitoneal glands. Among the rarer causes may be mentioned empyema, abscess of the liver, abscess of the ligamentum latum, cholecystitis, perforation of the bowel, and paratyphlitis. As might be expected, we do not, in this affection, find the multiple small abscesses so characteristic of suppurative nephritis, but rather a single large abscess, localized to one part of the organ. The process may assume the type of a gangrenous as well as a suppurative inflammation.

Besides the type of disease just described, paranephritis may result from infective processes originating in the kidney itself. Thus, suppurative pyelonephritis, with or without nephrolithiasis, is a most important cause.

Paranephritic abscesses are often large and usually single. Owing to the loose nature of the cellular tissue about the kidney, they extend rapidly. In some few cases, generally those due to pyelonephritis, multiple small abscesses develop, which may undergo absorption or fuse into larger ones. Where the patient survives long enough, a large amount of fibrous scar tissue is formed, so that the kidney becomes embedded in a dense cicatricial mass of almost cartilaginous hardness.

Orth has recorded a case of this kind which led to thrombosis of the renal artery and necrosis of the kidney. Where operative interference is not resorted to, a paranephritic abscess may burrow widely, and may rupture externally or into some viscus. It usually points in the loin or at Poupart's ligament. More rarely, it presents below the gluteus maximus, between the biceps and sartorius, or at the inguinal ring. When not discharging externally, the abscess may empty into the colon, pleural cavity, lung, peritoneal cavity, kidney, pelvis, urethra, bladder, and vagina. One of us (A. G. N.[1]) has reported a unique case in which rupture took place into the stomach.

Specific Nephritis.—Tuberculosis.—Tuberculosis of the kidney is by no means uncommon. The infection is usually hematogenic, but may be an ascending one, arising from other parts of the genito-urinary system. Occasionally, it is due to the extension of tuberculous disease from adjacent structures, as from the suprarenals.

The affection manifests itself in two forms, an **acute miliary tuberculosis** and a **chronic local tuberculosis.** The first variety is probably always secondary, and is usually but a manifestation of a generalized systemic tuberculosis. Occasionally, the primary focus is quite small, and the kidneys, either one or both, are the only organs presenting miliary involvement. The bacilli reach the organ through the renal artery and its branches and are often entangled in the glomerular capillaries. They may, however, get into the tubules, evidently as the result of an attempt at excretion (*elimination tuberculosis* of Cohnheim and Meyer). The lesions characteristic of this affection appear as minute tubercles, or milia, of a grayish-white color, at first somewhat pearly, later, dull and opaque, which appear usually as circumscribed nodules, but sometimes as indefinite streaks. These are generally bounded by a hyperemic zone. The tubercles may be few in number, perhaps restricted to a single arterial district, or, again, are abundant and scattered throughout the organ. They are most numerous in the cortical region. Occasionally, two or more may coalesce to form a larger focus.

Microscopically, the lesion is that typical of an acute tuberculosis. There is a small node of mononuclear or lymphoid cells, in or near a glomerulus, or in some part of the intertubular connective tissue. This may be the sole manifestation. The older and larger foci present in addition a small amount of central caseation. The vessels in the neighborhood of the tubercle are congested, while those within the node are obstructed by inflammatory products or by thickening of the intima. Inasmuch as the process is usually an acute and terminal one we do not find any attempt at healing in the form of fibrous hyperplasia. Giant cells are also absent or scanty.

Chronic local tuberculosis of the kidney is either hematogenic or ascending in its origin. One or both organs may be involved. It is usual at autopsies to find both kidneys affected, but not infrequently the disease is much more advanced in one than the other. The right kidney

[1] Montreal Med. Jour., 27: 1898: 119.

is affected as often as the left. A question that has given rise to some debate is whether genito-urinary tuberculosis is ever primary. Inasmuch as a tuberculous septicemia, without a local lesion, has been demonstrated as a possibility, it cannot be denied that primary genito-urinary tuberculosis can occur. It is, however, never safe to assume that this is the case, unless the most exhaustive search has failed to reveal tuberculous lesions elsewhere. The further point, whether in genito-urinary tuberculosis the affection begins in the kidney, subsequently extending and descending to the kidney pelvis, ureter, and bladder, or whether it originates in the genitalia or bladder and travels upward, is very difficult to decide. The preponderance of evidence at the present time favors the view that in most cases the infection is a descending one, the bacilli passing through the kidney and setting up disease elsewhere, as, for example, in the ureters and bladder. Later, the organisms are carried back and attack the kidneys.

FIG. 191

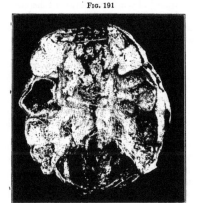

Chronic caseous tuberculosis of the kidney. (From the Pathological Museum of McGill University.)

Three main anatomical types have been described. The first and commonest is the *massive, caseous,* or *ulcerative* form. Here the process usually begins at one pole of the organ, generally the lower, and extends by local metastasis until the whole organ becomes involved. At first appearing as a small, grayish nodule, the tubercle enlarges, becomes caseous, and finally softens. In this way caseous abscesses are formed which in time open up communication with the pelvis. The kidney is thus converted into a series of loculi communicating more or less freely with its cavity and filled with a soft, pultaceous, or curdy necrotic material. These loculi are separated one from the other by septa formed of shreddy and disintegrating kidney substance. The organ is usually enlarged, although its shape is preserved. To the touch it presents in places a soft, fluctuating sensation. Occasionally, the surface will show a series of large bosses of doughy or elastic consistence, over which the capsule is firmly adherent. On section, the kidney is converted into a number of sacs, many of them communicating with the pelvis, and extending up into the cortex. When the necrotic material filling the spaces has been washed away, the walls appear either smooth or covered with a pyogenic membrane. In advanced cases the kidney may be totally destroyed, and is represented by a shrunken mass, consisting of a thin shell of kidney substance, or, perhaps, merely the capsule, enclosing inspissated caseous material. The inflammatory process frequently involves the kidney capsule (**tuberculous perinephritis**), or, again, may extend to the surrounding connective tissue (**tuberculous paranephritis**). The fibro-fatty tissue surrounding the kidney becomes thereby greatly indurated or the seat of abscess-formation. Another sequel of tuberculous nephritis is that the inflammation extends to the mucous membrane lining the pelvis and thence to the ureter and bladder. The process here is manifested by the appearance of scattered elevated tubercles of grayish color on the mucous surface. These are not uncommon in the mucosa of the bladder near the orifices of the ureters. In advanced cases the ureter may become obstructed either by swelling of the mucosa and thickening of the wall, or by the lodgement therein of detritus. If there be not complete destruction of the secreting portion of the kidney the organ becomes greatly enlarged and distended, owing to retention of the urine (**tuberculous pyonephrosis**). Finally, the destructive inflammation may open up the renal vein, and we then get a generalized miliary tuberculosis.

In the second type of renal tuberculosis, the process begins in the pyramids and leads to ulceration of the apices of the papillæ. Hematuria is an early and marked symptom in these cases.

The third variety is characterized by the fact that the organ is uniformly studded with numerous firm, grayish-white nodules, varying in size from that of a pinhead to that of a pea, which show little or no tendency to necrosis. The capsule is adherent, and when removed reveals small, elevated nodules upon the surface of the kidney. This is probably embolic in origin and merely a special form of miliary tuberculosis.

An affection of the kidney closely simulating tuberculosis, and due, as we know now, to a streptothrix, was described by Eppinger in 1891, under the name *pseudotuberculosis cladothricica*.

The final proof of the existence of tuberculous inflammation of the kidney and urinary passages is afforded by the detection of the Bacillus tuberculosis in the urine. This is by no means always an easy task. The germs may be quite few in number. It is then necessary to keep the urine for twenty-four hours, allowing it to deposit in a suitable vessel, centrifugalizing if necessary, and finally examining microscopically.

A further difficulty lies in the fact that the tubercle bacillus closely resembles morphologically certain other members of what are known as the "acid-fast" group of bacilli, of which the most important is the smegma bacillus, found in smegma, on the skin, in the mouth, and in lung cavities. One point of some assistance is that where the bacilli of tuberculosis are present in numbers they are apt to lie in fairly large and dense clumps, while the smegma bacilli are more scattered. It is possible, however, to differentiate the two organisms by means of certain staining reactions. It should be pointed out, however, in this connection that the time-honored Gabbett's method is absolutely unreliable, certainly in the examination of urine, and it would undoubtedly be safer to discontinue its use in the examination of sputum. A better method is to stain in the ordinary way with carbol-fuchsin, decolorize with 30 per cent. mineral acid for thirty seconds, and then with absolute alcohol for three minutes, finally counterstaining with methylene blue. Or, one may employ 1 per cent. rosolic acid in absolute alcohol for five minutes as a decolorizer. Even these methods have been shown recently to be open to objection. G. Basile recommends the use of a 2 per cent. solution of lactic acid in absolute alcohol. The tubercle bacillus will resist decolorization with this for half an hour, while the smegma and other acid-fast organisms lose their color in a few minutes.[1]

Another point of practical importance is that the urine to be tested should always be drawn off by catheter, after preliminary washing of the external genitalia. With this precaution, the entrance of the smegma bacillus is rendered much less likely.

Syphilis.—The manifestations of syphilis in the kidney are very variable. As in the case of most infectious diseases, we may get nephritis of an acute or subacute type, which may result eventually in chronic interstitial change. There may be nothing, however, but the history of the case to identify the lesions as syphilitic. Syphilitic endarteritis may lead to gradual occlusion of the branches of the renal artery with the formation of a typical arteriosclerotic kidney. According to Stroebe, intra-uterine syphilis may result in hypoplasia of the secreting substance of the kidney with a compensatory increase of the fibrous stroma. A striking feature is that the kidney is imperfectly developed. Immature glomeruli are to be seen in the cortex, apparently, in many cases, without proper communication with the secretory tubules.

The characteristic lesion of syphilis, the gumma, is rare in the kidney. Gummas do occur, however, and may be fairly numerous. They vary in size from that of a pin-head to that of a hazel-nut, and are surrounded by a grayish or hyperemic zone. Occasionally, they are soft, resembling abscesses. As they heal they give place to deep fissures, resulting from the contraction of the fibrous cicatricial tissue that is gradually formed. The kidney may thus be divided into a series of lobules, resembling closely the condition of things met with in the syphilitic liver (so-called *hepar lobatum*). Bowlby[2] has described a diffuse gummatous infiltration leading to a notable enlargement of the kidney. Miliary gummas occur but are extremely rare.

---

[1] Giorn. Internaz. d. Scien. Med., Naples, 30:1908:577.
[2] Trans. Path. Soc. of London, 48:1897:128.

Actinomycosis.—This affection in the kidney is usually secondary, the primary lesion being in some part of the alimentary tract, mouth, pharynx, or intestine. In the only instance we have met with, both kidneys contained small cavities filled with a thick, yellowish, homogeneous-looking material, resembling pus. In this the threads of the fungus were readily demonstrated. The primary lesion was in the liver, and the involvement of the kidneys was clearly embolic. Israel[1] has reported what he considered to be a case of primary renal actinomycosis.

FIG. 192

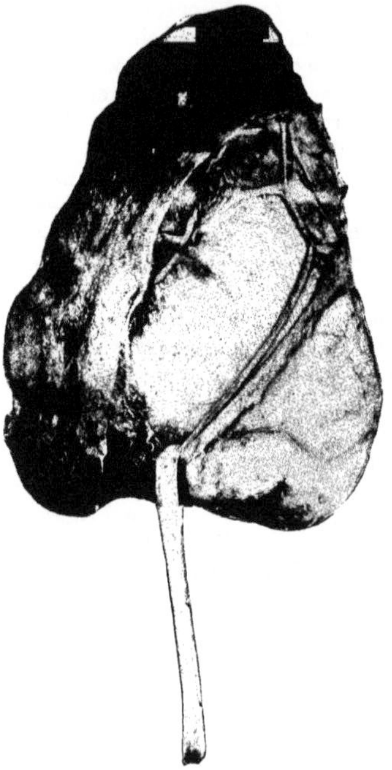

Hydronephrosis. The shell of kidney substance is seen to the left; the enormously dilated pelvis to the right. The ureter is kinked and obstructed by abnormally placed branches of the renal artery and vein. (From the Pathological Museum of McGill University.)

Glanders.—Glanders is rare in the human kidney. It is not uncommon in horses affected by the disease.

Leprosy.— Chronic parenchymatous and interstitial nephritis may be found in cases of leprosy, but are non-specific so far as their anatomical peculiarities are concerned. Amyloid degeneration has also been described. In one instance a leprous granuloma was found in the kidney of a leper (Hedenius; Babes[2]).

RETROGRESSIVE METAMORPHOSES.

Atrophy.—Atrophy of the kidneys occurs in general marasmus and as a senile change. In the former condition the organs are small, the perirenal fat is scanty, and the secreting cells are diminutive. In the senile form the kidneys are small, firm, dark colored, and the surface is finely granular. The capsule is thickened and somewhat adherent. The granulation is due to atrophy of the secreting structures and relative increase of the fibrous stroma. In many cases there is an actual proliferation of connective tissue, together with fibrosis and hyaline degeneration of the glomeruli, a condition no doubt to be attributed in great measure to the

---

[1] Chir. Klin. der Nierenkrank., 1901; Handb. der prakt. Chir.

[2] Untersuchungen uber den Leprabacillus, Berlin, 1898: 80.

arteriosclerosis so often present in advanced life. Retrograde changes incident to the involution period of life, no doubt, play a part also. Secondary atrophy of a kidney may follow obstruction of the ureter, as from stone or external pressure, nephrolithiasis, and chronic tuberculosis.

Hydronephrosis.—Hydronephrosis is the result of some obstruction to the free evacuation of urine. This usually depends upon the presence of a calculus impacted in the ureter, stricture of the ureter, or pressure exerted upon it by a tumor or fibrous band. Milder grades of the affection may be produced by an enlarged prostate, or stricture of the urethra.

The condition begins with dilatation of the pelvis and ureter, but as a result of the constantly increasing pressure, the kidney substance atrophies, the organ dilates, and is eventually converted into a large,

FIG. 193

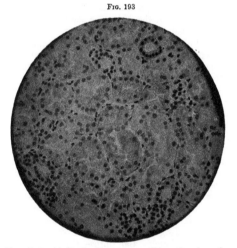

Cloudy swelling. Leitz obj. No. 7, without ocular. This section shows the swelling of the tubular epithelium, the stellate lumina, and the badly-staining nuclei. (From the collection of Dr. A. G. Nicholls.)

loculated sac, formed by a thin shell of kidney substance, containing clear, watery fluid. The function of the kidney is sooner or later destroyed. In this way a very large tumor may be formed in the flank, which is usually crossed in front diagonally by a coil of large intestine.

Degeneration.—**Cloudy Swelling or Albuminous Degeneration.**—Cloudy swelling, or albuminous degeneration, is a constant occurrence in all infective fevers, but particularly in diphtheria, scarlatina, typhoid, and variola. It is found also in certain forms of mineral poisoning, diabetes, hemoglobinemia, gout, and is invariably present in Bright's disease and all forms of local inflammation. Kidneys so affected are usually slightly enlarged, the consistency is relaxed, the cortex is a little swollen and somewhat paler than the pyramids, being of a dull, reddish-gray color. Microscopically, the secreting cells of the contorted tubules are the parts chiefly involved. They are somewhat swollen, turbid, and the nuclei frequently fail to stain. The lumina of the tubules are no longer circular but stellate or irregular. When a fresh section is examined, the cells are opaque and granular, being filled with minute refractile particles which obscure the nuclei. When treated with acetic acid the granules disappear, the protoplasm becomes clear, and the nuclei are again apparent. The condition is apt to pass into fatty degeneration and inflammation.

Fatty Degeneration.—Fatty degeneration is a common sequel of advanced cloudy swelling, and is met with frequently also in pernicious anemia, acute and chronic Bright's disease, amyloid degeneration of the kidney, and in poisoning by phosphorus and certain other mineral substances. In this condition the kidney is flabby, and in well-marked cases paler than normal. The cortex is the part chiefly affected. It is swollen and of a uniform pale, yellowish color, or, again, blotched with yellow, presenting a marked contrast to the darker red of the medulla. The fat may be detected microscopically by staining the tissue, which has previously been frozen or hardened in formalin, with Sudan III, or, again by placing it in Fleming's solution. By the first method the fat appears like granules or droplets of a golden-yellow or carmine-red color. By Fleming's solution, which contains osmic acid, the fat is stained black or brown. It is mainly to be seen in the secreting cells of the contorted tubules and the lining cells of Bowman's capsules.

Hyaline Degeneration.—Hyaline degeneration affects chiefly the glomeruli in chronic Bright's disease.[1] The globules of albumin and the desquamated cells within the tubules often fuse into hyaline masses, thus forming casts.

Hydropic Degeneration is met with in cases of Bright's disease.

Amyloid Degeneration.—This is a frequent accompaniment of general amyloid disease. A local amyloid transformation is occasionally met with in chronic Bright's disease. The condition is invariably associated with fatty changes and diffuse nephritis. The structures first involved are the capillaries of the glomerular tufts, the afferent arterioles, the interlobular arteries, and the vessels of the medulla. In advanced cases all the vessels of the cortex, and even the basement membranes of the tubules, are affected. The vessel walls are thickened, presenting a homogeneous translucent appearance, and the lumina may become impermeable. In advanced cases a whole glomerulus may be converted into a structureless mass. The specific secreting cells show cloudy swelling and fatty degeneration, while there is frequently an interstitial round-celled infiltration. In the tubules are to be seen cellular debris and hyaline-looking casts. It is doubtful whether the amyloid casts, so-called, are really composed of amyloid material.

The kidney is usually enlarged, very firm, and of a consistency sug-

---

[1] See *Landsteiner*, Ziegler's Beiträge, 33:1903:237.

PLATE VIII

FIG. 1

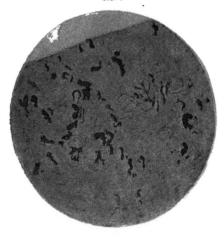

FIG. 2

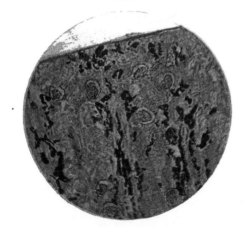

o Sections from the Same Kidney of a Rabbit Treated
with Injections of Corrosive Sublimate. (Klotz.)

1.—Section stained with Sudan 111 to demonstrate fatty degeneration of certain tubules.

2.—Section stained with silver nitrate to demonstrate calcareous deposits in the same groups of
{By combined staining it could be shown that the identical tubules took on both the fatty and
areous reactions.)

gesting india-rubber. When the cut edge is held up to the light it presents a grayish, translucent appearance. In some cases, the glomeruli are sufficiently enlarged to be recognized as small, grayish dots. Where there is much fatty change the kidney may be pale and present the gross appearance of the large white kidney, or, again, it may resemble the granular contracted kidney. The condition may be recognized in the postmortem room by the application of a watery solution of iodine to the cut surface of the organ. The glomeruli usually then appear as small, gelatinous-looking points of a mahogany brown color. The test may fail, however, in the early stages of the disease. In microscopic sections treated with anilin-gentian violet or methylviolet, the amyloid appears as pinkish masses on a dull bluish or greenish-blue background.

Necrosis.—Necrosis of the kidney is a common condition due to the destructive action of bacterial or mineral toxins or the products of disordered metabolism circulating in the blood. Among the infective diseases which bring it about may be mentioned diphtheria, scarlatina, variola, septicemia, typhoid, and tuberculosis. It is met with also in diabetes, gout, icterus, carcinoma, hemoglobinemia, and in poisoning with sublimate, phosphorus, arsenic, cantharides, pyrogallic acid, and salts of chromic acid. A local necrosis is also observed in acute or relapsing nephritis. The cells chiefly affected are those of the contorted tubules. The cytoplasm is swollen, the nuclei fail to stain, the lumina are irregular, and the whole cell has a diffuse, opaque, or ground-glass appearance. The condition closely resembles the coagulation necrosis found in infarction. In cases of sublimate poisoning, deposits of lime salts may be found replacing the cells of the degenerated tubules. The parenchymatous degeneration is often more marked than in the case of nephritis, but there is no infiltration of the connective tissue with inflammatory products.

Levaditi and Rehns, from Ehrlich's laboratory, have described a peculiar form of renal necrosis limited to the papillæ, brought about by vinylamin and tetrahydroquinoleïne.[1]

HEMATOGENOUS INFILTRATIONS.

These are of the nature of corpuscular elements, pigments, or salts, brought to the kidney by the blood and deposited either within the interstitial substance or within the lumina of the secreting tubules. Various soluble salts, the result of pathological processes within the kidney or elsewhere in the body, may through local chemical change be converted into insoluble products, forming the so-called "infarcts."

Hemorrhage.—Hemorrhage into the substance of the kidney is met with in severe passive congestion, embolism, trauma, certain forms of inflammation, and in the general hemorrhagic diathesis.

---

[1] Archives Internat. de Pharmacodynamie et de Thérapie, 8: 1901: 45 and 199.

The effusion takes place about the interlobular vessels or into the Bowman's capsules. Very frequently, the tubules become filled with blood so that blood casts are produced, or when destruction of the blood takes place, pigmentation of the secreting cells occurs.

In acute nephritis and in the hemorrhagic diathesis, small petechial spots are seen distributed over the cortex or throughout the kidney substance.

Leukocytic Infiltration.—Leukocytic infiltration, apart from inflammation, is met with in leukemia. The kidney is enlarged and pale, grayish-yellow in color, due, in part, to the leukocytic accumulation and in part to the associated fatty degeneration. The cortex is swollen. Whitish streaks, representing the overdistended straight vessels, are seen in the pyramidal portion, and more or less wedge-shaped or minute, rounded areas are to be made out in the cortex, the so-called "lymphomata."

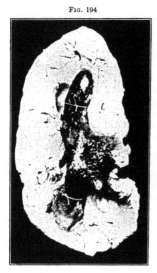

Fig. 194

A coral calculus in the pelvis of the kidney. (From the Pathological Museum of McGill University.)

Microscopically, the vessels of the interstitial substance are everywhere greatly distended with leukocytes, so that the secreting tubules are widely dissociated, and there may be extensive leukocytic infiltration about the glomeruli.

The secreting cells are found in all stages of cloudy swelling, fatty degeneration, and atrophy, owing to pressure and lack of nutrition.

Glycogen.—This is found in the epithelium of Henle's tubes in cases of diabetes.

Pigments.—The pigments found in the kidney are chiefly those derived from the blood, as hemoglobin, methemoglobin, hematoidin, hemosiderin; bile pigment; melanin; and extraneous substances, like carbon and silver.

Blood Pigments.—The blood pigments may be confined to the vessels or may be deposited in the interstitial substance and within the secreting cells.

Bile Pigments.—Bile pigments lead to a diffuse or streaky staining of the kidney of a greenish or greenish-yellow color. Bile pigment can be recognized in the secreting cells, which are often degenerated and cast off, so that a form of cast is produced. Crystalline deposits are seen.

Argyriasis.—Argyriasis, or the so-called "silver infarct," is now but rarely seen. The kidney has a dark gray or blackish tint, and the silver is deposited in the interlobular connective tissue. It may lead to fibroid changes.

Uric Acid.—Uric acid or urates may be precipitated within the kidney tubules or in the pelvis, especially in cases of gout and the uric acid diathesis, but also when the excretion of the urates is not beyond the normal.

Uratic infarcts, composed of acid sodium urate, are sometimes met with in cases of gout when they form whitish streaks in the dilated urinary tubules. Similar deposits are not infrequently found in the kidneys of infants dying between the second and fourteenth day after birth. Here the salts are deposited especially in the lumina of the collecting tubules of the papillæ in the form of doubly refractile spheroliths.

PROGRESSIVE METAMORPHOSES.

The kidney substance possesses considerable powers of regeneration. This might be inferred *a priori* from the fact that many cases of acute inflammation of this organ heal perfectly, and we have further proof of it in the fact that, in both acute and chronic nephritis and in the neighborhood of wounds and infarcts, the nuclei of the secreting cells of the tubules are to be found in different stages of mitosis. Whether these reparative powers are sufficient to reproduce whole tubules and glomeruli is still in question. It seems probable, however, that this may be possible in young developing individuals of certain of the lower animals. As age advances, the power of growth inherent in the cells becomes noticeably weaker.

Compensatory Hypertrophy.—Compensatory hypertrophy is found in cases where one kidney is congenitally defective, has been removed by operation, or is inefficient from disease. The remaining kidney resembles closely the normal organ save that it is much larger and its cortex is somewhat broader. It rarely, however, attains the weight of two normal kidneys combined. The pyramids are not increased in number. Such an organ is specially liable to disease, inasmuch as its reserve power is small. Whether the condition is a true hypertrophy, or not rather a hyperplasia, is still unsettled.

Tumors.—For purposes of description it is convenient to classify tumors of the kidney according to their histological appearance. On this basis we may recognize tumors of epithelial type, meaning by this the various forms of **adenoma** and **carcinoma**, and those of connective-tissue type, which would include such forms as the **fibroma, myoma, lipoma, myxoma, angioma,** and **sarcoma.** It should be remarked, however, that the various new-growths of the kidney have much more in common than have epithelial and connective-tissue neoplasms occurring elsewhere, inasmuch as the kidney, both in its secreting mechanism and supporting framework, is derived entirely from the mesoblast. We must, therefore, give the term carcinoma, if we apply it to the kidney, a histological sense, rather than a developmental one. In addition, not a few of the kidney tumors are of mixed type and may properly be classed as **teratoid** in nature.

The commonest tumors of the kidney are the sarcoma and carcinoma, the former being somewhat more frequently found than the latter. The benign growths are usually small and insignificant, though large lipomas have been described by Warthin and others.

Adenoma.—The adenoma, a benign tumor of epithelial type, varies in size from that of a millet-seed to that of a walnut, or even larger, and is usually found in the cortex. It forms single or multiple, soft, well-defined nodules of whitish color. Histologically, an *alveolar*, a *tubular*, and a *papillary* form can be recognized. The cells forming the tumor are of columnar type. Occasionally, the tubules are dilated into cysts—*cystadenoma.* Some of the tumors formerly classed with cystadenomas may possibly have been hypernephromas (q. v.).

FIG. 195

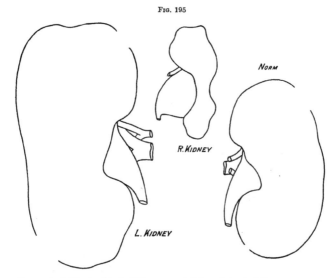

Compensatory hypertrophy: *R.* K*idney*, congenital hypoplasia: *L.* K*idney*, compensatory hypertrophy (length, 14.5 cm.); *Norm.*, a normal adult kidney (length, 11.0 cm.). (Outlines made to scale from specimens in McGill Medical Museum.)

Fibromas.—Fibromas are rather common in the kidney but are insignificant in importance. They form small masses, from a microscopic nodule to one the size of a pea, rarely larger.

Leiomyomas and Fibroleiomyomas.—Leiomyomas and fibroleiomyomas, composed of unstriped muscle, or an admixture of muscle and connective-tissue fibres, are met with, but are rare. They may be found both in the cortex and in the pyramids.

Rhabdomyomas are rare also.

Lipomas.—Lipomas are found beneath the capsule and in the cortex of the kidney. They are single or multiple, and usually of small size although exceptions to this rule occur. Histologically, they are encapsulated and consist of ordinary adipose cells. Some of them, when situated in the kidney substance, are occasionally combined with myoma and sarcoma (mixed tumors).

Besides these lipomas proper it must be noted that there is another very characteristic tumor whose cells of another type are also apt to be rich in fat—namely, the hypernephroma, to be described presently (p. 818).

Myxomas.—Myxomas are rare. Most of the growths described as myxomas are more probably to be regarded as connective-tissue growths that have undergone secondary mucinous degeneration. Bezold and Hollen, however, have each reported a case of true myxoma.

Chondromas and **osteomas** have been met with, but are extremely rare.

Angiomas, more correctly **teleangiectases,** are occasionally found. They may be situated in the pyramids or pelvis. When projecting into the cavity of the kidney they may give rise to serious hemorrhage.

Sarcoma.—Sarcoma is the most common tumor found in the kidney. It is met with both in childhood and in adult life. New-growths, often termed sarcomas, are comparatively common in early life and may even be congenital. Careful study of these, however, will show that the vast majority of them are of mixed type, containing striped muscle, cartilage, or bone. They are, therefore, more properly included under the teratoid new-formations.

Round-celled and *spindle-celled sarcomas* are described, the former being often highly vascular. *Alveolar angiosarcoma,* really either an endothelioma or perithelioma, is occasionally met with. Endotheliomas may arise from the lining cells of bloodvessels or lymphatics. Giant cells are at times found in renal sarcomas.

Carcinoma.—Carcinoma of the kidney is somewhat more common on the right side than on the left, and is more frequent in men than in women. It may arise from the secreting cells of the tubules or from the epithelium lining the pelvis. It is generally held that the adenoma has a distinct tendency to develop into carcinoma. Carcinoma of distinctly glandular type is known as *adenocarcinoma.*

It is somewhat difficult to draw the line between the simple adenoma and the carcinoma. Certain authors, notably Pilliet, Sottas, and Albarran, hold that tumors which histologically resemble pure adenomas behave at times like malignant growths, as evidenced by local infiltration and the formation of metastases. The same peculiarity has been observed in adenomas elsewhere.

Primary carcinoma may be nodular or diffuse, and is of the *scirrhous, simple,* or *medullary* type. The nodular forms are well-defined, and are provided often with a more or less perfect capsule. The diffuse forms lead to a generalized enlargement of the organ without much deformity. Carcinomas frequently attain a considerable size, but are not usually so large as the sarcomas. The growth may extend into the pelvis and ureter. Degenerative changes not infrequently occur in the centre of the growths, leading to hemorrhagic extravasation, cyst-forma-tion, and sometimes calcareous deposit. Hematuria is, therefore, a not uncommon manifestation of the disorder.

Carcinoma is much more often secondary in the kidney than primary. It may follow cancer of the testicle, liver, stomach, uterus, mamma, pancreas, or of the other kidney.

Sarcomas may also form metastatic deposits in the kidneys. The *melanotic sarcoma* is always secondary.

Teratoids.—The teratoid or embryonal mixed tumors[1] of the kidney form a most interesting study. They include the large majority of the so-called sarcomas and carcinomas found in childhood. Careful in-vestigations have shown, however, that they have distinct features of their own and should be placed in a class by themselves. Inasmuch as they have been found at birth or shortly after, it has been thought that they are due to developmental errors, probably being present in a latent form at a very early period of life, and being subsequently excited into activity under the influence of some stimulus, notably trauma. Very exceptionally, they are met with in adults. The left kidney is involved more often than the right, but both organs may be primarily affected. These tumors often attain a great size, one being on record which weighed thirty-six pounds. The general shape of the kidney is not greatly altered, though the surface may be somewhat nodular. The kidney substance proper usually forms a more or less complete shell about the tumor. On section, the growth may be homogeneous and of a grayish-pink color, but it is common to find areas of degeneration, cysts, and hemorrhagic extravasation into its substance. Extension usually takes place into the veins and the lungs are usually secondarily involved.

The histological structure is often highly complicated, and may vary considerably in different tumors, and in different parts of the same tumor. In general, it may be said that there are to be seen more or less abundant epithelial cells, arranged in masses or in tubules, and of glandular type, together with a somewhat cellular stroma, composed of round or spindle cells. This peculiarity of structure has led to these growths being termed *adenosarcomas*. According to the predominance of one or other type of cell, however, these mixed tumors may, at one time, closely re-semble the adenomas and carcinomas, with which they have often been confounded, and, at another, the sarcomas. In addition to the features mentioned, the majority contain fibres of striped and unstriped muscle (*rhabdomyoma, rhabdomyosarcoma, myosarcoma*), islets of hyaline carti-lage, and even, it is said, ganglion cells, thus indicating their teratomatous nature. Rarely, epithelial "pearls" surrounded by muscle-fibres have been observed.

Considerable divergence of opinion has been expressed in regard to the origin of these growths. The presence of striated muscle-fibres in

[1] See Hedrén, Ziegler's Beiträge, 40:1907:1.

many of them has suggested the idea that they are due to the development of misplaced embryonic tissue, notably portions of the Wolffian body. It is possible, however, as Wilms and others think, that the fibres in question are derivatives of the primitive myotomes of the embryo.

In the category, also, of tumors derived from embryonic "rests" is the form conveniently termed by Birch-Hirschfeld[1] the **hypernephroma**. This is a tumor believed by many competent pathologists to be derived from misplaced suprarenal tissue (Grawitz,[2] Lubarsch, Gatti, Kelly). Accessory suprarenals or misplaced portions of suprarenal tissue have been found in a great variety of situations, such as the immediate neighborhood of the normal site of the suprarenal, in or beneath the capsule of the kidney, about the renal vessels, in the spermatic cord, between the testis and epididymis, in the inguinal canal, in the broad ligament, in the solar plexus, the coeliac ganglion, and even in the liver and pancreas. Tumors may originate, conceivably, therefore, from the proliferation of suprarenal tissue in any of these situations.

The most common, and by far the most important, of such new-growths are those found in connection with the kidney. They are met with usually at the upper end of the organ, in the cortex just beneath the capsule. The tumor is well circumscribed, and usually bounded by a more or less perfect connective-tissue capsule. It is made up of a series of nodes, varying somewhat in size, divided one from the other by connective-tissue septa, and composed, in turn, of a series of smaller nodules, which contain, as a rule, but little connective tissue. Hypernephromas are moderately firm, of a yellowish, yellowish-white, or brownish-yellow color. There is a marked tendency to retrograde metamorphosis, necrosis, fatty change, hemorrhage, and cyst-formation. Rarely, there is calcification. As they grow they gradually replace the kidney substance, but are usually bounded by a zone of distorted and compressed renal cells. The connective-tissue capsule is often invaded by the proliferating cells, but the remains of it can generally be detected on careful examination. This constitutes one of the characteristic features of the hypernephroma. The larger growths tend to penetrate into the pelvis of the kidney and invade the renal veins. Metastasis thus takes place through the blood circulation.

Histologically, the structure of these tumors is highly complicated, and it is not surprising, therefore, that, until Grawitz pointed out their true nature, many of them had been described variously as lipomas, adenomas, carcinomas, sarcomas, adenosarcomas, angiosarcomas, endotheliomas, and peritheliomas. The microscopic examination will, as a rule, reveal a connective-tissue capsule, which in the smaller growths is often complete and in the larger ones, although more or less infiltrated, can usually be traced here and there. In brief, a hypernephroma may be described as a tumor composed of a stroma formed of a rather close meshwork of capillary vessels, and of cells arranged in rows, columns, or clusters closely associated with these capillaries. The character and arrangement

---

[1] Ziegler's Beiträge, 24:1898:343.   [2] Virchow's Archiv, 93:1883:39.

of the cells recalls more or less perfectly the appearance of the cortex of the suprarenal and of tumors arising therefrom. This resemblance is most striking in the case of the smaller hypernephromas. The larger growths are apt to be alveolar in type, the component nodules being separated one from the other by a small amount of connective tissue in the form of trabeculæ continuous with the capsule. The endothelium lining the capillaries is usually quite distinct and may even be proliferated. The alveolar appearance may cause the tumor to be mistaken for a carcinoma or a sarcoma. The tumor-cells proper, lying between the capillary vessels, are arranged in rows or double rows, like the cells of the zona fasciculata of the suprarenal cortex, and are directly continuous

FIG. 196   FIG. 197

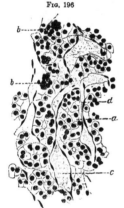 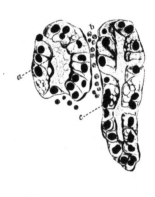

Section of portion of a hypernephroma of the kidney. A characteristic area showing columns of clear polygonal cells: *a*, lying in immediate apposition to the endothelium (*d*) of the capillary sinuses (*c*). At *b*, areas of infiltration and degeneration.

Section from another portion of the same tumor, more highly magnified, showing tubular arrangement: *a*, swollen translucent tumor cells surrounding a definite lumen *b*, capillary *c*, fat droplets in tumor cells. (Buday.)

with the cells of the vascular endothelium. They are of epithelial type, usually polygonal, but may be rounded, cubical, columnar, or irregular, and frequently contain multiple vacuoles, spaces which originally contained fat. The fatty infiltration of the cells is a noteworthy feature of the hypernephroma. Glycogen is also commonly present in relatively great amount. A black pigment is also to be found, similar to that normally present in the suprarenal gland.

Besides the alveolar form, a tubular or trabecular arrangement is occasionally met with; or, again, the type may vary in different parts of the growth. Tumors of great complexity may thus be formed.

Cysts.—The congenital so-called **"cystic degeneration"** of the kidney has been already referred to. **Single cysts,** often of large size, lined with flattened epithelium and containing a slightly albuminous fluid, are occasionally met with in otherwise healthy kidneys, especially in old people. They are possibly to be explained as the result of faulty development during foetal life or of retention of secretion. Small multiple cysts are common in chronic interstitial nephritis and the arterio-sclerotic kidney.

Dermoid Cysts have been found in the kidney, but are very rare.

Parasites.—Among the animal parasites described as at times infesting the kidney may be mentioned *Echinococcus, Cysticercus cellulosæ, Distoma hematobium, Eustrongylus gigas, Filaria sanguinis,* and *Pentastomum denticulatum.*

THE PELVIS OF THE KIDNEY AND URETERS.

CONGENITAL ANOMALIES.

These have been discussed above (see p. 778).

CIRCULATORY DISTURBANCES.

Œdema.—Œdema is found associated with passive congestion and inflammation.

Hyperemia.—**Active Hyperemia.**—Active hyperemia of the mucous membrane lining the pelves and ureters is met with in cases of inflammation and where irritating substances have been excreted by the kidneys.

Passive Hyperemia.—Passive hyperemia is observed in the condition of general systemic passive congestion, and also in obstruction to the outflow of blood from the renal veins.

Hemorrhage.—Hemorrhage results from inflammation, passive congestion, ulceration, traumatism, the hemorrhagic diatheses, parasites, and tumors. In certain cases, also, of acute and chronic nephritis, blood may escape into the urinary passages.

FOREIGN BODIES.

Nephrolithiasis.—When salts are deposited in the pelvis of the kidney they are found in the form of *uratic gravel,* or as *calculi,* varying in size from that of a pea to a large branched mass, the so-called "coral calculus," which may occupy the whole pelvis of the organ. The smaller calculi are not infrequently found within the calices, or may be impacted in the ureter.

The condition often leads to suppurative pyelitis or pyonephrosis, and the whole organ may be destroyed, being finally represented only by a fibrous sac inclosing the stones.

Deposits of *carbonate* or *phosphate* of *lime* are met with occasionally in old people when resorptive processes are going on in bone, and in cases of sublimate poisoning (see vol. i, p. 927).

ALTERATIONS IN THE LUMINA OF THE URINARY PASSAGES.

Narrowing of the lumen of the ureter may occur, and leads to a more or less complete obstruction to the outflow of the urine. A variety of causes may bring it about. Chief among these are, inflammatory thickening of the mucosa, the presence of granulomata, and fibroid induration of the ureteral wall. Owing to inflammatory changes, the mucous membrane lining the pelvis may encroach upon the orifice of the ureter after the fashion of a valve, and lead to obstruction. Swelling of the mucosa of the bladder may also shut off the opening of the ureter. Strictures of the ureter may, however, be congenital as well as acquired. Possibly both are inflammatory in their origin.

The lumen may be **obstructed** by foreign substances lodging within it. Calculi, blood clots, necrotic tissue, portions of tumors, and parasites are to be mentioned in this connection.

Pressure from without is also an important etiological factor. It may be due to tumors, enlarged glands, a retroflexed uterus, an overfilled rectum or bladder in a contracted pelvis, inflammatory bands, ligatures, a horseshoe kidney, an anomalous renal artery, or an accumulation of extravasated urine.

Traction upon the ureter, and kinking or torsion from a movable kidney, sometimes, also, bring about obstruction.

The effect of such obstruction is the same in all cases. The urine is dammed back, and that portion of the urinary passage proximal to the point of obstruction is dilated. When the pelvis of the kidney is distended with clear, watery fluid, usually a modified urine, the condition is known as **hydronephrosis**. Hydronephrosis is more likely to occur when the obstruction is brought about slowly or is due to intermittently acting causes. Both kidneys, but more often only one, may be affected.

In a moderately advanced case, the pelvis is dilated and the kidney substance is somewhat compressed and atrophic. The condition will, under ordinary circumstances, go on increasing until the external pressure is equal to that of the secretion. In time the kidney may be greatly enlarged, being converted into a thin sac containing, perhaps, several liters of fluid. The fluid in question is low in specific gravity (1002 to 1012), contains little or no albumin, and is deficient in urea, chlorides, and phosphates. Microscopically, it may contain leukocytes, red blood corpuscles, and cholesterin. Should infection take place the contents become intermingled with pus (**pyonephrosis**). (See also p. 765.)

Solutions of continuity of the ureters are usually due to traumatism, ulceration, or new-growths.

INFLAMMATIONS.

Inflammation of the pelvis of the kidney is called **pyelitis**; of the ureter, **ureteritis**.

Pyelitis.—Pyelitis most commonly results from an ascending infection, microörganisms reaching the pelvis of the kidney from the lower urinary passages by way of the urine. The possibility of this, in spite of the downward current of the urine, has been amply demonstrated. Any condition which interferes with the free outflow of the urine and brings about its decomposition would naturally aid in the production of pyelitis. Retention of urine, cystitis, enlarged prostate, and stricture of the urethra, are the conditions of most importance in this connection. It should be mentioned, however, that in these cases the inflammatory process need not progress by contiguity, for pyelitis may result from a preëxisting cystitis without the ureters being involved. Moreover, although the infecting agents may have developed within the bladder, they may infect the pelvis of the kidney without setting up a cystitis.

Pyelitis, again, may be the result of a hematogenous infection or of inflammatory processes involving the kidneys themselves. In this form the various infections and intoxications play an important role. Chief among these are typhoid, variola, diphtheria, pyemia, and agents like copaiba and cantharidin. Local irritation within the pelvis may also bring about pyelitis, such as may be produced by stones and parasites.

In rare cases, pyelitis may be due to the extension of inflammation from some of the parts about the kidney.

Although in many instances pyelitis is toxic or irritative in nature, it is usually not long before infection is superadded. The microörganisms most often at fault are B. coli, the various pyogenic cocci, Gonococcus, more rarely B. proteus.

Pyelitis is usually bilateral. Even if the process at first be localized to one kidney pelvis, as in the case of stone, it is not uncommon for the infective agents to make their way into the other ureter and attack the opposite kidney. According to the anatomical changes produced, we may recognize a **catarrhal**, a **suppurative**, a **membranous**, and a **gangrenous pyelitis**. The form produced depends largely upon the nature and intensity of the infection and the mechanical conditions subsisting.

In catarrhal pyelitis, the mucous membrane lining the pelvis is swollen, congested, and may present minute hemorrhages. The urine contains mucus, leukocytes, and desquamated epithelial cells.

In the purulent form, the inflammation is more intense and the urine is distinctly purulent. In some cases, as above mentioned, the pelvis, and even the kidney, may be distended with pus (**pyonephrosis**). In cases of stone, in which pressure is exerted upon the inflamed mucosa, ulceration and gangrene may result.

Membranous pyelitis is the result of a particularly virulent infection.

In cases of pyelitis that have lasted some time, the mucosa is reddened and thickened, and is studded with a number of grayish prominences.

These, according to some observers, are lymphadenoid in nature, and are due either to hyperplasia of previously existing lymph-nodes or to a new-formation of lymphoid tissue as a result of the inflammation. In other cases small cysts are present (**pyelitis cystica**). Polypoidal outgrowths are occasionally met with, particularly in suppurative cases. In very chronic pyelitis, and especially in the tuberculous variety, the lining membrane becomes thickened and horny (leukoplakia), and of a pearly white color, resembling cholesteatoma.

Ureteritis.—Ureteritis is, in most respects, similar to pyelitis, and its characters may, therefore, be inferred from what has just been said.

Tuberculosis.—**Miliary tuberculosis** of the pelvis of the kidney, apparently hematogenic in origin, has been met with, but is rare. The usual type is **chronic** and **caseating** in character. This form usually may be traced to the influence of a tuberculous kidney, but is sometimes, also, the result of an ascending infection from the lower urinary passages or genitalia. We find small, elevated tubercles in the mucosa which tend to coalesce. These are often found in the upper part of the ureter and near its entrance into the bladder. In time they lead to thickening of the mucous membrane with encroachment upon the lumen and more or less obstruction to the free outflow of urine. Ultimately the wall of the ureter becomes greatly thickened and ulceration takes place. In an advanced case, we have seen the whole of the urinary passages, from the point of the penis to the kidney, infiltrated and thickly studded with coarse tubercles tending to become confluent.

Parasites.—The more important parasites are *Filaria sanguinis hominis, Distoma hematobium, Eustrongylus gigas,* and *Ascaris lumbricoides.* Filaria in the urinary passages cause hematuria and chyluria, the latter being a characteristic symptom.

RETROGRESSIVE METAMORPHOSES.

The only condition worthy of note, coming under this category, is **ulceration.** This is sometimes the result of inflammation, but is perhaps more often due to the presence of a calculus (*pressure necrosis*).

PROGRESSIVE METAMORPHOSES.

Tumors.—The most frequently occurring tumor of the pelvis of the kidney is the villous **papilloma.**[1] It may give rise to serious, even fatal, hemorrhage. Squamous-celled **epitheliomas** have been met with, but are rare.[2] In such cases there must have been a metaplasia of the lining transitional epithelium. Primary **carcinoma** has been observed, but is

---

[1] Savory and Nash, Lancet, London, 2: 1904: 1699; Busse, Virchow's Archiv, 164: 1901:119; Matsuoka, Deutsche Zeitschr. f. Chir., 68:1903.

[2] Kelly, Proc. Path. Soc. Phila., (N. S.) 3: 1900: 217; also Kischensky, Ziegler's Beiträge, 30:1901:348.

also rare.[1]   It is occasionally found associated with the presence of stones, suggesting an etiological relationship.   **Lymphosarcoma** of the pelvis is described.[2]   Kaufmann[3] has met with a case of **sarcoma** containing smooth and striated muscle fibres (**teratoma**).   An **adenoma** of the ureter has been met with.   Inasmuch as this structure contains no glands, it has been supposed that the tumor originates from remains of the Wolffian duct.   Hektoen[4] has recorded an instance of primary carcinoma of the ureter.

Sometimes the mucous membrane lining the urinary passages is the site of multiple small cysts, a condition called, possibly erroneously, **pyelitis, ureteritis, cystitis, urethritis cystica**, as the case may be.   These have been thought by some to originate in downgrowths of the superficial epithelium.   Others think that they are due to proliferation of the subepithelial connective tissue, with elevation of the mucosa.   The cysts develop in the angle thus formed by the prominence and the general surface.   Still others would attribute them to the activity of parasites.

[1] Hektoen, Jour. Amer. Med. Assoc., 26: 1896: 1115.

[2] White, Trans. Path. Soc. London, 49: 1898: 178.

[3] Med. Gesellsch. Göttingen, 6:2:1908; also see Albarran, Ann. d. mal. d'organes gén. urin., 18:1900, and 21:1903.   (Lit.)

[4] Jour. Amer. Med. Assoc., 26: 1896: 1115.

CHAPTER XXXVI.

THE BLADDER AND URETHRA.

THE BLADDER.

CONGENITAL ANOMALIES.

THE development of the bladder may be interrupted at any stage of its progress. Complete defect of the bladder has been reported. In this case, the ureters discharge into the urethra. Occasionally, the septum dividing the rectum from the bladder is wholly or partially lacking, so that the ureters and the rectum empty into a large cloaca. This is sometimes associated with imperforate anus.

Doubling and bisecting septa are recorded. Aberrant prostatic glands have been found in the wall of the bladder (Henle).

Extroversion.—The most common anomaly, however, is extroversion. Here, there is failure of union between the two halves of the body along the median ventral line. The anterior wall of the bladder and the corresponding portion of the abdominal wall are wanting. The pubic bones are also often separated by a considerable interval. The condition is much more common in males than in females. Extroversion in the female is apt to be associated with prolapse or procidentia of the uterus. In rarer cases, the bladder is complete but prolapsed through an abdominal fissure (*ectopia vesicæ*).

Diverticula.—Diverticula may be found near the point of junction with the urachus.

Small cysts of the urachus are common.

DISLOCATIONS.

The bladder may be displaced upward, downward, or to one side. The pregnant uterus in the course of its enlargement, tumors of the pelvis and pelvic organs, and intestinal adhesions may carry or drag it upward.

Downward dislocation is the most common and important form. It is due to muscular relaxation, sagging of the pelvic floor, destruction of the perineal body, and malpositions of the uterus. *Cystocele* is a downward pouching of the floor of the bladder. *Extroversion* of the bladder through the urethra (female) is rare, and is met with chiefly in young children. It is sometimes caused by the prolapse of a tumor of the trigone, which passes into and through the urethra, eventually dragging the bladder after it.

Lateral dislocation may be caused by inflammatory infiltration or adhesions, tumors; in rare instances, the bladder has formed part of the contents of the sac in inguinal and femoral hernia. It is hardly necessary to say that, for anatomical and physiological reasons, dislocations of the bladder are almost confined to the female sex.

CIRCULATORY DISTURBANCES.

These are not of much practical importance.

Hyperemia.—**Active Hyperemia.**—Active hyperemia is nearly always an inflammatory manifestation, and is met with in cases where the urine contains irritating substances, as, for instance, cantharidin, or where there is extension of inflammation from the neighboring parts.

Passive Hyperemia.—Passive hyperemia is a frequent accompaniment of general systemic congestion. The vessels, particularly those of the trigone and neck of the bladder, are turgid or even varicose, standing out in marked contrast with the otherwise pale mucosa. This appearance is all the more characteristic since the normal vesical mucosa is strikingly pale. Passive congestion often leads to œdema of the bladder wall and finally catarrh of the mucosa.

Hemorrhages.—Hemorrhages, either in the form of **petechiæ** or **suggillations**, are met with in cystitis, ulceration, tumors, and the hemorrhagic diathesis.

Massive extravasations into the cavity may be due to extreme hyperemia, tumors, calculi, traumatism, and the hemorrhagic diathesis.

INFLAMMATIONS.

Cystitis.—Inflammation of the bladder—cystitis—is of frequent occurrence, and is due, in the vast majority of cases, to the extension of inflammation from other parts of the urinary passages (kidney, pelvis, ureter, etc.), or to abnormalities in the contents of the viscus. Gonorrhœal urethritis and pyelitis are examples of the first class. Of the second, decomposing urine, calculi, and foreign bodies may be cited. The irritation set up is usually aggravated by secondary infection.

Obstruction to the outflow of urine, as in stricture of the urethra or enlarged prostate, is a common cause, not only from the stagnation of the urine, but on account of infection which invariably takes place. A distended bladder is particularly liable to bacterial invasion, since its resisting power is diminished, and the retained urine, undergoing as it does marked chemical changes, acts as a direct irritant to the mucous membrane. Moreover, certain bacteria, which reach the bladder from outside, induce various forms of fermentation and chemical decomposition so that the original disturbance is aggravated and perpetuated. The microörganisms in question reach the bladder from the urethra, or from parts adjacent to the bladder. They are also introduced through careless instrumentation or the use of a dirty catheter.

The urine in cystitis is often alkaline and has a fœtid ammoniacal odor. The reaction and the fermentative processes going on depend, however, on the nature of the offending microörganism. The ordinary ammoniacal decomposition of the urine is brought about by Micrococcus ureæ. When B. coli is present alone, according to Schmidt and Aschoff, the urine is acid. If the urine contain staphylococci, either alone or associated with B. coli, the reaction is alkaline.

In a few instances, cystitis can be traced to hematogenic infection, to the action of a circulating toxin, or to the extension of an inflammatory process in adjacent organs, like the uterus and rectum.

Cystitis is acute or chronic.

Acute Cystitis.—Catarrhal Cystitis.—The mildest form of the acute affection is catarrhal cystitis. As people do not die from this disease, the condition is only discovered in the routine examination of those who have died from other causes. At autopsy, there may be surprisingly little evidence of its presence, even where the signs were clear during life. At most, there is slight redness and swelling of the mucosa, and any urine present contains a little mucus, with a few leukocytes and some degenerated epithelium. Small grayish blebs may be found about the neck and trigone (*herpes vesicæ*).

Acute Suppurative Cystitis.—A more serious disturbance is acute suppurative cystitis. Here, the mucous membrane is reddened and swollen, particularly about the fundus and trigone, and on the surface of the rugæ. If the urine has been alkaline, a macerating process has been going on and the epithelium is swollen, soft, and desquamating in large flakes. In this detritus phosphates, carbonates, and other urinary salts are often deposited, giving the mucosa a dirty whitish or whitish-brown, gritty appearance, not unlike mortar. Pus can frequently be squeezed out of the lacunæ, and hemorrhagic patches may be seen here and there.

The suppurative process may extend into the bladder wall, infiltrating the interstitial tissue and undermining the muscle, which may thus be dissected off and float free in the vesical cavity in the form of soft, friable tags. When the suppuration extends diffusely throughout the muscular wall, the condition may be spoken of as **phlegmonous cystitis**. The process may, however, extend still deeper to the surrounding connective tissue—**paracystitis**, or even to the peritoneum—**pericystitis**. Abscesses of considerable size may form in the perivesical cellular tissue. Provided that the patient survive, they may become circumscribed and heal, leading to fibrous induration. Perforation of the abscess into the peritoneal cavity, intestine, and vagina has been recorded.

Membranous Cystitis.—A third form is the so-called membranous cystitis. This, in many cases, is brought about by chemical changes in the urine, particularly by the action of ammonium carbonate, which produces swelling, desquamation, and maceration of the tissues. The condition, however, also occurs in certain of the infective fevers, typhoid, cholera, the exanthemata, pyemia, diphtheria, dysentery, and in secondary carcinoma derived from the uterus. The bladder is intensely congested and of a deep red hemorrhagic appearance, while upon the surface of the rugæ, particularly in the posterior part, there is a whitish-gray membrane, more or less firmly adherent. This membrane is liable to be infiltrated with urinary salts. Microscopically, the mucosa presents coagulation necrosis.

Emphysematous cystitis, an affection very similar to the so-called pneumatosis intestini and kolpohyperplasia cystica (q. v.), has been described.[1]

Chronic Cystitis.—Chronic cystitis may result from the acute form, or may be chronic from the start. Depending upon the cause, the bladder is distended and thin-walled, or contracted and hypertrophic. The secretion is mucopurulent. The mucous membrane is usually much thickened, and lies in deep folds, or polypoid outgrowths may be formed. The mucosa is sometimes greatly reddened, but more often is of a slaty color, showing incrustation with salts and slight superficial erosion. The lymph-follicles may be enlarged or increased in numbers, so that they become visible and give the surface a granular appearance.

Syphilis.—Syphilis but rarely affects the bladder; little or nothing is known of luetic ulceration in this locality.

Tuberculosis.—The mucous membrane of the urinary bladder is normally quite resistant to tuberculous infection. Active bacilli may, for a long time, be brought in contact with it without inducing lesions. A preëxisting cystitis will, however, lessen this relative immunity. Vesical tuberculosis is rarely hematogenic, but the infection is carried through the medium of the urine from the upper urinary passages, or, much more often, reaches the viscus by extension from the genitalia. That tuberculosis of the bladder is rarer in females than in males is explained by the fact that genital tuberculosis is not so often met with in the former. In the male, tuberculosis of the kidney or of the prostate is the usual cause. Only rarely is the tuberculosis primary, and in such cases the bacilli are, possibly, derived from the blood, but more probably from the outside through the urethra. That the urethra is uninvolved does not exclude this possibility, for it is particularly refractory to tuberculous infection.

Anatomically, there are two forms, **multiple milia** and the **caseous ulcer.**

The miliary variety takes the form of minute grayish nodules situated just beneath the epithelial layer of the mucosa. In descending infection these are usually most thickly grouped about the orifices of the ureters. In the ascending form they are found at the trigone and neck of the bladder. The milia are surrounded by a reddish zone. The larger ones present central caseation, but the smaller can only be distinguished from hyperplastic lymph-follicles by microscopic examination.

When the nodules coalesce, large granulomas are produced which undergo necrosis and ulceration. These tend to be restricted to the mucosa, and spread laterally rather than into the muscular wall. It may be difficult at first to recognize them as tuberculous, since the bases

[1] Ruppanner, Fortschr. d. Med., 2:1908.

may be quite clean and free from necrotic and caseous material. Only in the more extreme cases are large tuberculous masses produced, with irregular and fissured surfaces, which may undermine the mucosa. As in the case of other ulcers, the surface is often infiltrated with urinary salts.

Secondary tuberculosis of the bladd.r, derived from organs not in direct contact or communication with the viscus, is somewhat rare. It does, however, occur, through the mediation of the peritoneum. Tuberculosis of the small intestine, cecum, appendix, or Fallopian tubes, plays a leading role here.

Parasites and Abnormal Contents.—The urine which reaches the bladder may be abnormal in its secretion, or may become contaminated by contact with the urinary passages, or, again, may undergo chemical decomposition while retained within the bladder.

Erythrocytes or their derivatives may be found in the urine in certain cases of nephritis; in congestion of the urinary organs and passages; in acute inflammation or ulceration of the pelvis of the kidney, ureter, or bladder: in certain intoxications; and in the hemorrhagic diatheses. Tumors, like angiomas or carcinomas, may bleed freely. Blood clots or blood casts may be found.

Leukocytes result from inflammation in any part of the urinary tract. They may form casts.

Epithelium from the pelvis of the kidney and bladder is often met with, and is of considerable importance in diagnosis.

In ulcerative processes, simple or cancerous, necrotic tissue and detritus may be found.

Urinary casts are derived from the tubules of the kidneys in various forms of nephritis. They may be hyaline and colorless, amyloid (colloid), fatty, granular, epithelial, leukocytic, fibrinous, or composed of red blood cells. Casts should be carefully differentiated from cylindroids, which are of no practical importance.

Bacteria of various kinds are of frequent occurrence. They are derived either from the urethra, or are eliminated through the kidney. According to most authorities normal urine is aseptic. Enriquez[1] has made a careful study of this point. Whether a physiological excretion of microörganisms through the kidney is possible, in the absence of a lesion of the secreting epithelium, is still a moot question. The majority of observers, following Wyssokowitsch and Neumann and Konjajeff, seem to think it does not occur, but Schweitzer[2] and certain others hold that bacteria may pass the renal epithelium in the absence of any lesions that it is possible to recognize microscopically.

The chief pathogenic bacteria found in the urine in diseased conditions are B. coli, B. typhi, B. proteus, B. tuberculosis, staphylococcus, streptococcus, Diplococcus pneumoniæ, Gonococcus, and B. Friedländeri.

Yeasts have been met with in the urine of diabetics.

[1] Recherches bact. sur l'urine normale, Semaine médicale, No. 57: 1891: 468.
[2] Virchow's Archiv, 110: 1887: 255.

A variety of **foreign bodies** have been found in the urine. In fistulous communications with the rectum, feces and gas may enter the bladder. A dermoid cyst may open into the organ and hairs may be passed in the urine (*pilimictio*).

In the case of children and those addicted to masturbation, and in attempts to relieve itching, foreign bodies of all kinds have been passed into the urethra and may slip into the bladder. Among these may be mentioned catheters, hairpins, hatpins, needles, matches, straws, candles, handles of parasols or toothbrushes, glass. Foreign bodies may form the nucleus for the formation of concrements.

Concrements and calculi are produced in the pelvis of the kidney or in the bladder (see vol. i, p. 938). Stones in the kidney are usually composed of urates, uric acid, oxalates, or combinations of these with phosphates. Vesical calculi are commonly phosphatic. It is obvious, however, that stones of varying character may reach the bladder from the renal pelvis and form a nucleus for a much larger phosphatic calculus. Certain rare forms, cystin, xanthin, and silicates, may just be mentioned.

The **parasites** found are *Echinococcus, Filaria, Distoma,* the ova of *Bilharzia,* and, in cattle, the *larvæ* of certain flies.

RETROGRESSIVE METAMORPHOSES.

Atrophy.—Atrophy of the bladder is met with in old age, especially in women, and in marantic and cachectic states. The mucosa is thinned, but the muscular coat is the portion chiefly involved. The bladder wall is sometimes reduced to the thinness of paper. Long-continued distention, such as is met with in paralysis of the muscle, is an important cause of atrophy.

Necrosis.—Necrosis of the bladder wall, at times leading to perforation, is commonly due to injuries during parturition, either from instrumentation or the pressure of the fœtal head. It may also result from the pressure of a large calculus.

Fatty and **amyloid** changes are common.

PROGRESSIVE METAMORPHOSES.

Hypertrophy.—Hypertrophy of the vesical muscle is of frequent occurrence. According as the cavity of the bladder is contracted or dilated, we can recognize a concentric and an excentric hypertrophy.

The most common cause is some obstruction to the free outflow of urine, such as is brought about by an enlarged prostate, stricture of the urethra, the pressure of a prolapsed uterus, tumors of the uterus or bladder, or an impacted calculus. A second form, without urinary obstruction, is found in cases of chronic cystitis, vesical calculus, and tumors. Here, it is supposed that the constant irritation leads to increased activity of the motor nerves and functional overwork of the muscle. As in the case of the heart, hypertrophy may in time give place to dilatation, notably in the obstructive cases.

Dilatation of the bladder with hypertrophy of its wall is frequently met with in certain affections of the spinal cord, locomotor ataxia, mye-litis, and the like. In such cases there can be no question of obstruction or of reflex irritation. The dilatation might be accounted for on the score of diminished sensibility and consequent retention, but we may consider also that the hypertrophy is due to some trophic disturb-ance of the sympathetic nervous system or of the nerves in the muscular wall.

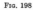

Fig. 198

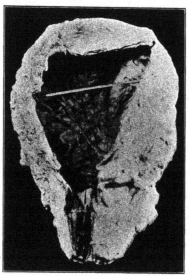

Hypertrophy and dilatation of the urinary bladder due to an enlarged prostate. The saccula-tion of the bladder is well shown and also the encroachment of the middle lobe of the prostate on the urethra. (From the Pathological Museum of McGill University.)

In pure hypertrophy the bladder wall is thickened and of firm con sistence. The muscular bands of the inner surface are greatly enlarged, recalling the columnæ carneæ of the cardiac ventricles. When obstruc tion has been operative, it is not uncommon to find smaller or larger sacculations or diverticula, either due to local weakening of the bladder wall, or to hernial protrusions of the mucosa through weak spots in the muscular coat. These diverticula are most frequent at the fundus of the bladder, while the trigone is usually free.

Tumors.—Primary tumors are not common. Benign vesical growths are rather more common than the malignant. In 640 cases given by

Watson,[1] 60 per cent. were non-malignant. Males are more frequently attacked than females, the proportion being about 3 to 2. As a rule the base, the posterior wall, or both, are involved.

Papilloma.—The most common growth is the papilloma, which is often benign but has a distinct tendency toward malignancy, and hence may develop into a papillary carcinoma. It appears as a soft, villous mass attached to the mucosa by a fibrous pedicle of varying thickness. When floated out in water the tumor has a shaggy, tree-like appearance. The growth is generally reddish, but may present paler areas, due to necrosis or superficial erosion.

Microscopically, the tumor consists in a number of connective-tissue cores, rather rich in bloodvessels, which are covered with simple or stratified polymorphous or columnar cells. If the tumor be malignant, the wall of the bladder is infiltrated with a soft, brain-like substance, from which a milky juice can be obtained on scraping. Under the microscope, the mucosa and muscularis are found to contain masses of epithelial cells, resembling those covering the papillæ of the original growth.

Fibroma.—Fibromas or fibrous polyps are rather more uncommon. They often show myxomatous degeneration.

Rhabdomyoma, Myoma, and Fibromyoma.—Myomas and fibromyomas are among the rarest of bladder tumors. They vary in size from that of a pea to that of a child's head, and may be pedunculated or sessile.

Adenoma.—Adenomas are quite rare. They are sessile or pedunculated, and have a smooth, lobulated, or papillary surface. They probably arise from the mucous crypts. Some of them, however, should possibly be traced to the aberrant prostates, before referred to (p. 820).

Angiomas and **teratomas** are excessively rare.

Carcinoma.—Carcinoma originates from the epithelium lining the bladder or that of the mucous crypts. It may form a rather superficial, diffuse growth, projecting only slightly into the cavity of the bladder, or presents a nodose, somewhat elevated surface (*medullary carcinoma*). The mucous membrane is sometimes intact, or may be eroded and ulcerated. Flattened ulcers with indurated edges may be formed. In other cases, as before mentioned, carcinoma takes the form of a papillary outgrowth, or cauliflower-like mass. *Squamous-celled epitheliomas* and *colloid carcinomas* (very rare) have been met with. Vesical carcinomas are, as a rule, somewhat slow growing, and do not tend to invade the deeper structures. Metastases, when present, are usually strictly local. Interesting, etiologically, is the carcinoma resulting from the action of Bilharzia.[2]

Sarcoma.—Sarcomas are commonly multiple, sessile, with a smooth surface. In color they are red, purplish, or almost black. They are extremely rare. *Myosarcoma, myxosarcoma, lymphosarcoma, chondrosarcoma,* and *osteoid chondrosarcoma*[3] have been recorded.

[1] Morrow's System of Genito-urinary Diseases, 1:1893:565.

[2] Goebel, Deuts. Zeits. f. Chir., 81:1906:288.

[3] Shattock, Trans. Path. Soc., 38:1887:183; also Beneke, Arch. f. path. Anat. u. Phys. u. f. klin. Med., 161:1900:70.

Secondary tumors, usually carcinomatous, are more frequent than primary ones. In the male they originate in the prostate; in the female, in the uterus or vagina. In both sexes, carcinoma of the rectum may extend to the bladder.

THE URETHRA.

CONGENITAL ANOMALIES.

Absence of the urethra is met with associated with other grave defects. The urethra may divide, so that it discharges by two or more openings. In the male the passage may open at the base of the scrotum instead of passing through the corpus spongiosum, and in the female it may empty into the vagina. Local **obliteration** of the urethra may be met with at the meatus and in other parts, due to defective development of the corpus spongiosum. **Valve-like membranes** also lead to partial or complete obstruction of the canal.

Diverticula are exceedingly rare.

CIRCULATORY DISTURBANCES.

What has already been stated with regard to the bladder applies with equal force to the urethra.

In females, **varices**, or **urethral hemorrhoids**, are met with, forming small caruncles or polypoid masses. They may give rise to serious hemorrhage or to submucous hematomas.

INFLAMMATIONS.

Urethritis.—Simple **Urethritis.**—Simple urethritis is commonly brought about by irritation from unclean habits, careless instrumentation, injections of fluids, foreign bodies, calculi, or direct violence. In the female, inflammations of the vulva and vagina not infrequently extend to the urethra.

A simple urethritis, analogous to inflammation of other mucous membranes, may arise in the course of the various infective fevers. It is also believed to be produced by coitus with a woman suffering from a leucorrhœal discharge, or who is menstruating.

Gonorrhœal Urethritis.—The most important affection is specific urethritis or gonorrhœa, which is due to a particular microörganism, the Gonococcus of Neisser. Gonorrhœal urethritis, as a primary disease, is more frequent in males than in females. In the latter it is more liable to spread by extension from a previous infection of the vulva or vagina. The condition is brought about by contact with infective secretion from a mucous membrane, usually by coitus, although instances

PLATE IX

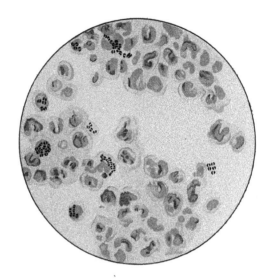

Gonococci in pus.

of mediate contagion are not uncommon. Thus the infecting agents may be carried by the fingers, towels, sponges, or bed-linen.

The specific microörganism is a micrococcus, usually lying in pairs, the opposed surfaces of which are slightly concave. Single cocci and tetrads are also met with. They are often intracellular, but are also found lying free. They stain readily with aniline dyes and are decolorized by Gram's method. Owing to the fact that certain other microorganisms, namely, Trichomonas vaginalis and some aberrant forms of B. coli, resemble Gonococci rather closely, diagnosis should not be made from stained films only, unless the history and clinical signs are clear. In doubtful and especially in medicolegal cases, culture methods should also be resorted to.

Gonorrhœa usually starts near the meatus and rapidly spreads to the rest of the anterior urethra. After the first week the inflammation may spread to the posterior urethra and the prostate.

The disease is a severe purulent catarrh, leading at first to intense congestion of the urethra, followed by the production of a profuse yellowish or greenish-yellow discharge, occasionally mixed with blood. The prepuce and glans are often inflamed (*balanoposthitis*), and there may be paraphimosis. In severe cases mild constitutional symptoms arise, together with painful erections of the penis (*chordeé*). The secretion consists of pus, blood, and desquamated epithelial cells, and contains the specific microörganisms.

Microscopically, the superficial epithelium is desquamating, and leukocytes can be seen passing between the cells to the surface, or infiltrating the periurethral connective tissue. The various lacunæ and periurethral glands are usually distended with pus.

After a few weeks the intensity subsides, as a rule, and the process may end, even in the absence of treatment, in healing. This is, however, not often the case, since the affection tends to become chronic, and certain complications may set in. If the inflammation extend to the prostatic gland, the disease becomes very obstinate. Ulceration or abscesses in the periurethral connective tissue occur, and the various glands —prostatic, Cowper's, Tyson's, and, in the female, Bartholin's glands— may retain infective pus long after the urethra is free. This local suppuration may be due to Gonococcus alone, or to other germs associated with it. More rarely, acute orchitis or epididymitis results. In the female, the vagina, particularly about the cervix uteri, is apt to be involved. Gonorrhœal endometritis is met with, but more often the uterus escapes, while the Fallopian tubes become diseased. A few cases of gonorrhœal peritonitis, due to extension of infection from the tubes, have been reported. In both sexes the bladder is not infrequently attacked, although the kidneys are but rarely involved. Among the most serious complications are conjunctivitis, adenitis and periadenitis (bubo), arthritis and tenosynovitis, endocarditis, and septicemia.

Gonorrhœal arthritis and tenosynovitis usually manifest themselves weeks or months after the first infection, and are most obstinate conditions. Suppuration in the joints and fibrous ankylosis are not uncommon.

Chronic gonorrhœa is usually the continuation of an acute attack in a less florid form. It may be catarrhal, hyperplastic, or indurative.

The catarrhal form resembles the acute. The exudation, however, is less, in parts there are superficial erosions of the epithelium, and the cylindrical cells may be converted into squamous ones. The various crypts and glands may contain pus or desquamated cells, and show evidences of deeply seated inflammation. Occasionally, in addition to catarrh, the mucosa is thickened and studded with warty or polypoid excrescences.

An important type practically is the indurative, in which dense fibrous tissue is produced, leading frequently by its contraction to stricture of the urethra.

Strictures may be single or multiple, and are usually found in the membranous urethra, although the penile portion may, at times, be affected. The condition is a slowly developing one and is important on account of the serious disturbances to which it gives rise, obstruction to the free discharge of urine, hypertrophy of the bladder with dilatation, hydronephrosis, pyonephrosis, rupture of the urethra, and extravasation of urine. Behind the stricture the urethra is generally in a state of chronic catarrh. In chronic urethritis there is usually a slight discharge, generally in the morning. It is not necessarily purulent, but is more of a mucous nature (*gleet*). In this form, the urine may contain a few flocculent shreds, upon which may be detected occasional leukocytes and gonococci.[1]

Membranous Urethritis.—Membranous urethritis is rare.

Of localized inflammatory lesions may be mentioned the **soft chancre** and the **primary syphilitic sore.** They are found, not rarely, just within the meatus, to which they give a peculiar square appearance in transverse section. These infections may be inoculated at the same time as a gonorrhœa.

Variolous pustules have been met with in the urethra.

Among the chronic inflammations may be mentioned polypoid or warty excrescences (**condylomas**), due to dirt or irritating discharges. They are usually found at the meatus.

Tuberculosis.—Tuberculosis of the urethra is not common. Local foci of caseous necrosis are sometimes met with in the prostatic portion, due to extension from the bladder and prostate, and in women, at the anterior portion, in cases of lupus of the vulva. We have seen the male urethra studded with coarse granular tubercles along its whole length, where the kidneys and urinary tract were extensively involved.

Foreign Bodies and Parasites.—What has already been remarked when dealing with the bladder applies also to the urethra. The most important **foreign bodies** are *calculi, colloid masses*, and portions of *bone*, all of which may lead to obstruction.

Of the **parasites** may be mentioned, by way of curiosity, *Penicillium*

---

[1] For pathology further see Finger, Ghon, and Schlagenhaufer, Arch. f. Dermat. u. Syphilis, 1894; and Finger, Die Blennorrhoea der Sexualorgane, Leipzig, 1896.

glaucum, Eustrongylus gigas, and the *larvæ* of certain flies. In females, especially in young children, *thread worms* may reach the urethra from the anus, and set up pruritus and marked irritation.

RETROGRESSIVE METAMORPHOSES.

Ulceration may take place from the action of caustics or from injuries inflicted during parturition or instrumentation.

PROGRESSIVE METAMORPHOSES.

Tumors.—Primary tumors are rare. They are more common in men than in women.

In females, small excrescences or **caruncles** are sometimes found, caused by thickening or hypertrophy of the normal folds of the mucosa.

Simple **retention cysts,** arising from the periurethral glands, are occasionally met with. They may also start from the Cowper's glands. Orth has recorded a **cystadenoma.**[1]

Fibrous polyps have been described.

Carcinoma is rare. It may originate in the Cowper's glands, or from periurethral fistulæ, which have become lined with squamous epithelium.

Sarcoma is still rarer. *Melanosarcoma* and *lymphosarcoma* are recorded.

As a rule, malignant growths arise by extension from the genitalia (glans penis, vagina, vulva).

INJURIES.

The urethra may be injured in various degrees through instrumentation, or parturition. Falls upon the perineum and fracture of the pelvis may produce **laceration.** When rupture of the urethra takes place and the urine cannot escape externally, extravasation of the urine occurs into the layers of the perineum and abdominal wall, leading to inflammation and, often, widespread necrosis and death.

---

[1] For literature see Pappel, Monatsschr. f. Geburtsh. u. Gynäkol., 27:1908.

SECTION VII.

THE REPRODUCTIVE SYSTEM.

CHAPTER XXXVII.

THE MALE SEXUAL ORGANS.

THE PENIS.

CONGENITAL ANOMALIES.

THESE are very rare. **Complete absence** of the penis, **doubling** of the organ, and **partial defects** in the corpora cavernosa may be mentioned.

A congenital **fistula** has been described, in which a duct connected with the prostate opens upon the dorsum of the penis or at the glans.

Cruveilhier[1] figures a case in which the ejaculatory duct took a course independently of the urethra and opened on the glans.

Somewhat more common than absence of the penis is **total defect** or abnormal **shortness** of the prepuce. **Hypoplasia** of the external genitalia is rare in men otherwise well developed, but is more frequent in crypt-orchids, cretins, idiots, and epileptics.

Hyperplasia has been observed. **Bifurcation** of the penis may simulate a double organ. A curious malformation is one in which the organ resembles the tongue of a bell. **Atresia** and **phimosis** of the prepuce are not uncommon. **Plates of bone** have also been noted in the penis.

CIRCULATORY DISTURBANCES.

Passive Congestion.—Passive congestion is met with in those suffering from valvular heart disease or other obstruction in the systemic circulation. The condition leads to enlargement of the corpora cavernosa. A similar effect is produced by the relaxation of the supporting structure of the corpora in those addicted to sexual excess. Occasionally a chronic congestion with erection (priapism) is encountered in leukemia, the result of leukocytic engorgement of the sinuses of the corpora. Passive congestion is sometimes also due to paraphimosis or other causes that lead to constriction of the organ, such as strings tied around

[1] Atlas, Lfg. 39: Taf. 2: Fig. 3.

it or rings slipped over it. The last-mentioned conditions are occasionally met with in young boys. The result is often serious, as gangrene may set in.

Gangrene.—Gangrene may also be due to embolism of the dorsal artery or to thrombosis in the corpora.

Varicosity.—Varicosity of the dorsal veins is not uncommon.

Hemorrhage.—Owing to the loose structure of the corpora and skin of the prepuce and penis, effusions of blood readily take place. These may be due to rupture of the corpora or the bloodvessels, and may attain considerable size (**hematoma**). This accident may occur during coitus. Dilatation of the larger lymph-channels is rare.

INFLAMMATIONS.

Inflammatory processes of various types affect the penis. The parts attacked are the skin, prepuce, glans, and corpora. We can thus speak of a **dermatitis, posthitis, balanitis,** and **cavernitis.** As a rule, both prepuce and glans are affected together (**balanoposthitis**). The preputial sac is particularly liable to inflammation, since there is a tendency to accumulation of smegma, pus, dirt, and urinary salts, which form a suitable culture medium for many germs. Chemical and mechanical irritation, however, also play a part. If the swelling of the parts be great, it may be impossible for the patient to draw the prepuce forward (*paraphimosis*). Passive congestion, ulceration, and even gangrene may then be the result.

Catarrhal Balanoposthitis.—Simple catarrh, which leads merely to slight reddening of the mucosa, swelling of the prepuce, secretion, and desquamation of cells is a trifling affection.

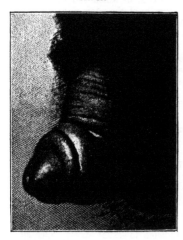

Fig. 199

Paraphimosis: penis curved nearly at a right angle. (Taylor.)

Suppurative Balanoposthitis.—More important is suppurative balanoposthitis, such as often occurs during the course of gonorrhœa and phimosis. Here there is an abundant purulent secretion, great redness and swelling, together with shallow erosions due to maceration and desquamation of the epithelium. The process sometimes leads to induration of the affected parts with fibrosis, and to union of the two layers of mucous membrane. Both acute and chronic forms may be the cause of phimosis.

Balanoposthitis Aspergillina.—A mycotic form—balanoposthitis aspergillina—has been met with in diabetics.

Membranous Balanoposthitis.—Membranous inflammation is due to the irritation of retained secretion or to wound infection, and occurs also in the infective fevers, diphtheria, typhoid, variola, scarlatina, and measles.

Herpes Progenitalis.—Herpes progenitalis begins with the formation of one or more groups of small vesicles that rupture and form superficial erosions, surrounded by a scanty, whitish border of epithelium. From infection larger ulcers may result. The condition is possibly neurotrophic, since in one case at least fibrosis of the nerves of the penis was discovered.

Cavernitis.—Cavernitis is either **acute suppurative** or **chronic productive** in character. It affects the corpora in whole or in part. Local abscesses may result which perforate into the urethra, or a diffuse affection with fibrous induration.

Syphilis.—The primary lesion of syphilis ("**hard**" **chancre**) is by far the most important affection. The initial sore makes its appearance on an average from three to four weeks after infection, usually upon the prepuce near the raphé, or on the corona, sometimes within the urethra or on the skin. It begins as a minute vesicle, which in time ruptures, leaving a superficial erosion surrounded by a reddish border. In a short time the ulcer becomes indurated and hard, so that when pinched between the finger and thumb it feels as if a small bit of parchment were inserted in the base. The amount of ulceration and inflammatory reaction is often trifling and the lesion is frequently overlooked. The sore is infective, but indolent and not auto-inoculable.

Microscopically, the part is infiltrated for the most part with small, round cells, but occasional epithelioid elements and giant cells are seen. The round cells are chiefly aggregated about the smaller vessels, the walls of which are also thickened and infiltrated. The endothelium of the capillaries is proliferated. In the periphery numerous "Mast-zellen" may be made out. The connective tissue shows a progressing fibrosis. The superficial epithelium presents a loss of substance that extends more or less deeply into the underlying strata.

By cleaning and then gently scraping the surface of the chancre and examining a drop of the removed material, mixed with distilled water, by the dark field or ultra microscope, it is a simple matter to detect abundant spirochetes of the typical size and appearance. These exist in the lymph-spaces and between the epithelial cells.

Sooner or later the infection becomes systemic, an early sign of which is hyperplasia of the inguinal lymphatic glands, forming what is known as the "*indolent bubo.*"

In the second stage of syphilis small, reddish, moist nodules form on the mucosa which may fuse together, and from the effect of warmth and moisture form the **broad condyloma.** As in the case of the primary chancre, these may ulcerate.

In tertiary syphilis, small **gummas** (syphilomata) may be formed in any part of the penis. They are usually deeply situated and may cause extensive ulceration. When they heal, dense and deforming scars may result.

Chancroid.—As contradistinguished from the primary syphilitic sore or "hard" chancre we have to recognize a non-specific sore or "soft" chancre (chancroid).

This develops in from one to five days after exposure, in the form of a small vesicle or pustule which rapidly breaks down into an ulcer, having a sharply defined or undermined edge and an angry reddish-yellow base secreting pus. A necrotic membrane is often formed on the surface.

The ulcer is usually found on the inner surface of the prepuce, especially about the frenum, and on the glans. It differs from the true syphilitic sore in the shorter incubation period, the more rapid and severe erosion, to a certain extent in its position, and on the fact that it is auto-inoculable, so that multiple ulcers are frequently observed. Secondary syphilides do not, of course, develop. A certain amount of inflammatory induration may be produced, but this is rarely to be confused with the parchment-like feel of the syphilitic sore, which may persist long after the ulcer has disappeared.

Microscopically, the vessels are dilated, the papillæ in the neighborhood are proliferating, and the base and edge of the sore are markedly infiltrated with inflammatory products. The exact cause of the soft chancre is not certainly known, whether it is due to the ordinary pus germs or to a specific microörganism acting with the pus germs. It should not be forgotten that a mixed infection with syphilis and soft chancre occasionally occurs. Here what appears to be an ordinary soft chancre, eventually becomes indurated and is followed by the ordinary secondary manifestations of syphilis. Soft chancre often leads to swelling of the prepuce, lymphangitis in the penis, and to suppurative inflammation of the inguinal glands (*virulent bubo*) and the neighboring tissues. In persons of low vitality it may become phagedenic.

Tuberculosis.—Tuberculosis is rare in adults, although caseous ulceration of the glans is recorded. Microscopically, it does not differ from tuberculosis elsewhere.

Tuberculous infiltration of the prepuce is commoner and is met with in children as a result of the ritual practice of circumcision, in cases where the saliva of the operator contained tubercle bacilli.

Foreign Bodies and Parasites.—Retained smegma and dirt may become inspissated and infiltrated with lime salts, so that a **concrement** is formed. Phimosis (tight prepuce) is a strong predisposing cause of this condition. Urinary calculi may also be arrested by a tight foreskin and form a nidus for further accretion (*preputial calculus*). Of parasites may be mentioned *bacteria, yeasts, spores of fungi,* and *mycelial threads.* The most important form is the smegma bacillus, inasmuch as, morphologically and tinctorially, it resembles closely the tubercle bacillus. As it is contained in most urines, it will be seen how important it is to differentiate between the two microörganisms (vide p. 802).

RETROGRADE METAMORPHOSES.

Senile' **atrophy** of the corpora is common. As the prepuce is less affected, it appears to be relatively long. **Necrosis** and **ulceration** may lead to deformity of the organ. In some cases, supposed to be due to a lack of resisting power on the part of the individual, ulceration may be rapid and destructive (**phagedena**). This is apt to occur in alcoholics, syphilitics, diabetics, and in tuberculous persons.

PROGRESSIVE METAMORPHOSES.

Condyloma Acuminatum.—Papillomatous outgrowths, due, for the most part, to inflammation or chronic irritation, are not uncommon on the glans and prepuce. The most frequent form is the condyloma acuminatum, which develops characteristically on an inflammatory basis, and is generally due to an irritating discharge (gonorrhœa) or retained secretion. Phimosis is a potent predisposing cause. Condylomas take the form of larger or smaller multiple papillary excrescences on the glans and prepuce not unlike a cock's comb. From the pressure of a contracted foreskin the growths are often somewhat flattened. In aggravated cases, large masses, the size of a fist, having a cauliflower appearance, may be produced.

Microscopically, the outgrowths consist of a fibrous vascular core covered with stratified squamous epithelium. The fibrous tissue is richly branched, so that papillomas are produced, although this arrangement is somewhat masked by the proliferation of the epithelial covering. Inflammatory infiltration is generally also to be observed. The diagnosis between condyloma and carcinoma is not always easy. Condylomas are usually soft and freely movable upon the subjacent tissues, unless ulceration has taken place. In this case, inflammatory induration is apt to impair the mobility. Carcinoma is usually hard and infiltrated.

Keratosis.—Another form of hypertrophy is seen in the heaping up of the superficial epithelium known as keratosis.

Elephantiasis.—Somewhat allied to tumor-formation is elephantiasis, which chiefly affects the prepuce, either alone or together with the whole penis, and sometimes the scrotum. The extent of the disease may be trifling or a large tumor may be produced. One is described that weighed more than 25 kilos. The growth is easily distinguished from elephantiasis of the scrotum in that the opening of the urethra is at the base of the tumor.

Microscopically, the mass consists chiefly of fibrous tissue, containing in the superficial layers many "Mast-zellen." In the preputial portion bundles of unstriped muscle have been noted. There may be diapedesis of leukocytes about the vessels. The superficial papillæ of the skin are often unaltered, but may show signs of overgrowth, and even may form papillomatous warts.

Tumors.—Carcinoma.—Carcinoma of the penis, usually *epithelioma*, forms, according to Orth, 2.8 per cent. of all cancers, and is met with generally between the ages of fifty and seventy. Phimosis, as it conduces to the retention of decomposing secretion, appears to be an important predisposing cause. Epithelioma may also arise in the condylomas just described and in keratosis. The growth may begin in any part, but usually at the edge of the prepuce, the sulcus, and the inner surface of the prepuce. It begins ordinarily as a small wart that gradually extends over the surface of the organ, forming a papillomatous mass that may erode through the prepuce. The surface is moist, the folds contain a foul, whitish, greasy secretion. Ulceration occurs in advanced cases.

Microscopically, processes of squamous epithelium are seen to extend deeply into the underlying structures from the superficial strata, often forming branching masses. "Cell-nests" of keratohyaline material are often present. When ulceration takes place the growth becomes very granular, owing to infiltration with inflammatory products. Extension takes place through the lymphatic system, and the inguinal glands are first and most strikingly involved. Much rarer is *medullary carcinoma* of the adenomatous type. Still rarer are *melanotic forms*.

Sarcoma.—*Melanotic sarcoma* occurs and is liable to be confounded with carcinoma. Unpigmented sarcoma has been found originating in the corpora, and also intravascular **endothelioma**. Secondary growths, carcinoma, and sarcoma, usually are metastatic or arise by extension from neighboring parts.

Fibroma, lipoma, and **neuroma** have also been described.

Cysts due to obstruction of the sebaceous glands are fairly common.

INJURIES.

The most striking injury is the so-called **luxation** of the penis, in which the main substance of the organ is separated from the prepuce and overlying skin and is found beneath the skin of the trunk, the original covering hanging like an empty sausage skin. **Fracture** of the penis, usually of the corpora cavernosa, occurs from striking the organ when in an erect condition against some hard substance. It is sometimes caused by intentional violence, as in the dangerous practice among the lower orders of "breaking the cord" in chordee. Injuries also occur during attempts at coitus, from falls, tying strings around the organ, or inserting foreign substances (catheters, etc.).

THE PROSTATE.

MALFORMATIONS.

These are not common. Complete **absence** of the prostate is met with in association with other grave defects of the genito-urinary apparatus.

Unilateral **aplasia** and **hypoplasia** are exceptionally observed in unilateral hypoplasia of the testes. **Aberrant prostates** have been found. Unilateral or complete **defect of the colliculus seminalis** and **dilatation of the prostatic sinus** have been described. **Cysts** are sometimes found along the course of the Müllerian duct, due to imperfect closure of the same.

CIRCULATORY DISTURBANCES.

Hyperemia is a common but comparatively unimportant condition. Repeated or continued congestion has been by some regarded as a cause of hypertrophy of the organ. The prostatic plexus is often found dilated, and *thrombosis* and *phlebolith formation* are comparatively common.

INFLAMMATIONS.

Prostatitis.—Catarrhal Prostatitis.—Simple catarrhal prostatitis is described, in which there is an accumulation of inflammatory products and desquamated cells within the tubules, together with hyperemia and œdema of the supporting structure. Little is known, however, about this affection.

Suppurative Prostatitis.—More important is suppurative prostatitis, in which the glands are filled with pus and abscesses are produced. This is not an infrequent sequel of gonorrhœa, but is also a result of severe cystitis and injuries to the urethra. The process in the first instance begins in the gland-tubes but soon spreads to the neighboring tissues where several foci may coalesce to form abscesses. The abscesses are multiple and are scattered irregularly through the gland, which may be almost entirely destroyed. They may perforate into the bladder, urethra, scrotum, perineum, rectum, or through the abdominal wall. A **paraprostatitis** may lead to general peritonitis. Should the abscesses heal, fibroid scars are the result or perhaps calcification. Suppurative prostatitis is, rarely, metastatic in septicemia.

Chronic Prostatitis.—In chronic prostatitis, prostatorrhœa may be a chief symptom, and Rokitansky has described a condition in which the secretion was quite milky from the presence of lecithin. The condition may be simple or suppurative. The organ is swollen and of a dirty brownish color. The gland-tubules are dilated and may coalesce, forming cysts.

Tuberculosis.—Tuberculosis takes the form of **multiple caseous nodules** in one, or, more frequently, in both lobes, which may lead to considerable enlargement of the gland. In advanced cases the whole prostate may be destroyed. The caseous foci sometimes soften, leading to the formation of abscesses which may burst into the urinary passages or into the rectum. As with suppurative inflammation, the process begins in the gland-tubules, both in tuberculosis of urogenital and hematogenic origin. As a rule, tuberculosis is part of an extensive urogenital infection. Primary tuberculosis of the organ is decidedly rare.

Foreign Bodies.—Concretions, corpora amylacea, are found commonly
in the prostate, especially of old people. On cutting into the gland

FIG. 200

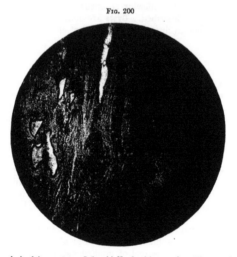

Caseous tuberculosis of the prostate. Leitz obj. No. 3, without ocular. The necrotic area is shown
to the right, with giant-cells toward the margin. (From the collection of Dr. A. G. Nicholls.)

FIG. 201

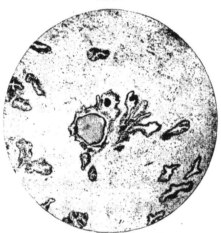

Corpora amylacea in the prostate. Leitz obj. No. 3. (From the collection of Dr A. G. Nicholls.)

they appear like grains of black pepper, but may be large and gritty, resembling grape-seeds. The latter peculiarity is due to infiltration with salts. The corpora are found chiefly in the neighborhood of the colliculus seminalis, but also throughout the gland.

Microscopically, the smaller ones are oval or rounded, more rarely triangular, showing concentric lamination, which gives them a general resemblance to starch granules, whence their name. In many cases two or three cells in process of fusion and disintegration may often be seen with beginning hyaline transformation, showing that the process has its origin in catarrh and degeneration of the lining epithelium. The larger granules show but little lamination, and are merely amorphous masses of brownish mineral matter. Posner has suggested that two bodies are present in the corpora, a hyaline, albuminous substance and lecithin. The condition is of little pathological significance.

Parasites.—*Echinococcus cysts* have been found in the prostate.

RETROGRADE METAMORPHOSES.

Simple atrophy of the gland occurs in from 20 to 30 per cent. of old men. It is, however, occasionally met with in young people, as a result of wasting disease, cachexia, castration, the impotence of the tuberculous, the pressure of retained urine, pent-up secretion, and concretions. In the form due to constitutional causes, the glandular portion is the one chiefly affected, while in that due to concrements the stroma suffers most. In the latter case, however, the epithelial cells may be flattened and fattily degenerated from pressure.

Pigmentation of the epithelial cells is found in advanced age and in the cachexias.

Hyaline degeneration of the muscle bundles and the glandular epithelium is met with. **Fatty degeneration** is also met with. The so-called **amyloid bodies,** above-mentioned, have nothing to do with amyloid disease.

PROGRESSIVE METAMORPHOSES.

Hypertrophy.—Hypertrophy of the prostate, a not uncommon condition in elderly men, while it may precede the development of definite neoplastic conditions within the organ, must, nevertheless, be sharply distinguished from the same. With the more recent authorities we would regard it as the outcome of a long-continued chronic inflammation, more particularly involving the urethral portion of the organ. Not a few writers ascribe this inflammation to the gonococcus, but proof is wanting of a constant association between previous gonorrhœa and prostatic hypertrophy. The results of such an inflammation may show themselves in several ways:

1. Interstitial fibrosis around the mouths of the prostatic ducts may lead to narrowing and partial obstruction, compensated by hypertrophy

of the plain muscle fibres, which constitute a characteristic feature of the prostatic stroma. We thus encounter cases in which a diffuse muscular hypertrophy is the main feature.

2. The obstruction may result in complete stenosis of sundry ducts, in which case the associated glands with their ramifications become greatly dilated and cystic with flattened epithelium. It is a mistake to speak of this condition as cystadenoma. Serial sections demonstrate that we deal with dilated gland tubules which can be traced to their urethral orifices.

Fig. 202

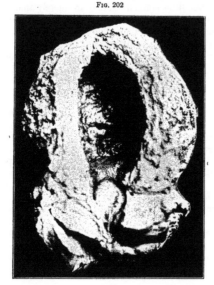

"Myomatous" enlargement of the prostate; obstruction to the outflow of urine caused by the overgrowth of the so-called middle lobe; consecutive hypertrophy of the walls of the bladder. (From the Pathological Museum of McGill University.)

3. Whether as a subsequent stage to the preceding or as the result of a continued mild catarrhal state, the glandular epithelium may exhibit indications of active proliferation (productive glandular hyperplasia), often accompanied by some degree of cystic dilatation.

4. Whether, again, as the result of progressive interstitial inflammation, or as the outcome of exhaustion and atrophy of the hypertrophic muscle fibres with replacement by connective tissue, we encounter a diffuse fibrous or mixed connective tissue and muscular hyperplasia.

None of these conditions, it will be seen, are blastomatous, but, while saying this, it would seem from clinical histories that (1) the productive glandular hypertrophy may favor the development of cells which take on carcinomatous properties, and (2) whether as an independent process or associated with previous interstitial inflammation, localized myomas and fibromas may, although rarely, undergo development in the organ.

While the enlargement of the organ may be generalized, more frequently it shows itself specially affecting the middle or Home's lobe, and doing this is the cause of the most frequent and serious sequels of prostatic hypertrophy. For this nodule or ridge, projecting upward, acts as a valve when the bladder contracts; obstructs the urethral orifice and impedes urination; brings about hypertrophy and subsequent dilatation of the bladder; causes the production of a bay or depression of the lower part of the bladder, which is not properly emptied in the act of micturiton and the "residual urine" is apt to become the seat of bacterial

FIG. 203

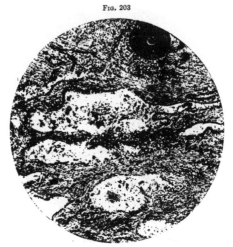

So-called "adenoma" of the prostate gland. An amyloid body can be seen at the upper right-hand edge of the section. Winckel obj. No. 3, without ocular. (From the collection of Dr. A. G Nicholls.)

growth; hence, cystitis and ascending inflammation, ureteritis, pyelonephritis, pyonephrosis, etc. The impeded urination leads to the employment of catheters and is a fertile source of infection, while, further, the projecting mass of prostatic tissue, in the hands of the patient or other amateur in the process of catheterization, may be pierced, leading to the formation of false passages.

It cannot be said that the exact nature of the middle lobe is yet positively settled. In the normal prostate of early life it is non-existent. Some have regarded it as an overgrowth of the postero-median portion of one or other lobe. Jores concludes that it is a development of accessory, or more accurately, free-lying prostatic glandules, which exist beneath the mucosa of the posterior portion of the prostatic urethra and adjacent mucosa of the bladder.

Tumors.—Of malignant growths **carcinoma** and **sarcoma** should be mentioned.

Carcinoma.—Primary carcinoma is not uncommon, and originates in many cases at least, in a previously existing glandular enlargement One case has come under our observation in which there were symptoms of urinary obstruction due to enlarged prostate for eleven years before the development of *adenocarcinoma*. Carcinoma of the prostate takes the form of a rather soft, nodular tumor in one or both lobes of the prostate, which rapidly infiltrates the capsule of the gland, the mucosa

FIG. 204

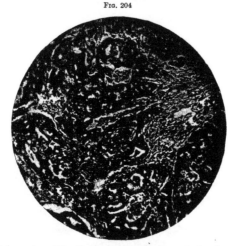

Carcinoma of the prostate. Zeiss obj. DD, ocular No. 1. (From the Pathological Laboratory of McGill University.)

at the neck of the bladder, and the prostatic urethra. It may, indeed, extend to the penis and rectum. Occasionally it assumes a *papillomatous* appearance.

Microscopically, the growth is composed of cylindrical or polyhedral cells, arranged more or less in glandular fashion or in solid bands or masses. The stroma is normal or infiltrated with round cells. Cases occur in which the growth, at first sight, resembles sarcoma closely until more careful study shows it to be carcinomatous (Adami). Metastases are insignificant, as a rule, and occur late. The retroperitoneal lymph-glands and, exceptionally, the inguinal glands and peritoneum are the parts attacked. A peculiar feature is the liability to form metastases in the bones—von Recklinghausen's "ossifying carcinosis." Carcinoma is found at all ages, but naturally much more commonly in old people.

Sarcoma.—Sarcomas are usually *round-celled* or *spindle-celled.* About 10 per cent. of all malignant tumors of the prostate, according to Orth, occur in childhood, and these are of sarcomatous type, or often in the form of "mixed tumors" with rhabdomyomatous and other indications of aberrant developmental origin. They may attain a large size.

Secondary tumors of metastatic origin are rare. More frequent are those due to extension from the bladder or rectum.

COWPER'S GLANDS.

These little bodies, which are situated behind the bulb, are apt to be involved in inflammatory conditions originating in the urethra. Of chief importance here is gonorrhœa. **Suppurative inflammation** and **abscess** may result. If the duct become blocked, **cystic dilatation** occurs. Very rarely **carcinoma** has been met with.

THE TESTES AND EPIDIDYMES.

CONGENITAL ANOMALIES.

These consist in defects of development and irregularities in the process of descent. An increase in the number of the testes—**polyorchidism**—is occasionally met with. Usually two on one side are found. One case is on record[1] where both testes were fused into one—**synorchidism**; complete absence of the testes—**anorchidism**—is more usual. The absence may be unilateral. In such cases, as a rule, there is defect of the epididymis and vas deferens on the same side. Incomplete development—**hypoplasia**—is not uncommon. The condition is bilateral or unilateral, and is due usually to retardation in the descent of the organ.

Hypoplasia is exceptionally met with in children and at the age of puberty. In such cases the testes may have descended properly but have lagged behind in the general growth of the sexual organs.

Abnormal position of the testis (**ectopia**) is not uncommon. The testis is either retained at some point in the canal or is actually dislocated out of its natural passage. The testis may be retained in the abdomen opposite the lumbar vertebræ, in the inguinal canal, or at the fold between the scrotum and thigh. Microscopically, a retained testicle shows a relative increase in the amount of the stroma, while the gland-tubes are atrophic or badly developed.

In dislocation, **dystopia**, the testis is outside its normal surroundings, and is found in the abdominal wall in a pouch, leading from the inguinal canal, at the femoroscrotal fold. The testis may also, as in a case once observed by us, be found in an artificial sac on the inner side of the thigh (**hernia cruralis testicularis**). A great rarity is the presence of both

[1] Cruveilhier, Traité d'anat. path. i: 301

testes in the same half of the scrotum. Dystopia is usually unilateral, but may be bilateral. A retained or dislocated testis is particularly liable to disease, and generally shows atrophy, fatty degeneration of the secreting cells, and fibroid induration. It may also be infarcted and inflamed. One of us (A. G. N.) has recently met with sarcoma involving a retained testicle. Dystopia is not always congenital, but may be due to trauma, as sometimes happens in gymnasts.

An interesting anomaly is the presence of aberrant adrenal tissue between the testis and the head of the epididymis.

CIRCULATORY DISTURBANCES.

Anemia of the testis is usually due to pressure, as in hydrocele and hematocele. Anemic and hemorrhagic **infarcts** are also occasionally met with. **Necrosis** is apt to supervene in such cases and when phlebitis or thrombosis of the pampiniform plexus is present. **Hemorrhage** into the testis is generally a result of traumatism, but is also met with in leukemia.

INFLAMMATIONS.

Orchitis and Epididymitis.—Inflammation of the testis—orchitis— and of the epididymis—**epididymitis**—may occur independently of each other, but are usually associated. The tunica vaginalis, vas deferens, and the spermatic cord are frequently involved as well.

As a rule, the condition is brought about by infection through the spermatic ducts (gonorrhœal) or from contiguity with the tunica and spermatic vessels. Trauma is the next most important cause. Hematogenic infection is not so common. In cases where the infection has spread from the spermatic ducts, the epididymis is usually first involved. The character of the inflammation varies somewhat in the case of the two organs. In the testicle the inflammation is at first interstitial, while in the epididymis it is more likely to be catarrhal and desquamative. Orchitis is often met with in gonorrhœa, less frequently in typhoid, mumps, and variola. It has also been observed after abdominal operations. The gonorrhœal form begins usually as a catarrhal and interstitial epididymitis which frequently extends to the testis. The affection, as a rule, arises from the second to the sixth week of the urethritis.

Macroscopically, the epididymis is enlarged and its consistency increased. On section it is reddened, the tubules are frequently dilated and filled with grayish-yellow material, composed of pus, mucus, and desquamated epithelium. The testis may show merely reddening and œdema, but may be actually inflamed. Here the inflammation tends to be interstitial, and abscess-formation is more common than in the epididymis.

Microscopically, in the epididymis, the vessels are congested, and the epithelial lining of the tubules is, in part, converted into goblet-cells secreting mucus. The connective tissue, the walls of the tubules, and the epithelium are all infiltrated with inflammatory products. The looser portions are œdematous. If the process last for a sufficiently long time, fibroid induration sets in, which may lead to obstruction and cystic dilatation of the tubules.

In suppurative orchitis the organ is swollen and its capsule tense. On section, it is of a yellow color, pulpy, and œdematous, the tubules showing as yellowish-white streaks. Large or smaller abscesses are often found. Microscopically, the tubules are distended with pus cells and the interstitial stroma is either diffusely infiltrated or presents foci of suppuration. In chronic cases fibrosis may result.

Chronic Fibroid Orchitis.—Chronic fibroid orchitis may, as has just been remarked, terminate a simple or suppurative inflammation, but is most strikingly found in syphilis.

Fig. 205

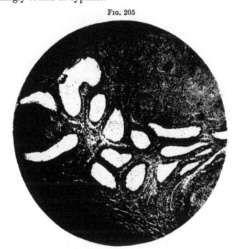

Tuberculosis of the epididymis. Zeiss obj. DD, ocular No. 1. (From the Pathological Laboratory of McGill University.)

Tuberculosis.—Tuberculous orchitis and epididymitis are fairly frequent. The affection is rarely primary, but is usually associated with tuberculosis of the seminal vesicles, vasa deferentia, prostate, bladder, and ureters. In adults the process generally begins in the epididymis and involves the testis secondarily. In children before the age of puberty the reverse is the case. The infection is either hematogenic or from extension along the vas deferens. Infection from the urethra is rare. Nakarai[1] has shown recently that tubercle bacilli may be found in the normal testicle and epididymis of a tuberculous person.

[1] Ziegler's Beiträge, 24: 1898: 327.

It is the rule for one or more large, caseous foci to be formed with subsidiary smaller tubercles, but occasionally there are numerous foci of about equal size. When the epididymis is involved it is converted into a caseous mass, often bounded by fibrous tissue. Here the process begins in the walls of the tubules in the globus major. Next to the epididymis, the corpus Highmori is the most seriously affected, being either filled with small, caseous nodules or totally destroyed. In time the infection spreads to the testicle, which contains a few small, gray or yellowish-white tubercles. These start in the tubules or, occasionally, in the interstitial tissue. Inflammatory infiltration takes place with catarrh and proliferation of the tubular epithelium, and the process gradually spreads along the lymphatics and tubules. Caseation rapidly

Fig. 206

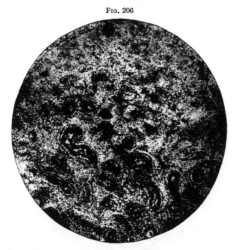

Healed syphilis of the testis. Leitz obj. No. 3, without ocular. There is a marked over-growth of connective tissue. Many of the tubules have disappeared entirely. Some are represented merely by rings of nuclei. Those still existing are compressed and atrophic. (From the collection of Dr. A. G. Nicholls.)

supervenes and giant cells are numerous. Later, the testis is filled with large caseous or caseofibroid masses tending to coalesce. The disease may gradually extend to the tunica propria and tunica communis, and finally to the skin. When softening occurs fistulæ may be formed. Fungoid granulations may appear externally. The fibrosis is never sufficient to overbalance the destructive process.

Syphilis.—Syphilis is not uncommonly found in the testicle in the later stages of the disease. As a rule, the process begins in the testis and spreads thence to the epididymis. Two forms are met with, a **diffuse fibroid induration** and **gumma.**

In the first type the testis on section presents delicate, pearly white bands of connective tissue, not infrequently extending from the rete to the tunica albuginea. These are pathognomonic of syphilis. Microscopically, the process is seen to be primarily an interstitial one, the intertubular stroma containing a few leukocytes and being greatly thickened, while the tubules are atrophic and hyaline. The arteries are also thickened. Federmann[1] has pointed out as a further diagnostic point that in syphilis the elastic tissue of the testis is preserved, while in tuberculosis it disappears even before caseation has set in.

In the gummatous form the testicle contains firm nodules enclosed in fibrous tissue. As a rule, only one organ is affected. In many cases the tunica albuginea becomes involved so that a serous or serofibrinous exudation is produced, which may lead to thickening and adhesion of the membranes. Occasionally, the skin is involved and gummy foci may discharge externally. Fungoid excrescences about the sinuses occur, as in tuberculosis, but are rare.

Lepra.—Leprosy occurs in the testis and epididymis in the form of granulomas, leading to necrosis. Should healing take place the organ remains permanently atrophic.

Glanders.—In the human subject glanders rarely affects the testicle. In guinea-pigs, however, that have been injected intraperitoneally with the B. mallei, the testes and scrotum become acutely and markedly infiltrated with inflammatory products (Straus' phenomenon). This fact is taken advantage of in the laboratory diagnosis of the disease.

RETROGRESSIVE METAMORPHOSES.

Atrophy.—The condition of atrophy, so-called, is found as a senile change and in wasting diseases. Pressure may bring it about, as in hydrocele, hematocele, varicocele, hernias, and tumors. A similar condition is met with in injuries to the cerebellum, concussion of the brain, and paraplegia.

The most common retrograde change is a diminution in the size of the testis, in which there is a more or less complete destruction of the secreting cells. It is not to be regarded entirely as an atrophic process, however, inasmuch as there is in many cases, although not in all, a progressive fibrosis of the stroma with thickening of the walls of the seminiferous tubules. Not infrequently, the walls appear swollen, transparent, and hyaline, so that folds project into the lumen of the tubules, which in advanced cases may be obliterated. The secreting cells show fatty degeneration, and, with the cells of the interstitial substance, are pigmented.

Calcification occurs in tumors, abscesses, and fibrous scars.

Gangrene of the testis occurs after trauma.

[1] Inaug. Diss., *Göttingen*, 1900.

PROGRESSIVE METAMORPHOSES.

Hypertrophy.—Compensatory hypertrophy of one testis, when the other is deficient, probably exists, although, contrary to what one would expect, it is very rare. A form of enlargement due to overgrowth of the connective tissue has been met with in the Tropics, associated with elephantiasis of the scrotum.

Tumors.—The tumors occurring in the testis are striking for their great variety and for certain special forms of a heterotopic nature. As a class they are apt to take on rapid growth, while recent studies show that a larger proportion than used to be held are truly mixed growths— **teratoblastomas**, or even **teratomas**. In other words, a full study of material from several areas of a testicular growth requires to be made before it can safely be described as a simple blastoma. It would seem that, in some cases at least, tumors of a highly malignant type originate from one order of cells in these teratoid growths, and with regard to more benign types, chondromas, for example, it is not yet regarded as settled whether, or to what extent, these originate from the testicular interstitial tissue or from the cartilaginous elements of a teratoid new-growth.

Teratoma.—The essential feature of these is the existence within them of cells originating from two or all of the primary layers of the embryo. Such tumors may exhibit epidermal elements, nerve cells (retinal), pigment cells, muscle fibres, bone, cartilage, and glandular spaces or cysts lined by columnar or other epithelium. Of late an increasing number of examples have been recorded of **chorio-epithelioma malignum**[1] in the testis, tumors which can only be ascribed to the preponderating growth of the syncytial and outer cell layers of the chorium of an aberrant heterotopic and atypical would-be embryo. The *teratoid* growths are simpler, containing cells of more than one type derivable from a single cell layer. The teratomas (dermoids) of the testes are more frequently of the solid type than are those of the ovary.

Fibroma, osteoma, and **angioma** are rare.

Myoma.—Myomas, composed of smooth or striated muscle, are occasionally observed. They arise from preëxisting muscle, as from the so-called "inner" cremaster, and from remains of the gubernaculum.

Chondroma.—This forms nodular growths or abundant cylindrical branching masses. In the last type there is a development of cartilage within the lymphatic vessels.

The tumor may reach a considerable size and form hard, warty masses. On section, softening, cystic degeneration, and calcification are frequently to be seen. The new-growth usually begins in the neighborhood of the rete. Microscopically, it consists of hyalin or fibrocartilage. A fibrous perichondrium is common.

These tumors are met with in children, and are therefore presumably due to congenital defects, probably cell-inclusion. A striking pecu-

---

[1] See Breus and Schlagenhaufer, Centrlbl. f. Gynäk., 27:1903:82; and Carey, Johns Hopkins Hospital Bulletin, 13:1902:275.

liarity is a tendency to form metastases, so that the tumor is to be regarded as relatively malignant.

Sarcoma.—Sarcoma is much less common than carcinoma, but also forms a rapidly-growing soft tumor. It is most frequently bilateral. It is commonest in childhood and in early manhood. On section, it is homogeneous, smooth, and grayish red in color, somewhat like bacon in appearance, and is often lobulated. The growth does not tend to infiltrate to the same extent as carcinoma and in the course of growth is apt to push the testis to one side. Microscopically, sarcoma is usually *round-celled*, but *spindle-celled* forms are seen. *Plexiform angiosarcoma* has been described.

A peculiar tumor, somewhat suggesting the intracanalicular fibroma of the breast, is the *intracanalicular cystosarcoma*, in which the interstitial tissue, in a state of sarcomatous proliferation, grows into the dilated tubules.

Chondrosarcoma and *myxosarcoma* are met with.

Carcinoma.—By far the most important malignant growth is carcinoma. It is most common between the ages of thirty and forty, but is met with in childhood. There is some difference of opinion as to whether it originates in the tubules or in epithelial cell "rests." The growth is usually *encephaloid*, but *scirrhous* forms occur. *Colloid* carcinoma is excessively rare.

Encephaloid carcinoma begins about the centre of the organ and infiltrates either as a diffuse growth or in the form of multiple nodules. The whole testis may be destroyed, but, while enlarged, may for long preserve a smooth surface, owing to the fact that the tunica albuginea is very resisting. On section, the growth is soft and brain-like and of a grayish or yellowish-gray color. Fatty degeneration, necrotic and hemorrhagic areas are often seen.

Microscopically, the cells are large, polyhedral, having a pale, delicate protoplasm. According to Langhans, glycogen is abundant. The vessels of the stroma are often numerous and dilated (*car. teleangiectaticum*). Cysts are also sometimes found.

Malignant glioma has been described.

Cysts may be (1) **developmental**, (2) of **teratoid origin**, or (3) due to **obstruction** of the ducts through fibroid induration or tumors. The seminiferous tubules and their discharging ducts are of independent development; hence if they do not unite in the normal manner, the tubules become distended into *retention cysts*. The cysts of the epididymis are similarly of developmental origin (see vol. i, Fig. 286, p. 853), due to persistence of aberrant tubules of the Müllerian duct and paradidymis. The cysts of teratomatous development vary considerably in their lining membrane and contents, having a ciliated, cylindrical, or stratified pavement epithelium. Their contents may be mucinous (*cystoma mucosum*), porridgy (*cyst. atheromatosum*) or cholesteatomous.

The Membranes of the Testes.

The membranes surrounding the testes and spermatic cords are formed by the evagination of the peritoneal sac (processus vaginalis peritonei).

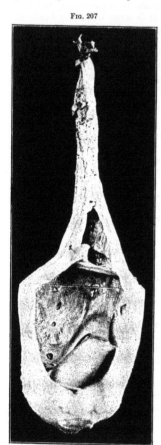

FIG. 207

Occasionally, from defective evolution, the portion about the testis does not become separated as it should, so that there persists a more or less perfect communication with the peritoneal cavity. This has an important bearing on the subject of hernia. In some cases fluid collects in the scrotum about the testicle, forming one variety of **hydrocele**.

Hemorrhage, usually between the tunica vaginalis and the tunica communis, may occur, forming a hematoma. It is usually due to external violence, heavy muscular work, coughing, or to the hemorrhagic diatheses.

Hydrops.—Simple hydrops may be found in general anasarca. In the Tropics, in association with filarial disease, a milky fluid is transuded into the cavity, the so-called "*galactocele,*" or, more correctly, *chylocele.*

Periorchitis.—By far the most important affection of the membranes is inflammation—**peri rchitis** or **vaginitis testis**. This may be acute or chronic, and is usually secondary to lesions of the testis or epididymis. Occasionally, it is primary and due to trauma but may occur apparently spontaneously. As might be supposed, periorchitis is more common during the earlier period of sexual activity. It is frequent in the Tropics. Congenital malformations predispose to the condition. According to the nature of the process, we can recognize an exudative and a productive form.

Hydrocele of the tunica vaginalis. The testicle is seen at the lower portion of the sac. (From the Pathological Museum of McGill University.)

Serous Periorchitis.—Serous or serofibrinous periorchitis is characterized by the exudation of a serous or serofibrinous fluid that often collects in considerable quantity, and leads to great distension of the sac. The process may be acute or, again, insidious in its onset. The fluid is clear or slightly turbid from the presence of leukocytes and epithelial cells (*acute hydrocele*), or may contain blood (*hematocele*). The fibrin that is formed tends to be deposited on the walls of the sac. Both the epithelium and the superficial layers of the sac may undergo fibrinoid transformation. The subserous connective tissue is usually œdematous. As the process goes on, fibrous adhesions may be formed, binding together more or less firmly the two layers of the sac (*adhesive periorchitis*). In long-standing cases the exudate is usually clear or tinged with blood. Not infrequently, it contains numerous crystals of cholesterin, giving it a milky, glistening appearance. The more fluid portions are in some cases absorbed, leaving behind a whitish or pigmented, mushy-looking mass, containing cholesterin.

Among the chief causes may be mentioned, gonorrhœa, traumatism, and the infectious fevers, such as scarlatina. Occasionally in children it appears independently of any of these causes.

A special form of fibrinous periorchitis is the *periorchitis villosa* or *verrucosa*, in which polypoid excrescences spring up, usually upon the epididymis. These may be torn off and form free bodies.

Suppurative Periorchitis.—Suppurative periorchitis is characterized by a purulent or fibrinopurulent exudation with much congestion of the membranes. Occasionally, putrid decomposition of the fluid occurs. The inflammation may extend up the spermatic cord to the peritoneum, or may involve the scrotum. In some cases healing takes place with adhesion of the two layers of the sac.

The process may be metastatic, but much more commonly is due to a preëxisting inflammation, to injuries, gonorrhœa, or to suppurative orchitis or epididymitis.

Chronic Serous Periorchitis.—Chronic serous periorchitis usually originates in an acute affection, but may begin insidiously. It leads to a considerable outpouring of fluid, as much as three liters in some cases, which contains about 5 per cent. of albumin and tends to clot on standing. It may contain blood and cholesterin. In some cases, where there is spermatocele or an aberrant vas deferens, spermatozoa may be found in the fluid (Roth). The walls of the sac are often thickened and pigmented (*productive periorchitis*). There may also be adhesions.

In all effusions into the tunica the testicle is usually situated in the posterior portion of the dilated sac, and while for some time it may retain fairly well its normal condition, it later becomes indurated and compressed, so as to be with difficulty recognizable. The testis and epididymis are frequently atrophic, not only from pressure, but often from preëxisting disease, the cause of the original hydrocele. When old adhesions are present a loculated collection of fluid results.

Tuberculosis.—This is by no means common, except when secondary to tuberculosis of the testis and epididymis. As a primary affection it takes the form of disseminated foci or large granulomas.

Syphilis.—Syphilis is, as a rule, met with as an adhesive periorchitis extending from the testicle. It may be complicated with hydrocele. Gummas are rare.

Tumors.—Primary tumors of the tunica vaginalis testis are rare. Among them may be mentioned **fibroma, leiomyoma, rhabdomyoma, lipoma, myxoma, chondroma, dermoid cysts,** and **sarcoma.**

Parasites.—*Echinococcus disease* is found in the membranes.

THE SCROTUM.

The scrotum is composed of modified skin, and the diseases affecting it, for the most part, resemble those of the skin. Only a few of the more important conditions, therefore, will be referred to here.

The structure is very elastic and contractile, owing to the presence of unstriped muscle fibres composing the tunica dartos. Subcutaneous fat is absent, but bloodvessels and lymphatics are abundant.

The most important **malformations** are the **fission** that occurs in hypospadias and hermaphroditism, and **hypoplasia.**

Owing to the elastic texture of the scrotum and its great vascularity, **hemorrhage** and **œdema** occur readily and are often of extreme degree. Œdema is frequently present in cases of chronic valvular disease of the heart. A local form is also described, which is possibly due to neuropathic influences.

INFLAMMATIONS.

The inflammations are usually due to external irritation, local infection, parasites, or extension from the testicle or epididymis.

RETROGRESSIVE METAMORPHOSES.

Gangrene.—Among retrogressive changes, gangrene is of frequent occurrence. It follows œdema, extravasation of urine, erysipelas, phagedena, and, rarely, infectious diseases.

PROGRESSIVE METAMORPHOSES.

Hypertrophy.—The most important progressive disorder is hypertrophy or **elephantiasis.** Frequently the penis and scrotum are involved together. Two forms exist, the one a **diffuse fibrosis,** and the other in which the more or less indurated tissue contains numerous dilated lymphatics, sometimes forming on the surface nodular tumors or vesicles (**lymph scrotum; pachydermia lymphangiectatica**). The disease is most common in the Tropics, and some of the cases, at least, are due to filariasis.

Tumors.—Of the tumors may be mentioned **fibroma, lipoma, fibromyoma, angioma, teratoma, sarcoma, carcinoma,** and various forms of **cysts.** The most important new-growth is carcinoma, interesting chiefly on account of its peculiar etiology. It is due apparently to irritation, and is found in chimney-sweeps and those working in tar and paraffin. *Melanotic carcinoma* is described, but is excessively rare.

Kocher[1] has described a remarkable *giant-celled sarcoma*.

Parasites.—The animal parasites found are *Filaria sanguinis hominis* and *Echinococcus*.

THE SPERMATIC CORD, VAS DEFERENS, AND VESICULÆ SEMINALES.

Œdema.—Œdema may lead to swelling of the cord or diffuse hydrocele.

Varicocele.—A common affection is dilatation of the veins, or varicocele. The disease is commonest in early adult life. It is occasionally due to the obstruction to the free outflow of blood by tumors or hernia, but frequently appears without obvious cause. It may be that there is some congenital weakness of the vessels that predisposes. The veins in question are poor in valves, and thus a long column of blood has to be supported. Among the causes to which the condition is attributed are prolonged standing, violent muscular exertion, sexual excess, gonorrhœa, and traumatism. The affection is usually found on the left side, owing to the facts that the left spermatic vein does not empty directly into the vena cava inferior but into the left renal vein, and, moreover, lies behind the rectum.

Funiculitis.—Inflammation of the cord—funiculitis—is due to the extension of a posterior urethritis or to traumatism.

Tumors.—Of primary tumors should be mentioned **lipoma, fibroma, myxoma, myxofibroma,** and **sarcoma.** They are rare. Metastatic deposits may occur in sarcoma or carcinoma of the testis.

Cysts are due to localized hydroceles of the cord, or develop from remains of the Wolffian body, (?) duct.

Deferenitis.—The most important affection of the vas deferens is inflammation, deferenitis or spermatitis. This is due to the extension of inflammation from the urethra, bladder, prostate, or epididymis. Rarely it is idiopathic or due to trauma. The usual cause is gonorrhœa. Obliteration of the vas and, if the condition be bilateral, sterility results.

Tuberculosis.—Tuberculous deferenitis arises by extension from the associated organs.

Syphilis.—Gummas have been occasionally observed.

The seminal vesicles may be **absent** on one or both sides, or may be **fused.** The first condition is usually associated with unilateral defect of the kidney, vas, and epididymis. **Hypoplasia** occurs in anorchidism.

Spermatocystitis.—Inflammation of the seminal vesicles, spermatocystitis, is usually an extension from the vas. Rarely, it occurs from trauma, or even without obvious cause. It is usually due to gonorrhœa. The inflammation may be simple, mucoid, mucopurulent, purulent,

---

[1] Deutsche Chir., 506: 1887.

hemorrhagic, or caseous. The walls of the vesicles are infiltrated inflammatory products, and the cavities are filled with leukoc chiefly mononuclear, desquamated epithelium, debris, and, if the be not occluded, with spermatozoa.

In **tuberculosis** there is a caseous detritus and the walls show tu culous infiltration.

In advanced cases of spermatocystitis the walls are thickened an cavities may be contracted. In old men who have suffered from chr gonorrhœa, hypertrophy of the prostate, vesical calculus, or strie diverticula are sometimes found, owing to irregular proliferatio fibrous tissue. Occasionally cystic dilatation is the result. The cont of the vesicles may in some cases become inspissated and infiltrated salts, so that *concretions* are produced.

CHAPTER XXXVIII.

THE FEMALE SEXUAL ORGANS.

THE female organs of generation include the vulva (external genitalia); the vagina, the uterus, Fallopian tubes, ovaries, and broad ligaments (internal genitalia). Inasmuch, however, as the mammæ are closely connected with the function of reproduction and attain their full development only in the female, it is convenient to discuss diseases of the breast also under this category. Affections of the placenta and fœtal membranes will also be treated here.

A great variety of malformations affecting the genital tract in whole or in part are described. **Hermaphroditism** is discussed in another place (see vol. i, p. 278). **Doubling** of the genital organs as a whole, including also the bladder and urethra, is recorded in one case.[1]

A more common anomaly is **hypoplasia**, either where the usual changes incident to puberty are retarded, or where the organs remain small or imperfect throughout life.

THE EXTERNAL GENITALIA.

These are the vulva, including the clitoris, labia majora, labia minora, the hymen, and certain associated glands—the Cowper's or Bartholini's glands.

CONGENITAL ANOMALIES.

Complete **defect** of the vulva is found in acephalic monsters and siren deformities. More common are defects of certain parts, either bilateral or unilateral. Such are absence of the labia minora, the labia majora, the clitoris, or the labia minora and clitoris together. Besides aplasia, **hypoplasia** exists, generally associated with retarded development of the internal organs. The vulva in the adult may present the characteristics of infancy (*vulva infantilis*).

Fission of the clitoris simulating reduplication has been met with. It is usually associated with epispadias. **Hypertrophy** of the clitoris affects the prepuce alone or the organ as a whole. The affection is more common in tropical countries. It is found occasionally in the black races, in pseudohermaphroditism, and, rarely, in prostitutes. In some cases, hypertrophy of the clitoris is combined with **hyperplasia** of the labia.

---

[1] V. Engel, Arch. f. Gynäk., 29:1887:43.

In certain races, as Bushmen and Hottentots, the labia, particularly the labia minora, are excessively enlarged, sometimes almost reaching the knees (*Hottentot apron*). Enlargement of the labia majora is said by some to be due always to new-growth.

An **increase** in the **number** of the labia is rare, less so in the case of nymphæ. Congenital **adhesions** of the labia, especially the labia minora, exist and may lead to interference with the function of urination.

Hernia into the labium majus through the inguinal canal may occur (*hernia inguinalis labialis*), or may extend from beneath the ramus of the pubes into the lower part of the labium (*hernia labialis inferior*).

The urogenital sinus may fail to develop naturally, and thus persistence of an embryonic condition may occur, such as **epispadias, hypospadias,** and **anus præternaturalis vestibularis.**

The hymen presents great variation in its form. It may be completely **occluded** or may possess merely a **small opening.** Or, again, the opening may be double (*hymen septus*), sieve-like (*hymen cribriformis*), or serrated (*hymen fimbriatus*).

CIRCULATORY DISTURBANCES.

Hyperemia.—**Active Hyperemia.**—Active hyperemia is due to inflammation, or to mechanical irritation, as in the sexual act.

Passive Hyperemia.—Passive hyperemia is commonly due to pregnancy, or to general blood stasis, as, for instance, in valvular disease of the heart.

If the condition persist, the vessels, especially those of the labia majora, become dilated and varicose. *Thrombosis* then may occur with possibly phlebolith formation, or a venule may burst, leading to large extravasations of blood (*hematoma*). Rupture of the veins may also take place from external traumatism or from parturition.

Hemorrhage.—Hemorrhage from tearing of the hymen at the first coitus is rarely dangerous. It is most likely to be severe when the orifice is small or the hymen thick and fleshy.

Œdema.—Œdema is common and may be associated with inflammatory hyperemia, passive congestion, or vascular changes. It is found especially in valvular heart affections and in nephritis.

INFLAMMATIONS.

The inflammatory affections of the vulva are practically those found on any skin surface. Among them may be mentioned **erythema, eczema, herpes, acne, furunculosis, hard** and **soft chancre, condylomas, impetigo, phlegmon, erysipelas, diphtheritis, gangrene,** and **lupus.**

Vulvitis.—**Acute Vulvitis.**—Acute vulvitis or vulvovaginitis is commonly due to gonorrhœa and occurs chiefly in children from mediate infection. It is, however, also met with in adults. Cases are sometimes due to uncleanliness or the irritation of thread-worms. The labia and clitoris are reddened, œdematous, and bathed in pus. The follicles may also be involved. Excoriation is common.

Catarrhal Vulvitis.—Simple catarrhal vulvitis may be due to dirt, mechanical irritation, or irritating discharges.

Phlegmonous Vulvitis.—Phlegmonous vulvitis has been known to follow injuries in labor.

Membranous Vulvitis.—Membranous vulvitis may be due to diphtheria, or may be merely diphtheroid. The latter form occurs in many of the infections, as puerperal sepsis, measles, typhoid, scarlatina, and cholera. It may also originate in the extension of inflammation from the bowel or vagina and may terminate in gangrene.

FIG. 208

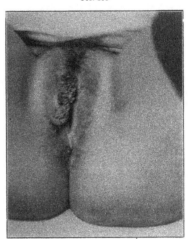

Condylomas of the vulva. (From the Gynecological Clinic of the Montreal General Hospital.)

Inflammation of the Bartholini's glands is commonly due to gonorrhœa, but may be an extension from vulvitis of other forms. It gives rise to catarrh of the duct, with retention of the secretion. Abscess frequently results. Induration also occurs. Inflammation, when of some standing, leads to productive changes and often adhesion of the nymphæ.

Condyloma.—Condylomas are inflammatory outgrowths on the mucous membrane of the vulva and vagina or the skin near by. They are either *acuminate* or *nodular*, and tend to be produced wherever there is heat and moisture. They are common in syphilis, but may also be due to irritating discharges, gonorrhœa, etc.

Chancroid.—Chancroid or **ulcus molle** is found upon the labia majora and minora, the fourchette, and meatus urinarius. The ulcers tend to be multiple, as they are auto-inoculable. They take the form of punched-out excavations secreting pus.

Syphilis.—The lesions of syphilis are protean. We may have the primary sore (**ulcus durum**), secondary eruptions, mucous patches, condylomas, and, rarely, gummas.

Tuberculosis.—Tuberculosis assumes the form of *lupus* or *rapid caseous ulceration.*

It should be mentioned that there has been described a form of chronic ulceration, very refractory to treatment, leading to inflammatory hyperplasia, that has been regarded by some as tuberculous, by others as syphilitic. Koch believes that it is due to lymph stasis following destruction of the inguinal glands. Microscopically, the appearances are those of simple inflammation.

Actinomycosis.—Actinomycosis of the vulva is very rare, only two cases being on record.[1]

RETROGRESSIVE METAMORPHOSES.

Atrophy.—After the climacteric the labia majora undergo atrophy, owing to the absorption of the fat, and become small and relaxed, tending to expose the vulvar orifice. Atrophy of the nymphæ also occurs.

Kraurosis Vulvæ.—A curious and rare form of atrophy and contraction of the vulva, first described by Breisky,[2] is the so-called kraurosis vulvæ. The etiology of the condition is still doubtful but it may be inflammatory in origin. The disease involves the vestibule, vagina, labia majora, clitoris, and the inner part of the labia minora. The mucous membrane is stretched, smooth, inelastic, glistening, dry, and pale reddish-gray in color. The surface is often fissured and enlarged bloodvessels can be seen.

Microscopically, according to Peter,[3] there is at first chronic inflammation with round-celled infiltration and inflammatory œdema of the corium and epidermis, and later atrophy of the upper layers of the corium, especially the papillæ. With this there is a marked tendency to contraction with hyperplasia of the connective tissue. Very little can be seen of the sebaceous and sudoriparous glands, and there is loss of the elastic tissue.

Gangrene.—Gangrene of the vulva results from simple or inflammatory œdema, hemorrhage, thrombosis, and from traumatism. It is found in certain infectious diseases, as typhoid, measles, scarlatina, and variola.

Certain special forms deserve mention. These are **phagedena** from chancroid, and **noma.** Noma vulvæ occurs under the same circum-

---

[1] Bongartz, Monatssch. f. Geb. u. Gyn., 3: 1896: 4.
[2] Zeit. f. Heilk., 6: 1885: 69.
[3] Monatsschr. f. Geb. u. Gynäk., 3:1896:297.

stances as noma of the cheek. It is found in anemic and debilitated children.

Concretions.—Concretions may form behind the prepuce of the clitoris.

SOLUTIONS OF CONTINUITY.

These occur during coitus and parturition. Small fissures may be produced, or, again, extensive lacerations. The most important form is laceration of the perineum during labor.

PROGRESSIVE METAMORPHOSES.

Hypertrophy.—Cutaneous horns due to hypertrophy of the epithelium have been met with on the clitoris.

Elephantiasis.—The most important and interesting of the hypertrophies is elephantiasis. The etiology is by no means perfectly understood and undoubtedly varies in different cases. Some cases are congenital, in the sense, at least, that at birth there is a hyperplastic enlargement of the parts that subsequently becomes excessive, or that there is an inherited predisposition to the disease (*pachydermatocele, eleph. mollis*). Other cases are undoubtedly due to chronic inflammation or to some affection of the lymph-glands and vessels. The latter is generally caused by obstruction to the outflow of the lymph and may be caused by filariæ and inflammatory fibrosis. The condition has been known to follow suppuration of the inguinal glands. The disease may be unilateral or bilateral, and affects the labia majora, less frequently the nymphæ and clitoris. The surface is either smooth (*eleph. glabra*) or nodular (*eleph. tuberosa*). The anatomical forms vary. In one type the parts, as a whole, are enlarged and the normal contour of the tissues is destroyed by a subcutaneous œdema or connective-tissue hyperplasia. In whatever way the process starts it is liable to be complicated by inflammatory changes, such as induration, ulceration, and gangrene.

Tumors.—Fibromas.—Fibromas have been found in the labia majora, less commonly in the labia minora and clitoris. They are either massive or pedunculated, and may weigh several pounds. They originate in the subcutaneous connective tissue, in the fascia, or in the periosteum of the pelvis (Kiwisch). Structurally, fibromas are composed of a loose, often œdematous connective tissue, or occasionally are in part mucoid (**myxofibroma**). Owing to hemorrhage or degeneration they may become cystic. **Myoma** and **fibromyoma** have also been described. Rarely, they arise from the end of the round ligament. **Lipomas** are rather uncommon, and develop in the mons veneris and greater labia. They may be combined with **angioma. Hemangioma** and **lymphangioma** are also met with. Among the greatest rarities is **chondroma** of the clitoris, occasionally associated with softening, calcification, or true bony growth. Pigmented *nevi* are met with in children on the labia. **Adenoma** of the Bartholini's glands is rare.

Carcinoma.—Carcinoma of the vulva is relatively common. It arises usually from the labia, clitoris, commissures, or urethra. It occurs as a papillary or nodular outgrowth or as a diffuse infiltration. Extensive ulceration may occur. The growth is, as a rule, of the type of horny *epithelioma*, but *scirrhous* and *soft* forms are also met with. Carcinoma is commonest in the later years of life, and appears to be related to chronic thickening of the epithelium, such as occurs in pruritus. Carcinoma may also arise from Bartholini's glands.

Sarcoma.—Much rarer than carcinoma is sarcoma, which usually takes the form of *melanosarcoma*. *Round-* and *spindle-celled* forms as well as *myxosarcoma* have been described.

A secondary **melanotic hypernephroma** of the labium minus has been described.[1]

Cysts are of various kinds, either **degenerative, retention, or developmental.** Some arise from a local collection of fluid in the canal of Nuck, or from remains of Gärtner's duct; others from obstruction to the duct of a Bartholini's gland. They may be found on the labia and hymen.

THE VAGINA.

The vagina in adults is a potential tube, the walls of which are normally in contact, composed of connective tissue in which are numerous bands of unstriped muscle. It is lined with a mucous membrane, consisting of stratified pavement epithelium, the cells in the lower layers of which, however, tend to be cylindrical. The mucous membrane is not smooth but thrown up into papillæ and transverse ridges or rugæ. As a rule, it contains no glands, but there are certain lacunæ or crypts opening between the papillæ and folds. In a few cases glands lined with ciliated epithelium have been observed (v. Preuschen[2]). In the submucous connective tissue small clumps of lymphoid cells are to be found.

By repeated coitus or the act of parturition the rugæ become gradually obliterated. As old age comes on involution takes place, the mucosa becoming atrophic and the lumen more or less contracted.

CONGENITAL ANOMALIES.

The vagina may be completely **absent** or represented only by a fibrous cord. In other cases it is more or less rudimentary and contracted for its full length (**total atresia**). **Partial atresia** also occurs in the lower portion of the vagina. It may consist in a membranous occlusion (**atresia vaginalis**) or in an imperforate hymen (**atresia hymenalis**). When the vagina is completely absent, there is defect of the uterus and generally of the adnexa. Partial atresia after the establishment of

---

[1] *Gräfenberg*, Virch. Archiv, 194: 1908:17. .
[2] Virch. Archiv, 70:1877:111.

puberty leads to retention of the menstrual discharge, which may collect in the vagina (**hematokolpos**), and may eventually lead to distension of the uterus (**hematometra**) and tubes (**hematosalpinx**).

Stenosis may be due to an arrest of development or to hyperplasia of certain portions of the vaginal wall. **Adhesion** of the walls may result from antenatal inflammation.

Doubling of the vagina occurs with reduplication of the whole genito-urinary tract, but is excessively rare. Owing to imperfect fusion of the lower ends of the Müllerian duct, a partial or complete septum may be formed in the vagina. A double vagina of this type is found in the condition of uterus septus, uterus duplex, and uterus didelphys.

CIRCULATORY DISTURBANCES.

These are comparatively unimportant. **Active hyperemia** is found physiologically during sexual excitement, and in acute inflammation. **Passive hyperemia** occurs, as elsewhere, from obstruction to the general circulation, and during pregnancy. **Hemorrhages**, either superficial or deep, are due to injury during parturition, and occasionally to violent coitus. Gangrene, varicose veins, tumors, and other pathological states predispose to the condition.

ALTERATIONS IN POSITION AND CONTINUITY.

With weakness of the structures forming the floor of the pelvis and consequent descent of the uterus there is more or less **prolapse** of the vagina. This may be accompanied by descent of the posterior wall of the bladder (**cystocele**) or of the anterior wall of the rectum (**rectocele**), or both. A torn perineum contributes largely to the latter event. Occasionally there is dilatation of the wall of the bladder or rectum without any defect in the vaginal support. Descending loops of bowel may distend the Douglas' pouch (**posterior enterocele**), or separate to some extent the bladder from the vagina (**anterior enterocele**). The same effect may be produced by prolapsed ovaries (**ovariocele vaginalis**), tumors, and fluid.

Contusions and Lacerations.—Contusions and lacerations are of frequent occurrence during labor. As a rule, they are situated on the posterior vaginal wall. Tears may extend into the connective tissue, the perineum, or even into the rectum. Lacerations have also occurred from violent sexual intercourse, especially when the female is in a constrained position, or where there is a disproportion between the male and female organs. Injuries, resulting in destruction of tissue, sometimes follow the use of the obstetric forceps, pessaries, and from carcinoma, syphilitic lesions, and the like. Not infrequently **fistulous communications** are opened up with the neighboring parts, as the bladder (*vesicovaginal fistula*), rectum (*rectovaginal*), and the urethra (*urethrovaginal*), or the several forms may be combined.

Dilatation.—Dilatation is due to the passage of some large body, such as a child, a tumor, or the like, or to the retention of fluid.

INFLAMMATIONS.

Vaginitis.—Inflammation of the vagina—colpitis, vaginitis—is brought about by a variety of causes, such as mechanical, chemical, or thermic insults, infection, or extension from the adjacent parts.

Catarrhal Vaginitis.—The commonest form is catarrhal vaginitis, which may be acute or chronic.

It is due to irritation of any kind, the decomposition of discharges from the uterus or from fistulæ, ulcerating cancers, or vulvitis. It may arise as a complication in the infective fevers, measles, scarlatina, typhoid, and variola. Gonorrhœa is not a common cause, for the squamous epithelium of the vagina is rather resistant to the action of the gono-coccus. Gonorrhœal vaginitis is, therefore, found chiefly in children and in elderly women where the mucous membrane is atrophic and the resisting power lessened.

In *acute catarrhal vaginitis* the mucosa is reddened, swollen, and œdematous, the epithelium more or less desquamated. These appearances are most marked upon the tips of the rugæ and papillæ. The exudation is at first scanty and serous, later may be abundant, milky, and purulent. The reaction is acid and the secretion contains pus cells, epithelium, and various kinds of bacteria. Microscopically, the mucosa is somewhat eroded, the vessels congested, and there is a round-celled infiltration of the underlying connective tissue.

In the *chronic form* the appearances produced are at first not greatly different from those of the acute stage, but eventually there is hyperplasia of the papillæ and connective-tissue proliferation in the deeper parts. The epithelium is thickened, except upon the papillæ, where it is eroded. There is also a tendency for inflammatory cells to become aggregated in little clumps resembling follicles, which project into the lumen, giving the mucosa a rough or granular appearance (*vaginitis granulosa* or *nodularis*). Narrowing of the vagina may result. Where also eroded surfaces come in contact fibrous adhesions may occur (*vag. adhesiva*). Adhesion is apt to occur in elderly women in whom the mucosa becomes denuded in the course of involution (*senile vaginitis.*) The secretion is sometimes thin, grayish-white, and flocculent, at other times purulent. Chronic catarrh may follow the acute affections or may develop independently. Common causes are excess in coitus, and the presence of pessaries or other foreign bodies.

Exfoliative Vaginitis.—A rare form is exfoliative vaginitis in which the mucous membrane is thrown off in one piece. It is liable to be found in certain forms of dysmenorrhœa.

Membranous Vaginitis.—Membranous vaginitis is met with as a complication of the acute infections, such as measles, variola, scarlatina, typhoid, cholera, and dysentery. Of local causes may be mentioned, injuries during parturition, the irritation of foreign bodies, puerperal sepsis, discharges from cancers or fistulæ, rarely gonorrhœa, polypi. True *diphtheria* is rare.

Phlegmonous Vaginitis.—Phlegmonous or erysipelatous vaginitis has been described. In this there is diffuse suppuration in the vaginal wall that may lead to exfoliation of tissue.

Aphthous Vaginitis.—Aphthous vaginitis is due to a micröorganism resembling Oïdium albicans. The mucosa is reddened and studded with white, elevated patches.

Emphysematous Vaginitis.—A curious affection is the so-called emphysematous vaginitis (*colpohyperplasia cystica, emphysema vaginæ*). This disease is met with usually in pregnant women or shortly after confinement, but has been found in others. In the vaginal wall are numerous small vesicles or cysts, varying in size from that of a millet-seed to that of a hazelnut. Otherwise the mucosa appears to be normal. Numerous opinions (Winckel, Schroeder, Eppinger, Zweifel, Klebs, Chiari) have been expressed as to the cause. The most recent investigator, Lindenthal,[1] finds that it is due to an anaërobic gas-producing micröorganism, belonging to the malignant œdema group. The bacillus coli is not a cause, except possibly in diabetic individuals.

Inflammatory processes may extend from the vagina or rectum into the perivaginal connective tissue and lead to abscess formation or fibrosis (*perivaginitis suppurativa, perivag. fibrosa*).

Chancroids.—Chancroids are not common in the vagina.

Tuberculosis.—Tuberculosis is uncommon, and as a primary affection, excessively rare. As a rule, it extends from the uterus, vulva, or anus, but, exceptionally, is metastatic. It takes the form of shallow ulcers with irregular edges and nodular bases that tend to coalesce. Less commonly, one finds grayish tubercles or caseating granulomas.

Syphilis.—The primary papule or sclerosis of syphilis is rare in the vagina. It is found at the entrance or near the posterior commissure. *Erythema, psoriasis, condylomas,* and *gummas* are also met with. Birch-Hirschfeld[2] has described a *perivaginitis gummosa*, in which the vagina is converted into a stiff, fibrous tube.

RETROGRESSIVE METAMORPHOSES.

Atrophy.—Atrophy of the rugæ and of the mucous membrane in general has already been referred to (p. 857).

In prolapse of the vagina the mucosa becomes converted into a structure closely resembling skin, with stratum granulosum and keratinization.

Gangrene.—Gangrene may result from traumatism, pressure, inflammation, carcinoma, etc.

---

[1] Beitr. zur Aetiol. u. Histol. der Colpohyperplasia cystica; Zeit. f. Geb. u. Gyn., 40: 1899: 375.

[2] Lehrbuch, 2: 1887: 794.

Circumscribed ulcers due to ischemic necrosis have been described by Zahn.[1]

PROGRESSIVE METAMORPHOSES.

These are rather uncommon.

Hypertrophy.—Hypertrophy of the vaginal wall from muscular overactivity is found in association with atresia and retained fluid. **Mucous polyps,** sometimes of considerable size, are met with. They are usually found on the posterior wall. The inflammatory new-growths, such as **hyperplastic papillæ** and **condylomas** have been referred to already.

Tumors.—**Myoma.**—Sessile or pedunculated myomas, composed either of smooth or striped muscle, grow occasionally from the anterior vaginal wall. They may be of several pounds' weight. In contradistinction to myomas of the uterus they are rarely multiple.

Sarcoma.—In young children multiple papillary or polypoid sarcomas or fibrosarcomas (see vol. i. p. 662), often containing muscle, are sometimes found.[2] They appear to be congenital. The neoplasms may remain latent for years and then take on rapid growth. Microscopically, the growths consist of round or spindle cells. In adults, *round-, spindle-,* and *giant-celled sarcomas* are met with, and also a *diffuse sarcomatous infiltration* of the vaginal wall. Myxomatous degeneration may occur. Secondary sarcoma has been observed.

Carcinoma.—Primary carcinoma (*epithelioma*) occurs not infrequently, and takes the form of a cauliflower-like mass starting from the posterior wall. Exceptionally, a more diffuse or ring-like infiltration of a *scirrhous* or *medullary* character is met with.

More common are secondary carcinomas that have extended from the uterus, rectum, bladder, urethra, or vulva. Metastatic growths originating from the uterus or ovaries are rare, as are the cases of implantation of cancer cells from the uterus.

Carcinoma of the vagina extends rapidly and is liable to ulcerate, so that fistulæ are quickly produced.

Cysts.—Cysts originate in remains of the Wolffian or Gärtner's ducts, from implantation of epithelium and from dilated lymphatics.

Foreign Bodies and Parasites.—Apart from bacteria, may be mentioned the *larvæ* of certain flies, *Oxyuris vermicularis, Ascaris, Trichomonas vaginalis, Oïdium albicans, Monilia albicans, Monilia candida,* and various *yeasts.*

Echinococcus cysts may penetrate the vagina from the intestine.

A variety of foreign bodies have been found in the vagina, as, for instance, feces, urinary calculi, calcified myomas from the uterus, pessaries, catheters, tampons, portions of instruments, and objects introduced for purposes of masturbation.

---

[1] Virch. Archiv, 95: 1884: 388; and 95: 1889: 167.
[2] Kolisko, D. polypöse Sarkom der Scheide im Kindesalter, Wien. klin. Woch., 6: 1889: 119.

Foreign bodies, if they cannot be absorbed or discharged, become encrusted with triple phosphates and carbonates.

THE UTERUS.

The uterus is a hollow viscus, composed chiefly of unstriped muscle, with a certain admixture of connective tissue, and lined with a mucous membrane of peculiar type. The organ is formed by the fusion of the Müllerian ducts and undergoes certain minor modifications of its form in passing from the infantile to the adult and functioning type.

In the adult nullipara, the uterus measures from 5.5 to 8 cm. in length, and in the parous woman, 9 to 9.5 cm. Its breadth varies from 3.5 to 4 and 5.5 to 6 cm. respectively. The organ contains abundant lymphatics, of which those of the cervix discharge into the iliac, and those of the corpus into the lumbar and inguinal glands. The mucosa is about 1 mm. thick, and is composed of a delicate, reticulated, fibrous stroma, containing numerous lymphoid cells. In this are abundant spiral and branching glands or crypts (glandulæ utriculares), composed, like the mucosa lining the cavity, of a single layer of ciliated, cylindrical cells. The mucosa of the cervix is thinner and more compact, containing short gland-tubes, many of the cells of which are mucin-producing. The vaginal portion is covered externally with squamous epithelium like the vagina. A submucosa does not exist in the uterus, but the glands pass directly down to the muscle, or even into it.

During menstruation the uterus, being to some extent an erectile organ, is congested. The mucous membrane is especially hyperemic, and hemorrhage takes place from its surface. Not only this, but there is hyperplasia both of the stroma and of the glands, which become larger and more elongated. Later, the superficial epithelium, and to some extent that of the glands, is cast off. Finally, the remaining cells proliferate and the mucosa is restored to its former condition.

In pregnancy the uterus becomes greatly enlarged, relatively more so in the corpus. In the first half of gestation there is said to be a true new-formation of muscle fibres, but later on there is simple hypertrophy. In the cervical portion, in addition to some hypertrophy, there is a notable increase in the elastic fibres. The vessels become thickened and greatly lengthened, and the veins and lymphatics are dilated. The mucous membrane is converted into decidua, which, in the later stages, undergoes fatty and necrotic changes.

After delivery the uterus becomes greatly reduced in size, at first from contraction, and later from atrophy of the muscle fibres, which also show cloudy, hyaline, and fatty degeneration. The process of involution usually takes about six weeks. The involuted uterus never quite regains its former appearance. The corpus remains relatively large and thick-walled, and the cavity is enlarged. The os is almost invariably fissured and the arteries show thickening of their elastic elements and are eventually, to a large extent, absorbed and replaced by new vessels (see vol. i, p. 896).

CONGENITAL ANOMALIES.

Two great classes of anomalies may be recognized, the first due to nutritive disorders (*dystrophies*), resulting in abnormality in the size of the organ; the second, due to eccentricities of development (*dysplasias*). To a certain extent both types may be associated.

Hyperplasia of the uterus is occasionally observed, and enlargement of the organ is described in connection with many of the dysplasias. The uterus may be completely wanting (**aplasia**) or diminutive in size (**hypoplasia**). Hypoplasia is symmetrical or asymmetrical, according as the Müllerian ducts are equally or unequally involved.

Transverse **fission** of the external os is sometimes met with and may be confused with that resulting from childbirth.

The dysplasias are to be divided into five classes: (1) partial or complete separation of the two Müllerian ducts; (2) imperfect fusion of the ducts; (3) imperfect development of the fundus; (4) anomalies of the cavity; (5) faulty relationship with neighboring structures.

Complete aplasia of the uterus is very rare. As a rule, on careful examination, scanty rudiments can be discovered. In these cases the vagina and external genitals may be normal. The tubes and ovaries may be present or absent. When the uterus is partly formed, the cervical portion is often absent or represented by a solid mass of muscle.

Another class of cases is that in which there is an unequal development of the Müllerian ducts leading to asymmetry of the uterus. The most marked example of this is where one duct almost completely fails to develop. This results in the **uterus unicornis**. On the affected side the ovary may be well-formed, but cases are on record where it was defective as well as the tube, together with absence of the ureter and kidney of the same side.

Development of the Müllerian ducts without fusion results in the formation of two separate uteri and vaginæ (**uterus didelphys**). In certain rare instances both uteri may open into one vagina.

In another class of cases, fusion of the two ducts takes place only in the lower portion of the uterus, while above the ducts remain separate (**uterus bicornis**). The amount of separation is very variable. The line of division may be indicated by a mere depression (**uterus arcuatus** sive **bifundalis**). In other cases it is anvil-shaped (**uterus incudiformis**). In the most extreme form the line of cleavage extends down to or even into the cervical portion. Sometimes between the halves there is found a vesicorectal ligament. Rudimentary and asymmetrical forms of uterus bicornis also exist. The uterine cavities may be entirely separate (**uterus bicornis duplex**) or may unite at the cervix (**uter. bicorn. unicollis**). In the first case there may be a double vagina or one with a septum, but this is not invariable.

When the cavity is more or less perfectly divided by a septum the condition is called **uterus bilocularis** or **septus**. The septum may vary in completeness. When it extends from the fundus only a short distance into the cavity we speak of **uterus bilocularis subseptus**; when it reaches the cervix, **uter. biloc. unicollis**; in other cases the septum is only found at the external os, **uterus biforis**; in still others, the septum is only present in the cervix, **uter. bicollis unicorporeus**.

Abnormalities in the formation of the cavity are common in the rudimentary uterus. The cavity may be completely absent or there may be one or more rudimentary cavities. It may be narrower than normal or obstructed (**stenosis uteri**).

There may be abnormal union with neighboring structures. Thus, the uterus may be connected with the bladder by a tube, or with the rectum, either directly or indirectly (**congenital uterorectal fistula; anus uterinus**).

Several forms of anomalous development that occur subsequently to birth should be referred to. The uterus may never progress beyond the stage to which it attained during fœtal life (**uterus fœtalis**), or it may preserve its infantile characteristics beyond the period of puberty (**uterus infantilis**). A peculiar form of hypoplasia is that in which the form of the uterus is normal but its muscular elements are greatly lacking. The uterine wall may be not more than 0.5 to 1 mm. thick (**uterus membranaceus**).

Precocious development of the uterus may also occur. This condition may be associated with the early onset of menstruation and enlargement of the breasts, while the rest of the body remains infantile in type.

The uterus is occasionally congenitally **retroflexed, retroverted, or anteflexed**. In children with spina bifida of the lumbosacral region the uterus had been found **prolapsed**. In some few instances the uterus has formed part of the contents of a crural or inguinal hernia (**uterocele; hysterocele**).

ACQUIRED MALPOSITIONS OF THE UTERUS.

In children and young women the uterus lies in contact with the posterior wall of the bladder. In the parous woman, it may occupy this position or may be inclined backward, so as to form almost a right angle with the plane of the posterior wall of the bladder. The latter position is, however, generally regarded as an abnormal one.

The uterus, as a whole, may be misplaced forward (**anteposition**), backward (**retroposition**), to the side (**lateroposition**), upward (**elevation**), downward (**prolapsus**). It may be turned inside out (**inversion**), or may form part of the contents of a hernial sac (**hysterocele**). The chief causes of these unusual positions are pressure, as from tumors, hemorrhage, and exudation; weight, as from uterine growths; and tension, from the contraction of ligaments or inflammatory bands.

Anteposition is usually due to the action of tumors in the posterior wall, collections of fluid or misplaced organs behind the uterus. Less commonly, it arises from the contraction of inflammatory adhesions between the uterus and the bladder or abdominal wall.

Retroposition is most frequently the result of contracting bands of adhesion traversing the Douglas' pouch. less frequently it is caused by tumors of the anterior wall or of the bladder, or a distended bladder.

Lateroposition is due to tumors or cysts in the broad ligament, to exudates in the parametrium pushing the organ to one side, or to the traction of inflammatory adhesions.

Another important class of malpositions is that in which there is an alteration in the direction of the axes of the uterus. The organ may be rotated in its transverse axis (**version**); forward (**anteversion**); backward (**retroversion**). Rotation on the anteroposterior axis leads to **lateroversion**; on its long axis, to **torsion**.

Retroversion is the most common form. The degree of retroversion varies. The long axis of the uterus may form an angle of 45° with the plane of the superior strait of the pelvis (first degree), or both cervix and fundus may lie in the same plane across the pelvis at an angle of 90° (second degree), or, again, the axis lies at an angle of 135° (third degree). The dislocation is commonly the result of childbirth or abortion, and is due to increase in the weight of the uterus, disturbance of its normal balance, or relaxation of its supports. Potent causes are subinvolution, relaxation of the round ligaments, laceration of the cervix and perineum, and tumors in the anterior wall of the uterus. The contraction of inflammatory bands in Douglas' sac may also bring it about. On account of the impairment of the circulation induced thereby, the uterus is congested, enlarged, and œdematous, and metritis and endometritis are frequently set up.

In the etiology of anteversion, pregnancy is not of such great importance, although pregnancy and subinvolution may play a part if the abdominal walls be lax. More important are inflammatory changes in the body of the uterus or in the neighboring connective tissue.

Lateral version is usually combined with torsion. It may be congenital, but is usually due to adhesions or tumors of the ovary.

Inversion of the uterus generally occurs in the puerperal uterus. Three grades exist: (1) *Incomplete*, where the invaginated fundus lies within the uterine cavity; (2) *complete,* where the fundus lies in the vagina; and (3) *inversion* with *prolapse,* where the uterus and vagina are turned completely inside out and the uterus appears at the vulvar orifice. In this position the puerperal uterus may undergo involution and become firm and hard. Often, however, it is soft, congested, the mucous membrane thickened, and there may be ulceration or polypoid outgrowths. The interstitial tissues show inflammatory hyperplasia, the glands gradually atrophy, at least in the more superficial parts, while they proliferate deeper down. In long-standing cases, the epithelium of the mucosa is converted into a horny layer of squamous cells resembling skin. As will readily be understood, circulatory disturbances may be extreme, so that ulceration, necrosis, and gangrene may result, with complete separation of the part.

Prolapse is the condition in which the uterus as a whole occupies a lower position in the pelvis than normal. Varying grades exist. When the external os reaches no farther than the floor of the pelvis, we speak of *descent;* when it protrudes through the vulvar opening, it is *incomplete prolapse;* when the uterus is entirely outside the body, it is *complete prolapse.* Some writers consider as prolapse a condition in which the corpus remains in its normal site but the cervix is elongated. It is more correct, however, to term this hypertrophy of the cervix. It **may exist** both with and without true prolapse or descent.

Fig. 209

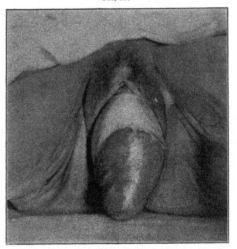

Complete prolapse of the uterus. From the Gynecological Clinic of the Montreal
General Hospital.)

The causes of prolapse are numerous and usually several are operative at the same time. The chief are, retroversion and retroflexion, with the conditions leading to them; lack of tone of or injury to the pelvic floor; relaxation of the uterine ligaments from frequent childbearing; increased weight of the uterus; weakness of the abdominal wall. Rarely, no obvious cause can be made out, as in a case occurring in a virgin, aged sixteen years, recorded by Duncan.[1]

In prolapse, the circulation is markedly interfered with, leading to congestion and œdema of the organ and hyperplasia both of the muscle and the endometrium, together with chronic metritis and endometritis. There may be ectropion of the mucosa, with erosion. As a rule, the bladder or rectum or both accompany the uterus in its descent (*cystocele, rectocele*).

Elevation of the uterus, apart from the general increase in size due to the presence of a fœtus or the accumulation of fluid in the cavity (hydro-

[1] Brit. Med. Jour., 1: 1899: 404.

metra, hematometra), may be caused by tumors growing in the cavity
or vagina, extravasations of blood in the Douglas' pouch, or by tumors
in the uterine wall, ovaries, and ligaments. The puerperal uterus may
also become attached to the abdominal wall, so that when parturition
takes place involution cannot take place normally and the uterus remains permanently in a high position. The uterus is also attached high
up in the operation of ventral fixation. The condition may lead to elongation of the organ, atresia of the cavity, and atrophy of the cervix.

One of the rarest anomalies of position is **hysterocele**. Not only may
the quiescent but also the pregnant uterus be involved. As a rule, the
tubes and ovaries are first engaged in the hernial sac and the uterus follows
owing to the traction. The uterus has been found in inguinal, crural, and
ventral hernias.

When the body of the uterus is bent upon the cervical portion we
speak of **flexion**. *Anteflexion, retroflexion,* and *lateral flexion* are described.

Retroflexion is the commonest, and is often associated with retroversion. In severe cases the fundus is found in the hollow of the sacrum.
When pregnancy occurs in such a uterus the organ may be incarcerated
in its false position. Retroflexion has been known to occur in nulliparæ
and newborn children, but pregnancy is the most important predisposing
cause. Relaxation of the ligaments, anterior fixation of the cervix,
tumors, inflammatory adhesions are also of importance. Retroflexion
is frequently combined with total prolapse.

Anteflexion is present when the uterus does not assume its ordinary
elevated position during the filling of the bladder and remains in part
of its length tilted forward, or when the angle between the axes of
corpus and cervix is 135° or less. When the angle is from 135° to 90°
it constitutes the first degree of anteflexion; when from 90° to 45°, the
second degree; 45° or less, the third degree. The chief causes are
traction on the cervix by adhesions in the Douglas' pouch·in the neighborhood of the os, or by bands between the fundus and the bladder.
In the infantile form, shortness of the anterior vaginal wall is of chief
importance In adults the weight of the abdominal contents, where
the abdominal wall is relaxed, plays the main role.

ABNORMALITIES OF THE UTERINE CAVITY AND OF ITS CONTINUITY.

Stenosis.—Narrowing of the uterine cavity may be congenital or
acquired. Partial narrowing (**stenosis**) usually occurs at either the external or internal os, rarely at both. Stenosis of the internal os is common
in elderly people. Complete obliteration, **atresia,** also occurs. The
chief causes in the acquired forms are mucus or tumors blocking the
cavity; inflammation and œdema of the endometrium; flexions or elongation of the uterus; and traumatism, such as arises from cauterization or
curetting.

Dilatation.—Dilatation of the cavity is produced by intra-uterine
growths or collections of fluid. In young and vigorous individuals the

muscular wall hypertrophies as well, but in elderly persons, in whom the uterus lacks tone, dilatation is often unaccompanied by hypertrophy.

According to the nature of the contained substances, we speak of **hydrometra, hematometra, pyometra, lochiometra,** and **physometra.**

Hematometra is the condition in which menstrual blood collects within the uterus owing to congenital or acquired atresia of the genital canal. When the occlusion is in the vagina, hematometra is combined with hematocolpos. In advanced cases the Fallopian tubes are dilated as well (**hematosalpinx**). Perhaps the commonest cause is imperforate hymen. In these instances the uterus may attain the size of the head. Rupture rarely takes place. The contents are thick, brownish-black blood, with cholesterin.

Hydrometra comes on after the menopause. Atresia is again the cause, or sometimes a tumor obstructing the cervical canal. The amount of fluid is rarely large. In appearance it is clear and colorless, grayish and cloudy, or possibly mixed with blood or mucus. The mucous membrane becomes atrophied from pressure and the epithelial cells are flattened. Pyometra is usually due to the suppuration of a tumor in the cervical canal.

Physometra, or gas in the uterine cavity, occurs most frequently in the puerperal uterus from the decomposition of blood, membranes, or placental remains. It may also be due to the decomposition of a malignant growth. Anaërobic bacilli of the malignant œdema class, B. Welchii, etc., may occasionally lead to the condition.[1]

Diverticula.—Diverticula may form in the uterine wall owing to irregular involution (Klebs[2]), or to the scarring of the wall following parturition or Cesarean section.

WOUNDS AND OTHER INJURIES.

Rupture.—Rupture of the uterus almost invariably occurs in connection with the pregnant or parturient state. The tearing of the cervix is one of the commonest events during delivery. All grades exist, from a slight fissure of the mucosa to a rent that extends into the muscle or even into the abdominal cavity. The laceration is unilateral, bilateral, or stellate, and usually runs in the long axis of the uterus. In rare cases the cervix is torn in its transverse axis. One or other lip, or even the whole cervix, may be torn off. Rupture may also take place in the later months of pregnancy, in cases where the uterus is abnormally soft from inflammation, thin-walled, or scarred from previous operations. It has been met with where pregnancy has occurred in a rudimentary horn or in an incarcerated uterus, or, again, where there has been obstruction to the progress of labor.

Bruising, laceration, and **perforation** of the uterus sometimes occur during operative measures (curetting) and in attempts at criminal

[1] See Lindenthal, Monatsschr. f. Geb. u. Gyn., 7: 1898: 269.
[2] Partielle Erweiterung. Handb., 1· 2: 1876: 900.

abortion. As a rule, the rupture is at or near the fundus. Besides this, perforation may be due to ulceration, pressure necrosis, and tumors. Fistulous communications may be opened up with the vagina (*cervicovaginal fistula*), the bladder (*uterovesical fistula*), or the rectum (*rectovaginal fistula*).

CIRCULATORY DISTURBANCES.

Anemia.—Anemia of the uterus is found in cases of generalized anemia, and, according to Rokitansky, in hypoplasia of the organ.

Hyperemia.—Hyperemia is found physiologically during menstruation, pregnancy, and for some time after full-term delivery and abortion. It is said to be caused also by sexual excitement.

Pathological **active hyperemia** is found in many of the infective fevers, as typhoid, influenza, and the exanthemata. As a rule, the mucosa of the corpus is affected, being reddened and swollen. Collateral hyperemia may occur when one part of the uterus is compressed from any cause.

Passive hyperemia is very common. It occurs in systemic venous stasis or from local causes, such as pressure of the distended rectum or bladder, prolapse, anteversion, retroversion, and inversion. Hyperplasia is not infrequently combined as well.

Hemorrhage.—Hemorrhage is one of the commonest occurrences in the uterus. This is not surprising when we bear in mind its physiological tendencies in this direction. The extravasation of blood takes place into the uterine cavity or into the endometrium. When retained within the uterus **hematometra** results. Hemorrhage occurs most frequently during or subsequent to parturition. It may also be due to traumatism, ulcerating new-growths, or to retrograde changes in advanced life.

Metrorrhagia.—Metrorrhagia is hemorrhage from the uterus at times other than those of the usual menstrual discharge. Apart from pregnancy and the parturient state, it occurs in hemophilia, scurvy, the hemorrhagic diatheses, typhoid, sepsis, the acute exanthemata, acute yellow atrophy of the liver, and phosphorus poisoning. Local disease of the uterus, such as endometritis, myomas, ulcerating cancers, also accounts for many cases. After abortion, and even full-term delivery, small portions of placenta may be retained and lead to hemorrhage. In some cases the blood clots upon the adherent tissue and forms a fibrinous polypoid mass (*hematoma polyposum*, Virchow). In extra-uterine gestation a special form of metrorrhagia with exfoliation of the decidua may occur. Hemorrhage into the mucosa may lead to the formation of large coagula (*hematomata*). A special form is the so-called *apoplexy* (Cruveilhier) of the uterus that occurs in old women. The uterus is atrophic and brittle, the vessels stand out as rigid, tortuous tubes, and the mucous membrane is swollen, friable, and infiltrated with blood. Hemorrhage may also occur in the muscular wall. The cervix and the portio vaginalis escape.

Menorrhagia.—Menorrhagia is an excessive menstrual discharge. It is due to a variety of causes, among which may be mentioned generalized passive congestion, endometritis, tumors of the uterus, and polyps. In some cases, in addition to menstrual blood, shreds of membrane are cast off (*dysmenorrhœa membranacea*). The entire lining of the uterus may be exfoliated in this way.

Microscopically, the membrane consists of a cellular mucosa with infiltrated connective tissue and remnants of glands. The epithelium may be unaltered or fattily degenerated and desquamating. In other cases the membrane consists simply of a fibrinous cast of the uterine cavity. A peculiar form of membrane is one consisting of squamous cells and containing the orifices of glands. As the cavity of the uterus does not normally possess such cells, it has been supposed that in these cases the epithelial lining of the vagina has extended farther than usual into the cervix and that the membrane is derived from the anomalous cervix. Such a condition of things, however, is much more likely to be due to metaplasia.

Œdema.—This is due to passive congestion and inflammation. The first type is well seen in cases of suddenly acquired malposition, as retroversion.

INFLAMMATIONS.

Inflammation may affect the serous covering of the uterus (**perimetritis**), the broad ligaments (**parametritis**), the myometrium (**metritis**), or the endometrium (**endometritis**).

Perimetritis.—Perimetritis is merely a local peritonitis, and will be dealt with under that head.

Endometritis.—Endometritis is due usually to an extension of inflammation from the vagina, but rarely is hematogenic. It may be confined to the cervix (*cervical endometritis*) or to the corpus (*corporeal endometritis*), or may involve the whole of the lining membrane. The affection arises most frequently during menstruation, and the puerperium. According to the mode of development we can recognize *acute* and *chronic* forms, or according to the morbid changes, *exudative* and *productive*.

Acute Catarrhal Endometritis.—In acute catarrhal endometritis the mucous membrane is reddened, swollen, and infiltrated with inflammatory products. The secretion from the cervix, which normally is scanty, viscid, and mucoid, becomes more abundant, more mucoid, or even mucopurulent. That from the corpus is thinner, serous, or seropurulent. A purulent exudate (fluor albus; leucorrhœa) is more common in cervical endometritis than in corporeal. In very severe cases the discharge may be mixed with blood. This is particularly the case in the form arising during the infective fevers, such as typhoid, cholera, and the exanthemata. Here we may perhaps speak of a *hemorrhagic endometritis*. This usually affects the corpus. Should the cervical canal become obstructed, the pus accumulates within the uterine cavity (*pyometra*). In some cases the retained material becomes inspissated, forming a granular, pulpy detritus resembling caseous matter. The disease is usually traceable to irritation and infection of the endometrium, the extension of inflammation from the myometrium or uterine adnexa, gonorrhœa, constitutional diseases, disorders of the circulation in the uterus, or the presence of neoplasms.

Microscopically, changes are found both in the glandular structures and in the stroma. The mucous membrane is infiltrated with inflammatory products, and the cells of the interstitial substance are more or less dissociated. The bloodvessels and lymphatics are dilated and there may be minute hemorrhages. The epithelial cells are swollen, granular, and desquamating, while the ducts may be blocked with secretion. In some cases the most marked changes occur in the stroma (*interstitial endometritis*), which is œdematous and infiltrated with round cells, so that the gland-tubules are dislocated. The epithelium here also shows degenerative changes.

Membranous Endometritis.—Another form of acute endometritis is the membranous. It occurs by far the most frequently in the puerperal uterus, but is occasionally met with in the infectious diseases, such as typhoid, cholera, and the exanthemata. True *diphtheria* of the endometrium has been observed, secondary to infection of the vagina. Membranous endometritis may also be found associated with ulcerating cancers or other tumors of the uterus. The process resembles that observed in other mucous membranes. A fibrinous exudate is thrown out which coagulates upon the surface and forms a membrane that may be exfoliated. Microscopically, this consists of interlacing threads of fibrin, including leukocytes, showing hyaline degeneration.

Chronic Endometritis.—Chronic endometritis assumes the guise of a catarrhal inflammation, inasmuch as it is accompanied by an abundant excretion, but the most important feature is the proliferation of tissue (productive endometritis).

Chronic productive or *proliferating endometritis*, as it affects the corpus uteri, takes the form of a new-growth of tissue (*endom. hyperplastica*), which later on gives rise to a form of atrophy of the mucosa (*endom. atrophica*). In the earlier stages the mucous membrane is thickened, its surface smooth or irregular, warty or villous (*fungous endometritis*). All grades exist from simple nodular elevations to polypoid or pedunculated outgrowths (*endom. polyposa*). The mucosa is also reddened and may show hemorrhages. At the menstrual period the lining of the uterus may be exfoliated in shreds or as a perfect cast of the cavity (*dysmenorrhœa membranacea; endom. exfoliativa*). The tissue is soft, loose, and friable, often porous.

Microscopically, in ordinary proliferating endometritis, the gland-tubules are enlarged, often lengthened and tortuous, and present numerous irregular dilatations even to the extent of cyst-formation. The overgrowth may be so great that papillary masses project from the surface. The epithelial cells have in great part lost their cilia, and are clear, swollen, and mucoid. Active mitosis is also going on.

The lumen of the ducts is filled with mucus, desquamated epithelium, and leukocytes. The interstitial stroma is infiltrated with leukocytes, and shows proliferation both of the cellular elements and fibrous tissue. This may lead to increased vascularity of the membrane with permanent induration and contraction. The enlarged tubules commonly penetrate between the muscle bundles of the uterine wall (*glandular heterotopia*, Cornil). This must not be mistaken for malignancy, for it should be remembered that the uterus possesses no submucosa, and the glands normally abut upon and occasionally penetrate the muscular layers. It is, however, doubtless true that such proliferation forms a ready starting point for malignant transformation. As distinguished from the above type, which is also termed chronic *glandular endometritis*, we have to recognize an *interstitial* form in which the morbid changes predominate in the interstitial substance.

In the later stages of the disease a form of atrophy may set in not unlike senile involution. The mucosa becomes smooth and thin, often pigmented, and is firmer and more fibrous than normal. Not infrequently, it contains cysts about the size of a pin-head, containing a clear or slightly turbid fluid (*endom. chronica cystica*). Microscopically, there is proliferation of the stroma with the production of dense fibrous or scar tissue. This leads to atrophy of the gland-tubules with contraction of certain sections of them, so that they become dilated.

As a result of the irritation, or perhaps to some extent from pressure, the cylindrical cells of the mucosa may become converted into squamous cells (*ichthyosis* or *psoriasis uteri*). This has an important bearing in view of the fact that squamous-celled carcinoma may occur in the corpus. It should be remarked in this connection, however, that while endometritis plays a most important part in this metaplasia, it is possibly not the only factor, for islets of squamous cells have been found in the decidua (Gottschalk and Winckler; Opitz and Gebhard), and in the uteri of fœtuses and infants (Meier and Friedländer).

The causes of chronic endometritis vary considerably. An important role is played by local disturbances of the circulation, such as are brought about by retroflexion and retroversion. Intra-uterine tumors and disease of the ovaries may lead to irritation of the endometrium. Endometritis may also follow the puerperium when portions of the products of conception are retained or when infection has taken place. Gonorrhœa is also another important factor.

Chronic Cervical Endometritis.—Chronic cervical endometritis is almost invariably accompanied by vaginitis. The mucosa is reddened and swollen, and polypoid outgrowths are not uncommon. It is not uncommon for small cysts to be produced, the so-called *ovula Nabothi*, which vary in size from that of a hemp-seed to a pea. They may project into the lumen of the cervix or may be concealed in the deeper layers. The contents are usually a clear viscid mucus, or may be cloudy from the presence of degenerating cells. The cysts may become infected and produce follicular abscesses. They are of the nature of retention cysts.

Microscopically, there is inflammatory infiltration with some enlargement of the glands. The epithelial cells are in many cases converted into goblet cells.

As a rule, there is an abundant mucoid or mucopurulent secretion (*leucorrhœa*). In women who have borne children, and in whom the external os is therefore large and fissured, the reddened and swollen membrane may be everted (*ectropion*). As a result of this ectropion erosions are frequently found in the portio vaginalis, which present as red, glistening patches that are moist and bleed at the slightest touch. The surface may be smooth and velvety (*simple erosion*), papillomatous (*papillary erosion*), or may present numerous cysts (*cystic erosion*). From suppuration and rupture of the cysts, follicular ulcers are produced.

Microscopically, there is superficial loss of substance, with congestion and the formation of granulation tissue. In old erosions one sees fatty degeneration or even calcification. A point of some importance in connection with the etiology and forms of carcinoma is the replacement of the eroded squamous epithelium of the portio vaginalis by a layer of cylindrical cells as well as the formation of glands similar to those of the cervical cavity.

Chronic cervical catarrh frequently gives rise to hyperplasia of the muscular structures, and occasionally to adhesion or obstruction of the canal near the internal os.

The most important causes of the condition are, traumatism during childbirth, and vaginitis extending to the cervix. Gonorrhœa is the most frequent infective cause. The erosion is brought about not only from the irritation of the inflammatory agents but also by the macerating action of the secretions that escape from the canal.

Metritis.—Inflammation of the muscular wall of the uterus is called metritis.

Acute Metritis.—Apart from the puerperium, acute metritis is rare and due generally to trauma or to hematogenic infection. The uterus is congested and œdematous, soft and doughy, while on section small hemorrhages may be observed in its substance and beneath the serosa.

Microscopically, one sees inflammatory leukocytes about the vessels, the interstitial tissue is œdematous, and the muscle fibres swollen and cloudy. In rare instances, abscesses are formed that may attain a large size. In such cases the pus may be discharged into the uterine or peritoneal cavities, vagina, rectum, bladder, intestine, or even externally. Septic peritonitis can be set up by the extension of a metritis.

Chronic Metritis.—Chronic metritis is usually attributable to chronic endometritis, traumatic insults, and subinvolution. Potent predisposing causes are repeated or chronic congestion, such as is brought about by dislocations. The disease occasionally follows the acute form. The uterus is more or less elongated, and the anteroposterior transverse diameter is increased. Both the overlying peritoneum and the endometrium are thickened. In the earlier stages the uterus is soft, congested, but later becomes firm and indurated. On section, in long-standing cases, the tissue is grayish in color, tough and fibroid.

Microscopically, there is an accumulation of leukocytes about the vessels, although this is not a marked feature. The interstitial connective tissue is increased. Numerous "Mast-zellen" may be seen in the interstices of the stroma. The condition of the muscle varies according to circumstances. It may be normal, or hypertrophied, where excessive uterine contraction has taken place, or, again, may be atrophic.

Tuberculosis.—Genital tuberculosis is rarer in women than in men. Tuberculosis of the uterus is almost invariably a descending infection originating in the Fallopian tubes. Not infrequently, the lungs, kidneys, and peritoneum are involved at the same time. Hematogenic infection is met with in the disseminated miliary form of tuberculosis. It is questionable whether primary tuberculosis ever takes place under ordinary circumstances. The affection has been found at all ages, from infancy to old age, but is most common during the period of greatest vitality.

The body of the uterus is the site of election. The disease begins at the orifices of the tubes and thence spreads throughout the endometrium, generally stopping abruptly at the internal os. It may, however, extend to the cervix and even to the vagina.

Several forms may be differentiated: (1) *Acute miliary tuberculosis;* (2) *chronic local tuberculosis;* and (3) *diffuse fibroid tuberculosis.* In the earlier stages the lesions produced are not unlike those of chronic productive endometritis. The mucosa is soft, swollen, and reddened, often nodular. Microscopically, the resemblance to productive endometritis is also close, with the addition, however, of giant cells in the neighborhood of the areas of cellular infiltration.

Sooner or later caseation sets in and the tubercles are recognizable as grayish elevations. The epithelium of the glands shows evidence of cloudiness and degeneration, and the tubules tend to disappear in the course of the formation of what amounts to tuberculous granulation tissue. Caseation rarely remains local, and the rule is for neighboring tubercles to coalesce until the whole endometrium is converted into a caseous mass. The surface of the uterine wall becomes uneven, nodular and eroded, and the uterine cavity is more or less completely filled with a caseopurulent detritus. The walls of the uterus are often distended. The destructive process gradually extends into the muscularis, and small, caseous foci may be found along the margin of the destroyed zone, or simply areas of cellular infiltration with giant cells.

Tuberculosis of the neck of the womb as a primary disease is excessively rare. The cervix may be enlarged and the lesions produced are similar to those in the corpus.

Syphilis.—The indurated primary sore may be found on the portio vaginalis and within the cervical canal. The cervix may be swollen and hypertrophied, and there is frequently a complicating endometritis. The ulcer does not differ materially from those found on other mucous surfaces. Secondary lesions are also met with.

Parasites and Foreign Bodies.—Bacteria and yeasts of various kinds are found in the cervical secretion. The most important parasite is *Echinococcus.* The cysts are usually submucous, but have been found also in other situations. The disease may form a hindrance to childbearing, as in a case recorded by Birch-Hirschfeld.[1] A calcified round-worm has been found on the posterior wall of the uterus.

Among foreign bodies may be mentioned tents, catheters, needles, fœtal remains, clots, bits of tumors, and free myofibromas.

RETROGRESSIVE METAMORPHOSES.

Atrophy.—Simple atrophy of the uterus is of common occurrence, and is found more especially in women past the climacterium. It may also be found in what has been called premature senility, where, either from operative interference (castration), tumors, or inflammation, the normal function of the ovaries is markedly inhibited. The process affects first and chiefly the portio vaginalis, in contradistinction to what occurs in congenital hypoplasia, where the corpus is the part mainly involved. The uterus is small, thin-walled, the muscle fibers wasted, so that the connective tissue appears to be increased. The vessels are atheromatous. The mucous membrane is thin, flattened, and infiltrated, while the lining cells have in great part lost their cilia. A form of atrophy is also met with in Addison's disease and exophthalmic goitre. Retained secretion leads to atrophy of the wall through pressure. Occasionally other local causes are at work, as, for instance, the pressure of a tumor within the cavity.

PROGRESSIVE METAMORPHOSES.

Hypertrophy.—Apart from that form which occurs during the puerperal period, pathological hypertrophy affects the uterus either in whole or in part. In partial hypertrophy, the corpus, cervix, or the endometrium may be involved. Many cases are associated with inflammation, and it is not always easy to draw the line between what is inflammatory and what is not. Not only the muscle but the connective tissue may be affected. One important type is hypertrophy from overwork, found in cases of retained secretion and tumors within the cavity. Muscular hypertrophy may also be seen in many cases of chronic endometritis.

A remarkable form of partial hypertrophy, said to be due to chronic inflammation, leads to a proboscis-like elongation of the whole cervix. An exceedingly common form of hypertrophy of the endometrium is seen in the formation of polyps as a result of inflammation. Some of these are cystic. A form known as follicular hypertrophy or cystic glandular hypertrophy is found at the os. A special form of hypertrophy of the endometrium should also be mentioned, namely, the formation of a decidua in cases of extra-uterine gestation.

[1] Lehrbuch, 1887: 789.

Tumors.—Among the benign tumors we have **fibroma, leiomyoma, fibromyoma, myxoma, lipoma, adenoma, adenomyoma,** and **chondroma.**

By far the most common tumor of the uterus is the **fibroma** (see also vol. i, p. 744). This is almost invariably a mixed tumor, containing a variable quantity of muscular elements (**myofibroma, uterine fibroid**). The appearance of the growth varies according to the amount of muscle it contains. The purer myomas are usually submucous and start from the fundus. They are soft, vascular, and of a reddish, flesh-like appearance. They are apt to be indefinitely bounded. The more fibrous the tumor is, however, the firmer and paler it becomes. Myofibromas are generally multiple and may vary in size from that of a pin-head to that of an adult man's head, or even larger. Most of them originate in the posterior wall of the corpus; next in frequency, in the anterior wall and the fundus. From 5 to 8 per cent. begin in the cervix.

FIG. 210

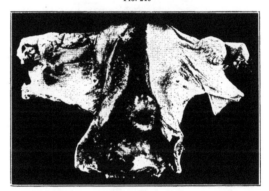

Submucous polyp of the uterus.   (From the Pathological Museum of McGill University.)

In a well-marked example of a myofibroma the mass is hard, possibly more or less nodular, and well-defined. On section, it is hard, grating somewhat under the knife, and of a pale, grayish color. On closer inspection, the cut surface is seen to be glistening and has a sheen like watered silk, the substance being formed of interlacing fibrillæ. Very often nodules or whorls of fibrous tissue can be made out. In the middle of the smaller nodules a bloodvessel can often be seen. In some forms (*teleangiectatic* and *cavernous myofibromas*) the vessels are abundant and form large sinuses.

Microscopically, both muscular and fibrous elements are to be made out, the proportion varying in different cases. The connective tissue tends to be grouped about the bloodvessels. In many cases the tumor consists of little else but interlacing fibrillæ of connective tissue, forming strands, whorls, and nodules. Epithelial remains and nerve-fibres have been demonstrated.

According to the site of the tumor we can recognize four types: (1) the intramural or interstitial; (2) the subserous; (3) the submucous; and (4) the intraligamentous.

Intramural myofibromas, on account of their favorable position, whereby they receive an abundant supply of blood, grow rapidly, and may attain a relatively large size. They are often encapsulated and surrounded by a plexus of large venous sinuses. In other cases, they are directly, though loosely, attached to the uterine musculature and may form diffuse growths. They occur in simple nodules or aggregations of nodules, which are often more or less compressed.

Fig. 211

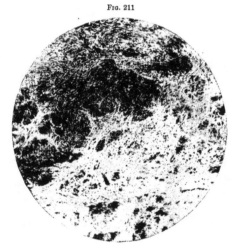

Fibromyoma of the uterus. The dark area to the left is composed of muscle bundles; the lighter, to the right, is dense fibrous tissue. Winckel obj. No. 3, without ocular. (From the collection of Dr. A. G. Nicholls.)

Subserous myofibromas form either sessile nodules, appearing beneath the peritoneal investment of the uterus, or pedunculated growths. Owing to torsion of the pedicle, grave circulatory disturbances are liable to supervene, such as infarction, necrosis, and gangrene, unless the tumor receives an adequate blood supply through the formation of secondary adhesions. Occasionally, the mass becomes separated from the uterus and forms a free body in the peritoneal cavity. When situated low down and posteriorly, compression of the cervix and elongation of the uterus may take place. The tumor may also grow out between the layers of the broad ligament (intraligamentous myofibroma).

Submucous myofibromas are found most frequently at the fundus, but occasionally arise from the internal os and cervical canal. They are not lobulated, but form sessile nodes or pedunculated outgrowths. They are usually small, but may attain the size of a child's head. Considerable dilatation of the uterus may take place.

Histologically, these growths consist of a core of fibrous and muscular tissue, enveloped in mucous membrane. Owing to contraction of the uterus, together with retrogressive changes, submucous tumors may become entirely detached or in some cases shelled out from their mucous investment and be discharged through the genital passages. Occasionally such growths are calcified.

The etiology of uterine myofibromas is still obscure. Certain points are, however, fairly well established. Fibroids do not occur before the age of puberty, and are found chiefly in elderly women. The part that the sexual activities play is doubtful. A relatively high percentage of unmarried persons is said to have these growths. Cohnheim[1] has advanced the view that the uterus contains "germ centres" that remain more or less in abeyance while the sexual functions are in operation, and that some irritation, apart from the physiological one, leads to the atypical and excessive development of these centres. Virchow also attributed fibroids to an irritative cause. Race plays a part, for it is said that the condition is more common in black peoples. With regard to the site of origin opinions also differ. Virchow held that myomas originate in the muscle fibres of the myometrium. Other views are that they grow from the walls of the bloodvessels, or from certain round cells that are said to exist about capillaries that are undergoing involution. Some have held that certain cases are the result of endometritis. A parasitic theory has also been advanced.

Myofibromas, particularly the intramural and submucous forms, but also to some extent the subserous, lead to generalized hypertrophy of the myometrium with dilatation of the cavity. Where multiple tumors exist, atrophy from pressure in some instances takes place. It is not uncommon for the endometrium covering a large submucous growth to be thinned and atrophic. Secondary inflammatory changes are frequent. The Fallopian tubes often show changes, the mucosa being œdematous, hemorrhagic, and infiltrated with inflammatory products, while productive manifestations are not uncommon. The ovaries are said always to show some alteration. They are enlarged from hypertrophy and hyperplasia of the follicles and proliferation of the connective tissue. The interstitial stroma is infiltrated with round cells and the vessels present signs of endarteritis.

Myofibromas are subject to secondary changes that should be mentioned. Fatty degeneration occurs usually in patches but may sometimes be so extensive as to convert the tumor into a soft, yellowish material resembling pus. It is, however, more common to find areas of softening and degeneration cysts in these tumors. In rare instances the growth

[1] Allg. Path., 1: 1882: 744.

may entirely disappear. Pregnancy and the puerperal state are potent influences in bringing about these retrogressive changes. The tumor may participate in the involution process of the puerperal uterus.

Hyaline degeneration and necrosis may affect the muscular elements to such a degree that the muscle tumor is gradually converted into a fibrous one. The fibrous tissue, in turn, may undergo hyaline and myxomatous transformation. In the latter event, the tumor increases rapidly in size, and may contain numerous cystic areas filled with mucin (*myxomyoma*). Amyloid infiltration has also been observed. Calcification is relatively more common in the subserous variety. The lime salts form a porous network that may be compared to the siliceous skeleton of a sponge, or else form an external hard covering. In rare cases the entire tumor becomes calcified. Transformation into cartilage (*chondromyoma*) and into bone (*osteomyoma*) has been recorded.

Inflammation of the growth, both acute and chronic, is met with. Suppuration and gangrene may lead to complete disintegration of the tumor, or, if the inflammation be more chronic, to fibroid induration. In the large growths œdema is of common occurrence, giving the structure a soft, gelatinous appearance. This may lead to the formation of cystic cavities filled with clear fluid. These can, however, be readily distinguished from true cysts in that they are not lined with epithelium, and are often traversed by shreds or bands of tissue. Cysts may also be due to dilatation of the lymphatics (*myofibroma lymphangiectaticum*) or bloodvessels (*m. cavernosum*). Rarely, cysts are found lined with cylindrical epithelium. Some of these are believed to be due to pinching off of portions of the uterine glands that thus become included in the myomatous overgrowth, but others, notably in the subserous forms, were said to be derived from embryonic epithelial "rests." According to Cullen, the forms in which there are epithelial inclusions are apt to be diffused throughout the uterus. The "rests" have been definitely shown to be derived from the mucosa.

An important modification, that should be referred to, is *sarcomatous* transformation of uterine myomas,[1] of which five or six cases are now on record. The condition gives rise to metastatic myomatous deposits in the various organs. The tumor grows rapidly and on section presents a more homogeneous appearance than the ordinary myofibroma. It is liable to undergo degenerative changes, necrosis and extravasation of blood. Microscopically, the cells are large, spindle-shaped, or irregular, containing large nuclei rich in chromatin. Giant cells may also be seen. Two forms are to be differentiated, the first in which the sarcomatous elements arise from more or less undifferentiated and embryonic muscle cells (*myosarcoma*), and the second, in which there is transformation of the interstitial fibrous tissue into sarcoma (*myoma sarcomatodes*).

---

[1] See Mastuy, Zur Kenntniss der malignen Myome des Uterus, Zeit. f. Heilk., 22; Abth. f. Path. Anat; also Schlagenhaufer, Myoma teleangiectodes Uteri, Wien. klin. Woch., 15:1902:523.

The so-called *adenomyoma uteri* is a distinctly less common condition. It is characterized in general by a diffuse rather than a nodular overgrowth of the muscle elements, with inclusions of more or less cystic or dilated gland tubules, lined by a single layer of columnar epithelium. These tubules, it is true, are out of place, but beyond the fact that they may exhibit a somewhat striking pectinate branching there is no indication that they undergo active independent growth. As we have pointed out in vol. i, p. 748, the studies of Cullen[1] and others have conclusively demonstrated that in the vast majority of cases it is possible by serial sections to demonstrate that these tubules are abnormal downgrowths of the uterine glands, and not remnants of the Gärtner's ducts as held by von Recklinghausen. We deal here with a myomatosis uteri with glandular inclusions, not with a true adenomyoma. True adenoma primary in the myometrium may occur, but if so it is excessively rare. So also, at times, the dilatation of the included tubules may be so great as to make the cystic change the main feature ("adenomyoma cysticum").

In a few cases striated muscle tumors, **rhabdomyomas,** have been described. They form polypoid excrescences in the cervical canal, and are very malignant, owing to the fact that the component cells are intrinsically immature and endowed with great vegetative force. In one such tumor glycogen and amyloid material have been found.

Myocarcinoma probably only occurs in the form of a carcinomatous transformation of the glandular elements in an adenomyoma. The condition may, however, be simulated closely by the secondary invasion of a myofibroma with carcinoma, either by metastasis, which is rare, or by direct extension.

Lipoma.—Lipomas have been found growing as polypoid excrescences from the cervical canal. They are excessively rare.

Chondroma.—Chondromas occur generally as metaplasias of other tumors, notably rhabdomyoma and sarcoma.

Cystic Growths.—Besides cystic polyps, cystadenomas, cystic myomas, and sarcomas, the only form that need be mentioned is the **dermoid cyst,** which may form polypoid outgrowths.

The malignant tumors of the uterus are the **malignant adenoma, carcinoma, sarcoma, endothelioma,** and **rhabdomyoma** (above described).

Malignant Adenoma.—Here, as elsewhere, it is difficult to decide with certainty what is a neoplastic overgrowth of glandular tissue and what is merely an inflammatory hyperplasia. Some would regard the inflammatory polyps to be referred to later as adenomas. The difficulty arises from the fact that in inflammation the glandular elements are increased, both in numbers and in size, forming branching and often communicating tubes, with, sometimes, cystic dilatation. The gland-tubes also tend to invade the muscular layers. The existence of cellular infiltration, again, affords no clue, since it is present alike in new-growths and in inflammation. There can be no doubt, however, that the so-called *malignant adenoma* is a true tumor. It consists almost entirely

---

[1] Adenomyoma of the Uterus, Philadelphia and London, 1908:194.

of glandular elements in the shape of branching and intercommunicating
tubules, which may present dilatation or intraglandular invagination,
held together by a scanty stroma. The tubules in question are lined
with a single layer of more or less distorted and closely packed, long,
cylindrical cells, sometimes ciliated, and showing mitotic figures. The
muscular wall of the uterus may be extensively infiltrated. This tumor
is found usually about the menopause or later. The importance of
the growth lies in the fact that it is infiltrating and may give rise to
distant metastases, also of the simple adenomatous type.

Carcinoma.—The uterus is a favorite place for carcinoma. In about
30 per cent. of women suffering from this disease, the growth is located
in the uterus (Orth). With few exceptions, carcinoma of the uterus is
primary in that organ. The affection may be found at any time after
puberty, but is generally met with about the menopause or later. In
nulliparæ, cancer of the uterus is rare, and when it does occur is usually
in the corpus. In parous women it is usually at the cervix. The
etiology is obscure, but, so far as we can judge, the most important factor
is chronic endometritis leading to glandular hyperplasia. Whether
traumatism, as laceration of the cervix, has much to do with it is perhaps debatable, yet it seems probable. Tears or fissures in this
situation, if they do not heal in complete apposition, often become
covered with epithelium, either squamous from the vagina, or columnar
from the cervix. Such epithelium, being in an abnormal situation, is
likely to be unstable and more susceptible to irritation. Granular
erosion of the portio vaginalis is possibly a factor also in some cases.
Race plays some part, for the disease is said to be more frequent in the
white peoples.

Carcinoma may affect any part of the uterus, but in the vast majority
of cases is met with in the cervix. We have to recognize three points of
origin, the portio vaginalis, the cervical endometrium, and the mucosa
of the corpus. With regard to the forms occurring in the cervix, it is
only possible to differentiate between them macroscopically in the
earlier stages.

Carcinoma of the cervix presents at first a smooth, slightly reddened
surface, quickly becoming uneven, granular, warty, and eroded. The
outgrowth is not always so marked as the infiltration, but very commonly
polypoid or papillomatous excrescences are formed giving to the tumor
the well-known "cauliflower" appearance. In cancer of the corpus and
cervical cavity such outgrowths are not so common. The tumor takes
the form of *squamous epithelioma, adenocarcinoma, scirrhous,* and *colloid*[1]
carcinoma. The last two varieties are excessively rare.

A frequent type is the squamous-celled carcinoma, which arises almost
invariably from the portio vaginalis. It forms flat or papillomatous
outgrowths originating in the superficial layers of the mucosa. It is,
moreover, liable to spread to the vagina, and may extend into the parametrium with extensive destruction of tissue. In very rare instances, as

---

[1] Waldeyer, Virch. Archiv, 55: 1872: 110.

v. Rosthorn[1] and Zeller[2] have pointed out, a metaplasia of the cylindrical epithelium of the uterine cavity into squamous cells may take place, and three undoubted cases (Gebbard,[3] Kaufmann,[4] Fleischlen[5]) are on record where squamous-celled carcinoma has developed in the body of the uterus. This form may also originate in the cervical canal in cases of erosion where the pavement epithelium of the portio has invaded the cavity.

Histologically, the squamous-celled carcinoma presents an overgrowth of epithelial processes, more or less branching, which invade the deeper layers. The stroma is infiltrated with round cells, and cell-nests are occasionally to be seen. In some cases the overgrowth of epithelium and stroma is so great that papillomatous excrescences are produced. Erosion often takes place, and the surface presents granulation tissue together with masses of fibrin. Rarely, the growth assumes the type of a rodent ulcer, being of slow growth, with merely superficial loss of substance, and separated from the underlying structures by a zone of round cells.

The most common form of cancer is the adenocarcinoma, which is found usually in the portio and cervix, much less often in the corpus. The growth originates in an atypical proliferation of the glandular elements of the endometrium. The explanation probably is that it arises from portions of glands or cysts (ovula Nabothi) that have become pinched off from the superficial mucous membrane. The tumor is definitely of the glandular type and penetrates deeply into the muscle. The cells are cylindrical and may be grouped like glands about a central lumen, or heaped up into several layers, forming solid masses or strands. Cavities may be formed through softening and necrosis of the central portion of the growth. According to the amount of stroma present we can differentiate *carcinoma simplex* and *c. medullare*. The tissues in the neighborhood of the growth show an abundant round-celled infiltration. Myxomatous degeneration of the stroma is occasionally observed.

Palmer Findley[6] has recorded a case of cancer of the body of the uterus which was both adenocarcinomatous and squamous in type. A peculiar and apparently unique form of adenocarcinoma is one recorded by Cullen,[7] where the tumor formed dome-like elevations affecting both corpus and cervix alike, in which the epithelium of the glandular elements resembled closely that of the normal glands.

---

[1] Ueber Schleimhautverhornung der Gebärmutter, Zeit. zur Feier des funfzigjährigen Jubilaums der Gesselsch. f. Gyn. Wien, 1894: 319.

[2] Plattenepithel im Uterus, Zeit. f. Geb. u. Gyn., 11: 1884–85: 56.

[3] Zeit. f. Geb. u. Gyn., 24: 1892: 1.

[4] Jahresbericht der Schlesischen Gesselsch f. vaterländische Cultur. Jahrg., 72: 1894: 52.

[5] Ueber den primären Hornkrebs des Corpus Uteri, Zeit. f. Geb. u. Gyn., 32: 1895: 347.

[6] Squamous Cell Carcinoma of the Body of the Uterus, Trans. Chicago Path. Soc., 5: No. 6: 1902.

[7] Cullen, Tumors of the Uterus, 1900: 588, D. Appleton & Co., N. Y.

Primary *melanocarcinoma* is described.[1]

Numerous secondary changes are associated with carcinoma. The surface may become ulcerated and almost gangrenous, with consequent enlargement of the uterine cavity. Obstruction in the cervical canal often leads to retention of secretion and necrotic material and dilatation of the uterus. Chronic endometritis, either of simple or membranous type, may complicate the condition also. Hypertrophy of the uterine wall may occur.

Extension of the disease to neighboring parts is common. Cancers of the portio tend to invade the vagina, while those of the cervix extend to the parametrium. Both the bladder and the rectum may be involved and fistulous communications established. In the former case, cystitis may be set up with obstruction of the ureters, leading to hydro- and pyonephrosis. In exceptional cases the bony pelvis may be attacked. The peritoneal membrane is often involved, especially in cases of carcinoma of the corpus, but also of the cervix. Local peritonitis with adhesion may occur. Metastases develop relatively late and are never extensive. Most frequently the lumbar, retroperitoneal, and inguinal lymphatic glands are first and chiefly involved, and also the ovaries. Secondary carcinoma is rare in the uterus. Orth has observed a metastatic polypoid melanocarcinoma in a case of generalized melanocarcinosis.

Sarcoma.—Sarcomas originate either in the connective tissue of the endometrium, possibly as a sequel of chronic productive endometritis, or in the myometrium. In the latter case the tumor is frequently associated with myofibroma, forming a mixed growth.

Sarcomas developing in the endometrium are found relatively early in life as compared with carcinomas, even before puberty. They are common relatively in nulliparæ.

Microscopically, sarcomas are large or small *round-celled, spindle-celled, oat-shaped, giant-celled,* or *mixed.* In some cases they are very vascular (*angiosarcoma*), or the vessels may show hyaline thickening (*cylindroma*). Sarcomas originating in the mucosa are found in the corpus, rarely in the cervix. They form local or more or less diffuse growths having a lobulated, warty, or papillomatous appearance. Ulceration is apt to occur early. In the cervix they form polypoid or cauliflower-like growths in the canal or on the lips of the os. In consequence of congestion and œdema, they may present an appearance not unlike an hydatidiform mole. The substance of the tumor is whitish, soft and brain-like, friable, and shows evidences of degeneration.

The sarcomas of the myometrium form usually single or multiple nodules of varying size, more rarely a diffuse infiltration leading to marked enlargement of the uterus. As a rule, they are met with in the corpus, but may occur also in the cervix. Pure sarcomas of this type have a pale homogeneous appearance and are of soft consistence.

As before mentioned sarcoma may be associated or combined with myofibroma and adenoma.

[1] Haeckel, Arch. f. Gyn., 32: 1888: 400.

Sarcoma of the uterus may for a long time remain latent and then suddenly take on rapid action, infiltrating and penetrating the uterine wall, and extending to the peritoneum, broad ligaments, tubes, ovaries, intestines, and abdominal parietes. Implantation metastases are rarer than with carcinoma. Distant metastases are also rare. When they occur, they are found first and chiefly in the lungs. The retroperitoneal lymphatic glands are commonly implicated.

Degenerative changes, particularly hemorrhagic extravasation, necrosis, fatty degeneration, and liquefaction, are apt to be present in sarcomas.

Secondary sarcoma of the uterus has been met with. There is in the pathological institute at Prague an interesting specimen of a uterus with multiple fibroids in which there are secondary nodules of melanosarcoma.

Endothelioma.—Endotheliomas originating in the lining cells of bloodvessels and lymphatics have been met with in rare instances.[1]

The uterus, it should moreover be mentioned, is a favorite site for multiple and independent primary growths. The association of uterine fibroids with carcinoma is, of course, so common as scarcely to excite remark, but instances are on record of associated malignant growths. A case, for example, is described[2] of carcinoma and sarcoma of the body of the uterus.

THE FALLOPIAN TUBES.

CONGENITAL ANOMALIES.

Congenital defects of the tubes are usually associated with anomalies of the uterus, although exceptions occur. The tube may be almost completely **absent**, being represented by a mere tag. Not infrequently the **fimbriæ** are **imperfectly developed**, a persistence of the infantile condition. Another anomaly is an **unusual position**, as prolapse or a vertical course. In about one-fifth of autopsies on women a small **cyst** (hydatid of Morgagni), filled with clear fluid, is found at the end of the fimbriæ or attached by a long pedicle.

Diverticula occasionally are met with caused by a hernial protrusion of the mucosa through the muscular wall. **Accessory openings** may be found near the fimbriated extremity of the tubes.

ALTERATIONS IN POSITION AND CONTINUITY.

Apart from the congenital anomalies of position, above referred to, the position of the tubes depends mainly on pathological changes in the neighboring structures, uterus, ovaries, and peritoneum. Displacements of the uterus, ovarian tumors, and inflammatory adhesions frequently

---

[1] See Elizabeth Hurdon, Johns Hopkins Hosp. Bull., 9:1898:187.
[2] Emmanuel, Zeitsch. f. Geb. u Gynäk., 34:1896:1.

drag the tubes out of their normal position. When prolonged tension is put upon a tube it atrophies at some point, usually near the uterus, and may even be separated from the uterus. The tube may also be twisted spirally upon its axis. The tube has been found forming part of the contents of a hernial sac (**salpingocele**).

Stenosis and Atresia.—Stenosis and atresia of the lumen are comparatively common. The abdominal and uterine ostia are the parts most likely to be involved. When both tubes are affected sterility results. A slight grade of the affection is said to be one of the causes of extrauterine gestation. The cause is usually salpingitis or pelvic peritonitis. In such cases secretions and fluids of various kinds, blood, pus, or serum, may distend the tube into a form of cyst (*hemato-*, *pyo-*, and

FIG. 212

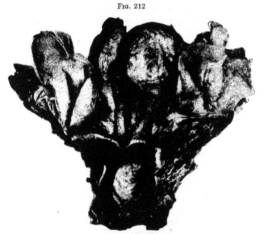

Double hydrosalpinx. The specimen shows also an intramural "fibroid" of the uterus.
(From the Pathological Museum of McGill University.)

hydrosalpinx). In cases where the abdominal end only of the tube is closed, there may be a periodical discharge of clear or bloody fluid into the uterus, which may simulate menstruation (*hydrops profluens*). When secretions are retained the mucous membrane is flattened, the cells have lost their cilia, while the muscle bands are compressed, atrophic, and more or less dissociated. The tube in this condition may be converted into a semitransparent, thin-walled sac. No fimbriæ can be seen, as in some curious fashion they become inverted.

Tuboövarian Cyst.—A brief reference should be made here to a special form of tubal hydrops, the so-called tuboövarian cyst. The wall of the cyst is composed in part of tube, in part of ovary. It is usually brought about by the bursting of an ovarian cyst into the tube, and is of the nature either of a true cystoma, a hydropic Graafian follicle, or a cystic corpus luteum. According to Bland Sutton, there is in some cases an accessory fold of peritoneum forming a sort of covering about the ovary, analogous to the tunica of the testis, in which fluid collects (*ovarian hydrocele*).

Rupture of the tube is rare, except in cases of tubal gestation.

Ulceration is also rare. It may occur in tuberculosis and carcinoma.

CIRCULATORY DISTURBANCES.

These are similar to those occurring in the uterus. **Hyperemia** is found in infective diseases and in obstruction of the inferior vena cava. Small **hemorrhages** into the mucosa are met with not infrequently in cases of burns, phosphorus poisoning, and in the hemorrhagic diatheses.

An accumulation of blood within the tube (**hematosalpinx**) may be due to retention of menstrual or extravasated blood, owing to atresia in some part of the genital canal. It may be associated with chronic inflammation and hypertrophy of the muscular wall of the tube.

INFLAMMATIONS.

Salpingitis.—Inflammations of the tubes (salpingitis) are, for the most part, comparable to those of the uterus. The mucous membrane may be chiefly affected, or all the coats may be involved.

Acute Catarrhal Salpingitis.—In simple acute catarrhal salpingitis the mucous membrane is reddened, swollen, and infiltrated. The secretion is scanty, grayish or grayish-white in color, and contains small masses of desquamated and degenerated epithelium.

Chronic Catarrhal Salpingitis.—More common is chronic catarrh, where the most important feature is productive change in the mucous membrane. The folds of the mucosa are thickened and infiltrated, and, owing to the loss of the epithelium, become adherent or connected by fibrous bands. In this way small, gland-like structures are pinched off from the general cavity, which may, in time, be converted into cysts. In this feature there is a striking similarity to glandular endometritis. Under the designation of *salpingitis productiva glandularis*, Chiari[1] has described a special form of chronic catarrh, in which small nodular outgrowths are found at the uterine end of the tube, composed of hyperplastic muscle and gland-like structures from the mucous membrane, often cystic in appearance, which contain a clear serous fluid and are lined with non-ciliated epithelium.

In cases of chronic catarrh the muscular coat may be relatively unaffected, showing either hypertrophy or atrophy, but at times it is also infiltrated with inflammatory products. Productive hyperplasia of the connective-tissue elements, chiefly along the bloodvessels, often supervenes (*interstitial salpingitis*).

[1] Zeit. f. Heilk., 8: 1887: 457.

Apart from the simple forms of salpingitis, we have to recognize, according to the character of the exudate, suppurative and membranous varieties.

Suppurative Salpingitis.—There is no marked difference, etiologically or anatomically, between simple and suppurative salpingitis. In both there is the same infiltration and adhesion of the mucous folds. In the suppurative form, however, the secretion is more abundant, seropurulent or purulent, and tends to collect in the ampulla. The amount of degeneration of the epithelium is also greater and sets in earlier. In this way most of the mucous membrane may be destroyed. In some cases the mucosa is greatly infiltrated with cells, and becomes fibrous and indurated. The condition of the muscular coat varies. Cellular infiltration, the formation of multiple small abscesses, and productive changes are common. In many cases, owing to the inflammation, both the uterine and the abdominal openings of the tube become blocked, and the pus accumulates until the tube assumes a sac-like appearance (*pyosalpinx*). The tube may thus become greatly distorted and present irregular swellings, owing to the sacculation of the contents through adhesions (*pyosalpinx saccata*). Mauclaire[1] has recorded a curious case of purulent salpingitis where gas was produced (physopyosalpinx), the exact cause of which was not determined.

Membranous Salpingitis.—Membranous salpingitis is of relatively little importance; it is characterized by necrosis with the formation of an adherent fibrinous or fibrinohyaline exudation.

The causes of salpingitis are various. Among ordinary sources may be mentioned, "catching cold" or traumatism during the menstrual period, inflammation of the uterus or ovaries, tumors of the uterus, dislocations, and general systemic infection. The majority of cases are bacterial in origin. Some cases are extensions of septic endometritis and metritis. The most frequent cause, however, is the Gonococcus.

Gurd,[2] from bacteriological and histological studies, concludes that a much larger percentage of cases of salpingitis than is usually supposed (at least 80 per cent.) is due to the Gonococcus. He obtained cultures of this organism in 35 per cent. of his series and confirms Schridde and Amersbach in the conclusion that every case of salpingitis can be diagnosed as gonorrhœal, which in the thickened folds of the mucosa shows a marked infiltration with plasma cells, lymphoblasts and lymphocytes, these same cells also predominating in the pus.

A number of serious results may follow salpingitis. A frequent event is the extension of the inflammation to the serous membrane (**perisalpingitis**) and to the pelvic peritoneum (**pelvic peritonitis**), leading to dislocations of position and distortion of the tubes from the formation of adhesions. When pyosalpinx is present the pus may escape into the peritoneal cavity, setting up a general peritonitis, or it may be walled off by adhesions so as to form a pelvic abscess. Abscesses of this kind

[1] Bull. et. mém. de la Soc. anat. de Paris, April, 1901
[2] Jour. of Med. Research, 23:1910:151.

may discharge into the vagina or rectum. In the cases that undergo involution, the pus is often absorbed, becoming inspissated into a thick whitish, putty-like material that may be mistaken for caseation, or the contents may become calcified.

Syphilis.—But little is known of syphilitic lesions of the tubes. So far as we know, only one case, that of Bouchard and Lépine,[1] is recorded, where the tubes were thickened and dilated to the size of the finger and contained gummas.

Tuberculosis.—This is much more common, and is primary or secondary. It is said (Orthmann) that primary tuberculosis occurs in about 18 per cent. of all cases of genital tuberculosis in the female. The infection is almost always hematogenic, although it is conceivable that some cases may arise from the presence of sperm containing tubercle bacilli. Secondary tuberculosis may arise by the extension of disease from the peritoneum, the ovaries, or the uterus. In both types the peritoneum and the rest of the genitalia are apt to be involved as well. As a rule, both tubes are affected, although not always to the same degree.

Judging from the extent of the lesions usually found, the Fallopian tubes form a particularly good soil for the development of the tubercle bacillus. What constitutes this special predisposition is not exactly known, but it would seem that previously existing inflammatory or circulatory disturbances, and disorders arising during menstruation and the puerperium play an important part. Rokitansky pointed out that the disease was particularly common after the puerperium. While, however, it is true that the disease is commonly met with during the period of greatest sexual activity, it is nevertheless found in old women and children.

Tuberculosis generally begins in the mucous membrane of the ampulla and spreads rapidly to the adjacent parts. The affected tube is greatly thickened, firm, more or less tortuous, and the muscular wall is hypertrophic. The fimbriæ are short, thick, and firm. As a rule, the tube is bound down by inflammatory adhesions. On opening the tube, in the early stages the mucosa is swollen, reddened, and the folds are adherent, while the lumen contains a small amount of grayish or yellowish secretion. The appearance is similar to that in simple chronic productive salpingitis. In more advanced cases grayish points can be seen in the mucosa, or, again, caseous nodules or streaks. Later, the mucosa may be converted into a dense caseous mass. The lumen may be obliterated, or enlarged when the necrotic material has been evacuated.

Microscopically, the mucosa is swollen, infiltrated with round and epithelioid cells, while here and there can be seen remains of the gland-follicles, frequently showing cystic dilatation. Definite tubercles are to be seen near the lumen with central caseation. In the more advanced cases the mucosa is largely caseous, and the process can be seen advancing into the muscular and serous coats. In the more chronic forms giant cells can be made out.

---

[1] Gaz. méd. de Paris, 1866: 726.

The caseous detritus in some cases becomes liquefied and puriform, and may be retained and sacculated (*tuberculous pyosalpinx*). Some of these cases are examples of mixed infection. Ulceration and perforation of the tube is rare. Usually the abscess produced is walled off by adhesions. The tube may become adherent to the uterus, the appendix, or to other portions of the intestinal tract, or may be bound down in Douglas' sac.

Actinomycosis.[1]—This is rare and generally is due to extension of the disease from the peritoneum. The tube is thickened, studded with granulomata, and the puriform exudate and detritus contain the actinomyces "grains."

Foreign Bodies and Parasites.—These are of little importance, apart from bacteria. Orth records a curiosity in the form of a roundworm that had made its way into a tube from a ruptured intestine.

RETROGRESSIVE METAMORPHOSES.

Simple atrophy affecting the muscular wall and mucosa is met with after the menopause. It may also be due to the pressure of retained secretions, and the pressure or traction of tumors. In some cases the tube may be actually separated from the uterus.

PROGRESSIVE METAMORPHOSES.

Hypertrophy.—Hypertrophy of all the tissues of the tube is not uncommon. Overgrowths of the mucosa are met with as a result of inflammation or possibly as a true hyperplasia, for instance, in association with myofibromas of the uterus. Polyps of the mucosa are very rare. Hypertrophy of the muscle results from overwork, such as is met with in stenosis of the ostium and in retention of blood or secretion.

The fimbriæ are occasionally thickened, fibrous, or club-like.

Tumors.—Tumors of the tube, at least the primary ones, are rare. **Fibromas** and **myxomas**, often multiple, are met with.

Warty or papillomatous outgrowths of fibrous nature are described, at times containing a clear fluid or dilated into cysts. Subserous **lipomas** have been met with. Benign **papillomas** have also been reported, and a **cystoma papilliferum** (Eberth).

Sarcoma is excessively rare. **Carcinoma** is usually secondary to carcinoma of the uterus or ovary. As a rule, it takes the form of a diffuse growth in the mucosa, or forms nodules in the muscle and serosa. It is usually of the soft type, but may be scirrhous. Primary carcinoma of the tube generally takes the papillary form. Le Count[2] has discussed the nature of these growths.

---

[1] Zemann, Wien. med. Jahrb., 1883: 477.

[2] The Genesis of Carcinoma of the Fallopian Tubes in Hyperplastic Salpingitis, Johns Hopkins Hosp. Bull., 12: 1901: 120.

THE OVARIES.

The ovaries are ovate glands situated on the posterior aspect of the broad ligaments. They are attached by a reduplication of the peritoneal membrane—the mesovarium, which, however, ends abruptly without forming a complete covering for the organs. In the adult the ovaries measure 2.5 to 5 cm. in length, 2 to 3 cm. in breadth, and 1 to 2 cm. in thickness. Their weight ranges from 5 to 7 grams. From the inner end within the layers of the broad ligament runs a fibrous cord containing unstriped muscle—the ligamentum ovarii.

Microscopically, the ovary consists of two parts: a medullary portion composed of strands of connective tissue, unstriped muscle, abundant bloodvessels, and in some cases rows of cells of embryonic type derived from the Wolffian body, which are in relationship with the epoöphoron (Markstränge-Kölliker); and a cortical part composed of rather cellular connective tissue, containing the Graafian follicles. The outermost layer of the cortex, called the tunica albuginea, is more condensed and contains fewer follicles, but does not form a definite membrane.

The Graafian follicles measure 0.04 to 0.15 mm. in diameter. They are formed externally of a connective-tissue membrane—the theca folliculi—which is composed of an outer layer of fibrous character (tunica fibrosa), an inner softer, more cellular, and vascular layer (tunica propria), and a stratified layer of epithelial cells (membrana granulosa). At a certain point, about the ovum, these cells are heaped up into the discus proligerus.

The cavity of the follicle is filled with fluid, the liquor folliculi. The ovum possesses an outer layer of hyaline appearance, the zona pellucida, presenting radiating striæ; a nucleus, and a germinal spot.

The ovary is developed from the Wolffian body by the ingrowth of connective tissue into a mass of epithelial cells derived from the cœlom. The follicles are by most authorities believed to be derived from the downgrowth and subsequent separation of the superficial mesothelial cells of the body cavity. The ovary is thus entirely mesoblastic. Therefore, tumors arising from it, even if histologically of epithelial or carcinomatous type, are from the point of view mesothelial (mesotheliomas).

The ovary is particularly liable to circulatory disturbances; indeed, these are largely physiological, for congestion accompanies the functions of ovulation and menstruation, and hemorrhage takes place into the follicles after the ovum is discharged. The changes in the follicles incident to pregnancy and ordinary involution are somewhat striking and should not be mistaken for pathological conditions. Neither circulatory disturbances nor inflammations, however, are of so much importance, either clinically or anatomically, as are cysts and tumors, which form a large proportion of the pathological conditions found in these organs.

CONGENITAL ANOMALIES.

Complete absence of the ovaries is rare and generally associated with absence or rudimentary development of the uterus. **Unilateral defect,** associated with the condition of uterus unicornis, is more frequent. In such cases the kidney on the same side is sometimes absent or dislocated. In exceptional instances a uterus of normal type may be present. The condition is not due to aplasia then, but rather to some condition that exerts traction or torsion on the Fallopian tube. In this way, from atrophy, a portion of the tube with its attendant ovary is completely separated from the uterus and in time disappears. It may, however, become attached in some other situation or form a free body in the abdominal cavity.

Unilateral and bilateral **hypoplasia** is described. The ovaries may either be small, with, however, normally developed follicles, or the follicles may be rudimentary or absent. In bilateral hypoplasia the individual often presents the secondary male characteristics of development.

Accessory ovaries have been observed.[1] They are usually of small size, multiple, and situated at the hilus of the normal ovary at the free margin of the peritoneum. It is possible that they are not always true accessories, for some hold that they are simply portions of the main ovary that have been pinched off through peritoneal adhesions. Winckel reports a case where a third ovary was found in front of the uterus.

The ovary may occupy an **abnormal situation,** for instance, in the canal of Nuck.

DISLOCATIONS.

Hernia.—Malpositions of the ovaries are congenital or acquired. Hernia of the ovary (**ovariocele**) is usually congenital and due to patency of the processus vaginalis. The condition is often bilateral. The ovary may be found in any part of the inguinal canal (*hernia ovarica inguinalis*), even in the labium (*hernia ovarica labialis*). The acquired form is usually met with during confinement. *Hernia ovarica cruralis* is also acquired. Rare varieties are the *hernia ischiadica, h. abdominalis* (into the scar of a Cesarean section), *h. umbilicalis,* and that into the obturator foramen. The dislocated ovary is often congested and inflamed, rarely, cystic, carcinomatous, or sarcomatous.

Prolapse.—The ovary may also be prolapsed when for any reason the uterus is dislocated. Another cause is increase in the weight of the ovary, as from congestion, œdema, cysts, and tumors, in some instances combined with diminished elasticity of the ligaments or the traction of fibrous bands. The prolapsed organ is generally swollen and congested.

---

[1] For literature see Falk, Berl. klin. Woch., 44: 1891: 1069.

CIRCULATORY DISTURBANCES.

Hyperemia.—Active Hyperemia.—Active hyperemia, apart from the physiological congestion that occurs in the course of the various sexual functions, coitus, menstruation, ovulation, and pregnancy, is of little importance. It occurs in the early stages of inflammation.

Passive Hyperemia.—Passive hyperemia may be a part of a general systemic condition, or localized to the ovary. In the latter case it is due to any cause that interferes with the proper discharge of blood through the veins. Among these may be mentioned, torsion of the pedicle, prolapse of the ovary, the pressure of fibrous adhesions, and the presence of cysts or tumors. The ovary is enlarged, reddened, and œdematous, and in long-standing cases may be fibroid. **Phlebectasia** of the veins of the medulla is described by Kaufmann.

Hemorrhage.—Hemorrhage into the ovary may occur in any of the foregoing forms of hyperemia, and in the infectious fevers, such as typhoid, diphtheria, and cholera, in the hemorrhagic diatheses, in phosphorus poisoning, and in severe burns. The effusion of blood may be local or diffuse, and may involve the stroma (interstitial hemorrhage) or the follicles (follicular hemorrhage).

When extravasation takes place into a follicle, the follicle is enlarged, sometimes to the size of the fist. The blood may be normal in appearance, clotted, or resembling tar. Frequently, from degeneration and reactive inflammation, a yellowish zone is formed at the periphery. The distended follicle may give way and lead to fatal bleeding or to retro-uterine hematocele. Hemorrhage into a follicle is generally due to the rupture of a distended vessel, but the possibility of ovarian pregnancy must also be borne in mind. Should rupture not take place, the theca becomes thickened, the blood is gradually absorbed, and a pigmented, fibrous scar is the result. Small hemorrhages are sometimes seen in the stroma, usually about the follicles. These may coalesce, forming large extravasations, or the hemorrhage may be extensive from the first, leading to a diffuse infiltration of the organ. In such cases the ovary is greatly enlarged and the tissue more or less destroyed, so that it resembles a sponge filled with blood (**hematoma ovarii**). This is not infrequent in children.

Leukemia.—In leukemia the vessels of the ovaries are filled with leukocytes and there is also infiltration of the stroma with white cells, which are found along the course of the vessels or else form definite nodules.

INFLAMMATIONS.

Oöphoritis.—Inflammation of the ovary—oöphoritis—is usually secondary, being caused by the extension of inflammation from the uterus, tubes, broad ligaments, or peritoneum. The infection may be immediate or through the bloodvessels and lymphatics. The majority of cases arise from the uterus during the puerperium, or from gonorrhœa. In some cases, as in typhoid, measles, septicemia, pneumonia, influenza diphtheria, and cholera, the infection is hematogenic. In rare instances oöphoritis is primary, due to reactive inflammation about areas of degeneration or hemorrhage in the ovary. Among the germs regarded as exciting causes may be mentioned Gonococcus, Streptococcus, B. coli, Diplococcus lanceolatus, and B. typhosus.

According to the portion of the ovary chiefly affected, we can divide cases into **follicular** or **parenchymatous** and **interstitial**.

Slavjansky[1] has described a degenerative form of follicular oöphoritis occurring in the acute infective diseases. The cells of the membrana granulosa are swollen, cloudy, and later undergo fatty degeneration. The ovum may be affected in a similar way, and the whole follicle may be destroyed, so that the cavity becomes filled with a whitish, granular detritus. The follicle in some cases undergoes cystic change. Some extravasation of blood may be found about the follicles, especially in cholera. In more severe cases the follicles or the corpora lutea may become filled with pus (**suppurative foll. oöphoritis**). Occasionally the infection travels along the lymph-channels of the broad ligament to the ovary (**oöph. lymphangitica**) or takes the form of thrombophlebitis (**oöph. thrombophlebitica**). The ovary is enlarged, softened, and infiltrated with inflammatory products. When suppuration occurs, which frequently happens, one can make out yellowish streaks running from the hilus to the cortex along the lymphatics or veins.

It is by no means always possible to draw a hard and fast line between the follicular and interstitial forms of oöphoritis, for in many cases the inflammation is diffuse. In the milder grades the ovary is enlarged, reddened, and œdematous, being infiltrated mainly with serum (**oöph. serosa**). In other cases suppuration occurs (**oöph. purulenta**) or extravasation of blood (**oöph. hæmorrhagica**). In the most severe forms the entire ovary may become purulent and necrotic.

The suppurative form of oöphoritis is usually due to Gonococcus or to septic microörganisms that gain an entrance after parturition. In such cases, as a rule, the infective agents spread from the broad ligaments or from the peritoneum, less commonly from the tube.

The results of suppurative oöphoritis are various. Frequently the inflammation extends outward to the surface of the ovary, to the peritoneum, or tubes (**perioöphoritis**), or a **tuboövarian abscess** may form. A local pus collection may burst into the peritoneal cavity, setting up a serious and often fatal peritonitis, or may burst into the rectum, bladder, more rarely into the vagina, or even externally. Should the patient survive, the abscess may become encapsulated and partly absorbed. The ovary in such cases is usually tied down by firm adhesions. As a result of secretion from the walls of the abscess the cavity may attain a considerable size. The largest abscesses occur where a previously existing cyst has become infected. The commonly resulting

---

[1] Arch. f. Gyn., 3: 1872: 183, and 23: 1890.

perioöphoritis may result in the attachment of the ovary to the tube, the uterus or to the Douglas' pouch. Sterility is a common result of oöphoritis and salpingitis.

Chronic Oöphoritis.—Chronic oöphoritis is, in the main, due to the same causes as the acute form. Thus, it may supervene upon the subsidence of an acute attack or after repeated relapses. It may also result from prolonged or repeated congestion, as from excessive sexual excitement or venous stasis. The main characteristics of this form are those of a productive inflammation affecting the interstitial tissue, though the follicles usually show degenerative changes.

The ovary is possibly at first somewhat enlarged, but diminishes in size as the process becomes established. The surface is often nodular but may be even, and is covered with bands or tags of adhesion. The tunica albuginea is thickened and of a pearly-white or grayish appearance. On section, the organ is cirrhotic and contains numerous small cysts, due to the dilatation of the follicles.

Microscopically, in the early stages, there is a small-celled infiltration in the stroma, principally about the vessels. Later, this is less marked, and fibrous hyperplasia predominates. The vessels usually show hyaline thickening. The follicles in some parts may be normal, but many of them manifest degeneration. The membrana granulosa is cloudy or fattily degenerated and often stripped off from the theca, while the ovum is destroyed. In other cases the follicles are atrophic and represented only by corpora fibrosa, or are converted into cysts.

Syphilis.—Gummas analogous to those found in syphilitic orchitis have been observed (Lancereaux[1]).

Tuberculosis.—Tuberculosis is more common and takes the form of milia, large caseous foci, or areas of colliquative necrosis. As a rule, the disease is bilateral. It is rarely primary in the ovary, but originates in the uterus, tubes, or peritoneum. Sometimes, however, the ovaries are alone affected. Occasionally, the follicles (Heiberg, Schetlander) or cysts of the ovary are secondarily infected. A tuboövarian abscess may be formed or the ovary may be enveloped in a caseofibroid mass.

Actinomycosis.—Actinomycosis is excessively rare, and is invariably secondary. Small abscesses containing the actinomyces "grains" are found in the stroma.

Parasites and Foreign Bodies.—*Echinococcus disease* has been found in the ovary (Schatz, Péan), and in a dermoid cyst (Freund[2]).

Needles have been discovered in the ovary, having reached it from the uterus or bowel.

RETROGRESSIVE METAMORPHOSES.

Atrophy of the ovary occurs as a senile change, or results from chronic oöphoritis. The senile ovary is smaller than normal, firm, nodular, and of a grayish or pearly white color. The albuginea is hard and may

[1] Traité hist. et prat. de la syph., 1874: 228.　　　[2] Gyn. Klin., 1885.

be several millimeters thick. The follicles are in all stages of atrophy and degeneration and for the most part are converted into minute fibrous nodules (*corpora fibrosa*) with marked thickening of the theca. The arteries show hyaline change and often calcification.

Cloudy and **fatty degeneration** are found in the ovum and the membrana granulosa in the various forms of atrophy, as well as **hyaline change** in the vessels and connective tissue.

PROGRESSIVE METAMORPHOSES.

As has been frequently remarked with regard to other organs, so with the ovaries, it is difficult to draw a hard and fast line between developmental overgrowths of tissue and certain forms of inflammation.

An increase in the number of the follicles, or a precocious ripening of the same, is met with in young children, associated with precocious menstruation and puberty, and by many is regarded as a form of **hypertrophy (hyperplasia)** of the follicles. In a certain number of these cases the ovary presents, also, a number of small cysts. These, as Leo Loeb has shown, may originate in follicles that have atrophied prematurely (atresia of the follicles). This atrophy is common in early life. In some cases of uterine fibroids the ovaries are hypertrophic, showing not only cystic dilatation of the follicles, but also round-celled infiltration, proliferative changes in the stroma, and hyaline thickening of the vessels.

Besides, however, the cysts just mentioned, there are certain others that must, like them, be differentiated from the large, developmental cysts or cystadenomas. Such are the small cysts that are commonly found in the ovaries in cases of chronic oöphoritis, perioöphoritis, and salpingitis, originating in the follicles or corpora lutea. These are to be regarded as "retention" cysts (**hydrops follicularis**). Here it is probable that there is a thickening or condensation of the theca or tunica albuginea, which prevents the bursting of a follicle and the discharge of its contents.

Usually there are more cysts than one, but eventually one or two predominate. A thin-walled sac is produced, reaching in size from that of a walnut to that of the fist or a man's head. The smaller cysts are lined by cylindrical epithelium, but in the larger ones this is more or less altered from pressure. The contained fluid is usually clear, transparent, and serous, resembling the normal liquor folliculi, but may contain blood, degenerated epithelium, and pigment. In the larger cysts, as a rule, the ovum degenerates and disappears. The remaining stroma of the ovary presents but little change, except that in the case of the larger cysts it becomes fibroid and atrophied from pressure. Occasionally the wall becomes calcified. Ovarian cysts of this type are unilateral or bilateral.

Analogous to follicular hydrops, are the retention cysts sometimes originating in the corpora lutea. They are usually single, though two or more may be found. In size they do not often exceed a walnut, but have been found as large as a child's head. The cyst wall is composed of a loosely attached corrugated membrane of reddish or reddish-yellow color, containing capillaries, leukocytes, and pigmented round cells (lutein cells). The cavities contain a thin, ropy fluid of reddish or yellowish color, containing more or less altered blood. There is no epithelial lining in this type.

Tumors.—In the attempt to arrive at an adequate scientific classification of ovarian tumors we are beset by many difficulties. The older writers boldly cut the Gordian knot by dividing them into cystic and solid growths. This, while a fairly good practical division from a clinical point of view, must, however, be regarded, pathologically speaking, as unscientific and misleading, inasmuch as under the term "cystic tumors" are grouped not only the true "proliferation" cysts, or cystadenomas, but also "retention" cysts which are, of course, not properly neoplasms. Farther, certain growths are separated that, embryologically speaking, should be classed together. Still, when all is said, it may be questioned whether we have much better to propose for it. The difficulty is that the etiology of many of the ovarian growths is still in doubt. Thus, with the important class of the cystomas, leaving out of the account the simple retention-cysts, and confining our attention to the developmental cysts (cystadenomas), we know that certain of them tend to be unilocular, others multilocular, while the fluid contents of cysts that appear in the main to be the same vary considerably, being at one time serous, at another ropy and mucinous. Other cysts again are papillomatous. These striking variations suggest differences in origin, but what these are we are not able to say positively.

Theoretically, it is possible to get cystadenomas developing (1) from the follicles, (2) from invagination of the original germinal epithelium (Keimepithel), (3) from remains of the Wolffian body, and (4) from extra-ovarian tissues. The ideal classification would be along embryological and developmental lines, but in the state of our present knowledge, or, rather, ignorance, it is perhaps better to fall back on morphological differences, at least in the main. This is the basis of Pfannenstiel's classification, in which three groups are recognized: (1) The parenchymatous growths, divided into (a) those derived from the epithelium and (b) those derived from the ovum; (2) growths arising from the stroma; and (3) mixed types. This is not entirely satisfactory, as it brings teratomas into the same class as the cystadenomas, with which they have little in common, either in structure or in origin.

We would suggest the following classification, not as having finality or being scientifically accurate, but as having at least the advantage of grouping like things together and separating unlike ones.

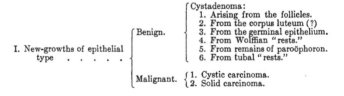

I. New-growths of epithelial type

Benign.
  Cystadenoma:
  1. Arising from the follicles.
  2. From the corpus luteum (?)
  3. From the germinal epithelium.
  4. From Wolffian "rests."
  5. From remains of paroöphoron.
  6. From tubal "rests."

Malignant.
  1. Cystic carcinoma.
  2. Solid carcinoma.

II. New-growths of connective tissue type . .

Benign.
1. Fibroma.
2. Papilloma.
3. Hemangioma.
4. Lymphangioma.

Malignant.
1. Endothelioma
2. Perithelioma.
3. Sarcoma.

III. Teratomas . . . .
1. Epidermoid cysts.
2. Pure dermoid cysts.
3. Compound dermoids.
4. Compound teratomas.

IV. Mixed tumors. . . .

Combined and cognate forms:
Benign.
1. Myofibroma.
2. Adenofibroma.
3. Cystic fibroma.

Malignant.
1. Myosarcoma.
2. Adenosarcoma.
3. Sarcocarcinoma.
4. Cystadenomatous carcinoma.
5. Cystic sarcoma.
6. Cystadenomatous sarcoma.

Teratogenous blastomas:
Benign.
1. Cystadenoma developing in a teratoma.

Malignant.
1. Sarcoma developing in a teratoma.
2. Carcinoma developing in a teratoma.

Cystadenoma.—Of the epithelial growths, the most important are the cystadenomas, which, indeed, are the commonest neoplasms found in the ovaries. They may be unilateral or bilateral. Nowadays they rarely reach a large size, inasmuch as they are usually operated upon somewhat early, but in former times cases have been met with in which the weight of the cyst actually exceeded that of the patient affected. Several varieties are recognized, according to the number of cysts, the character of the lining epithelium, and the nature of the contents. As the main type, we may take the common ovarian cyst or *simple cystoma.* This is generally unilateral, and consists of one main cyst of proportionately large size, with several subsidiary or daughter cysts. The smaller cysts may exist more or less independently in the fibrous stroma or may encroach upon the cavity of the major cyst. On examining the inner surface of the wall, one can generally make out ridges representing the remains of former divisions between the cysts. Hence, the major cyst is evidently developed from the confluence of smaller cysts. A multilocular cyst may thus be converted into a unilocular one. The cyst-wall is often tough, thin, and translucent, but in some cases thick. The blood supply is by means of large vessels that enter in the pedicle and ramify over the surface. The fluid found within the various cysts differs somewhat in character, being thinner in the larger cavities. The specific gravity varies from 1010 to 1030. It is often viscid, mucinous, or stiff like honey. In color it may be clear and glassy, in other cases turbid, brownish, or, rarely, tinged with blood. The character of the fluid is due to the presence of certain bodies, regarded by Scherer and Eichwald as paralbumin and metalbumin, but which, according to Hammerstein and Pfannenstiel, are more nearly related to mucin. They term them pseudomucins.

The cyst-wall is composed of two layers of fibrous tissue, an outer firmer and more fibrous, an inner cellular and vascular. The lining membrane of the cyst is usually composed of a single layer of high cylindrical cells. In the larger cysts the lining cells are short, columnar, cuboidal, or even occasionally flattened. The lining epithelium forms downward evaginations, so that simple or compound gland-tubules are produced in the wall of the cyst. Some of these may become pinched off and form minute, intramural cysts. It is rare for the epithelium to be stratified. Some cysts are lined with ciliated cells, either wholly or in part. In many cases the cells of the lining epithelium present colloid change and discharge their contents into the cavity. The cells, also, from pressure, frequently show fatty degeneration, atrophy, and necrosis.

Microscopically, the fluid content contains fat globules, leukocytes, degenerating cells, detritus, blood, and cholesterin. In many cases the typical ovarian structure has completely disappeared, but occasionally some more or less flattened and atrophied remains can still be made out containing active follicles.

A second but rare form of cystadenoma is a *pedunculated, multilocular cyst* of moderate size, usually unilateral, lined with ciliated cylindrical epithelium. The cyst-contents are thin, more serous than in the last form, and light yellow or greenish in color. The fluid is rich in albumin and contains no pseudomucin. The cyst-wall usually contains gland-tubules in considerable numbers, especially near the pedicle.

A third and important type is the *papillary cystoma* (*cystadenoma papilliferum*). This is a multilocular, or occasionally unilocular, cyst,

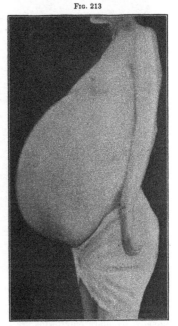

Fig. 213

Ovarian cyst. (From the Gynecological Clinic of the Montreal General Hospital.)

and is liable to be bilateral. The growth may extend between the layers of the broad ligament or form a pedunculated mass springing from the surface of the ovary. The cysts are usually smaller than in the case of the simple cystadenoma. In this variety, the cavities are more or less completely filled with warty, villous, or tree-like excrescences derived from the proliferation of the connective-tissue stroma of the cyst-wall, which are covered with ciliated cylindrical epithelium. In some few cases, the cilia are absent or only to be observed on the papillæ. The stroma is composed of fibrous tissue containing

Fig. 214

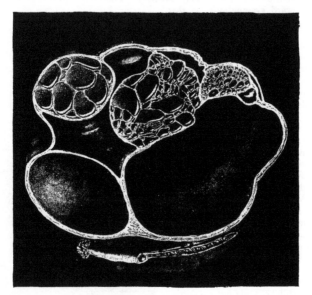

Cystadenoma. Multilocular ovarian cyst. (Dudley.)

numerous bloodvessels. It may show mucinous degeneration. Exceptionally, papillary outgrowths are found on the external aspect of the tumor. This is due, for the most part, to the fact that the cyst-wall, through atrophy, has given way and the originally intracystic outgrowths appear on the surface. More rarely, there is a true invasion or infiltration of the cyst-wall by the papillæ. It is not unusual to find granules of lime (sand bodies, psammoma) in the wall and in the papillæ. The fluid contained is thin, watery, and more serous than in the simple cystadenomas. It contains little or no pseudomucin. The color is often dark like coffee. The tumor is clinically of great importance, since in time it invariably develops malignancy, and secondary nodules are found scattered over the peritoneal membrane. According to Pfannenstiel, one-half of the ovarian papillary cystadenomas are in reality carcinomatous from the start.

With regard to the origin of these cystic growths much has been written and much remains to be learned. It is not likely that they are all derived from the same elements. Theoretically, cystadenomas may arise from the epithelium of the follicles, from the corpus luteum, from the superficial germinal epithelium, from certain tubules of the paroöphoron (Waldeyer), from displaced "rests" of the ciliated tubal epithelium (Kassmann), from remains of the Wolffian body (Kölliker's Markstränge).

FIG. 215

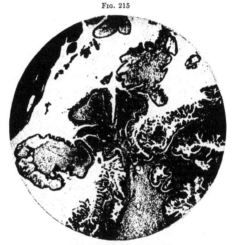

Cystoma papilliferum of the ovary. Zeiss obj. A, without ocular. (From the collection of Dr. A. G. Nicholls.)

Attempts have been made to assign a particular origin to the cysts according to the character of the contained fluid, but this is a small point to decide upon, since, as is well known, the fluid varies considerably in different parts even of the same growth. As much depends upon absorption as upon secretion. Again, differentiation has been made on the ground of the presence or absence of papillary outgrowths and of ciliated epithelium. As Orth points out, however, it is difficult to draw a hard and fast line between the simple and the papillary cystadenomas, inasmuch as all sorts of transitional forms have been met with. It has been shown, moreover, that under certain circumstances non-ciliated epithelium may acquire cilia, and in man the existence of ciliated germinal epithelium has been proved. This being the case, it will readily be seen how difficult it is to come to any satisfactory conclusion as to the etiology of these cysts. A developmental origin for many of them is supported by several facts. Cystadenomas are usually met with during the period of sexual activity and not infrequently in both ovaries. Again, cases have been recorded where sisters, or mother and daughter, have been similarly affected, indicating an hereditary vitium. Perhaps even more suggestive is the not uncommon event of the combination of a cystadenoma with a dermoid. In some multilocular cysts certain of the cysts are lined with cylindrical epithelium and present a glandular character, while others resemble dermoids.

The origin of the papilliferous cystadenomas has been variously referred to the follicles, the germinal epithelium, Wolffian "rests," or, bearing in mind their frequent situation between the layers of the broad ligament, the parovarium. Authorities are divided whether to assign the same etiology to the simple cystadenomas and the papillary forms. Orth is inclined to attribute the majority of them to the same origin— the germinal epithelium.

From the cystadenoma there is a natural transition to the **carcinoma**, for the epithelial benign tumors of the ovary, especially the cystic forms, are particularly liable to undergo malignant metamorphosis. This is borne out by the fact that, like the cystadenoma, carcinoma of the ovary has been found in early life, even before the age of puberty.

Carcinoma.—Carcinomas may be conveniently divided into *cystic* and *solid* growths. The former arise commonly in the simple cystadenomas, but still more frequently in the papillomatous variety. The cystic carcinomas in general resemble their non-malignant prototypes, but seldom attain such a large size. In the malignant cystadenomas, the walls and septa are found to be infiltrated with nodules that histologically are composed of masses of epithelial cells. In many places the lining epithelium has proliferated, so that a stratified layer of cells has taken the place of the original single row. The fluid contents of the cysts are clear, or cloudy from the admixture of cells and blood. The material may also be viscid or even colloid. In the latter case the metastases are also colloid, as in a case recently under our observation.

In the papillary type (*cystadenoma papilliferum malignum*) there is an exuberant growth of the excrescences, which are more cellular than usual, and the septa are infiltrated with secondary cancerous nodules of papillomatous appearance. In many cases the papillæ extend through the septa and appear externally, giving rise to peritoneal and other metastases. The stroma frequently presents mucinous degeneration, and occasionally sarcomatous transformation. As in the benign form, psammoma bodies may be found. In some few cases it has been thought, that simple cystadenoma and cystic carcinoma have arisen independently in the same ovary.

The solid carcinomas of the ovary are also unilateral or bilateral. They form smooth or nodular growths, sometimes attaining the size of a child's head. The ovarian tissue is frequently diffusely infiltrated and destroyed, or the main mass of the organ may be pushed to one side in the course of growth. As a rule, the tumor is of the medullary or scirrhous type, but may be colloid. A curious form is the so-called *superficial papillary carcinoma*, in which papillomatous outgrowths develop on the surface of an otherwise fairly normal non-cystic ovary.

Histologically, carcinoma is made up of cylindrical, cuboidal, or polymorphous cells, either arranged in more or less perfect alveoli, or forming a diffuse infiltration, and not infrequently showing mucinous change.

The mode of origin of the solid carcinomas is obscure. They are supposed to arise from any of the following sources: the superficial germinal epithelium, Pflüger's tubules, the follicles, the corpus luteum (Rokitansky), or remains of the Wolffian body.

Ovarian carcinomas of all kinds spread readily over the peritoneum, owing to grafting in the Douglas' pouch. They also may extend to the broad ligaments and produce distant metastases by invasion of the lymphatics and bloodvessels. Metastases in the opposite ovary are recorded. Secondary growths are formed in the tubes and ovaries either by local implantation or, in the case of the tubes, by direct infiltration or by a method similar to the transportation of the normal ovum.

Secondary cancer may arise by extension from the neighboring parts, as the uterus or rectum. The primary growth may also be in the breast or stomach. A curious fact is, that in some cases the ovaries are the only seat of secondary growths, and this, together with the additional fact that a considerable length of time (some years) may elapse between the occurrence of the primary tumor and the appearance of the secondary growths, has led to the suspicion that some, at least, of these cases may not be examples of metastasis, but rather of multiple independent neoplasms. This possibly has also to be thought of in those cases where in primary carcinoma of one ovary cancerous nodules have been found in the other. It is not always easy to decide whether they are independent growths or not, but it is quite probable that many are so, when we remember the decided tendency of ovarian growths, benign as well as malignant, to be bilateral.[1] Metastatic deposits originating in distant organs develop through the blood stream, or in cases of abdominal growths, by means of the peritoneum.

Of the connective-tissue tumors, the only ones worthy of note are the **fibroma** and the **sarcoma.**

Fibromas usually form diffuse growths leading to uniform enlargement of the ovary, but circumscribed nodules are occasionally produced. They may be unilateral or bilateral, and may attain a considerable size. Multiple, warty, nodular, or papillary fibromas are occasionally met with, arising from the surface of the ovary. Occasionally fibromas arise from the corpora lutea from overgrowth of the theca and form tumors the size of a walnut. The theca is thickened and thrown into deep folds, while the centre is composed of loose connective tissue of

[1] See Woolley, Boston Jour. Med. and Surg., January 1, 1903: 1; and Nicholls, Montreal Med. Jour., 32; 1903: 326.

soft consistence and grayish or grayish-brown color. Occasionally, these growths contain cavities filled with serous fluid and altered blood pigment. Leo Loeb[1] has recently described a curious fibrocystic tumor, containing numerous cells derived from the lutein tissue, occurring in the ovary of a calf.

Several modifications of fibromatous tumors are described, such as *myofibroma, fibrocystoma, adenofibroma,* and *fibro-adenocystoma.* In some cases osteoid tissue is formed (*fibroma osteoides*) or true bone (*fibroma osseum*). It is doubtful, however, whether true **osteoma** or **chondroma** are ever found in the ovaries. The bloodvessels and lymphatics may be abundant and greatly dilated. Suppuration, gangrene, and calcification may occur in fibromas.

A simple **hemangioma** has been met with by Orth[2] in both the ovaries of a child, associated with angiomas in the skin and internal organs.

Lymphangioma has been described by Leopold[3] and others.

The malignant growths arising from the stroma are **endothelioma, perithelioma,** and **sarcoma.** Marchand[4] was the first to describe endotheliomas, or tumors arising from the lining membrane of bloodvessels and lymphatics, in the ovary. Some originate in the lining cells of the perivascular lymphatics, one form of perithelioma. These tumors vary considerably in appearance. They attain a considerable size, are unilateral or bilateral, and are often soft, spongy, and friable. Occasionally they are cystic.

Histologically, they resemble carcinoma or sarcoma, or one of the many forms of mixed growth. One may see masses of cuboidal, cylindrical, or polyhedral cells, arranged in bands or alveoli, or often more or less definitely enclosing a lumen, which may contain blood or lymph. In these masses giant cells may sometimes be seen. Hyaline degeneration often occurs. The nests of cells are separated by fibrous tissue, occasionally presenting a myxomatous appearance. In some cases the fibrous tissue penetrates the lumina so as to form intracanalicular papillomas. Amann has also described a form of sarcoma (perithelioma) arising from the adventitia of the vessels. The most recent writer, Ribbert, however, it may be said, doubts the existence of tumors arising from the endothelium, and sees no reason for separating peritheliomas from other sarcomas. It should be remarked in this connection that the so-called endotheliomas may in some cases arise from the mesothelial lining of the cœlom, a possibility that does not seem to have suggested itself to the systematic writers.

Sarcoma.—Sarcomas are relatively rare, constituting, according to Schröder, only 1.5 per cent. of all ovarian tumors. They are frequently bilateral, but also unilateral, and may be found in quite young children. The affected ovary may be uniformly enlarged or present a nodular surface. The tumor is moderately hard, and is usually covered with a

---

[1] Virchow's Archiv, 166: 1901: 157.   [2] Lehrb., 2: 1893: 572.
[3] Die soliden Geschwülste der Ovarien., Arch. f. Gyn., 6.
[4] Beitr. z. Kenntn. d. Ovarialtumoren, 1879: 47.

serosa-like membrane. The growth originates in a single focus that gradually enlarges until the whole ovary is involved. Nodular forms are, however, met with.

Histologically, ovarian sarcomas are *spindle-celled* and *round-celled*. *Mixed forms*, however, occur, with or without giant cells, and sometimes containing much fibrous tissue—*fibrosarcoma*. Myxomatous change may often be observed. The growth is usually isolated, although peritoneal adhesions and metastases may occur. Metastasis in distant organs is rare, and is found chiefly in the round-celled variety. In all forms, hyaline and fatty degeneration, necrosis, hemorrhage, and thrombosis may be seen. Martin and Hamilton[1] have recorded an apparently unique case in which there was bilateral mixed-celled sarcoma of the ovaries, with fairly generalized sarcomatosis and purpura. The blood showed a marked leukocytosis of lymphocytic type. The metastases seem in the main to have formed along the perivascular lymphatics, and spindle-celled emboli were found in the vessels of the skin, thus accounting for the purpura.

In some cases the sarcoma cells are seen to be grouped about the small and middle-sized bloodvessels. Von Rosthorn would classify this form with endothelial peritheliomas above mentioned. It should be noted that sarcomatous change may be found concomitantly in adenoma, cystadenoma, carcinoma, and myoma.[2] This, it may be added, is only what is to be expected if the tumors are mesotheliomas, *i. e.*, transitional lepidomas (see vol. i, p. 807).

Teratomas (Embryomata).—Under the term "embryomata," on the ground that they contain, more or less abundantly, structures similar to those found in the embryo, Wilms includes that class of tumors that we generally call dermoids and teratomas. These tumors are generally cystic, and may be simple, composed of structures resembling skin (hence the term "dermoid"), or compound, where in addition to epidermal tissues there are others derived from the mesoblast and hypoblast, teeth, bone, cartilage, muscle, glands, nerve tissue, and mucous membrane.

It should be remarked, however, that the term "dermoid," which has had such extensive vogue, in the light of recent researches has lost much of its significance, if, indeed, it is not now actually misleading. It was commonly held, for example, that the dermoids are cysts composed of more or less modified skin with other structures of epidermal origin. Careful study has shown, however, that even the simplest of them contain structures from the other primitive germ layers. Consequently, the distinction between "dermoid and teratoma" is an artificial one, and had better be discontinued. It is simpler and more correct to class all the growths of this kind under the one generic term "teratoma." If the word "dermoid" be retained at all, it should be employed simply for convenience of description.

<hr>

[1] Jour. Exper. Med., 1: 1896: 595.
[2] Wilms, Die Mischgeschwülste, Leipzig, 1899 and 1902.

Teratomas are rather frequent in the ovaries. They are generally unilateral, sometimes bilateral. More rarely, multiple separate
teratomas are found in one or both ovaries. These tumors are of slow
growth, remain latent for a long time, and usually give rise to symptoms
first during the period of sexual activity. The growths are in the vast
majority of cases cystic, and range in size from that of an apple to a
man's head or larger. They are usually pedunculated and project into
the peritoneal cavity. More rarely, they extend partially between the
layers of the broad ligament.

It is difficult to draw up an entirely satisfactory classification of ovarian
teratomas. Authorities differ somewhat in their conceptions of the condition, and the terminology that has been at times proposed is entirely

FIG. 216

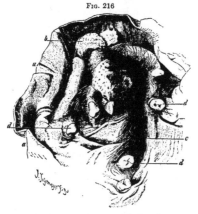

Interior view of an ovarian teratoma ("dermoid cyst"), showing Rokitansky's island
bearing *c*, hairs with *d*, teeth surrounding. (Schwalbe.)

confusing. The nature of teratomas, their relationships to other forms
of growth, the question of monogerminal or bigerminal derivation, have
been fully dealt with elsewhere (vol. i, p. 652 et seq.), and we will not,
therefore, repeat here. The simplest and most direct way of regarding
the question is to group what have been variously known as epidermoids,
dermoids, teratoids, teratomas, and embryomas, under the general term
teratoma. We may then recognize two main types, the *solid* and the
cystic.

1. Solid teratomas may be described in general terms as "mixed"
growths composed of a variety of cells and tissues, which do not, however, tend to form completed organs. Cysts may be present, but are of
small size and are inconspicuous. These tumors are much rarer in the
ovary than are the predominantly cystic forms, but may attain a considerable size (that of a man's head). They are more common in the
testis.

2. Cystic teratomas may be divided into simple and compound. The former include what Orth and Kaufmann term the epidermoids and the true dermoid cysts; the latter include what are variously known as compound dermoids, simple and compound teratomas. The epidermoids possess a wall formed in a general way of modified epidermal elements, while the pure dermoids contain accessory structures of similar nature, such as hair-follicles, sudoriparous and sebaceous glands, hair, and inspissated sebum. The compound dermoids, in addition, contain teeth and bone. Still more complicated forms are met with, presenting structures such as mucous membranes, glands, muscle, brain and nerve substance, rudimentary eyes, intestine, mammæ, fingers, ribs, and extremities. The most complex forms approximate closely to the *fœtus in fœtu*. It should be remarked, however, that such classifications are more or less artificial, for the numerous and careful studies published of late show that even in the simplest forms indications of their development from the three primitive layers are definitely to be made out, thus proving their essential unity.

Teratomas are particularly liable to complications. The pedicle may be twisted, causing anemia and necrosis. Hemorrhages may occur into the substance or into the cavity. The cyst often becomes inflamed and suppurates. It is common to find it more or less bound down by inflammatory adhesions. Peritonitis may result, or the dermoid perforate into the bladder, rectum, vagina, or through the abdominal wall. In the last connection it may be mentioned that Amann[1] has reported a melanotic sarcoma developing in an ovarian dermoid.

Mixed tumors of the ovary usually constitute merely a variation of the forms hitherto described. They may be divided into two classes: (1) those in which two distinct types of tissue develop independently and simultaneously (mixed tumors proper), and (2) those in which we have a modification or transformation occurring secondarily in a previously existing new-growth.*(tumor in tumore)*.

In the first class, of the benign growths may be mentioned **myofibroma, adenofibroma, cystofibroma**; of the malignant, **myosarcoma** (?), **cystosarcoma, cystadenosarcoma**, and **sarcocarcinoma**. In the second group, we may recognize **myxosarcoma, cystadenoma carcinomatodes, cystadenoma sarcomatodes, cystadenomatous, carcinomatous**, or **sarcomatous transformation** of teratomas.

Owing to their structure and position, ovarian tumors, particularly the cystadenomas, are liable to undergo important secondary changes.

Carcinomas show frequently œdema, fatty or mucinous degeneration, hemorrhagic infiltration, or necrosis. Many of these retrogressive changes result in the formation of pseudo- or degenerative cysts. When the tumor is pedunculated, torsion leads not infrequently to strangulation of the bloodvessels and its well-known consequences. The growth becomes swollen and œdematous, the veins are overdistended with blood, and the tissue is often infarcted and necrotic. In such cases infection

---

[1] Monatssch. f. Geb. u. Gyn., January, 1903.

and suppuration readily take place. Sometimes the pedicle is completely severed and the growth lies free in the abdominal cavity, where it will necrose unless it become vascularized through new adhesions forming about it.

Peritonitis is also not uncommon. Should the cyst-wall rupture, the contents, if unirritating, may be absorbed, but if infected, set up septic peritonitis. In the case of rupture of a cystadenoma, the pseudomucinous material is only imperfectly absorbed, and part of it may become encysted through the formation of inflammatory adhesions, giving rise to a structure resembling at first sight a tumor (*pseudomyxoma*).

Hyaline and calcareous degeneration in the wall have also been observed. Secondary tuberculous infection of an ovarian cyst has been recorded.

THE UTERINE LIGAMENTS: THE PELVIC PERITONEUM AND CONNECTIVE TISSUE.

CONGENITAL ANOMALIES.

In cases of complete defect of the uterus the ligaments are also **absent**. When, however, the tubes and ovaries are present the round ligaments are often well-formed. One round ligament may be **shorter** than the other, leading to dislocation of the uterus. **Reduplication** of the round ligaments has been observed. A comparatively common anomaly is the **persistence**, either partial or complete, of the **canal of Nuck**, causing hernia and hydrocele. **Remains** of the **parovarium** and its attendant ducts may give rise to disturbance.

CIRCULATORY DISTURBANCES.

The veins of the round and broad ligaments and those in the neighborhood of the ovaries may be dilated and tortuous (**varicocele**). **Thrombosis** frequently occurs, with the formation of phleboliths.

Hemorrhage.—Of more importance is hemorrhage, which may be intraperitoneal or extraperitoneal. This usually takes place between the layers of the broad ligament or in the round ligament. The most common causes are, the rupture of a vessel during parturition, more rarely during menstruation; the giving way of a varicose vein; and tubal gestation. The extravasation may be extensive and remain more or less localized, forming a tumor-like mass (**hematoma**). In other cases it infiltrates the connective tissue about the uterus, bladder, and rectum, and exceptionally may be discharged into the vagina or rectum. In other instances the blood is effused into the abdominal cavity (**hematocele**). The usual site for this is the Douglas' pouch (*hema-*

tocele retro-uterina). Rarely it is into the uterovesical pouch (*hema-tocele ante-uterina*). This form is due to an extensive effusion, or to the fact that the Douglas' pouch has been obliterated by inflammatory products. The most frequent causes are, ruptured tubal gestation and hemorrhagic peritonitis, where there is a formation of new vessels. Less commonly, it may be due to the rupture of a vein in the broad ligament, a ruptured Graafian follicle, a cyst or varicose vein of the ovary, hematosalpinx, the operative ablation of an ovary, and the discharge of blood through the abdominal ostia of the tube. The blood is not necessarily free in the cavity, for it may happen that it is extravasated into a sac formed of previously existing adhesions. In many cases, from reactive inflammation, a fibrous limiting wall is produced. Provided the patient survive, the blood may be absorbed or the resulting clot may become organized after the fashion of a thrombus. In this way a pigmented mass of fibrous tissue may be produced. In less favorable cases, where infection has occurred, the mass may be converted into an abscess. This may discharge into the bowel or, rarely, into the abdominal cavity, bladder, or vagina. In this way fecal fistulæ are produced that often lead to extensive disorganization of the pelvic connective tissue. Some few cases, after the discharge of the pus, may heal.

INFLAMMATIONS.

Inflammation about the uterus and its appendages, both in the overlying serous membrane and in the loose connective tissue of the pelvis, is not uncommon. According to the localization of the process to the serosa covering the uterus, tubes, and ovaries, we can speak of a **perimetritis, perisalpingitis,** and **perioöphoritis.** When the connective tissue is involved the condition is termed **parametritis.**

Parametritis.—In **simple exudative parametritis,** the tissues are œdematous and sodden. No clear line can, however, be drawn between this and the suppurative form, where the tissue is diffusely infiltrated with pus or presents abscess-formation. In very severe cases the structures become gangrenous. The pus may remain localized or may burrow along the ligaments to the abdominal wall, into the thigh, into the pelvis, or behind the rectum. In this way caries of the bony parts may be produced. Perforation may occur in the inguinal region, in the ischiadic fossa, the vagina, rectum, or bladder. Should healing take place, the abscess becomes encapsulated and more or less absorbed, or the whole of the affected area may be converted into a dense mass of fibrous tissue.

The commonest causes of parametritis are injuries during parturition, and puerperal sepsis. The inflammation occasionally spreads from the rectum. An actinomycotic form is also described.

A fibrinous or fibrinopurulent inflammation is frequently observed in the Douglas' pouch (**pelvic peritonitis**). It is due to the extension of inflammation from any of the pelvic organs, and is met with also in carcinoma, tuberculosis, and ovarian cysts. Abundant adhesions may form so that the pus is completely walled off from the abdominal cavity (*retrouterine pyocele*). As in the case of suppurative parametritis, the pus may be discharged into the rectum, vagina, bladder, the general peritoneal cavity, or externally. The causes are the same as those of parametritis, except that here gonorrhœa plays an important role. The process results in the formation of dense, fibrous masses or adhesions between the various parts (*productive pelvic peritonitis*). This may lead to the occlusion of the tubes and dislocation of the tubes and ovaries. When the adhesions are extensive, pockets may be formed, filled with clear, seropurulent, or colloid-looking fluid.

Tuberculosis.—Tuberculosis of the ligaments is always secondary to tuberculosis of the Fallopian tubes or general peritoneum.

RETROGRESSIVE METAMORPHOSES.

Atrophy of the round ligaments accompanies atrophy of the uterus, or may follow parametritis and rapidly recurring pregnancies.

After the menopause the vessels of the broad ligaments frequently become tortuous, thickened, and **calcareous.**

PROGRESSIVE METAMORPHOSES.

The round ligaments are often **hypertrophied** in cases of hypertrophy of · the uterus. Hypertrophy of the muscle of the broad ligaments occurs in connection with ovarian and parovarian cysts.

Tumors.—The majority of the tumors found in the broad ligaments are due to the extension of growths of the uterus and ovaries between the layers. Subserous myofibromas of the uterus sometimes grow out into the broad ligament and may be eventually detached from the uterus. **Lipomas, leiomyomas,** and **myxofibromas** have been found both in the broad and round ligaments. Cullen[1] has recorded an example of **adenomyoma** of the round ligament, and three cases have been described since (Pfannenstiel, v. Heuff, Blumer). The growth is composed of non-striated muscle fibres, together with glandular elements strongly resembling the glands of the uterine mucosa. The tumor has been found also within the groin and in the vagina. It is thought to be derived from remains of the Wolffian body (v. Recklinghausen), or possibly from the Müllerian duct.

Cysts.—By far the most common tumor-like masses in the uterine ligaments are the cysts. These may be cysts of the ovaries that have

---

[1] Johns Hopkins Hosp. Bull., 62–63: 1896: 112; Ibid., 87: 1898: 142.

extended into the broad ligament, cysts derived from the parovarium, or, very rarely, from the paroöphoron between the parovarium and the uterus.

Parovarian cysts vary greatly in size, but may be as large as a man's head. The growth lies at first between the abdominal end of the tube and the ovary. The tube may to some extent encircle it, but in the case of the larger growths is, of course, elongated, more or less flattened, and atrophic. The ovary is also much flattened so that it may be difficult if not impossible to find it. As the cyst develops between the two layers

FIG. 217

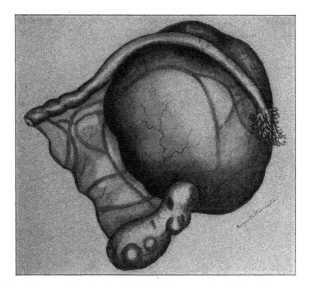

Cyst of the parovarium; there is no distortion of the ovary; the Fallopian tube has been much elongated. (BeYea.)

of the peritoneum, it is covered externally by loose connective tissue and serosa, which can usually be readily stripped off. As a rule, it possesses no pedicle and the wall is thin, being composed of connective tissue and more or less hypertrophic muscle derived from the muscle of the broad ligament. The wall internally sometimes presents flattened or papillary outgrowths, in some part, at least, of the surface. The contained fluid is clear and watery with relatively little albumin, no pseudo-mucin, and few cells. Its specific gravity is low, 1004 to 1005.

In other cases it is more viscid and may be mixed with blood. wall is lined with ciliated cylindrical cells, although in some cas cells are somewhat flattened and the cilia lost.

Rarely, **teratomas** have been found in the pelvic connective tiss

Primary **sarcoma** has been recorded occasionally in the broad lig and on the surface of the uterus (Sänger).

Carcinoma is always secondary and generally arises by extension the cervix uteri or ovary. Occasionally it is produced by lym metastasis.

CHAPTER XXXIX.

AFFECTIONS OF THE PUERPERAL UTERUS.

CIRCULATORY DISTURBANCES.

DURING the act of parturition, and for some time subsequent to it, a certain amount of blood is lost, chiefly from the placental site. Occasionally, this passes physiological limits, and the bleeding may be so severe as to endanger the life of the individual (**postpartum hemorrhage**). Bleeding also takes place from the lacerations of the cervix normally produced during labor, or from actual rupture of the corpus uteri.

Placental remains that have been retained within the uterus give rise frequently to **menorrhagia** and **metrorrhagia**. Such placental tissue may become crusted over with fibrin and form large polypoid masses (fibrinous placental polyps). A noteworthy form of metrorrhagia is that where in extra-uterine gestation the decidua is cast off with discharge of blood.

INJURIES. (See also p. 873.)

Lacerations of greater or less extent occur commonly in the cervix during labor. Rarely, the fundus of the uterus is ruptured. The uterus may be perforated by instruments during operations and in attempts at criminal abortion. It may also be injured by contusions of the abdomen, bullet wounds, and the horns of animals.

INFLAMMATIONS.

Inflammations of the puerperal uterus may be purely local, but frequently give rise to systemic manifestations (**puerperal fever**). The endometrium, the muscular wall, or the serosa may be involved (**endometritis puerperalis, metritis puerp., perimetritis puerp.**).

The process usually begins, as one would expect, at the point of primary injury, such as the cervix and the placental site, and may extend to any part of the uterus.

Endometritis.—Two main types of puerperal endometritis are to be recognized, the **putrid** and the **septic**. The former is characterized by the decomposition of the lining membrane of the uterus with the production of foul gases; the latter, by various forms of necrosis, coagulation, or suppuration. The two are not infrequently combined.

Putrid Endometritis.—Putrid endometritis originates in retained fœtal products, stagnated blood, pent-up lochia, or sequestrating portions of the uterus, to which putrefactive microörganisms have gained access, either directly through manual or instrumental manipulation, or by extension from the vagina and vulva.

The uterus in advanced cases is enlarged, the wall thickened and œdematous, and in parts congested. The endometrium is converted into a dirty green or brownish-black, pulpy mass having a very offensive odor. The process may extend to the muscle which, in time, becomes soft and rotten (**putrid metritis**). Physometra may be produced.

Microscopically, the affected tissue, when decay is advanced, is cloudy and the nuclei stain badly, while numerous bacteria of many kinds are present. At the periphery the necrotic portion is bounded by a zone of inflammatory leukocytes.

The process leads to the sequestration of uterine tissue and sometimes to the formation of fistulæ between the uterus, or the uterus and vagina and the bladder. Perforation into the peritoneal cavity is rare. Masses of clot at the placental site may be involved in the necrotic process (*putrid thrombosinusitis*). When a strong line of demarcation is formed, portions of the endometrium or even of the muscle may be exfoliated (**metritis diseccans**). Complete cure may result with the formation of scars and contraction.

Septic Endometritis.—Septic endometritis, in its simplest expression, consists in superficial suppuration, which is particularly liable to involve the site of the cervical lacerations, converting them into discharging ulcers. More commonly there is the formation of a grayish adherent membrane, perhaps limited to the eroded surfaces, although at times it may extend over the greater part of the uterine cavity. When affecting the placental site, the membrane is most marked on the top of the prominences of the uneven uterine wall and may be slight or absent in the fissures. It can, in some instances, be peeled off, but, as a rule, the necrotic process extends some little distance into the deeper tissues. The surface of the affected area is usually dry and of a dirty grayish- or brownish-green color.

Microscopically, the superficial layers of the placental site show necrosis, the cells staining badly, while there is a thick network of fibrin often presenting a certain amount of hyaline transformation. Upon the surface is an exudate of similar appearance. Small masses of lenkocytes can also be seen both in the membrane and in the underlying necrotic tissue. The glands show more or less erosion, with degenerative changes, and the lumina may contain fibrin. Bounding the necrotic area is a zone of inflammatory leukocytes with great hyperemia. Small clusters of micrococci can generally be demonstrated. The process often spreads to the uterine muscle, and cases occur where the wall is affected from the start (**septic metritis**).

Endometritis Decidualis.—A variety of inflammation affecting the lining membrane of the uterus, that should be mentioned, is that involving the decidua (endometritis decidualis). This rarely occurs except when the patient is suffering from some infectious disease, notably cholera or measles. As a rule, it is traceable to preëxisting endometritis, but may be due to infection in cases of abortion. The process may occur in all parts of the decidua and is of the nature of a productive fibrosis. The decidua is thickened and often presents nodular or polypoid out-growths (*endometritis decidualis polyposa*). The tissue is dense and firm and has lost the normal yellowish-white appearance. In some cases the surface may be covered with pus. Occasionally, secretion collects between the deciduæ and gives rise to discharge (*hydrorrhœa gravidarum*).

Microscopically, the large decidual cells are increased in size and numbers, and present fatty degeneration. The tissue is infiltrated with round cells and shows marked productive change. The glands in the deeper parts are rarely increased and still more rarely dilated. In the lower strata, the lymph-channels may be considerably distended, giving to the tissue a cavernous structure. Hemorrhage readily occurs so that abortion is frequent, or there is the formation of a blood or fleshy mole. The placenta sometimes also becomes adherent.

Septic Metritis.—Septic metritis may be diffuse (*m. phlegmonosa*), or again the infective process may extend along the lymphatics (*m. lymphangitica*) or veins (*m. thrombophlebitica*).

Phlegmonous Metritis.—In phlegmonous metritis, the uterine muscle is relaxed, soft, swollen, and œdematous, and has a doughy feel. The interstices of the muscle contain an abundant thin, blood-stained fluid, or actual pus. The condition is generally best marked in the outer layers of the wall.

Microscopically, there is a more or less abundant accumulation of leukocytes in the interstitial stroma, which is also œdematous. The muscle fibres are swollen, cloudy, and vitreous. Clusters of micrococci may be seen. This form is frequently combined with lymphangitis.

Lymphangitic Metritis.—In lymphangitic metritis one can recognize in the uterine wall and adjacent parts, dilated lymph-channels containing detritus and pus. On cross-section, the lymphatics appear as cavities, the size of a pea or larger, filled with yellowish material composed of fibrin, pus cells, and bacteria. The walls of the lymphatics show various grades of degeneration and may give way, so that irregular abscesses are formed by the extension of the infection. These abscesses are often very numerous, and may sometimes be seen projecting upon the serous surface. This form of metritis is liable to occur in cases of infection that are running a not very acute course.

Thrombophlebitic Metritis.—Thrombophlebitic metritis is somewhat rarer, and begins generally at the placental site. Atony of the uterus predisposes strongly to the condition, but not infrequently membranous endometritis is present as well. Large thrombi are found in the veins, presenting all grades of softening, necrosis, and purulent infiltration.

The appearances are analogous to those in lymphangitis of the uterus. The process may spread to the para-uterine veins and even to the spermatica interna.

In all forms of septic metritis the process may extend widely from its original starting point. The inflammation may reach the parametrium and the retroperitoneal tissues. Large abscesses in the connective tissue may result. Lymphangitis sometimes extends to the ovaries and along the vertebral column to the diaphragm. Thrombophlebitis may extend to the femoral veins and the inferior vena cava. Peritonitis (*perimetritis*) is not uncommon, and may spread to the pleura and pericardium. *Septicemia* is a not infrequent sequel. *Ulcerative endocarditis* and *abscesses* in the various viscera have been observed.

Puerperal Perimetritis.—Puerperal perimetritis is characterized by the formation upon the serosa of the uterus of an exudate that is fibrinous, fibrinopurulent, or purulent, according to the nature and intensity of the infection. In the more chronic cases, the deposit becomes gradually organized, adhesions form, and the exudation may be walled off. In acute cases, general peritonitis may occur. When healing takes place, bands of adhesions may dislocate the uterus from its normal position.

With regard to the etiology of puerperal sepsis, the exciting cause is the presence of septic or putrefactive microörganisms. The most important offenders, in order of frequency, are, Streptococcus pyogenes, Staphylococcus albus and aureus, and Diplococcus pneumoniæ.

PROGRESSIVE METAMORPHOSES.

Tumors.—Pregnancy may of course occur in a uterus that is already the site of tumor growth. Among these may be mentioned myofibroma and carcinoma, but the only tumor that need specially be discussed here is a very remarkable one—the **chorio-epithelioma malignum**—first described by Sänger.

Many differing opinions have been advanced as to its nature, as may be gathered from the variety of names that have been proposed for it—deciduoma malignum (Pfeiffer), syncytioma malignum, deciduosarcoma, chorio-epithelioma, syncytial carcinoma, sarcoma deciduochoriocellulare. It is now, however, practically settled that it is a new-growth originating in the fœtal epiblast of the chorionic villi. Consequently, being a tumor of fœtal origin, growing in the tissues of another individual—the maternal organism—it should be classed with the teratomas, or at least as a teratogenous blastoma (vol. i, p. 664). Inasmuch as it grows rapidly, infiltrates, and forms metastases in distant parts, it is of malignant character.

The tumor only develops after pregnancy. It may occur after normal parturition, after abortion, after the expulsion of a hydatidiform mole, and in extra-uterine gestation. The growth may remain latent for a considerable time after delivery. It usually begins in the chorium frondrosum, but may arise from any part of the uterus to which chorionic villi are attached. It is said by Schmorl that chorionic villi may be detached and carried to distant parts where the cells may proliferate and form a primary chorio-epithelioma extra-uterine in situation.

Chorio-epithelioma tends to form polypoid or fungating growths projecting into the uterine cavity, but eventually invades the muscle beneath the endometrium and may infiltrate more or less deeply. The mass is of reddish color, frequently hemorrhagic, and is of a soft, friable, and spongy nature.

Microscopically, according to Webster,[1] three types are to be differentiated: (1) Where the primary growth and metastases are of sarcomatous or carcinomatous type, or both; (2) where, in addition, to the appearances just mentioned, syncytial or plasmodial masses may be recognized; and (3) where in addition to the structures of the second group, there are cell-masses resembling placental villi.

Fig. 218

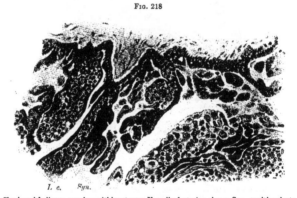

Chorio-epithelioma growing within uterus: *V*, wall of uterine sinus; *Syn.*, multinucleate cells of syncytial type; *L.c.*, cells of Langhans' type. (Teacher.)

The growth is seen to originate in the proliferation of the syncytium and Langhans' layer of the chorionic villi. The normal relationships are disturbed, the syncytium is thickened, and the cells of the Langhans' layer tend to extend through to the surface. The superficial area is generally necrotic and covered with a deposit of fibrin. The deeper parts present an alveolar structure, the spaces possessing no epithelial lining and containing blood and fibrin. The resulting tumor has no stroma and no bloodvessels.

The so-called syncytial elements, when present, are large, irregular, or elongated plasmodial masses, containing numerous deeply-staining nuclei. The protoplasm is finely granular and may contain vacuoles.

[1] Canadian Practitioner, 22 : 1897 : 714.

The plasmodia are well defined but their protoplasm may, in certain parts, pass imperceptibly into that of the surrounding tissue.   It must be admitted that these plasmodial cells are not necessarily of syncytial origin, for identical appearances are to be found in other malignant growths, notably sarcomas, originating in other parts of the body.

The cells derived from Langhans' layer form groups of varying size. They are irregular in shape, long, spindle, or spherical, with pale protoplasm.   When not pressed upon, they have an epithelial appearance. The nuclei often show mitosis.   In many cases the cells of Langhans are grouped about the plasmodial masses, but in other cases the latter

FIG. 219

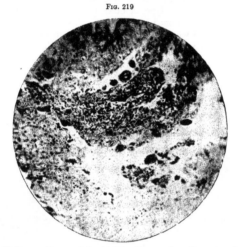

Chorio-epithelioma malignum.   Zeiss obj. DD, without ocular.   (From the collection of
the Montreal General Hospital.)

are in excess and arranged in more or less parallel rows with their long axes at right angles to the base of the tumor.   As in the normal chorion, these cells tend to erode and grow within the uterine vessels.   Hence, hemorrhages and necroses are common, as also are metastases along the course of the bloodstream, in the vagina, lungs, and occasionally in the ovaries, liver, and spleen.   The most frequent site for the secondary deposits is the vagina, which is involved in half the cases.   The lining of the uterus in the neighborhood of the growth takes the form of a decidual membrane or a normal or more or less inflamed endometrium.

THE PRODUCTS OF CONCEPTION.

Apart from the decidua, these are the placenta, the cord, the amnion the amniotic fluid, and the fœtus.

The Placenta.

An abnormally large placenta is found when the child·is large. The placenta may be unusually thin, although the villi may be hypertrophied. (**placenta membranacea**). Instead of one placenta, from one to seven have been observed, even in the case of only one child (**p. duplex, triplex,** etc.). When in addition to a large placenta, several subsidiary ones are met with, the smaller are called **placentæ succenturiatæ**.

An otherwise normal placenta when in an abnormal position, that is in the lower uterine segment, is called **placenta prævia**. Several varieties of this may be recognized. *Placenta prævia centralis* is the form in which the centre of the placenta lies over the internal os. In *partial* placenta prævia the internal os is covered, but the margins of the placenta are not equidistant from the central axis. In *lateral* placenta prævia the edge of the placenta reaches nearly to the internal os. When the placenta projects slightly over and into the internal os it is termed *placenta prævia marginalis*. The condition is not common, and is especially rare in primiparæ. Various theories have been advanced to account for the condition, such as fructification of the ovum when in a false position, and irregular growth and vascularization of certain parts of the decidua, with atrophy of others (Hofmeier,[1] Kaltenbach[2]).

The predisposing cause seems to be endometritis. Not infrequently, myofibromas of the uterus are present and the placenta usually presents some abnormality also.

Ischemia.—Ischemia is produced by the obstruction of the circulation in the umbilical arteries, and in those cases where at birth the umbilical vessels have been severed without tying them.

Hyperemia.—Torsion, looping, compression of the cord, and thickening of the umbilical vein lead to hyperemia.

Hemorrhage.—By far the most important circulatory disturbance is hemorrhage, inasmuch as it is one of the most important causes of abortion. Hemorrhage may occur in the decidua serotina, or in the placenta and membranes and leads to more or less complete separation of the maternal and fœtal organisms.

Hemorrhage into the placenta takes the form of dark red nodules of coagulated blood in the intervillous spaces and blood sinuses. It comes on suddenly and leads to compression of the villi, with some destruction of tissue. The pigment is gradually absorbed, leaving a pale, brownish or brownish-yellow area which finally undergoes organization. with the formation of a fibrous patch (*placental infarct*).

Œdema.—Œdema of the placenta is found in cases of syphilis, hydramnios, and in hydremia. The placenta is large, pale, juicy, and somewhat friable.

Syphilis.—Syphilis of the placenta usually takes the form of a cellular infiltration and œdema of the villi. Widespread gummatous degeneration is unknown. Endarteritis is rarely a marked feature, but may

[1] D. menschl. Placenta, 1890.   [2] Zeitschr. f. Geb. u. Gynäk., 18:1890:1.

lead to obstruction of the circulation with infarction and fibrin deposit in the intervillous spaces (see also vol. i, p. 223).

Degenerations.—Hyaline Degeneration and Necrosis.—Hyaline degeneration and necrosis occur in the chorionic villi as a result of grave circulatory disturbances, such as infarct.

Fatty Degeneration.—Fatty degeneration is also largely due to circulatory disturbances.

Calcification.—Calcification often follows fatty degeneration, and is found in the villi. It is met with early in syphilitic embryos.

Hypertrophy.—Hypertrophy of the chorionic villi may occur as a result of increased demands of function, or in association with inflammation. It is possible that in cases of extensive destruction of the chorion certain villi undergo compensatory overgrowth. A form of hypertrophy, or rather hyperplasia, is found in cases of abortion. and also after normal labor, where portions of the placenta or chorion are retained and take on overgrowth, leading to the formation of the so-called placental polyps. Malignant transformation may take place in such cases (chorioepithelioma malignum).

FIG. 220

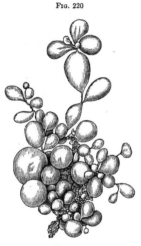

A small portion of an hydatidiform mole; natural size.

A peculiar and striking manifestation allied to hypertrophy is the **cystic** or **hydatidiform mole** (myxoma chorii—Virchow). Here, in addition to hypertrophy of the villi, there is cystic metamorphosis. The villi become extraordinarily lengthened and branched, and are converted into numbers of round, oval, or elongated vesicles containing a clear, viscid, or slightly blood-stained fluid. The appearance produced bears a general resemblance to a bunch of grapes. The condition is due to the infiltration of the enlarged chorionic villi with abundant gelatinous fluid not unlike the Wharton's jelly. The extent of the change varies. In very young embryos the whole chorion may be affected, but it is more common for the placenta alone to be involved. On liberating the fluid, a delicate meshwork or supporting stroma is disclosed.

Microscopically, one finds a delicate, connective-tissue framework with but few cells, covered by an epithelial layer. Sometimes the growth is very vascular.

It is an important practical point that these moles occasionally take on malignant action and invade the wall of the uterus. Neumann[1] has

---

[1] Ueber Blasenmole u. malignes Deciduom. Verhandl. d. deutschen Gesellsch. f. Gynäk., 1897:304.

reported eight cases of hydatidiform mole in three of·which chorio-epithelioma subsequently developed. Pestalozza[1] has also met with a case where one of these moles eroded into the vessels and gave rise to numerous metastases.

Apart from the ordinary mole of the placenta just described, Virchow recognized a form in which the nodules present a connective-tissue character, rather than the usual myxomatous appearance (*myxoma fibrosum*). Increase in the embryonic connective tissue that normally is present between the chorion and the amnion gives rise to the so-called *diffuse myxoma* of the chorion.

Tumors.—Fibroma, fibromyoma (Alin), and angioma have been described. The occurrence of true sarcoma is not proved. The sarcomas of the placenta described by Hyrtl and Waldeyer are probably to be classified as chorio-epitheliomas.

Small cysts of doubtful origin are occasionally seen in the placenta.

The Cord.

The cord may be abnormally long or short. In the first case it may be encircled about the neck of the foetus and cause strangulation; in the latter it may be a hindrance to birth and be torn off violently.

The cord may be inserted eccentrically in the placenta (insertio marginalis), or the umbilical vessels pass first to the membranes before reaching the placenta (insertio velamentosa). The cord may also divide into several trunks. The omphalomesenteric duct at the attachment of the cord may be imperfectly closed leading to hernial protrusion of the intestines or other organs (hernia of the cord).

The cord may be twisted or looped about the neck, trunk, extremities, or breech of the foetus (Fig. 221). In the earlier stages of the development it may cause amputation of certain parts. It may also become knotted, with resultant arrest of the circulation and death of the foetus.

Thrombosis of the umbilical vein and hemorrhage into the cord has been described.

Fatty degeneration and calcification are occasionally observed.

Septic infection of the foetal end of the cord is sometimes met with, leading to arteritis and phlebitis.

Periarteritis and endarteritis, with cellular infiltration and fibrous induration, may occur.

Syphilis.—According to Thomsen[2] the most common syphilitic manifestation is an extensive small-celled infiltration.

Chorionic and allantoic cysts are found at both the foetal and placental ends of the cord.

Myxoma and angioma are met with, but rarely.

[1] Il Morgagni, October, 1891.
[2] Ziegler's Beiträge, 38:1905:524.

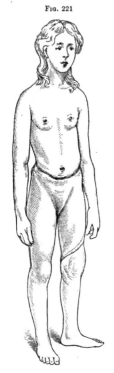

FIG. 221

Girl, aged ten years, showing cicatricial grooves due to constriction of umbilical cord. At birth, according to the mother, the grooves in the abdominal wall and left thigh were occupied by the cord. (Hawthorne.)

The Amnion.

The amnion may be **imperfectly formed** and **fuse** with the fœtus in certain regions. It may thus form bands and adhesions. These are important, inasmuch as they may produce arrest of development and malformation in the affected parts, or again, by obstructing the circulation may produce giant growth.[1]

Little is known with regard to the inflammatory affections of the amnion. **Amnionitis** (Ahlfield) is mentioned, as well as **periarteritis** and **endarteritis**.

The Amniotic Fluid.

The amniotic fluid is sometimes increased in amount (**hydramnios, polyhydramnios**), or it may be diminished (**oligohydramnios**). From contamination with meconium or putrefactive germs, the fluid may become foul, cloudy, discolored, and full of bubbles of gas. The amniotic fluid also becomes altered in cases of maceration of the fœtus, although generally without putrefaction. Various drugs administered to the mother may appear in the fluid.

The Fœtus.

Death of the fœtus may arise from a variety of causes and leads to several curious results. If it be not discharged prematurely (*abortion*), it may be retained within the uterus for weeks or months, leading to atrophy and necrotic changes in the various structures. In some cases the fœtus becomes **macerated** or undergoes a form of **mummification**. Should pressure be exerted upon it, it may be flattened out to the thinness of paper (**fœtus papyraceus**). Rarely, calcification takes place (**lithopedion**). In the event of microörganisms gaining access to the uterus, putrefaction of its contents and sepsis may occur.

[1] Klaussner, Ueber Missbildungen der menschlichen Gliedmassen, Wiesbaden, Bergman, 1905.

The most potent cause of death of the fœtus is syphilis, either by producing a generalized weakness of the system, or by cutting off the blood supply through placental disease. In a macerated fœtus it is often possible to find evidences of syphilis at the epiphyses of the bones and in the viscera. Other causes that should be mentioned are pathological changes in the membranes, placenta, or cord, and constitutional disease in the mother (Bright's disease; eclampsia).

Malformations.—Malformations, apart from developmental anomalies, may arise from mechanical causes. Such are, too small an amount of the amniotic fluid, adhesion of the membranes, and the pressure of bands traversing the amniotic sac. (See vol. i, p. 215 et seq.)

Fig. 222

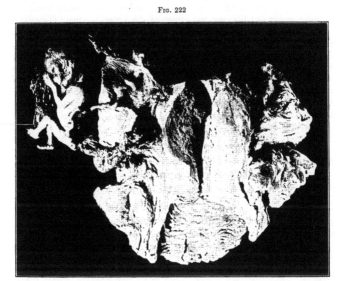

Tubal ectopic gestation. The uterus and vagina are opened from the front. The right Fallopian tube is greatly distended and is ruptured. The fœtus and cord are also shown. (From the Gynecological Clinic of the Montreal General Hospital.)

The developmental anomalies are of great interest. Such conditions as dwarfism, gigantism, chondrodystrophia, micromelia, osteopsathyrosis are discussed elsewhere (p. 1051 et seq.; also vol. i, p. 224).

Ectopic Gestation.—When the embryo develops in an abnormal situation, the condition is called ectopic gestation. Of this there are several varieties.

Intra-uterine Ectopic Gestation.—Gestation may occur within the cavity of the uterus but in an abnormal position (intra-uterine ectopic gestation). Thus, the embryo may lie in a rudimentary horn of the uterus or in a diverticulum from its wall. The embryo has also been found in the lower uterine segment, in the cervical canal, and even in the vagina. The latter cases are, however, more correctly to be regarded as forms of abortion than of ectopic gestation.

Interstitial Ectopic Gestation.—A second form is interstitial ectopic gestation. Here in most cases pregnancy occurs in the uterine portion of a Fallopian tube (*interstitial tubal gestation*).

Extra-uterine Gestation.—The third, and most frequent form, is extra-uterine gestation. This takes place in the free portion of the tube, as a rule about the middle. In these cases it generally happens that some time between the second and fifth month the tube ruptures and the fœtus is extruded into the peritoneal cavity. Very rarely, tubal pregnancy may go on to full term. This occurs most commonly when the embryo grows out between the layers of the broad ligament (*intraligamentous tubal gestation*). Occasionally, pregnancy occurs in the infundibulum, and the embryo may project into the abdominal cavity (*tubo-abdominal gestation*). In this case discharge of the fœtus into the abdominal cavity readily takes place (*tubal abortion*). In those cases where the fimbriæ closely embrace the ovary, so that it lies in close contact with the abdominal opening of the tube, or where a tuboövarian cyst has existed into which a ripe follicle has ruptured, we may speak of a *tuboövarian gestation*.

Ovarian Gestation.—Ovarian gestation is excessively rare, but undoubtedly occurs. The first case was reported by Katherine van Tussenbroeck at the Third International Congress of Gynecology and Obstetrics at Amsterdam (1899). Others have been described since by Thompson and Clarence Webster.[1] True ovarian gestation may occur, or the ovario-abdominal form.

Abdominal Gestation.—The last variety of extra-uterine gestation is the abdominal. It is open to question whether a pure form of abdominal gestation exists, that is, where an ovum has been discharged into the abdominal cavity and has been fertilized, either while within the ovary or after its liberation. Possibly, a more critical analysis of the cases reported would show that they were primarily tubal or ovarian. Gutierrez[2] has, however, recently reported a case that is almost convincing. He found, in a woman aged thirty-four years, a mature fœtus in a sac within the abdomen attached to the great omentum and parietal peritoneum. The placenta was inserted on the great omentum.

Cases of what may be termed *secondary* abdominal pregnancy occur, where through rupture of the sac the fœtus is discharged into the abdominal cavity. So long as the placenta remains *in situ* and communication is kept up with the mother, development is possible.

In ectopic gestation the uterus undergoes changes in kind, although not in degree, strictly comparable to those occurring under normal conditions. The muscle hypertrophies, a decidual membrane is formed, and the cervix may partially dilate. The decidua in time may be cast off.

[1] Amer. Journ. of Obstetrics, 50: 1904: 28.
[2] Révista Ibero-Americana de Ciencias Medicas, March, 1904.

Apart from those rare cases of interstitial pregnancy where delivery takes place *per vias naturales*, the fœtus invariably dies. When small, the products of conception may be completely absorbed, but usually this is not possible, and the fœtus, when discharged into the abdominal cavity, becomes encapsulated and degenerates. Mummification, maceration, or calcareous infiltration may occur. Occasionally, the membranes alone become calcified (*lithokelyphos*). With regard to the effects on the mother, tubal gestation is the most dangerous, as rupture of the tube almost invariably takes place after the earlier months, and may lead to sudden and fatal hemorrhage. Blood may be effused freely into the abdominal cavity (hematocele) or may become more or less encapsulated owing to reactive peritonitis (hematoma).

The causes of extra-uterine gestation are various. The most potent are all conditions that interfere with the natural passage of the ovum down the Fallopian tube to the uterus. Fructification may occur in a tube and the ovum be retained owing to salpingitis, kinks, tubal polyps, compression, diverticula, or defects in the ciliated epithelium. Among inflammatory causes, gonorrhœal salpingitis plays an important part.

CHAPTER XL.

THE MAMMARY GLAND.

FROM the point of view of development and structure there is no essential difference between the male and female breast. In the male, however, with rare exceptions, the organ remains rudimentary and, therefore, functionless, throughout life. In the female, with the onset of puberty, certain developmental forces are set in motion, looking toward the preparation of the breast for its important function of lactation, and resulting in a peculiarity of type which, among other things, differentiates the one sex from the other. The breast in the case of both sexes is susceptible to the same diseases, with the qualification that owing to the greater functional activity in the female the organ is much more frequently involved than in the male. Particularly is this true of inflammation.

The breast is formed by a downward proliferation of the epidermis, according to Minot, from the sudoriparous glands; according to others, from the sebaceous glands. At birth the organ is at most 2 cm. across by 1 cm. thick. The glandular portion consists in from ten to twenty ducts, arranged radially, which discharge in a small depression in the nipple. These ducts are lined by cylindrical epithelium or stratified pavement cells, and end in club-like enlargements. During the first few weeks after birth the proliferative activity may be so great that the ducts become distended with masses of epithelial cells and granular detritus. The breast becomes enlarged and possibly somewhat painful. Frequently a milk-like fluid can be expressed, to which, in some countries, the popular name of "witch's milk" is given. The dilatation may in some cases be so extreme that a cavernous structure is produced (Kölliker). In both sexes up to the age of puberty there is only a slight further development.

As puberty is approached, the various ducts produce a few side branches, which to some extent bifurcate and form in turn club-like terminations. In the male, complete development, so far as it goes, is reached about the twentieth year, when the breast measures from 4 to 5 cm. in breadth. Only rarely does it develop further, as in pseudo-hermaphroditismus masculinus. In the female, however, the formation of side branches and end bulbs is more extensive, especially in the deeper parts of the organ, although the transition to a perfect acinous gland is still incomplete. The glandular elements are composed of a structureless basement membrane lined by short cylindrical cells, and are surrounded by a zone of firm, almost hyaline, connective tissue. Besides the regular ducts, in the lobules are to be seen solid masses of epithelial cells bounded by a basement membrane. These various parts are held together by a firm connective-tissue stroma containing elastic fibrils and fat; about the larger ducts in the nipple fibres of unstriped muscle are present. The changes incident to the onset of puberty may be so marked, both in boys and girls, that the breasts become swollen and tender and a milk-like secretion is produced.

It is only, however, at the onset of lactation that the breast attains its full development. Numerous side branches and end bulbs are produced, so that regular acini are formed, which now present a definite lumen. The lining epithelium is a single layer of cylindrical cells more or less flattened from the accumulation of secretion. The basement membrane is composed of subepithelial flat cells, that about the end bulbs assume a stellate appearance, but about the ducts are more spindle-like, with their long axes the way of the ducts. Outside the membrane is the hyaline zone, and then a kind of adventitia composed of a cellular and vascular connective tissue. The stroma, as a whole, is softer, more juicy, and congested. After the cessation of lactation the gland-tubules collapse and diminish somewhat in size, while the connective-tissue stroma is again relatively increased. It never again, however, attains its former firmness and consistency.

After the menopause the acini atrophy and the tubules collapse, while the epithelium shows degenerative changes. The tubules gradually revert to the infantile condition. It is not uncommon to find cystic dilatation of the ducts with accumulation of a brownish or grayish, thin, or mucoid fluid. Ultimately, the acini entirely disappear and only the ducts remain.

ANOMALIES OF DEVELOPMENT.

Absence of the breasts (**amastia**) is a rare condition and only found in association with grave developmental defects. Sometimes only one organ is defective, usually the right. The ovary on the same side may also be absent in such cases. Abnormal smallness, either of the gland as a whole (**micromastia**) or of the nipple (**microthelia**), is more common. Micromastia, like amastia, is more frequent on the right side and becomes in evidence first at puberty.

Of more importance is an increase in the number of nipples (**polythelia**) or of the glands themselves (**polymastia**). The supernumerary organs may be found on both sides or only on one, usually the left. The redundant nipples are often defective in size or abnormally formed, and may be situated on one and the same gland or may be connected with accessory glands. As a rule, in polymastia there are only one or two supernumerary breasts, but as many as ten have been observed. The additional organ is usually below and to the inner side of the normal breast, rarely above and external. Exceptionally, breasts have been found on the acromion, the thigh, or the labium. As a rule, these supernumerary structures are imperfectly developed, but occasionally have been known to functionate. The condition is met with in males

as well as in females We have discussed the significance of this phenomenon in the first volume (p. 181), showing that it must be regarded as
a mutation and not, as commonly held, as a reversion to an ancestral
condition.

CIRCULATORY DISTURBANCES.

Hyperemia.—Hyperemia of a physiological character is met with
during menstruation, the breast becoming swollen and tender. This
condition may, however, go on to **hemorrhage**, which may take place into
the skin, the interstitial substance, or, rarely, into the ducts. In the last
event, which is more liable to occur in cases of dysmenorrhœa and
amenorrhœa, the blood may be discharged through the nipple (*vicarious
menstruation*). The blood is, as a rule, absorbed, but may form tumor-
like nodules of a yellowish-red, fibrinous substance or a chocolate-like
debris. It is possible that such areas may soften and be converted into
cysts. Hemorrhage from the nipple may also be due to the development
of a papilloma within the ducts.

A remarkable affection is one sometimes met with in hysterical women,
where there are single or multiple nodules the size of a hen's egg, that
on palpation give the sensation of tumors. They are nothing more than
local areas of œdema of neuropathic origin (**angioneurotic œdema**, hysterical or blue œdema—Charcot).[1]

INFLAMMATIONS

Inflammation of the breast may begin in the skin, the superficial
connective tissue, the nipple or areola, or in the substance of the gland
itself. It is acute or chronic.

Acute inflammation of the areola begins in the sebaceous glands and
may lead to local abscess-formation or a diffuse phlegmon involving the
skin and subcutaneous tissue. The appearances do not differ materially
from those of ordinary erysipelas of the skin elsewhere.

Inflammation of the connective tissue behind the breast is of more
importance (**paramastitis**). It is rather a rare condition, and may be
caused by extension of inflammation from the substance of the breast,
by carious ribs, by the bursting of an empyema through the chest wall,
or by an axillary abscess. Fever and constitutional disturbance are
marked. The breast is pushed forward, but retains its normal shape, is
tense, and feels as if it were resting on an elastic cushion. Pain is severe
and increased by the movements of the arm and chest. Generally an
abscess forms (**retromammary abscess**), which may burst into the thoracic
cavity or dissect through the breast, forming numerous sinuses or external
fistulæ. Orth[2] records an extraordinary case where the entire breast

---

[1] See Fowler, Medical Record, 1 : 1890 : 179 and 191.   [2] Lehrbuch, 1893: 654.

became sequestrated owing to the dissection of an abscess in the connective tissue surrounding it.

Thelitis.—Inflammation of the nipple (thelitis) is not uncommon in nursing women, and originates in small cracks or fissures caused by the irritation of the mechanical act of sucking and the macerating action of the milk and saliva. In such cases infection readily takes place, especially with the staphylococcus, less commonly the streptococcus, or the thrush fungus. The process readily spreads to the substance of the gland by means of the lymphatic channels or along the galactophorous ducts.

Mastitis.—Acute Mastitis.—Acute inflammation of the breast proper —acute mastitis—occurs at all ages. It is found in the first few days of infancy, where, as has been before remarked, swelling and inflammation of the breasts is not uncommon. This would rarely, however, cause much trouble were it not for the meddlesome practice among nurses of "rubbing out the milk." It is also seen in girls about the time of the first menstruation, particularly in those of a strumous disposition, and is met with as a complication of the infectious fevers. These forms rarely go on to suppuration. Acute mastitis is, however, by far the most frequently found during the first month after delivery, and especially in primiparæ. Here the process is in immediate relationship to the function of lactation. Traumatism, as, for instance, erosions or fissures of the nipple, is the direct exciting cause, as it leads to the infection of the breast with microörganisms. The old view that retention or oversecretion of milk is the cause is, of course, incorrect, except in so far as these conditions predispose to the occurrence of infective processes.

Puerperal Mastitis.—In puerperal mastitis the inflammation is of the exudative type, and may either be uniformly disseminated throughout the breast (*diffuse mastitis*) or, as is most frequently the case, affects a circumscribed area, usually the lower and outer portion of the organ. Sometimes multiple isolated foci are produced. The inflammatory process in most cases originates in the connective tissue between the lobules (*interlobular mastitis*), which is hyperemic, infiltrated with inflammatory products and round cells. The epithelium of the acini shows merely secondary degenerative changes. The process may resolve or go on to abscess-formation. Multiple foci of suppuration are produced, which often coalesce to form large pus cavities. The pus frequently burrows around and between the lobules, until the breast is practically disorganized. Perforation may take place, usually through the skin, or into a milk duct, or, again, into the pleural cavity. When the abscess is large we get a cavity with irregular nodular walls, unless in the case where the pus is contained within a dilated milk duct, when the wall is smooth. Fistulæ are often formed externally, which may, in some cases, communicate with the milk ducts (*milk fistulæ*). Occasionally the abscess does not perforate, the pus becomes more or less absorbed, and only a fatty, granular, and calcareous detritus remains. In other cases the process assumes a chronic course with the formation of contracting scar tissue and discharging sinuses.

Acute Galactophoritis.—Acute galactophoritis, or inflammation of the milk ducts, is found, as a rule, a considerable time after the puerperium, usually in anemic patients. It apparently originates in a catarrh of the larger ducts, and is again the result of infection. Occasionally it is secondary to interstitial or interlobular mastitis. There is spontaneous pain in the breast, increased during the active function of the gland, tenderness on pressure over the duct, and during the quiescent period pus may be expressed from the nipple.

According to Orth, the Staphylococcus is the most common offender in this affection, and the Streptococcus in interstitial mastitis.

Chronic Mastitis.—Chronic mastitis, as has just been hinted, may follow the acute form, and abscesses may remain more or less latent for a long time, accompanied by local fibrosis. Besides this, however, we have to recognize a chronic *productive* inflammation in which the overgrowth of fibrous tissue is much the most prominent feature. As in the case of the acute forms, here again, we have a diffuse and a local variety.

The diffuse form (*cirrhosis mammæ*, Wernher) is very rare. Beginning with pain and other signs of inflammation, the breast at first swells, but later gradually shrinks in size, owing to the formation of contracting scar tissue. The skin becomes attached to the deeper structures, with some dimpling, and the nipple is often drawn in so that the resemblance to certain cases of scirrhus is striking. Only a careful examination will suffice to differentiate, and not always then. The axillary glands are swollen and tender, but in mastitis the enlargement is not permanent. Sometimes a compensatory overgrowth of the surrounding fatty tissue of the breast occurs, so that the total volume of the breast need not be diminished.

Microscopically, together with the formation of scar tissue, the acini are atrophic and the ducts dilated into cysts.

The local form of productive mastitis is much more common. This gives rise to the formation of multiple hard nodules, sometimes in both breasts.

Microscopically, the appearances do not differ from the former type, except that the condition is circumscribed and not diffuse. In spite of the fact that atrophy of the acini is the rule, carcinomatous transformation has been known to occur (*mastitis carcinomatosa* of some authors[1]).

Tuberculosis.—This affection of the mammary gland occurs at all ages and in both sexes. The occurrence of pregnancy and the puerperal state favor the extension of the disease. The lesions may be unilateral or bilateral. The disease was first described by Sir Astley Cooper[2] in 1836, and since his time several careful studies have appeared.

Primary tuberculosis, so far as we know, does not occur, but the

[1] See Reclus, Maladie cystique des mamelles, Rev. d. Chir., 1865: 761; and Gaz. des Hôp., 1887: 673; also König, Centralbl. f. Chir., 3 : 1893 : 49.

[2] Diseases of the Breast, 1836. See also Sabrazes and Binaud, Arch. gén. de médecine, 1896, for the pathological anatomy.

affection originates in the extension of infection from other parts, most frequently by retrograde metastases from the axillary glands or thoracic cavity, from a carious rib, or occasionally through the blood stream.

Three forms may be differentiated—the **acute miliary**, the **discrete**, and the **confluent**.

The first type is similar to the miliary affection elsewhere and does not call for an extended description. It is, of course, hematogenic.

In the discrete form one or more nodules are to be found, varying in size from a hemp-seed to an almond. When a single mass is present it is usually in the upper and outer portion of the breast. The multiple nodules are disseminated throughout the organ. The breast is not, as a rule, enlarged, the skin is intact, and the nodules are firm, distinct, and usually immovable. On section the lesions are composed of a central, grayish or whitish caseous material, or sometimes contain a puriform fluid, and are surrounded by a more reddish-gray, semitranslucent zone. There is also often a certain amount of fibrosis in the immediate neighborhood.

In the confluent form, which originates in the condition just described by the coalescence of neighboring foci, the breast is often considerably enlarged, and usually asymmetrically so. The organ is firm and appears to contain a solid mass. On section, the affected area is made up of cavities irregularly spherical with lateral pouches. In the adjacent parts may be seen apparently separate cavities, which, however, are found to communicate with the main abscess by small channels. The whole, therefore, frequently has an areolar appearance. The cavities are lined by a soft, pyogenic membrane presenting yellowish points. Radiating from the central area of softening are dense, fibrous bands, and in the immediate vicinity can be seen small secondary tubercles. The larger cavities frequently communicate with the exterior by fungous-looking sinuses. As a rule, one breast only is affected. The process begins in the connective tissue surrounding the lobules and acini, but it may spread into the ducts.

Microscopically, the tubercles have the ordinary composition of epithelioid, round, and giant cells, with central caseation, and peripheral fibrosis. A point worthy of note, however, is that tubercle bacilli are remarkably scanty.

A rare variety of the confluent form is the *cold abscess*. It is essentially chronic and insidious in its development, and is found only in the adult, and generally after pregnancy. The cavity is sharply defined, lined by a fungous pyogenic membrane of a reddish-purple color, and contains thin pus and grumous material.

Syphilis.—Secondary syphilitic manifestations in the skin of the breast are of course common and need only be mentioned. The most important lesion is the primary **chancre** or sclerosis, which is found starting in the nipple, but may lead to destruction of this organ, and extend to the skin of the breast. The lesion is ordinarily due to suckling a syphilitic child. The ulcer is of the characteristic type, chronic and indurated, and accompanied by indolent bubo of the axillary glands. **Gummas**

are rare. They have been met with both in the male and the female breast. More common is said to be **diffuse mastitis.**

Actinomycosis.—Actinomycosis is excessively rare. It may be due to the extension of pulmonary actinomycosis through the thoracic wall. One or two cases have occurred superficially which were attributed to the application of poultices.

RETROGRESSIVE METAMORPHOSES.

Atrophy.—It is debatable whether retrogressive changes properly so-called are ever met within the mamma. Simple atrophy of the glandular elements is found as an involution process after the menopause, and occasionally, although by no means invariably, after removal of the ovaries. The atrophy is often masked by an excessive overgrowth of fat. Atrophy is also said to follow the prolonged use of iodine or its derivatives. Bollinger and others have described a curious atrophy from inactivity among the people of Upper Bavaria that appears to be a family vitium.

Cysts.—Cysts, usually multiple and of small size, filled with greenish or brownish fluid, are not uncommon in the breast during the involution period. They are due to the obstruction of the ducts, and from their size and hardness may simulate scirrhus.

PROGRESSIVE METAMORPHOSES.

It is perhaps a little difficult to know exactly what conditions ought to be discussed under this section. As is well recognized, there is a physiological relationship between the breasts and the genital organs, and this interdependence is still to be observed in various pathological conditions, of which, indeed, it may be a cause. There are also certain states of overgrowth and functional overactivity that are perfectly natural in certain individuals at certain times, which in other persons, at other times and under different circumstances, must be regarded as abnormal. Thus, the active and excessive growth associated with lactation, if found in the non-pregnant or non-parturient woman, before the age of puberty or after the menopause, or, again, in the male, must be regarded as distinctly pathological. We shall not perhaps greatly err if we refer to such conditions in this place.

Hypertrophy.—An hypertrophy of the breasts, simulating that found in pregnancy, is found associated with tumors of the uterus or ovaries. Repeated stimulation, as from the application of a child to the breast, has sometimes established the function of lactation in virgins and in old women. Occasionally, in males, the breasts assume the female type (**gynecomastia**), and milk may even be secreted. The condition is often associated with pseudo-hermaphroditism or atrophy of the testicles.

A peculiar form of hypertrophy is that not infrequently found in tuberculous individuals.

Compensatory Hypertrophy.—Compensatory hypertrophy of one breast after the removal of the other may be produced in experimental animals, as Ribbert has shown, but it is doubtful if it occurs in the human subject under ordinary conditions.

A *vicarious overgrowth* of the fatty tissue of the breast has been observed in cases of atrophy and contraction, as in some forms of scirrhus (cancer atrophicans), whereby the total volume of the breast is not altered materially. An overgrowth of fat is also common in simple cases of obesity.

Exceptionally, after the menopause, and therefore after the normal stimuli are removed, the breasts may not involute, but remain large and may even continue to secrete.

FIG. 223

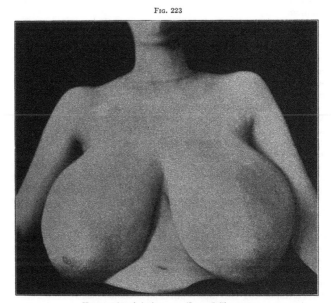

Hypertrophy of the breasts. (James Bell's case:)

Diffuse Hypertrophy.—Of more importance are the cases of diffuse hypertrophy of the breast, of which a number of instances are now on record. The affection is usually met with in young girls at or shortly after the time of the first menstruation. The growth may, for a time, remain latent, being lighted up again only with the occurrence of pregnancy, or may be continuous from the first. Both breasts are involved in a uniform enlargement of the tissues, in which, however, the nipple does not participate, but is gradually flattened out over the mass. Large veins are generally to be seen beneath the skin, and necrosis from pressure or interference with the circulation may result. The breasts have a soft, baggy feel, or may contain hard, more tumor-like masses, as in a case recorded by James Bell.[1] The enlarged organ has been known to attain the weight of from four to seven kilos or more. Durston[2] and Williams have each recorded a case in which a breast reached the enormous size of sixty-four pounds. Different pathological conditions appear to be included under the term "diffuse hypertrophy." In some cases there is what is practically a diffuse fibromatosis, in others the glandular elements may be increased as well, and in still others true adenomatous masses may be found throughout the organ. The condition seems to be associated with some disorder of the genital functions.

Care should be taken not to mistake a retromammary lipoma for this condition.

Tumors.—Much difficulty is experienced in distinguishing between the various conditions that lead to the formation of new tissue in the breast. As all clinicians are aware, retention cysts and the hyperplasia incident to chronic mastitis may at times closely resemble the true neoplasms so that diagnosis is apt to be difficult. And pathologically speaking, the same difficulty confronts us in differentiating between what is true tumor-formation and that neoplastic overgrowth which is so often secondary to inflammatory irritation. In the breast we have both fibrous and glandular elements, and it is usually easy to say whether the latter are in excess of the normal amount for the individual or not, but the further question whether this overgrowth is primary, "active," and independent, or secondary and what might be termed "passive," must sometimes remain in doubt. This passive hyperplasia is at one time the result of inflammatory or mechanical irritation and at another a secondary manifestation concomitant with the development of a tumor in the related tissues. The appearances are still further complicated when cysts are produced. In some cases the newly-formed glandular structures become dilated, partly it is probable from obstruction, but also from excessive secretion (cystadenoma), while in others there is merely a retention of secretion within the normal or approximately normal acini (retention or simple cyst).

The breast being in the main composed of three distinct types of tissue, the integument, the glandular elements, and the fibro-fatty stroma, we have, corresponding with these, epithelial, adenomatous, and connective-tissue tumors. With the exception of the epithelial new-growths, these are not always pure in type, for, as a rule, both fibrous and glandular elements partake in the proliferation, and from modifications of their structure give rise to a considerable variety of forms. The breast, in fact, is a common site for the development of mixed growths. As an illustration of this we may take the case of the adenoma, which is rather a rare tumor, while various combinations with fibroma (adenofibroma;

[1] Montreal Med. Jour., 28: 1899: 772.
[2] Quoted by Labarraque, Thèse de Paris, 1875.

fibroadenoma) or modified connective tissue (adenomyxoma; adeno-sarcoma; myxoadenoma, sarcoadenoma) are much more common.

The exact point of origin for many of the breast tumors is still in doubt. With regard to the fibromas and sarcomas, Billroth[1] and Dreyfuss[2] believed that they took their rise in the hyaline connective tissue surrounding the acini, but this undoubtedly does not explain all forms. Again, in the case of the adenomatous and carcinomatous new-growths, it has usually been taught that they develop from the epithelial cells of the acini, but Creighton[3] has published an elaborate study in which he promulgates the view, which, indeed, appears to be supported by many facts, that the majority of the glandular tumors originate not in the acini of the breast proper, but in sudoriparous glands which are to be found deep down in many normal breasts in a more or less perfect state. Some of them are possibly to be explained as originating in a reversion to the more embryonic condition. This work of Creighton's, while most suggestive, as yet lacks confirmation, and, like other theories, cannot explain all cases. However, this may be, the ultimate causes of tumor-growth in the breast are as obscure as they are in the case of neoplasms of other regions.

It is a well-known fact that the breast is one of the most frequent sites for tumor-formation. This is perhaps to be explained in view of the fact that this organ, like the uterus, where new-growths are also common, is in the majority of individuals for a prolonged period in a state of both physiological and anatomical unrest. The truth of this is evident when we consider the various vicissitudes to which it is liable in the course of pubescence, gestation, lactation, and senility. Normally, then, we must conclude there is a predisposition to rapid proliferation of tissue, which a great variety of apparently trifling stimuli are competent to bring about. Besides this, inflammatory changes of all grades, with their associated irritation and morphological changes, are particularly common in the breast, so that it is not extraordinary that the natural balance of things should frequently be upset. Many writers lay stress upon hereditary influences, trauma, race, and sex. Hereditary predisposition is found only in the case of malignant growths, and has been variously estimated as being present in from 9 to 21 per cent. The influence of trauma is still a matter for debate. A history of injury or inflammation is given in from 12 to 40 per cent. of cases of carcinoma, while in sarcoma the influence of trauma is said to be much greater. Whether this is of etiological importance or is a mere coincidence, we are not as yet in a position to say. With regard to race, it is a remarkable fact that fibrous tumors of the breast are rare in negresses, while, on the other hand, fibroids of the uterus are particularly common. With regard to sex, practically all the tumors found in the female breast may be met with in the male, but with much less frequency, a fact which goes a long way to support the view just enunciated that dis-

[1] Virch. Archiv, 18: 1860: 51.   [2] Ibid., 113: 1888: 535.
[3] Cancers and Other Tumors of the Breast, Williams & Norgate, London, 1902.

turbance of functional and structural equilibrium is an important etiological factor.

Tumors of the breast may be conveniently divided into benign and
malignant forms. Apart from simple cysts, among the former we
may recognize **fibroma, adenoma, fibroadenoma, adenofibroma, cystadenoma, lipoma, myxoma, myoma, angioma, osteoma, chondroma**; among the
latter, **epithelioma** and various types of **carcinoma** and **sarcoma**. Many
of the cysts are merely "retention" cysts and, therefore, properly not
tumors, while some are either benign or malignant **cystadenomas, cystic
fibromas, or sarcomas**. An overwhelming proportion of mammary growths,
variously estimated by White, Williams, Gross, and Senn at from 80
to 95 per cent., are carcinomas. An analysis of cases from the records
of the Royal Victoria Hospital gives the following proportions for the
various forms: Total number of cases, 184; fibroma, 1; adenoma, 31;
fibroadenoma, 11; cystadenoma, 1; sarcoma, 3; epithelioma, 5; carcinoma,
132. These figures agree fairly well with those of Williams,[1] who reports
2430 cases divided as follows: fibroadenoma, 15.3 per cent.; myxoma,
0.16; sarcoma, 3.9; carcinoma, 77.5. The great preponderance of malignant forms renders it imperative that all mammary tumors should be
removed early. Even the fibroadenoma has been known to give rise
to metastases not withstanding the fact that the histological picture has
been that of a non-malignant growth. Hanseman[2] has recorded a case
of this type, and many German pathologists, therefore, speak of "carcinoma in the guise of adenofibroma." In any case, before giving an
opinion it is necessary to examine every portion of the tumor, and even
then one may be deceived. An adenofibroma is rarely mistaken for a
carcinoma, but no doubt the reverse frequently occurs.

Fibroma.—The most common of the benign new-growths is the
fibrous tumor. This is composed of more or less dense, fibrous tissue
in which are embedded glandular elements, differing but little from
those of the normal gland (**fibroma**), though in some cases, while
there is an overgrowth of the connective-tissue elements, there is a
preponderance of glandular structures (**fibroadenoma**). All possible
variations between the two extreme types may occur (**adenofibroma**).
In this connection it should be remarked that considerable confusion in
the nomenclature has arisen from the loose way in which these various
growths have been regarded. In other words, authorities have not been
clear as to what constituted an adenoma and what a fibroma. A
little thought would have avoided the difficulty A fibroma is a tumor
composed of fibrous tissue. In the course of its formation it naturally
may include certain ducts and acini of the breast. The glandular
structures may further be considerably altered from traction or pressure,
and frequently present proliferative or degenerative changes, owing to
the irritation produced by mechanical or inflammatory causes. These
changes are, however, obviously secondary and in no respect to be con-

---

[1] Brit. Med. Jour., 2: 1892: 576.
[2] Die mikroskopische Diagnose der bösartigen Geschwülste.

sidered as evidences of independent growth. Such a tumor can only be a fibroma, not a fibroadenoma. It, of course, takes considerable practice to decide whether the glandular changes in any given case are secondary or are really an adenomatous new-formation, but an attempt should be made in every case to settle the point. An adenoma, on the other hand, is a tumor composed chiefly of glandular elements derived from the acini or ducts, but varying notably from those characteristic of the normal gland. The epithelial cells forming the acini and ducts have proliferated considerably, so that solid epithelial-cell masses are produced or lumina enclosed by several layers of cells, in contradistinction to the normal acini, where, at least in the passive condition, the acini are composed of a single row of cells. Farther, in adenoma, and it is this that constitutes the main difference between the tumor and those secondary changes which have just been mentioned, the ducts and acini are not grouped into lobules, nor are they mere offshoots from the lobules, but are arranged in an erratic way differing more or less widely from the orderly arrangement of the normal gland. The diffuse enlargement of the breasts, referred to above under the name of "diffuse hypertrophy," is in some cases associated with great increase of the glandular elements, and hence has been called by some "diffuse adenoma." It is in no sense, however, a tumor, but a form of hyperplasia. A true adenoma is unilateral, circumscribed, and encapsulated. Such a tumor may be associated with fibromatous overgrowth (**fibroadenoma, adenofibroma**), or the fibrous tissue may undergo mucoid or sarcomatous transformation (**adenomyxoma, adenosarcoma**, etc.). It is the imperfect apprehension of these considerations that has led to the multiplicity of names that have been proposed for these tumors, such as adenoid, fibroadenoma, and adenocele.

Pure fibromas without any admixture with glandular structures are rare. As a rule, certain ducts and acini become entangled in the fibrous overgrowth and appear as compressed and atrophied remnants, or, again, become distorted and dilated. In some cases the dilatation amounts to cyst-formation, so that clinically we can differentiate solid and cystic fibromas. Fibromas are met with, as a rule, in early adult life, from the age of sixteen to thirty, although cases have been met with as early as twelve and as late as fifty-six. The cystic forms are found somewhat later than the others. The tumor usually first comes in evidence during menstruation or the puerperium, owing to the discomfort it causes at such times. The growth, as a rule, forms a circumscribed, rounded, and nodular mass, firm and elastic, projecting under the skin. The most frequent site is at the periphery of the breast above the nipple, although the intracanalicular variety is apt to be more deeply situated. When cysts are present they may often be recognized as fluctuating bosses. A capsule is usually formed, so that the growth is freely movable. Fibromas are generally solitary, but may be multiple, or even affect both mammæ. The rate of growth is slow and the tumor rarely attains a large size. Cystic forms tend to enlarge more rapidly. Cysts are more likely to be found in the older patients. After removal local recurrence has been observed in some few cases, but there is no tendency to infiltration. Besides the nodular form just described, there is a diffuse variety

FIG. 224

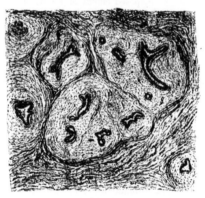

Pericanalicular fibroma of the mammary gland. The glandular acini and ducts are prominent and show some irregular overgrowth of the epithelium, but the main feature is the development of connective tissue both periacinous and interstitial, the latter not sharply defined. (Ribbert.)

FIG. 225

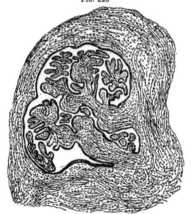

Intracanalicular fibroma or intracystic papilloma of breast. (Orth.)

in which the whole breast is liable to be involved. Here, the fibrous tissue forms cylindrical sheaths along the ducts and acini, the so-called *plexiform fibroma* of Nordmann.

On section, fibromas are firm, fasciculated, and of a grayish or grayish-red color, and, if of the pericanalicular variety, made up of an agglomeration of hard nodules. Should there be dilatation of the ducts this is evidenced by the presence of numerous minute fissures, or even cysts.

Histologically, we may differentiate two main types, the *pericanalicular* or *periglandular* and the *intracanalicular*.

In the former there is proliferation and often hyaline transformation of the adventitial connective tissue about the gland-tubes, which are usually altered by mechanical pressure. The newly formed fibrous tissue surrounds the glandular elements as a well-defined sheath. This produces on section the appearance of a nodular or granular surface. The condition of the interlobular connective tissue varies, at one time partaking but little or not at all in the hyperplasia, while at others it is increased and merges almost imperceptibly into the adventitial sheaths, thus giving rise to a more diffuse fibrous growth. The glandular tissue preserves more or less completely the ordinary arrangement into lobules. Should the various ducts become obstructed, as not infrequently happens, irregular fissures or actual cysts are produced (*fibroma cysticum*). The fibrous tissue may be dense or cellular, giving rise to hard and soft fibromas.

In the intracanalicular form there is a remarkable overgrowth either of the periglandular adventitia or of both this and the interstitial stroma into the lumina of the ducts and acini, so that a kind of cystic tumor is produced, the cavities of which are filled with conical, nodular, or leaf-like projections, giving the tumor a warty, papillomatous, or cauliflower appearance. These papillæ are covered with epithelium similar to that of the normal glands.

Fibroadenoma and Adenofibroma.—Here we have a combination in varying proportions of hyperplastic connective tissue and adenomatous new-formation. Should the glandular elements predominate, we have a fibroadenoma; if the fibrous tissue is more developed, then we have an adenofibroma. The glandular structures recall in appearance both the acini and the ducts, but differ considerably from those of the normal gland, being more numerous, wider, and irregular, with proliferation of their epithelial lining. With this there is a more or less marked increase of the fibrous elements.

Taking the intracanalicular fibroma as a prototype, we have a *cystadenofibroma intracanaliculare* corresponding to it. In this the papillary excrescences are present as before, but the fibrous tissue is much reduced, forming merely a delicate central core, while the epithelial cells have actively proliferated and are heaped up into masses. In other cases adenomatous structures are found within the substance of the fibrous outgrowths (*adenocele*, Virchow). Owing to the rapid development of the papillary processes, the cavities of the gland become greatly dilated, so that cysts would be produced were it not for the fact that the spaces are practically filled up with cauliflower-like masses, reducing the cavities to fine, collapsed, and ramifying fissures. The growth may be so exuberant that papillomatous excrescences appear at

the nipple externally or burst through the skin.   When this occurs th
cyst-walls are perforated, and, owing to the dislocation of the ou

FIG. 226

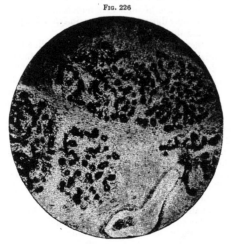

Fibroadenoma of the mamma of the acinous type.   Winckel obj. No. 3, without ocular.
(From the collection of Dr. A. G. Nicholls.)

FIG. 227

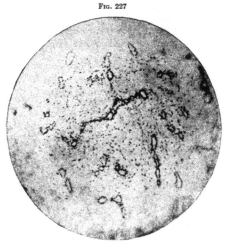

Adenofibroma of mamma.   Zeiss obj. DD, without ocular.   (From the collection of the
Royal Victoria Hospital.)

growths from their original position, their place is left free, and distinct cystic cavities make their appearance. The resemblance to the papillary cystadenoma of the ovary is striking. The cysts when present are filled with a serous, mucinous, and viscid fluid, often stained with blood, and sometimes containing fat-globules and cholesterin. Rarely, keratinized epithelial masses (cholesteatoma) are found. Both the fibromas and the fibroadenomas are liable to undergo secondary mucoid or even sarcomatous change, while hemorrhagic infiltration and œdema are also common. This gives the tumors on section a very variable appearance, here firm and fibrous, there soft, grayish, gelatinous, and transparent.

The adenomatous mixed tumors are found at all periods of life, but are most common about the third and fourth decade. They may be quite small or may attain a considerable size. A weight of twenty kilos has been recorded. The rate of growth is sometimes slow, sometimes rapid. The growths are hemispherical, definitely lobulated, and somewhat warty on the surface. At first they are freely movable, but later become attached to the skin. While they tend to grow rapidly and produce considerable disturbance in the neighborhood, they are in general to be regarded as benign growths, as when removed they do not tend to recur and do not form metastases. When they do return, it is generally because of the subsequent development of a small, independent growth that has been overlooked. This statement is not without exceptions, however. A suspicious feature is when the tumor masses are multiple or when both breasts are affected.

Adenoma.—Pure adenoma is a relatively rare tumor in the breast. It consists of a fibrous stroma in which are embedded glandular elements of the type of acini or of ducts lined by cylindrical epithelium. Thus, we can recognize two forms, the *adenoma acinosum* and the *adenoma tubulare*. In the first form there is a great numerical increase of the acini, which deviate considerably from the normal in that they are not arranged into lobules. In the tubular variety the duct-like structures are evenly scattered throughout the tumor or are aggregated into groups. In both forms the interstitial fibrous stroma is looser and more cellular than that of the normal breast. The tumor is usually small, circumscribed, and encapsulated. It occurs in young women, and starts as a small nodule in the upper and outer quadrant of the mamma. As it enlarges it becomes round or oval. On section it is firm, smooth, and grayish-white in color, and a milk-like fluid may sometimes be expressed.

Lipoma.—Lipoma does not occur in the breast proper, but in the connective tissue behind or above it.

Myxoma.—The myxoma is rare as a pure tumor without admixture with glandular elements, but mucinous transformation of fibromas and sarcomas is not uncommon.

Myoma.—Myomas are also rare. They start from the unstriped muscle in the skin or about the nipple.

Chondroma and Osteoma.—Chondromas and osteomas, either as pure growths or associated with sarcoma or carcinoma, are decidedly uncommon. Chondromas are more frequent in dogs. Care should be taken not to mistake cysts with calcified walls for these growths.

Angioma.—Angioma is so rare as only to need mention.

Sarcoma.—Sarcoma of the breast is a comparatively rare affection, forming scarcely 4 per cent. of the tumors found in this situation. Clinically, as in the case of the fibromas, we may have *solid* and *cystic*

FIG. 228

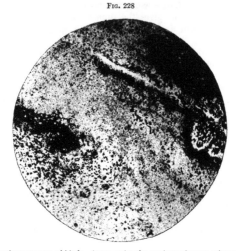

Chondroma from mamma of bitch. At one point the specimen shows a calcareous deposit. Winckel obj. No. 3, without ocular. (From the collection of A. G. Nicholls.)

forms. Cystic sarcoma is said to be peculiar to the breast. Sarcomas form, when pure, unilateral, circumscribed, and movable nodules, and occur by preference in girls and youngish women, being rarely found after the menopause. In this respect they differ from carcinomas. Occasionally, they form diffuse masses and are found in both breasts. Sarcomatous transformation is not uncommon in fibromas and in fibrous and adenomatous mixed tumors.

Histologically, the solid sarcomas are composed of mixed cells, some of them giant cells, round or spindle cells. Myxomatous degeneration, hemorrhage, necrosis, calcification, are not infrequent complications. Sometimes the component cells assume an alveolar arrangement.

Angiosarcoma (perithelioma malignum) has been described, starting from the adventitia of the vessels. As curiosities, may be mentioned *melanotic sarcoma* and *round-celled sarcoma* containing *striated muscle*.

Cystic sarcomas are strictly comparable to the cystadenofibroma intracanaliculare before referred to, which they greatly resemble. These tumors are found in early adult life, and form large bossy, succulent growths imperfectly encapsulated. On section they present irregular clefts or spaces filled with mucoid or blood-stained fluid, into which project numerous villi or papillary excrescences (*cystosarcoma phyllodes*).

Microscopically, these papillæ have a central core, not of ordinary fibrous tissue, but of a highly cellular and vascular tissue composed of round and spindle cells. Myxomatous and degenerative changes may be found.

Involvement of the chest wall and the skin is much less frequent than in the case of carcinoma, although the pectoralis major is occasionally infiltrated. Lymphatic enlargement is rare in sarcoma, and when it occurs is due usually to inflammatory or other irritation and not to sarcomatous invasion. The metastases arise through the blood stream and the lungs are early affected.

Carcinoma.—The breast is one of the most frequent sites for carcinoma, 40 per cent. of all cases of carcinoma being found in this region (Williams). The average age at which it is first discovered is forty-eight, most cases being met with shortly before the menopause. It is rare before the age of thirty-five and in advanced life. Instances have, however, been recorded under twenty (Boussereau) and as late as ninety-four (Coley[1]). When not operated upon the average duration of the disease is 27.1 months (Gross). Some cases have been known, however, to run a chronic course of from five, ten, fifteen, or more years. One authentic case is recorded where the disease lasted more than thirty years. The scirrhous type is the one most likely to run a prolonged course.

Carcinoma may commence in any part of the breast, being found deeply seated or immediately under or about the nipple. A favorite position is in the lateral portions of the gland. It occurs both as a circumscribed nodule or as a diffuse infiltrating growth. Clinically, we recognize superficial and deep-seated forms. In the former class are included epithelioma and miliary carcinosis (squirrhe disseminée); in the latter, hard and soft forms, such as scirrhus, carc. medullare, adenocarcinoma, carc. gelatinosum.

A rare form of carcinoma is *squamous epithelioma* (Paget's disease of the nipple;[2] malignant papillary dermatitis; superficial carcinoma of the skin). This affection at first assumes the appearance of a chronic eczema of the nipple. There is a thickening of the epithelium of the nipple, followed by an inflammatory infiltration of the subepithelial layers. After a long time the proliferating epithelial cells reach the galactophorous ducts and form a more deeply invading growth of the usual squamous type, with epithelial cell nests (Perlkugeln). In time the nipple is destroyed and the disease spreads over the surface of the breast and eventually invades the deeper parts. The ulcer produced is slightly raised, with sharp edges, and is of a bright red, raw appearance. Secretion is scanty.

Another rare variety is the *acute miliary carcinosis*, or disseminated

---

[1] Refer. Handb. Med. Sci., 2: 1901: 629.
[2] St. Bartholomew's Hosp. Rep., 1874: 87.

scirrhus. In 170 cases recorded by Williams only 2 were of this type.
It begins superficially and appears to spread by means of the lymphatics.

The deeper forms of carcinoma are conveniently divided according to
the amount of connective tissue they contain into scirrhous carcinoma,
c. simplex, and c. medullare. The clinicians are in the habit of classifying them into hard or scirrhous and soft forms. It should be remarked,
however, that many tumors that have all the characters of scirrhus on
physical examination, when examined microscopically are really simple
cancers. In fact, a pure scirrhus, histologically considered, is one of
the less common types of carcinoma. Consequently, there is a liability
for some confusion to arise in the use of the term. A further point of
considerable importance is that any given carcinoma is rarely of one type
throughout. It may be scirrhous in one part and simple carcinoma in
another, proving the necessity of a careful examination of all parts of
the growth.

The forms just mentioned conform more or less perfectly to an acinous
type of growth, but there are other forms in which the epithelial cells
are arranged in a tubular fashion somewhat resembling ducts (*adenocarcinoma*), and still others that are *cystic*.

Scirrhous carcinoma begins as a small nodule within the breast. It is
not so sharply defined as a fibroadenoma, as it is not encapsulated, and
soon becomes more or less immovable. It is knotty on the surface and
somewhat flattened, with rounded outgrowths from the margin. In
consistency, it is extremely hard, without much elasticity, and conveys
to the examining hand a suggestion of weight rather than size. Later,
fixation to the skin occurs, which becomes immovably adherent with
some dimpling. Only when advanced does the tumor project above
the general level of the breast. In many cases, where the larger ducts
are implicated, it is impossible to draw the nipple forward, and later
on the nipple is actually retracted. In cases that are neglected the
tumor becomes attached to the chest wall and may ulcerate on the
surface. The breast, as a whole, is often flattened and its volume
diminished. When cut into, the growth is hard, nodular, and fibrous,
often showing radiating bands of connective tissue and yellowish patches.
In elderly people it is not uncommon to find small involution cysts filled
with a yellowish-green fluid, resembling pus or colostrum.

Histologically, the carcinoma cells proper are small, mononuclear,
and atrophic looking, arranged in small islets or elongated rows. The
fibrous tissue is relatively greatly increased, so that the epithelial cells
have the appearance of being compressed. Undoubtedly, there is a
proliferation of the interstitial stroma as well. At the periphery the
type of growth is apt to be softer and more cellular than in the centre.
Consequently, in scirrhus the metastases are frequently of the simplex or
medullary type. The amount of fibrous tissue may, in some cases, be
so great that at first sight the new-growth resembles scar tissue rather
than a tumor. In the most advanced forms of this type the carcinoma
cells are largely degenerated and reduced to debris, while the tissue
around is atrophic and sclerosed (*cancer atrophicans*).

PLATE X

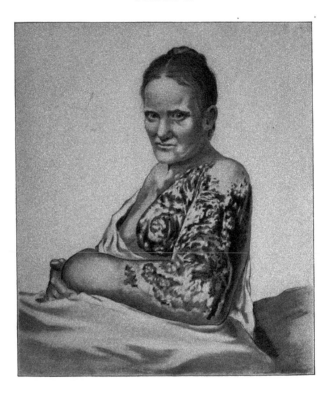

Neglected Carcinoma of Breast. (Brewer.)

In *carcinoma simplex* the clinical features are practically the same as in the case of scirrhus, except that the growth is more rapid. The tumor is rounded, nodular, very hard, and is apt to be much larger than in the scirrhus, causing marked prominence of the breast.

Microscopically, however, the appearances differ considerably. The epithelial cells are larger, more rounded, and with relatively more protoplasm. They are also much more abundant, both actually and relatively, so that cells and stroma are about equal in amount. As a rule, the growth tends to assume an alveolar type.

The *medullary* or *encephaloïd carcinoma* is much more rapid in its development than the scirrhous form, and may attain a large size. It is soft, vascular, rounded in form, and cannot be differentiated on palpation from the breast substance. It offers to the hand a sensation of fluctuation. Retraction of the nipple does not occur.

Histologically, the epithelial elements are abundant and the stroma is reduced to fine delicate fibrillæ. In all the softer carcinomas the interstitial tissue is looser and more cellular than in the scirrhous form. It is common, therefore, to find a marked cellular infiltration at the periphery of the growth and round about it. These cells do not suggest the character of exudate cells or leukocytes, but are of the granulation type, with a single round nucleus.

Macroscopically, the softer, more acinous carcinomas are somewhat nodular on section and of a grayish-red color. A milky juice may be obtained on scraping. The connective tissue between the cancerous masses appears as grayish, glistening bands. The medullary form, however, is pulpy and brain-like.

Occasionally, the carcinoma simplex undergoes a colloid or gelatinous degeneration (*c. gelatinosum*). This occurs chiefly in the older portions of the growth, while the periphery presents the ordinary features of carcinoma. Here, too, there are nodular and diffuse forms.

In the larger masses of epithelial cells it is not unusual to find fatty degeneration and even extensive necrosis of the central portions. Hyaline degeneration of the fibrous stroma and calcification are rare.

Adenocarcinoma.—This is a term applied to a growth having a special histological structure. The general resemblance to the acinous and lobular arrangement of the normal gland may be fairly well preserved. The epithelial cells, however, have proliferated into the lumen of the ducts and into the lymphatic spaces. The appearances vary in different portions of the tumor. In one part there may be normal gland-tissue; in another, numerical increase of the ducts with enlargement and dilatation and some proliferation of the connective tissue. The amount of carcinomatous invasion of the stroma varies considerably in different cases. At times there may be scarcely any. In other cases the epithelial elements extend into the lymph-channels and form small clusters. The stroma is never so dense and fibrillar as in the case of the scirrhus. The epithelial cells are similar to those of the normal acini, but are, as a rule, larger and polymorphous.

Clinically, the growth is rather hard, and a serous discharge from the nipple is not uncommon.

One or two cystic forms of carcinoma should be mentioned, although they are rare. In the first variety, there is a single main cyst with smooth walls, varying in size from that of a walnut to that of an apple. At one point of its surface there crops out a grape-like or papillomatous mass sometimes provided with a pedicle. The warty excrescences may be œdematous and juicy and on microscopic examination prove to be carcinomatous, being composed largely of columnar cells. Orth thinks that the growth originates in a milk-duct, which then becomes dilated and finally hypertrophied. In other cases we have a carcinomatous growth combined with numerous small cysts of the proliferation type (*cystadenocarcinoma*).

There can be little doubt that, with the exception of epithelioma and the columnar-celled variety, carcinoma of the breast in many instances originates in the lobules of the gland, for in the older portions of the growth the acinous arrangement can still often be recognized.

The epithelial cells proliferate, filling up the lumina and leading to dilatation of the spaces. The hyaline membrane of the tunica soon disappears, although the spindle-celled layer is longer preserved, and finally the glandular elements break through the membrane and appear in the stroma, when extension continues along the lymphatics. Once this process is well established it soon extends into the neighboring lobules, which thus become infiltrated with carcinoma. While only a portion of the lobules are likely to be involved in the cancerous overgrowth, it is usual for both the glandular and the interstitial structures of the rest of the mamma to proliferate.

Carcinoma of the breast, if left alone, does not remain confined to the glandular substance, but gradually extends to the neighboring structures. The skin becomes involved and is found to be fixed to the tumor mass. It is reddened, inflamed, and in time the growth bursts through, forming a foul, excavated, and suppurating ulcer. Secondary nodules form also in the pectoralis fascia; the pectoralis itself, and in time invade the thoracic wall and even the pleural cavity and the lung. Thus, the tumor becomes attached firmly to the thoracic wall. This extension takes place by means of the lymphatics, and distant metastases are produced also through the dissemination of small masses of cancer cells through the same channels. Occasionally, small, secondary nodules form in the skin and subcutaneous tissues followed by diffuse carcinomatous infiltration, whereby the anterior thoracic wall becomes converted into a stiff, swollen, sclerœdematous mass (*cancer en cuirasse;* Panzerkrebs), which, in time, may show superficial ulceration. This is rare, being only observed in two cases of our series. Some writers have taught that the condition is here confined to the skin, but this is undoubtedly not the case.

The distant metastases are met with first in the lymph-glands in closest anatomical relationship with the part of the breast affected. As a rule, the axillary, infraclavicular, and supraclavicular glands are involved in the order given, and become hard and shotty. It should be noted, however, that the enlargement is not invariably due to metastatic deposit, for, in the early stages at least, it may be caused by inflammation or some other as yet undetermined irritation. We have more than once seen caseous tuberculosis of the axillary glands in association with carcinoma of the breast. When the growth originates in the inner portion of the breast the glands of the anterior mediastinum are liable to be involved, or even those of the opposite axilla. In the former case extension to the liver may follow. The carcinomatous invasion begins at the periphery of the nodes, which may become fused together, and may, in time, extend to the neighboring tissues. The type of growth produced in the glands is not necessarily identical with that of the original tumor. Visceral metastases rarely arise until after the involvement of the lymphatic glands is well marked. They occur usually in the lungs, liver, and brain, and are most probably hematogenic in origin. Metastatic involvement of the bones also is hematogenic, and is relatively more common in the scirrhous or sclerosing cancer. The bones affected are the head of the humerus on the same side as the original tumor, the vertebræ, the sternum, and the upper end of the femur. The growth begins in the medulla, but the shaft may in time be eroded, so that spontaneous fractures or compression of the spinal cord sometimes occur.

It might further be remarked, as a matter of interest, that the mammæ are not infrequent sites for multiple independent growths. We have twice observed simple carcinoma attacking both breasts simultaneously. These multiple growths are not always of the same type, however; epithelioma has been observed in one breast and glandular carcinoma in the other. Two cases also have been reported of carcinoma in one breast and angiosarcoma in the other.

Caseous tuberculosis, with epithelioid, giant cells, and tubercle bacilli, has been found in mammary carcinomas (Warthin[1]).

Cysts.—The simple cysts found so often in the involution period of the breast and the cysts associated with sarcoma and carcinoma have already been referred to. Besides these, we have as rarities *Echinococcus, Cysticercus,* and *Dermoid* cysts.

Of more importance are those dilatations of the milk ducts and acini that contain milk (**galactocele**). These occur, of course, only in the functioning breast. When obstruction takes place in a large duct near the nipple, a cord-like swelling can be felt beneath the areola which gradually extends toward the periphery of the breast. In the event of obstruction in the lobules the enlargement is more deep-seated. There is no inflammation and but little pain. The increase at first is rapid, but diminution in size may occur after lactation has ceased. In some cases single large cysts are produced having an oval shape and smooth outline. Occasionally, if the wall of the cyst has given way at some part and its contents have escaped into the surrounding tissues, the cyst is more lobulated. Scarpa has recorded a well-known case in

---

[1] Amer. Jour. Med. Sci., 118 : 1899 : 25.

which the cyst contained ten pounds of milk.   After a time absorption
of the more fluid parts of the milk may occur, and the cyst is found to
contain a creamy or butter-like substance.   Occasionally these cysts
suppurate or hemorrhage occurs into the cavity.

The male breast is liable to the same affections as the female, but, of
course, much less frequently, having regard to its ordinarily rudimentary
condition.   Chronic mastitis and many forms of tumors have been
met with.

In relative frequency as compared with those of the female breast they
are as 3 to 100.   The most common tumor is carcinoma, generally of the
simple type.[1]

From what has been said with regard to the various forms of inflammation and tumors it will readily be gathered that there must often be
great difficulty in making a differential diagnosis between the various
conditions.   The difficulty is not so great for the morbid anatomist, who
will rarely be in doubt, and in any case will have the microscope to help
him, but during life the most careful investigation is in all cases necessary
and even then in many cases the clinician will often be at fault.

Warfield, Carcinoma of the Male Breast, Johns Hopkins Hospital Bulletin,
12 : 1901 : 305.

SECTION VIII.

THE TEGUMENTARY SYSTEM.

CHAPTER XLI.

THE SKIN AND ASSOCIATED STRUCTURES.

THE SKIN.

THE skin is a somewhat complicated structure, composed, as it is, of an outer epidermal layer of flattened and horny cells resting upon a subcutaneous cushion of fat and fibrous tissue, in the deeper parts of which are the bloodvessels, nerves, tactile corpuscles, hair-follicles, sudoriparous and sebaceous glands.

In accordance with its structure, the skin performs numerous and important functions. It is the organ of tactile, painful, and thermic sensation. It acts as an external protective covering, regulates the bodily heat, and to some extent exercises excretory and respiratory functions.

As one would expect from its structure and exposed position, as well as from the fact that it is in close physiological relationship with many of the internal organs, such as the heart, kidneys, nervous system, and, indirectly, the liver and sexual apparatus, the skin is susceptible to a great variety of disturbing influences, and its disorders are consequently numerous.

CONGENITAL ANOMALIES.

A remarkable and rare affection is **ichthyosis congenita,** a condition characterized by overgrowth of the epidermis with a marked tendency to cornification of the superficial layers (keratosis). The disease usually involves the whole or the greater part of the body, but may be localized. In the mildest form, there are merely small, papular elevations about the hairs, due to proliferation and keratosis of the cells at the mouths of the follicles (*xerosis, xeroderma*), and all intervening grades may be found up to the production of large, flattened plaques and scales of horny texture, so that the skin resembles that of a fish or alligator (*ichthyosis sauroderma*). As the growth of the body goes on, these scales become separated more and more one from the other, and the skin becomes lined with fissures and furrows, while the scales turn up somewhat at the edges. The fine hairs are implicated in the overgrowth. The fingers and toes may be so affected that they remain stunted.

Microscopically, the epidermis is greatly thickened, the plaques being composed of dense, laminated, keratinous material, which extends to the papillæ and even into the dilated hair-follicles. The cells in the deeper layers of the cutis are shrunken looking. Fragmentary and atrophied hairs may be found embedded in the horny substance.

Absence of the normal pigment of the skin is a not uncommon congenital peculiarity, known as **leukoderma** or **leukopathia congenita** or **albinism**, as opposed to **leukopathia acquisita** or **vitiligo**.

Fig. 229

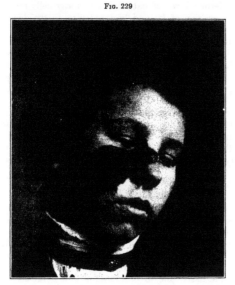

Pigmented nevus. (Hyde.)

Albinism may affect the pigmented structures of the body as a whole, skin, hair, iris, and choroid. The affected persons, called albinos, have clear, white or rosy transparent skins, white or yellowish-white silky hair, and pink eyes. In partial albinism there may be whitish streaks on the skin in various parts of the body. The condition is said to be hereditary.

An excess of pigment is found in certain of the nevi or birthmarks (**nævi pigmentosi**). They vary in color from pale brown to black.

Congenital **hypertrophy** of the nails (**hyperonychia**) is found associated with ichthyosis. **Absence** or **imperfect development** of the nails is also met with.

The hair may be abnormally scanty or, rarely, completely absent (**alopecia congenita universalis**). This is often accompanied by imperfect development of the teeth and nails.

Excess of hair, **hypertrichosis** (hirsuties, polytrichia), may be local or involve the body as a whole. Universal hypertrichosis is usually inherited and affects several individuals in the same family. The whole body, except perhaps the palms of the hands and the soles of the feet, may be covered with long hair, giving the individual a striking resemblance to certain of the lower animals (hairy men, dog-faced or baboon men). Local hypertrichosis is met with in the *nævus pilosus*, and on the sacrum in association with concealed spina bifida.

FIG. 230

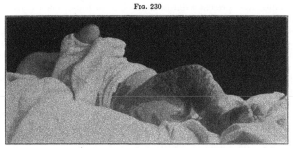

Extensive verrucose and "port-wine" nevus: macrodactyly and microdactyly.
(Dr. A. E. Vipond's case.)

A common anomaly of the skin is the so-called "**birthmark**" or nævus, which is met with in the form of large or small, well-defined, reddish or purple patches (*nævus vasculosus*, port-wine stain), soft, nodular excrescences or warts (*nævus verrucosus*), or local diffuse thickenings of the skin (*elephantiasis*). In all these there is a local anomaly in the arrangement and development of the bloodvessels. Some nevi, again, are level with the skin (*nævus spilus*); others hairy (*nævus pilosus*).

Seborrhœa, or excessive secretion of the sebaceous follicles, is occasionally met with at birth and afterward. Here, the vernix caseosa or smegma, which is normally present on the skin of the newborn infant, persists into later life.

CIRCULATORY DISTURBANCES.

The amount of blood in the skin varies, of course, widely at different times, even under physiological conditions, as, for instance, under the influence of exercise, heat, cold, and emotion. Pathological hyperemia occurs as a diffuse blush over an extended area, or in small spots and patches.

Hyperemia.—Active Hyperemia.—Active hyperemia is found in the first stage of inflammation, in vasomotor disturbances, exposure to excessive heat or cold (erythema pernio), and as a result of slight injuries, such as are caused by mechanical or chemical irritation. Large patches of hyperemia are termed *erythema;* small spots, *roseola.* The color is a pale rose pink, and disappears on pressure, only to return instantly when the pressure is removed. Erythema is not infrequently associated with exudation of plasma and swelling (inflammatory œdema), and when long-continued or repeated may lead to pigmentation of the skin, owing to diapedesis of the red cells and metamorphosis of the hemoglobin.

Passive Hyperemia.—Passive hyperemia is well seen in chronic valvular disease of the heart and other conditions which favor blood-stasis, such as pneumonia, toxic states, and sunstroke. The lips, face, neck, and the extremities often present a diffuse dusky blue or leaden color (*cyanosis*). A small spot of cyanosis or lividity is termed *livedo.* After death the blood stagnates to the dependent parts of the body (*postmortem lividity*).

Local passive congestion of the skin may be brought about by the pressure of tumors or inflammatory products on the efferent vessels of a part.

Teleangiectasis.—Dilatation of capillaries (teleangiectasis) is due to obstruction to the free outflow of blood from any part, as, for instance, from the pressure of tumors or contracting fibrous tissue on the efferent vessels.

Rosacea, a condition due to the dilatation of the superficial capillaries, is met with more especially in those addicted to alcohol, or who are exposed to wind and weather.

Œdema.—The natural result of prolonged passive congestion is œdema. This is found more especially in connection with chronic stasis in the blood- or lymph-systems. The skin and subcutaneous structures are infiltrated with plasma, are firmer than normal, and pit on pressure (*anasarca*). The skin is commonly tense and shiny. In severe cases blisters are formed, or the skin may burst through overdistension and the fissures weep clear, watery fluid. Secondary infection and inflammation are not uncommon sequels.

Angioneurotic Œdema.—Angioneurotic œdema is a vasomotor disturbance of the skin and subcutaneous tissues found in neurotic individuals. It is notably a hereditary affection, reappearing in several generations. It is characterized by the sudden onset of local swellings, generally about the eyelids, ears, lips, or cheeks, but which may also be found in the hands, feet, breast, genitalia, or back. The attack may be preceded by slight itchiness and redness of the skin. The condition may shift about from one place to another, and usually passes off as suddenly as it came. According to Osler, giant urticaria is the same disease.

Myxœdema.—In this disease the skin is pale, dry, wrinkled, and firm to the touch. It is elastic and does not pit on pressure. This condition is due to an interstitial infiltration with a mucinous fluid, giving place in later stages to diffuse hyperplasia of the subcutaneous connective tissues.

Hemorrhage.—Hemorrhage into the skin is commonly the result of traumatism, or is a symptom in certain of the infectious fevers. Not infrequently, too, it comes on spontaneously or "idiopathically."

Hemorrhages vary greatly in size, are of reddish or purplish-red color, and do not disappear on pressure. Small, irregular spots about the size of a pin-head are termed **petechiæ**. Elongated streaks or branching lines are called **vibices**. Large, irregular patches of considerable superficial extent are known as **ecchymoses**. Occasionally, the amount of blood effused is sufficient to produce nodules (**purpura papulosa**) or actual tumor (**hematoma**). In some cases the epidermis is elevated, forming a blood blister. The blood may also be effused into the sweat glands, causing bloody perspiration (**hematidrosis**). The extravasation takes place into the corium or papillary layer.

FIG. 231

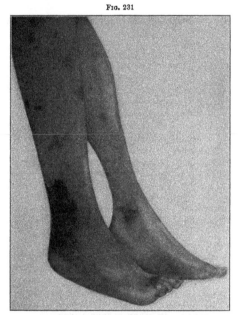

Purpura rheumatica. (From the Montreal General Hospital.)

In course of time the effused blood, which is at first reddish, is transformed, and, as in the familiar instance of the "black" eye, the affected patch passes through all stages of reddish-brown, brown, yellowish-green, and yellow. In many cases, the blood is completely absorbed and the only trace of its presence may be a little pigmentation of the skin, due to the deposit of hemosiderin.

Purpura.—Spontaneous hemorrhage is usually included under the general term purpura. By this is meant a condition in which there are multiple hemorrhages in the skin, either petechial or ecchymotic, sometimes associated with bleeding from the various mucous surfaces, such as the nose, lips, gums, stomach, intestines, kidneys, or uterus.

Purpura may be conveniently divided into the following types:[1]

1. *Essential purpura,* including peliosis rheumatica, morbus Werlhofii, purpura simplex, purpura urticans, and, possibly, scorbutus.

2. *Symptomatic purpura,* such as is found in the infectious fevers, typhus, variola, scarlatina, measles, bubonic plague, sepsis, typhoid fever, and icterus gravis.

3. *Cachectic purpura,* in pernicious anemia, Bright's disease, leukemia, and carcinoma.

4. *Toxic purpura,* as in snake bite and poisoning with phosphorus, antipyrin, copaiba.

5. *Multiple sarcomatosis* of the vessels.[2] To which may perhaps be added,

6. *Neuropathic purpura,* as in hysterical "stigmata."

No doubt, "purpura" ought to be regarded merely as a symptom, for it may be produced by a variety of causes. As a rule, more than one cause is at work. It is safe to say that in all cases, save possibly the neuropathic, there is some abnormal condition of the walls of the smaller vessels and capillaries, such as fatty degeneration, which leads to hemorrhage *per diapedesin* or *per rhexin.* Actual rupture of the vessels is probably rare, but has been demonstrated. The importance of diseased vessels in the production of these hemorrhages is well seen in elderly persons with arterial sclerosis, who sometimes develop purpuric spots on the lower extremities. In some cases thrombi and emboli have been found obstructing the vessels. The ring-shaped petechiæ, occasionally seen, are of this nature. Or, again, as in a case of purpura complicating acute endocarditis, which one of us (A. G. N.) studied, the condition is due to hematogenous infection (mycotic infarct), the minute vessels of the parts being filled with bacteria and surrounded by leukocytic infiltration.

The majority of cases, including all the symptomatic and probably some of the essential purpuras, are the result of infective processes. Some of the cachectic forms, notably those occurring in nephritis, cancer, and leukemia, are possibly to be attributed to terminal infection. The toxic forms are most likely due to profound changes in the blood, which lead to rapid disintegration of the vessel walls, or to slower hyaline and fatty degeneration. In many instances, however, a combination of factors is at work. Circulating toxins, of whatever kind, may cause degeneration of the vessel walls, with consecutive dilatation, together with a diminution of the coagulating power of the blood. Local obstruction, as from thrombosis or embolism, will tend to damage the vessel walls and raise the blood pressure at that point, so that dilatation and rupture readily take place.

[1] Nicholls and Learmonth, The Hemorrhagic Diathesis in Typhoid Fever and its Relationship to Purpuric Conditions in General, Lancet, London, 1:1901:305.

[2] Martin and Hamilton, Jour. Exper. Med., 1:1896:4.

Anemia.—Anemia of the skin is manifested by pallor. General anemia is one of the commonest pathological conditions, being found in chlorosis, pernicious anemia, leukemia, hemorrhage, after fevers, and in all chronic wasting diseases. Local anemia is due to exposure to cold pressure, or may be neuropathic, as in neuralgia and fainting.

INFLAMMATIONS.

Owing to its exposed position and its function as a protective covering, the skin is liable to a great variety of insults, not only from mechanical trauma, but from variations in temperature, the effects of light, and the irritation of chemical and other toxic substances. Again, interference with its action as an excretory organ sometimes results in inflammation. The vascular system conveys to it various microörganisms, microbic and other toxins. Lesions of the nervous system often result in congestive hyperemia and sometimes inflammation, or, again, in disorders of nutrition.

An entirely satisfactory classification of the various forms of dermatitis, or inflammation of the skin, has yet to be made. This is accounted for by the fact that authorities have not always agreed as to the lesions present in any given case, nor as to the interpretation of the appearances. Inflammations of the skin are of the most protean character. One and the same cause may, on occasion, give rise to the most diverse clinical manifestations, and, conversely, one definite clinical picture may be the result of widely differing etiological factors. Again, inflammation may originate not only in the skin, but in its appanages, and in the subcutaneous tissues. In the rarer affections, moreover, the exact sequence of events has not always been made out. In many cases, finally, the cause or causes is obscure or quite unknown. The classification which we here present is simple and convenient, and, we believe, in harmony with the facts as they are at present known.

We may divide dermatitis, or inflammation of the skin, into two main varieties: **primary** or **essential dermatitis**, in which the lesions originate in the skin or its associated structures, and are confined to it; and **secondary** or **symptomatic dermatitis**, in which the cutaneous manifestations are simply one phase of a generalized systemic disorder.

Primary or Essential Dermatitis

(a) *Traumatic*, from
    1. Mechanical injury.
    2. Physical agents, such as light, heat, cold, moisture, filth, chemical and other external toxic substances.
(b) *Infectious*, from
    1. Bacteria, yeasts, and moulds.
    2. Animal parasites.
(c) *Neuropathic.*
(d) *Of unknown or doubtful etiology.*

Secondary or Symptomatic Dermatitis

(a) *Exanthematous eruptions.*
(b) *Toxic*, from the internal administration of medicinal and other poisonous substances.

⌐ The lesions produced by dermatitis are extremely variable, depending upon the nature, extent, localization, and chronicity of the disease. The cardinal features of inflammation, namely, redness, swelling, heat, and pain, are particularly well exemplified in the case of the skin. Diffuse redness and swelling is termed *erythema*. The color is bright and vivid, quite in contrast with the dull lividity of passive congestion, disappearing momentarily on pressure. The more circumscribed areas of infiltration are known as papules, wheals, nodes, or tubercles. *Papules* are small elevations, due to infiltration in the skin, which vary in size from that of a millet-seed to that of a pea. Larger elevations, up to a hazelnut in size, are called *nodes, nodules,* or *tubercles*. Still larger ones are sometimes termed *phyma*. *Wheals* are broad, flattened elevations, quite well defined, which appear and disappear rapidly. They are dull reddish in color, or, in the case of the larger ones, with whitish, anemic-looking centres. Histologically, one finds in such mild forms of dermatitis, infiltration of the tissues with serum, together with diapedesis of leukocytes and, occasionally, of red cells. The epithelium is usually but little affected, although certain of the cells may be swollen and hydropic, and there may be slight proliferation.

Where the serous exudation is more intense, local collections of fluid occur, which, provided that the superficial epidermis remain intact, lead to the separation of the outer layers from the underlying portions, thus forming elevations commonly known as *blisters, blebs,* or *vesicles*. Such vesicles may be single or lobulated. They contain a clear, translucent serum, almost devoid of cellular elements. In other cases, the fluid is slightly turbid from the admixture of leukocytes, or reddish from extravasation of blood (blood blisters). Not infrequently, also, the exudation is turbid, whitish, and purulent, the vesicle then being known as a *pustule*. When the pustule dries it forms a *crust* or *scab*.

In other cases, where the corium is markedly infiltrated with fluid, the exudation spreads to the papillary layer, and finally to the epidermis. The cells involved are swollen, vacuolated, and hydropic, to some extent compressed, and eventually dissociated. When cornification is not marked the fluid exudes upon the surface, where it may coagulate or dry, giving rise to crusts or scabs. This exudate may be gelatinous, fibrinous, mixed with leukocytes or red cells. A diffuse purulent infiltration is known as *phlegmon*. Superficial defects in the epidermis, *fissures* or *excoriations*, are not uncommon under such circumstances, or even cracks or *rhagades*, extending through the entire thickness of the skin. In more extreme conditions, especially where the circulation is much interfered with, we get actual *ulcers, abscesses,* or *gangrene*.

▶ Acute inflammation, if mild. may quickly pass off, leaving little or no traces behind. Frequently, however, even after so trifling an affection as erythema, the superficial epidermis is cast off or desquamates. The loosened cuticle may come away in the form of a fine white powder composed of minute dry scales (*desquamatio furfuracea*), or as larger, but still delicate, whitish, silvery flakes, or, again, as thick, dirty white shreds or membrane (*desquamatio membranacea*). The scales are, for the most part, exfoliated, horny epithelium, but in many instances are pathologically altered as well. *Pigmentation* is also a common sequel of dermatitis, due to the deposit of blood coloring matter.

In cases where there has been a loss of substance, as, for instance, in vesicles, pustules, or fissures, there is a regeneration of the epithelium from the cells at the periphery of the lesion, from any remnants of the epidermis that remain, and even from the epithelium of the hair-follicles sweat and sebaceous glands. A thin, bluish, semitranslucent covering is thus produced, which ultimately is converted into ordinary horny epithelium. Should, however, the papillary layer or the corium be damaged, regeneration is not so perfect, and the loss of substance is made good by the production of new fibrous tissue. The papillæ are commonly not reproduced or are stunted, while the superficial epithelium is smooth, shiny, and largely or entirely devoid of hair-follicles and glands. A pigmented *scar* is a common result.

In chronic inflammations atrophy and hypertrophy may be combined. The formation of epithelium may be in abeyance, inadequate, or excessive, and the normal process of cornification may be interfered with in various ways. The papillæ frequently hypertrophy, becoming elongated and branched, while the corium and subcutaneous tissues are thickened. In other cases the papillæ are atrophic and flattened, while the corium is thinned.

Primary or Essential Dermatitis.—Traumatic Dermatitis.—Traumatic dermatitis in its widest sense, may be taken to include all those forms of inflammation of the skin due to mechanical injury, exposure to light, heat, or cold, and the action of chemical and other irritating substances. Not infrequently, several etiological factors are combined. Owing to the exposed position of the lesion, secondary infection is apt to be superadded. Thus, for example, in the moist condylomas found so often about the genitals we have the combined effects of moisture, heat, dirt, toxic irritation, and infection. Dermatitis is often met with in contusions, abrasions, and lacerations.

Under the heading of dermatitis from the effects of light may be mentioned the well-known *x-ray dermatitis*. In the mildest grades we get little more than a transient irritation, which, in time, after repeated application of the rays, is followed by pigmentation, glossiness of the skin, atrophy of the glands, and loss of hair. Of the frank inflammations, perhaps the commonest is a simple erythema, which appears after a variable period, from a few hours to some days. Vesicular, bullous, and hemorrhagic forms are more frequently met with than are the papular and pustular varieties. Occasionally, deep ulcers or eschars are formed which are exquisitely painful and difficult to heal. Weeks, or months or even one or two years may elapse before cicatrization is complete. Among other effects may be noted, canities, and, rarely, leukoderma. Occasionally the ulcers become malignant.[1]

Histologically, our knowledge is incomplete. Darier, in the milder

[1] See Porter and White, Publications of the Mass. Gen. Hosp., 2 : 1908; also Wolbach, Jour. Med. Research, 21:1909:415.

grades of the affection, found marked thickening of the stratum corneum; the stratum granulosum showed both hypertrophy and hyperplasia of its cells, which contained numerous eleidin granules; the cells of the stratum spinosum were also hyperplastic and hypertrophic, presenting mitoses, while the hair papillæ, arrectores pilorum, and sebaceous glands had disappeared.

The simplest form of dermatitis due to heat (*dermatitis calorica*), and, perhaps, to some extent also, to light, is the erythema caused by exposure to the sun (*sunburn*). Here, the injury has not been sufficient to destroy the tissue, but has led to relaxation of the bloodvessels, congestive hyperemia, and slight exudation. After the process has subsided, desquamation, and more or less pigmentation is apt to follow. The susceptibility to "sunburn" varies greatly in different individuals, being dependent apparently to some extent on the amount of pigment normally in the skin. People of fair complexions and those with leukoderma suffer more than others.

In all respects similar is the inflammation due to *burning* in its mildest degree (*dermatitis ambustionis erythematosa, burn of the first degree*). Where the injury has been more severe, owing to a higher temperature or a more prolonged contact, considerable exudation takes place from the papillary bodies beneath the epidermis, which is thereby elevated into vesicles (*dermatitis ambustionis bullosa, burn of the second degree*). Again, where there is loss of substance of the cutis, we speak of a *burn of the third degree*, or in the case of charring, of a *burn of the fourth degree*. Burns of the second degree heal, provided infection does not take place, with simple regeneration of the epithelium. In the cases where there is actual loss of substance, the burn heals by granulation and the formation of a scar.

Closely allied to dermatitis calorica is the dermatitis due to frost-bite (*pernio, dermatitis congelationis*). Here, again, there may be merely erythema, with swelling, and later desquamation, vesiculation (*dermatitis congelationis bullosa*), or even gangrene (*dermatitis congelationis gangrænosa*). In the severer form, the affected part is red and livid, later dark red, and finally becomes surrounded by a line of demarcation.

Inflammation of the skin may, also, be caused by contact with a great variety of chemical and other toxic agents (*dermatitis venenata*). A great number of substances, derived from the vegetable, animal, and mineral kingdoms, may on occasion be at fault. A few that may be mentioned are the poisons of poison-ivy and poison-oak, the nettle, the venom of certain reptiles and insects, various dyes, caustic alkalies and acids, and certain substances used in medical practice, such as cantharides, croton oil, turpentine, mustard, iodoform, formalin, and carbolic acid. Some of these substances may be absorbed into the system and produce dermatitis elsewhere.

Infectious Dermatitis of Bacterial Origin.—Under this heading we may conveniently and properly include all those inflammations of the skin and subcutaneous tissues, due to vegetable parasites, which are not dependent on constitutional disease. Dermatitis in this sense may be local or diffuse.

A local dermatitis, involving all the elements of the skin and its related structures, is common as a result of wounds, bruises, blisters, and abrasions, particularly when they have become infected.

Hospital gangrene, a disease probably never met with now, but common under the unhygienic conditions of former days and before the advent of antiseptic surgery, was a form of gangrene which was liable to attack even the most trifling wounds. The tissues at the edge and in the immediate neighborhood of the wound assumed a dirty yellowish-gray color and were converted into a foul, slimy mass. The destruction of tissue was rapid, and the necrotic material was cast off in the form of an offensive, shreddy, serous discharge.

FIG. 232

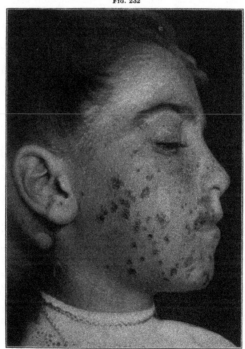

Impetigo contagiosum. (Hyde.)

Impetigo, formerly divided, but erroneously so, into *impetigo simplex* and *impetigo contagiosum,* is a pustular dermatitis, found in badly nourished children who live under unhygienic conditions. It is due to infection with pyogenic cocci. The pustules are found in the derma. They do not tend to infiltrate, but the infection may be carried from one part to another by scratching. Uncomplicated cases heal without scarring. The disease may become chronic, and may result in the formation of vesicles, pustules, and crusts, with desquamation of the epidermis. It chiefly affects the head and extremities.

Ecthyma is a more severe form of impetigo. The pustules are larger, the infiltration is more extensive. It is rare to have scarring, but pigmentation may result.

The *soft chancre* (ulcus molle, chancroid, venereal ulcer) is a local infectious inflammation of the skin and mucous surfaces, transmitted from one person to another by immediate contagion, usually by coitus. Within twenty-four hours of the infection there appears on some part of the genitalia a small vesicle or pustule, which rapidly breaks down into an ulcer. The base and edge are yellowish, soft, and purulent, and the ulcer is bounded by a reddish hyperemic zone. Exceptionally the chancroid may be found on some other part of the body, such as the legs, arms, hands, or face. The lesions are apt to be multiple, and the virus may be transplanted from one part to another. A small bacillus, described by Ducrey, has by some been regarded as the specific cause of the affection. Pyogenic cocci are, however, to be found in the ulcer as well, and are present exclusively in the buboes.

Microscopically, one sees extensive infiltration of the tissues with inflammatory round cells, the more superficial of which are in various stages of degeneration and molecular disintegration.

Under suitable treatment, soft chancre heals with the formation of a small scar. Lymphangitis and inguinal lymphadenitis (bubo) are not infrequent complications of this form of ulceration. Syphilis does not result except in instances where there is mixed infection. In such cases the chancroid does not disappear, but in three or four weeks is converted into the true chancre (hard chancre, ulcus induratum). Other complications are erisipelas, diphtheria, and gangrene (phagedenic ulcer).

Chancre (true chancre, hard chancre, ulcus induratum) is the primary manifestation of syphilis in the skin and mucous membranes. Most commonly it is found on the genitals or some adjacent part, but exceptionally may be found elsewhere, as on the finger, breast, scalp, lip, nose, eyelid, or tonsil. It appears usually from ten to thirty days after infection, and may assume several forms. In some cases a sharply defined, firm area of infiltration is found beneath the superficial epithelium, composed of an accumulation of small round cells, and sometimes large epithelioid and giant cells. In other instances, the lesion begins as a papule, the size of a shot or larger, of dark bluish or pale red appearance. At first it is hemispherical, but tends gradually to spread laterally. When on parts of the body that are kept dry the superficial epidermis is heaped up and desquamates, while the surface may be covered with a scab. On moist situations the chancre is soft and moist also. The typical hard chancre begins as a papule or vesicle. Very soon the superficial epithelium is cast off and a shallow erosion is the result. The ulcer extends into the corium, is sharply defined, with smooth base and clean-cut edges. Infiltration is usually marked and so that when the ulcer is palpated laterally, it feels as if there were a bit of parchment in the base. The ulcer is quite indolent, and does not tend to spread. It is single in the vast majority of cases, and after the tenth day the virus cannot be inoculated in any other part of the body. The secretion is scanty, consisting of thin pus. Rarely, granulation tissue forms in abundance and small papillary excrescences are found on the base. Occasionally, when the ulcer is infected secondarily with pus cocci, it resembles closely the soft chancre, but the course of the affection and the sequelæ will distinguish. The hard chancre heals with formation of a scar, but induration persists for a long time. Recently, the Spirochæta pallida, the specific organism of syphilis, has been detected repeatedly in scrapings from chancres and in the tissues about them.

Tuberculosis of the skin is primary and secondary. Primary tuberculosis includes the "postmortem wart" (verruca tuberculosa) and lupus vulgaris. The secondary forms are the so-called scrofuloderma of the older writers, and certain ulcers of the skin and mucous surfaces about the various orifices of the body, found sometimes in tuberculous subjects.

The *verruca tuberculosa*, or anatomist's wart, is occasionally found in those who are brought into close contact with the bodies of individuals affected with tuberculosis, such as morbid anatomists, surgeons, and butchers. Washerwomen have also been known to become infected from handling infected linen. Human beings are usually infected with bacilli of human derivation, but, as Ravenel has shown recently, butchers may be infected from bovine tubercle. The bacilli enter through punctures and incised wounds, or through abrasions. The wart appears as a small, rough, elevated papule, of purplish color, which is extremely indolent in its development.

Microscopically, there is overgrowth of the papillæ, with hypertrophy and desquamation of the epidermis. Tubercles are found in the rete and in the subepithelial tissues. Bacilli are particularly scanty.

Should infection with pyogenic cocci take place at any time, a deeper, more widely-spreading, ulceration takes place, with, possibly, a lymphangitis. Systemic infection with death from disseminated tuberculosis has been known to occur. The skin, however, appears to be a particularly unfavorable soil for the growth of the tubercle bacillus, so that the resulting lesion remains for a long time strictly localized.

Lupus vulgaris has now been demonstrated beyond question to be a chronic tuberculosis of the skin and subcutaneous tissues. Two processes are at work, one of destruction of tissue, and one of hyperplasia, and the disease assumes several clinical forms according to the relative predominance of one or the other. The affection usually begins in early childhood, is commoner in females, and may last for many years. The lesion is single, more rarely multiple, and is oftenest found on the face, less frequently on the extremities and trunk.

The process begins in the lower layers of the corium with the formation of multiple minute tuberculous granulomas. These in time undergo necrosis and may become absorbed, but commonly fuse and extend through to the surface, so that open ulcers discharging pus and covered with crusts are produced. The older foci show central caseation, and the process spreads by the coalescence of neighboring granulomas and the formation of new ones at the periphery. Some of the granulomas may be absorbed, while others, after the discharge of the necrotic material, heal with the formation of dense fibrous scars. Thus, the picture is presented of scarring and more or less distortion of the parts at the centre of the lupus patch, while at the margin the disease is active and progressive. The connective-tissue hyperplasia may be so extreme that a form of elephantiasis results.

Fig. 233

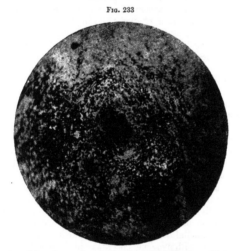

Tuberculous granulation tissue. A node of round-celled infiltration with two giant cells. An early stage. Zeiss obj. A, without ocular. (From the collection of the Royal Victoria Hospital.)

Microscopically, there is marked infiltration with round cells. Giant cells are fairly numerous, but epithelioid cells are scanty. Tubercle bacilli are but few in numbers. The sebaceous glands are often filled with inflammatory cells, and the various glands and follicles show varying grades of atrophy and destruction. The epithelium is involved secondarily, the cells of the rete being swollen, degenerated, or in other cases proliferating. The papillæ are frequently enlarged and extend downward, suggesting in appearance an epithelioma, which, indeed, in some cases is superadded. In other parts the epithelial layer is thinned, atrophic, and even destroyed.

According to the gross appearances presented, several clinical forms have been recognized. In the early stages, before there is destruction of tissue, the tubercles in the cutis may be indicated by reddish or yellowish-brown, smooth or scaly spots (*lupus maculosus*). Later, several foci are in close proximity, the central portion of the area, owing to absorption, becomes depressed, and the skin over it is brownish-red or brownish-yellow, fissured, and desquamating (*lupus exfoliativus*). When loss of substance has taken place, so that an open ulcer secreting pus and covered with crusts is produced, we speak of *lupus exulcerans*. In many cases the process tends to heal at the centre, with the formation of smooth, stellate scars, while it extends at the periphery (*lupus serpiginosus*). Or, under the epithelium and in the base of the ulcer

FIG. 234

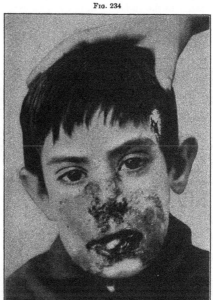

Ulcerating lupus of the face. (From the Skin Clinic of the Montreal General Hospital.)

papillary excrescences may form (*lupus frambœsioides, papillaris, verrucosus*), or nodules (*lupus nodosus, tuberosus, tumidus, hypertrophicus*), covered with crusts and epithelial scales. In the course of time, the disease extends to the deeper structures, even to the bone, and the larger part of the face, eyes, and lips may be destroyed, while from the extensive scarring marked deformity is produced. Carcinoma may develop in the base of such ulcers or even in the resultant scar.[1]

Secondary tuberculosis is not uncommon in tuberculous subjects, in parts of the body which are liable to be contaminated with infective

[1] Sequeira, Brit. Jour. of Derm., 20:1908:40.

discharges. Small superficial ulcers, of oval or rounded shape, with slightly infiltrated edges, and surrounded by minute granulomas, are found usually about the orifices of the body, the lips, genitalia, anus, but also on the head and other parts.

The so-called *scrofuloderma* (*tuberculosis subcutanea*) is found in cases of widespread chronic tuberculosis of various organs, and is found particularly in children the subjects of tuberculous lymphadenitis. The affection takes the form of well-defined, isolated, nodular granulomas, usually in the subcutaneous tissues. The disease may burrow deeply, or gradually extend to the surface. In this way an excavated ulcer is produced with livid undermined edges, having its base covered with granulations and necrotic material, and discharging a thin yellowish-white fluid.

FIG. 235

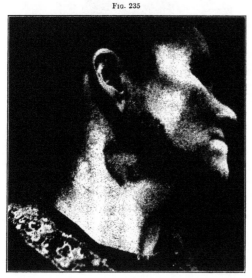

Serpiginous lupus of the face.   (From Dr. Shepherd's Skin Clinic, Montreal General Hospital.)

Miliary tuberculosis of the skin has been observed in cases of generalized hematogenic infection.

Rhinoscleroma is a rare disease, which appears to be practically confined to the continent of Europe. Its distinguishing feature is that it is an inflammatory granuloma possessing little or no tendency to necrosis. The generally accepted etiological factor is Bacillus rhinoscleromatis of v. Frisch, which is a short capsulated bacillus with rounded ends, not unlike Friedländer's organism.

The disease affects the skin of the nose and the mucous membrane of the throat and larynx. Large tumor-like growths, which are hard, grayish-red in color, and covered by relatively but little altered epithelium, are produced. These, microscopically, consist of cellular connective-tissue, arranged in rounded masses or strands, enclosing cells of varying appearance. Some are large, swollen, reticulated, and stain badly. Others are colloid or hyaline in appearance and contain bacilli, which are also to be found scattered throughout the tissues. Lymphatic channels are numerous. The disease remains strictly local and extends extremely slowly.

Lepra.—Leprosy is a disease, which, with tuberculosis, syphilis, actinomycosis, and rhinoscleroma, is classed among the infectious granulomas. The specific cause is Bacillus lepræ of Hansen, which is found in great numbers in the lesions. The affection is feebly contagious, being, so far as is known, only transmitted by close personal contact, or inoculation with infectious discharges.

Two main forms are recognized, identical in pathogenesis, and differing only in localization, namely, *lepra tuberculosa, tuberosa,* or *nodosa,* and *lepra anæsthetica.*

Tubercular leprosy usually affects the face, the extensor surfaces of the knees and elbows, the extremities, and especially the prepuce and scrotum. The lesion consists in the formation of granulomas, similar to those in tuberculosis and syphilis. These are composed of the usual lymphoid and epithelioid cells, with the addition of large granular and vacuolated cells known as "lepra cells." Giant cells are also present. The bacilli are found both in the lepra cells and in the lymphatics. A scraping in the skin lesions, stained with carbol-fuchsin, as shown by the late Wyatt Johnston, reveals the specific bacilli in abundance and affords a ready means of diagnosis. The process begins in the corium and gradually spreads through it to the subcutaneous tissues and to the surface. The various glands and follicles at first show hyperplasia but eventually are destroyed. The papillæ are gradually obliterated, and the epidermis is thinned or exfoliating. In the more advanced cases ulceration takes place. Objectively, the disease manifests itself at first by reddish patches on the skin, which may retrograde, leaving merely a pigmented spot, or are gradually transformed into discolored nodules or tumor-like masses. The disease may for a long time remain stationary, but in many cases the infiltration becomes extreme and the various nodules coalesce, so that the tissues of the face are greatly thickened and deformed (*elephantiasis Græcorum, facies leontina*). Redness and swelling of the skin, of erysipelatoid type, are found about the lesions, indicating the onset of fresh leprous infiltration.

In the anesthetic form the nodules form upon the nerves, in the peri- and endoneurium. The lesions affect at first the distal portions of the smaller nerves and spread centripetally. As a result, trophic changes become manifest in the skin in the form of whitish or brownish streaks (*lepra maculosa, morphœa nigra* et *alba*). Anesthesia of the part is a prominent symptom, resulting from the disintegration of the nerve fibres. As a result of the trophic disturbance, or of traumatism, ulcers readily form, which penetrate deeply and lead to the loss of portions of the body, such as the fingers and toes (*lepra mutilans*).

Leprosy has been recovered from, but, as a rule, the disease remains stationary for years, or, at most, is slowly progressive. As a consequence, those affected commonly die, not of leprosy, but of some intercurrent disease. Secondary septic infection of the ulcers may occur.

FIG. 236

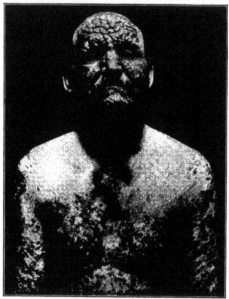

Case of nodular leprosy (from a patient of Dr. John V. Shoemaker's in the Medico-Chirurgical College, Philadelphia). The leonine expression is well shown. (McFarland.)

Actinomycosis of the skin may be primary, but is usually secondary to disease of the deeper parts. In man the affection most often begins somewhere in the buccal mucous membrane, usually at the alveolar process, and extends to the cervical lymphatic glands and the skin of the face and neck. The lesion is a chronic destructive granuloma, the skin being ulcerated or penetrated by discharging sinuses. Nodular foci with central cicatrization or diffuse infiltration may also occur. In the necrotic material and the discharge the specific organism—the actinomyces—is usually to be found. It may, however, be few in numbers and difficult to detect. Primary actinomycosis of the skin over the mamma has been noted, due to the application of a poultice.

Closely allied to actinomycosis is the *Madura foot disease* (*mycetoma pedis, fungous foot of India*), found in India and other tropical countries. It is rare in America,[1] only 5 cases having been recorded to date. The disease usually begins in the ball of the great toe, and is generally believed to result from trauma, such as the pricking of the toe with a thorn. The injured part begins to swell, and a firm, nodular mass forms beneath the skin, which assumes a purple color, and becomes indurated and adherent. The progress of the disease is excessively slow, and, curiously enough, painless. Secondary nodules form in other parts of the foot, which in the course of a year or so break down, and finally discharge externally, producing numerous intercommunicating sinuses. The discharge is a thin pus containing numerous spherical grains, which have been compared to salmon roe. Two varieties of these are described, the first pale yellow or pinkish in color, the second black. Etiologically, they are different. The pale variety is due to Actinomyces Maduræ of Vincent; the black or melanoid, to a hyphomyces.[2] The foot may be converted eventually into an enormous distorted mass, full of necrotic material and riddled with cavities while the skin on the surface presents numerous button-like nodules corresponding to the orifices of the fistulæ.[3]

Anthrax of the skin (*malignant pustule*) is a local inflammation produced by the anthrax bacillus. It is an affection of sheep, horses, and cattle rather common in certain countries. Human beings become infected through contact with infective discharges, or from handling the hides or wool of diseased animals. The virus enters usually through a scratch or abrasion, or, occasionally, from insect bites. The lesion takes the form of a pustule or carbuncle at the site of inoculation. The affected area is elevated above the general surface of the skin, and of a reddish or yellowish, often hemorrhagic appearance. On the surface of this are often to be seen vesicles, bullæ, or pustules. Slight erosion may take place with the effusion of a small amount of blood and serum, which dries into crusts. Consequently, the margin of the area is higher than the centre. The skin in the neighborhood is swollen, reddened, and œdematous, and may present small blebs. General infection and death often result, but where this does not occur, a gangrenous slough is formed which gradually separates. Occasionally, instead of a carbuncle being formed, there is a diffuse œdematous swelling.

Histologically, the papillary layer and the corium are infiltrated with inflammatory cells and exudate, together with hemorrhagic extravasation, and contain numbers of the specific bacilli. The superficial epidermis is in places elevated into vesicles. The deeper layers are also more or less infiltrated.

Glanders is a disease, occasionally involving the skin, due to infection with Bacillus mallei, which enters through some small cut or abrasion. The disease is usually derived from horses. At the site of inoculation an area of inflammatory swelling is formed, which quickly breaks

[1] Adami and Kirkpatrick, Trans. Assoc. Amer. Phys., 10: 1895: 92.

[2] Wright, Jour. Exper. Med., 3: 1898: 421.

[3] See also Dübenhofer, Arch. f. Derm., 88: 1907.

down into an ulcer, secreting thin pus, and having ragged eroded edges. The bacilli are apt to extend from the primary lesion along the lymphatics, producing diffuse erysipelatoid inflammation, or, again, secondary pustules and ulcers. Along the lymphatics, and in the glands, inflammatory nodules may be formed (*farcy buds*), which break down, giving rise to deep ulcers. When systemic infection occurs, abscesses may form in the internal organs, and, in fact, in any part of the body.[1] Pustular areas, resembling the pocks of variola, or pemphigoid blebs, may be formed in the skin, which break down and discharge a viscid bloodstained pus, often having an offensive odor.

Glanders may run an acute course of from two to four weeks, or, again, may last for many months. Acute glanders is almost invariably fatal. The chronic form may be recovered from. It may be associated with amyloid degeneration of the viscera.[2]

Oriental furuncle (tropical ulcer, Aleppo evil, Delhi boil, bouton de Biskra) is a local inflammation of the skin, which is contagious and due to a protozoön, similar to the Leishman-Donovan body found in kala-azar. The affection begins as a papule, which soon becomes a pustule. ·This breaks down into an ulcer. Healing takes place with the formation of a bluish-white cicatrix. Histologically, the lesion resembles a tubercle.[3]

Tropical phagedena is a rapidly progressing gangrenous ulceration of the skin found in certain tropical regions. The disease is supposed to be due to some germ which enters the skin through a slight wound.

Frambesia (Yaws) is a curious affection, found chiefly among negroes in some tropical countries. The disease is endemic and infectious and has some analogies with syphilis. It begins with a local manifestation at the site of inoculation, which after a variable time is followed by lesions of the skin, some constitutional disturbance, and often general enlargement of the glands. The disease may be acute or chronic. The skin lesions are found in the upper part of the cutis, and, histologically, resemble the other infectious granulomas. The later manifestations present the appearance of fungoid nodules covered with a scab, which when removed leaves a warty surface resembling a raspberry or cauliflower. The causal agent is a spirochete not unlike that of syphilis, the Spirochæta pertenuis of Castellani.

Erysipelas.—The chief diffuse dermatitis is erysipelas, an acute infectious and contagious disease, due to infection of the skin by Streptococcus erysipelatis of Fehleisen, believed to be a variety of Streptococcus pyogenes. The affection begins suddenly, with chill, fever, and considerable constitutional disturbance. It is often primary, but may complicate other diseases. Previously existing chronic skin diseases and previous attacks predispose. The infection spreads along the

---

[1] For literature see Arzt, Wiener klin. Woch., 5:1909.

[2] See Robins, Studies from the Royal Victoria Hospital, Montreal, 2: 1906: No. 1.

[3] See Wright, Jour. Med. Research, 10 : 1903; also Reinhardt, Zeitsch. f. Hygiene, 62:1908.

lymphatics. It is usual to classify the disease under three heads, according to the severity of the lesions, namely, *cutaneous erysipelas*, *cellulocutaneous erysipelas*, and *cellulitis*. The last-mentioned form should not, however, be regarded as necessarily due to the same etiological factor that is at work in the other types.

In the first form the skin is smooth, shiny, and of a vivid red color, the blush disappearing momentarily on pressure. Later, the color changes to a dusky bluish- or brownish-red. To the feel the affected part is hot, painful, and brawny. The spreading margin is sharply defined and more elevated than the remainder of the patch. The amount of exudation varies according to the intensity of the inflammation and its situation. In the case of loose tissues the œdema may be extreme. Frequently, the effused fluid collects beneath the superficial epidermis, which it raises into blisters or bullæ (*erysipelas vesiculosum et bullosum*). Occasionally, the vesicles contain seropus (*erysipelas pustulosum*). The exudation may dry into a scab upon the surface (*erysipelas crustosum*). As the inflammation subsides, the skin becomes less swollen and indurated, the color gradually disappears and desquamation of the epidermis occurs.

Histologically, one finds in the corium, and even in the deeper structures, evidences of a cellulofibrinous exudation. The bloodvessels and lymphatics are congested. Inflammatory leukocytes are found in clusters about the vessels. The cells of the epidermis are swollen, cloudy, vacuolated, or may have undergone colliquation necrosis. The vesicles, if present, contain fibrin, and a few inflammatory cells. Streptococci are found chiefly in the lymphatics, but also to some extent in the tissues.

In cellulocutaneous erysipelas the subcutaneous tissues are involved as well as the skin. The parts are greatly swollen, œdematous, and of a dull red color. When incised the tissues suggest the appearance of wet washleather. The skin may present numerous blebs or may actually slough. Abscesses form in the subcutaneous structures which often point and discharge externally. Gangrenous necrosis of certain areas may result, and the process spreads laterally and to the deeper parts, advancing along the lymphatics. General pyemia sometimes follows.

Most cases of erysipelas heal. Meningitis is an occasional sequel of the disease. Repeated attacks may lead to a form of elephantiasis.

Besides the forms of dermatitis of frankly bacterial origin, there are others due to the action of various kinds of moulds. These are generally known as the *dermatomycoses*. Chief among these are the affections called favus, ringworm, pityriasis, erythrasma, and blastomycetic dermatitis.

Favus (tinea favosa) is an affection of the skin due to the activity of a vegetable parasite, Achorion Schönleinii. The hairy parts of the body, notably the head and beard, are those usually affected, but other regions may be attacked, as, for instance, the nails. The disease is common in certain of the lower animals, and is readily transmitted to man and from man to man. The fungus takes the form of a mycelium, composed of threads, frequently branching, which vary considerably in length and breadth. Some are thin, delicate, and homogeneous; others larger, moniliform, or divided into compartments by transverse divisions, and contain spores. The spores also vary considerably in appearance, some being round or oval, others irregular, polyhedral, or oblong. They are found chiefly at the ends of certain of the mycelial fibres, but are also free or in little clumps. The organism is found chiefly in the shaft and bulb of the hairs and in the hair-follicles. It insinuates itself between the horny cells of the epidermis, forming a small, yellowish area just beneath the surface, penetrated by a hair. As it grows, a sulphur-yellow, concave or cup-like disk (*scutula*), the size of a lentil or larger, is produced. This disk is convex below and

Fig. 237

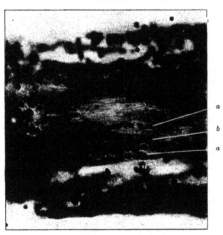

Portion of a hair invaded by the trichophyton, endoectothrix. × 500. *a, a,* chains of spores in focus. *b,* a chain situated farther within the hair, and hence not in focus. (From a photomicrograph.) (Hyde.)

lies in a corresponding excavation in the skin. When the growth is removed the underlying skin is moist and red, owing to reactive inflammation. In long-standing cases, atrophy of the hair-papillæ and various glands, and of the rete and upper part of the corium results. Loss of hair and scarring may be permanent. When exposed to the air, the favus clump becomes dried into a dirty, yellowish-white, crumbling mass, which is readily broken up. The hairs of the affected part are dry, lustreless, and easily pulled out. The fungus by suitable methods can be demonstrated in the hair-sheaths.

In favus of the nails—*onychomycosis favosa*—the fungus grows between the keratinous layers of the nail-plate, which is thickened, brittle, and infiltrated with yellowish masses. Complete disintegration of the nail may result.

Ringworm is a dermatomycosis of which several forms are recognized according to the nature of the parasite at work. At least two distinct varieties of fungus have been demonstrated, one with small spores— Microsporon Audouini; the other with large spores—the Trichophyton. In the first case the mycelium is developed within the hair itself, and the filaments after division terminate on the outer aspect of the hair shaft. The spores are entirely external to the hair. In the case of the trichophyton the spores are found in rows, parallel to the long axis of the hair. The mycelium is not produced within the hair. Three subvarieties of the trichophyton are now recognized, according to the position of the spores within or without the hair, viz., the endothrix, the ectothrix, and the endoectothrix.

Several forms of ringworm (tinea) are recognized clinically, according to the localization of the lesions.

Tinea tonsurans (ringworm of the scalp) is due to the presence of the microsporon, less often of the endothrix, within the hairs and hair-follicles. The affection results in the formation of an area of slight inflammation on the scalp, in which the hairs are brittle and readily break off, leaving brush-like stumps projecting just above the surface of the skin. This is due to the distortion of the bulb and shaft of the hair, together with its separation into fibrils. The disease is commoner in children than in adults, is, of course, contagious, and is liable to appear in epidemics.

Tinea circinata is found on the hairless portions of the body and is due to the presence of the trichophyton in the deeper parts of the horny layer and in the upper parts of the rete. The fungus extends centrifugally, forming the characteristic circinate lesions of ringworm. A reactive inflammation, marked by hyperemia, is also present, and varies in severity according to the amount of moisture, warmth, and irritation to which the part involved is subjected. In parts of the body where two surfaces rub upon one another, and the epithelium is macerated from retained and decomposing sweat, a severe inflammation with the formation of vesicles and scabs (*eczema marginatum*) results.

Tinea sycosis (barber's itch) is a ringworm of the hairy parts of the face, caused by the trichophyton, usually the ectothrix variety, or, possibly, the endoectothrix. The lesion is a folliculitis and perifolliculitis. The hairs become loosened and fall out. The inflammation is more intense than in other forms of ringworm. The hair-follicles and sebaceous glands are destroyed, and small abscesses may form here and there in the deeper parts. This is possibly the result of secondary infection with pyogenic microörganisms.

Tinea imbricata (Tokelau ringworm) is found in tropical countries and is due to a form of trichophyton. The fungus is found only in the epidermis and the follicles are unaffected.

Tinea versicolor (pityriasis versicolor, dermatomycosis furfuracea) is a mycotic disease of the skin, affecting chiefly the covered parts of the body. The organism at work is Microsporon furfur, which is found in the upper portion of the stratum corneum. It produces desquamation, but the reactive inflammation is practically nil. The hair-follicles are not involved. The affected part presents an irregular, yellowish-brown, blotchy appearance, with slight desquamation of the epidermis.

Erythrasma is a somewhat similar affection, believed by some to be due to Microsporon minutissimum, although others think that it is produced by bacteria. The disease is found in parts of the body which are warm and moist, as, for instance, in the groins and axillæ, where two skin surfaces come together. The patches are fairly well defined, and present slight redness and desquamation.

FIG. 238

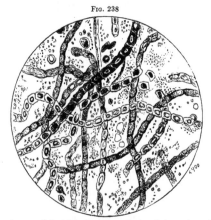

Filaments and spores of the trichophyton from the beard of a patient affected with tinea sycosis. (Hyde.)

Blastomycetic dermatitis is a curious and rare affection of the skin, first described by Gilchrist,[1] due to a fungus related to the yeasts. When fully developed, the lesion bears a somewhat close resemblance to verrucose tuberculosis, and occasionally to superficial papillary epithelioma. With care, however, differentiation is possible. The affection begins with the formation of a papule or pustule, which gradually spreads until, in the course of months or years, considerable areas of skin are involved. A warty, tumor-like outgrowth, presenting occasional superficial ulcerations covered with crusts, is the result. The lesions may be extensive and are apt to be multiple.

Histologically, the appearances are those of an inflammatory granuloma. The most marked changes are found in the rete, the epithelium of which shows hyperplasia in the form of extensive, elongated and branching, downgrowths of its cells, producing finger-like processes

[1] Johns Hopkins Hosp. Rep., 1 : 1896 : 269.

PLATE XI

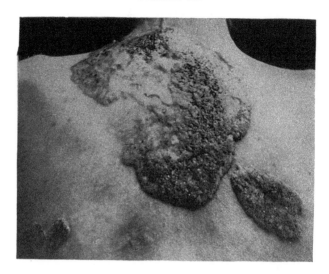

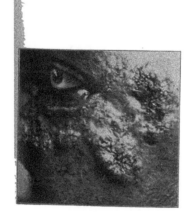

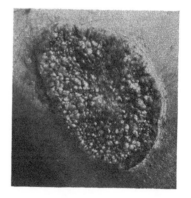

Clinical Types of Cutaneous Blastomycosis.

practically identical with those seen in epithelioma. Polymorphonuclear leukocytes are found scattered about, both between and within
the cells, or in small clumps which are really minute abscesses. These,
according to Montgomery, are characteristic of the process. When
disintegration is complete, the abscesses contain degenerating leukocytes,
red-blood cells, epithelial cells, particles of chromatin and other cell-
detritus, the specific microörganism, and, usually, giant cells. The
rete-cells are large and swollen, somewhat dissociated, and the prickles
are particularly well defined. Those in the immediate neighborhood
of the abscesses are more or less flattened. Single giant cells are occasionally to be observed, surrounded by a few leukocytes. Isolated cells,
or groups of cells, show pathological keratinization. A layer of columnar
cells, occasionally showing mitoses, can usually be traced, more or
less perfectly between the epithelium and the corium.

In the corium inflammatory infiltration may be very marked. Leukocytes, endothelial cells, and plasma cells are to be observed. Miliary
abscesses may occur here also. Mast-cells and giant cells may be
found in varying numbers.

The horny layer of the skin varies much in thickness. In some
places it is eroded, in others thickened, penetrating downward between
the papillæ, which are thereby dislocated and distorted. On the surface can be seen scab-like masses of dried secretion, composed of pus,
blood, desquamated epithelium, and bacteria.

The specific organism can readily be demonstrated by placing portions
of tissue or pus in a strong solution of caustic potash. In stained
sections the parasite is a round, oval, or slightly irregular body, possessing a highly refractile, doubly contoured, homogeneous capsule. The
protoplasm is somewhat granular, and separated from the capsule
by a space of varying width. In the cell-body, a clear vacuole can
often be made out. The parasite lies singly or in pairs, and budding
forms in all stages can usually be seen. It is found in the abscesses,
between the epithelial cells, and in the giant cells.

The organism has been successfully cultivated, although it grows
with some difficulty, and when inoculated into the lower animals has
produced abscesses or inflammatory granulomas. It seems fairly well
established now that the parasite is specific, although it is possible that
there may be several subvarieties.[1]

Dermatitis Due to Animal Parasites.—The most important disease
to be considered here is *scabies*, an inflammatory affection due to the
action of the itch-mite or Acarus scabiei. The impregnated female
mite penetrates the epidermis and burrows its way into the rete, or
even as far as the upper layers of the corium, forming a curved, somewhat sacculated track. In the early stages the parasite can usually
be recognized at the blind end of the burrow as a whitish speck the size

---

[1] For a very full consideration of this form of dermatitis, see Ricketts, Oidiomycosis,
(Blastomycosis) of the Skin and its Fungi, Jour. of Med. Research (new series)
1 : 1901 : 373.

of a pin-point. In the burrow are also to be found brownish or blackish granules, the feces, and sometimes more or less numerous immature mites. Owing to the irritation caused by the presence of the parasites, and also from the scratching induced thereby, considerable inflammation is set up, so that an eczematous eruption is usually the result, characterized by the formation of pustules and vesicles. In long-standing cases the skin may undergo a marked change. The stratum corneum is hypertrophied, the cutis is thickened and infiltrated with inflammatory products, and the papillæ are increased in length.

Pediculosis is an inflammatory affection of the skin produced by the agency of lice upon the skin or in the hair. The inflammation is usually a mild one, and is produced, in part, by the irritation caused by the insect, and, in part, by scratching. Three different forms are described. In pediculosis capitis the parasite is found upon the scalp or on the hairs, while the ova can be detected attached to the hairs by a chitinous sheath. In long-standing cases marked inflammation results. Pustules or even small abscesses may form in the scalp. There is notable exudation and the hair may be considerably matted together (plica polonica). This is seen most often just above the nape of the neck. The irritation in the case of pediculosis corporis is less marked. The lice infect the clothes and wander on the skin to feed. Owing to the long-continued mild inflammation, the skin becomes somewhat thickened and pigmented and scored with scratches (vagabond's disease). Pediculosis pubis is usually found in the pubic region, but may affect the other hairy parts of the body. The ova are similar to those of the head-louse, but are smaller. The secondary inflammatory disturbance is trifling in this variety.

A somewhat similar disturbance is caused by certain other parasites, among which may be mentioned Pulex irritans, or common flea, Cimex lectularius, or bedbug, Pulex penetrans, or sand-flea. The larvæ of certain diptera are sometimes found beneath the skin. The most common offender is the gad-fly (Æstrus bovis).

Cysticerci and Echinococci have been found in the skin.

Filaria medinensis (Guinea-worm) is a parasite, found in warm countries, which gains access to the body through the ingestion of water containing the larvæ. The female worm, which is the one causing the disease, is from fifteen to forty inches long, and one-tenth of an inch in diameter. For ten to fifteen months the worm remains lodged in the muscles and then gradually works its way to the surface of the body, where it can be felt as a soft coil under the skin. The skin over the worm ultimately gives way and a small ulcer is produced. Abscess-formation may result in some cases in lymphangitis, septicemia, and gangrene.

Craw-craw is a rare disease, in the form of an acute superficial dermatitis, which affects principally the negroes of the west coast of Africa. It is supposed to be due to a worm, allied to Filaria medinensis.

Dermatitis of Neuropathic Origin.—It is a well-known fact that in certain disorders of the central nervous system and of the peripheral nerve-trunks the skin may undergo striking changes. These may be simply minor alterations in the appearance and texture of the skin, or may amount to actual inflammation or other profound disturbance. Thus, in cases of rheumatoid arthritis, the skin over the affected joints is often found to be soft, velvety, and of smooth, glistening appearance. In certain organic diseases of the spinal cord, gangrene of the skin and subcutaneous tissues (bedsores) often comes on with great rapidity. So also in tabes dorsalis, penetrating ulcers on the extremities, usually over the great toe, are occasionally met with. Besides these, there is a considerable number of disorders of the skin, which, with more or less certainty, may be attributed, either wholly or in part, to neurotrophic influences.

FIG. 239

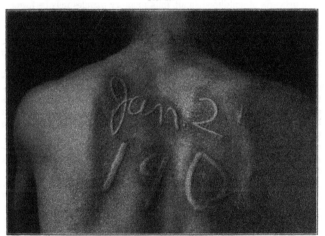

Urticaria factitia (angioneurosis). (Hyde and Ormsby.)

Among the conditions which may, in some instances at least, be attributed to nervous disturbances should be mentioned *urticaria*. This is an angioneurosis in which an idiosyncrasy of the individual plays an important predisposing role. The disease is found in those of a neurotic temperament, and has been known to follow upon mental worry. In other cases, disorders of digestion, gastro-intestinal intoxication, are at work. Thus, some persons are intolerant of certain foods, such as cheese, shellfish, fruits, or, again, certain drugs. In those predisposed, external irritation, even of the slightest description, may precipitate an attack. For example, in *urticaria factitia* (dermatographia) the simple drawing of the finger-nail over the skin is followed in a few moments by the production of a wheal, exactly conforming to the region of irritation.

The exact pathogeny of the condition is not altogether agreed upon. Most seem to think that there is a preliminary brief contraction of the vessels. This is followed by paretic dilatation with exudation of plasma, and local stasis. At first there is produced an elevated, somewhat firm nodule, of dull red color, which soon becomes paler in the centre (the wheal). This last change is attributed to the compression of the capillaries of the part by the increasing exudation. The effusion of plasma may be so great as to elevate the superficial epidermis, thereby forming blisters (*urticaria bullosa*). Or, again, the œdema may be followed by extravasation of blood (*urticaria hemorrhagica, purpura urticans*). In still other cases there is an accumulation of pigment in the deeper layers of the rete, with persistence of papules and nodules after the wheals have disappeared (*urticaria pigmentosa*). In the obstinate urticaria of childhood small, inflammatory papules may be formed, apparently follicular in origin (*urticaria papulosa, lichen urticatus strophulus*).

A closely allied, if not identical, condition, is *angioneurotic œdema* (see p. 113). This probably does not depend upon external irritation and is believed to originate in the subcutaneous tissues.

Prurigo.—The term "prurigo" is rather loosely employed by dermatologists to designate any pruritic dermatitis associated with the formation of more or less persistent papules. The prurigo of Hebra is an affection of early childhood, which persists mostly throughout life. It begins with the formation of urticarial nodes on the extensor surfaces of the extremities, associated with the most intense itching. In course of time, owing to the irritation produced by scratching, small inflammatory nodules are formed, over which the skin is excoriated and often covered with scabs. It may be complicated by eczema and erysipelas. Auspitz, v. Hebra, Schwimmer, among others, class it among the neuroses.

Herpes[1] is an affection of the skin characterized by the formation of papules, which are soon converted into vesicles, and after some days into pustules. The efflorescence corresponds fairly accurately with certain nerve tracts. Various parts of the body may be involved, the face (*herpes facialis*), the forehead (*herpes frontalis*), the conjunctiva (*herpes ophthalmicus*), the lip (*herpes labialis*), the genitalia (*herpes progenitalis* and *preputialis*), and the trunk (*herpes zoster*). The exact cause is not known, but is believed to be some local or reflex nervous disorder. Herpes of the face and lips is found in certain infectious diseases, notably pneumonia, and gastro-intestinal derangements. Herpes progenitalis may be reflex or the result of some local irritation.

In herpes zoster the lesions are found along the course of one or more intercostal nerves. They are usually unilateral. The affection is believed by some to be bacterial in origin. Others consider it an angioneurosis. It may be sporadic or epidemic. The pathological condition most frequently found is inflammation of the posterior ganglion and of the nerve-trunk supplying the affected portion of the skin. Changes of various kinds have also been reported in the central nervous system.

---

[1] For literature see Hedinger, Deutsche Zeitschr. f. Nervenheilkunde, 24 : 1903.

PLATE XII

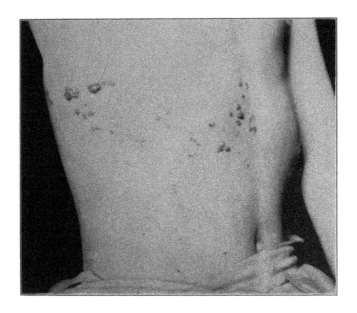

Herpes Zoster.

Histologically, the rete cells undergo rapid proliferation and certain of them degenerate, forming small cavities. The papillary bodies in turn become inflamed and the cavities coalesce to form vesicles. Gilchrist[1] found in the papular stage, before the formation of the vesicle, a notable multiplication of the nuclei in the rete without any increase in the mitotic figures.

Herpes iris is, according to Kaposi, identical with erythema iris. The vesicles are found on the hands and feet.

Dermatitis herpetiformis (dermatitis multiformis, herpes gestationis, hydroa herpetiforme, Duhring's disease, pemphigus pruriginosus) is an obscure affection, regarded by Duhring as intermediate between pemphigus and erythema multiforme. It is most likely neuropathic in nature. It has been attributed to many causes, neurasthenia, general debility, renal and other organic disease, and pregnancy. The process is an acute inflammation of the papillary layer. There is a marked exudation of plasma, leukocytes, and red blood-cells. The exudate is fibrinous in nature. Large numbers of eosinophiles are found in the blood and in the local lesions.

Dermatitis of Unknown and Doubtful Etiology.—*Dermatitis exfoliativa* is the term rather loosely employed to designate any inflammation of the skin associated with desquamation of the epidermis. The condition sometimes complicates eczema, psoriasis, lichen ruber, and other varieties of dermatitis. Occasionally, it arises idiopathically.

In the early stages there is, according to Crocker, a superficial inflammation of the corium, characterized by congestion, œdema, and cellular infiltration. The rete is thinned and there is separation of the upper portion of the stratum corneum. Later, there is proliferation of the rete cells with some connective-tissue hyperplasia. In the most advanced forms the horny layer is thickened and there is more or less atrophy of the rete and corium and of the hair-follicles and sebaceous glands. The *pityriasis rubra* of Hebra is by many considered to be a severe form of dermatitis exfoliativa. It is a rare affection, which may continue for many years, and is usually fatal from marasmus. Histologically, it seems to correspond fairly accurately with the more advanced form of exfoliative dermatitis. Exfoliative dermatitis has been found in young infants (Ritter) and may be epidemic (Savill).

Pityriasis rosea (herpes tonsurans maculosus, pityriasis maculata et circinata) is a somewhat similar disease, a simple superficial inflammation running an acute course, and associated with branny desquamation of the epidermis. Kaposi believed it to be due to the local action of a parasite, but it is more probably due to a systemic infection. According to Unna, there is a superficial inflammation with œdema and cellular infiltration of the cutis and lower portions of the rete, œdema of the upper rete cells, acanthosis and parakeratosis, together with the formation of minute "subcorneal pressure vesicles."

Eczema is perhaps the most common form of inflammation of the skin. The disease may be acute but is often chronic, and has a notable tendency

[1] Johns Hopkins Hosp. Rep., 1.

to relapse. The lesions are strikingly polymorphous. The skin is more or less reddened and swollen, and may be covered with papules, vesicles, pustules, and crusts. The affected part is very itchy, may be exfoliating, and often is moist from exudation. In the chronic cases the skin is thickened and often fissured.

Although the condition has been frequently and carefully studied, the etiology is still to a great extent, obscure. Many cases are to be attributed to external irritation, such as may be caused by parasites, scratching, moisture, or acrid discharges. Some individuals are more susceptible to the action of these causes than are others. Other cases are the result of some systemic disorder or of disturbed metabolism, such as gout, rheumatism, toxemias, gastro-intestinal derangements, and malnutrition. In still other instances there seems to be a neurotic agency at work.

In the mildest form, where the irritation is not extreme or the skin is not particularly sensitive, small nodular elevations are found in the skin (*eczema papulosum*). In somewhat more severe cases vesicles may be produced (*eczema vesiculosum*). When the contents of the blisters are absorbed or dry up the superficial epidermis may be exfoliated. When the inflammation is more intense, considerable areas of skin may become painful, red, and swollen (*eczema erythematosum*). On this inflamed base may be formed blisters, which subsequently may become purulent (*eczema pustulosum*). Should the epidermis be lost, as from rubbing or scratching, we get a weeping surface (*eczema madidans*). Where considerable patches of epidermis are lost, the underlying surface presents a dusky red appearance (*eczema rubrum*). Frequently, the serous or purulent discharge dries upon the surface into yellowish crusts (*eczema crustosum*). Under the crusts pus may accumulate (*eczema impetiginosum*). In other cases the epithelium may proliferate beneath the scabs, so that the surface appears to be reddened, thickened, and scurfy (*eczema squamosum*). Eczema characterized by somewhat larger pustules covered with crusts is often called *impetigo*. When the pustules and crusts are still larger the condition is known as *ecthyma*.

Histologically, in acute eczema, one finds congestion of the blood and lymphatic vessels in the corium, with exudation of plasma, and diapedesis of leukocytes. The connective-tissue fibres are swollen and compressed, and there is to some extent proliferation of the connective-tissue corpuscles. In the milder forms, the process is chiefly confined to the papillary regions and upper layers of the corium, but in severer cases extends to the subcutaneous tissues. The cells of the rete are swollen, and there is effusion of fluid, with more or less numerous wandering cells. The rete-cells may also undergo a colliquative necrosis with the formation of cavities. When the exudation is marked, vesicles or bullæ may form between the rete and the horny layer, which contain serum, fibrin, leukocytes, and detritus. In the pustular variety the number of leukocytes is very considerable. Desquamation of the superficial epidermis takes place in many instances and is a characteristic change in eczema squamosum and rubrum.

In chronic eczema, proliferation of connective tissue in the corium, with deposit of pigment, together with hyperplasia of the rete, dominate the picture. The process may extend to the subcutaneous tissues, producing atrophy of the fat, hair-follicles, and glands. Occasionally, owing to the obstruction of veins and lymphatics, a form of elephantiasis results. The acute form, however, may heal without producing much permanent change, save, possibly, a little pigmentation.

Erythema exudativum multiforme is an affection of unknown etiology, the characteristic features of which are congestion, œdema, and sometimes hemorrhage in the skin. It is found usually in young persons and those of a rheumatic tendency. In some cases the disease is symptomatic, being found in such affections as rheumatism, typhus, syphilis, and gonorrhœa. Here, it is possibly of the nature of an infective metastatic dermatitis. In other cases it is thought to be an angioneurosis caused by some reflex disturbance or a circulating toxin.

In the mildest form of the affection there is simple congestion of the skin. In others, there is an inflammatory exudation into the papillary and middle layers of the corium, and sometimes even into the deeper portions of the corium and the subcutaneous tissues. The cells of the rete may show proliferation. Where the serous exudation is marked it may lead to the accumulation of fluid in the rete, or the elevation of the epidermis into blisters (herpes iris, herpes circinatus, erythema bullosum, hydroa vesiculosum). There is always more or less extravasation of the red blood-cells.

In *erythema nodosum*, rather deeply seated painful nodes are formed in the cutis and subcutaneous tissues. These often project slightly above the surface as firm, dusky red infiltrations. As the process subsides, the color changes to bluish-red, green, and yellow. In exceptional cases the inflammation is so intense as to result in gangrene. The disease is usually associated with inflammatory rheumatism, but may occur without arthritic manifestations. It is found also as a complication of scarlatina, measles, typhoid fever, and pyemia. It is probably a sporadic and embolic myositis of infective origin.

Pemphigus[1] is a somewhat obscure affection of the skin, the chief feature of which is the efflorescence of numerous vesicles, varying in size from that of a pea to that of a goose egg. The vesicles appear occasionally on apparently healthy skin, but, as a rule, develop in patches of erythema or urticaria-like nodes. They contain a clear watery fluid, or sometimes blood, which eventually becomes cloudy and purulent. The vesicles then dry up with the formation of crusts (*pemphigus vulgaris*). In some cases the superficial epidermis is cast off so that the corium is exposed over considerable areas (*pemphigus foliaceus*). A red weeping surface is thus produced. In such cases the corium is more or less infiltrated and there may be a certain amount of necrosis (*pemphigus diphtheriticus*). Fresh granulations may be formed, which in their turn are destroyed. In the so-called *pemphigus*

---

[1] For literature see Luithlen, Arch. f. Derm. u. Syph., 40:1897.

vegetans, which is the most severe form of the affection and progresses
rapidly toward death, the inflammatory phenomena are more marked.
The vesicles appear at first on the skin of the genitals, on the inner side
of the thighs, the axillæ, and the mucous membrane of the mouth,
eventually spreading to the other mucous surfaces and the skin of the
whole body. When the superficial epidermis is exfoliated, numerous
polypoid or warty excrescences, closely set together, are produced,
which become bounded by an excoriated zone, and later, are surrounded
by other blisters. A foul-smelling discharge is the result, which dries
into crusts.

The histological appearances in pemphigus have been variously
interpreted. Some think that the process is a primary dermatitis.
Auspitz, among others, believes that there is first a sudden liberation
of fluid from the vessels of the derma, which mechanically separates the
cells of the rete. Spaces are thus formed which coalesce to form the
vesicles. The vesicles or bullæ may originate between the rete and
the superficial horny layers, but, according to Crocker, may also be
found entirely within the rete. Later the signs of a secondary inflammation set in.

Numerous etiological factors have been held to be the cause of
pemphigus. Many cases are attributable, directly or indirectly, to
disorders of the central nervous system and peripheral nerves, so that
such cases may be regarded as trophoneuroses. Chills (Crocker),
hysteria (Dumesnil), traumatism, and local wound-infection (Pernet
and Bullock) have also been assigned as causes. A curious point is
the marked increase of the eosinophile cells in the blood and in the
fluid of the vesicles. There is some evidence in favor of a microbic
origin for the disease.

Closely related to pemphigus is the disease known as *pompholyx*
(cheiropompholyx, dysidrosis). Here the vesicles are more deeply
seated in the palms of the hands and soles of the feet. The condition
is an inflammatory one. The vesicles form in the upper layers of the
rete, the cells of which are compressed and pushed apart, and are filled
with serum, fibrin, and later with leukocytes. The sweat-glands,
almost without exception, are unaltered. The upper layers of the corium
show slight inflammation. The affection is found most often in those
of a nervous temperament, or who suffer from worry or overwork.

In *hydroa vacciniforme* vesicles form upon the skin, not unlike those
found in variola. They present a central dark depression and ultimately heal, forming a scar. The disease is a rare one, beginning
usually in infancy, and appears to follow exposure to the sun's rays,
and to heat and cold. The process seems to begin with inflammation
of the upper layers of the corium, followed by the formation of vesicles
in the middle portion of the rete. This gives place to a sharply defined
necrosis, involving the rete, the upper part of the corium, and the lower
layers of the stratum corneum.

Psoriasis is a rather common affection of the skin which begins with
the formation of small brownish-red papules that in the course of a

few days become topped with a whitish silvery scale. This when removed leaves a somewhat reddish-brown surface on which may be seen a small bleeding point. In some cases the patches may be of considerable size. As the process heals, the scale is exfoliated and the epidermis returns to its normal condition, save that a certain amount of pigmentation usually remains. Sometimes the patches heal at the centre while extending at the periphery (*psoriasis annularis* sive *gyrata*). The lesions of psoriasis usually affect chiefly the extensor surfaces of the limbs in the neighborhood of the joints, the sacral region, and on the hairy parts of the head. Any part of the body, however, may be involved, even the nails.

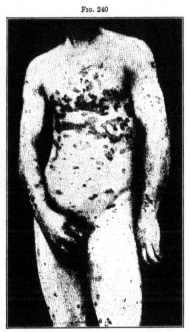

FIG. 240

Psoriasis. (From Dr. Shepherd's Skin Clinic, Montreal General Hospital.)

Histological examination shows the horny layer to be considerably thickened, the cells being more or less dissociated from each other, so that spaces are formed which contain cell-debris, bodies that are thought by some to be micrococci, and air. This presence of air gives the scales their characteristic silvery sheen. Cornification is imperfect. The stratum granulosum is in places thickened, in others, thinned or absent. The cells of the rete show proliferative changes. There are effusion of serum and extravasation of cells into the corium. In advanced cases there is overgrowth of the papillæ, together with hyperplasia of connective tissue, and the process may spread even to the subcutaneous structures. These appearances have been variously interpreted. Some have held that the inflammation in the corium is primary, but later observers think that it is secondary to the changes in the rete and the deeper layers of the epidermis.

The disease is an obstinate one, and certain individuals seem to have a special predisposition to it. In such persons slight external irritation may precipitate an attack. It is common also in those of a rheumatic or gouty tendency.

Lichen ruber acuminatus (Kaposi) is characterized by the formation of minute, hard, reddish papules, covered at their summits with thickened epidermis. These enlarge by peripheral growth, until large, diffuse, reddish, scaly patches are produced. Eventually the whole body may be involved.

Histologically, one finds overgrowth, and imperfect cornification of the horny layer, involving the outlets of the sebaceous follicles. There is a cellular infiltration about the vessels of the corium, the sweat-glands, and the papillary bodies. The rete is thickened and the inter-papillary processes are irregularly hypertrophied. The disease is now generally believed to be the same as the *pityriasis rubra pilaris* of the French school. The cause is not known.

FIG. 241

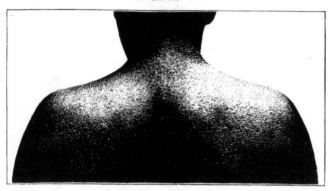

Lichen ruber acuminatus in a negro. (Howard Fox's case.)

In *lichen ruber planus* the nodes are flat, somewhat concave, and of a glistening, pale or reddish waxy appearance. Crocker[1] holds that the process is an inflammation of the upper layers of the corium with secondary involvement of the epidermis.

The disease is said to occur most frequently in those of a neurotic disposition or who are suffering from some derangement of the nervous system.

Hypertrophic and verrucous forms are described.

Lupus erythematosus is a rather uncommon affection of the skin, found most often in women, and during the third decade of life. The etiology is quite obscure. Some believe the disease to be a form of tuberculosis, but this view is not supported by a study of the lesions.

According to Kaposi, lupus erythematosus begins with the formation of small, elevated, reddish patches from the size of a pin-head to that of a lentil. These are somewhat depressed in the centre, which has a glistening scar-like appearance or is covered with thin adherent scales. The process may heal at the centre and advance at the periphery (*lupus*

Diseases of the Skin, second edition, 1893.

erythematosus discoides). In other cases the disease progresses by the formation of secondary foci (*lupus erythematosus disseminatus*). The lesions may be found on the face, the fingers, toes, knees, and elbows. When on the face a somewhat characteristic appearance is produced in the form of a butterfly-shaped patch of redness extending across the bridge of the nose over both cheeks.

The lesion appears to consist in an inflammation of the upper layers of the corium, in the neighborhood of the hair-follicles, sebaceous glands, and bloodvessels. This is shown by the presence of a more or less extensive infiltration of the tissues with leukocytes, and hyperplasia of the connective tissue. The specific cells of the glands show some overgrowth, but in course of time, owing to retrograde changes and the fibrous-tissue overgrowth, the glands tend to atrophy and disappear. The papillæ and interpapillary process also are destroyed. Small hemorrhages may be observed, and the vessels show some endarteritis, with occasionally, thrombosis or embolism. The epidermis is swollen, heaped up into scales, or elevated into vesicles. Later, it becomes thin and atrophic. The caseous nodes with giant cells, characteristic of lupus vulgaris, are not met with here.

Secondary or Symptomatic Dermatitis.—The Exanthemata.—There are a number of systemic diseases, some of them certainly and others probably of the nature of infections, in which skin lesions are a more or less constant and characteristic accompaniment. The cutaneous manifestations may be comparatively trifling, as in the diffuse erythemas which are occasionally met with in sepsis, or, again, may be so striking as to dominate the clinical picture. The diseases belonging to the latter group are known as the exanthemata. Chief among them are measles, scarlatina, varicella, variola, typhoid, and typhus, to which may perhaps be added secondary syphilis.

The pathogenesis of such manifestations is, possibly, to be explained as the effect of circulating toxins upon the bloodvessels, either directly or through the vasomotor system, and by the local action of the toxins upon the epidermis.

The exanthem of *measles* is met with first on the mucous membrane of the lips and mouth in the form of small bright red spots, in the centre of which are minute bluish-white points (Koplik's spots). These may appear from twenty-four or forty-eight hours to three or even five days before the eruption appears on the skin. Occasionally, they may be found before any catarrhal symptoms manifest themselves. The skin lesions appear upon the neck, face, forehead, trunk and limbs, in the order named.

The spots are dull red blotches in the skin, or sometimes slightly raised above the general level. They are irregular, often crescentic in shape, and in places may become confluent. The skin and subcutaneous tissues are in parts somewhat œdematous. In the course of a few hours, or two or three days, the eruption begins to pale, and gradually disappears, leaving a slight yellowish pigmentation, with fine desquamation of the epidermis. Rarely, the eruption may be hemorrhagic.

Histologically, one finds usually congestion of the bloodvessels and lymphatics with œdema of the corium. In the papular form there is in addition slight diapedesis of leukocytes about the vessels, around the glands, and in the papillary bodies. Minute hemorrhages are also occasionally met with. In the most severe forms there may be necrosis of the epithelium.

The eruption in *scarlatina* makes its appearance first upon the neck and upper part of the thorax in front, extending rapidly to the rest of the trunk, and finally to the extremities. The skin presents, at first, the appearance of a fiery, reddish-pink blush. When examined more closely, the rash is found to consist of innumerable fine reddish points closely set together. Occasionally, the exanthem is more distinctly papular (*scarlatina papulosa*), or may be associated with the formation of vesicles and blebs (*scarlatina vesicularis* et *pemphigoides*). Hemorrhages into the skin may also occur (*scarlatina hemorrhagica*). After a variable period, from one to seven days, the eruption assumes a more dusky red or livid appearance and gradually fades, leaving a slightly pigmented surface. Finally, the epidermis desquamates in the form of fine impalpable scales (desquamatio furfuracea) or in large flakes (desquamatio membranacea).

Histologically, the bloodvessels of the skin are found to be congested and in a state of paralytic dilatation. It is said by most, although this is denied by Unna, that there is an inflammatory exudate in the interstitial tissues, consisting of plasma, leukocytes, and extravasated red blood-cells. The rete cells appear also to be rapidly proliferating.

Recently, Mallory[1] has described certain bodies in and between the epithelial cells of the epidermis and free in the superficial lymph-vessels and spaces of the corium, which he is inclined to think are protozoa and the specific cause of scarlatina. It should be noted that Field has been unable to confirm this.[2]

In *variola* the eruption appears about the fourth day in the form of small, firm, shotty papules of a reddish color. The papules are met with first on the wrists and on the forehead about the border of the hair, but scattered papules quickly form elsewhere on the face and on the trunk (*discrete smallpox*). On the fifth or sixth day the papules are transformed into vesicles, which are elevated, rounded, and depressed in the centre or umbilicated. About the eighth day the vesicles become pustules. These are rounded, have lost the central umbilication, becoming thereby more spherical, and are bounded by a zone of hyperemia. The intervening skin is usually somewhat swollen. In the course of ten or eleven days, in favorable cases, the pustules gradually dry up, forming crusts, under which regeneration of tissue gradually goes on. After the crusts are cast off there does not usually result any scarring unless the papillary layer has been involved.

In the form of smallpox modified by vaccination, known as *varioloid*,

[1] Jour. Med. Research, 10: No 4: 1904: 483.
[2] Jour. Exper. Med., 7:1905.

vesiculation and maturation take place more rapidly, and the pocks are much fewer in number.

Much more severe is *confluent smallpox*. Here the papules are very numerous and closely set, and while at first they may be discrete, they soon become more or less fused, so that large areas of the skin are transformed into practically an extensive superficial abscess. The skin is greatly swollen and œdematous. The separation of the scabs, in the cases that recover, is a slow process, and scarring is often extreme.

Occasionally, the eruption assumes a hemorrhagic type. Of this, two varieties are recognized; the first, *purpura variolosa*, in which the hemorrhagic extravasation appears early, and the second, in which the effusion of blood occurs after the vesicles and pustules have been formed, *variola pustulosa hemorrhagica*.

The process, as studied histologically, begins with local hyperemia of the papillæ with exudation of inflammatory products into the rete. The exudation leads to œdema of the cells, which are also, from the pressure of the out-poured fluid, dissociated more or less from each other, and compressed into a filamentous meshwork. In this way, owing in part to interstitial exudation, and in part to colliquative necrosis of the rete cells, a vesicle is formed which is peculiar in that it is traversed by a number of delicate bands composed of the compressed epithelial cells. The vesicles contain plasma, cell detritus, nuclear fragments, and fibrin. The superficial epidermis is in this way elevated above the general level. About the periphery the tissues are congested and more or less infiltrated with leukocytes. These gradually work their way into the vesicle, and, gradually increasing in numbers, convert it into a pustule. The delicate septa, before referred to, give way and the pustule assumes a more spherical, elevated appearance. The papillary layer is usually intact, but in the more severe cases there may be infiltration of the corium with necrosis, resulting in the formation of a scar in the process of healing. Certain spherical bodies, believed to be sporozoa, have been described by numerous observers as occurring both within the nucleus and in the protoplasm of the epithelial cells in the pock, which have been held to be the specific cause of the disease. The most recent and important work on these lines is that of Councilman, Magrath, and Brinckerhoff,[1] who conclude that they have discovered the specific cause of variola. The life history of their organism has been studied by Calkins,[2] who identifies it with the cytoryctes of Guarnieri. Inasmuch as it has hitherto proved to be impossible to cultivate the sporozoa on artificial media, the determination of the etiological importance of these organisms is rendered excessively difficult, and we feel that until further light is forthcoming the whole subject must remain *sub judice*. The present indications favor rather the view that we are dealing with an ultramicroscopic organism.

---

[1] The Pathological Anatomy and Histology of Variola, Jour. Med. Research, 80: 1904: 12.

[2] The Life-history of Cytoryctes Variolæ, Guarnieri, ibid., 136.

The lesions of *vaccinia* are in all respects comparable to those of variola, both in their clinical progression and in histological structure.

Varicella bears a general resemblance to variola, but the pocks are formed more rapidly, are usually more scanty than in unmodified smallpox, and the disease altogether is attended with but trifling discomfort. The pocks begin as reddish papules, which rapidly are converted into clear, pearly vesicles. They quickly become slightly turbid, or occasionally, pustular, and finally dry up. Each vesicle is sharply defined, considerably elevated, and surrounded by a hyperemic zone. Scarring, as a rule, does not take place.

Histologically, the lesion somewhat closely resembles that of variola, but is more superficial. The vesicle formation both in varicella and in zoster is attributed by Unna to a peculiar form of cell-degeneration which he terms "ballooning colliquation." Certain multinucleated cells have been found in the vesicles in both the diseases just mentioned, and have been regarded by some as parasites, although this is believed by Gilchrist[1] to be erroneous.

The rash in *typhoid fever* is characterized by the formation of isolated, slightly elevated papules, of a rose pink color (rose spots), which appear first upon the abdomen and the lower thoracic zone. As a rule, the spots are rather few in number, but in some cases the eruption is abundant, involving the back, and even the extremities. The papules come out in successive crops after the end of the first week and in two or three days gradually disappear, leaving a slight brownish stain. The spots are from 2 to 4 mm. in diameter, are palpable, and disappear momentarily on pressure. Occasionally, the rash is sudaminal in character. Rarely, it is hemorrhagic.[2] After the rash has disappeared the skin may desquamate. The spots are largely congestive in character and contain the specific bacillus.

In *typhus fever* the rash is rather characteristic. It appears usually between the third and fifth days, and in the course of two or three days more is completely out. The eruption is composed of two elements, papular rose spots and petechiæ. The rose spots and the petechiæ appear together, or else many of the rose spots become hemorrhagic. The skin between the spots presents a curious, apparently deep-seated or subcuticular mottling of a dusky-red color. Sudamina are not common. In the case of children the disease has been mistaken for measles. The rash does not disappear after death.

Syphilis.—In the secondary stage of syphilis, that is to say, after the infection has become systemic, skin eruptions are an almost constant feature. It is characteristic of syphilitic exanthemata that they are extremely polymorphous; so much so that the lesions may simulate almost any of the ordinary skin eruptions. Consequently many writers speak of syphilitic roseola, lichen, .eczema, psoriasis, impetigo, herpes, pemphigus, and so on.

[1] Johns Hopkins Hosp. Rep., 1.
[2] See Nicholls and Learmonth. The Hemorrhagic Diathesis in Typhoid Fever, Lancet, London, 1 · 1901: 305.

The most common efflorescence upon the skin occurring in secondary lues is the so-called *syphilitic roseola*, or maculopapular syphilide. This appears usually upon the trunk, but may extend to the arms and other parts of the body. The face may be exempt. The patches are reddish-brown in color, somewhat elevated above the general surface, varying in size from that of a lentil to that of a bean, and tend to be symmetrically distributed. After one or two weeks the spots become a dirty brown or gray color and gradually disappear.

FIG. 242

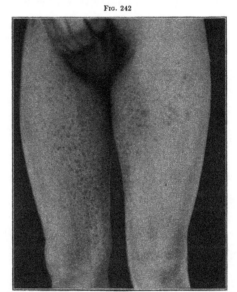

Secondary macular syphilide. (From Dr. Shepherd's Skin Clinic, Montreal General Hospital.)

Microscopically, the superficial vessels are dilated and show both endothelial and perithelial proliferation. There is more or less extravasation of leukocytes about the vessels and glands, together with some œdema. Veiklon and Girard, among others, have found Spirochæta pallida in this lesion.

The papular syphilide assumes various forms. It begins with the formation of reddish patches, the size of a pin-head or larger, within which acuminate or flattened papules develop. When the papules are small the condition bears a general resemblance to lichen ruber, and is known as *lichen syphiliticus*. In some cases, vesicles or pustules form upon the papules (*herpes syphiliticus, impetigo syphilitica*), which dry up into scales or crusts. This is less common than the acniform eruption. Where the lesions involve the soles of the feet and palms of the hands, the papules are flattened, and when involution has taken place are attended with the production of abundant scales (*psoriasis plantaris et palmaris syphilitica*).

In regions where warmth and moisture are complicating conditions the papules are converted into the so-called *condylomas*, which are flat elevations, of a grayish color, with a moist, shiny surface, sometimes secreting an offensive discharge.

Microscopically, in the papular syphilide the process is chiefly to be observed in the papillary layer, but may also extend to the deeper parts of the corium.

Spirochæta pallida has repeatedly been found in secondary papules (Levaditi,[1] Buschke, and Fischer), and in the condyloma (Blaschko[2]).

FIG. 243

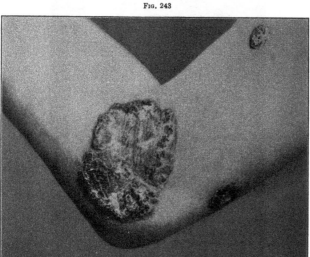

Syphilitic rupia on the arm.   (From the Skin Clinic of the Montreal General Hospital.)

The *tubercular syphilide* is slower in development and more inveterate than the papule.   The process may be diffuse but is more often circumscribed.   There may be more or less absorption in the centre of the nodules, or, again, central necrosis may result in the formation of an ulcer.   In the transition period from the secondary to the tertiary stage, the lesions may be covered with extensive crusts, presenting a curious and characteristic concentric arrangement, something like an oyster shell—*rupia*.

[1] Comptes rend. Soc. de. Biol., Paris, 59: 1905: 527.
[2] Blaschko, Med. klin. Woch., 1906.

The lesion results in some destruction of tissue so that more or less scarring results.

Gummas frequently originate in the subcutaneous structures and later involve the skin. They sometimes result in much destruction of tissue and are followed by scarring and pigmentation.

Dermatitis from the Ingestion of Drugs or Other Toxic Substances.—A great variety of skin lesions have been described as the result of the ingestion of certain drugs and allied substances, taken either unwittingly or for medicinal purposes. In some cases these are due to the direct action of the drug; in others, to certain toxic principles elaborated in the process of absorption and elimination. The character of the lesion attributable to any one drug is by no means constant. Acniform eruptions are fairly characteristic of the iodine and bromine compounds; scarlatiniform rashes, of belladonna, antipyrine, and quinine, and diphtheria antitoxin. Purpura has been described after the exhibition of copaiba, quinine, belladonna, ergot, mercury, and iodide of potassium. Salicylic acid and its compounds may produce erythema, purpura, or even necrosis.

It should be mentioned that these results sometimes follow doses of the drugs well within therapeutic limits, and do not always imply careless or extravagant dosage. Personal idiosyncrasy must often be taken into account.

Ergotism results from the use of grain infested with the ergot fungus. Two forms are described, the convulsive or spasmodic, and the gangrenous. In the latter variety the fingers and toes, less commonly the nose and ears, become gangrenous.

Allied to ergotism is *pellagra* (maidismus; erythema endemicum[1]), a disease found in certain parts of Europe among the peasantry who eat decomposing grain, usually maize. An increasing number of cases has been observed within the last few years in the United States. According to an Italian observer, Ceni,[2] the specific cause is a fungus belonging to the aspergillus family. This has not been positively settled, however. The earliest symptoms are referable to the alimentary tract, anorexia, epigastric pain, vomiting, severe diarrhœa, and thirst. Anemia soon sets in with palpitation on exertion and sometimes œdema. Next, those regions of the skin exposed to the sun manifest a diffuse or patchy erythema. Petechial spots, bullæ and œdema may be observed. Later, the skin becomes rough, thickened, scaly, cracked, and finally exfoliates. It remains shrivelled and atrophied. In the terminal stages of the disease we get various paraplegias, delirium, mania, and melancholia. The disease may last for years.

[1] See Crocker, Diseases of Skin, 1893; Lombroso, Lehre von der Pellagra, Berlin, 1898.

[2] Riv. sper. di fremat., Reggio-Emilia, 33: 1907: 1.

RETROGRESSIVE METAMORPHOSES.

Atrophy.—Simple atrophy of the skin is characterized by the wasting of almost all its elements. The condition may be local or generalized. It may be primary or the result of some preëxisting pathological state. As a type, may be taken the physiological atrophy found in old age. Here the cutis becomes thinner, and the papillæ tend to be flattened and may disappear, while the epidermis becomes dry and brittle. The subcutaneous fat is to some extent absorbed, and the skin is thus thrown into folds. The elastic tissue involutes and the superficial vessels undergo degeneration. It is not uncommon to find granules of pigment of brownish color in the cells of the rete and about the vessels of the cutis. The deeper layers of the epidermis are atrophied, so that the stratum corneum is less widely separated from the papillary layer. The hair-follicles also partake in the process and the hairs become downy and eventually fall out. The openings of the follicles not infrequently become blocked, owing to the accumulation of epidermal scales, and they may be dilated into cysts. The sebaceous glands similarly are obstructed, and the hair-follicles and sebaceous glands are distended into one cavity containing hairs, fat, and epithelial debris, the so-called *atheroma.* Eventually, the sebaceous glands atrophy and finally disappear. Not infrequently the superficial epidermis is heaped up here and there into branny scales (*pityriasis simplex*).

Local atrophy is often brought about by distension of the skin from whatever cause. The regions usually affected are the breasts, abdomen, and thighs. The commonest cause is pregnancy, but similar effects are sometimes produced ·by tumors, lactation, ascites, and anasarca. During pregnancy the abdomen is covered with reddish livid streaks, which after delivery are transformed into whitish silvery lines or scars (lineæ albicantes). On examining such a scar, the papillæ are seen to be flattened or absent, the connective-tissue fibres of the corium are dissociated, the elastic fibres and bloodvessels are atrophic.

A somewhat similar local atrophy of the skin is found after the absorption of the subcutaneous fat in the course of chronic wasting diseases (**marantic atrophy**), and even in certain acute febrile processes, notably typhoid (Osler). Lineæ atrophicæ are also met with on the thighs and abdomen as the result of the pressure of corsets or other articles of apparel.

Idiopathic diffuse symmetrical atrophy has been reported by several observers (Bronson,[1] Elliott, and Fordyce).

Neurotrophic Atrophy.—In certain nervous affections, such as leprosy, neuralgia, and neuritis, the skin supplied by the nerves involved is often found to be thin, smooth, and shiny, and there may be wasting of the glands and hair-follicles (Paget, Weir-Mitchell).

Ulceration.—Bedsores.—Bedsores (decubitus) are a form of necrosis of the skin and underlying parts due largely to pressure in those who are

---

[1] Jour. Cutan. and Genito-urinary Dis., 13: 1895: 1.

greatly reduced in health. Impoverished blood, a weak heart, and the recumbent position are the most important predisposing causes. Neurotrophic influences, however, often play a part, for bedsores are apt to develop with exceptional rapidity in nervous affections, such as tabes dorsalis and myelitis. The regions usually involved are the sacrum, trochanters, heels, and scapulæ. The affected part becomes bluish-black or black in color, the skin cracks, and then, owing to infection with putrefactive germs, a spreading ulcer or gangrenous patch is formed, which extends to the subcutaneous soft tissues and even to the bone.

Perforating Ulcer.—Somewhat allied to this is the perforating ulcer of the foot, met with in *locomotor ataxia* and other diseases of the spinal cord. A deeply-penetrating ulcer, which extends rapidly, is produced, usually at the metatarsophalangeal joint of the great toe. The process may lay bare and erode the bone. It may possibly be due to pressure, but in the majority of instances is of neurotrophic origin.

Small ulcerations are also found on the hands in *syringomyelia*, an affection of the spinal cord in which the sensory fibers are largely interfered with. These ulcers are probably, to some extent at least, to be referred to trauma or irritation, which more readily occur in cases where sensation is impaired.

Varicose Ulcers.—Ulceration also occurs as a result of impaired circulation, as, for example, in the lower extremities in consequence of varicose veins.

Gangrene.—Gangrene of the skin and other tissues is met with in chronic ergotism, frost-bite, and infection with B. Welchii.

Senile Gangrene.—Senile gangrene is a form occurring in old persons who have advanced arteriosclerosis. It generally begins in one of the toes and may spread gradually upward. It is usually of the dry variety, and is often induced by some slight injury, such as may be caused by paring a corn, or a rag-nail. Gangrene also is met with occasionally in diabetes mellitus. Buerger[1] has studied cases of so-called "pre-senile" or "juvenile" gangrene, found in persons between the ages of twenty and forty years, often of the Jewish race, which he holds are due not to endarteritis obliterans, but to an organizing thrombosis.

Raynaud's Disease.—Raynaud's disease, when extreme, leads to symmetrical gangrene of the extremities, supposed by some to be due to a primary nervous disturbance. It is also attributed to anemia brought about by repeated spasm of the arterioles.

Ainhum.—Ainhum is a rare disease of unknown etiology, first described by Clark[2] and found especially in the African races. A circular groove is formed, usually on the fourth or fifth toes, at the point where the toe joins the foot. The toe swells, and the affected part becomes rough and scaly. Finally spontaneous amputation of the member takes place.

[1] Amer. Jour. Med. Sci., 136:1908.
[2] Clark, Trans. Epidemiol. Soc., Lond., 1860.

Histologically, it has been regarded by several observers, notably Unna, as a form of scleroderma, in which the epidermis is thickened, the papillæ are narrowed and lengthened, and the overgrowth finally leads to strangulation of the deeper layers with consecutive necrosis. The vessels of the cutis are dilated and there is some round-celled infiltration, with obstruction to the lymphatics. Cases have been reported in this country by F. J. Shepherd.

Colloid Transformation.—Colloid transformation of the skin (colloid milium) is a rare disease in which the cells of the derma and the connective tissue undergo colloid changes. The degeneration is most marked about the bloodvessels, nerves, and sebaceous glands.

ABNORMAL PIGMENTATION.

The anomalies of pigmentation fall into two classes: the first, in which there is a diminution or increase in the amount of the normal coloring matter of the skin, and the second, in which there is a deposit of pathological or extraneous pigments.

Congenital absence of the pigment, leukopathia congenita or albinism has already been referred to (p. 954).

Acquired leukopathia, leukoderma, or **vitiligo** occurs spontaneously, or, occasionally, as a sequel of the infectious fevers. It is apt to begin in early life, and is commoner in the black races. In certain regions, as in Turkestan, it is said to be endemic. The disease is characterized by the production of whitish, pigment-free, blotches, often symmetrical, usually on the face, neck and hands. The condition tends to spread, and by the confluence of the patches large areas of skin become white. The hair upon the affected regions also becomes bleached (*poliosis circumscripta*).

Histologically, one finds lack of pigment in the decolorized areas with occasionally an increase of that in the surrounding more normal skin, usually in the corium.

The etiology is unknown. Leloir was of the opinion that the affection should be referred to nervous influences. Perhaps less obscure are those cases of local symptomatic leukoderma resulting from inflammation, such as the forms which occur in boils, eczema, lupus, leprosy, and syphilis. Here, the skin is smooth and sometimes cicatrized.

Lentigo.—Lentigo is a term somewhat loosely employed to designate sharply defined spots, of yellowish or brownish-black color, varying in size from that of a pin-head to that of a lentil. They somewhat resemble small nevi, appear shortly after birth, and persist throughout life.

Ephelides.—Ephelides, or freckles, are small, irregularly shaped yellowish-brown blotches, which are found usually on the face, hands, and arms, but occasionally on other parts of the body. They are most common in childhood and early life, and are due to the action of the light, which causes an increase of the pigment.

Chloasma.—In women who are pregnant, menstruating, or who are suffering from disease of the genital organs, it is not uncommon to get

PLATE XIII

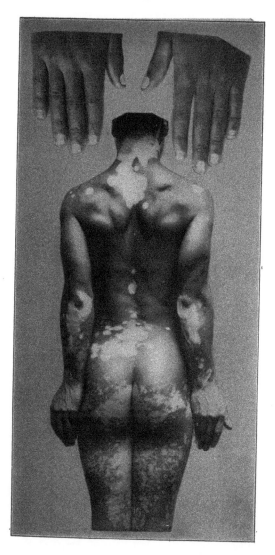

Leukoderma and Leukonychia in a Negro. (Howard Fox.)

pigmentation of the skin, usually on the forehead, temples, cheeks, abdomen, and breasts. Bright brown or blackish-brown patches of varying size, often becoming confluent, are produced. This is termed *chloasma uterinum*. A similar coloration is sometimes found in those suffering from chronic wasting disease, especially tuberculosis (*chloasma cachecticorum*), and is a result of the irritation produced by heat, toxic agents, and scratching.

Addison's Disease.—In Addison's disease the skin and mucous surfaces, especially of the face, mouth, throat, hands, breasts, and genitalia, assume a dark bronzed appearance. Microscopically, all that is seen is an increase of pigment in the corium. (See also vol. i, p. 358.)

Hemochromatosis.—A curious dull, brownish, or bluish discoloration of the skin is that known as hemochromatosis, which is a symptom associated with some cases of cirrhosis of the liver and diabetes (diabète bronzé). (Cf. p. 486.)

Pigmentation of the skin also results from a variety of **thermic, chemical,** and **mechanical** insults, which, owing to their nature, produce chronic irritation. Such are sunburn, scratching, parasitic diseases and parasites, and the application of mustard or fly-blisters.

The exact nature of the increased pigmentation in these cases is quite obscure. It seems generally accepted now that the normal pigment of the skin is produced through the metabolism of the epithelial cells (Loeb[1]), and it may be inferred that we are dealing with increased or, at least, disordered metabolism in cases such as have been mentioned.

Icterus.—Icterus is a yellowish, yellowish-green, or olive discoloration of the skin and external surfaces, due to the presence of bile in the blood and lymph.

Pigmentation is frequently found about varicose veins, chronic and healed ulcers, and is due to **hemorrhage**, the effused blood being transformed into hemosiderin and in some cases into hematoidin.

Pigmentation may also be due to the deposit of silver in the vessel-walls and fibrous tissue (**argyriasis**) in persons who have been taking nitrate of silver for prolonged periods, or, similarly, to arsenic (**arsenical melanosis**). Among the extraneous pigments sometimes found, also, in the skin may be mentioned **Indian ink** and **carmine** (in tattooing) and **gunpowder.**

PROGRESSIVE METAMORPHOSES.

Hyperplasia.—Hyperplasia of the skin is met with under widely differing conditions and in a variety of forms. The congenital hyperplasias, such as ichthyosis congenita, elephantiasis, and nevi have already been dealt with (p. 953 et seq.). The acquired forms are in great measure due to inflammation and irritation, although in some the etiology is obscure or unknown. Certain of them, again, are on the borderland between simple hyperplasia and inflammation.

[1] Transplantation of Skin and Origin of Pigment, Medicine, Detroit, 5:1899:286; also, Journ. Amer. Med. Assoc., 31:1898:1362.

Callus.—The simplest form of hyperplasia is *callus* (callositas, tyloma), so commonly met with as the result of intermittent pressure. It is found usually on the palms of the hands and soles of the feet. The outer layers of the epidermis are compressed into a dense homogeneous mass. As a result, the middle layers are thickened, while the rete and papillæ are atrophied. In advanced cases the cells of the rete extend deeply into the corium, where they become fused together to form a sort of core, giving rise to the well-known *corn*. As a rule, there is more or less secondary inflammation in the neighboring tissues, which are swollen and hyperemic.

Cornu Cutaneum.—Cornu cutaneum is a remarkable outgrowth of the epidermis, forming a horn-like excrescence, which often reaches a considerable size. The usual situation is on the forehead, breasts, and hands. The horns may develop on otherwise healthy skin, or in connection with scars, atheroma, or tumors. According to Unna, the process is a combination of acanthosis with hyperkeratosis. The cells of the rete grow downward between the papillæ, some of which become narrowed and elongated, while others undergo atrophy. As the process advances the horny layer becomes thickened and the cells are heaped up until a hard outgrowth is the result.

Palmar and Plantar Keratodermia.—Palmar and plantar keratodermia (tylosis, keratosis palmæ et plantæ) is a local keratosis, believed to be the result of disordered nerve function. It is a rare disease, and is congenital or acquired early in childhood, but has been known to follow hyperidrosis and the prolonged use of arsenic.[1] A somewhat similar condition is found in eczema, lichen planus, syphilis, and other inflammations of the parts.

Ichthyosis.—The so-called acquired form of ichthyosis develops shortly after birth, and is met with in all degrees of severity, from a simple thickening of the skin, scarcely if at all to be distinguished from lichen pilaris, to *ichthyosis simplex*, and finally to *ichthyosis sauroderma* and *ichthyosis hystrix*, in which the skin is thick, scaly, or warty.

In the milder grades there is, according to Unna, a marked hyperkeratosis of cells derived directly from the rete without the interposition of the granular layer. The cells of the rete are small and hypoplastic, the papillæ broad and flat. Excess of pigment is found, chiefly in the palisade cells. In the cutis the collagenous fibres are thickened, the elastic fibres and fat tend to disappear, and the lymph-channels are obliterated. Secondary inflammation is not uncommon. In the so-called ichthyotic eczema, there is more reaction on the part of the rete, as shown by proliferation and hyperplasia, with reappearance of the granular layer. A moister process with the heaping up of crusts is produced. When the hyperplasia affects the papillæ as well, a granular or nodular surface, and even actual warts, may be the result. One form is associated with elephantiasis.

---

[1] Romberg, Klin. Wahr. u. Beobach, Berlin, 1851   228   Erasmus Wilson, Jour. of Cut. Med., 1: 1868: 355.

Scleroderma.[1]—Scleroderma is an affection of doubtful etiology. It is most common in females and in those of a neurotic disposition.

Anatomically, it may be *diffuse* and widespread, or give rise to local lesions of a peculiar clinical type, known as *morphœa.* The diffuse form, less often the circumscribed, occasionally comes on after exposure to cold, erysipelas, and acute rheumatism. In some cases of morphœa it is possible that some disorder of the nerve centres is at work, but in the majority of cases the nature of the scleroderma is quite obscure. In a few cases the thyroid gland has been found to be diminished in size (Singer and Beer). The disease is met with on the trunk, face, or extremities, and is characterized by a peculiar brawny induration of the skin and subcutaneous tissues, which feel much as if they were frozen. The disease may come on quickly and extend rapidly, it may remain stationary, or, again, may finally retrograde.

The histological changes are confined almost exclusively to the corium and underlying parts. At most there may be slight pigmentation in some cases in the deeper parts of the rete. The vessels are thickened, the lymph-channels are narrowed, and there is hypertrophy of the elastic and fibrous tissue. There is a certain amount of cellular infiltration. The newly-formed connective tissue finally undergoes cicatricial contraction and atrophy of the various glands results.

A peculiar form occurs in children, usually in those of low vitality, known as *sclerema neonatorum.* It is congenital or begins in the earlier months of life, and usually affects the legs and feet. According to Langer it is due to the solidification of the subcutaneous fat, produced by the lowering of the temperature.[2]

Elephantiasis.—Elephantiasis (elephantiasis Arabum, pachydermia acquisita) is a condition characterized by the most extreme hyperplastic thickening of the skin and subcutaneous tissues. The disease is endemic in certain tropical and subtropical countries, as Arabia, Egypt, Central America, and Brazil, but sporadic cases are occasionally met with in the temperate climes. Some cases begin with the clinical manifestations of a local inflammatory process, as, for instance, erysipelas and lymphangitis, together with fever. Repeated attacks add to the thickening of the tissues, which finally becomes extreme. Others, again, are more sluggish and insidious.

The etiology is not altogether clear. Many cases, although not all, are due to the presence of Filaria sanguinis hominis and its embryos. These accumulate in the lymphatic channels, usually of the lower extremities, scrotum, or abdomen, where they cause stasis of the lymph, with consecutive inflammation and fibrous hyperplasia. Obstruction of the lymphatics from other causes, such as the pressure of inflammatory exudates or tumors, removal or destructive disease of the lymphatic glands, predispose to the condition, if they do not actually cause it.

---

[1] For literature see Luithlen, Art. Sclerodermie in Mraçek's Handbook of Dermatology, vol. iii.

[2] See Luithlen, Die Zellgewebshärtungen der Neugeborenen, Wien, Hölder, 1902.

Sporadic cases are not infrequently attributable to passive congestion, or to chronic and relapsing inflammations, such as erysipelas, eczema, tuberculosis of the skin or bones, varicose ulcers, prurigo, and syphilitic

Fig. 244

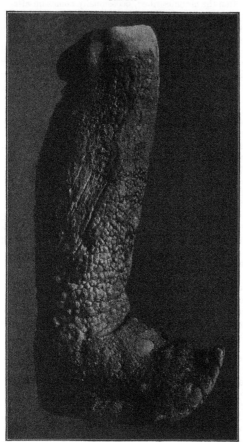

Elephantiasis of the leg.   Enormous enlargement of the limb, with ichthyosis.
(From the Pathological Museum, McGill University.)

periostitis.   Those cases which develop insidiously, without inflammatory manifestations, are of more doubtful nature.   Some are supposed to be due to inherited peculiarities or intra-uterine pathological conditions.

In acquired elephantiasis the tissues involved present more or less thickening, resulting in some cases in enormous enlargement of the part, with obliteration of the normal contour. The skin and subcutaneous tissues are thickened, firm, and indurated. They may be hard (*elephantiasis dura*), or soft and grayish-white (*E. mollis*). In some cases the lymphatics are dilated and on section abundant serous fluid exudes (*E. lymphangiectatica*). The skin surface is smooth (*E. glabra*), warty (*E. verrucosa*), nodular (*E. tuberosa*), or papillomatous (*E. papillomatosa*). In some cases the horny layer is thickened, forming scales or plates (*acquired ichthyosis, keratosis*).

Microscopically, in the severer forms, the connective tissue of the cutis is hyperplastic, with some atrophy of the fat. The bloodvessels are dilated and thickened, but not invariably so, and there is often perivascular leukocytic infiltration. In the tropical variety the lymphatics are dilated, their walls thickened, and the subcutaneous tissues are œdematous. The epidermis presents varying degrees of keratosis.

Besides the diffuse form, local tumors of similar appearance are described as occurring on the scrotum, prepuce, vulva, and, rarely, on the breast.

Keratosis Pilaris.—Keratosis pilaris (lichen pilaris) is characterized by the formation of small papules about the hair-follicles. The process may be simple (*keratosis pilaris alba*), or complicated by inflammation (*keratosis pilaris rubra*). Various grades and modifications of the disease exist. In well-marked cases there is hyperkeratosis in and about the follicles, which become occluded by horny plugs at their orifices. The simple variety is usually found on the extensor surfaces of the limbs, while the inflammatory form is apt to involve the flexor surfaces as well.

Keratosis Follicularis.—Keratosis follicularis, or Darier's disease, is a peculiar affection of the skin, first described by Darier[1] under the name "psorospermose folliculaire," since he thought that certain cell-inclusions in the rete were of the nature of psorosperms. These are now generally thought to be peculiar forms of cell-degeneration. The disease usually begins in childhood. The etiology is unknown. The lesion consists in a primary keratosis and parakeratosis of the sebaceous follicles and hair-bulbs. The process apparently begins at the orifices of the follicles and, later, extends to the interfollicular tissues. The mouths of the follicles are dilated and occluded by imperfectly cornified cells. It is believed, also, that the lesions may at times originate in the epidermis and about the openings of the sweat ducts. In the rete are to be seen certain rounded bodies that closely resemble psorosperms, and at the bottom of the follicle-plugs are compressed homogeneous masses, which Darier called "grains." Fissures or lacunæ are observed between the cells of the rete. The rete generally shows marked proliferation, and may extend deeply into the corium. The stratum granulosum is absent. There is slight cellular infiltration in the corium, and a deposit of pigment at the periphery of the lesion.[2]

[1] Internat. Atlas selt. Hautkrankh., 8.
[2] For literature see Bizzozero, Arch. f. Derm., 93:1908.

Condyloma.—Local outgrowths, resembling papillomas, are not infrequently found in situations where the skin is subjected to chronic irritation, as, for instance, the presence of inflammatory processes, discharges, dirt, and friction. Warmth and moisture predispose to their formation. We find, therefore, that they are most commonly present about the external genitals and near the anus, where they form what are usually known as *condylomata acuminata.* Gonorrhœa, venereal ulcers, and decomposing secretions play the most important part. They begin as small papillary excrescences, and may increase until extensive warty or cauliflower-like growths, of firm consistence and whitish color, are produced. The process is essentially an overgrowth of the papillæ, which increase in length and usually become branched. Histologically,

Fig. 245

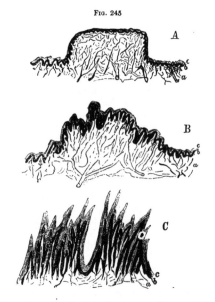

The various grades of warts and cutaneous papillomas. (Perls.)

the outgrowths consist of vascular connective tissue, containing collections of round cells here and there. The lymphatics are frequently packed with inflammatory round cells, which are also numerous in the immediate neighborhood. The epithelium over the hyperplastic papillæ is markedly increased in thickness.

Warts.—Warts (verrucæ) are of various kinds, hard, soft, or papillomatous. The common wart is found usually upon the hands. They are often multiple, a fact suggesting a possible contagious nature. The

:d, and the overlying epithelium is hyperplastic.

.mors.—**Fibromas.**—Fibromas are not infrequently found in the
   They are often multiple and may attain considerable size.   The
fibroma (*fibroma durum*) is much rarer than the soft form (*fibroma*
).

FIG. 246

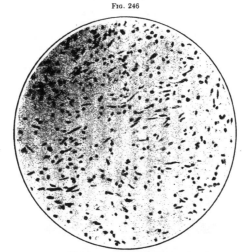

fibroma.   Winckel obj. No. 6, without ocular.   (From Dr. A. G. Nicholls' collection.)

croscopically, it is composed of interlacing bands of dense fibrous
:, with relatively few nuclei, and but few elastic fibrils and blood-
ls.

e soft fibroma (*fibroma molle, fibroma molluscum, molluscum simplex,*
:*scum pendulum*) is composed of a loose meshwork of connective
:, often œdematous or myxomatous. The new-growth begins in
ubcutaneous tissues and corium, and projects secondarily into the
rmis.   The papillæ are flattened from pressure, and the epidermis
forms a uniform thin layer over the tumor.   Possibly of the same
e is the soft wart or *acrochordon*.

:ording to v. Recklinghausen,[1] the soft fibromas arise from the
ıs sheaths of the subcutaneous nerve filaments, which proliferate

[1] Ueber die multiplen Fibrome der Haut., Berlin, 1882.

and form connective-tissue growths of rather cellular type. He consequently termed them *neurofibromata*. These tumors may be restricted to the area supplied by a particular nerve, or may be disseminated.[1] In the local form a large soft tumor is produced (*molluscum elephantiasticum*). In other cases a complicated meshwork of connective tissue arises from the endoneurium (*plexiform neuroma; "Rankenneurom," q. v.*). These in the course of their development sometimes lead to diffuse fibrous thickening of the skin and subcutaneous tissues (*elephantiasis neuromatosa*). This form is often congenital and developmental in nature and gives rise to curious lobulated folds of the skin, recalling the appearances in certain pachydermata. In the case of

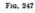

Fig. 247

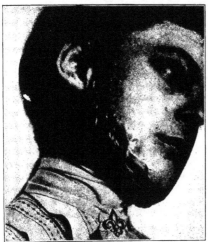

Keloid.

dermatolysis or *cutis laxa*, found in the so-called "India-rubber" men, the connective tissue has been found to be transformed into myxomatous material, while the elastic fibres were normal.

Diffuse fibromatosis of the skin (*elephantiasis fibrosa*) is met with as well as an abnormal overgrowth of the fat, leading to thickening of the skin (*elephantiasis lipomatosa*).

Gerhardt, Baerensprung, and Simon have described a multiple pigmented papilloma or nevus, which is supposed to develop in connection with the nerve trunks (*neuropathic papilloma, nervennevus, nævus unius lateris*). Little is known about it.

[1] For another possible mode of origin see p. 634.

A peculiar form of fibroma is the *keloid* (cheloid), which forms flattened, round, or irregular masses, plaques, and elevated streaks over which the skin is smoothly stretched. In general it may be said that the new-growth resembles scar tissue. The disease is not common, and is said to be more frequent in the negro race. It is usual to divide the cases into *true* or *spontaneous* and *false* or *cicatricial* keloid. Both varieties are probably of the same nature, although it is not always possible to get evidence of a previously existing scar. Keloid usually follows traumatism, as a scar, a vesicle, a pustule, a burn, or even a blow. Occasionally, no etiological factor can be made out. The growth is apt to be multiple, and while not malignant, in the usual sense, commonly recurs after removal, owing probably to a persistent tendency toward overgrowth manifested in the new scar.

FIG. 248

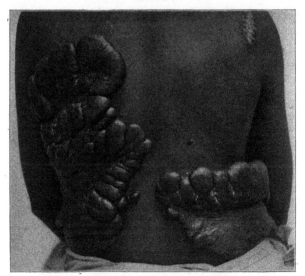

Keloid in a negro   (Howard Fox's case.)

Histologically, keloid in the earlier stages is made up of numerous spindle cells, but later of dense fibrous tissue fibrillæ, which in general are arranged parallel to the long axis of the tumor. The adventitia of the vessels, even beyond the limits of the growth, shows signs of proliferation, and it is probable that this is the primary change. The corium to some extent becomes involved in the growth.

Papilloma —Papillomas are not infrequent.

Lipoma.—Lipomas, or fatty tumors, are of frequent occurrence, and arise from the subcutaneous tissue. They form round, flattened,

FIG. 249

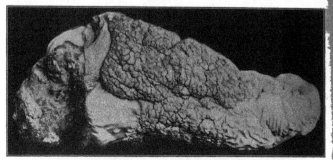

Extensive papilloma of the foot. (From the Pathological Museum, McGill University.)

[FIG. 250]

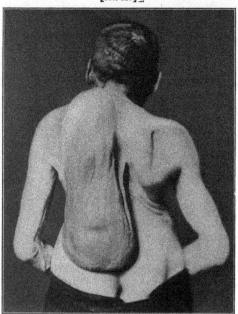

Pendulous lipoma of the shoulder. (From the collection of the Montreal General Hospital.)

and lobulated growths, often multiple and symmetrical, which are met with commonly on the arms and about the shoulders. They may be associated with fibrous overgrowth (*fibrolipoma*), mucoid tissue (*myxolipoma*), sarcoma (*liposarcoma*), or with new formation of vessels (*lipoma teleangiectodes*). Rarely, the tumor may *calcify* or become *bony*. The exact cause is not understood. Some are congenital, and in some there appears to be an inherited peculiarity. They may attain a considerable size. Rarely, they become inflamed and necrose, giving rise to foul ulcers.

Fig. 251

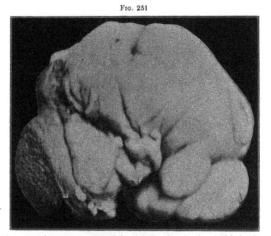

Lipoma from the subcutaneous tissues of the gluteal region, showing the lobulated structure. (From the Pathological Museum of McGill University.)

Xanthoma or **Xanthelasma.**—Xanthoma or xanthelasma is a peculiar pigmented tumor found on the eyelids and other parts of the body, but occasionally in the internal organs, such as the trachea, pericardium, the capsules of the liver and spleen.

Histologically, it is a new-growth of connective tissue, between the fibres of which are to be seen cells of epithelioid type, which vary considerably in size and are multinucleated, so that they resemble the giant cells in sarcomas. These cells are grouped about the vessels and are often markedly infiltrated with fat. They may be regarded as immature fat cells. The growth forms lobulated masses in the deeper layers of the corium, which occasionally reach as high as the rete. The epidermis may be slightly thinned. The characteristic yellow color of the tumor is due to a pigment called lipochrome, found chiefly in the fat-containing cells or "xanthoma bodies," but also in the cells of the rete and corium.

Xanthomas form yellowish growths in the skin (*xanthoma planum*) or projecting above it (*xanthoma tuberosum*), and are commonly multiple. The etiology is obscure. Cases are occasionally met with in diabetics and in those suffering from jaundice, but are more usually spontaneous. Some observers attribute the growth to a preceding inflammation, while others (Ziegler) regard it as a lipomatous lymphangioma or endothelioma. Politzer[1] believes that the xanthomas found on the eyelids are different from those occurring in other places, and are not really tumors, but are due to fatty degeneration of the fibers of the orbicularis muscle with proliferation of the nuclei.

Fig. 252

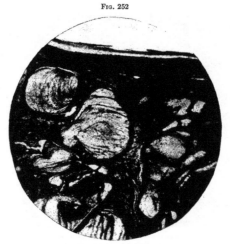

Hemangioma of the skin. The large blood sinuses are well shown. Zeiss obj. DD, without ocular
(From the collection of Dr. A. G. Nicholls.)

Myoma.—Myomas occurring superficially in the skin are rare. They form growths varying in size from that of a pin-head to that of a walnut. They are often multiple, and arise either from the arrectores pilorum, the walls of the arterioles, or, again, the muscle fibres of the sweat-glands. The tumors are composed of interlacing smooth-muscle fibres, with a few elastic fibrillæ, and are sometimes definitely encapsulated. They are generally found in the skin of the face and arms. They are apt to recur. Herzog[2] has collected about a dozen cases from the literature and reports one of his own. In some instances the vessels are dilated (*angiomyoma*). *Rhabdomyomas* are very rare (Schmorl). Zieler[3] has described a *myoma sarcomatodes*.

[1] Trans. Amer. Derm. Assoc., 1897.
[2] Jour. Cutan. and Genito-urin. Dis., 16 : 1898 : 527.
[3] Pathol. Gesellsch., 12 : 1908.

Myxomas, chondromas, and **osteomas** are rare in the skin. The myxomas are more properly myxosarcomas, and are found usually on the external female genitalia.

Angioma.—No hard and fast line can be drawn between certain birth-marks composed of dilated or newly-formed vessels (*nævi vasculosi*) and true tumors. The congenital forms are commonly found on the face and neck, but occasionally also on the extremities, and are sometimes related to the branchial clefts (*fissural angiomas*). All grades exist from a simple dilatation of thin-walled vessels resembling capillaries, and generally restricted to a particular arterial district (*teleangiectasis, angioma simplex*), or a congeries of dilated anastomosing vessels, leading to some enlargement of the part (*cavernoma, angioma*

FIG. 253

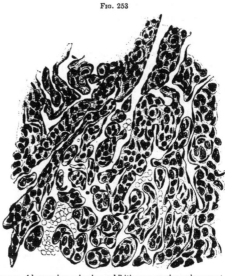

Section from a case of hemangioma simplex, exhibiting progressive enlargement and extension. (Borrmann.)

cavernosum), to a tumor-like outgrowth (*angioma hypertrophicum*). In the last-mentioned form, soft warts are produced containing thick-walled vessels and often solid cell-masses. They are pale or purplish-red in color, and are covered with smooth skin. They are commonly multiple. Pigmented nevi are not infrequently of this type.

Secondary changes are common in angiomas. Thus, the intervening fibrous stroma may be noticeably increased, and the epidermis or horny layer may be thickened (*kerato-angioma*).

Lymphangioma.—Lymphangioma is, anatomically speaking, strictly comparable to hemangioma and occurs in the form of simple local dilatations of the lymph-vessels, elephantiasis, or elevated nodules. Lymphangiomas are found in almost any part of the body and may arise either in the skin or in the subcutaneous tissues. The cause is unknown, but from the fact that many cases arise in infancy it may be inferred that they are often due to some developmental anomaly of the lymphatics. Certain cases of lymphangiectasis in the genitalia or lower extremities are often associated with proliferation of fibrous tissue, and are properly to be regarded, in the majority of instances at least, as due to obstruction of the lymph-channels with hyperplasia rather than as true tumors. In all forms there is dilatation of the lymphatics, and, in the lymphangioma proper, a new-formation of lymph-vessels. Frequently with this is associated round-celled infiltration about the vessels with connective-tissue hyperplasia. There may also be keratosis of the superficial epidermis. As a rule, the blood-vessels show dilatation and overgrowth as well.

Some of the warts of the skin are pure lymphangiomas, while others are composed of solid masses of cells in the corium, and have been called hypertrophic lymphangiomas, or endotheliomas. Certain pigmented nevi are also to be included in this group.

Xeroderma Pigmentosum.[1]—Under the name xeroderma pigmentosum (*atrophoderma pigmentosum, melanosis lenticularis progressiva*, Pick), Kaposi has described a rare affection of the skin, beginning a few months after birth. It is at first manifested by the repeated efflorescence of reddish spots, which, later, disappear with some scaling of the skin. As the spots fade, pigmented areas, not unlike freckles, are left, and the vessels dilate. The skin becomes smooth and atrophic, and later, warty outgrowths are produced, which have a striking tendency to develop into carcinoma.

Multiple Benign Cystic Epithelioma.—Multiple benign cystic epithelioma is a rather rare disorder of the skin, which has led to considerable difference of opinion. It was first described by Jacquet and Darier[2] under the name "hydradénome eruptif," and somewhat later by Brooke,[3] who termed it "epithelioma adenoides cysticum," and by Fordyce.[4] The lesion consists in the formation of multiple small papules, nodules, or tubercles in the skin, usually on the face, eyelids, forehead, trunk, or arms. In some cases superficial erosion takes place, so that something like "rodent" ulcer is the result. In a few instances the lesions are restricted to a small district, but, as a rule, numerous widely disseminated growths are observed. The disease usually manifests itself in the first two decades but has been found also in advanced life.

Histologically, the tumors are composed of irregular, oval, or elongated masses and strands of epithelial cells, resembling those of the deeper layers of the epidermis. In some cases the epithelial cells form a uni-

[1] For literature see Adrian, Derm. Zentralbl., 7:5.
[2] Ann. de dermat. et de syph., 8: 1887.
[3] Brit. Jour. of Derm., 4:1892:269.
[4] Jour. Cutan. and Genito-urin. Dis., 10 : 1892 : 459 and 501.

form diffuse growth, while in others there is an intricate interlacing and anastomosis of the various bands. Occasionally the growth presents an alveolar arrangement. "Cell-nests," identical with those met with in malignant epithelioma, are often seen. Many of these have undergone central necrosis and liquefaction, forming globular cysts. It is probable that the appearances described under such a variety of names are due to a number of growths differing in their nature. Some have their starting point in the deeper layers of the epidermis and the outer parts of the hair-sheaths—*true benign cystic epithelioma;* others, again, begin in the sebaceous glands—*cystadenoma sebaceum;* others, again, in a proliferation of the endothelium of the bloodvessels—*hemangioendothelioma;* while still others, according to Kaposi and his school, are due to a new-formation and dilatation of lymph-vessels in the skin—*lymphangioma tuberosum multiplex.* Some cases, like the one reported by Pick,[1] are of mixed type, combining the peculiarities of the first and second forms.

Fig. 254

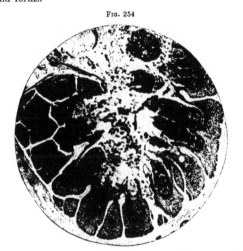

Molluscum contagiosum. Zeiss obj. DD, without ocular. (From the collection of Dr. Oskar Klotz.)

Molluscum Contagiosum.—Molluscum contagiosum (epithelioma contagiosum, molluscum epitheliale, endocystic condyloma—"Schumwartze"), like the last-mentioned, is a disease that has given rise to much difference of opinion. It appears in the form of elevated nodules about the size of a pea or bean, which have a peculiar shiny and waxlike appearance and present a small central depression. The affection

[1] Arch. f. Derm. u. Syphilis, 58: 1902. For literature, see Hartzell, Benign Cystic Epithelioma, Proc. Path. Soc., Philadelphia, October, 1902.

is found most commonly in children who live under unhygienic conditions. It occurs sometimes in small epidemics and is believed by many (Virchow, Liveing, Bollinger, Klebs, Stellwagon) to be contagious, although this is denied by others (Erasmus Wilson, Rokitansky, Hebra, Kaposi, G. H. Fox).

In general terms, the tumor may be said to consist of a series of radially arranged masses of epithelial cells, separated from each other by fibrous septa and converging toward a common centre. The centre of the new-formation is broken down and a soft tallowy substance can be expressed. According to White and Robey,[1] the most recent investigators, the new-growth begins in the rete. The lowest layers of cells resemble the normal prickle-cells, with the addition that many of them contain one or more nucleoli. Some of the cells have lost their nucleus and are composed of a fine fibrillary protoplasm. The cells of the layers above become more or less distorted, are often devoid of nuclei, and contain clear rounded spaces which give the characteristic appearance to the structure (molluscum bodies). Toward the upper regions of the growth the cells become more or less keratinized. The significance of the changes has been interpreted variously. Some think that the peculiar vacuolated appearance is due to amyloid infiltration of the cells, while others attribute it to the presence of protozoa. Repeated attempts have been made to cultivate the organism, but without success so that the majority of observers are now agreed that the so-called "molluscum bodies" are examples of cell-degeneration and not parasitic. The older views of Engel, Rokitansky, and Hebra, that the growth originates in the sebaceous follicles, and that of Virchow, that it arises from the hair-follicles, have now practically been given up, and it is believed to be more probable that the new-growth is due to a peculiar and characteristic transformation of the rete cells into keratin.

Sarcoma.—Sarcomas of the skin are relatively rare, and may be conveniently divided into pigmented and non-pigmented forms. They are primary or secondary.

Melanotic sarcoma[2] (melanoma, chromatophoroma) may arise, though rarely, from apparently normal skin. In about half the cases, however, it is secondary to sarcoma of the uvea. The majority of the remaining 50 per cent. originate in pigmented and unpigmented nevi or warts. The tumor is recognized by its color, which is brownish or brownish-black, either diffuse or patchy in distribution. The primary tumor may be single and remain latent for years. It may then form local metastases rapidly. This form of new-growth is met with also in horses, and curiously enough only in white horses, in the dark skin around the anus.

Melanomas are tumors of connective-tissue appearance, originating in the proliferation of certain cells which are identical with the pigment-bearing cells (chromatophores) of the normal skin. The newly-formed chromatophores do not always reach adult development, for many are found to possess shorter processes or are actually rounded. The

[1] Molluscum Contagiosum, Jour. Med. Research, (N. S. 2): 1902 : 225.
[2] For a general discussion of the nature of melanomas see vol. i, p. 825.

young cells, again, are often devoid of pigment. The growth commonly begins in the deeper layers of the skin and gradually insinuates itself through the epidermis, so that small warts, rarely larger than a pea, are produced which eventually form a fungating mass. Unna, Gilchrist, and others regard these tumors as originating in the epithelium, and hold, therefore, that they are epitheliomatous rather than sarcomatous. The most recent investigations, however, do not appear to support this view, for as Ribbert[1] points out, melanotic growths frequently start in the choroid of the eye, where the chromatophores are undoubtedly of connective-tissue origin.

Morphologically, the melanomas are spindle-celled or alveolar sarcomas. The latter is the common form of the primary melanomas of the skin. They are often very vascular and may contain extravasations of blood.

The pigment—melanin—is found in fine particles or irregular clumps within and about the cells. Its exact composition is not known, possibly varying according to the nature and position of the growth, but it is peculiar in that it contains sulphur. Melanomas are very malignant, frequently recurring after removal, and forming metastases rapidly in the various viscera. The secondary growths may at times be devoid of pigment.

Under the term *idiopathic multiple pigment sarcoma*, Kaposi[2] described a new-growth, which is pigmented and highly vascular, owing to the presence of numerous thin-walled capillaries. It is not now believed to be a true pigmented sarcoma, for the color is due to the vascularity and the deposition of altered blood pigment. The growth may last for years, and finally becomes malignant, although spontaneous resolution sometimes takes place. The exact nature of this tumor is not known. Some hold that it belongs to the infectious granulomas.

FIG. 255

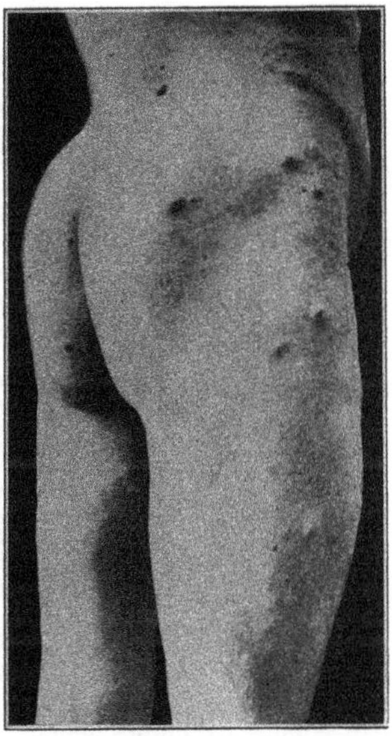

Multiple pigmented sarcomas in the skin.
(From the collection of Dr. F. J. Shepherd.)

Non-pigmented sarcomas also occur. They are primary and secondary, single or multiple, and form nodular or papillomatous masses

[1] *Lehrbuch der speciellen Path.*, 1902: 784.
[2] Path. u. Therapie der Hautkrankheiten, Wien, Urban u. Schwarzenberg, 1893.

projecting above the skin. Histologically, they are round-, spindle-, or mixed-celled.

Fibrosarcoma and *angiosarcoma* are sometimes met with. *Angioma serpiginosum* is a rare affection, which appears to be a form of angiosarcoma dependent on some congenital anomaly of the vessels.[1]

Sarcoma-like new-growths are found in the skin in certain cases of *leukemia* and *pseudoleukemia*.

Diffuse sarcomatosis of the skin (Kaposi), also called *mycosis fungoides*, occurs under the form of a round-celled sarcoma, which produces flattened, knotty masses of new-growth in the skin. It extends slowly until considerable areas are involved. The cells composing it resemble young connective-tissue cells and form diffuse masses, or are separated

FIG. 256

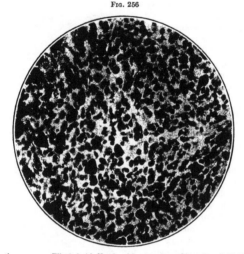

Melanotic sarcoma. Winckel obj. No. 6, without ocular. (From Dr. A. G. Nicholls' collection.)

into clumps by fibrous septa. The vessels are dilated and there is œdema of the cutis and rete. This is the stage of erythema and infiltration. Later, the cells are more numerous, more uniform in shape and size, and tend to be arranged in columns, while the connective tissue is reduced to a minimum. Fungating and ulcerating masses are ultimately produced. The tumor finally takes on malignant action, although occasionally it involutes spontaneously. It is not yet settled whether the new-growth is properly to be regarded as a sarcoma or whether it is inflammatory.

[1] White, Jour. Cut. and Genito-urin. Dis., 12 : 1894: 468.

Acanthosis Nigricans.—Another rare condition of doubtful nature is acanthosis nigricans, described by Politzer, Darier, Morris, and others. Deeply pigmented, warty, and papillomatous nodules are found in various parts. Histologically, there is hyperplasia of the papillæ and epidermis, dilatation of the blood- and lymph-vessels, with increase of the pigment in the palisade cells. There is also an imperfect attempt at the formation of "cell-nests." The disease has been found associated with carcinoma of other structures. Darier thinks that it is due to some lesion of the sympathetic nerve.[1]

Carcinoma.—Carcinoma is of frequent occurrence in the skin. It is found on the lip, nose, eyelids, prepuce, scrotum, and vulva, but may occasionally develop in other regions. It is in this form of carci-

FIG. 257

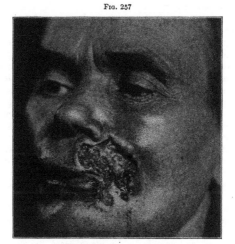

Epithelioma of the lip. (Hyde.)

noma that long-continued irritation appears to play an important role. Thus, it is met with on the lower lip in smokers, at the margins of indolent ulcers, in lupus, in patches of chronic dermatitis caused by soot, tar, paraffin, and irritating discharges, and about warts or nevi, which have been frequently rubbed or excoriated.

Carcinomas may develop from the epidermis or from the epithelium of the glands and hair-follicles, but it is not always possible to determine the point of origin in fairly advanced cases. Certain of them, not connected with the epidermal layer, may originate in cell-inclusions, derived from the epidermis (dermoids), or from the branchial clefts (branchiogenic carcinoma).

[1] For literature see Janovsky, Mraçek's Handb. d. Hautkr., vol. iii.

Thiersch has divided skin carcinomas into *superficial* and *deep* forms, which, however, merge imperceptibly one into the other.

Among the superficial forms may be mentioned rodent ulcer and Paget's disease of the nipple. These form shallow ulcers with infiltrated, slightly elevated edges, which from necrosis may assume a somewhat nodular appearance.

Rodent ulcer occurs most frequently at the corner of the nose, near the eyelids, or upon the forehead. The growth is excessively slow in its development, sometimes lasting many years. Under surgical measures it may heal up for a time, but sooner or later, as a rule, breaks out again. The tumor is quite superficial and spreads slowly at its margin, but, owing to the relatively large amount of necrosis, presents the clinical picture of an ulcer rather than a neoplasm. Histologically, it is an epithelioma.

Paget's disease begins at the nipple and apparently originates in a very chronic form of inflammation (see p. 947).

The deeply-penetrating carcinomas originate in nodules of new-growth, which, when necrosis has taken place, present the appearance of ulcers with nodular bases and irregular edges. When growth is active, fungating papillomatous masses are produced. This form is very malignant, growing rapidly, and producing metastases more quickly than the superficial varieties. All sorts of intermediate grades exist between the superficial and the deeply-penetrating carcinomas, and epithelial proliferation, connective-tissue overgrowth, and necrosis may be combined in a variety of ways.

The microscopic appearances of epithelioma of the skin vary according to circumstances. In a well-marked example of a not too rapidly growing epithelioma, the rete sends out downgrowths into the underlying tissues in the form of processes which divide, subdivide, and anastomose. The outermost cells of these downgrowths correspond in structure with the lowermost cells of the normal rete. As they approach the central portion they become more cuboidal, being practically identical with the prickle-cells, while at the centre they are more or less flattened and cornified. In many cases the cornified areas present the appearance of flattened, concentrically arranged spindles or plates, which may be compared to the stratification of an onion, the so-called "cell-nests" (Perlkugeln). The central portion occasionally becomes fatty, colloid, granular, or in rare instances calcified. The connective tissue enveloping the growth is normal, or, as in most cases, thickened, and shows infiltration with small round cells, either the result of cell-proliferation, or, possibly, inflammation. In the more rapidly growing varieties the cells are of the more primitive type and present little or no tendency to cornification, so that cell-nests are lacking. In cases where pressure has been exerted upon the processes, the cells become flattened and spindle-shaped, resembling somewhat those of a sarcoma.

Certain rare forms of carcinoma deserve a passing notice. One of these is the so-called *"lenticular"* carcinoma. It is usually found in the mamma, where it is secondary to a deeper seated carcinoma of the gland, but is occasionally met with as a primary growth in other parts of the body. The affected skin and subcutaneous tissues are diffusely infiltrated with new-growth, and are swollen, hard, and resistant, resembling washleather. On section the structure is tough and gristly, and may contain considerable fluid, due to pressure upon the lymphatics. Thus a form of elephantiasis, "cancer en cuirasse," is the result.

Alveolar carcinoma may be found in the deeper layers of the skin and subcutaneous tissues.

Apart from the local metastases that form in the skin about an epithelioma, secondary carcinoma is not common. Both connective tissue and epithelial tumors may form metastases in the skin. Carcinoma of the breast is perhaps the most frequent cause.

Cysts.—Apart from the cysts originating in the glandular elements of the skin should be mentioned **dermoids** and **implantation-cysts**. The former are congenital; the latter are due to trauma.

THE ACCESSORY STRUCTURES AND APPENDAGES OF THE SKIN.

The Hair.

The congenital anomalies of the hair, **hypertrichosis, alopecia, adnata canities**, have already been referred to (see p. 955).

Alopecia.—The acquired form of alopecia, or falling of the hair (alopecia acquisita, clavities acquisita), may be a senile manifestation (**alopecia senilis**), usually associated with atrophy of the skin and absorption of the subcutaneous fat, or may occur early in life (**alopecia prematura**).

Alopecia Prematura.—Alopecia prematura may come on without any obvious cause (idiopathic), but is often associated with disease of the scalp or of the general system. Thus, eczema, erysipelas, syphilitic eruptions, seborrhœa, favus, and ring-worm are common causes of loss of hair. The hair also not infrequently falls out after acute and other infective diseases, such as typhoid, scarlatina, syphilis, and tuberculosis, and during lactation in weakly individuals.

Alopecia Areata.—Alopecia areata (**porrigo**[1]) is characterized by the formation of one or more areas of baldness, which may be found on any region of the body normally covered with hair. The scalp and the beard are the parts usually involved. The patches are round or oval, sharply defined, and become quite devoid of hair. The skin of the affected part is soft, smooth, depressed, at first slightly reddened, later white and glistening. The hair at the periphery shows no obvious change, but gradually falls out in turn. The sharp line of demarcation between the round bald spot and the normally covered scalp is a characteristic feature. The spots may gradually increase until the hair of the scalp,

---

[1] See Behrend, Haarkrankheiten, Eulenberg's Realenzyklop., 1895.

beard, and eyebrows, and even of the whole of the body, has entirely disappeared.

Microscopically, the hairs and hair-follicles are atrophied, there are diapedesis of lymphocytes with accumulation of mast-cells, and absence of pigment in the rete.

The exact cause is not altogether understood. Perhaps the majority of observers consider the disease to be a trophoneurosis, inasmuch as it in many cases follows injury to the nerves, shock, or other disturbance of the nervous system. On the other hand, the occasional occurrence of the disease in epidemic form, together with some evidence of contagion, suggests a parasitic cause in some, at least, of the cases. Sabouraud regards as the specific cause a bacillus, which is present in the hair-follicles, and identical with a bacillus which he finds in seborrhœa. Rarely ringworm gives rise to similar appearances, and has been mistaken for alopecia areata by competent observers.

Atrophy.—Atrophy of the hair is due to disease of the scalp, such as seborrhœa, eczema, and psoriasis, or to some systemic disorder associated with poverty of nutrition. The hair is dry, brittle, and lacks lustre.

Trichorrhexis nodosa[1] is a rare form of atrophy, in which the shafts of the hairs, usually of the beard, present nodular swellings, through which the hair readily breaks. In **monilethrix**, an affection which is generally congenital, the shaft of the hair presents ring-like constrictions through which the hair is apt to fracture.

Hypertrichosis.[2]—Hypertrichosis, apart from the congenital and developmental forms, occasionally results in areas that have been subjected to irritation, pressure, inflammation, or other cause which leads to congestion. In women, hair upon the upper lip, or other parts of the face, is occasionally due to an hereditary peculiarity or to some abnormality of the sexual functions It is not uncommon after the menopause.

Canities.—Canities, or blanching of the hair, occurs physiologically in old age, but is not infrequently met with in younger people. It is sometimes an inherited peculiarity, or may follow mental overwork, nervous shock, or prolonged disease. Local blanching has been noticed in migraine and neuralgia. The condition is due not only to loss of pigment, but to the presence of air in the substance of the hair.

The Nails.

Congenital absence and **developmental anomalies** of the nails are rare and usually associated with defects of the hair and teeth.

White spots upon the nails (**leukopathia unguis**) are not infrequent, due to the presence of air between the layers of the keratin. They

---

[1] See Sack, Haarkrankheiten in v. Mraçek's Handbook, 4:1907.

[2] Friedenthal, Die Behaarung des Menschen, Jena, 1909.

are the result of slight injuries or of impairment of nutrition. **Transverse furrows** are often found upon the nails of those who have suffered from acute disease or other cause which has lowered their vitality.

The nail may be **dislocated** from its bed by traumatism or the collection of pus or blood beneath it. This may lead to complete **exfoliation**. The nails may also be shed in alopecia areata, syphilis, diabetes mellitus, and hysteria.

Inflammation of the matrix of the nail (**onychia**) and of the surrounding soft parts (**paronychia**) may be the result of traumatism or local infection, or, again, may be occasionally seen in syphilis and tuberculosis. Favus and ring-worm sometimes attack the nail (**onychomycosis**) and give rise to onychia and paronychia.

In **atrophy** the nail is thinned and softened, becomes brittle, and is often traversed by ridges or furrows.

Simple **overgrowth** of the nails, which may perhaps be regarded as a physiological condition, since it is due to the omission of the customary cutting of the nails, is met with among certain races, such as the Chinese, and among some of the fakirs of India. In the forms of overgrowth found in other nations, however, there is evidence of disease as well. The nail substance is thickened (**hyperonychia**), irregular, roughened, brittle, and discolored. The nails may in time become twisted, bent, and project like talons beyond the finger-tips (**onychogryphosis**). It is not uncommon to find inflammation and even suppuration going on in these cases beneath the nail. The condition is met with in old persons who are dirty, debilitated, and uncared for, in syphilis, eczema, psoriasis, and, occasionally, in tuberculosis, leprosy, myxœdema, acromegaly, neuritis, and neurotrophic disorders. A common form of simple enlargement is the so-called "*ingrowing toe-nail,*" in which the nail increases in breadth and penetrates the flesh of the toe, giving rise to inflammation and suppuration (*paronychia*).

The Sweat-glands.

Hyperidrosis and Anidrosis.—These are functional disorders of the sweat-glands, and are either an evidence of some inherited peculiarity or the result of systemic or local disease. No gross changes are found in the glands, but it is probable that in most cases the conditions are due to some disturbance of the innervation of the part, or to the direct action of a toxin upon the secreting cells in the process of elimination. Complete absence of sweat secretion (**anidrosis**) probably does not occur, except locally in cases where the glands have been destroyed by disease. Diminution in the amount of sweat (**hyphidrosis**) is found in many acute fevers, in Bright's disease, in myxœdema, and in such conditions as eczema, psoriasis, and pityriasis. **Hyperidrosis** is most common in the palms, soles, axillary and pubic regions. Unilateral or local hyperidrosis is met with in some nervous diseases and in neurotic individuals.

Bromidrosis.—Bromidrosis, or offensive perspiration, is usually associated with hyperidrosis, and generally affects the same parts. There is a certain amount of odor connected with ordinary perspiration, and this is more evident in some individuals and races than in others. In stout persons or those who perspire freely the sweat often emits a sour smell shortly after it is excreted. In true bromidrosis the odor is penetrating and disgusting. The condition may. of course, be assisted by uncleanly habits, but is often met with in those who are scrupulously clean. In such we have to look for the cause in some neuropathic disturbance. The fœtid odor is by many attributed to the decomposition of the sweat by microörganisms.

Uridrosis.—Uridrosis, or the excretion of urinary salts through the sweat, is met with occasionally in Bright's disease, cholera, and some serious constitutional disorders. It has been recorded also after the administration of jaborandi. In marked cases scales of urea may be deposited on the skin.

Chromidrosis.—Chromidrosis, or colored sweat, is an excessively rare condition. It is possibly in some cases neurotrophic in nature. More often, coloration of the sweat is due to the elimination through the skin of such substances as copper, or the application of dyes to the skin. One form, red sweat, which affects the axillary and genital regions, is due to concretions upon the shaft of the hairs (*leptothrix*), resulting from bacterial activity.

Hematidrosis.—Bloody sweat (hematidrosis) is a rare condition due to hemorrhage into the sweat-glands. It has occurred in neurotic individuals.

Phosphorescent Sweat.—Phosphorescent sweat has been described.

Sudamina.—Sudamina (**miliaria crystallina**) are not infrequently met with in febrile conditions, especially those associated with profuse sweating. Small, clear vesicles, often abundant, form in the horny layer of the skin, which disappear after a few days. The condition is due either to blocking of the duct and consequent retention of the sweat, or, according to some, rupture of the duct and escape of the sweat into the horny layer. The disease, rarely, is epidemic (*miliaria epidemica*).[1]

Hidradenitis Suppurativa.—Hidradenitis suppurativa (*furunculosis*) is, as its name implies, a suppurative inflammation of the sweat-glands. It is most often found in the axillary and pubic regions. The process begins deep in, involves the surrounding structures, and eventually leads to destruction of the glands. Less often furuncles originate in the hair-follicles or sebaceous glands.

Carbuncle is a more intense form of infection; anatomically an aggregation of furuncles. It tends to spread peripherally, is slowly progressive, and tends to lead to a phlegmon of the skin and subcutaneous tissues and to gangrene. The affected part is swollen, reddened, brawny, and intensely painful. When incised it is necrotic and often riddled

---

[1] Weichselbaum, Zeitschr. f. klin. Med., 62:1907.

with suppurating sinuses. It only occurs in marantic individuals and especially in connection with diabetes mellitus. It may lead to death by septicemia.

Hidrocystoma.—Hidrocystoma is a rather rare condition, usually affecting the face. One or more clear, deep-seated vesicles are formed, apparently the result of dilatation of the sweat-ducts in their course through the corium. Papillary outgrowths into this cyst may occur (*cystadenoma papilliferum*). **Adenomas** may also arise from the sweat-glands.

The Sebaceous Glands.

Seborrhœa.—The sebaceous glands normally secrete an oily substance, which is elaborated in the glandular epithelium and dis charged upon the surface of the skin, where it acts as a sort of lubricant. Excess of this secretion gives rise to the condition known as seborrhœa. In one form, **seborrhœa sicca,** minute, dry, filmy scales are produced, composed in part of dried sebum, but also of desquamated horny epithelium and dirt or dust. In the other, there is excessive secretion of the sebum, so that the skin is kept constantly oily (**seborrhœa oleosa**).

Seborrhœa may be a local or a general condition. The former is usually met with on the scalp or in the genital region. Generalized seborrhœa is rather rare, and is most frequently found in young children where the greasy secretion which normally covers the skin during intrauterine life (smegma, vernix caseosa) persists for some time after birth. It is not uncommon to find in infants dirty crusts upon the scalp, composed of sebum, dirt, epithelial scales, and hairs. In mild cases of seborrhœa sicca there is only a trifling exfoliation of the epithelial scales (*dandruff*), with slight increase of secretion, but in others there may be considerable heaping up of material into larger scales and crusts (*pityriasis furfuracea capillitii*). Seborrhœa, if long-continued, leads to atrophy of the hair-follicles and loss of the hair. It is not infrequently, also, accompanied by inflammatory phenomena (*seborrhœal eczema, seborrhœal dermatitis*).

The cause is obscure, since many cases occur in apparently healthy people, but some are connected with digestive disturbances or poor nutrition. Anything which tends to keep the scalp warm and moist would predispose to the affection.

Asteatosis.—Asteatosis, absence or lack of the sebaceous secretion (xeroderma), is rare as a primary disease, but is usually an accompaniment of other disease, notably where the skin is dry and scaly. Thus, it is found in psoriasis, prurigo, pityriasis rubra pilaris, leprosy, and ichthyosis. The skin becomes dry, fissured, and the epithelium scales off.

There are several allied conditions that are due to the accumulation of the sebum within the sebaceous glands or their ducts. This accumulation and retention of secretion is brought about by obstruction to the ducts from dirt or overgrowth of the lining epithelium, or, in some cases, by alteration in the character of the secretion itself.

Comedo.—Comedo is a condition in which the excretory duct of a sebaceous gland and sometimes that of a hair-follicle are obstructed. This results in the formation of a minute nodule in the skin, which presents externally as a blackish point, the size of a pinhead or less. On squeezing this, a fine worm-like or thread-like substance is extruded, having a blackish or brownish spot at the end. This substance is composed of inspissated sebum, fattily degenerated and keratinized epithelial cells, and not infrequently lanugo hairs. The dark spot at the end of the plug is largely composed of dirt and dust, and, according to Unna, a particular pigment—ultramarine.

The anatomical condition appears to be overgrowth of the epithelial cells lining the duct, with, possibly, parakeratosis of the external cells, in this way leading to obstruction to the free discharge of the sebum, which consequently becomes altered in character. It is also possible that the irritation of fine hairs or inspissation of the secretion may be the exciting cause of the cellular proliferation. Not infrequently, the obstructed glands become inflamed, forming small red, elevated papules and pustules (one form of *acne*). Comedones are found usually upon the face near the nose, on the forehead, and occasionally upon the shoulders. They may be very numerous. The affection has been regarded as having some connection with gastro-intestinal disturbances, but is often enough met with in healthy people. It is, however, most common about the age of puberty, when the skin and its associated glands are particularly active.

Milium.—Milium is a form of obstruction of the sebaceous glands in which the lumina become somewhat dilated, forming small nodules the size of a pin-head or smaller, of a whitish or yellowish color, which project slightly above the general surface of the skin. On incising one of these, a smooth or warty lobulated mass can be expressed consisting of fat and epidermal cells surrounded by concentric layers of keratinized cells. Milia are found usually upon the eyelids. Where a group of sebaceous glands are enlarged and distended with secretion and proliferated cells the condition is known as *acrochordon*. This is met with most frequently in elderly people, usually on the eyelids, throat, and neck.

Inflammations.—Acne Vulgaris.—Acne vulgaris is an inflammation of the sebaceous glands, which is liable to involve the hair-follicles and surrounding tissues as well. Not infrequently the trouble is to be traced to comedones. In the early stages small, elevated, reddened papules are formed, usually upon the face, but occasionally also on the neck, shoulders, trunk, and extremities (*acne simplex*). Where there is a central blackish point the condition is called *acne punctata*. The process often goes on to suppuration, so that elevated, reddish pustules are produced, varying in size from that of a pin-head, or smaller, to that of a pea, presenting a yellowish centre (*acne pustulosa*). On incising this a small drop of pus can be evacuated. In the so-called *acne indurata* comparatively large purplish-red and hard nodules are produced which are much indurated and persist for a considerable time.

They leave considerable staining of the skin and more or less scarring. Occasionally acne spots present central necrosis and resemble variola pocks. In very aggravated and prolonged cases the vessels of the skin become dilated, the sebaceous glands are greatly enlarged, and the fibrous tissue is increased, so that a form of elephantiasis results. When affecting the nose the condition is called **Rhinophyma** (*Pfundnase*).[1] Acne is most common in persons about the age of puberty or in early adult life. Those who have poor circulation or who are the subjects of gastro-intestinal disorders are supposed to be more liable. Acne may also be caused by external irritation.

A mycotic folliculitis and perifolliculitis, involving the hair-follicles and sebaceous glands, due to the trichophyton, is well known (*tinea sycosis*) (see p. 975).

Cysts.—**Atheroma**, or sebaceous cyst, is a cystic dilatation of a sebaceous gland or hair-follicle, due to the accumulation of secretion within its cavity. There is usually a smooth, connective-tissue capsule, lined by stratified pavement cells. The contents are liquid, semi-solid, or cheesy, and are composed of fat, epithelial debris, cholesterin, and fine hairs. The cysts may be all sizes up to that of a fist. They are usually found upon the scalp, but occasionally also in the skin of the neck and face, of the trunk and extremities. The contents of sebaceous cysts may undergo extensive horny transformation or even calcification, so that bone-like nodules result.

Tumors.—Somewhat similar cysts, but more deeply seated, present a different structure, being lined by modified skin, and therefore are of the nature of **dermoids**. Others, again, are more or less completely filled with papillary outgrowths, so that they may be properly regarded as **papillary cystadenomas**. Occasionally they become malignant.

Adenoma of the sebaceous glands is a rather rare affection, met with usually in persons mentally ·defective. Small, round or oval, sessile tumors are found usually on the chin, forehead, or about the nose.[2] They may simulate nevi. The growth may become in part cystic. Transitional forms, midway between adenoma and carcinoma are described. The *Epithelioma adenoides cysticum* of the dermatologists is possibly of this nature (see p. 1010).

Carcinoma may develop from the sweat-glands.

---

[1] For literature see Egger, Zur Kasuistik d. Rhinophyma, Inaug. Diss., Basel, 1905.

[2] See *L*. Pick, Virch. Archiv, 175:1904:312.

SECTION IX.

THE MUSCULAR SYSTEM.

CHAPTER XLII.

THE SKELETAL MUSCLES.

THE MUSCLES.

THE skeletal muscles belong to the voluntary group, and are there-fore of the striated order. They are composed of fibres averaging about 4 to 5 cm. long and from 10 to 55 μ broad. On finer analysis, these fibres consist of a soft protoplasmic ground-substance, presenting a distinct transverse striation and a fainter longitudinal fibrillation, inclosed in a clear, structureless, and elastic sheath (the sarcolemma). The nuclei of the muscle-fibres are situated upon the surface of the muscle-cylinder, are ellipsoidal in shape, with their long axes parallel to that of the fibre. The number of the nuclei varies considerably, being more numerous in the young and smaller muscles. Increase in size of the fibre is not necessarily associated with numerical increase of the nuclei.

The muscle-fibres are grouped into fasciculi, and these again into larger bundles, which together constitute the complete anatomical muscle. The various components are held together and supported by a connective-tissue stroma, that inclosing the larger bundles being called the perimysium, while the delicate interstitial substance envelop-ing the individual fibres is termed the endomysium.

The muscles are highly vascular, the larger vessels being found in the perimysium, and these break up into a freely anastomosing network of capillaries within the endomysium. The terminations of the nerves supplying them are highly specialized arborizations or end-plates.

Under normal conditions, the length and breadth of the muscles vary within wide limits, according to the degree of relaxation or contrac-tion incident to their functioning for the time being. When at rest, the muscles are held in a condition short of complete relaxation, called tonus, apparently the result of a succession of slow sub-minimal nervous stimuli. Under pathological conditions the degree of contraction and of tonus may be greatly altered.

Muscles are not liable to a great variety of primary disease processes. Owing to their exposed position and their close association with the skeleton in regard to the function of locomotion, they are particularly liable, however, to direct and indirect traumatism. Again, owing to their abundant blood supply they are readily brought under the influence of various circulating toxins and infective microörganisms. The effect of these is somewhat minimized, owing to the inherent protective powers of the muscle juices. And, further, they may present grave changes as a result of defective innervation.

The pathological lesions are manifested not only by qualitative changes in the fibres themselves, but also quantitatively by an increase or diminution of the muscle-substance, either absolutely or relatively to the amount of the connective-tissue stroma.

CONGENITAL ANOMALIES.

These are so numerous that it is impossible to enter adequately into the subject here. Many of the anomalies are interesting, not only from the point of view of development, but also because they have a practical bearing on surgery.

In general terms it may be said that there is no anomaly of the muscles in man which does not have its prototype in one or other species of the lower animals. Briefly, these consist in irregular origin and insertion of the muscles; complete or partial defect of certain muscles or groups of muscles; reduplication; while again, certain muscles may b present in man which, though normally present in other species, are no regularly found in the human subject.[1]

One of the most important of these peculiarities about which a wor or two may be spoken is defect of the **diaphragm,** which sometimes give rise to serious clinical manifestations. The diaphragm may be defectiv to an extent varying from a small opening to one involving half th structure. The deficiency is usually on the left side and in the muscula portion somewhat posteriorly. The condition is often associated witl other grave developmental errors, such as anencephaly, hemicrania, an anomalies of the fingers and toes. In many such cases prolonged con tinuation of life is of course impossible, but where the diaphragm alon is involved persons so affected have been known to reach a fairl advanced age. Owing to the deficiency in this structure, it is usual a some time or other, to find certain of the abdominal viscera, such a the stomach, omentum, intestines, liver, spleen, and kidney in th thoracic cavity. In such cases there is usually marked dyspnœa an embarrassment of the heart's action, with physical signs of displacemen of the heart and lungs, and the presence of a solid organ or hollow viscu containing air in the chest cavity (see p. 410).

---

[1] Those desiring more detailed information are referred to Dr. F. J. Shepherd' article on The Anomalies of Muscles, in the Reference Handbook of the Medica Sciences, 6: 1903: 42, second edition. Wm. Wood & Co., New York.

CIRCULATORY DISTURBANCES.

Owing to the free anastomosis of the vessels, local disorders of the circulation are not readily brought about. Any such changes are caused only by extensive disease of the bloodvessels or systemic affections of the blood and circulatory apparatus. Except in the case of the grosser lesions, it is difficult to recognize circulatory disturbances post mortem.

Anemia.—Anemia may be **local** or **general.** The local form is brought about by obstruction of a main arterial trunk or compression of the muscle. Toxic substances acting upon the blood, various blood diseases, and weak driving power of the heart lead to general anemia. Muscles so affected are pale, soft, drier than normal, and deficient in coloring matter, although in some cases this is increased.

Hyperemia.—**Active hyperemia** is found in the neighborhood of inflammatory processes. **Passive hyperemia** is present in all conditions of general vascular stasis.

Œdéma.—Microscopically, here, the muscle-fibres are vacuolated, owing to hydropic infiltration, while the connective tissue appears to be looser than normal. In the severer forms the fibres degenerate or even liquefy. The causes are inflammation, hydremia, and vascular stasis.

Hemorrhage.—Hemorrhage into the muscles is not infrequent. It may be extensive, minute or petechial. The larger extravasations (**hematoma**) are the result of trauma; rupture of the muscle from excessive contraction, as, for example, in tetanus; increased blood pressure, and certain degenerative changes in the vessel walls. **Petechiæ** are most probably due to defective nutrition of the walls of the capillaries and smaller bloodvessels, leading to fatty changes which predispose to rupture, or, as some think, to diapedesis. These small hemorrhages are met with in certain of the infectious fevers, the hemorrhagic diatheses, pernicious anemia and leukemia, poisoning from phosphorus and various drugs, and multiple sarcomatosis.[1] When the extravasation is extensive the muscle-fibres are pushed apart and compressed, and eventually undergo coagulation necrosis or even disintegrate. Should the process go on to healing, the blood is absorbed, or in part absorbed and in part organized, with the formation of a pigmented scar in which there is an imperfect attempt at restoration of the fibres. In rare instances, as in traumatic myositis ossificans, the connective tissue may undergo metaplasia into cartilage and bone.

Infarction.—Infarction is occasionally brought about by obstruction to the blood supply, as, for instance, in arteriosclerosis, endarteritis, local compression, weak circulation, thrombosis, and embolism. For the reason mentioned, the condition is not common. It is most

[1] For a critical examination of the forms of hemorrhage here referred to, see Nicholls and Learmonth, The Hemorrhagic Diathesis in Typhoid Fever, and its Relationships to Purpuric Conditions in General, Lancet, London, 1: 1901: 305.

likely to be met with in those weakened by prolonged disease. When extensive, large areas of muscle may present what is known as Zenker's necrosis, but more commonly multiple minute hemorrhages into the connective tissue are produced. The larger areas of anemic necrosis are often bounded by a zone of secondary hemorrhagic exudation. Should such an area become infected, abscess may result. Certain cases of bedsores and senile gangrene are of the nature of infarcts. Total or partial ischemic necrosis of the psoas, usually the left, has been noted in patients who for a long time have kept the recumbent position.

INFLAMMATIONS.

Myositis.—Myositis, or inflammation of muscle, usually arises by the direct extension of an inflammatory process from some adjacent part, or from trauma. Affections of the bones, joints, skin, and mucous surfaces play an important role, as do also pleurisy, peritonitis, peri- and paranephritis.

In other cases, myositis is hematogenous, the result of bacterial invasion or circulating toxins. This form is met with in septic infection of wounds, puerperal septicemia, osteomyelitis, malignant endocarditis, acute rheumatism, typhoid fever, and glanders.

In general terms it may be stated that the inflammation largely affects the connective tissue and bloodvessels, while the changes in the muscle-fibres are mainly degenerative and secondary.

Acute Myositis.—Acute myositis assumes several forms. The simplest type is characterized by a slight exudation of inflammatory products into the perimysium with diapedesis of leukocytes. The muscle-fibres may be practically normal (*acute interstitial myositis*) or may show various grades of degeneration, such as cloudy swelling, fatty degeneration, and coagulation necrosis (*acute diffuse myositis*). The condition is met with in typhoid fever, after slight trauma, about intramuscular hemorrhages, in the neighborhood of local inflammatory foci, and is usually a temporary condition of trifling import. The process may heal, and, provided that the organization of the muscle be not destroyed, *restitutio ad integrum* may be complete.

In more severe cases the muscle-fibres may to some extent be destroyed and replaced by fibrous tissue.

In still more severe forms, where there is, for instance, infection with pyogenic microörganisms, diffuse suppuration may occur in the muscle, or abscesses may form (*acute purulent myositis*). This is seen in such conditions as infected wounds, erysipelas, septic arthritis, ulcerative colitis, septicemia, and glanders.

In the early stages the muscle is greatly reddened and swollen, gradually becoming grayish, grayish-yellow, or, if hemorrhage occur, brownish or grayish-green in appearance. It is soft, friable, and quickly breaks down, so that numerous cavities of varying size, containing pus and shreddy debris, are produced. The abscesses may remain localized or the pus may burrow widely along the fascia and intermuscular septa.

In very severe infection, or where the resisting power of the tissues is slight, gangrene may occur, the muscle turning greenish-black or black, and becoming converted into a dirty, evil-smelling mass, which quickly undergoes liquefaction and disintegration. In the neighborhood of the abscesses the muscle-fibres are found to be in various stages of degeneration, and where there is a tendency to heal, there is a zone of granulation tissue. If the patient survive, small abscesses may disappear after the pus has been absorbed, while larger ones may heal when the contents have been discharged, either externally, or into some cavity. Others become encapsulated by active granulation and the formation of connective tissue. In time the abscess contracts, the contents gradually disappear, become inspissated, or infiltrated with lime salts. When large portions of the muscle are destroyed, repair by proliferation of the muscle cells is very imperfect. Where the irritation is comparatively slight, though continuous, or where repeated attacks of acute myositis have taken place, there may be marked proliferation of the connective tissue, so that the muscle looks as if traversed by whitish bands or membranes.

A curious affection, the etiology of which is still somewhat obscure, is the so-called *primary acute polymyositis*, described by Wagner,[1] Unverricht, Hepp, v. Strümpell,[2] and Levy. It is characterized clinically by fever, pain, and swelling of the muscles of the tongue, back, and extremities. Voluntary movement is usually completely lost. There is generally some redness of the skin, with the production of rashes of various sorts, so that the disease has been called *dermatomyositis*. The resemblance to trichinosis is close, and at times a microscopic examination is necessary to make the diagnosis.

Post mortem, the muscles are brownish-red in color, with areas of waxy yellow appearance, and present punctate and linear pigmentation. The fibres are separated by hemorrhagic (polymyositis acuta hæmorrhagica[3]) or purulent exudation. Marked extravasation of blood between the muscle bundles may be found.

Microscopically, one finds granular degeneration of the muscle-fibres, with vacuolation, loss of striation, proliferation of the muscle-nuclei, and round-celled infiltration in the intramuscular connective tissue.

The disease may be of mild intensity, but is apt to become chronic, and usually terminates fatally after weeks or months. It is almost certainly of an infective nature. Senator was probably the first to advance the view that polymyositis is in the main due to auto-intoxication. Since the affection has been observed after the use of improper food, it has been suggested that the toxin is derived from the gastro-intestinal tract. Von Strümpell regards it as due to bacterial toxins circulating in the blood, derived from some local focus of infection.

A condition of great interest is the so-called **myositis ossificans**, which,

[1] Acute Polymyositis, Deutsches Archiv f. klin. Med., 40: 1887: 241.
[2] Zur Kenntniss der primären akuten Polymyositis Deutsch. Zeitschr. f. Nervenheilk., 1: 1891: 479.
[3] See Struppler, Deut. Archiv f. klin. Med., 68: 1900: 407.

as its name implies, is an inflammation of the muscles accompanied by the formation of bone. The disease is a rare one, although it has been known since 1740, when the first case was reported by Freke in the *Philosophical Transactions*. Since this date only about 85 examples have been recorded. The etiology is still quite obscure. Following Cahen,[1] it is usual to divide the disease into two forms, a localized or *stationary* and a *progressive* form.

In the first-mentioned class of cases the disease appears to be dependent upon trauma or irritation, and is found particularly in muscles which are overexercised (exercise bones). The muscles affected are usually the deltoids and pectorals in soldiers, the adductors of the thighs in riders, occasionally the arms in gymnasts, and the legs in dancers. The bone is present in the form of splinters, plates, or bosses, either attached to the bones and tendons, or forming movable masses in the intramuscular connective tissue.

More obscure still is *myositis ossificans progressiva*, which is distinguished from the first-mentioned form by the fact that it begins in early life and successively involves one muscle-group after another. The disease is most commonly found in males, according to Münchmeyer, 9 out of 12 cases, and Roth, 30 out of 39. The affection comes on idiopathically or follows slight trauma. After a somewhat acute onset with local swelling, pain, and slight febrile reaction, it subsides in intensity, but usually advances steadily by a series of relapses. The disease generally begins in the muscles or fasciæ of the neck, back, and thorax, gradually spreading to other parts of the body. It invariably ends fatally.

In the first stage the muscles contain areas which are swollen, painful, and doughy, due apparently to inflammatory infiltration within the intramuscular connective tissue. In the next stage there is an overgrowth of the intramuscular connective tissue with leukocytic infiltration. The muscle-fibres lose their striation and show fatty or other degeneration, the muscle-nuclei are increased in many cases, suggesting giant cells, and the fibres finally disintegrate. In the third stage, ossification takes place in the affected areas. The bone is found in the form of spicules, plates, nodules, or arborescent masses in the connective tissue of the muscles, the fascia, and tendons. In some cases the muscle-bundles are chiefly involved; in others, the tendons and fasciæ; and in a third class the newly-formed bone is so associated with the old that the disease presents the picture of multiple exostoses, or, in parts, hyperostoses. In course of time large areas of muscle are replaced by bone, leading to marked deformity and immobility of the joints. Ultimately the patient becomes perfectly helpless. The only muscles which escape are those of the hand and the muscles which are not attached to bone at both ends, although even in the latter case immunity is not absolute. The "ossified man" seen in circuses is usually an example of this terrible disease.

[1] Ueber Myositis Ossificans, Deut. Zeit. f. Chir., 31: 1890: 372.

The newly-formed bone is formed directly from connective or granulation tissue after the fashion of periosteal bone-formation, or indirectly from newly-formed cartilage cells. The muscle-bundles remain passive throughout the process and the degenerative changes present in them are usually regarded as secondary to the pressure of the enlarging bony masses and to ankylosis.

Many different opinions have been expressed as to the true nature of myositis ossificans. Virchow placed it on the border-line between tumor-formation and inflammation. Mays and Cahen, among others, regard it as a true tumor. Nicoladoni advances the hypothesis that the disease is a trophoneurosis. Eichhorst thinks that it is secondary to some disease of the spinal cord.

Among the predisposing causes may be mentioned exposure to cold, unhygienic surroundings, and rheumatism. The most important exciting cause is trauma, either a single injury or repeated irritation. This plays the most important part in the local form of the disease. We have an analogous formation of bone in the choroid of the eye in chronic inflammation, and it is supposed that there is here a metaplasia of the newly-formed granulation and connective tissue due to a constant mild stimulation. Warthin is inclined to favor the view that in the localized form, in which he includes inflammatory ossification and the "exercise bone," there is an atavistic reversion to the splint-bones of the lower animals.

With regard to the progressive form of the disease, the fact that it is so commonly found in early childhood and that it is usually symmetrical has suggested that there is some congenital anomaly at work. This view is supported by the observation of Florschütz, who noted the frequent association of microdactyly with ankylosis of the phalanges of the thumb and the absence of one phalanx of both great toes. This malformation has since been found in about 75 per cent. of the cases. Hallux valgus, malposition and hypoplasia of certain organs of generation, have also been reported. If we take this view, we may assume that portions of the osteogenic layer of the periosteum or its forerunners, or possibly bone-corpuscles, have become isolated in the course of growth from their proper environment, forming "rests" within the muscles, which have subsequently taken on abnormal activity. Or, it may be that undifferentiated mesenchymal cells have remained dormant until, under some sufficient stimulus, they have developed into masses of connective tissue, cartilage, or bone in abnormal situations.[1]

Tuberculosis.—Tuberculosis of the muscles is usually secondary to tuberculosis of neighboring parts, such as the joints, bones, skin, mucous and serous membranes. It is met with commonly in the muscles of the thorax, back, pelvis, and hip-joint, as a result of tuberculosis of the pleura, spinal column, pelvic bones, and hip-joints. The iliopsoas and gluteal muscles are commonly involved in tuberculosis of the lumbar vertebræ and the sacro-iliac synchondrosis.

---

[1] For a discussion of the nature of myositis ossificans and a full bibliography, see *Lydia M. De Witt, Amer. Jour. Med. Sci.*, 120: 1900: 295

The intermuscular connective tissue in such cases presents chronic thickening, and there may be the formation of numerous granulomas, which by their confluence lead to the production of large caseous nodules and, when they soften, to the so-called "cold" abscesses. The abscess cavities are lined by tuberculous granulation tissue. The puriform material often burrows extensively through the muscle and along the fascia, and may burst externally, leaving discharging fistulæ or sinuses. Large areas of muscle and connective tissue may be destroyed in this way. The process spreads through the formation of new tubercular foci in the neighborhood of the abscesses, which in their turn enlarge, become confluent, and break down. In the more chronic cases there is a considerable proliferation of fibrous tissue, which invades and replaces the muscle-bundles and in its turn becomes caseous.

Microscopically, the tuberculous nodules consist of a caseous necrotic centre, bounded by a zone of lymphocytes and epithelioid cells, with possibly occasional giant-cells. The smaller bloodvessels may be obliterated by proliferative endarteritis. The muscle-fibres in the neighborhood of the destructive process are usually atrophied, while the nuclei are increased in number. In many places all that remains is the sarcolemma sheath with nuclei. Where the muscle has disappeared, its place is taken by connective tissue, which may be seen in places to be infiltrated by tuberculous granulation tissue.

Primary tuberculosis,[1] so far as is known at present, is rare. It is always hematogenous. The rarity of the affection is believed by some to be due to the bactericidal action of the muscle fluids, which Trya states is more powerful than that of other tissue juices. Primary tuberculosis may be a manifestation of general miliary infection, or may be purely local. Multiple miliary foci of tuberculous granulation tissue may be found, or larger single or multiple nodules, which in time may soften and break down into abscesses. In certain cases these abscesses become delimited by connective tissue. In others there is a more infiltrating or diffuse process at work, which at first, or until caseation sets in, bears a general resemblance to sarcoma.

Syphilis.—Syphilis of the muscles takes the form of chronic proliferative inflammation of the connective tissue (**myositis fibrosa syphilitica**) or of **gummas**. The muscles usually affected are the biceps and those of the neck, back, throat, tongue, and sphincter ani. The gummas are often of large size, and are surrounded by dense connective tissue. In the early stages the vascular granulation tissue may easily be mistaken for sarcoma, but the course of the case and the therapeutic test will generally differentiate. The muscle-fibres in the neighborhood undergo secondary atrophy and the extensive fibrosis frequently leads to marked contractures.[2]

Gonorrhœal Myositis.—Gonorrhœal myositis is occasionally hematogenic, but usually arises by extension from the joints or bones. In

---

[1] For literature see Saltykow, Centralbl. f. allg. Path. u. path. Anat., 13:1902; also Kaiser, Inaug. Diss., Bern, 1905.

[2] For further information see Busse, Arch. f. Chir., 69:1903.

this form interstitial proliferation of the connective tissue is a marked feature.

Glanders.—Glanders may be acute or chronic. It produces multiple abscesses throughout the muscle. The infection is hematogenic or lymphogenic. The muscles of the calves are those chiefly involved. The abscesses contain a thin, greasy, puriform fluid of grayish color, in which the specific microörganisms can usually be demonstrated.

Actinomycosis.—Actinomycosis is metastatic or produced by direct extension from some neighboring part. Sluggish granulomas are formed, showing fatty degeneration and liquefaction. In this way abscesses are produced which may heal with the formation of fibrous nodules.

Fig. 258

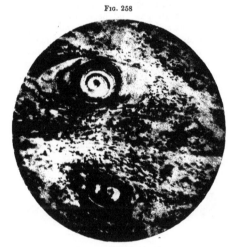

Trichinæ encysted in muscle. Zeiss obj. DD, without ocular. (Collection of McGill University, Pathological Department.)

Parasites.—The chief parasites are *Trichina spiralis, Cysticercus cellulosæ,* and *Echinococcus.*

The most common is *Trichina spiralis,* which enters the human organism through the ingestion of imperfectly cooked, infected, or "measly" pork. The parasite is found encysted in great numbers in the diaphragm, tongue, muscles of the neck, larynx, thighs, the intercostals, and to some extent in other parts. The embryos are produced in the intestine and make their way along the lymphatics to the various muscles. At first the organism is found in the sarcolemma sheath, but soon invades the muscle-fibre, which in time degenerates and disappears. When the condition is fully developed there is found a clear, chitinous cyst in which the parasite lies coiled up amid a granular detritus. These cysts are large enough to be easily recognized by the naked eye. In the early stage there is more or less acute inflammation with round-celled infiltration of the intermuscular connective tissue the formation of fibroblasts, and multiplication of the muscle-nuclei. Later, the acute manifestations pass off and the cyst becomes infiltrated with lime salts.

RETROGRESSIVE METAMORPHOSES.

The physical state of a muscle is conditioned by the degree of its functional activity, the nature of the nervous impulses reaching it, and the character of the metabolism going on within it. In cases where the functional demands are diminished or altogether lacking the muscle undergoes atrophy and degeneration. Where there is an increased call upon its activity, hypertrophy and hyperplasia result. If, however, the demand be excessive or too prolonged, hypertrophy in time gives way to atrophy. Again, so long as the normal relationship between the muscle and the nervous system is maintained, the muscle retains its natural tonus. Where this relationship is disturbed, as in certain disorders of the central nervous system and peripheral nerves, the tonus is gradually impaired, nutrition is defective, and the muscle eventually undergoes wasting and degeneration.

FIG. 259

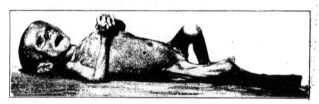

Generalized marantic (toxemic?) atrophy, from "summer diarrhœa." (Dr. A. E. Vipond's case.)

Atrophy.—Atrophy of muscle may be divided into four main varieties, simple degenerative, neuropathic, and primary myopathic or dystrophic atrophy.

Simple Atrophy.—Simple atrophy is found typically in old age (*senile atrophy*) and in athrepsia and inanition from any cause (*marantic atrophy*). In many cases the condition is a transient one, provided that the exciting cause be removed, and the muscle returns to its normal condition. In other instances, however, when the condition is long-continued, degenerative changes are superadded. Atrophy from disuse may be brought about by fracture of a muscle, tendon, or bone, ankylosis of joints, fixation by splints, or even by voluntary inactivity. The last-mentioned form is met with in certain fakirs in India, who retain a limb in some fixed position for prolonged periods. Overwork, by excessive contraction of the fibres and exhaustion of nutrition, will, after a preliminary stage of compensatory hypertrophy, also give rise to atrophy.

Perhaps more common are **degenerative atrophies**, such as those met with in infections and intoxications, chronic cachexias, anemia, arteriosclerosis, and pressure.

In general, atrophic muscles are small, pale, and flabby, or sometimes brownish from a deposit of pigment (*brown atrophy*). In simple atrophy the changes are not striking. The fibres are thinner than normal, are losing their striation, and occasionally are fragmented. The connective tissue between the bundles may be relatively or absolutely increased, and may present a deposit of fat—*lipomatoid atrophy*. In many cases, however, and possibly the majority, these changes are combined with others of a degenerative nature, such as Zenker's degeneration, cloudy swelling, lacunar erosion, hydropic and fatty changes. In both the simple and degenerative forms of atrophy, rows or clusters of nuclei are met with along the atrophied fibres, upon which they abut, due possibly to a more or less abortive attempt to reproduce the damaged structures. When the atrophy is complete, sarcolemma sheaths are found containing pigment, nuclei, and multinucleated cells.

Neuropathic Atrophy.—Of great practical importance are the neuropathic atrophies. Here the process is confined to certain muscles or groups of muscles, and is due to a lesion in the central or peripheral nervous system. In the first case one finds a degeneration of the ganglion cells of the anterior horns of the spinal column, in the pyramidal tracts, the medulla, and the motor areas of the cerebral cortex. This results in what are called respectively *progressive spinal, bulbar,* and *cerebral* atrophies. The extent of the atrophy resulting is dependent upon the degree of the disease present in the trophic centres, and its localization is governed by the particular centres involved. In certain diseases with a comparatively localized lesion, such as anterior poliomyelitis, myelomalacia, certain forms of sclerosis, tumors, and compression myelitis, the atrophy is confined to those small groups of muscles deriving their nutrition from the affected cells, but some of the affections are progressive, leading to extensive muscular wasting and in some instances to the involvement of nearly all the principal muscles of the body. In some cases, as in amyotrophic lateral sclerosis, the primary degeneration is not confined to the trophic ganglion cells but extends to the pyramidal tracts and other regions near by.

The neuropathic atrophies usually attack persons who have previously been well and strong, and specially affect those muscles which are most used. In manual laborers the muscles of the thenar and hypothenar eminences, the lumbricales and the interossei, are liable to be first involved (Aran-Duchenne type). In other cases the disease begins in the muscles of the shoulder and arm. The disease is often, although not invariably, symmetrical, and gradually extends from one group of muscles to another, until, unless the disease be arrested, most of the muscles are involved and the patient becomes almost, if not entirely, helpless. In cases where the medulla is first involved there is diffi-

culty in articulation and deglutition, with drooling of saliva and feebleness of the voice (*progressive bulbar paralysis*). The muscles of the
lower extremities are involved late, if at all. Irregular forms are also
met with in which the wasting begins in the lower extremities and
extends gradually upward.

Secondary muscular atrophy is also met with in certain affections
of the peripheral nerves, such as multiple neuritis, chronic lead and
arsenical poisoning, injuries to the motor nerves.

FIG. 260

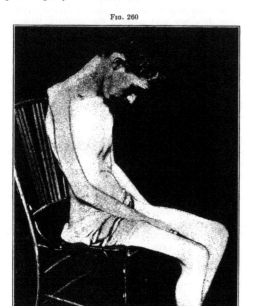

Progressive muscular dystrophy (family type, showing the characteristic pose). (From
the clinic of the Royal Victoria Hospital.)

Bearing a somewhat close resemblance to the progressive spinal
atrophies is the so-called *primary myopathy* or *progressive muscular
dystrophy*.[1] This affection frequently begins in childhood, but is also
met with in adults. The cause is quite obscure, but it is characteristically a familial disease, so that it has been suggested that some
congenital anomaly of development is at work.

Three clinical types are recognized: the infantile, juvenile, and adult.
The first-mentioned form usually begins in the muscles of the face,

[1] For literature see Lorenz, Die Umskelerkrankungen, Nothnagel's spez. Path.
u. Therap., Wien, 1904.

giving rise to a peculiar expressionless appearance pathognomonic of the disease—the myopathic facies. The juvenile form involves the muscles of the calves, thighs, back, shoulder-girdle, and arms. The adult variety begins either in the lower extremities or in the upper extremities and face.

In this affection no constant changes have been found in the cord or peripheral nerves, although some observers have described atrophy of the ganglion-cells of the posterior roots and cytoplasmic changes in the ganglion-cells of the spinal cord. Kollaritz has described atrophy of the motor cells and fibres of the central gray matter of the cervical and dorsal cord. The majority of observers seem to think that the disease originates in the voluntary muscles. It is quite possible, however, that the changes in the central nervous system and the muscle are related, and that both are dependent on errors of development. For it is obvious that developmental errors affecting the ganglion cells and motor fibres would necessarily be associated with imperfect development of the corresponding muscles. Others again would regard the nerve changes as secondary to the degeneration of the muscle-fibres. Clinically and anatomically there are two forms, the *atrophic* and the *pseudohypertrophic*.

In the former the changes in the muscle do not differ materially from those found in the spinal form. There are vacuolation, fragmentation, atrophy, and finally disintegration of the muscle-fibres. The transverse striation is lost and the fibres appear to be either homogeneous or finely granulated. Numerous cells may be met with containing many nuclei, thus resembling giant cells. There is also a certain amount of proliferation of the connective tissue forming the endomysium. These appearances have been variously interpreted. Hoffmann and Waldeyer hold that the striated muscle cells are a syncytium produced by the fusion of spindle-shaped mesodermic cells. Some, like Durante and Kroesing, regard the longitudinal fibrillation of the muscle-fibre as a reversionary degeneration. They believe that these fibrillæ are competent to form new muscle-fibres, but usually degenerate into connective tissue. The increase of the connective tissue may, therefore, be due to this degeneration rather than to proliferation of the old connective tissue. It is more generally believed, however, that the increase of the connective tissue is owing to the well-known tendency of connective tissue to replace destroyed structures. The large multinucleated cells referred to are usually regarded as evidence of an attempt at regeneration, but Fujinami holds that they are identical with the myoblasts of growing muscle and that therefore they indicate a return to an embryonic condition—a reversionary degeneration.

The pseudohypertrophic form presents, in addition to the changes just described, a formation of fatty tissue resulting in a notable increase in the bulk of the affected muscle. The muscle-fibres here again are more or less atrophied. A true hypertrophy of the fibres, accompanying the increase of connective and adipose tissue, has been observed by Durante. In most cases the fatty transformation follows the atrophy

and is compensatory, in a manner somewhat analogous to the produc
tion of fat about a contracted or fibroid kidney, although in some few
cases it is possibly the precursor and the cause of the muscular atroph
from simple pressure. The fat is produced probably from the proliferating cells of the endomysium, although Kroesing believes that ther
is a direct metaplasia of the muscle into fat.

Degenerations.—Cloudy Swelling.—Cloudy swelling (parenchymatou
degeneration, albuminous degeneration, parenchymatous myositis) is
common accompaniment of acute febrile diseases, and is also brough
about by inflammation, circulating toxins, and disturbances of circulation
The affected muscle is pale, swollen, and doughy.

Microscopically, the fibres are swollen, the striation indistinct, an
the cytoplasm contains innumerable minute globules of an albuminou
nature, which render it somewhat opaque. These are readily dissolve
out by the application of dilute alkali or acetic acid.

Fatty Degeneration.—In severe cases the condition passes by eas
stages into fatty degeneration. This is also met with in phosphoru
poisoning. In this condition the muscle is soft, friable, and of a pal
yellow, streaky appearance.

Microscopically, the fibres are swollen, paler than usual, somewha
reticulated, and the nuclei show degenerative changes. When the tissu
is treated with osmic acid the fatty droplets within the fibres stai
brown or black, and with Sudan III, yellow or carmine.

Fatty Infiltration.—In fatty infiltration there is a deposit of fat in
the connective tissue of the endomysium. In the earlier stages there
is sometimes a proliferation of the cells of the endomysium. In many
instances the infiltration, or metaplasia, whichever it may be, is only
microscopic in amount, but in some cases, as in pseudohypertrophic
muscular paralysis, the amount of fat is excessive and leads to enlargement of the muscle bundles.

Hydropic or Vacuolar Degeneration.—Hydropic or vacuolar degeneration is met with in œdema of the muscle and some forms of inflammation. The muscle appears to be pale and watery.

Colliquative Necrosis.—Colliquative necrosis occurs in chronic œdema
and suppurative inflammation. The fibres at first are enlarged, granular,
or vacuolated, and finally melt away.

Lacunar Erosion.—Lacunar erosion is a process analogous to the
lacunar erosion of bone. Here certain cells, derived possibly from the
internal perimysium or the sarcolemma sheath, attack the fibres and
lead to atrophy. This is seen most frequently in the neighborhood
of metastatic cancerous nodules.

Zenker's Degeneration.—Vitreous, waxy, or hyaline degeneration is a
form of coagulation necrosis affecting the protoplasm of individual
fibres, first described by v. Zenker[1] as occurring in typhoid fever,
and hence called Zenker's degeneration. It is, however, met with in
a great many other conditions, such as sepsis, variola, intoxications,

---

[1] Ueber d. Veränderung. d. willkurl. Musk. bei Typhus abdom., Leipzig, 1864.

inflammation, traumatism, burns, freezing, bedsores, tetanus, and in the neighborhood of carcinomas. The muscles usually affected are the recti abdominis, the adductors of the thighs, and psoas.

When the condition is extensive, the affected muscle is soft, doughy, pale, and semitranslucent like raw fish.

Microscopically, the fibres are swollen, the striations have disappeared, and the protoplasm has a structureless, waxy, somewhat opaque appearance. In the milder forms the whole fibre is not involved and regeneration may occur, with active multiplication of nuclei, but in severe cases the nuclei disappear. There is usually to be seen a small-celled infiltration of the endomysium. In the most advanced cases the swollen fibres fragment and coalesce into irregular hyaline masses. The hyaline substance, as a rule, stains badly, although at times it presents the micro-chemical reactions of fibrin or colloid. Disintegration is occasionally so extreme that hemorrhages, often of large size, may take place into the muscle.

Fig. 261

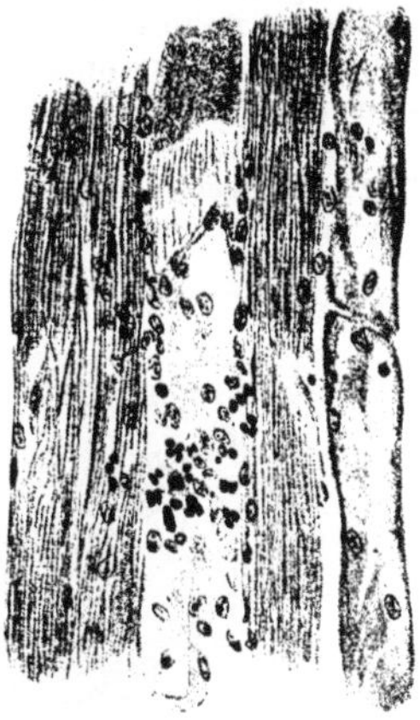

V. Zenker's, or wax-like, degeneration of muscle fibres (*a*, *b*) seventeen hours after temporary ligation of the same. In *b* there is already some accumulation of leukocytes. (Oberndörffer.)

Amyloid Transformation.—Amyloid transformation is rare and apparently always a local condition, being found in situations where there has been previous inflammation. According to Ziegler, amyloid disease is met with in the tongue and larynx. The process begins in the perimysium internum and the sarcolemma sheaths, which are converted into a thick translucent material encroaching upon the muscle-fibres and eventually leading to their atrophy. In time, neighboring deposits become confluent and form nodular masses.

Calcification.—Calcification has been observed in the muscles in the neighborhood of old encapsulated abscesses, in certain other chronic inflammatory processes, trauma, and as a sequel of marked atrophy. The condition may follow, for example, suture of a wound of the muscle. According to Schujeninoff, calcification takes place after the fibres have undergone colloid degeneration.

Gangrene.—Gangrene occurs in severe infective processes, decubitus, burns, freezing, electric discharges, sclerosis of the nutrient arteries, or results from pressure exerted on tissues of low vitality. The affected muscles become brownish, grayish- or greenish-black, break up into shreds or liquefy (*moist gangrene*). In cases where the blood supply to the part is scanty and the tissue is exposed to the air, the part dries up (*mummification*).　Owing to the presence of putrefactive germs, noxious gases are produced and the tissues become very foul and offensive.　A very rapid and malignant form of gangrene, associated with the production of gas in the subcutaneous tissues, is the so-called *emphysematous gangrene,* or "gangrène foudroyante," due to the B. Welchii or to the bacillus of malignant œdema.

Microscopically, in the moist form, the muscle-fibres show simple or coagulation necrosis, vacuolation, and liquefaction, while there is a deposit of blood-pigment, cholesterin, and triple phosphates.　In dry gangrene the cells shrink and dry up into a keratinoid substance.　As a rule, the dead tissue is delimited from the healthy part by a zone of reactive inflammation in which the vessels are congested, and there is an exudation of inflammatory leukocytes.

FIG. 262

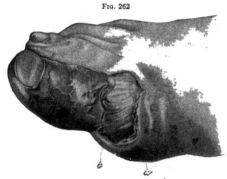

Senile gangrene of the great toe, from a case of arterial thrombosis.　The toe is shrunken and its epidermis is being exfoliated.　At the line of demarcation the skin has retracted (a) and the deeper parts are separating (b).

Pigmentation.—Pigmentation is a constant accompaniment of that form of atrophy known as *brown atrophy.*　The pigment, generally called hemofuscin, is found in the form of minute, yellowish-brown granules in the cytoplasm about the poles of the nuclei, but in advanced cases is scattered throughout the greater part of the fibre.　In some cases the increase in pigment is possibly only a relative matter, due to atrophy of the cytoplasm with retention of the normal muscle pigment.　In other cases there seems to be a transformation of the myohematin into granular material, leading to an absolute increase.

In cases of hemorrhage, *hematoidin* and *hemosiderin* may be deposited in the muscle-bundles and connective tissue.

PROGRESSIVE METAMORPHOSES.

The repair of injury to muscles, such as that produced by disease or mechanical trauma, may be perfect or imperfect according to the character and extent of the lesion.　Provided that the muscle-nuclei and the sarcolemma be not destroyed, slight injuries to the contractile substance are repaired by the production of new muscle-fibres exactly as in the cases of the embryonic formation of muscle. Volkmann states that regeneration is functionally important only after typhoid fever and freezing, while in injuries function is not restored unless the wound is small. Where large areas of muscular tissue are destroyed, as by inflammation or severe mechanical trauma, regeneration of muscle is incomplete and a large part of the deficit is made good by the formation of granulation and ultimately connective tissue. In all cases the repair is brought about by the proliferation of the preëxisting cells of the part. Where a fibrous scar has been produced, after a more or less prolonged period, it is replaced to a limited extent by the invasion of new muscle-fibres derived from the uninjured muscle in the neighborhood. The muscle-nuclei divide either directly or by mitosis, while at the same time there is a local increase of the sarcolemma substance. At the end, or at some point along the course of the fibre, multinucleated buds of protoplasm are produced which grow out into the granulation tissue. At first these present no striation, but soon become fibrillated, and the bud, or myoblast, as it is called, becomes striated. Besides the myoblasts, free multinucleated cells may be seen which are known as sarcolytes. The majority of these probably undergo fatty degeneration or necrosis and ultimately disappear, although some of them may form new fibres or fuse with preëxisting ones. The sarcolytes are probably derived from free muscle-corpuscles, and, where there has been an actual loss of substance in the muscle, are apt to be rather numerous. They are phagocytic and may be seen to contain pigment, bits of necrotic muscle, and detritus.

Hypertrophy.—True hypertrophy of muscle probably does not occur except in the case of individual fibres. It is true that under conditions of increased work the muscle-fibres increase both in length and breadth, but there is practically always a numerical increase as well, so that the condition, more correctly speaking, is a combination of hypertrophy and hyperplasia. Hypertrophy, so-called, may be congenital as well as acquired, as in the cases of general and local gigantism and hemihypertrophy.

In **myotonia congenita**, or Thomsen's disease, Erb[1] has described a marked increase in the size of the affected muscle-fibres, with proliferation of nuclei, loss of striation, and vacuolation. Koch describes longitudinal cleavage of the fibres, producing numerical increase. He observed amitotic division of the nuclei resulting in the production of narrow elongated cells, which contained rows of nuclei similar to those found in degenerative and regenerative processes. It is doubtful whether the disease is not a degenerative process rather than true hypertrophy.

In certain cases of muscular atrophy, the myopathies, local trauma, and certain infectious diseases, like typhoid, isolated fibres may show hypertrophy, apparently compensatory.

[1] Die Thomsen'sche Krankheit, Leipzig, 1886.

Tumors.—Primary tumors of the muscles are quite rare and generally arise from the fascia or intermuscular connective tissue. Among the benign growths may be mentioned the **fibroma, lipoma, myxoma, chondroma,** and **angioma.**[1] Hard fibromas have been observed in the fascia of the recti abdominis, and myxomas in the muscles of the thigh. **Myomas** may originate from the arrectores pilorum.

Sarcoma.—The most frequent growths are the various forms of sarcoma, *fibrosarcoma, myxosarcoma,* and *myxoliposarcoma.* These form large tumors and are soft and cellular, being composed of round or spindle cells.

Various forms of degeneration are common, and there may be metaplasia into bone or cartilage.

Fig. 263

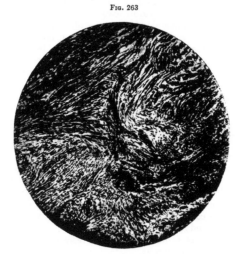

Myoma from the arm. Winckel obj. No. 3, without ocular. (From the collection of Dr. A. G. Nicholls.)

Myosarcoma, that is to say, a sarcoma originating from embryonic muscle cells, is theoretically possible, but little is known as to its actual occurrence.

Rhabdomyoma and *rhabdomyosarcoma* have been described by Billroth[2] and Buhl,[3] but are excessively rare. We have met with one case (Fig. 264) of a rhabdomyosarcoma, in a trout.[4] It is thought that such tumors arise from preëxisting muscle-cells, possibly of embryonic inclusion.

Secondary sarcoma of the muscle is common.

[1] Porcile, Il Policlinico, Rome, 15: 1908: 289.

[2] Rhabdomyom, Virch. Arch., 9: 1856: 172.

[3] Rhabdomyom, Zeit. f. Biol., 1: 1865.

[4] Adami, Montreal Med. Journ., 37: 1908: 163.

Carcinoma.—Carcinoma is always secondary and due to direct extension or lymphogenic invasion from a growth in some neighboring part, as, for example, in the breast, lips, skin, or stomach. Hematogenic metastasis is rare.

The growth is usually diffuse or in the form of minute miliary nodules, arranged in clusters or rows in the interstices of the tissues. The sarcolemma sheath may be invaded by the cancer cells, so that absorption of the fibres takes place with the formation of indentations

FIG. 264

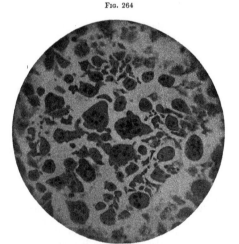

RhabdomΥosarcoma in a brook trout.   Reichert obj. No. 7, without ocular.   (From the collection of Dr. J. George Adami.)

similar to Howship's lacunæ.   Owing to pressure, the eroding action of the cancer cells, and the influence of the soluble toxins, the muscle-cells undergo atrophy, coagulation necrosis, liquefaction, and ultimately disappear.   There is usually a certain amount of interstitial inflammation, and the endothelial lining of the neighboring vessels proliferates, leading gradually to their obliteration.

Small **teratomas** and **dermoid cysts** have been found in the muscles of the cheek, tongue, neck, abdominal wall, and lumbar region.

THE TENDONS, TENDON-SHEATHS, AND BURSÆ.

The tendons are composed of a peculiar dense, avascular connective tissue, arranged as an aggregation of small bundles which are embedded in a looser connective tissue provided with bloodvessels.   They are inclosed in a sheath containing a small amount of synovial secretion, thus allowing movement of the tendon backward and forward. Owing to the peculiarly dense and resistant character of these structures and the fact that the bloodvessels are scanty, primary affections, particularly the infective and inflammatory ones, are infrequent. Much more commouly, the tendons and their sheaths are secondarily involved from disease processes in the neighborhood.

CIRCULATORY DISTURBANCES.

Hemorrhage into the sheath of a tendon may follow trauma and result in the formation of a hematoma.

INFLAMMATIONS.

Tendinitis.—Inflammation of a tendon is called **tendinitis**; of a tendon sheath, **tendovaginitis** or **tenosynovitis**. The two conditions are more often than not associated one with the other.

In general, tendinitis and tenosynovitis bear a close resemblance to inflammation of the joints. The condition usually follows trauma or arises by extension from neighboring structures. It is rarely primary. Wounds, fractures, and strains may set up inflammation and also circulating toxins and bacteria, such as the pyogenic cocci, Micrococcus gonorrhœæ, and Diplococcus pneumoniæ. Tendinitis and tenosynovitis may be serous, fibrinous, or purulent in character.

Simple Tendinitis.—Simple tendinitis and tenosynovitis may occur in those of a rheumatic or gouty disposition after strain of the tendons, exposure to cold, and rarely in certain infective diseases, such as syphilis, typhoid, and scarlatina. There is usually little exudate, but owing to the deposit of fibrin upon the surfaces of the tendon and sheath, a rough, grating sensation or crepitus is felt when the tendon is put in action (*tenosynovitis sicca acuta*). It is, perhaps, most frequently met with in the tendo Achillis, and next in the extensor tendons of the forearm.

Acute Purulent Tendinitis.—Acute purulent tendinitis and tenosynovitis arise after traumatism where a wound has become infected, or by extension from neighboring parts, as, for instance, in erysipelas, infected wounds and abscesses. It may also be hematogenic, due to the action of gonococci or other pyogenic microörganisms.

The tendon and its sheath become œdematous, the interfascicular connective tissue is congested and infiltrated with round cells, while there is an accumulation of pus within the cavity. In mild cases recovery may take place without much or any interference with function. In severe cases there is liable to be adhesion between the tendon and its sheath, or the tendon may become cloudy, soften, and finally necrose. Where the tendon has been destroyed regeneration and repair may take place.

Chronic Tendinitis.—Chronic tendinitis may occur alone, but is usually associated with tenosynovitis. It may follow the acute forms or repeated acute attacks, or, again, may come on insidiously.

In this form degeneration of the tendon is common. Mucinous and hyaline changes take place. The interfascicular connective tissue is increased in amount, and calcification or metaplasia into bone or cartilage is sometimes met with. In certain diseases, as senile arthritis and rheumatoid arthritis, small nodosities, varying in size from that of a pinhead to that of a bean, may form in the interfascicular connective tissue, arranged often like a string of beads.[1] They usually disappear spontaneously in a few months, but may undergo hyaline change or calcification.

In chronic tenosynovitis there may be a serous exudate, or, again, but little fluid may be present. The exudate, when present, contains mucin and pseudomucin. It may be so great in amount as to cause marked distension of the tendon sheath (*hygroma* of the tendon sheath, *hydrops tendo-vaginalis*). This usually occurs in the palms and in the sheath of the flexors of the carpus. At times the accumulation is so great that cyst-like swellings are produced. Owing to the fact that the sheath is contracted at the annular ligament of the wrist, fusiform or hour-glass-shaped swellings result. More rarely, the tendon sheaths of the finger, the back of the hand, or other parts may be involved. The sheath in time becomes thickened and there is a deposit of fibrin within its cavity. This finally may become organized, so that papillary or polypoid excrescences are formed, at first hyaline, but later fibrous, or even cartilaginous or bony. These, when in the partially organized condition, may break loose, forming free bodies in the sac, the so-called "rice-bodies," or "*corpora oryzoidea.*"

Microscopically, they consist of homogeneous or laminated masses of hyaline appearance, in which but few cells are seen. Giant cells and leukocytes, however, are at times in evidence. They are particularly common in tuberculous tenosynovitis. In fact, hygroma of the type just described is held by some to be commonly tuberculous.

Gout.—In gout, the tendons and their sheaths are frequently involved. There is a deposit of uratic salts in the stroma of the tendon, the peri- and interfascicular connective tissue proliferates and becomes cellular, the tendon bundles are dissociated, and the various tissues may finally undergo degeneration and necrose. The salts are surrounded by granulation tissue which sometimes contains giant cells.

Tuberculosis.—Tuberculosis of the tendons and their sheaths is rarely primary, but usually follows tuberculosis of the bones or joints. Primary tuberculosis occurs most frequently in the forearm (Schuchardt[2]). The tubercles are formed chiefly in the tendon sheaths and are accompanied by an exudative process. The sheath in time becomes thickened from the production of numerous tubercles within its substance, as well as by the formation of new fibrous tissue. In the advanced

---

[1] See Hirschsprung, Jahrb. f. Kinder., 16: 1881.
[2] Virch. Archiv, 135: 1894: 394.

stages the tendons and sheaths may be incrusted with fungous granulations covered with fibrin or puriform exudation. The amount of the fluid is often large, and "rice-bodies" are common.

Syphilis.—Gummas may be found in the tendons and tendon-sheaths in the tertiary stage.[1]

RETROGRESSIVE METAMORPHOSES.

Degenerative disturbances are apt to be slight and unimportant.

Atrophy.—Atrophy may occur where the muscle belonging to the tendon has previously undergone atrophy, but this result is usually long delayed. The structure peculiar to the tendon is lost and it is converted into scar-like connective tissue. The supporting stroma is increased through proliferation of its cells, and may be converted into fat.

Degenerations.—**Hyaline** and **mucinous** degeneration have been observed in some cases of inflammation.

After injuries or severe inflammation the tendons may **necrose**.

Calcification has been observed in chronic inflammations, and **uratic deposits** in the tendons and tendon sheaths are frequently met with in gout.

PROGRESSIVE METAMORPHOSES.

When a tendon is severed, provided that suppuration do not occur, function is restored by the union of the divided ends. This takes place, not by the formation of new tendon, but by the production of dense scar-tissue, more grayish and less glistening than tendon, derived mainly from the proliferation of the connective-tissue matrix.

Metaplasia.—Metaplasia of the tendinous material into mucin, fat, cartilage, or bone is met with in many forms of chronic inflammation.

Tumors.—Tumors are rare.[2] **Sarcoma** may, possibly, develop from the tendon or its sheath. A very rare growth is the **lipoma arborescens**, in which branching papillary excrescences of fatty tissue are formed within the tendon sheath.

According to Ledderhose,[3] the so-called **ganglion** of the wrist, back of hand, and foot, which used to be considered a form of hydrops of the sheath, is a new-formation of a myxomatous, gelatinous, or colloid nature.

Under the misleading term "myeloma" has been described (Bonjour,[4] Malherbe, and others) a rare tumor of the tendon-sheaths, which in

---

[1] Ullmann, Lubarsch und Ostertag's Ergebnisse, 3: 1897.

[2] See Bellamy, Jour. of Path. u. Bact., 7: 1901.

[3] Zeitsch. f. Chir., 37 : 1893.

[4] Contribution à l'étude des tumeurs fibro-tendineuses et des tissus fibreux, Thèse de Paris, 1897.

general has the appearance of a sarcoma. It is peculiar, however, in that, in addition to spindle cells, it contains enormous giant-cells, an iron-containing pigment, and nests of cells having the appearance of xanthoma-cells.

The Bursæ.

The bursæ are connective-tissue sacs containing clear synovial fluid. The structures forming the wall resemble in general the tendon sheaths. Bursæ are usually found in well-defined situations, wherever muscles or tendons play over bones, or where the tissues are subjected to pressure. They are not constant in number or in situation, but may be developed by friction or pressure, in the course of certain occupations, in places where they ordinarily are not present. The pathological processes affecting them are analogous to those occurring in the tendon sheaths.

Hemorrhage into bursal sacs occurs from trauma or circulatory disturbances. Large blood tumors or **hematomata** may be produced.

Inflammations.—**Acute bursitis** or **acute hygroma** is due most commouly to wounds, bruises, or contusions, or, more rarely, to hematogenic infection (notably in gonorrhœa). It may give rise to a serous, serofibrinous, or purulent exudation. A painful fluctuating swelling is produced. Common examples of this are the so-called "*housemaid's knee*" and "*miner's elbow.*" *Suppurative bursitis* may extend to the adjacent tissues.

Chronic bursitis takes the form of an accumulation of fluid in the cavity—*hydrops* or *hygroma bursæ*. The exudation is at first viscid and mucinous, but later becomes thinner and more watery. The swelling may be as big as an apple or larger. The wall of the bursa is not at first much altered, but sooner or later becomes thickened, or may be covered with shaggy fibrous outgrowth or even cartilaginous or bony plates and excrescences. Frequently "rice-bodies" are observed. In some cases these may be so large and numerous that the sac is filled, and on palpation gives rise to a peculiar crepitus—*ganglion crepitans*.

Tuberculous bursitis is primary or secondary. The wall of the sac becomes thickened and infiltrated with tuberculous granulomas, while the surface is covered with fungous granulations. There is usually considerable exudate (*hygroma tuberculosum*).

Tumors of the bursæ are rare. **Sarcoma, endothelioma, fibroma, myxoma,** and **papilloma** have been described.[1]

---

[1] For literature see Adrian, Beiträge zur klin. Chir., 38 : 1003; also Martina, Deutsche Zeitschr. f. Chir. 83 : 1906 : 317

SECTION X.

THE OSSEOUS SYSTEM.

CHAPTER XLIII.

· THE BONES, JOINTS, AND CARTILAGES.

THE BONES.

INTRODUCTORY.

THE bony skeleton subserves two important purposes in the organism. It affords a more or less rigid scaffolding for the support of the organs and soft tissues generally, and contributes to the important function of locomotion, with the secondary circulatory and respiratory functions which this mechanical act connotes. Bone is, perhaps, the most resistant and indestructible tissue in the body, but, in spite of its hardness and apparent solidity, it is not the permanent, unchangeable structure that one would at first sight suppose. Like other tissues it exhibits the various anabolic and katabolic processes that are characteristic of all vital activity. Breaking down and building up are continually going on even in health, and may be much exaggerated and perverted under various pathological conditions.

Bone is normally produced in two ways. It is derived from osteo-genetic centres within a but slightly differentiated connective-tissue matrix (intramembranous formation) or from cartilage (endochondral formation). The first mode of origin is well exemplified in the case of the calvarium, and the second, in the spinal column and long bones generally.

In the intramembranous form of osteogenesis, bony spicules containing lime salts, together with bone-corpuscles and cells, are formed within a proliferation-tissue consisting partly of cells and partly of a more or less perfectly developed homogeneous or fibrillar ground substance. These bony masses gradually increase in size, and, when they finally coalesce to form plates, gain in thickness through the activity of the external connective-tissue layer, which is henceforth known as the periosteum. Much in the same way, the earliest manifestations of ossification begin in the preëxisting cartilage that is eventually to become the bony skeleton. In certain regions in the surrounding fibrous investment or perichondrium bony processes are formed which gradually extend inward. This method of growth from the peri-chondrium, or from what later becomes the periosteum, is found to some extent throughout life, and accounts more especially for the increase in thickness of bone.

Besides this, there is what is called the endochondral ossification, which is brought about by the marrow tissue of the primitive bone proliferating and invading the calcifying cartilage, which it extensively destroys. As soon as the marrow spaces begin to appear, endochondral bone forma-tion proper commences. In the neighborhood of the medullary spaces,. where they are bounded by the solid cartilage, the cartilage cells enlarge and proliferate, forming small clusters, which ultimately become arranged in rows parallel to the long axis of the bone that is to be. It is through the proliferation of these cells that the increase in the length of bone is brought about. When the cartilage cells have attained their full size, there occurs a deposit of lime salts in the ground substance and the capsules of the cartilage cells. In this way is formed a narrow line of demarcation in the deeper layers of the intermediate cartilage, which, however, does not remain perfect, inasmuch as the vascularized marrow gradually dissolves it away in places and penetrates through it, leaving only islets of cartilaginous ground substance and calcified tissue. These are, in time, converted into bone proper through the agency of certain cells derived from the bone-marrow, called osteoblasts. The cartilage in this way is gradually replaced by bone.

If one examines a growing bone after it is completely blocked out, the following condition of things will be found. The shaft, or diaphysis, is completely ossified. At the end is the cartilaginous plate called the epiphysis. Between the diaphysis and the epiphysis is the so-called intermediate cartilage. The epiphysis contains within it more or less complete centres of ossification. The intermediate cartilage is com-posed of two layers, a bluish, translucent one, the zone of proliferation, and another of a thin, opaque, yellowish-white appearance, the zone of calcification. The centre of ossification in the epiphyses gradually enlarges until the structure is completely transformed into bone. As soon as the shaft and the epiphysis are firmly united into a bony mass growth in the length of the bone ceases. This normally occurs between the ages of twenty and twenty-seven, but under certain pathological conditions may take place prematurely, or, again, may be delayed. Similarly, the synostosis of a synchondrosis or suture arrests further growth at that point. Synostosis may be delayed or may occur in places where ossification does not normally take place. In the case of the skull premature ossification of one or more sutures may be found and leads to various forms of asymmetry and, in extreme conditions, to micro-cephaly. Premature synostosis of the intersphenoid and sphenobasilar synchondroses causes shortening of the base of the skull and a deeply set nose. This is to be observed in cretinism and some forms of chondro-dystrophia. Premature synostosis of both sacro-iliac synchondroses leads to a uniform contraction of the pelvis; of one, to an obliquely con-tracted pelvis.

ANOMALIES OF GROWTH AND DEVELOPMENT.

These are numerous and important, and are manifested in the forms of deficiency or excess in growth, or in some peculiarity in the quality of the bone. The causes that bring these about may be inherited, or acquired during intra-uterine or extra-uterine life. As a rule, imperfections of the bones are associated with analogous abnormalities in the soft parts connected with them, although exceptions occur. The term applied to complete defect of a bony or other structure is **agenesia** or **aplasia**, but these names are applied sometimes, though incorrectly, to a less extreme degree of the condition, a partial deficiency. This is more properly styled **hypoplasia**.

Agenesia, in the stricter sense, is always local, and is found usually in the calvarium and vertebral arches, less frequently in the extremities and bodies of the vertebræ. The skull, as a whole, may be practically absent, as in acephaly, or partially defective, as in anencephaly, cyclops, and other grave malformations. The spinal column may be rudimentary, as in iniencephaly and spina bifida. or one or more of the vertebræ may be lacking. The sternum may be cleft into two longitudinally. The distal ends of the radius, tibia, and fibula may be absent in malformations of the hands and feet. Occasionally the clavicles are absent, or the fibula.

In another class of cases the primitive "Anlagen" have been laid down, so far as we know, in a normal manner, but the structures arising from them have failed to reach their complete development—**hypoplasia**. This condition may be local or general. In the local form the head may be abnormally small (one form of **microcephaly**), an arm or a leg may be deficient in size (**microbrachius, micropus**), or, again, all four extremities may be affected (**micromelus**). In such cases the most important etiological factor seems to be pressure upon the fœtus from a contracted amnion or from bands or adhesions, although it is not impossible that in some instances the primitive "Anlagen" may be at fault.

Dwarfism.—When the body as a whole is diminutive we may speak of dwarfism (**microsomia, nanosomia**). An allied condition is **infantilism**, with which dwarfism is usually, but not invariably, associated. Dwarfism implies a diminutive structure, while infantilism connotes delayed or imperfect function, whereby an individual retains the characteristics of the child long after these should have disappeared. In other words, dwarfism bears the same relation to vegetative growth that infantilism does to function.

There are two forms of dwarfism: *essential dwarfism*, in which the individual is to all intents and purposes normal save in the one particular of size, and *symptomatic dwarfism*, where, in addition to diminutive size, there are evidences of more serious disturbance, such as the stigmata of infantilism, cretinism, rickets, syphilis, cardiovascular anomalies, or actual malformations and deformities. In the combination of dwarfism and infantilism, to which the name **ateleiosis** has been applied, the process of ossification is greatly delayed, and the genital organs are imperfect in structure and function. Perfection may in time be reached, but the size remains small.

The most important etiological factors in the production of essential dwarfism are peculiarities of the germinal cells, which may be inherited or acquired *de novo*. In the latter case, tuberculosis, alcoholism, and syphilis appear to play a part. Intra-uterine malnutrition of the fœtus, due to hardship or ill-health on the part of the mother, and anomalies of placentation should also be mentioned in this connection. Circulatory disturbances and disorders of internal secretion in the fœtus itself are of importance. Virchow long ago pointed out the close connection between infantilism and cardiovascular hypoplasia, and more recently, Gilbert and Rathery[1] have noted a tendency to dwarfism in certain cases of mitral stenosis. The dependence of some forms of dwarfing on athyroidism is also well recognized. According to Küster, Eiselsberg,[2] and others, removal of the thyroid in growing animals is followed by inhibition of growth, and defect of the thyroid secretion is now generally admitted to be the cause of that interesting congenital affection called cretinism, in which stunting of the growth is a conspicuous feature. Inferentially, athyroidea may be a factor in the production of the true dwarfs.

In secondary dwarfism, in addition to general hypoplasia, there are evidences of disease or malformation, and the changes in the tissues are qualitative as well as quantitative. Many cases of this type have been regarded as syphilis, rickets, or cretinism, and the lines of demarcation have not always been closely drawn. In fact, the exact nature of these conditions is one of the most difficult problems in etiology, and further study is still needed to finally clear up the subject. We have to consider in this connection the affections known as cretinism, rachitis, chondrodystrophia fœtalis, osteogenesis imperfecta, and osteopsathyrosis.

Cretinism.—In cretinism the head is usually large, the vertex flattened, and the occiput prominent. The fontanelles and sutures remain open for a long time. The nose is retracted at the root and is short and thick, with large, wide nostrils. The lips and tongue are enlarged. The teeth appear late, and the first dentition usually persists throughout life. The limbs and trunk are disproportionate and the stature is stunted. Maffei, in 22 cases out of 25, found the height to be less than 140 cm., while several were under 95. The hair on the pubes and in the axillæ is scanty or absent, and the sexual organs are poorly developed. Puberty, if it occur at all, is late.

The disturbance is associated with delayed ossification of the cartilages. Hofmeister,[3] studying a case with the x-rays, found that the epiphyseal ends of the bones grew slowly, while the epiphyseal plates persisted for a long time. Periosteal ossification may be normal or in excess.

---

[1] Presse méd., May 7, 1900.   [2] Langenbeck's Archiv, 49: 1895: 207.
[3] Fortschr. auf dem Gebiete der Röntgen-Strahlen, 1: 1897.

Microscopically, Langhans[1] found that at the ends of the bones the cartilage cells were small, spindle-shaped, and anomalously arranged, being longitudinal to the long axis of the columns. The rows were interrupted and irregular. The bony trabeculæ were shortened and the marrow spaces in the youngest portions of the bones were large and widely separated.

Cretins may continue to grow until they are thirty to forty years of age, and ossification may, in time, be completed. The cause of the disorder, namely, defect of the thyroid secretion, may be due to a variety of pathological conditions, such as atrophy, fibrosis, or cystic degeneration of the gland.

Fig. 265

Fig. 266

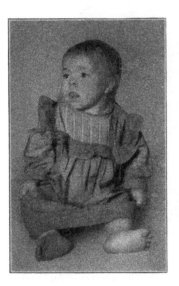

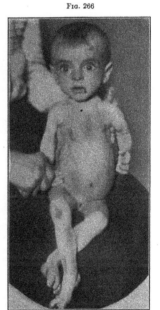

Sporadic cretinism.

Rickets. Fractured clavicles: prominence of frontal eminences; Harrison's groove; and pot-belly. (Dr. A. E. Vipond's case.)

Rachitis.—The exact place which rachitis or rickets should occupy in the scheme of pathology is still somewhat debatable. The condition is thought by some to be due to infection or auto-intoxication, and, therefore, to some extent is possibly inflammatory (Kassowitz[2]). This view is somewhat supported by the character of the lesions in the bones, and

---

[1] Virch. Archiv, 128: 1892: 318.   [2] Zeit. f. klin. Med., 7: 1884: 36.

by the experimental work of Morpurgo,[1] who showed that rachitic changes could be produced in young white rats by the injection of a certain diplococcus. The condition is, however, so closely dependent on malnutrition, brought about by improper diet, overcrowding, and general unhygienic surroundings, that in default of more information we may perhaps be justified in regarding it, for the present, simply as a disorder of growth. Rickets probably is not hereditary, although it cannot be denied that intra-uterine influences may play a part to a limited extent.

The disease, first described by Glisson,[2] usually makes its appearance after the sixth month, during the first or second year. The lesions are characteristic, and, if severe, lead to serious deformity and stunting of the

Fig. 267

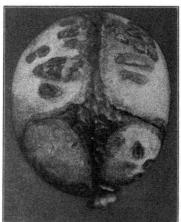

Craniotabes in the newborn child. Supposed cause, rickets. (From the Pathological Museum, McGill University.)

growth. The skull is large, although the face is relatively small. The forehead is square and prominent, owing to the presence of flat hyperostoses on the frontal eminences. The sternum projects, while the sides of the thorax are drawn in (*pectus carinatum*). The abdomen is protuberant. The spine is often curved and the extremities greatly deformed, owing to the weight of the body and muscular traction acting on the imperfectly calcified bone. The pelvis is deformed and contracted. Dentition is delayed and the teeth are small and badly formed. In the milder cases deformities are not so extensive, but swellings at the ends of the long bones and at the costochondral junctions (*rachitic rosary*)

[1] Centralbl. f. Path., 13: 1902: 113.
[2] Tractatus de rachitide, London, 1650

are a noteworthy feature., Periosteal as well as epiphyseal bone-formation is interfered with. The periosteum is readily stripped off and the underlying bone is softer and more spongy than normal. The epiphyseal zone of proliferation is thicker than usual, irregular in outline, soft, and hyperemic.

The pathological changes may be summed up in the statement that there is excessive absorption of the bone with impairment of the process of calcification. The normal process of lacunar bone-absorption is much exaggerated, so that the solidity of the greater part of the skeleton is more or less destroyed. The external denser layer of the bones becomes osteoporotic and the trabeculæ of the spongiosa are attenuated and may even disappear. This is well seen in the bones of the skull, which

Fig. 268

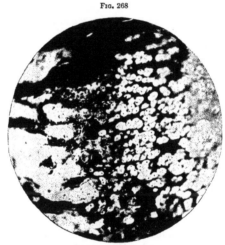

Rickets. The section is taken longitudinally at the junction of a rib with a costal cartilage. The irregularity of the columns of cartilage cells and the zone of congestion are easily seen. Zeiss obj. A, without ocular. (From the collection of Dr. Oskar Klotz.)

sometimes become soft and give way under the pressure of the finger (*craniotabes*). Deformities and even fractures may thus be brought about. Not only this; there is quite early a formation of new bone which is poor in or quite devoid of lime salts (osteoid tissue). This is laid down in the neighborhood of the remains of the trabeculæ, and may also form new trabeculæ. The newly-formed osteoid tissue is derived from the periosteum and the bone-marrow, which are extremely vascular. The proliferating tissue is composed not only of epithelioid osteoblastic cells, but also of spindle and stellate cells within a fibrillar matrix. When arising from the marrow the new substance is strictly comparable to the internal callus found in recent fractures. The trabeculæ derived from the periosteum are formed in much the same way also as the outer callus, and are composed of a cellular or cellulofibrous material. In the periosteum of the long bones cartilage is often laid down, which in turn undergoes the characteristic transformation. In this way it comes about that the external surface of the bones is covered with a vascular spongy layer, which offers some resistance to the finger, but is readily cut with the knife. In extreme cases, the original compact bone becomes porotic.

The endochondral ossification is also seriously interfered with. In the more marked cases there may be no deposit of lime salts in the zone of calcification, and in the milder forms there are merely spicules scattered here and there. At the same time there never fails to be an enlargement of the proliferation zone of the cartilage, manifested principally in the long columns of hypertrophic cartilage cells. With this, vascular marrow spaces are formed here and there which gradually encroach upon the solid cartilage. The more severe the disease, the more marked is the absorption of the cartilage. Somewhat behind the zone of hypertrophic and vascularized cartilage a zone of osteoid tissue is formed, which may be from 5 to 15 mm. in thickness. As the disease heals, lime salts are deposited, beginning in the central portions of the trabeculæ of osteoid substance and gradually extending, until the bone becomes solid again, and even, in fact, much more dense and ivory-like than normal bone.

Chondrodystrophia Fœtalis.—Somewhat allied to cretinism and rickets, at least in outward appearance, is the affection known as chondrodystrophia fœtalis (Kaufmann) or **achondroplasia** (Parrot). We owe our knowledge of this disease chiefly to the researches of Kaufmann,[1] whose work has enabled us to differentiate it from a variety of other conditions with which it was formerly confused. The obscurity involving the condition is well indicated by the numerous names that have been proposed for it: namely, rachitis fœtalis, pseudorachitism, pseudorachitis fœtalis micromelica, cretinoid dysplasia, chondrodystrophia fœtalis, achondroplasia, chondritis fœtalis.

The disease begins in fœtal life, running its course, as it is believed, from the third to the sixth week. Consequently, the parts chiefly affected are the base of the skull, the long bones, ribs, and pelvis. The bones that are formed in membrane and those that in late fœtal life are mainly cartilaginous commonly escape. The individuals thus affected are usually stillborn but may survive to adult life.

In a typical case the body as a whole is dwarfed, the type being micromelic, and the lesions are generally symmetrical. The head is large and the trunk plump, approximating normal size. The micromelia is rhizomelic, and the hands exhibit what is called the "trident" deformity. There are, however, notable variations in the configuration of the skull, and in the length, curvature, and consistence of the bones of the extremities. In regard to the first-mentioned particular, Kaufmann recognizes

[1] Untersuchungen über die sogennante foetale Rachitis, Berlin, 1892, and Ziegler's Beiträge, 13: 1893: 32.

PLATE XIV

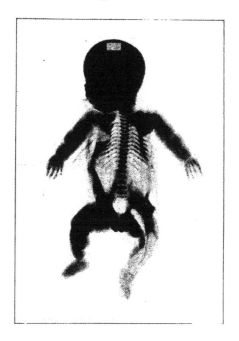

Osteogenesis Imperfecta, with Multiple Antenatal Fractures of
Ribs, Long Bones, etc.

The fractures show themselves as nodosities with abnormal
curvatures of the bones.

two main groups: one in which there is a cretinoid conformation of the head, that is to say, a deeply sunken nose, prominent eyelids and lips, thick cheeks, and a large mouth; and a second, in which the nose is flattened and retracted as a whole. In the former group the bone is of good consistence, although somewhat more vascular than normal, while in the latter its texture is soft. Some cases are associated with craniotabes (Klein), and there may be beading at the costochondral sutures. Defective development of the pelvis, cotyloid and glenoid cavities, has also been noted. The vertebræ may be involved (Regnault), so that lordosis results. Growth in the length of the bones is seriously interfered with, owing to faulty ossification at the epiphyseal lines, but periosteal ossification is practically normal, with the result that the bones become short, plump, and thick. An ingrowth of the periosteum into the epiphyseal sutures has been observed in many cases.

According to the character of the changes in the long bones, Kaufmann differentiates three forms—*chondrodystrophia malacica, c. hypoplastica*, and *c. hyperplastica*. In the first variety the cartilages at the ends of the long bones are to some extent increased in size, but no columns of cartilage cells are formed. The cartilage in places is softened and in others is irregularly calcified and ossified. In the hypoplastic form the ossification of the cartilage is appreciably behind the normal in extent, the columns of cartilage cells are small, the cells themselves are deficient in growth, being spindle-shaped, irregularly arranged, and having the appearance of being compressed. The hyaline matrix is more or less soft and homogeneous. The third type presents a marked overgrowth of the cartilage leading to notable thickening at the epiphyseal ends of the bones. Ossification is extremely irregular.

The etiology of this disease is quite obscure, and it is by no means certain that Kaufmann's three types are different phases of the one affection. Heredity seems to play a part in some cases. There is some evidence for believing that the cretinoid variety is really a form of cretinism and due to athyroidea. With regard to the other types, it is possible that defects in the primitive "Anlagen" are at fault, or, again, intra-uterine pressure (Klebs[1]). In view of the fact that obvious errors in development are sometimes associated with chondrodystrophia, as, for instance, polydactylism and cleft palate, and that the condition imperceptibly shades off into a pronounced developmental abnormality which is finally represented by phocomelia, Virchow has objected to the term chondrodystrophia, which is certainly open to criticism in that it localizes the disturbance, and, moreover, attributes it to a nutritional defect.

Osteogenesis Imperfecta.—The exact relationship of the disease, called by Vrolik and Stilling, osteogenesis imperfecta, to chondrodystrophia is still *sub judice*. The studies of Stilling,[2] Hildebrandt,[3] and Harbitz[4] go to show that it is a definite intra-uterine process. Although the

---

[1] *Lehrbuch d. allg. Path., Jena*, 2.   [2] Virch. Archiv, 115: 1899: 357.
[3] Virch. Archiv, 158: 1899: 426.   [4] Ziegler's Beiträge, 30: 1901: 605.

affection has been described only in newborn or very young infants, it is not necessarily fatal, and Harbitz suggests that certain of the cases of dwarfism that have been regarded as fœtal rickets may have been osteogenesis imperfecta.   There is, undoubtedly, some defect in the process of ossification, inasmuch as the bones are soft and brittle, so that deformities and fractures readily occur.   Like chondrodystrophia, porosity of the bones is occasionally inherited, and, as Bircher[1] has shown, the two conditions may be combined.   It is interesting, also, that borderland cases, presenting in one and the same individual some of the features of chondrodystrophia, osteogenesis imperfecta, and rickets, have been recorded (Hektoen[2]).

FIG. 269

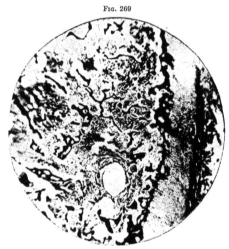

Fragilitas ossium.   Section is taken transversely through the femur of a newborn infant with chondrodystrophia and osseous fragility.   To the right is periosteum with a layer of cartilage; to the left a portion of the shaft.   Bone-formation is deficient, as evidenced by the scanty and attenuated trabeculæ.   Zeiss obj. DD, without ocular.   (Case of Dr. Oskar Klotz.[3])

In osteogenesis imperfecta a cardinal feature is the extraordinary manner of ossification of the skull.   The calvarium is not formed of continuous bony plates with regular sutures, but of a multitude of small mosaics, sometimes touching one another, but more often united by bridges of membrane.   In a remarkable case, described by Stilling, the vault of the skull consisted of a membranous sac in which were scattered spicules of bone.   So far as is known, synostosis of the os tribasilare does not occur in this disease.

Microscopic study shows that the trabeculæ **are** few in number,

[1] Lubarsch u. Ostertag's Allg. Aetiol., Wiesbaden, 1896: 53.
[2] Amer. Jour. Med. Sci., 125:1903:751.   [3] Jour. Path. and Bact., 13:1909·467.

irregular, and imperfectly (formed. There is no continuous system of trabeculæ with Haversian canals, and lamellæ as in normal bone. The cause is absolutely unknown. In one case hydramnios was present in the mother.

As has been mentioned, the condition of brittleness of the bones, **osteopsathyrosis** or **fragilitas ossium**, is an occasional feature in the curious affections just described, but is sometimes found as a distinct entity. The etiology of the so-called "idiopathic" or primary fragility is quite obscure. It comes on quite early in life and may even be congenital. The disease runs, also, in families.[1] Apparently there is an insufficient apposition of bone, though the normal process of resorption is not interfered with. The final result is a rarefaction of the bones which predisposes to fracture on the slightest provocation. Looser[2] regards it as an *osteogenesis imperfecta tarda*. The exact connection between osteopsathyrosis and osteogenesis imperfecta, however, is by no means clearly made out. A remarkable instance is on record also of dwarfism and osseous fragility occurring in the same family throughout three generations (Ekmann[3]).

The sum total of these collective studies serves to show that there are a number of anomalies of growth and development, more or less distinct, but shading off imperceptibly one into the other. That there is such a thing as "fœtal rickets," in the sense of rickets that has run its complete course during intra-uterine life, may well be doubted.[4]

Gigantism.—In many respects the antithesis of dwarfism is the remarkable condition known as gigantism, or more correctly **macrogenesia**, in which there is a notable increase in the length and thickness of the bones, with concomitant changes in the soft tissues. We have here evidences of increased proliferation of the cartilages in the process of endochondral ossification, together with excessive deposit of bone by apposition. The condition may be congenital or may develop in later life.

Partial or Local Gigantism.—Local forms, affecting chiefly the bones of the face (*leontiasis ossea*, Virchow), the fingers, and toes, have been observed. The exact nature of leontiasis ossea is obscure, but it appears to be a diffuse hyperostosis, somewhat analogous to the local exostoses and hyperostoses found in certain degenerative disturbances and chronic inflammations. The local gigantism of childhood affects usually the upper limbs, and may be unilateral or bilateral. Other developmental anomalies may be associated with the overgrowth. Thoma,[5] for example, has observed defective formation of the genital organs in a youth the subject of hemihypertrophy.

---

[1] Gurlt, Handb. der Lehre von den Knochenbruchen, 1 : 1862 : 147.

[2] Pathologische Gesellsch, 11:1907.

[3] Dissertatio medica descriptionem et casus aliquot osteomalaciæ sistens, Upsalæ, 1788.

[4] Those interested will find the subject more fully discussed in an article by one of us (A. G. N.) in the Reference Handbook of the Medical Sciences (2d edit.) 8:1904:419, N. Y., Wm. Wood & Co.

[5] Text-book of General Pathology, London, 1: 198, A. & C. Black.

General Gigantism.—When the body as a whole is hypertrophic we speak of general gigantism or **macrosomia**.

This is excessively rare as a congenital anomaly. According to the law of "deviation" formulated by Thoma,[1] we can assume the existence of giant growth in cases where the length of the body exceeds 57 cm. and the weight is above $4\frac{3}{5}$ kg. The largest newborn infant on record is one reported by Dubois,[2] which weighed 11.3 kilos (twenty-four pounds thirteen and one-half ounces). As a rule, giant children are stillborn. When they survive, the excessive size may be compensated by slow growth subsequently, but occasionally such infants grow very fast and attain puberty early.

More often, however, general macrosomia first makes its appearance between the tenth and the twentieth year, usually with the onset of puberty. The abnormality manifests itself chiefly by an increase in the length of the long bones, mainly of the lower extremities, but to some extent in the trunk, so that the height is notably increased. The increase in weight is less apparent, being never more, and usually less, than the increase in height would warrant. In giants the head is relatively small and the overgrowth is disproportionate. Stigmata of infantilism, such as knock-knee and genital hypoplasia, may be present. Some cases are associated with other developmental defects, facial hemihypertrophy, local exostoses, or curved bones. These may be regarded as examples of *symptomatic* gigantism.

Much rarer is *essential* gigantism, in which the overgrowth is uniform and symmetrical, and the affected individuals are strong and in every way perfect.

The causes of gigantism are obscure. It has been attributed by some to peculiarities in the germ cells. This view is supported by the fact that the condition is sometimes inherited, and, also, by the observations of Engel-Reimers,[3] who has emphasized the view that excessive muscular development, the so-called "athletic" habit, is often due to an abnormal predisposition and not to functional overactivity. In this connection increased intra-uterine nutrition appears to play a leading role.

Several facts, also, would indicate that irritation or excessive stimulation of the epiphyseal ends of the bones tends to produce overgrowth. This can be brought about experimentally by driving ivory pegs into the ends of the bones or by feeding young animals with phosphorus or arsenic (Wegner[4]). Elongation of the bones has also been noted in connection with osteomyelitis, fractures of the shaft, tuberculosis of the joints, superficial ulcers, and dilated veins. Local hyperostoses of the head have been known to follow trauma and erysipelas.

Giant growth also has been met with after the acute infective fevers in childhood, which were apparently the exciting cause.

---

[1] Untersuchungen über die *Grösse* u. das *Gewicht* der anatomischen Bestandtheile des menschlichen Körpers im gesunden u. im kranken Zustande, *Leipzig*, 1882.

[2] Les gros enfants au point de vue obstétrical, Thèse de Paris, 1897.

[3] Jahrb. der Hamburg Staatskrankenanstalten, 3: 1894.

[4] Ueber den Einfluss des Phosphors au den Organismus, Virch. Archiv, 55:1872:11.

Other cases, again, appear to be dependent on disorders of internal secretion. A tendency to exaggerated growth, particularly of the lower extremities, has been observed in eunuchs and castrated animals.

There is considerable ground for believing, further, that a large proportion of the cases of gigantism (42 per cent. according to Sternberg[1]) are really acromegaly. Brissaud and Meige[2] have upheld the view that

Fig. 270

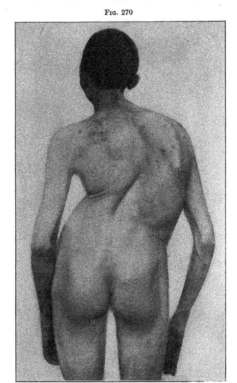

Lateral scoliosis. (From the Surgical Clinic of the Montreal General Hospital.)

the two affections are essentially the same thing. The same pathological process at work during the growing period of life will produce gigantism; at a later period, when epiphyseal ossification is completed, acromegaly. It is possible that some at least of the cases of gigantism which do not

[1] Beiträge zur Kenntniss der Akromegalie, Zeit. f. klin. Med., 27: 1894: 85, ibid., 1895:86.

[2] Jour. de méd. et chir. prat., January 25, 1895.

present the characteristics of acromegaly are nevertheless dependent on abnormal function of the pituitary body (acromégalie fruste[1]).

Besides the peculiarities of growth and development just considered, there are others more localized which are brought about by abnormal static and mechanical influences exerted upon the organism during the developmental period of life. These may arise both before and after birth and frequently cause most pronounced deformities.

Fig. 271

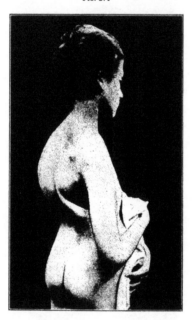

Scoliosis with marked posterior deformity (kyphosis).

While many of these congenital anomalies are probably to be attributed to peculiarities of the germinal cells, others are, at least in many instances, more closely connected with intra-uterine pressure. Among these conditions may be mentioned **microcephaly, micromelia,** the **fusion of bones,** and the **amputation of limbs.** The factors usually at work are a contracted amniotic sac, bands or adhesions traversing the sac, the weight of superimposed limbs, or a knotted umbilical cord.

[1] For a full discussion of the general subject of gigantism, and references to the literature, see Nicholls, article *Gigantism,* Reference Handb. of the Med. Sci., second edition, N. Y., Wm. Wood & Co., 8 : 1904 : 457.

To a large extent, also, the development of the bony cavities, such as, for instance, the cranium, the orbits, and the thorax, is dependent upon the state of development of the contained organs. Should these be small or otherwise defective, the corresponding bony parts are hypoplastic or defective. In this category may be placed such conditions as **cranioschisis, craniorachischisis, anencephaly, spina bifida,** and the like. Increased pressure within the bony cavities will also lead to enlargement of the same. Thus, **hydrocephalus** is an enlargement of the cranium, often with separation of the bones and flattening of the brain substance, caused by excess of the cerebrospinal fluid.

FIG. 272

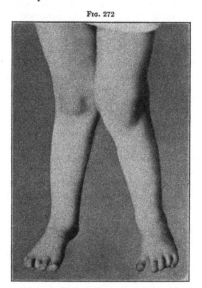

Knock-knee. (From the Surgical Clinic of the Montreal General Hospital.)

In later life, too, owing to external influences, bones that were originally well-formed and developed may become deformed, and this the more readily occurs should the bone from any cause become soft and yielding.

Scoliosis.—One of the most common of these deformities is scoliosis, or lateral deviation of a portion of the vertebral column. As a rule, there is curvature of the dorsal spine to the right, with a compensatory deviation of the lumbar, and sometimes the cervical, portion to the left. This may be brought about by excessive distension of one thoracic cavity, as from an exudate or new-growth, or by contraction of the cavity from fibroid induration of the lung, the inspissation of a pleuritic exudate, or, again, by fixation of the pelvis in an oblique position. It is also met with in Friedreich's ataxia and the progressive myopathies. Perhaps the commonest causes are faulty methods of standing or sitting in childhood. In the more severe cases the deformity comes on quickly and becomes extreme, being often combined with posterior curvature—**kyphosis**. There is often with this more or less rotation of the vertebræ on their vertical axes. The ligaments become stretched and may calcify, owing to the production of osteophytes. Curvature forward, or **lordosis**, is also frequently met with.

Coxa Vara.—Coxa vara is a condition of the hip-joint brought about by imperfect development of the acetabulum, or changes in the head or neck of the femur. It is met with where there is abnormal yielding of the bone, as in rickets, and leads to dislocation.

Genu Valgum.—Genu valgum is met with in children from the second to the fourth year, or at puberty. In this condition the leg forms an obtuse angle with the thigh at the knee-joint. It may be unilateral or bilateral, and is often met with also in those who are a great deal on their feet and who do heavy manual labor. It may occasionally be due to traumatic separation of the epiphyseal cartilages with dislocation of the fragments and subsequent union in the faulty position, to carious processes in the external condyle of the femur, or, again, to arthritis deformans.

Talipes Valgus.—Talipes valgus (**pes planus**), or flat-foot, is a condition in which, owing to the stretching of the internal lateral and plantar ligaments, the arch of the foot is more or less completely destroyed. In severe cases the normal concavity on the under side of the foot may give place to actual convexity. The result is that the foot as a whole is turned outward, the soft tissues are often reddened and swollen, while more or less pain is complained of. The trouble is usually brought about by much standing or by carrying weights, in the case of those whose health is not robust. It may also be caused by knock-knee or rachitic disease of the ankle-joints. Rarely it is congenital.

Hallux Valgus.—Hallux valgus is to be regarded as a pressure deformity due to the use of improperly fitting boots. The great toe often is forced to assume a position beneath the other toes.

Abnormal positions of the articular surfaces of bones may also be brought about by faulty positions of the limbs, as in certain forms of paralysis, contractures of neuropathic origin, or, again, by the contraction of scar-tissue in fascia or tendons. The nature of **talipes varus, t. equinus, t. calcaneus, cubitus valgus** and **varus**, is sufficiently indicated by their names and calls for no extended description.

CIRCULATORY DISTURBANCES.

Hyperemia.—Active Hyperemia.—Active hyperemia is met with in the periosteum and medulla in growing bone, and, pathologically, in various forms of regeneration and inflammation.

Passive Hyperemia—Passive hyperemia is found in general venous stasis and whenever the free outflow of blood from the bone is interfered with. Chronic passive congestion appears to favor the growth of the bone and soft tissues, as is well seen in the clubbed fingers of chronic pulmonary and cardiac disease. Whether the peculiar disease, first described by Marie,[1] and called by him *hypertrophic pulmonary osteo-arthropathy*, is of this nature cannot at present be settled.

Hemorrhage.—Hemorrhage into the periosteum or marrow is not very uncommon. It rarely attains serious proportions, and the blood effused is, as a rule, quickly absorbed. It may follow traumatism, and occurs in new-growths and other destructive processes. The so-called **cephalhematomata** are localized extravasations of blood beneath the periosteum, usually of the parietal bones. Rarely, they are found

Fig. 273

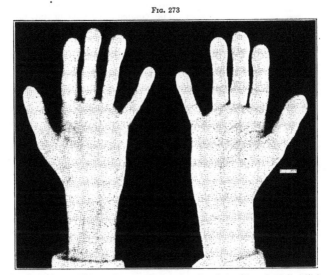

Spatulate (Hippocratic) fingers in a case of pulmonary tuberculosis. (From the Medical Clinic of the Montreal General Hospital.)

in the interior of the bone, leading to elevation of the external plate. Petechial hemorrhages are found also in the hemorrhagic diatheses, Barlow's disease, and scurvy. In Barlow's disease[2] the periosteum of the long bones may be dissected off from the shafts owing to the extensive extravasation of blood.

Embolism.—Embolism as a rule produces little effect on account of the abundant anastomoses that are present, but, according to Gussen-bauer, end-arteries are to be found at the ends of the diaphyses, obstruction of which might lead to ischæmic necrosis.

[1] Révue de Médecine, 10: 1890: 1.
[2] Barlow, Med.-chir. Trans., London, 66: 1883: 159; also Schmorl, Jahrb. f. Kinderheilk., 65: 1907: 50.

Thrombosis.—Thrombosis of the vessels is common after trauma and fractures, and in the neighborhood of hemorrhages, inflammatory and necrotic processes. It is of no practical importance.

INFLAMMATIONS.

The inflammatory processes occurring in bone affect first and chiefly the vascular structures, that is to say, the periosteum and bone-marrow.

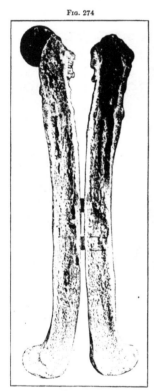

FIG. 274

Femur cut longitudinally, to show rarefaction, osteosclerosis, and new-growth of bone from the periosteum. Case of osteomyelitis. (Pathological Museum, McGill University.)

We may therefore distinguish two forms: **periostitis** and **osteomyelitis** The compact material of the bone may be involved secondarily (**osteitis**) in either of these conditions and usually in the form of erosion and disintegration.

Periostitis and Osteomyelitis.—Periostitis and osteomyelitis are not infrequently combined.

Inflammation of bone may be brought about by local or systemic causes. As a rule, infective microorganisms are at work, but toxic agents and local trauma may play a contributory and sometimes a leading role. The causal agents reach the affected part either directly or through the blood stream. The most characteristic form of inflammation is the acute osteomyelitis and periostitis due to pyogenic cocci (*osteomyelitis et periostitis purulenta*), but an analogous condition is occasionally met with as a complication of some of the infectious fevers, such as acute articular rheumatism, scarlatina, measles, typhoid, variola, relapsing fever, dysentery, and epidemic parotitis. Here the condition may, in some cases, be due to the action of the specific microorganism of the primary disease, but perhaps more frequently is the result of secondary or mixed infection with some of the pus-forming cocci.

The results are various. Mild grades of inflammation and those that are early and efficiently treated may heal with little or no perceptible effects. Much more frequently, however, the sequelæ are serious. These may be grouped under two main heads, disintegration and proliferation. In many forms of acute and chronic inflammation *necrosis* of bone is a marked feature, either in the form of a slow eroding process of resorption—*caries*—or as an exfoliation of larger or smaller portions of the bone *en masse*—*sequestration*. Short of this extreme result, the bone may become porotic, owing to lacunar resorption. This results from the destructive action of the granulation tissue in the medullary spaces (*rarefying osteitis*). In other cases, on the contrary, the function of new bone formation appears to be stimulated. Thus, in the neighborhood of abscesses, sequestra, and tuberculous areas, the bone becomes denser and more compact, owing to the deposit of new bone upon the trabeculæ (*osteosclerosis*). This may be a primary condition in some cases of syphilis and phosphorus poisoning. Not infrequently, there is a new-formation of bone in the shape of osteophytes, or a diffuse concentric deposit, owing to excessive activity of the periosteal osteogenetic layer (*periostitis ossificans*). This may lead to increased thickness of the bone and to more or less perfect restoration of its contour after extensive destruction. In growing bones, inflammation of the shaft of the bone, provided that it be not too severe and not too near the epiphyseal cartilage, may result in a marked increase in the length of the bone. Should, however, the inflammatory process occur near or at the zone of ossification, irregularity in growth will occur, and should the epiphyseal cartilage be separated or destroyed, growth will come to a standstill.

It is not uncommon, also, under the influence of chronic irritation, to find the periosteum thickened and attached firmly to the underlying bone (*periostitis fibrosa*). This is seen as a result of local trauma and in the neighborhood of necrotic foci and chronic ulcers of the soft tissues.

It is hardly necessary to state that inflammatory affections of bones may extend to the adjacent tissues such as the veins, muscles, tendons, aponeuroses, and skin. In this way local abscesses and fistulæ are produced. Thrombophlebitis is a dangerous complication, inasmuch as it frequently leads to a dissemination of the infective agents and may thus produce systemic septicemia.

A rather peculiar form of inflammation of the periosteum has been described by Ollier and Berg. The disease occurs more particularly in young persons and usually runs a mild course. There is a subperiosteal exudation, clear and serous, or sometimes viscid, containing fibrin, fat globules, and relatively few corpuscles. It may be combined with osteomyelitis. The exact etiology of the condition is not as yet definitely made out.

Acute Infectious Osteomyelitis.—Acute infectious osteomyelitis belongs to the group of septicemic infections and occurs spontaneously or as a complication of various fevers. The spontaneous, or so-called "idiopathic," form is most commonly due to Staphylococcus pyogenes aureus or albus, and is met with usually in young persons. It is a severe affection characterized by great pain, fever, and symptoms of constitutional involvement. The infection is hematogenous, the original point of entrance of the germ being usually in the skin or mucous membranes. The primary wound may have been so trifling that all trace and recollection of it may have disappeared.

The process begins either in the periosteum or in the medullary canal, and is characterized by an intense suppurative and necrotizing inflammation. The disease involves usually the periosteum and the neighboring parts. The affected region is swollen, tense, reddened, and intensely painful. The bone-marrow is at first congested, presenting, later, areas of hemorrhagic extravasation, and later still, numerous small foci of suppuration. Owing to the confluence of these foci larger or smaller abscesses result, and the suppurative process may extend throughout the medullary canal to the Haversian canals and periosteum, and even to the surface. Sometimes the epiphyses and the joints are involved. In milder cases the process may terminate without such marked disturbance, but usually, owing to the interference with the circulation due to the pressure of the inflammatory products, larger or smaller portions of the bone may become necrosed and in time exfoliated. This takes place both within the bone and at places where the periosteum has been separated from the underlying structure. Large masses of bone and, in fact, the whole central portion of the shaft, may be thus sequestrated and necessitate surgical interference. Owing to the occurrence of septic venous thrombosis, metastatic abscesses may form in various parts and death is a not infrequent result. The bones are involved primarily in the following order: femur, tibia, the bones of the upper extremities, the flat and short bones.

In cases where a bone is injured, as by crushing, splintering, or fracture, a moderate amount of inflammation is set up which may readily heal. Should, however, infective microörganisms be circulating in the blood-stream the injured region is liable to become infected and a condition similar to infective osteomyelitis and periostitis is produced (locus resistentiæ minoris). In cases of compound fracture, infection may also take place from the external air.

Chronic Osteomyelitis.—Chronic inflammation may be the result of a preëxisting acute process or may be chronic from the start. The latter is apt to be the case in tuberculosis, syphilis, typhoid, and actinomycosis. All the changes just described as occurring in the acute form may occur here, but the process is more gradual and long-continued. Granulation, suppuration, and necrosis are marked features and both osteoporosis and hyperostosis occur. Chronic inflammation may also arise by the extension of inflammatory processes from the neighboring parts, as, for example, from ulcers of the skin. Osteophytes may be produced or diffuse hyperostosis.

A peculiar form of chronic inflammation that should be here mentioned is the *phosphorus necrosis*[1] which attacks the jaw bones of those working in match factories. The process usually begins in the lower maxilla and may extend to the upper jaw and, rarely, to the bones of the face.

[1] v. Stubenrauch, Sammlung f. klin. Vorträge, 303:1901; also Perthes, Deut. Chirurgie, 33a, 1907.

The condition is brought about by the fumes of the yellow phosphorus, which, being dissolved in the saliva, attack the gums, and, if carious teeth be present, invade the alveolar processes. Infection with micro-organisms from the buccal cavity also plays an important part. In the early stages there is a slight inflammation, in consequence of which the periosteum and bone-marrow are stimulated and produce new bone, so that the jaw becomes thickened and sclerosed. Later, suppuration and necrosis set in, and larger or smaller portions of the bone are sequestrated and cast off. In this way the whole of the lower jaw may be destroyed. Rarely, the process runs a much more acute course.

FIG. 275

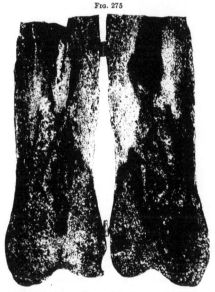

Chronic osteomyelitis of the femur. The specimen shows great thickening of the shaft of the bone, with the formation of abscesses. On the left a sequestrum is well shown. (From the Pathological Museum of McGill University.)

We come now to discuss two rare and striking affections the etiology of which is quite obscure.

Paget's Disease[1] (**Osteitis Deformans**).—Paget's disease is a rare affection found after middle life and usually in advanced age. In brief, there are two opposing pathological processes at work, absorption and osseous hyperplasia. In some cases, owing to the absorption of the

[1] Med. Chir. Trans., 60: 1877:37, and 65:1882; also Stilling, Virch. Archiv, 119 1890:542; Waston, Johns Hopkins Hosp. Bull., 9:1898; and Prince, Amer. Jour. Med. Sci., 124:1902:796.

bone, the affection bears a close resemblance to osteomalacia. The disease begins with pains of a rheumatic character, which are quickly followed by pathognomonic changes. The bones, especially those subjected to the weight of the body, as the spine and leg bones, become curved and otherwise deformed, while there may also be a considerable and irregular hyperostosis. The parts chiefly affected are the bones of the lower extremities, the spine, clavicles, and the calvarium. The process of absorption goes on both in the spongy and compact parts of the bone, and leads to more or less complete destruction of the bony plates, which are replaced by a fatty, gelatinous, or fibrous tissue, poor in cells (*osteomyelitis fibrosa*). Or the tissue may liquefy, forming cysts. Besides this, proliferation and new-formation of bone take place both in the periosteum and in the marrow, leading to great increase in the mass and density of the bone (osteosclerosis). As a consequence of this, irregular nodular enlargements are formed in various parts of the bones, which may also be enormously thickened. Eventually, calcification may set in, and as it becomes dominant the disease comes to an end. Richard and Ziegler regard the disease as being strictly comparable to arthritis deformans while v. Recklinghausen believes it to be allied to osteomalacia.

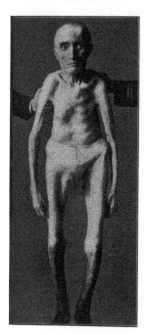

Fig. 276

Osteitis deformans. (Packard.[1])

Hypertrophic Pulmonary Osteo-arthropathy.[2]—The nature of the second disease referred to, hypertrophic pulmonary osteo-arthropathy, is, if possible, still more obscure. Attention was first directed to it by Marie[3] and shortly after by Bamberger.[4] It was precisely described by the former, who differentiated it from acromegaly, to which it bears a strong general resemblance. In the vast majority of cases the disease is found in those suffering from chronic pulmonary or cardiac affections.

In a typical case the hands and feet are considerably enlarged and the bones of the forearm and leg are also increased in size toward their distal ends. The finger tips are clubbed. The cartilages of the joints are eroded and the synovial fluid is increased. The process in the affected

[1] Amer. Jour. Med. Sci., 122:1901:552.

[2] Alexander, St. Bartholomew's Hosp. Rep., 42:1907:41.

[3] Révue de Médecine, 10: 1890: 1.   [4] Zeit. f. klin. Med., 18: 1890: 193.

bones is a periostitis with sclerosing hyperplasia and a rarefying osteomyelitis. The face and head are not involved. Cases are often complicated with tuberculosis of the spine, thus giving rise to deformities.

So far as is known, the disease appears to be a chronic inflammation,
brought about possibly by the absorption of infective agents and products,
assisted by venous stasis. The analogy with Hippocratic fingers should
be remarked in this connection.

Tuberculosis.—Tuberculosis is the most common and important
disease of bone. The affection attacks by preference children and young
persons, but is not unknown in middle life. This is probably to be explained in that the bones of young growing individuals are more vascular

Fig. 277

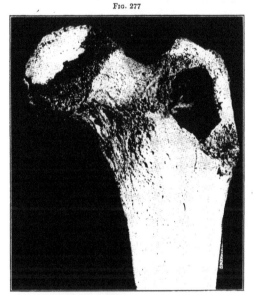

Tuberculous caries of the upper end of the femur: abscess in the great trochanter.
(Pathological Museum, McGill University.)

and susceptible to relatively slight injuries, while the comparatively slow
circulation in the vessels of the medulla also predisposes. Although
tuberculosis of the bones often appears to be a primary affection in so
far as the clinical manifestations are concerned, yet the disease is probably
always secondary and an expression of metastasis from some distant
focus, usually in the lungs or lymphatic glands. This focus may be so
minute as to escape observation, or may even appear to have healed.
As a rule, the infective germs are brought to the part by the blood, but
occasionally the disease arises by extension from a joint or other structure
in the immediate neighborhood. Possibly also infection may take place

through the lymph-stream.   The disease may be acute, in the form of a disseminated miliary infection, but this is always a terminal event and of less interest than the more frequent chronic forms.

The tuberculous process begins either in the bone-marrow or periosteum, and manifests a preference for the cancellous structure and epiphyses.   The bones most frequently involved are the vertebræ, femora, the bones of the tarsus and carpus, the ribs, and occasionally the skull.   The disease does not tend to attack the medulla except in the case of the phalanges, metacarpal and metatarsal bones.

The process begins with the formation of one or more areas of tuberculous granulation, which gradually extend by erosion of the bony structure until they finally fuse.   At the same time new foci of infiltration are

FIG. 278

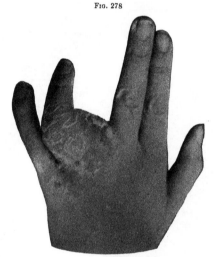

Tuberculous dactylitis (spina ventosa).   (From the Surgical Clinic of the Montreal General Hospital.)

being formed in the neighborhood of the older areas.   The bone trabeculæ become gradually involved in a process of resorption and caseation, and finally disintegrate, and in certain cases considerable portions of bone may be exfoliated *en masse*.   In this way in the later stages caseous abscesses of varying size result.   To the naked eye these appear as rounded or elongated yellowish, necrotic areas surrounded by grayish or grayish-red, gelatinous-looking, granulation tissue.   In other cases there may be seen large areas of necrotic bone of a yellowish-white or reddish color infiltrated with inflammatory cells and surrounded by granulation tissue or caseopurulent exudation and detritus.   A much rarer form than this is the one in which the process is so rapid that there is very little attempt at the formation of granulation tissue. Instead, there is a diffuse caseating process which extends rapidly throughout the bone-marrow. Occasionally wedge-shaped areas of necrosis and caseation are found, the broad base of the wedge being situated toward the articular surface. This suggests that the condition is brought about by infarction, a view that is supported by the experiments of Müller. The articular surfaces of bone have been shown to contain end-arteries, and these probably become occluded by infective emboli or by a combination of embolism and thrombosis.

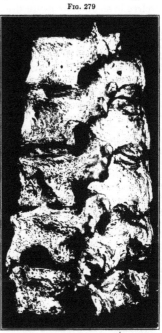

FIG. 279

The results of the process are various. Small foci undoubtedly may heal by the softening and absorption of the destroyed tissue, which is gradually replaced by connective tissue, marrow, or bone. The larger cavities may, however, remain and become delimited by dense, fibrous tissue or a zone of tuberculous granulation tissue. In nearly all cases a compensatory process of the nature of a new-formation of bone by apposition takes place. In other cases rarefaction occurs in the central portion of the bone, so that the central canal becomes enlarged, and with this there is a deposit of new bone externally from the periosteum (*spina ventosa*). This resorption and concomitant apposition of bone may also be localized to a particular place. In many instances, especially in the larger bones, the structures become thickened and sclerosed.

Tuberculous erosion of the vertebræ. (From the Pathological Museum of McGill University.)

Tuberculous Periostitis.—Tuberculous periostitis may be primary or secondary to tuberculous osteomyelitis and arthritis. The process may be localized in the form of an area of tuberculous granulation or a caseous node, or may extend over the whole surface of the bone. Where the inflammation has started in the deeper parts there may be direct communication with the exterior. If the process do not tend to heal, it goes from bad to worse, the tuberculous foci caseate and soften, and the infective agents are carried along the tissue spaces and lymphatics, to invade the muscles and the bloodvessels and possibly the joints by a steadily advancing process of granulation and caseation. In this way large cold abscesses or caseofibroid nodules are formed. In advanced cases the process may reach the surface, giving rise to tuberculous sinuses and fistulæ which discharge caseous pus. With this there is, as a rule, more or less extensive superficial erosion of the bone with formation of new bone from the osteogenetic layer of the periosteum. In the case of the carpus and tarsus more than one bone and several joints are usually involved in an extensive destructive process.

In tuberculosis of the vertebræ those from the seventh dorsal to the second lumbar are more commonly involved. The process begins superficially and tends to invade the bodies of the vertebræ, the ligaments are destroyed, and, owing to the weight of the body, the spine may collapse, forming an angular curvature (*Pott's disease*). The vertebral canal may be opened up and compression of the cord from tuberculous deposit or pressure of the dislocated bones may result, giving rise to a spastic paralysis. Large prevertebral cold abscesses are occasionally formed, which may burrow most extensively. The usual course is for the abscess to extend retroperitoneally downward into the pelvis. It tends to point below Poupart's ligament, or lower in the thigh (*psoas abscess*), or, again, may excavate the gluteal region and extend backward, dissecting the soft tissues away from the sacrum. In one case which we sectioned the abscess discharged into the trachea. Here, amphoric breath sounds and metallic tinkling were heard in a limited area near the spine, evidently due to the presence of air in the abscess cavity. A tuberculous abscess may extend through the sacrosciatic notch, giving rise to symptoms of obstinate sciatica. Should the disease heal, the deformity usually remains. Tuberculosis of the atlas, axis, and the base of the skull is rare, but is of importance, since, when the ligaments are destroyed, a sudden strain may cause dislocation and the odontoid process of the atlas is then driven forcibly into the medulla, causing instant death. The process more often than not does not completely heal, but gradually extends, giving rise to secondary infection, amyloid disease and exhaustion. In some cases the tubercle bacilli become disseminated, reaching the lungs and other distant parts.

Syphilis.—The syphilitic manifestations in bone vary considerably, according as the disease is congenital[1] or acquired. In the first case, the affection manifests itself at the line of ossification of the long bones, usually the femora. The lesion is really a specific osteochondritis. The line of calcification is broader than normal, more irregular, and of a whitish or whitish-yellow color.

Microscopically, the zone of ossification is irregular, the bone-trabeculæ vary in thickness, sometimes containing islets of cartilage, and the medullary spaces are irregular in size. In other cases the process of ossification is still further interfered with; the cartilage is soft and swollen; the epiphyses may be enlarged, owing to proliferation of the cartilage, and may be separated from the shaft by an extensive soft, grayish-yellow, or reddish zone, in which are necrotic areas. In advanced cases the epiphyses

---

[1] For literature see Herxheimer, Lubarsch und Ostertag's Ergebnisse, 12:1908.

FIG. 280

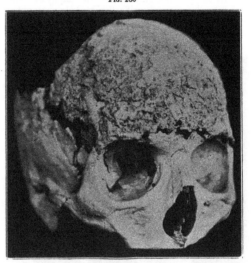

Periostitis with destructive inflammation (osteoporosis) affecting the frontal and temporal bones, due to syphilis. (From the Pathological Museum of McGill University)

FIG. 281

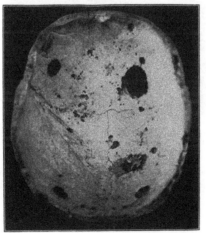

Syphilitic osteoporosis of the calvarium with perforation, due to multiple gummas. (From the Pathological Museum of McGill University.)

may be more or less completely separated from the diaphysis. The interference with the normal process of ossification leads to a somewhat characteristic form of dwarfing.[1]

Fig. 282

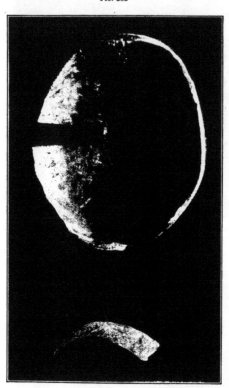

Sclerosis of the calvarium, of syphilitic origin. Note the thickness of the segment of bone (at the lower part of the picture), which is also dense and ivory-like. (Pathological Museum, McGill University.)

In the acquired form of the disease the characteristic lesion is the **gumma,** which may be situated in the periosteum or marrow. Periosteal gummas are much the commoner. Here, at first, we see a localized,

[1] It is possible that some cases of productive osteomyelitis of the long bones, hitherto regarded as tuberculous in nature, are of late congenital syphilitic origin. One such case, observed by R. P. Campbell and one of us (A.), gave the Wassermann reaction, and became painless and arrested in development with "606."

somewhat flattened, swelling of gelatinous appearance and elastic consistency. Later, this may assume a more grayish appearance and become firmer, owing to the presence of granulation tissue. Dry, whitish, necrotic areas, not unlike caseation, with more or less fibrosis, are frequently met with. As the process heals it leaves a dense, fibrous scar. At the points where the periosteal gummas are situated there are considerable erosion and caries of the underlying bone. This process may occur in any part of the skeleton, but is most commonly met with in the calvarium. It begins in the external layer, may extend to the diploë and the inner table, finally reaching the dura. According to the extent of the disease, the destruction of the bone may be almost microscopic, or furrows and excavations may be produced, or, again, large portions of the calvarium may become exfoliated.

Fig. 283

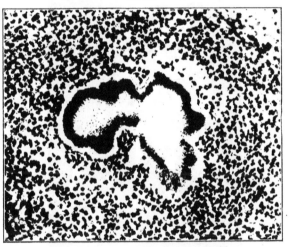

Mycetoma. Fungus surrounded by a dense accumulation of leukocytes. × 300.
(Dr. Hyde's case; from a photomicrograph.)

Osteomyelitis.—Syphilitic osteomyelitis is rare in the long bones but is met with occasionally in the phalanges and the diploë of the cranial vault. Gelatinous or fibrogelatinous-looking foci, often of a somewhat purulent character, are formed, of a grayish-yellow color, in which the bone is becoming necrotic. In the neighborhood, the less affected bone shows a tendency to hyperostosis. Under proper medication the disease may come to a standstill and finally heal. The granulation tissue disappears, the caseoid detritus is absorbed, dead bone is sequestrated and cast off, and any defects are either filled up by new bone or bridged over by connective tissue. The bone in the neighborhood frequently becomes dense and sclerotic, and of a texture and hardness resembling ivory. In all forms of this affection osteoplasia is a marked feature, and, in fact, in one type of periostitis, may dominate the anatomical picture. It should be mentioned that, where large masses of bone are being sequestrated, inflammation may extend to the soft tissues and skin, so that inflammatory exudation and necrotic material are discharged externally with the formation of suppurating sinuses.

FIG. 284

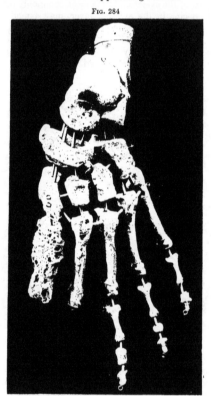

Osseous lesions in mycetoma. (Hyde.)

Actinomycosis.—This is usually found in the maxillæ, vertebræ, and bones of the thorax. Infection usually takes place through the alimentary tract. The infective agent is the ray-fungus (Actinomyces bovis), which seems to be frequently present on grass and hay. The disease has been known to follow pricking the gums with a needle, or may invade the alveolar process through decayed teeth. The infection may also enter from the cecum and appendix, whence it spreads to the retroperitoneal tissues, thence to the ilium. At first a periostitis is produced and the fungus gradually extends into the interior of the bone, which is rarefied and infiltrated with granulation tissue. There is considerable destruction of the bone. Macroscopically, the affected structures are involved in a granulating necrotizing process. By proper methods the ray-fungus can be detected in the inflammatory tissues.

Madura Foot.—Madura foot is a disease of the bones of the tarsus closely resembling actinomycosis. The infective agent is a fungus, in some cases, the Streptothrix Maduræ, an organism allied to the actinomyces; in other instances an aspergillus has been found. The disease is most common in India, but a few instances have been met with on the American continent. One case has been reported in this country which is remarkable in that it occurred in a person who had spent his whole life in America.[1] The lesions produced are similar to those in actinomycosis, leading to rarefaction and destruction of the affected bones, with numerous discharging sinuses, the pus from which contains the specific organism (vide also p. 970).

Lepra.—In leprosy, granulomas containing bacilli may be found in the periosteum and bone-marrow,[2] causing more or less osteoporosis and, where an extremity is involved, mutilation.

Variola.—According to Chiari, in variola an osteomyelitis may be found characterized by the formation of multiple minute, yellowish foci with gray centres, varying in size from that of a millet-seed to that of a split pea.

Microscopically, these consist of epithelioid cells, a few leukocytes, and a fibrinous exudate with central necrosis.

Parasites.—*Echinococcus* and *Cysticercus cellulosæ* have been met with, forming cysts.

RETROGRESSIVE METAMORPHOSES.

The structure of the bony framework of the body is in health undergoing constant change. In the child, while there is a certain amount of breaking down of the substance of the bone, vegetative and productive forces are predominant, with the result that the bone increases in size and strength until it attains its perfect structure. In the adult, breaking down, or resorption, as it is called, also goes on, but is compensated by a continuous deposit of bone by the process of apposition. In the aged, however, resorption is in excess, so that the bone becomes smaller, lighter, and more fragile. Lacunar resorption, both under normal and pathological conditions, is brought about by the agency of large, multi-nucleated cells, the osteoclasts (myeloplaxes), situated in the periosteum and bone-marrow. These take up their position upon the bony trabeculæ and gradually erode their way into the structure, forming excavations, called Howship's lacunæ.

[1] Adami and Kirkpatrick, Trans. Assoc. Amer. Phys., 10 : 1895 : 82.
[2] Sawtschenko, Ziegler's Beiträge, 9:1891:241.

Atrophy.—In the rapid resorption of the bone characteristic of certain diseases, the osteoclasts are greatly increased in number and lie closely packed together. The result of this is that the surface of the bone becomes rough, eroded, and irregular. Should the process come to an end, the projecting ridges are absorbed, there is a deposit of new bone in the hollows, and the surface of the bone again becomes smooth. Should the resorption be most marked next the medullary cavity, the external appearance of the bone is not altered, but the cavity is enlarged, the trabeculæ become gradually thinner, and may, in parts, disappear (*eccentric atrophy*). When the process begins externally, the bone

Fig. 285

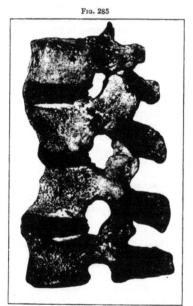

Atrophy of the bodies of the vertebræ from the pressure of an aneurism. (Pathological Museum, McGill University.)

becomes gradually thinner and local defects are manifested (*concentric atrophy*). In other cases the compact substance of the bone becomes porous, owing to the widening of the Haversian canals. This is known as *osteoporosis*. According to Pommer,[1] atrophy of bone may be a relative matter, that is to say, the amount of lacunar resorption does not exceed the normal, but there is a diminished deposit of new bone by apposition, so that the bone becomes smaller, or, again, the atrophy may be absolute.

[1] Ueber die Osteoklastentheorie, Virch. Archiv, 92: 1883: 449.

Atrophied bones are light and fragile, easily broken or sawn. The medullary substance will vary in appearance according to the extent of, the affection. It may be hyperplastic, presenting the appearance of, lymphoid marrow, fatty, or the fat may be replaced by a semitranslucent, gelatinous-looking substance (*serous atrophy*). As a consequence of the excessive resorption of the solider portions, the bones become brittle, and unable to support their accustomed burden, and may readily fracture (*symptomatic osteopsathyrosis, fragilitas ossium*). Atrophy of bone may arise as a senile or marantic change, from pressure, disuse, or from neurotrophic disorders.

Fig. 286

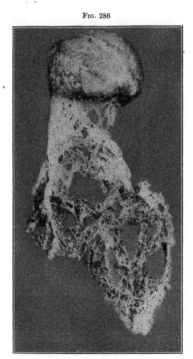

Rarefaction of the shaft of the humerus, due to sarcoma. (Pathological Museum, McGill University.)

Senile and Marantic Atrophy.—Senile and marantic atrophy may affect the skeleton as a whole, but the former is apt to involve more extensively the flat bones, the calvarium, the scapulæ, and the pelvis. The process begins at the points which are devoid of muscular attachments. The atrophy may be concentric or eccentric, and the bone may

also become more porous. The facies so characteristic of old age is
due to atrophy of the maxillæ, the alveolar processes of which may
disappear entirely. In the case of the calvarium, the whole of the outer
table and the diploë, or even portions of the inner table, may be destroyed.
In some instances there is a deposit of new bone on the surface of the
inner table. This is most frequently seen in the frontal bone. The
vertebræ become porous and diminished in size, so that the bodily height
is diminished. The dorsal curvature, so often seen in elderly people, is
due largely to the absorption of the anterior portion of the intervertebral
disks.

Fig. 287

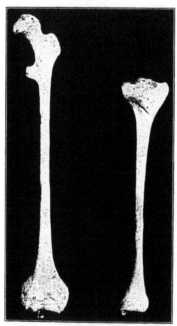

The femur and tibia of an idiot, showing the simple atrophy of disuse. The contrast in size
between the shaft and the extremities of the bones is marked. (From the Pathological Museum
of McGill University.)

Pressure Atrophy.—Atrophy from pressure is of course local. A
familiar instance is the depression in the bones of the calvarium due to
the Pacchionian bodies. Hydrocephalus and intracranial growths lead
to atrophy of the calvarium. Pressure atrophy is also brought about by
aneurisms, tumors, scars in the skin and subcutaneous tissues, the pressure
of the umbilical cord on the embryo.

Inflammatory Atrophy.—Atrophy may also follow inflammation.

Atrophy from Disuse.—Atrophy from disuse is met with especially in the limbs, as in amputations, fractures, anterior poliomyelitis, joint and bone inflammations.

Neuropathic Atrophy.—The neuropathic forms result from some disorder of the central nervous system, as dementia paralytica, tabes dorsalis, syringomyelia, anterior poliomyelitis. In many cases, however, the atrophy is attributable to disuse as well as to disease.

Death.—Death of bone takes two forms—**caries** and **necrosis**. Caries is a slow disintegration of the bone into fine and almost imperceptible particles, and is analogous to suppuration of the soft tissues. Necrosis may be compared to gangrene and is death of bone occurring *en masse*. Caries is practically always due to inflammation. Necrosis may be due to inflammation, interference with the proper circulation of the part, traumatism, or chemical and thermic agencies. As a rule, when a portion of a bone dies it becomes separated from the healthy part by a zone of reactive inflammation, where resorption and exfoliation is actively going on. In such cases the necrotic portion is termed a *sequestrum*.

Halisteresis.—A striking and important retrogressive change sometimes found in bone is halisteresis, a condition in which, while the organic substance of the bone remains comparatively unaltered, there is a notable diminution in the amount of lime salts, so that the bone becomes soft and yielding. The process may be restricted to a small area in a bone, as, for instance, in the neighborhood of a tumor, or may be more widely spread throughout a whole bone, or even the greater part of the skeleton. The more extensive affection is commonly known by the name of **osteomalacia** (mollities ossium, malacosteon).[1]

The pathological changes, here, consist in the main of decalcification of the old bone, with, at the same time, a tendency to the formation of new bone, which, however, remains imperfectly calcified. The process of decalcification begins at the periphery · of the bone-trabeculæ and gradually extends to the deeper parts. The line of demarcation between the normal and the altered bone is sometimes even and continuous, or may be irregular with excavations, like Howship's lacunæ. Frequently there is formed an intermediate zone, where the lime salts are not completely absorbed but remain in the tissue in the form of a crumbling detritus preliminary to their removal. In the course of the disease the original bone canals become enlarged, and, following upon the absorption of the salts, new canals are formed in the ground substance. The matrix itself may appear to be homogeneous, or may present a finer or coarser fibrillation. Some of the bone-corpuscles may be preserved but many are atrophied or have disappeared, leaving small cavities. In some cases there is a formation of new osteoid tissue,

---

[1] For literature and complete study see Weber, Virch. Archiv, 38:1867:1; v. Recklinghausen, Naturforschervers., Braunschweig, 1897; Anschütz, Mittheil. aus d. Grenzgebiete d. Med. u. Chir., 9; Bassett, Arch. d. Med., 18:1907.

which for a long time, or perhaps permanently, remains uncalcified. This new tissue may be quite dense, containing only a few spaces, or it may present a laminated or fibrillated structure with large corpuscles. Osteoclasts and Howship's lacunæ are not more numerous than in normal bone. The condition of the marrow varies. It may be reddish, with giant cells, yellowish and fatty, gelatinous, or even fibroid. Hemorrhages and pigment are commonly found in the marrow.

As would be expected, such changes in the structure and consistence of the bones lead to marked interference with their function. The bones are no longer able to support the weight of the body or oppose muscular contractions, so that curvatures, fractures, and indentations are not uncommon. The bone becomes so soft that it is wax-like and is readily cut with the knife (*osteomalacia cerea*). In other cases resorption of the bone is so excessive that there is a huge medullary cavity with a mere shell of bone beneath the periosteum, so that the bone is light and brittle (*osteomalacia fragilis*). When the vertebral column is involved, lordosis, kyphosis, and scoliosis are frequently met with, with all that this implies. The clavicles and ribs may be much deformed, and the thorax is flattened from side to side, the anteroposterior diameter being increased. In the pelvis, owing to the weight of the body and the pressure of the femora, the acetabular regions are driven in, the pubes is pushed forward, while the promontory descends. The tuberosities of the ilia are more or less approximated. The cavity of the pelvis is thus greatly reduced, a deformity which is of the greatest importance in regard to the question of parturition. Not only is there deformity, but the bones actually shrink, so there is a double reason for the production of a contracted pelvis. In the lower extremities there is at first an exaggeration of the natural curves of the bones, but later there are more acute curvatures or twists. In the femur the greatest deformity is found just below the trochanter. Where bending or fractures have taken place there is an attempt at repair by the formation of new osteoid tissue along the concave side of the curvature or at the site of the fracture.

The true cause of osteomalacia is quite obscure. The disease is found both in the old (*senile osteomalacia*) and in the young, but is most common between the third and fourth decade. It is usually met with in women, especially in those who are pregnant (*puerperal osteomalacia*) or unusually prolific, while it is only rarely found in men. It is noteworthy that the affection is endemic in certain localities, such as the Rhine valley, Westphalia, Flanders, and northern Italy, although cases are not unknown in other parts of Europe. It appears to be rare on the North American continent, Dock[1] only finding record of ten cases. Among the direct exciting causes the most important is pregnancy, which in the majority of instances initiates the affection or leads to relapses and exacerbations.

Numerous theories have been advanced to explain the condition. Some, like v. Winckler, think that unhygienic surroundings and modes

[1] Amer. Jour. Med. Sci., 109: 1895: 449.

of life, unsuitable or poor food, insufficient clothing, repeated pregnancies, or prolonged lactation, are the important predisposing causes.
Hanau's observation, that in 25 to 30 per cent. of puerperal women,
osteophytes and osteoid tissue are present in the cranial bones, suggests
that osteomalacia, at least in puerperal cases, may be due to an exaggeration of a physiological process. That there is some connection
between the disease and the genital apparatus would seem to be indicated by the fact that it is sometimes cured by removal of the ovaries.
On these grounds Fehling has enunciated the theory that osteomalacia
is a trophoneurosis due to reflex irritation from the ovaries. In view
of the frequent existence of hyperemia of the bone-marrow, v. Recklinghausen is of the opinion that the disease is due to a local irritation and
stimulation of the bloodvessels of the bones. Virchow also believed the
condition to be of an inflammatory or hyperemic nature. Others, like
Volkmann, think that in addition to circulatory disturbances there is
some abnormality of the nerve-supply in the medulla. Examination of
the central nervous system, however, does not reveal any special evidence of this. It used to be thought, too, that an excess of lactic acid
in the blood was the cause of the solution of the calcareous salts of the
bone. It is, however, not the case that there is an excess of this substance in the blood in osteomalacia, nor has it been found possible to
produce the disease in experimental animals by feeding them with
it. Others, notably Morpurgo,[1] look for the cause in bacterial infection.

PROGRESSIVE METAMORPHOSES.

While under ordinary circumstances bone may be regarded as the most
stable and unchanging tissue of the body, waste and repair are to some
extent always going on. In the adult these two opposing processes
are almost perfectly balanced, so that for a time at least the volume
and the texture of the skeleton remain constant. On occasion, however,
regenerative processes may become more active, as, for example, in the
process of repair of bone after injuries, and sometimes result in an excess
of growth over and above the obvious needs of the organism.

Hyperplasia.—The causes underlying hyperplasia of bone are often
obscure. Some forms, such as leontiasis ossea, local and generalized
gigantism, are *congenital* and *primary,* being apparently due in the main
to excessive or disordered nutrition during prenatal existence. Much
more commonly the process is *acquired* and *secondary*. A common
example of this is the repair that takes place after fractures, and the
increase in length and thickness of bones in certain cases of inflammation and traumatism. Experimentally, increase in the length of bones
has been produced by driving ivory pegs into the growing end of the
bone. In other cases, hyperplasia seems to be due to chemical substances circulating in the blood. Thus, the exhibition of phosphorus

[1] Ziegler's Beiträge, 28:1900:620.

and arsenic (Gies,[1] Kassowitz,[2] Maas,[3] Wegner[4]) stimulates bone production in experimental animals.

In this category also may be placed those hypertrophies of the bone and soft tissues associated with disorders of internal secretion, as, for example in acromegaly. An increase in the length of the bones, particularly those of the lower extremities, is frequently observed also after castration.

Fɪɢ. 288

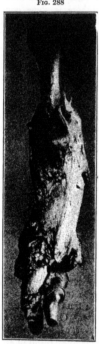

Fracture of the humerus with the formation of an enormous permanent callus. The patient from whom this specimen was taken was a lunatic, who kept his arm in almost constant motion. As a consequence, splints could not be kept properly applied. (From the Pathological Museum of McGill University.)

Prolonged passive congestion seems also to favor overgrowth of tissue, as in the clubbed fingers of those suffering from chronic pulmonary and cardiac affections.

Bony hyperplasia is sometimes also compensatory, for example, the well-known enlargement of the fibula in ununited fracture of the tibia.

The overproduction of bone may manifest itself in several ways. When a bone becomes enlarged, either as a whole or in part, the condition is termed *hyperostosis*. Again, when the density of bone is increased owing to the formation of new trabeculæ and the deposit of an excess of lime salts, so that the structure becomes more compact, we speak of *osteosclerosis*. Both conditions may be combined. Local outgrowths of bone are called *osteophytes* or *exostoses*. These may be seen in the neighborhood of inflammatory processes, and at the points of insertion of the tendons where these are subjected to excessive muscular traction. *Enostoses* are local new-formations of bone within the spongiosa. It is hard, however, in some cases to draw the line between local hyperostoses and true tumor-formation.

Callus (see vol. i, p. 612).—When a bone is fractured or splintered, as from some traumatic cause, regenerative processes are initiated in

[1] Einfluss des Arsens auf den Organismus, Arch. f. exper. Path., 8: 1877.
[2] Zeit. f. klin. Med., 7: 1884: 36.
[3] Tageblatt d. Leipsiger Naturforschervers., 1872.
[4] Ueber den Einfluss des Phosphors auf den Organismus, Virch. Archiv, 55: 1872: 11.

the periosteum and bone-marrow, which, provided that the process be not complicated by infection or senile or other cachexia, lead in the

Fig. 289

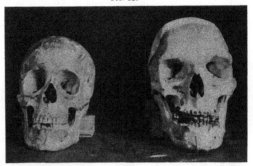

Normal skull.   Skull from a case of acromegaly. (Osborne.)

Fig. 290

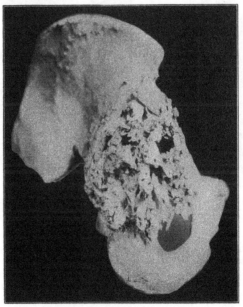

New-growth of osteophytes about the hip-joint, the result of chronic arthritis. (From the Pathological Museum of McGill University.)

course of a few weeks to consolidation and more or less perfect repair
of the injury.

In the ordinary course of events, immediately on receiving the fracture,
there are more or less tearing and bruising of the neighboring soft
tissues, together with extravasation of blood. A moderate amount of
inflammation sets in, with effusion of fluid and infiltration of leukocytes

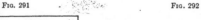

Fig. 291   Fig. 292

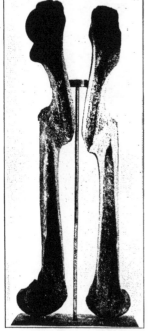 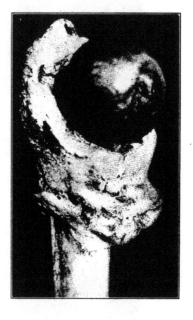

A badly-set fracture of the femur, showing
union with interruption of the central canal.
(From the Pathological Museum of McGill
University.)

Femur; ununited fracture through the great
trochanter; excessive growth of callus. (From
the Pathological Museum of McGill University.)

into the structures in the neighborhood of the injury. This subsides in
from five to six days. About the second day the cells of the periosteum
and bone-marrow show signs of proliferation in that they are enlarged
and their nuclei are undergoing karyokinesis. In the next few days
the number of the proliferating cells is greatly increased and the endothelium of the bloodvessels now begins to take part in the process,
so that about the fourth day the osteoblastic layer of the periosteum is

converted into a vascular germinal tissue. Under the microscope this consists of large polymorphous cells, containing frequent mitotic figures, embedded in a partly homogeneous, partly fibroid, stroma. After the fourth day, the germinal layer begins to be differentiated into chondroid and osteoid tissue, which, in turn, is rapidly converted into bone. After the lapse of a week, the ends of the fractured bone are embedded in a large number of young osteophytes and osteoid spicules. In this way is produced about the injured region a spindle-shaped sheath, or natural splint, called the *external callus*. A prolongation of this between the ends of the fractured portions constitutes the *intermediary callus*. Similarly, a callus is formed within the cavity of the bone, if one of the hollow bones, constituting the *internal* or *myelogenic callus*. This is produced by the osteoblasts which are grouped into masses and are transformed into osteoid and eventually into osseous tissue. In the neighborhood of the fractured portion the periosteal germinal layer may be converted in part into hyaline cartilage and in part into fibrous connective tissue, which, in time, is transformed into bone. In the course of from two to three weeks the fractured ends are more or less completely reunited. The amount of callus resulting from this process varies considerably at times, being dependent on individual idiosyncrasy, the condition of the bone, the nature of the fracture, and the amount of deformity.

In addition to the formation of new tissue, and to some extent synchronous with it, an opposite process is at work, namely, resorption. The fractured ends become somewhat rounded off and splinters of bone separated from the main mass are absorbed. The callus, which, at the end of the sixth or seventh week, consists of a rather soft and porous bony substance, is gradually converted into denser bone by means of lacunar resorption, the formation of medullary spaces, and the thickening of the trabeculæ through the agency of the osteoblasts. In this way the *permanent* or *definitive callus* is substituted for the *temporary* one. In the course of months or years, according to the amount of traumatism and deformity, the permanent callus is still farther modified. Excess bone is removed and the weak spots are strengthened until a more or less perfect return to functional, if not anatomical, integrity is complete. In severe dislocations of the parts the medullary cavity of the bone is not usually restored (Fig. 291).

The process as just described may be materially modified by certain untoward factors. Thus, infection, inflammation, or necrosis may delay the union of the fragments, or, again, the condition of senility or cachexia may prevent it. The absence of a nutrient artery in one of the portions also renders union impossible. When two bones are in close proximity and one only is broken, the resulting callus may involve the uninjured bone, producing a *synostosis*. In fractures near or involving a joint an exuberant formation of osteophytes may lead to *ankylosis* of the joint. Should the separated fragments be improperly replaced, be too far apart, or should a large amount of bone be destroyed, or, again, should muscle or fascia intervene, the parts may fail to unite. Should the fragments be united immovably by fibrous tissue, the condition is known as *patho-*

logical syndesmosis. In other cases fibrous union takes place, leading to the establishment of a false joint, *pseudarthrosis.* In still other cases a true joint, with a more or less perfect approximation to the ball and socket type with a capsule, may be formed—*nearthrosis.*

As might be expected, the process of healing is completed more quickly in children, taking place in from two to three weeks in those under two years of age, while in adults it may take six to eight weeks. As we have already seen, it may be much prolonged and even fail to occur.

FIG. 293

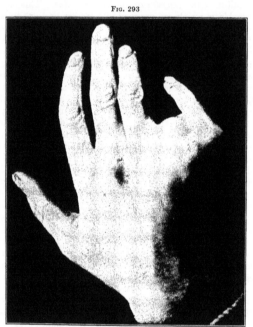

Spindle-celled periosteal sarcoma of the hand. (From the surgical clinic of the Montreal General Hospital.)

Tumors.—The tumors that develop primarily in the bones belong to the connective-tissue group and originate from the periosteum, the bone-marrow, or the cartilage. In accordance with their genesis they assume the type of **fibroma, myxoma, lipoma, angioma, chondroma, osteoma, myeloma, sarcoma,** and various admixtures thereof. The secondary tumors are usually forms of **carcinoma.**

Like that of tumor-growth generally, the etiology of the neoplasms of bone is somewhat obscure. Traumatism, however, such as a fracture or blow, seems to play a relatively important part (callus tumors), as does also inflammation. Irregularities in ossification were believed by Virchow to account for the chondromas, especially those arising in the neighborhood of the epiphyseal sutures.

The primary tumors are usually solitary, but occasionally assume the form of multiple, isolated, and independent growths. The presence of tumors in bones, especially when of the malignant type, leads usually to considerable lacunar resorption of the structure, so that the bone may become greatly deformed. Besides this, there is often a production of new bone from the periosteum, owing to the stimulation of the osteogenetic layer, with the result that the new-growth may be more or less completely enclosed within a bony shell. Not only so, the cells of the

FIG. 294

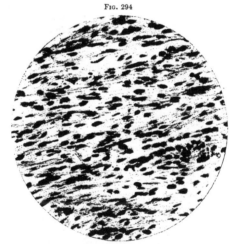

Spindle-celled sarcoma of the periosteum. Winckel obj. No. 6, without ocular. (From the collection of Dr. A. G. Nicholls.)

tumors and of their supporting stroma show a peculiar liability to undergo metaplasia into bone, and a more or less perfect osseous framework may be produced within the growth. Sarcomas and carcinomas are most likely to manifest this tendency. The ground substance in some cases also undergoes petrifaction.

Sarcoma.[1]—The most important and frequent of the primary tumors of bones is the sarcoma. Of this there are two varieties, the *central* and the *peripheral*.[2] The former are rapidly growing tumors which tend to produce great rarefaction and expansion of the shaft of the affected

[1] Buerger, Surgery, Gynecology, and Obstetrics, Oct., 1909 : 431; also Amer. Jour. Med. Sci., 142:1910.

[2] Ribbert, Beiträge z. Entstehung der Geschwülste, 1906.

bone. Microscopically, they are giant-celled, round-celled, spindle-celled, and alveolar. They are dealt with more at length elsewhere (see p. 234 et seq.).

The peripheral sarcomas are usually of spindle- or mixed-celled type, but occasionally are composed of round cells. They may be found in any part of the skeleton, but are most frequent near the ends of the long bones, in the upper maxilla, and on the shoulder girdle. The denser forms are closely allied to the fibromas, and the two conditions may pass almost imperceptibly one into the other. The term *epulis* is applied clinically to either a fibrous or fibrosarcomatous periosteal new-growth in the buccal or nasal cavities.

Peripheral sarcomas arise at first on one side of the bone, and tend gradually to envelop it. The underlying bone becomes rarefied and destroyed, or may, on the contrary, be transformed into very dense tissue. These tumors frequently produce bone in the form of plates and spicules of osteoid tissue without calcification (*osteoid sarcoma*). In other cases a denser anastomosing framework of bony processes is produced from which finer spicules and plates grow out in a radiating manner into the substance of the softer tissues (*osteosarcoma, ossifying sarcoma*). Cartilaginous and sarcomatous growths may be combined (*chondrosarcoma*), or cartilage, bone, and sarcoma (*chondroösteosarcoma*).

An important clinical type is the *giant-celled sarcoma*, which originates on the alveolar process or in the antrum of Highmore. It is small, firm, and relatively slow growing, and is one of the least malignant forms of the sarcomas, since when removed it does not always recur. The relationships of this form have been discussed in vol. i, p. 733.

Macroscopically, it is dense and fibrous and of sessile form. On section it is of a brick-red color, owing to the fact that hemorrhage into its substance is common. Microscopically, it consists of fibrous tissue, with masses of spindle and multinucleated giant cells.

The **myeloma** (**myelomatosis**) is a peculiar and interesting blastomatoid formation, described at length elsewhere (p. 235 and vol. i, p. 734).

Osteoma.—Of the benign growths, perhaps the commonest is the osteoma. It is not always possible to draw the line between osteophytes and hyperostoses of inflammatory origin and tumors proper. The true osteomas are usually found in early childhood or during the developmental period of life, and may even be inherited. Especially when the exostoses are multiple, or derived from cartilage, it is likely that they are due to some aberration in the growth of the skeleton, for in such cases other disturbances of development are apt to be present. Osteomas are formed from the periosteum (*exostoses*) or from the bone-marrow (*enostoses*). They may arise also by metaplasia from fibrous tissue or cartilage.

According to their structure, osteomas may be divided into two forms, one composed of dense compact bone—*osteoma eburneum;* the other formed of cancellous bone—*osteoma spongiosum*. Small exostoses are rounded, conical, nodular, or fungoid in appearance, while the larger ones are bulbous, warty, irregular, or even pectinate. The fibrous exostoses develop especially in connection with the bones of the skull and the flat bones of the trunk, and the cartilaginous ones at the diaphyseal ends of the long bones. Occasionally, in the case of exostoses near a joint one sees a closed membranous sac resembling a bursa, and structurally similar to the synovial membrane, associated with the tumor (*exostosis bursata*). This, rarely, contains free bodies, and is supposed to be derived from the cartilage of the joint or a misplaced "rest."

The enostoses are found most frequently in the diploë of the calvarium and in the bones of the face.

Fig. 295

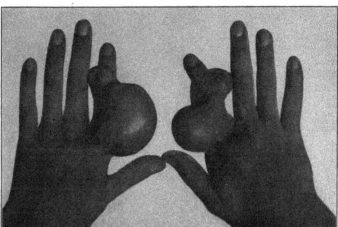

Multiple chondromas. (From the surgical clinic of the Montreal General Hospital.)

Chondroma.—Chondromas are lobulated tumors, composed usually of hyaline cartilage, and are enveloped in a fibrous capsule which sends prolongations into the substance of the growth. They are usually due to some disturbance in the development of the growing bone whereby portions of the primitive cartilage become displaced. They may originate in the periosteum and medulla as well as from the cartilage. According to their position on the surface of the bone or within its interior, we may make a division analogous to that of the osteomas, into *ecchondromas* and *enchondromas*. They are found most frequently in children and young growing persons, and may be congenital. As a rule, they are multiple, and are met with most commonly on the bones of the hands and lower extremities, less frequently on the trunk, and still more rarely on the calvarium. They are particularly liable to undergo retrogressive manifestations, such as fatty and mucinous degeneration (*myxochondroma*) calcification, and liquefaction, with the formation of cysts. Metaplasia into bone not infrequently takes place (*osteoid-chondroma, osteochondroma*). Sarcomatous transformation is also rather apt to occur (*chondrosarcoma; osteochondrosarcoma*) which may be associated with metastasis. Simple chrondromas, it should be remembered, may occasionally produce metastases also. In this case the secondary growths reproduce all the features of the primary growth, but do not tend to invade or destroy the neighboring tissues.

Fibroma.—Fibromas are derived from the periosteum, or, more rarely, from the bone-marrow. They are found most frequently in connection with the bones of the face and skull. Those occurring in the nasal and buccal cavities form one variety of nasopharyngeal polyps and of the growths known clinically as epulis. They are met with less commonly on the bones of the trunk and still more rarely in the extremities.

Fig. 296.

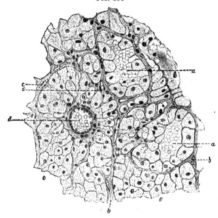

Section from a hemangio-endothelioma of bone. *a*, large vascular spaces filled with erythrocytes and surrounded by large, clear, cubical endothelial cells, which in parts, as at *e*, form solid masses; *b*, stroma; *d*, larger and *c*, smaller bloodvessels. (Driessen.)

Fibromas form nodular tumors of varying consistency, which under the microscope may be densely fibrous or more cellular, so that they may not be easily distinguished from sarcomas, into which they imperceptibly merge. Occasionally, they are more vascular and contain large blood channels and spaces (*fibroma teleangiectaticum*). Again, they may undergo metaplasia into bone (*osteofibroma, ossifying fibroma*).

Myxoma and Fibromyxoma.—Myxoma and fibromyxoma are, on the whole, rare. They originate from the periosteum or bone-marrow. They frequently undergo liquefaction, and may form bone (*osteomyxoma*), or, again, present sarcomatous transformation (*myxosarcoma*). They may be single or multiple.

Lipoma.—Lipomas are extremely rare. They have been known to arise from the periosteum, and are often associated with striated muscle fibres (Sutton).

Angioma.—Pure angiomas are also excessively rare, but have been described in connection with the vertebræ (Virchow), the calvarium, femur, sternum, and palate (Péan). Combinations of angioma with endothelioma, chondroma, and osteoma have also been recorded.

The secondary tumors of bone are the **carcinoma** and **sarcoma**. The latter are rare and usually of the *melanotic variety*. The *perithelial angiosarcomas*, more especially those of the thyroid, kidney, and suprarenal, are particularly liable to produce metastases in the bones which take the form of vascular pulsating growths, strongly suggesting aneurisms.

Fig. 297

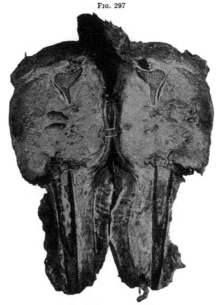

Secondary carcinoma of the head of the humerus. (From the Pathological Museum of McGill University.)

Carcinoma arises by the direct extension of a carcinoma of the adjacent soft parts or by metastasis, and forms either a *diffuse infiltration* or a *nodular* growth. Metastatic carcinoma is said to be most frequently secondary to carcinoma of the breast, prostate, thyroid, and bronchi. The bones involved, according to v. Recklinghausen, are, in order of frequency, the vertebræ, femur, ribs, sternum, humerus, and cranium. The secondary deposits are usually to be found in those parts of the bones which are subject to the greatest traction or pressure. Retrograde metastasis to the head of the humerus is occasionally met with in carcinoma of the breast.

Carcinomatous infiltration is usually associated with a marked proliferation of the periosteum and bone-marrow, while the bone itself undergoes lacunar resorption and finally disintegration. Occasionally, the process of lacunar resorption is associated with the formation of new osteoid tissue devoid of lime salts (*carcinomatous osteomalacia*) or true bone. In this case the medullary spaces of the osteoid or bony substance are infiltrated with carcinoma cells.

Cysts.[1]—Cysts are sometimes due to softening of portions of solid tumors, as the chondroma, myxoma, and sarcoma. Colliquative cysts are sometimes also found in osteomalacia, arthritis, and ostitis deformans. Most cases are associated with periostitis or ostitis. Rarer factors are hematoma, aneurism, cholesteatoma, and parasites.

True cystomas are rare except the variety known as the **dentigerous cystoma** found in the maxilla. This is supposed to originate in the misplaced matrix of a tooth.

THE JOINTS AND CARTILAGES.

A joint, or diarthrosis, is an association of two or more bones in such a way that, while they are closely approximated and held together by a capsule, they are separated by a space so as to permit a certain amount of movement. The capsule is composed of dense, unyielding, fibrous tissue, lined by a soft, thin, and vascular membrane covered with flattened cells, known as the synovial membrane. The cavity contains a small quantity of limpid fluid, the synovia.

Pathological changes affecting the joints may originate in the synovial sac and extend to the articular cartilage, the ends of the bones, and even to the surrounding soft tissues, or arise by extension from the neighboring structures. They are important in that they may produce functional disability through pain, deranged mechanism, or limitation of movement.

CONGENITAL ANOMALIES.

The anomalies of development occurring in the joints are practically those of the bones themselves. When certain bones are absent or abnormal the associated joints are necessarily affected. Of interest from the point of view of orthopedic surgery are such conditions as **genu valgum** and **varum, morbus coxæ, club-foot, spinal curvatures,** and **dislocations.** Some, at least, of the cases of club-foot appear to be due to antenatal affections of the spinal cord, *e. g.,* anterior poliomyelitis. Genu valgum is occasionally a stigma of general infantilism.

[1] See Bloodgood, Annals of Surgery, 44:1910:145.

Congenital Luxation.—Congenital luxation most frequehtly involves the hip-joint. It is due to hypoplasia of the acetabulum and head of the femur, or to abnormal positions of the limbs and excessive pressure during intra-uterine life.[1]

CIRCULATORY DISTURBANCES.

These are comparatively unimportant. **Active hyperemia** is met with in the early stages of inflammation. **Passive hyperemia** occurs under the same conditions as elsewhere.

{ Fɪɢ. 298

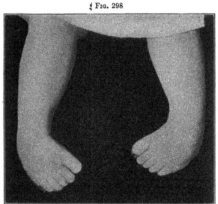

Double club-foot (talipes varus). (From the surgical clinic of the Montreal General Hospital.)

Hemorrhage into a joint cavity is usually due to trauma, such as a sprain, contusion, dislocation, or fracture. It may also occur in the hemorrhagic diatheses and as a neuropathic manifestation. Small effusions quickly disappear, larger ones are partly absorbed, and the remaining portions are substituted by fibrous tissue derived from the proliferation of the cells of the synovial membrane. The cells lining the synovial sac also proliferate and may extend over the clot. In severe cases the clot may not be entirely absorbed and may break loose, forming one variety of "floating body" in the joint. Not infrequently, considerable reactive inflammation is set up, leading to the production of adhesions and fibrous ankylosis.

INFLAMMATIONS.

Inflammation of the joints may involve first and chiefly the synovial membrane—**synovitis**—the cartilages—**chondritis**—etc. In severe cases not only the joint, but the bones and soft tissues may be involved—**osteitis** and **periarthritis**.

[1] For literature see Joachimsthal, Enzyk. Jahrb. v. Eulenberg, 2:1904.

Acute Arthritis and Synovitis.—These disorders may be produced by direct *trauma* or the *extension* of inflammatory processes from structures near the joints.   In many cases there is a *hematogenic* origin. As examples of the first form, punctured wounds, gunshot injuries, and the like may be cited; of the second, the joint changes in infective osteomyelitis; of the third, the polyarthritis of acute inflammatory rheumatism.   The hematogenic forms are in the vast majority of cases due to infective microörganisms, and are found in such conditions as inflammatory rheumatism, septicemia, gonorrhœa, scarlatina, measles, typhoid fever, pneumonia, erysipelas, and dysentery.   In the diseases

FIG. 299

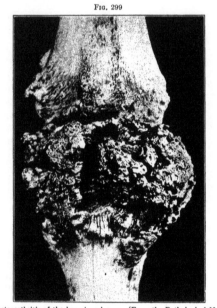

Chronic osteoarthritis of the knee in a horse.   (From the Pathological Museum McGill University.)

just mentioned, the inflammation of the joints is in some cases due to the specific microörganism of the disease in question, but not infrequently to secondary infection with pus-producing cocci.

In the milder grades of inflammation, and in the early stages of the severe forms, the synovial membrane is congested and swollen, especially about the folds, and there may be occasional small extravasations of blood, with exudation of thin yellowish fluid containing a few delicate flocculi of fibrin (**serous synovitis, hydrops articuli**).   This form is apt to be lighted up by trauma, such as sprains or contusions, floating bodies

in the joints, and occurs also in the lighter grades of inflammatory rheumatism, gonorrhœa, and osteomyelitis. Swelling of the joint results,
with possibly some redness. In more severe cases the exudate is more
abundantly fibrinous (**synovitis serofibrinosa**), and in some instances
the exudate may be mainly fibrin, with but little fluid (**synovitis fibrinosa
sive sicca**). In other cases the effusion may become purulent or may
have been purulent from the start (**synovitis purulenta, empyæma articuli**).
Here the synovial membrane is thickened and swollen, infiltrated
with inflammatory products, and covered with a fibrinopurulent or
purulent deposit, while the cavity of the joint contains a variable quantity
of turbid fluid. In the severest forms the synovial membrane may be
partially destroyed, and the articular cartilages undergo fatty degeneration, fibrillation, and ultimately necrosis. The whole joint may in time
become disorganized (**panarthritis purulenta**). The process frequently
extends to the exposed ends of the bones, the soft tissues, and along the
lymphatics. The pus may burrow widely along the lines of least resistance, and general infection may be set up. ·Osteomyelitis or lymphangitic abscesses sometimes also result. This form is the one most
commonly seen as a complication of pyemia, measles, scarlatina, and
puerperal infection.

Acute synovitis and arthritis frequently heal, leaving little or no
trace, or may pass on into a chronic condition. Not infrequently,
where there has been necrosis of the structures composing the joint,
more or less fibrous proliferation takes place in the process of repair,
and osteophytic outgrowths may form about the joints, so that ankylosis
occasionally results.

A peculiar form of polyarthritis is occasionally met with in children,
which is apparently of an infective nature. It runs a low febrile course,
and the joint manifestations are accompanied by enlargement of the
lymph-nodes and spleen. It is known as **Still's disease.**

Arthritis Urica.—Arthritis urica (**gout, podagra**) is a form of acute
inflammation due to the deposit in the joint and adjacent structures
of salts of uric acid, together with phosphate and carbonate of lime
and hippuric acid. These salts are precipitated in the form of fine
needles and granules, not only in the cells and matrix of the cartilages,
but also in the synovial membranes, ligaments, and soft tissues. This
leads to irritation and inflammatory infiltration, with the exudation
of a serous fluid into the joint. The metatarsophalangeal joint of the
great toe is first involved, but other joints, as those of the fingers, hands,
and knees, may be involved. It is characteristic of the disease that
it tends to relapse and in time leads to chronic changes in the joints
Between the acute paroxysms the pain and swelling subside, but the
chalk-like deposit still remains upon the cartilages. In severe or prolonged cases the articular cartilages eventually undergo necrosis and
disintegrate, the synovial membrane becomes thickened, and the salts
may be deposited in such quantities as to form concretions (*chalk-
stones, tophi*). The tendons, periosteum, and bones may be similarly
involved. The deposit may be so great that the soft parts necrose

and the chalk presents externally.   Ulceration and abscess-formation
are common.   While the joint-changes constitute a striking picture
in the disease, they form only one aspect of the affection, which is a
systemic one, due to disordered metabolism.   Arterial sclerosis, digestive
disorders, skin eruptions, and degenerative changes in the kidneys
are frequent accompaniments.

Chronic Inflammations.—In the present state of our knowledge it is
impossible to make an entirely satisfactory classification of the chronic
morbid processes affecting the joints.   There are, it is true, certain
broad generalizations which enable us to differentiate anatomically
several forms in a rough way, but all possible combinations and intermediate gradations exist.   Moreover, we are often in the dark as to the
etiological factors at work in certain cases, and even when these are
known, they at times give rise to widely differing anatomical pictures.

In general we may, perhaps, divide these processes into the *inflammatory* and the *degenerative*.   The former group includes those due to all
forms of infection, traumatism, gout, and toxic causes.   The latter
embraces the senile and neurotrophic forms.   Inasmuch as in the second
group the inflammatory features are comparatively trifling and, indeed,
sometimes in abeyance, it is open to debate whether they are properly
to be regarded as inflammatory or whether they should not be classed
with the retrogressive metamorphoses.   The leading forms will be
found in the accompanying table:

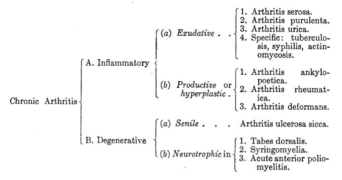

Chronic Serous Arthritis.—Chronic serous arthritis is a somewhat
sluggish disease characterized by the effusion of a thin serous exudate.
The affection results from an acute or, more often, a recurring synovitis.
The knee is attacked most frequently, and next, the shoulders, hips,
and elbows.   The lesions may be bilateral or unilateral.   The effusion
in some instances may be so great that the synovial membrane is forced
out through the fibres of the capsule in the form of hernial protrusions.
The changes in the synovial membrane and the cartilages are often
comparatively trifling, but in long-standing cases the capsule may be-

come thickened and the cartilages fibrillated. The folds and fringes of the synovial membrane are enlarged and vascularized, and sometimes extend as a pannus (*synovitis pannosa* sive *prolifera*) over the articular surfaces. The affection frequently follows exposure to cold in those of a rheumatic tendency, but often also traumatism, as in contusions, sprains, and the incarceration of synovial fringes or free bodies in the joint.

Chronic Suppurative Arthritis.—Chronic suppurative arthritis results from hematogenic infection, traumatism; or the extension of disease from the adjacent parts. The cavity of the joint is filled with purulent or seropurulent fluid, and there is a deposit of fibrin and pus on the synovial membrane and the surface of the cartilages. The cartilages show cloudiness, fibrillation, and various grades of degeneration, amounting sometimes to necrosis. The synovial membrane and the capsule are infiltrated with inflammatory products. Not infrequently, the inflammation extends to the bone and the surrounding soft tissues. In this way caries and necrosis may be brought about and abscess-formation in the capsule and its neighborhood. Healing takes place by the exfoliation of dead bone and cartilage, the absorption of the exudate and its discharge, the production of new bone from the periosteum and bone-marrow. Fibrous and bony ankylosis not infrequently result.

Chronic Gouty Arthritis.—Chronic gouty arthritis has been sufficiently referred to in discussing the acute form.

Arthritis ankylopoetica chronica is a peculiar anatomical form of arthritis due to various etiological causes. The main features are the formation of adhesions between the cartilages with vascularization and fibrous transformation of the cartilages. The condition may result from acute exudative inflammation, and tuberculosis or other chronic destructive affections.

In the early stages the synovial membrane is somewhat injected and thickened, while the surface of the cartilages is rough and fibrillated. The cartilages are here and there vascularized and the opposing surfaces are more or less adherent. The deeper layers of the cartilages are also gradually converted into medullary spaces through resorption brought about by the encroachment of the subchondral medullary substance. Some of the islets of cartilage thus isolated may in time be converted into bone. Thus, the cartilages are gradually transformed into a vascular fibrous or fibroösseous tissue. The joint cavity is traversed by dense fibrous bands and is converted into a number of small spaces, bounded by dense fibrous tissue and containing synovial fluid. In very advanced cases the whole of the articular cartilage may disappear and be replaced by fibrous tissue, so that the original structure of the joint becomes well-nigh unrecognizable. Not only so, but the newly formed fibrous tissue may in time be converted into a mass of spongy bone and complete osseous ankylosis result.

Polyarthritis Chronica Rheumatica.—The disease commonly known as chronic rheumatism, or polyarthritis chronica rheumatica, is of somewhat uncertain etiology. It is found commonly in old persons, and may result from repeated attacks of acute rheumatism or may come on insidiously. It usually begins in the phalanges or metacarpal and carpal bones, but the larger joints, such as the knees and ankles, are not infrequently involved. The disease is usually steadily progressive, chronic in its course, occasionally with acute exacerbations, and leads to more or less limitation of movement. Proliferation of bone is rather marked, so that the affection presents a close resemblance to arthritis deformans.

Arthritis Deformans.—Arthritis deformans (rheumatoid arthritis, rheumatic gout, arthrite séche) is a rather common disease of the joints, characterized, on the one hand, by degenerative changes in the articular cartilages and bone, and, on the other, by a marked production of new bone. The disease may be monarticular, but is more usually polyarticular. It has been known to follow repeated traumatic insults, fractures, or infectious disease, or, rarely, is spontaneous. The affection begins usually in the third decade of life or later, and may run a chronic course for many years, with occasional acute exacerbations. It has been known, however, to attack young children.[1] Women are more commonly affected than men (1 to 5). The etiology is quite obscure. Some have regarded it as neuropathic in nature, on the analogy of Charcot's joints. This is supported by the fact that muscular wasting, contractures, glossiness of the skin, and paresthesiæ are frequently observed. Others regard it as a degenerative process, a mark of actual or premature senility. Certain recent observers have found in the synovial fluid of these cases cocci, which they, on experimental grounds, believe to be specific. The proof of this, however, is not as yet conclusive. Considering the fact that certain cases begin acutely or present acute exacerbations, it is not impossible that some at least are infective in nature. The close relationship to gout, which used to be insisted upon, is now no longer accepted. Lately, the view has been advanced that arthritis deformans is due to a toxin of enterogenous nature.

Anatomically, the lesions produced may be summed up as degeneration of the cartilages, together with the formation of new bone-marrow and osteophytes. Considerable deformity of the joints results, with more or less complete limitation of movement. The superficial layers of the articular cartilages become fibrillated and fissured, while in the deeper parts there are areas of necrosis and softening. Further, owing to some stimulation, the bone-marrow begins to proliferate and a new vascularized marrow invades the deeper layers of the cartilage and grows into the degenerated areas just referred to. The intervening cartilage that remains is gradually converted into osteoid tissue and eventually into bone. Sometimes there is an overgrowth of the cartilage, leading to the formation of nodular excrescences, which may in time project into the medullary spaces. Coincidently with the changes just described, the joint capsules and the synovial membranes become

---

[1] Nicholls, Rheumatoid Arthritis in Young Children, Montreal Medical Journal, 25: 1896–97: 97.

PLATE XV

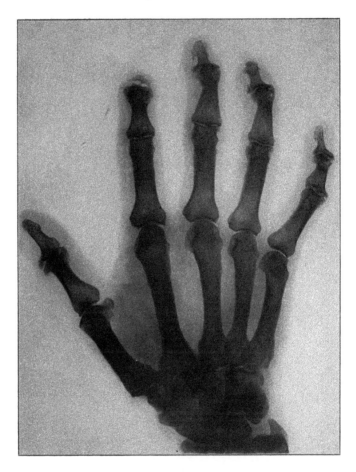

**X-ray Photograph of the Hand, showing the changes in the
bones resulting from rheumatoid arthritis.**

The dislocation of the phalanges with erosion and osteophytic
outgrowths are well seen.

(From Dr. Finley's Clinic, Montreal General Hospital.)

thickened. Occasionally, the folds and fringes of the latter encroach upon the joint cavity and are infiltrated with fat, forming the so-called *lipoma arborescens*. Small portions of the altered synovial membrane may be converted into cartilage or bone. Should these break loose, they form free bodies in the joint. In the bone itself noteworthy changes take place, in the form of resorption of the trabeculæ, resulting in considerable loss of substance and alterations in the shape of the bone.

Fig. 300

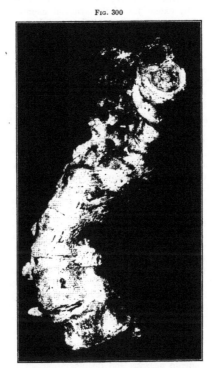

Spondylitis deformans; curvature of the spine, with ankylosis due to subperiosteal osteogenesis. (Pathological Museum, McGill University.)

In course of time the newly formed osteoid tissue in its turn undergoes similar retrogressive changes. The marrow of that part of the bone near the joint loses much of its fat and is converted into gelatinous or lymphoid marrow. If the resorption of the bone be extensive, it may be more or less substituted by gelatinous fibrous tissue. In other cases the marrow softens and liquefies, producing small cysts. The tissues bounding these cysts may proliferate and produce new bone by metaplasia.

In course of time extensive changes in the size and contour of the bone take place., In the case of the hip-joint, for example, the neck of the femur is more or less shortened, the head is enlarged, and nodular excrescences or osteophytes form about it and around the edge of the acetabulum. Where the cartilage is completely absorbed the exposed bone, owing to pressure and friction, becomes flattened, smooth, and eburnated. Where cysts in the bone are laid bare by erosion, irregular grooves and depressions are formed and the bony surfaces not in contact are covered by extensions of the synovial membranes. In this way marked deformity of the articulations results. Ankylosis is a common event due to thickening of the capsule and the formation of bony outgrowths in the capsule and along the edge of the bone. A common deformity is the ulnar deflection seen in the fingers. Dislocations of various kinds occur.

Arthritis deformans oftenest attacks the hip-joint and the knees, but is frequently found in the shoulders and elbows and in the smaller joints of the hands and feet. When the vertebral column is involved the condition is known as *spondylitis deformans*. This often leads to bowing of the trunk forward, with limitation of movement.

Arthritis Chronica Ulcerosa Sicca.—Arthritis chronica ulcerosa sicca, or **senile arthritis,** is in some ways not unlike arthritis deformans, but the degenerative side of the process is more marked while the proliferation of bone and cartilage is less obtrusive. As its name implies, it is found in advanced life, and is to be regarded as a degenerative process resulting from deficient nutrition. It occasionally follows rheumatic and other inflammatory disturbances, and has been known to occur where the bones have been kept for a long time in one position. In other cases it is a neurotrophic disturbance. Most commonly the hip-joint is affected (*morbus coxæ senilis*), but the shoulder, elbow, finger-joints, and patella may be attacked.

The lesions found consist in fibrillation and fissuring of the articular cartilages with some superficial erosion. At the periphery, where the synovial membrane is attached, the cartilage undergoes gelatinous and fibrous transformation, and may even disappear. In advanced cases the whole of the articular cartilages may be lost, so that the underlying bone is laid bare. This in turn may be eroded, or become compacted and eburnated. The capsules and synovial membranes are frequently thickened, leading to capsular ankylosis. Occasionally, instead of this, the fibrous bands undergo necrosis and disintegration. Calcification and amyloid transformation are sometimes to be noticed in the degenerating cartilage, in the fibrous capsule, and adhesions.

Tuberculosis.—Tuberculous arthritis, in so far as the clinical features are concerned, may occur as a primary disease. In this case the infection is hematogenic in origin. How this is brought about is not clear, but it is possible that the bacilli of tuberculosis may enter at some point in the respiratory or alimentary tracts, and, without causing a local lesion at the point of invasion, may on occasion be carried to some distant point, as, for instance, a joint. It is much more probable, however, that there is some local focus, either obvious or concealed, from which the infection proceeds. As has been demonstrated conclusively by the experiments of Schüller and Krause, among others, a slight injury to a bone or joint will determine the localization of the germs at that point. In the majority of cases, two-thirds according to Krause and König, the affection of the joints arises by the extension of previously existing tuberculous disease of the bones. In discussing tuberculosis of bone, it was pointed out that the disease most frequently occurs at the ends near the epiphyseal junction, so that involvement of the joint is readily brought about. In other cases it is probable that infection takes place by way of the lymphatics. The progress of the affection is characteristically sluggish, and, while often unattended by distressing subjective symptoms, may in time lead to destruction and complete disorganization of the joint. The disease is preëminently one of the developmental period of life, for, according to Gibney, about 84 per cent. of cases are found in persons under fourteen years of age.

· It usually begins by the production of minute tubercles, which in course of time increase considerably in size and number. In **acute miliary tuberculosis** of the synovial membrane, which is but one mani- festation out of many of a systemic distribution of the bacilli, comparatively few tubercles may be produced, and there may be little or no inflammatory reaction of any moment in the joint.

In other cases, where the foci are more numerous, the synovial membrane is reddened, swollen, infiltrated with inflammatory products, and is converted into a soft grayish-red granulation tissue containing abundant tubercles (**arthritis granulosa**). There is frequently an exudation into the joint cavity of a serous (*hydrops articuli tuberculosus*), serofibrinous, fibrinopurulent, or purulent exudate (*empyæma tuberculosum*). More or less abundant shreds and flakes of fibrin cover the granulation, and the so-called "rice-bodies" (*corpora oryzoidea*) may be found in the joint. These bodies are smooth, soft, and rather elastic, of a gelatinous, whitish or grayish-white appearance. On section they present a concentric lamination. They are supposed to be derived from fibrin or bits of synovial fringe that have become detached and have undergone hyaline degeneration. The synovial membrane may undergo a simple inflammatory proliferation and may extend into the joint in the form of folds or villi of an œdematous or gelatinous appearance. Or, again, there may be papillary or polypoid thickenings of the membrane. Tubercles situated beneath the synovial membrane may in the course of their growth invade the cavity of the joint (**arthritis nodosa** or **tuberosa**). In other cases the tubercles are extremely minute, perhaps not visible to the naked eye, and the membrane is only slightly thickened. A layer of vascular granulation tissue is formed from the synovial sac and spreads gradually over the articular surfaces, converting the cartilage into connective tissue (*synovitis pannosa*). In cases where the granulation tissue extends to the cartilages and remains in contact with them, disintegration and absorption of the cartilage takes place, with destruction of the cartilage cells and the invasion of the cell capsules with inflammatory leukocytes. Later, the cartilage may be invaded by vessels; and undergoes a patchy and mucinous degeneration or is converted into loose fibrous tissue. Simultaneously, resorption of the neighboring bone may take place. The advancing layer of the granulation tissue encroaches upon the interior at the edge of the cartilages, gradually dissecting them away from the deeper structures and finally extending to the bone and the medullary cavity. The medullary substance loses its fat and is converted into a vascular lymphoid marrow.

As a consequence of these changes, the joint becomes enlarged and presents a pale, smooth, rather shiny appearance (*white swelling*). Sooner or later, the process extends from the cartilage and bone to the surrounding soft tissues. Caseous nodules are formed which coalesce and break down into tuberculous or "cold" abscesses. These may enlarge and burrow their way to the surface, and fistulæ result. The joint may be disorganized to such an extent that dislocation of the bones takes place. When the process tends to heal, numerous osteophytes are produced in the neighborhood of the diseased part, and fibrous or fibroösseous ankylosis may result.

Comparatively few bacilli are to be found in the effusion, but it is usually possible to produce tuberculosis in susceptible animals by the injection of the fluid. Further, as the studies of Lartigau have demonstrated, bacilli may be detected in a joint, even where the disease has apparently healed, and may be of a comparatively high grade of virulence. Thus, the disease may be disseminated to distant parts or break out again after months or years. The joints usually affected are the hip, vertebræ, knee, ankle, shoulder, elbow, tarsus, and carpus.

Syphilis.—In congenital syphilis an **exudative arthritis**, associated with thickening of the capsule and disintegration of the cartilages, occurs as a primary affection or follows osteochondritis. **Gummas** in neighboring parts may extend to the joint.

In acquired syphilis the joint changes may appear during the period of eruption or in the later stages. In the first event there is produced a **diffuse serous synovitis**, not unlike that of acute rheumatism. Rarely, a similar state of things may be observed in late syphilis, but it is more common to find **gummatous infiltration** of the capsule with thickening of the capsule and synovial sheath, together with erosion and fibrillation of the cartilages. These changes may be primary or may be secondary to specific inflammation of the periosteum and bone-marrow.

Actinomycosis.—Primary actinomycosis of the joints is unknown. The affection usually arises by metastasis or extension from neighboring parts. The cervical vertebræ, the elbow, the tibiotarsal, and hip-joint have been found involved.

Neuropathic Joints.—The neurotrophic changes in joints are of considerable clinical interest and importance. They are found chiefly in tabes dorsalis (**Charcot's joints**), syringomyelia, anterior poliomyelitis, compression and destruction of the spinal cord, and after the severance of nerves. As a rule, the condition comes on quickly, without pain, and leads to great enlargement of the joints, owing to the accumulation of fluid within the synovial sac. Degenerative changes are in excess and quickly bring about disintegration of the joint. Besides this, there are atrophy of the ends of the bones, and sometimes osteoporosis, with erosion and thickening of the membranes. Spontaneous luxation is common. In tabes, the lesion is found chiefly in the lower extremities, in the knee or

Fig. 301

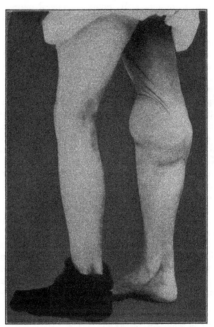

Charcot's joint. The illustration shows also very well the hyperextension of the leg on the thigh from laxness of the joint. (From the Medical Clinic of the Montreal General Hospital.)

hip, but the shoulder, elbow, and smaller joints of the hands and feet do not escape. The condition is single or multiple. In syringomyelia the lesion occurs chiefly in the upper extremities, depending upon the site of the disease in the cord.

Parasites.—*Echinococcus* disease may invade the joints from the neighboring parts.

RETROGRESSIVE METAMORPHOSES.

Degenerative changes may affect the articular surfaces or the investing membranes.

Degeneration. — Fatty Degeneration. — Fatty degeneration of the cartilages is not uncommon. It occurs in general marasmus and as a senile change, in interference with the circulation, and in inflammation. The fat-globules are deposited within the cells.

Hyaline Degeneration.—In hyaline degeneration the capsule may be involved as well as the cartilage and its cells. The cartilage is converted into a homogeneous semitranslucent mass, or breaks up into flakes.

Amyloid transformation is also met with.

Mucoid Degeneration.—The so-called mucoid degeneration is a peculiar change found principally in the costal cartilages of old persons and also upon the articular surfaces of the long bones. The cement substance of the cartilage liquefies and the fibrillæ of the matrix are dissociated or separated into bundles, giving the cartilage a curious fibrillated structure. In advanced cases the cartilage may break up into clumps or fine granular detritus. The cartilage cells are in part destroyed, but those remaining proliferate, so that small clusters may be seen lying within the same limiting membrane. At first the tissue is gray and transparent, but later becomes streaked, opaque, or, if calcification occur, dense and white. The softening may proceed to such a degree that cysts filled with fluid are formed. The process of softening is frequently met with in old age, and is an important feature in connection with chronic arthritis. If the degenerated areas are near the medullary cavity or the perichondrium, vessels may grow into them with proliferation of cells, so that the destroyed parts are substituted by fibrous tissue, bone-marrow, and eventually, in some cases, with bone. Besides the mucinous changes, cartilage may undergo a retrograde metaplasia into fibrocartilage and fibrous tissue. This is common in connection with chronic inflammation.

Necrosis and Caries.—Necrosis and caries of the cartilage occur with suppurative and other forms of inflammation.

Pigmentation.—Pigmentation of the cartilages is usually due to the absorption of the hematoidin from blood effused within the cavity.

Ochronosis is a peculiar and rare condition, in which the cartilage assumes a brownish or blackish hue. The cause is unknown.

Infiltration.—In gout there is a deposit within the cartilages and the capsule of needles of **urates**.

Calcium carbonate and **phosphate** are often precipitated in the cartilages in old age, and as a result of the previously mentioned degenerative processes.

The capsule of the joints may undergo all the degenerative changes just described as affecting the cartilage.

INJURIES AND THEIR REPAIR.

When a cartilage is injured there is invariably more or less degeneration of the specific cells in the form of swelling, vacuolation, albuminous and fatty degeneration, and even necrosis. The regenerative power of cartilage is slight, and only in rare cases and in young persons is new cartilage formed. In the event of fracture, restoration is brought about by proliferation of the cells of the perichondrium producing fibrous tissue and bone. In the case of the articular cartilages, any loss of substance is, as a rule, only imperfectly made good. Here repair takes place by means of fibrous tissue. Portions of the articular and semilunar cartilages, if they break loose, may become free in the joint cavity.

Joints may be injured by **puncture, contusion, torsion, dislocation, subluxation,** or **fracture** of the bones within the capsule. The amount of injury, of course, varies. The capsule may be crushed, pulled upon, or actually torn.

In a dislocation the end of one of the bones forming a joint is found in an abnormal position outside the capsule. In subluxation the dislocation is only partial. In some cases, the articular cartilages or the end of the bone, may be injured or fractured (complicated dislocation).

The results of such accidents depend largely upon whether infection takes place or not. In the more trifling injuries recovery takes place, and restoration of function is eventually complete. In severer traumatism the changes initiated are not unlike those occurring in fracture of the bones. Immediately following a dislocation or intracapsular fracture there is more or less abundant hemorrhage into the joint. Later, inflammation sets in. The capsule and surrounding parts become swollen, œdematous, infiltrated with inflammatory products, and there may be effusion into the synovial cavity. In simple non-infected cases the inflammation rapidly reaches its height and then resolves. The effused blood and the inflammatory exudate are absorbed. In rare cases it happens that portions of the coagulum may persist and become organized, forming one variety of "free bodies" in the joints. When the dislocation is reduced, the tear in the capsule is repaired by the formation of a cellular material which in time becomes differentiated into dense connective tissue. Should fracture have taken place, it heals, as do ordinary fractures of bone and cartilage. In time the joint may return to its normal anatomical condition and function be perfectly restored. Should reposition not be effected, the capsule and ligaments contract, the articular surfaces waste away, the joint-cavity is invaded by fibrous tissue, and the disused muscles atrophy. The end of the dislocated bone will atrophy or become attached in its abnormal situation by fibrous tissue. Should it rub against a bony surface, a new articulation in the form of a shallow socket is in time produced. This is in part due to pressure atrophy. Round about the newly formed groove the bone proliferates and forms a ring. In this way a more or less perfectly functionating joint is produced. Useless muscles atrophy, others become elongated, and the soft tissues in time adapt themselves to the altered condition of things. In some cases a new capsule is formed by the proliferation of cells derived from the original capsule or from the soft tissues in the neighborhood. If the dislocated bone be not movable, partial or complete fibrous or fibrous and osseous union takes place (ankylosis).

Where a joint is resected the result varies according to circumstances. The ends of the bones at the point of injury become rounded off and a proliferation of connective tissue from the periosteum and bone-marrow takes place, so that the two ends are united by fibrous bands, in which bone sometimes develops. If the parts be kept at rest, a strong immobile union takes place. If, however, motion be kept up, designedly or otherwise, a new joint results. In young persons articular cartilages may be formed. In time, the parts return in a considerable degree to their normal appearance and a capsule secreting synovia may even be produced.

As a result of injuries and some forms of inflammation a joint may become fixed—*ankylosis*. If completely immobile, the condition is called *true* or *complete* ankylosis; if partially movable, *false* or *incomplete* ankylosis. Ankylosis is usually brought about by the proliferation of fibrous tissue into or around the region of injury. Should the intra-articular cartilages be preserved in whole or in part, they sometimes undergo direct metaplasia into fibrous tissue or fibrocartilage, or into mucinous tissue, which gradually becomes fibrous. In some cases the newly formed fibrous tissue is trifling in amount and the ankylosis is produced mainly by cartilage or bone. In other cases the ankylosis is due to fibrous tissue or cartilage and bone intermingled. In still another class of cases, the interference with mobility is due to some cause outside the capsule (*extracapsular ankylosis*), such as, abundance of osteophytes, for example, in arthritis deformans; thickening and contraction of the capsule; adhesions of tendons; the formation of bony bridges; contractions and paralyses of muscles.

PROGRESSIVE METAMORPHOSES.

Metaplasia.—The phenomenon of metaplasia is frequently exemplified in the case of cartilage. Cartilage is rather an inert tissue, and when destroyed is apt to be replaced by fibrous tissue or occasionally bone. Ordinary hyaline cartilage in the joints may be transformed into fibrocartilage or fibrous tissue in certain cases of inflammation. **Mucinous metaplasia** is very common. **Ossification**, particularly of the costal cartilages and larynx, is met with as an expression of senility and as a result of inflammation.

Hyperplasia.—Hyperplasia, both of the cartilages and the connective tissue of joints, is a frequent event in most forms of chronic inflammation, especially in tuberculosis and arthritis deformans. Not only may the fibrous capsule and its synovial lining be diffusely thickened, but new cartilage and bone may be developed. The cartilages may also be diffusely thickened, or nodular and papillary excrescences may be formed. Overgrowth of the cartilage is seen also in the hyperplastic form of that rare disease called by Kaufmann chondrodystrophia fœtalis.

Solutions of continuity are usually made good, not by new cartilage, but by fibrous tissue or bone.

Tumors.—Primary tumors of the joints are rare. A curious form is the so-called **lipoma arborescens,** which is rather common in cases of tuberculosis and arthritis deformans. Here the synovial membrane becomes thickened and hypertrophic, and is thrown into numerous folds and papillæ, in which fat is subsequently deposited. **Sarcoma** may originate in the capsule. **Angioma** and **chondroma** are also recorded.

The secondary involvement of a joint by tumors of the adjacent parts is not uncommon.

APPENDIX.

PROFESSOR GREENFIELD has pointed out to me while this work has been passing through the press that the statement in the last paragraph on page 43 does not accurately set forth his results upon infarct formation, and has referred me to his "Chapters upon Pathology"[1] for fuller statement of his teaching. That work he had been so good as to send me some years ago. I fear that while writing this work I had treated it like pathological text-books in general, namely, had but glanced through it, lest willingly or unwillingly I should find myself copying my fellow writers' text-books. The result was that when I came to write upon infarct formation I hunted for Professor Greenfield's observations and never recalled that I had encountered them in this little book of 113 pages, written for his students. To my knowledge they have not been published *in extenso;* the nearest I could approach to them was in the work published by his pupils, Beattie and Dickson. I regret this all the more because Greenfield has conscientiously repeated the various classical experiments upon infarct formation, and doing this has not only harmonized the findings of the original observers, but also has given so clear a picture of the whole matter that it will be serviceable to note rapidly his main conclusions.

Phenomena following Artificial Obstruction of Arteries.—1. **Entire Renal Artery.**—(*a*) In two hours after ligation of the renal artery, in the dog or the rabbit, the engorgement and swelling of the kidney is very distinct, reaching a maximum in sixteen to eighteen hours, when the organ may be nearly twice as large as its fellow. During the earlier stages this engorgement is most marked *in the region of the pelvis and calices and in the superficial part of the cortex under the capsule.* (*b*) If both renal artery and vein be tied the engorgement is *greater* than when the artery alone is tied. (*c*) Ligation of the ureter and stripping off of the capsule entirely prevent the engorgement, and this when the renal vein is patent. The organ remains bloodless and does not enlarge. It is clear, therefore, that the hyperemia cannot be due to reflux of blood through the renal vein; it is of arterial and collateral origin, due, that is, to blood entering the organ through anastomoses (1) between the minute vessels of the ureters and pelvis and the vessels of the medulla, and (2) between branches from the lumbar arteries supplying the perirenal fat

[1] Greenfield and *Lyon*, "Chapters upon Pathology, being an Outline of *Lectures* upon Some Points in the Pathology of Elementary Nutritive and Circulatory Derangements." Edinburgh, Waterston & Sons, 2d edit., 1907.

and the capsular vessels of the kidney. (*d*) Any blood supply which comes through the vessels in the capsule is mainly distributed by capillaries which unite with those of the intertubular plexus. It is perhaps possible that it may pass into the glomerular arteries and follow the normal course. But it is more likely to fill some of the capillaries of the intertubular plexus, and if it passes through the glomerular capillaries, does so in reverse order, through the efferent vessel. As under such conditions the blood cannot escape, the result will be distension of the glomerular vessels and, often, consequent rupture. This rupture is what we find actually occurring.

2. **Obstruction of Branches of the Renal Artery.**—By repeating Vulpian's experiment of taking a suspension of tobacco seeds and injecting this forcibly upward through the crural artery of the dog into the aorta (or in the rabbit, employing begonia seeds) it is possible to produce infarcts in the kidney (and in the spleen). The presence of the seeds blocking the arteries of the affected areas shows their relationship to the effects produced.

(*a*) There is an early and progressive effort to replace the obstructed blood supply by collateral afflux. The congestion is most marked in the medulla if a seed block one of the arterioles supplying the pyramids, and here there may be rupture of many of the capillaries. In the more typical obstruction of a cortical artery there is rapid filling of the vessels through the capsular anastomoses, and here after some hours there may be hemorrhages between capsule and cortex. So also at the lateral margins of the infarct there is rapid filling of the intertubular capillaries and of the nearby glomeruli. After eighteen hours there are often hemorrhages from these capillaries of the marginal glomeruli into the capsule space.

(*b*) "The extent to which the blood penetrates into the capillary system of the obstructed area varies considerably." Sometimes it refills a considerable part (red infarcts). At other times the occurrence of secondary degenerative changes in the tubular epithelium with swelling and transudation of lymph would seem to occur before the capillaries can be refilled (white infarct).

(*c*) Here also there is no evidence of refilling of the capillaries through the veins. What is more, the collateral engorgement continues after the veins have become blocked by thrombi. Such thrombosis in the veins of the affected area develops gradually and most often is complete in from twenty-four to thirty hours.

3. **Obstruction of Branches of the Splenic Artery.**—While all renal infarcts experimentally produced have from the first a peripheral zone of hyperemia and hemorrhage and the majority have a pale main central area (white infarct), experimental splenic infarcts, whether produced by embolism or ligature, are invariably red or hemorrhagic throughout from the first. The difference from the kidney conditions appears to be that the blood can easily penetrate the meshes of the spleen pulp. A paler coloration of the splenic infarct is an after-result, due to escape of the hemoglobin and partial absorption.   J. G. A.

INDEX.

Spermatic cord, tumors of, 855
   varicocele of, 855
Spermatocystitis, 855
Spina bifida, 552, 1063
   ventosa, 1073
Spinal cord, 597, 601
   anemia of, 602
   circulatory disturbances of, 601
   degeneration of, 610
   glioma of, 627
   gliomatosis in, 627
   hemorrhages of, 601
   hyperemia of, 601
   inflammations of, 602
   ischemia of, 602
   leprosy of, 609
   meningo-myelitis of, 607
   in pellagra, 620
   pernicious anemia of, 624
   retrogressive metamorphoses of, 609
   softening of, 603, 608
   syphilis of, 609
   tuberculosis of, 608
   tumors of, 627
   dura mater, 597
   meninges, 597
   muscular atrophy, progressive, 615
   paralysis, spastic, 616
   pia-arachnoid, 599
Spirochæta pallida, 965, 992
Splanchnoptosis, 412
Spleen, 221
   accessory, 222
   actinomycosis of, 229
   alteration of position of, 223
   anemia of, 223
   anomalies of, congenital, 222
   atrophy of, 229
   "bacony," 229
   carcinoma of, 231
   circulatory disturbances of, 223
   cirrhosis of liver and, 227
   cyanotic induration of, 223
   cysts of, 231
   degeneration of, hyaline, 229
   dislocation of, 223
   echinococcus disease of, 229
   function of, 221
   glanders of, 228
   hemorrhage into, 225
   hyperemia of, 223
   hyperplasia of, 230
   infarction of, 223
   infiltration of, 229
   inflammations of, 225
   leprosy of, 228
   necrosis of, 230
   parasites of, 229
   "sago," 229
   sarcoma of, 231
   syphilis of, 228
   tuberculosis of, 228
   tumors of, 231
   "wandering," 223
Splenadenoma, 230

Splenitis, 225
Splenization of lungs, 305
Splenocytes, 221
Splenomegaly, 226, 227
Spondylitis deformans, 1104
"Spotted fever," 571
Spring catarrh, 642
Staphyloma of cornea, 650
   scleræ, 656
Status lymphaticus, 209
Stauungspapille, 676
Steapsin, 367
Stenosis of aorta, 145
   of aortic valve, 169
   congenital hypertrophic, of pylorus, 411
   of Eustachian tube, 694
   of Fallopian tubes, 890
   of intestines, 427
   of mitral valve, 169
   of œsophagus, 403
   of pulmonary valve, 145, 168*
   of tricuspid valve, 168
   of uterus, 869, 872
Stertor, 243
Still's disease, 1099
Stomach, 410
   actinomycosis of, 418
   adenocarcinoma of, 425
   anemia of, 413
   anomalies of, congenital, 410
   atrophy of, 419
   carcinoma of, 423
   circulatory disturbances of, 413
   contraction of, 412
   degeneration of, 420
   dilatation of, 350, 412
   diphtheria of, 416
   displacements of, 412
   diverticula of, 410
   echinococcus disease of, 418
   erosion of, 422
     hemorrhagic, 414
   foreign bodies in, 418
   hair-balls in, 418
   hemorrhages of, 414
   hernia of, 410
   hour-glass, 410, 412
   hyperemia of, 414
   hypertrophy of, 422
   inflammations of, 414
   lumen of, alterations in size of, 412
   motor insufficiency of, 350
   œdema of, 413
   overactivity of, 350
   parasites of, 418
   phytobezoar in, 419
   pylorus of, congenital hypertrophic stenosis of, 411
   syphilis of, 418
   thrush of, 417
   trichobezoar in, 418
   tuberculosis of, 417
   tumors of, 422
   typhoid of, 418
   volvulus of, 413 *5*